NURSING STUDENT'S
GUIDE TO
DRUGS

CONTENTS

FUNDAMENTALS OF DRUG THERAPY

THERAPEUTIC CLASSES AND GENERIC DRUGS

Antimicrobial and Antiparasitic Agents

Cardiovascular System Drugs

Central Nervous System Drugs

STAFF

Executive Director, Editorial
Stanley Loeb

Editorial Director
Helen Klusek Hamilton

Clinical Director
Barbara F. McVan, RN

Art Director
John Hubbard

Drug Information Editor
George J. Blake, RPh, MS

Clinical Project Editor
Marlene Ciranowicz, RN, MSN, CDE

Clinical Editors
Diane Schweisguth, RN, BSN; Galene Sellers, LPN; Patricia Holmes, RN (aquisitions)

Copy Editors
Jane V. Cray (supervisor), Mary T. Durkin, Traci A. Ginnona,
Christina A. Price

Designers
Stephanie Peters (associate art director), Julie Carleton Barlow
(book designer), Maryanne Buschini, Don Knauss

Typography
David C. Kosten (director), Diane Paluba (manager),
Joyce Rossi Biletz, Phyllis Marron

Manufacturing
Deborah C. Meiris (manager), Anna Brindisi

Production Coordination
Maree DeRosa

Editorial Assistant
Mary Madden

Indexer
Janet Hodgson

© 1993 by Springhouse Corporation. All rights reserved. No part of this book may be used or reproduced in any manner whatsoever without written permission except for brief quotations embodied in critical articles and reviews. Printed in the United States of America. For information write Springhouse Corporation, 1111 Bethlehem Pike, P.O. Box 908, Springhouse, PA 19477-0908.
IDT-010692
ISBN 0-87434-389-5

Library of Congress Cataloging-in-Publication Data
Nursing student's guide to drugs.
   p. cm.
  Includes index.
  1. Pharmacology. 2. Chemotherapy.
   3. Nursing.
  [DNLM: 1. Drug Therapy—handbooks.
2. Drug Therapy—nurses' instruction. 3. Pharmacology—handbook. 4. Pharmacology—nurses' instruction. QV 39 S933]
RM300.S765 1992
615.5'8—dc20
DNLM/DLC
ISBN 0-87434-389-5   92-2324
                            CIP

NURSING STUDENT'S
GUIDE TO
DRUGS

Springhouse Corporation
Springhouse, Pennsylvania

Hematologic Agents

Antineoplastic Agents

Immunomodulation Agents

Eye, Ear, Nose, and Throat Drugs

Dermatomucosal Agents

Miscellaneous Drug Categories

APPENDIX AND INDEX

CLINICAL CONSULTANTS AND PHARMACY REVIEWERS

At the time of publication, the clinical consultants and pharmacy reviewers held the following positions:

Clinical Consultants

Sandy R. Conover, RN, MS, GNP-C
Associate Professor of Nursing
Cerritos College
Norwalk, Calif.

Betty M. Hanson, RN, MN
Coordinator, First Year
Associate of Science in Nursing Program
Sante Fe Community College
Gainesville, Fla.

Jeannine L. Hayduk, RN, PhD, CS
Director of Nursing and Allied Health
Southern Illinois Collegiate Common Market
Carterville, Ill.

Sandra S. Huddleston, RN, MSN, CCRN
Assistant Professor of Nursing
Berea (Ky.) College

Rita S. Monahan, RN, MSN, EdD
Associate Professor
Oregon Health Sciences University School of Nursing
Eastern Oregon State College
LaGrande

Mary D. Naylor, RN, PhD, FAAN
Associate Dean and Director of Undergraduate Studies
University of Pennsylvania, School of Nursing
Philadelphia

Deborah P. Nelson, RN, MS, CCRN
Cardiovascular Clinical Specialist
LaGrange, Ill.

C. Lynne Ostrow, RN, EdD
Associate Professor
West Virginia University, School of Nursing
Morgantown

Sandra C. Pendergraft, RN, MSN
Professor of Nursing
Valencia Community College
Orlando, Fla.

Patricia Peschman, RN, MS, CNN
Renal Clinical Nurse Specialist
Abbott Northwestern Hospital
Minneapolis

Lois Piano, RN, C, MSN
Assistant Professor
Gwynedd-Mercy College
Gwynedd Valley, Pa.

Sue Svoboda, RN, MEd
Coordinator of Non-Traditional Programs
St. John's School of Nursing
Springfield, Mo.

Dolores Vaz, RN, MSN, MEd
Professor of Nursing
Bristol Community College
Fall River, Mass.

Anita L. Wynne, RN, PhD
Associate Professor
School of Nursing
University of Portland (Ore.)

Pharmacy Reviewers

Paula Castor, RPh, MHA
Director of Pharmacy Services
Moss Rehabilitation Hospital
Philadelphia

Bruce M. Frey, RPh, PharmD
Assistant Professor of Clinical Pharmacy
Philadelphia College of Pharmacy and Science
Clinical Pharmacist in Pediatrics and Neonatology
Thomas Jefferson University Hospital

Jill A. Hoffman, RPh, BS
Staff Pharmacist
Presbyterian Medical Center of Philadelphia

Susanne P. Mulligan, RPh, BS
Staff Pharmacist
Presbyterian Medical Center of Philadelphia

Kathleen A. Piontkowski, RPh, BS
Staff Pharmacist
Cooper Hospital University Medical Center
Camden, N.J.

David Pipher, RPh, PharmD
Assistant Director for Clinical Services
Forbes Regional Health Center
Monroeville, Pa.

Joseph F. Steiner, RPh, PharmD
Professor of Clinical Pharmacy
University of Wyoming
Casper

HOW TO USE THIS BOOK

The *Nursing Student's Guide to Drugs* represents the efforts of nursing educators and pharmacists to develop a drug handbook that addresses nursing students' special needs. To that end, this volume integrates both clinical and pharmacologic aspects of drug therapy within the framework of the nursing process. It emphasizes information useful at the bedside and organizes it in an easy-to-use format that clarifies the relevant pharmacologic and therapeutic classifications.

Fundamental Information

The first four chapters provide an introduction to pharmacotherapy. Chapter 1, Understanding Drug Action, explains pharmacodynamics—how drugs produce their effects—and pharmacokinetics—how they act within the body (absorption, distribution, metabolism, and excretion). Chapter 2, Drug Administration, describes the various routes of drug administration and available dosage forms and explains when and why each is appropriate. Chapter 3, Adverse Reactions and Interactions, explains drug reactions and the factors that influence them and summarizes the mechanisms whereby drug effects are changed by other drugs, foods, or other substances (such as histamine) within the body. Chapter 4, Drug Therapy and the Nursing Process, explains how the individual steps of the nursing process apply to the care of patients who require drug treatment.

Therapeutic Classes and Generic Drugs

In subsequent chapters, generic drugs are organized according to their approved therapeutic uses. Organization by therapeutic use relates drug information easily to bedside teaching and allows comparison of drugs that share the same clinical application. Drugs that have multiple uses are classified according to their most common use and are also listed among drugs that share their secondary uses. For example, nadolol, a beta-adrenergic blocker, is described among the antianginals because its major therapeutic application is the management of angina pectoris; because it is also used to treat hypertension, it is listed in Chapter 22, Antihypertensives.

Each drug chapter lists all relevant generic drugs and describes their pharmacologic characteristics: major uses; mechanisms of action; absorption, distribution, metabolism, and excretion; onset and duration; and adverse reactions. A glossary defines important related terms. Within each chapter, prototype entries provide comprehensive information for representative drugs of the major pharmacologic groups. For example, Chapter 22, Antihypertensives, includes detailed drug information for six representative prototypes: captopril, representing the angiotensin-converting enzyme (ACE) inhibitors; atenolol, representing the beta-adrenergic blockers; phentolamine mesylate, representing the alpha-adrenergic blockers; trimethaphan camsylate, representing the ganglionic blocking agents; methyldopa, representing the centrally acting sympatholytics; and hydralazine, representing the vasodilators.

Each prototype entry includes generic and trade names, pronunciation, pharmacologic classification, Drug Enforcement Administration (DEA) schedule of control, pregnancy risk category, available dosage forms and strengths, indications and dosage, contraindications and precautions, adverse reactions, interactions, and nursing considerations.

In each prototype entry, the generic name (with alternate generic names following in parentheses) precedes a phonetic guide to pronunciation and an alphabetically arranged list of current trade names. A single dagger (†) identifies drugs available only in Canada; a double dagger (‡), drugs available only in Australia; an open diamond (◊), drugs available without a prescription. A single asterisk (∗) identifies drugs whose liquid formulation may contain alcohol. This is particularly important for persons taking disulfiram (Antabuse) as part of a treatment program for alcoholism; it is also important for persons taking drugs that may elicit a disulfiram-like adverse effect (such as metronidazole). A double asterisk (∗∗) indentifies drugs that contain tartrazine dye (F, D&C Yellow No. 5), a coloring agent that can provoke a severe allergic reaction in susceptible persons. Although the incidence of tartrazine sensitivity is low (about 1 in 10,000 persons), persons with asthma or aspirin sensitivity may be at higher risk. Several drugs available solely as combinations (for example, pyrimethamine with sulfadoxine) are listed according to the first generic in the combination.

Classification identifies the drug's pharmacologic group. If appropriate, the next line identifies any drug the Food and Drug Administration (FDA) lists as a controlled substance and specifies the DEA schedule of control as II, III, IV, or V.

Pregnancy risk category identifies the potential risk to the fetus. These categories, labeled A, B, C, D, or X, define a drug's potential to cause birth defects or fetal death. They are listed and explained below. Drugs in category A are usually considered safe to use in pregnancy; drugs in category X are contraindicated.

A: Adequate studies in pregnant women have failed to show a risk to the fetus in the first trimester of pregnancy—and there is no evidence of risk in later trimesters.

B: Animal studies have not shown an adverse effect on the fetus, but there are no adequate clinical studies in pregnant women.

C: Animal studies have shown an adverse effect on the fetus, but there are no adequate studies in humans, or there are no adequate studies in animals or humans. Pregnancy risk is unknown.

D: There is evidence of risks to the human fetus, but the potential benefits of use in pregnant women may be acceptable despite potential risks.

X: Studies in animals or humans show fetal abnormalities, or adverse reaction reports indicate evidence of fetal risk. The risks involved clearly outweigh potential benefits.

How supplied lists the preparations available for each drug (for example, tablets, capsules, solution, or injection), specifying available dosage forms and strengths.

Indications and dosage presents all approved indications for use, with general dosage recommendations for adults and children. Specific recommendations for infants, elderly patients, or other special patient groups are included when appropriate.

Contraindications and precautions lists conditions that are associated with special risks in patients who receive the drug.

Adverse reactions lists the undesirable effects that may follow use of the drug; these effects are arranged by body system: blood, central nervous system (CNS), cardiovascular (CV), eyes, ears, nose, throat (EENT), gastrointestinal (GI), genitourinary (GU), hepatic, metabolic, respiratory, skin, local, and other. Local effects occur at the site of drug administration (by application, infusion, or injection); adverse reactions not specific to a single body system (for example, the effects of hypersensitivity) are listed under "Other." For easy identification by the reader, common reactions are listed in italic type; life-threatening reactions, in boldface type.

Interactions specifies the clinically significant additive, synergistic, or antagonistic effects that result from concomitant use with other drugs.

Nursing considerations follow and are organized strictly according to the nursing process—from assessment to evaluation—and include nursing diagnoses, detailed recommendations for supportive care, and patient teaching. The Implementation section contains action-oriented recommendations for monitoring the effects of drug therapy; for preventing and treating adverse reactions; for promoting patient comfort; for preparing, administering, and storing the drug; and for teaching patients.

Nursing considerations emphasize specific recommendations for each drug. Universal recommendations, such as "assess the five rights of drug therapy (patient, drug, dose, time, and route) before administration" and "assess the patient's compliance with drug therapy," which apply to all drugs, are not repeated in the prototype entries. Review such fundamental questions in detail in Chapter 2, Drug Administration.

Supplementing the prototype entries, charted summaries guide clinical use of other major drugs listed in each chapter. As appropriate, additional charts summarize pharmacokinetics, adverse reactions, and selected commercially available combination products.

At the end of each chapter, a *Self-Test* containing questions based on clinical situations aids the student's review and reinforcement of chapter content.

The *Appendix* includes answers to the self-test questions.

The *Index* lists generic and trade names (including Canadian and Australian usage, and drug combinations), pharmacologic and therapeutic drug classes, charts, and introductory pharmacotherapeutic concepts.

GUIDE TO ABBREVIATIONS

The following abbreviations are used repeatedly in this book:

AIDS	acquired immunodeficiency syndrome
ALT	alanine aminotransferase
AST	asparate aminotransferase
ATP	adenosine triphosphate
AV	atrioventricular
b.i.d.	twice daily
BUN	blood urea nitrogen
cAMP	cyclic 3′, 5′ adenosine monophosphate
CBC	complete blood count
CHF	congestive heart failure
CMV	cytomegalovirus
CNS	central nervous system
COPD	chronic obstructive pulmonary disease
CPK	creatine phosphokinase
CPR	cardiopulmonary resuscitation
CSF	cerebrospinal fluid
CV	cardiovascular
CVA	cerebrovascular accident
CVP	central venous pressure
DNA	deoxyribonucleic acid
ECG	electrocardiogram
EEG	electroencephalogram
EENT	eyes, ears, nose, throat
FDA	Food and Drug Administration
g	gram

G	gauge
GI	gastrointestinal
GFR	glomerular filtration rate
GU	genitourinary
G6PD	glucose-6-phosphate dehydrogenase
h.s.	at bedtime
I.M.	intramuscular
IND	investigational new drug
IPPB	intermittent positive pressure breathing
ID	intradermal
IU	international unit
I.V.	intravenous
kg	kilogram
L	liter
M	molar
m^2	square meter
mm^3	cubic millimeter
MAO	monoamine oxidase
mcg or μg	microgram
mEq	milliequivalent
mg	milligram
MI	myocardial infarction
ml	milliliter
Na	sodium
NaCl	sodium chloride
ng	nanogram (millimicrogram)

NSAID	nonsteroidal anti-inflammatory drug
OTC	over the counter
PABA	para-aminobenzoic acid
P.O.	by mouth
P.R.	by rectum
p.r.n.	as needed
q	every
q.d.	every day
q.i.d.	four times daily
RBC	red blood cell
RDA	recommended daily allowance
REM	rapid eye movement
RNA	ribonucleic acid
RSV	respiratory syncytial virus
SA	sinoatrial
S.C.	subcutaneous
SGOT	serum glutamic oxaloacetic transaminase
SGPT	serum glutamic pyruvic transaminase
SIADH	syndrome of inappropriate antidiuretic hormone
S.L.	sublingual
t.i.d.	three times daily
UCE	urea cycle enzymopathy
USP	United States Pharmacopeia
WBC	white blood cell

CHAPTER 1

UNDERSTANDING DRUG ACTION

Understanding the complex processes a drug undergoes in the body can improve your patient care. For example, knowing how a drug achieves its therapeutic effect helps you evaluate a patient's response to it.

To achieve a desired effect—curing or preventing a disease or disorder, relieving symptoms, or aiding diagnosis—a drug interacts biochemically or physiologically with body tissues. It may change, interrupt, replace, or intensify an existing physiologic process; it does not cause tissues or organs to take on new functions.

Most drugs produce their effects by inhibiting or augmenting the action of cellular elements called *receptors*. However, some drugs act by local effects (for instance, antacids neutralize gastric acid in the stomach) or by altering cell membrane activity (for instance, local anesthetics). Moreover, most drugs exert multiple widespread actions rather than a single local action. Consequently, drugs may produce both beneficial and adverse effects.

Pharmacotherapeutics is the study of drugs used to treat disease. It encompasses selection of drug therapy, understanding the disease process, and factors that influence a patient's response to drugs.

PHARMACODYNAMICS
The study of the mechanism of action of drugs is called pharmacodynamics. Theories of drug action identify three mechanisms:
• drug-receptor interaction—the drug combines with cellular receptors
• drug-enzyme interaction—the drug interacts with cellular enzyme systems
• nonspecific drug interaction—the drug alters physical and chemical properties of the outer cell membrane and intracellular structures in some undetermined way.

Drug-receptor interaction
The mechanism of drug-receptor interaction hinges on the concept that a drug is selectively active and has a high affinity for a specific receptor. This means that a certain part of the drug molecule, the active site, selectively interacts or combines with a part of a cell or cell surface (the reactive site) to produce a pharmacologic effect. In other words, the tissue receptor provides a reactive cellular site with which the drug interacts to produce a pharmacologic response. A cell altered by a drug-receptor interaction to produce a pharmacologic response is called an *effector cell*.

GLOSSARY

Affinity: force causing certain atoms to combine with others.
Catalyst: a substance that promotes a chemical reaction without being permanently altered in the reaction.
Enzyme: an organic catalyst produced by living cells, which induces chemical changes in other substances without being changed itself.
Idiosyncratic reactions: unusual and unpredictable drug reactions probably linked to genetic enzyme deficiencies. They include abnormal resistance, hypersensitivity, and paradoxical reactions.
Receptor: a cell component that combines with a drug or hormone to alter cellular functions.
Substrate: a substance acted upon by an enzyme.

Some researchers suggest that a chemical bond or other special force accounts for drug-receptor binding. Presumably, a drug gains access to the receptor after leaving the bloodstream and being distributed to tissues containing receptor sites. Here, drug molecules combine with their receptors like a key fits into a lock. The drug molecule that best fits the receptor probably elicits the greatest response from the cell.

Like a key that fits into a lock but cannot turn the tumblers, some drugs fit the receptor site but cannot elicit a pharmacologic response. Called blocking agents, these drugs prevent the effects of other drugs or substances that *would* elicit a pharmacodynamic response by occupying the receptor site.

The drug-receptor interaction mechanism explains why drugs that are chemically similar usually have similar actions. More than one drug may interact with a given receptor, provided each drug fits the receptor site. Drugs with similar chemical and structural features that produce the same pharmacologic response probably do so by acting on the same set of receptors.

Drug-enzyme interaction

Drug-enzyme interaction involves an interaction between a drug and a cellular enzyme, a biologic catalyst that controls the cell's biochemical reactions. By inhibiting the enzyme's action, the drug alters a physiologic response. For example, neostigmine, used to improve muscle strength in patients with myasthenia gravis, combines with the enzyme acetylcholinesterase to prevent it from inactivating acetylcholine at the neuromuscular junction.

A drug combines with an enzyme because it structurally resembles the enzyme's *substrate* molecule, the substance the enzyme acts on. Such a drug may directly block normal enzymatic action or may trigger production of other interacting substances.

Nonspecific drug interaction

Some drugs exert nonspecific effects, acting through more general effects on cellular membranes and processes. By penetrating cells or accumulating in cell membranes, these drugs interfere physically or chemically with a cellular function or basic metabolic process, such as adsorption, solubility, or permeability. General anesthetics, for instance, probably produce a pharmacologic response by altering conductive properties of nerve cell membranes rather than by acting on specific receptors.

Other structurally nonspecific drugs may act biophysically in ways that do not affect cell or enzyme functions. For instance, edetate calcium disodium (EDTA), used to treat heavy-metal intoxication, forms irreversible bonds with certain metals (such as lead), facilitating their excretion. Osmotic diuretics, such as mannitol and glycerin, increase glomerular filtrate osmolarity and reduce water reabsorption, thereby increasing urine volume.

Purely chemical actions, such as gastric pH neutralization by antacids, also reflect nonspecific drug interactions. Other drugs that act by chemical means alone include plasma expanders, cathartics, adsorbents, astringents, and chemical antidotes.

DOSE-RESPONSE RELATIONSHIPS

A basic pharmacologic principle holds that the degree of a drug effect reflects the administered dose—the amount needed to produce a particular biologic response. By determining dose-response relationships, pharmacologists can identify the dosage required to produce various effects; this, in turn, permits evaluation of a drug's safety and efficacy.

Dose-response relationships include the therapeutic index (TI). This measurement, reflecting a given drug's relative safety, represents the ratio of two factors:
- lethal dose (LD_{50})—the dose (usually expressed in mg/kg) that is lethal in half the laboratory animals tested
- effective dose (ED_{50})—the dose (usually expressed in mg/kg) required to produce a therapeutic effect in half the subjects in a similar population.

The formula below shows this ratio:

$$TI = \frac{LD_{50}}{ED_{50}}$$

The closer the TI is to 1, the greater the drug's risk to humans. Thus, if 30 mg/kg of a drug killed half the animal subjects studied and 10 mg/kg produced the desired effect,

$$TI = \frac{30 \text{ mg/kg}}{10 \text{ mg/kg}} = 3$$

Conversely, the higher the TI, the safer the drug. The calculation of TI is made long before a drug is used clinically.

FACTORS AFFECTING PHARMACOLOGIC RESPONSE

Individual responses to drugs can vary markedly. One patient may have an unexpectedly intense response to a drug, whereas another receiving an identical dose of the same drug has little, if any, response. A patient may even respond differently to the same drug each time he takes it.

Such variations may reflect influence by any of the following factors: individual characteristics; age; weight; sex; genetic, pathologic, or immunologic factors; psychological factors; environmental factors; time of administration; tolerance; cumulative drug effects; and drug interactions.

Age

Children and elderly patients commonly experience variations of drug effects—usually because of underdeveloped or impaired ability to absorb, distribute, metabolize, or excrete drugs. Typically, the most marked variations occur with drugs affecting the CNS. Elderly patients, for example, frequently become disoriented after receiving a standard dose of a sedative. Children seem more vulnerable to drug-induced seizures than adults.

Pregnancy poses special problems. Drugs taken by a pregnant woman can cross the placental barrier, possibly causing adverse effects on the uterus and fetus. If the drug alters uterine motility, a miscarriage can result. Some drugs exhibit direct toxic effects on the developing fetus.

Weight (body mass)

Because a drug must pass through body tissues and fluids for distribution and dilution, the drug dosage must take into account the patient's weight. Generally, the heavier the patient, the less drug is delivered to target tissues and the weaker the drug effect. Overweight patients therefore may need increased dosages. Another factor is drug distribution to body fat. Some drugs (short-acting barbiturate anesthetics, for example) redistribute from the bloodstream into fat stores. Higher doses of these drugs may be necessary in obese patients.

Dosages of some drugs usually are calculated according to the ratio of milligrams of drug to kilograms of body weight. The average adult drug dosage is based on the drug quantity that will produce a particular effect on half the population between ages 18 and 65 weighing approximately 150 lb (70 kg). Most formulas used to adjust adult drug dosages for a child are based on the child's weight or body-surface area rather than age.

Sex

Because women have a smaller average body size than men, they may experience a higher drug concentration from the same dosage. They also have less muscle perfusion and a higher ratio of adipose tissue to muscle mass. Consequently, they may absorb I.M. drugs more slowly and thus experience delayed and prolonged drug effects.

Certain drugs may be extremely toxic to a developing fetus. Such drugs must be avoided in women who are capable of becoming pregnant.

Genetic factors

Genetically determined deficiencies in receptor sensitivity or metabolism may alter a patient's response to certain drugs, sometimes causing idiosyncratic reactions. Succinylcholine provides an interesting example of such genetic influence. Normally this drug is so rapidly hydrolyzed by plasma and liver enzymes (cholinesterases) that its action ends a few minutes after administration. But in rare patients (about 1 in 3,000), this drug produces muscular relaxation and apnea that persist for several hours. Such patients have been found to have atypical cholinesterase as a genetically determined trait.

Pathologic factors

An underlying pathologic condition may cause an unusual response to a drug. Hepatic or renal dysfunction, for example, may impair detoxification or excretion of a drug, causing it to accumulate and produce toxicity or unexpectedly severe drug reactions. Certain other pathologic states may alter tissue responsiveness to drugs and cause toxic reactions or resistance to drug therapy.

Circulatory and metabolic disorders and fluid and electrolyte imbalances commonly interfere with drug effects. For example, a patient with metabolic acidosis resulting from excessive bicarbonate and sodium loss may respond poorly to the diuretic acetazolamide (Diamox). A high basal metabolic rate may cause a patient to metabolize or excrete drugs more rapidly than normal.

Immunologic factors

Certain drug molecules may stimulate a patient's immune system to produce antibodies. The next time the patient receives the drug, he may experience anaphylaxis—an immediate life-threatening immune response. Penicillin, for example, is notorious for inducing anaphylactic reactions.

Psychological factors

An optimistic outlook may enhance a patient's response to drug therapy. The placebo effect is a prime example. Defined as a drug or other treatment used for its implicit or explicit therapeutic *intent* rather than its chemical or physical properties, a placebo may work by reducing anxiety or by triggering a biochemical mechanism in which expectation of relief stimulates production of endorphins, the body's natural pain-relieving substances.

A caregiver who maintains an upbeat attitude may improve the chance for a positive patient response to both placebos and active drugs. A patient who senses that his nurse or doctor is optimistic about his treatment is more likely to experience the desired therapeutic effect.

Environment

Some circumstances or settings may promote—or hinder—a positive patient response. Consider that a warm room temperature may intensify the effects of vasodilatory drugs by relaxing peripheral vessels, whereas a cold temperature has the opposite effect. High altitude may increase sensitivity to some drugs by causing oxygen deprivation.

Time of administration

A drug administered between meals may produce a faster pharmacologic response because some drugs are absorbed more rapidly when taken on an empty stomach (however, a patient may better tolerate a drug that irritates the GI tract by taking it with food).

Biological rhythms may play an important role in patient response to drugs. Rhythms governing sleep and wakefulness, drug-metabolizing enzymes, hormone production and secretion, and blood pressure—as well as circadian (24-hour) variations in drug absorption and renal excretion—may alter pharmacologic response and could predispose a patient to adverse or toxic drug effects.

A circadian rhythm also may contribute to drug-receptor sensitivity. For example, a hypnotic or sedative drug is much less effective when administered in the morning, presumably because circadian rhythms make the CNS less responsive to depressant drugs early in the day.

Tolerance

Prolonged or frequently repeated drug administration may lead to tolerance or reduced responsiveness. In this phenomenon, a dose no longer produces the anticipated effect—or produces it only briefly. Thus, the patient needs a progressively increasing dose to experience the desired effect. Tolerance most commonly occurs with opium alkaloids, nitrates, barbiturates, and ethyl alcohol.

Cross-tolerance may occur between related drugs. In this phenomenon, the drugs act at the same cellular sites to produce similar effects. A patient who develops tolerance to nitroglycerin's vasodilatory effects, for instance, will probably develop a tolerance to other nitrate and nitrite vasodilators. Addicts who become tolerant to heroin are also tolerant to morphine and other opiate and opioid drugs. Because alcohol and certain general anesthetics may produce cross-tolerance, alcoholics may also have a reduced responsiveness to anesthetics that depress the CNS in the same way that alcohol does.

Quickly developing tolerance to the repeated administration of a drug is known as *tachyphylaxis*. When this occurs, the patient's initial response to the drug cannot be reproduced even with larger doses.

Physical dependence

With certain drugs (opiates, for example), the brain adapts to the drug and fails to function normally when the dose is reduced. Thus, the patient must continue to receive the drug to preserve equilibrium. Discontinuance of the drug causes a characteristic *withdrawal,* or abstinence, syndrome.

Cumulative effects

Drug accumulation can occur if a patient receives a new dose before the body has metabolized the last one. Drug absorption then exceeds drug excretion, with each new dose adding more to the total drug concentrations in the blood and tissues than the body can excrete over the same period. Without compensatory adjustment of the dose or frequency of administration, drug concentrations may reach toxic levels.

Cumulative toxicity can occur quickly, as in alcohol intoxication, or gradually, as in heavy-metal poisoning. Lead, for example, is stored in many body tissues and deposited in bone, leading to prolonged effects while accumulation continues.

Drug interactions

When two or more drugs are administered to a patient simultaneously, one drug may modify the effects of the other, causing an abnormal pharmacologic response. Although many drug interactions cause adverse—or potentially fatal—effects, some can be used for the patient's benefit.

A drug interaction can result from summation, antagonism, synergism, or potentiation. *Summation* (additive effect) occurs when the combined effects of two drugs yield a response equaling the sum of the drugs' separate effects (1+1=2). For example, when taken together, codeine and aspirin usually provide greater pain relief than when either drug is given alone. Additive drug therapy usually reduces the risk of adverse reactions by allowing lower doses of each drug.

Antagonism occurs when the combined effect of two drugs is *less* than the sum of the drugs acting separately (1+1=<2).

Synergism, also called potentiation, describes an interaction in which two drugs' combined effects exceed the sum of their separate effects (1+1=3). For example, two antihypertensives may produce a combined blood pressure decrease that exceeds the sum of the decreases these drugs produce when given alone.

PHARMACOKINETICS

Pharmacokinetics—the study of drug movement through the body over time—helps predict drug action (therapeutic and adverse drug effects). It encompasses the four basic processes a drug undergoes after it enters the body: absorption, distribution, metabolism, and excretion.

A fundamental pharmacologic principle holds that the magnitude of a drug's effect depends on the drug concentration at the site of action. With few exceptions, a drug must move from the administration site to the target tissues in which it will act by distributing through numerous tissues. Some tissues, such as the liver, may biotransform (metabolize) the drug as it moves through them. After metabolism, the drug is eliminated.

Absorption

The first process, absorption, takes the drug from the administration site into the bloodstream (systemic circulation). However, a drug administered I.V. or intra-arterially enters the bloodstream directly and therefore does not undergo absorption; the entire dose is 100% bioavailable immediately, ready for distribution to its receptor site. (Bioavailability refers to the rate at and extent to which a drug reaches the systemic circulation and thereby becomes available to the site of action.)

Drugs administered by all other routes (oral (P.O.), I.M., rectal (P.R.), subcutaneous (S.C.), sublingual (S.L.), buccal, nasal, intratracheal, intradermal, and topical) must be absorbed before they can become available to target tissue. (See *How administration route affects drug absorption* for more information on drug absorption and these other routes.) Before a drug can be absorbed, it must be in solution; therefore, an orally administered drug is available most rapidly for absorption in liquid form. However, special formulations of oral drugs (such as sustained-release tablets) can change the rate at which a drug dissolves in the stomach or small intestine, and therefore slow the rate of absorption.

How drugs move across membranes

To be absorbed when given by a route other than the I.V. or intra-arterial route, a drug first must pass through cellular membrane barriers. These barriers (called semipermeable membranes) are biomolecular lipoidal sieves composed of lipid, protein, and carbohydrate, which allow drug molecules with different characteristics to diffuse across membranes. A drug must have some hydrophilic (water-soluble) properties to dissolve in blood or in gastric or intestinal fluid and to pass through a lipoidal membrane.

Semipermeable membranes offer selective permeability to drugs, allowing some to pass through easily and others to pass through with some difficulty, and preventing still others from penetrating at all. The degree of permeability depends on the structural and physiochemical properties of both the barrier membrane and the migrating drug molecules—for example, the relative size of membrane pores and drug molecules and differences in pH, electrical potential, and concentration.

An important influence on the transport of a drug across a membrane barrier is the degree of a drug's ionization. Most drugs cross tissues by passive diffusion. This process requires that drugs dissolve in and pass through biologic membranes, moving from an area of high concentration to one of low concentration. Most drugs are weak electrolytes—organic compounds that are electrically charged (separated into ions) when in solution. As a result of the electrical charge, they cannot cross membranes. Weak acids are non-ionized (uncharged) in an acidic medium, such as gastric contents; weak bases are non-ionized in a basic (alkaline) medium such as the small intestine. Non-ionized drugs are more lipid-soluble and thus more readily absorbed than ionized (charged) drugs, which are lipid-insoluble. Acidic drugs are better absorbed in the stomach, an acidic environment; basic drugs are better absorbed from the intestine, an alkaline environment.

GI absorption

The following factors influence drug absorption from the stomach and intestines:

HOW ADMINISTRATION ROUTE AFFECTS DRUG ABSORPTION

A drug's administration route plays a key role in its absorption.

Oral administration

For many drugs, the oral route is the safest and most convenient method of administration. However, various factors may alter the amount of oral drug available to the systemic circulation, including pH changes, destruction by enzymes, the presence of food, and fluctuations in GI motility.

I.M. administration

Muscle perfusion and the degree of the drug's lipid solubility affect drug absorption from the I.M. route. Muscle movement determines perfusion to the involved area; usually, the rate of drug absorption from a moving muscle exceeds that from a resting muscle. Massaging a muscle or applying heat also increases circulation to the muscle, thereby speeding drug absorption.

S.L. or buccal administration

Drug administration by S.L. or buccal routes results in rapid and substantial absorption through these highly vascular areas. Drugs absorbed through the oral mucosa enter the venous system and empty into the superior vena cava, avoiding hepatic first-pass metabolism. Only non-ionized drugs pass through the oral membrane, so salivary pH, which affects drug ionization, proves extremely important.

Inhalation and intratracheal administration

Drugs are absorbed into the bloodstream from alveolar sacs when administered by these routes. The pulmonary tree's large surface area provides an extensive, highly perfused region for enhanced absorption.

Rectal administration

Administering drugs rectally eliminates the risk of drug destruction by digestive enzymes in the stomach and small intestine. The degree of a drug's ionization and lipid solubility determine its absorption across the rectal mucosa.

Because approximately half of the hemorrhoidal circulation empties into the systemic, rather than portal, venous system, rectally administered drugs avoid first-pass metabolism. However, variable suppository placement may account for inconsistent absorption and bioavailability with this drug form.

Topical (percutaneous) administration

Drugs are absorbed through the skin or mucous membranes to subcutaneous sites. In general, highly lipophilic and non-ionized drugs are best suited for topical administration.

Because topically administered drugs must have a higher affinity for the skin than for the pharmaceutical vehicle, appropriate vehicle selection proves crucial. The greater the skin hydration, the faster the absorption rate. Application of a physical barrier, such as plastic wrap or an occlusive bandage over the topical preparation, also enhances skin hydration. Increasing drug concentration in the vehicle or the surface area over which the preparation is applied increases the amount of drug absorbed.

Until recently, drug absorption through the skin has been variable and hard to control. However, the transdermal patch now provides a controlled, consistent means of administering certain drugs topically.

Surface area

The amount of drug that can be absorbed depends on the amount of surface area available for absorption. The long, convoluted GI tract offers a large surface area for drug absorption. Most drug absorption occurs in the small intestine, which has a greater surface area than the stomach and large intestine.

GI tract pH

The GI tract's chemical environment varies. Stomach fluid, with a pH of about 2.0, is highly acidic. Intestinal fluid becomes progressively alkaline, with a pH ranging from 5.0 or 6.0 in the duodenum to 8.0 in the terminal ileum. This pH variation affects drug ionization, which, in turn, affects lipid solubility as drugs move through the GI tract.

Drugs and other substances that alter the pH in the GI tract may enhance or impair absorption of certain concomitantly administered drugs. Some oral drugs, including drugs that can be destroyed by acid (such as penicillin) and those that irritate the stomach (such as erythromycin), have an enteric coating that prevents tablet contents from dissolving in the acidic stomach. When given with an antacid (which raises gastric pH), the drug's enteric coating is destroyed in the stomach, exposing the drug to an acidic environment and altering its absorption.

GI tract motility

The length of time a drug remains in the GI tract also can influence the absorption rate. Usually, slower gastric emptying time and reduced GI tract motility slow absorption because the drug takes longer to reach the small intestine, which is the main absorption site for most drugs. Food in the stomach, especially a large fatty meal, also slows gastric emptying, thereby slowing drug absorption. However, delayed absorption usually does not affect the *extent* of drug absorption if the drug remains stable in acidic gastric juices.

Factors that increase GI motility (for example, administration of antacids containing magnesium) typically speed absorption. Factors that decrease motility slow absorption. For instance, morphine derivatives, anticholinergics, and antacids containing aluminum slow GI motility, possibly decreasing absorption of concomitantly administered drugs by decreasing drug transit time through intestinal regions where absorption takes place.

First-pass metabolism

An orally administered drug must cross the hepatic portal system and the liver before reaching the bloodstream. If the drug is significantly metabolized (eliminated) by the liver, only a small fraction of the unchanged drug will reach the systemic circulation and exert its effects. This process is known as first-pass metabolism. Drugs subject to extensive first-pass hepatic elimination may be ineffective after oral administration.

Significant first-pass hepatic metabolism explains why an equally potent I.V. dose may be much smaller than an oral dose.

DISTRIBUTION

Once a drug reaches the bloodstream, it is distributed throughout the body. Blood flow plays a key role in drug distribution and may determine how quickly a drug reaches its receptor site. Highly perfused tissues, such as the heart, liver, kidneys, and brain, receive most of the available drug before it distributes to other tissues. Distribution to other tissues (for example, skin, fat, muscle, and viscera) is slower.

A drug's ability to cross a lipid membrane affects its distribution to various body sites. Because some drugs cannot pass through certain cell membranes, they have limited distribution. Conversely, other drugs, such as ethyl alcohol, can pass through virtually all cell membranes.

Plasma protein binding

Through its effect on distribution, plasma protein binding proves crucial to the effectiveness and duration of drug action. Plasma contains many proteins. Some drugs are highly bound to these proteins, many are moderately bound, and others are not bound at all. All bound drugs have a ratio of free, or unbound, drug to bound drug. Only the unbound portion is available for action at a receptor site; therefore, the degree of plasma protein binding determines how much drug is available to exert a pharmacologic effect. Highly protein-bound drugs distribute mainly to the plasma, resulting in a lower drug concentration available for distribution to other tissues.

Plasma protein binding is a process of dynamic equilibrium: as tissue concentrations of the free drug decline, the protein-drug complex begins to dissociate, releasing more free drug for distribution. Thus, proteins act as drug storage sites, slowing the rate at which a drug reaches its receptor site.

Because albumin accounts for a large portion of plasma proteins—4 to 5 g/dl of plasma—changes in the amount of albumin available for binding also alter the amount of unbound drug. Fewer albumin binding sites mean higher concentrations of free drug. Thus, in patients with hypoalbuminemia from malnutrition, proteinuria (loss of protein through the urine resulting from kidney disease), reduced hepatic synthesis, or leakage of protein into interstitial fluids, a given dose may exert an exaggerated pharmacologic effect. Patients with conditions marked by loss of plasma proteins may need significantly lower doses to compensate for fewer binding sites.

Compartmentalization

To better understand drug distribution, think of the body as a system of physiologic compartments based on blood flow. Highly perfused organs and blood make up the central compartment; areas receiving less perfusion form the peripheral compartment, which, in turn, consists of the tissue compartment (muscle and skin) and the deep compartment (fat and bone). These compartments act as drug reservoirs throughout the body, releasing their stores as plasma concentrations decline. With some drugs, such accumulation may prove beneficial because it permits a sustained pharmacologic effect. However, chronic accumulation of drugs may lead to adverse reactions. Compartmentalization factors affecting distribution include storage in fat, bone, and skin; fetal transfer; and the blood-brain barrier.

Storage in fat, bone, and skin

Highly lipid-soluble drugs distribute readily to fat cells (adipose tissue), where they are stored, because adipose tissue lacks receptors for drug action. This proves beneficial with such drugs as anesthetic barbiturates, which are released from fat stores to provide a sustained anesthetic effect during surgery. In some cases, though, such prolonged action is undesirable and may be dangerous.

A few drugs are deposited in bone. Tetracycline, for instance, distributes throughout bone and eventually may crystallize there. In a growing child, this may cause permanent tooth discoloration. Lead and certain other toxic agents also may accumulate in bone, resulting in prolonged, harmful exposure to these agents. The skin also may store drugs and may cause photosensitivity, increasing the risk of skin damage from ultraviolet light.

Fetal transfer

Transport of drugs to the fetus represents a uniquely important form of drug distribution. A drug administered to a pregnant patient may pass through the placental membrane by passive diffusion or active transport. If the drug gains access to the fetal side of the placenta, it may cause teratogenic effects. Alkaline drugs are generally more ionized on the fetal side; acidic drugs, less ionized. Thus, because the fetus tends to be acidotic, weakly alkaline drugs (such as lidocaine) are more likely than weakly acidic drugs to accumulate in the fetus.

Blood-brain barrier

Separating the CNS from the blood, the blood-brain barrier consists of specialized capillary walls in the CNS and surrounding glial membranes. Usually, only non-ionized drugs can cross this barrier and gain access to the brain—a fact that proves important in drug therapy for certain CNS disorders. For instance, dopamine, which is ionized, does not cross the barrier and therefore cannot be used to treat Parkinson's disease—a disorder caused by lack of dopamine in certain brain regions. Levodopa, a metabolic precursor to dopamine, readily enters the CNS and is commonly used in the treatment of this disease.

METABOLISM

By changing drugs chemically, the body biotransforms (metabolizes) them so that it can eliminate them. It does this through the action of enzymes that change a drug's structure to a more water-soluble form. This makes the drug less likely to cross semipermeable membranes and more likely to remain in the plasma to undergo filtration by the kidneys. The products of drug metabolism, called metabolites, may or may not be pharmacologically active.

Unlike food metabolism, in which the body breaks down complex proteins and starches to their component amino acids and carbohydrates, drug metabolism usually leaves the drug's parent molecule relatively intact while adding more ionized molecules to it. Drug metabolism usually implies drug inactivation, but some pharmacologically inactive drugs must be activated during metabolism to be effective. Such drugs, known as pro-drugs, include the sedative-hypnotic chloral hydrate, which is metabolized to its active metabolite, trichloroethanol.

The primary site of drug metabolism is the liver, but metabolism takes place in many other tissues, including the lungs, kidneys, skin, muscle, blood, placenta, and blood-brain barrier. Each of these sites contains special enzymes that can act on a wide range of chemical substances.

Factors affecting drug metabolism

Physiologic, life-style, genetic, and dietary factors, as well as concomitantly administered drugs, may increase or decrease drug metabolism.

Physiologic factors

Hepatic blood flow, the most important physiologic determinant of drug metabolism, may decrease with such conditions as reduced cardiac output. Age also influences metabolism. For example, neonates lack the hepatic microsomal oxidase enzyme P-450, essential to the metabolism of many drugs; elderly patients have less efficient hepatic metabolic pathways, resulting in slower elimination of most drugs and greater risk of toxicity.

Life-style

A person's life-style or habits, such as smoking, may affect drug metabolism. Drug metabolism may be more rapid in smokers because cigarette smoke contains certain aromatic hydrocarbons, which induce hepatic enzyme activity. For example, this reaction increases metabolism of theophylline, a drug commonly prescribed for asthma. For this reason, smokers who must take theophylline require higher dosages to maintain therapeutic blood levels.

Genetic factors

The study of genetic variations in drug response has been gaining increasing recognition. At least some of the variation is caused by genetic differences in drug metabolism. Researchers studying the activity of the enzyme N-acetyl-transferase divided the American population into fast (autosomal-dominant) and slow (autosomal-recessive) acetylator status. (Acetylation refers to the addition of an acetyl group into the molecule of an organic compound.) The study concluded that about half of all Black and Caucasian Americans are slow acetylators, whereas over 80% of Americans of Japanese, Chinese, and Inuit ancestry are fast acetylators. In slow acetylators, drugs requiring acetylation, such as isoniazid, may undergo slower metabolism, possibly leading to excessive accumulation and toxic blood levels.

Diet

A diet high in carbohydrates or fat may slow metabolism of certain drugs. Conversely, a diet high in protein may speed some drugs' metabolism.

Concomitant drug use

Certain drugs induce hepatic enzymes responsible for drug biotransformation. For example, long-acting barbiturates (such as phenobarbital) or the antibiotic rifampin speed the metabolism of other hepatically metabolized drugs, possibly leading to subtherapeutic blood levels. Conversely, cimetidine, a histamine$_2$ antagonist used to treat peptic ulcer disease, inhibits hepatic metabolism of many concomitantly administered drugs, possibly causing excessive accumulation and subsequent toxicity.

EXCRETION

Excretion—drug removal from the body through an eliminating organ—usually occurs via the kidneys into the urine. However, some drugs are excreted hepatically (via the bile into the feces) and a few by minor routes (the lungs, saliva, sweat, and breast milk).

Renal excretion

Renal excretion is most efficient with ionized, water-soluble drugs and metabolites. Drugs first undergo glomerular filtration, in which free, non-protein-bound drug filters through endothelial pores in the glomerular capillaries.

After filtration, a drug may undergo passive reabsorption in the proximal and distal tubules, then be returned to the bloodstream to extend the drug's duration of effect. Only lipid-soluble, non-ionized drugs can be reabsorbed.

pH

Urinary pH serves as an important excretion variable. A weakly acidic drug can be reabsorbed in an acidic pH; a weakly alkaline drug can be reabsorbed in an alkaline pH. The proximal tubule has a neutral pH—7.0. Administration of acidifying agents (such as ascorbic acid) or alkalinizing agents (such as sodium bicarbonate) may change renal tubular fluid pH and thereby alter drug ionization, and may reduce drug excretion by increasing reabsorption.

Molecular weight

High-molecular-weight compounds, such as the plasma protein albumin, do not pass through the glomerular membrane. Therefore, highly protein-bound drugs can only end up in the urine through a process of active secretion.

Patient factors

Various patient factors may influence renal excretion. These include sex, age, and renal function status.

Females have a lower average creatinine clearance than males. Consequently, they excrete drugs more slowly and have a higher risk of drug accumulation and toxicity.

Because renal function commonly declines with age, elderly patients may have impaired drug excretion.

Renal status

Such renal disorders as pyelonephritis, nephrosclerosis, and renal failure may decrease renal clearance markedly, causing slower renal excretion. Some drugs (NSAIDs, for example) alter renal blood flow and may decrease renal function, especially after prolonged use.

Hepatic (biliary) drug excretion

The liver extracts some drugs and metabolites dissolved in blood and secretes them into the bile via active transport. The amount of each drug concentrating in the bile varies. Drugs and metabolites that enter bile usually have a high molecular weight and are highly ionized.

Because bile is secreted into the duodenum, many drugs and metabolites excreted by the liver ultimately enter the feces. However, some drugs may return to a non-ionized, lipid-soluble form, either by the influence of intestinal pH or the action of bacterial flora. Non-ionized drugs may undergo enterohepatic recycling, returning to the bloodstream after reabsorption from the intestine. This process prolongs the drug's presence in the blood.

OTHER FACTORS AFFECTING DRUG ACTION

A drug's blood concentration, latency, half-life, and accumulation in the body also affect drug action.

Blood concentration

The processes of absorption, distribution, metabolism, and excretion continuously affect a drug's blood concentration. Absorption of an oral drug exceeds its excretion until the peak blood level is reached. After this, more drug is excreted than is absorbed and the blood drug level falls. On the other hand, a drug administered by I.V. bolus is immediately bioavailable. Blood levels peak immediately after the infusion and then fall until the next dose is given.

For most drugs, blood concentration at equilibrium correlates with magnitude of effect and can be used to predict therapeutic efficacy or toxicity. The minimum drug amount that must be present in the blood to produce a therapeutic effect is called the minimum effective concentration. The level at which the greatest blood drug concentration occurs is called peak concentration.

With I.V. or intra-arterially administered drugs, peak concentration occurs immediately. With drugs administered by any other route, peak concentration is delayed until the drug is absorbed.

Latency

Also known as time to onset, latency refers to the interval between administration and the onset of action, minimum effective concentration, or measurable response.

Half-life

Defined as the time required for the blood drug concentration to decrease by half, this important characteristic helps establish a drug's optimal dosage regimen, including loading dose, maintenance dose, and the interval between doses (dosing interval). For most drugs, half-life remains constant regardless of the drug's plasma concentration.

Remember that a drug administered in a single dose is eliminated almost completely after five half-lives; a drug administered repeatedly reaches its maximum blood level after about five half-lives. Knowing a drug's half-life helps determine its dosing interval, which in turn affects the drug's accumulation. For example, a drug with a short half-life, such as penicillin G, must be given several times a day to maintain therapeutic effectiveness. A drug with a long half-life, such as digoxin, can be given once daily.

Accumulation

Many drugs reach a therapeutic blood level after several doses. When an immediate response is required, a large loading dose is given, followed by smaller maintenance doses. Giving each successive dose before the previous dose has been completely excreted causes the drug to accumulate until the dose given equals the amount of drug being excreted. At this point, called a *steady state*, the blood level remains stable as long as the patient receives consecutive doses and other variables (bioavailability, renal function, and metabolism) do not change.

Accumulation explains why a drug's full effect may not appear for days to weeks after therapy begins. It also explains how toxicity occurs. When drug absorption exceeds excretion, the amount of drug within the blood and tissues increases; if dosage is not reduced, cumulative toxicity follows.

SELF-TEST

1. Amanda Snow, age 53, is diagnosed with Type II diabetes mellitus. After a 6-month trial of dietary therapy, her blood glucose level is not well controlled. In addition to her 1,500-calorie diet, her doctor prescribed glyburide (Diabeta, Micronase) 2.5 mg P.O. daily to be taken with breakfast. When explaining the pharmacodynamics of this drug, Ms. Snow's nurse will be explaining the drug's:
   a. therapeutic use.
   b. mechanism of action.
   c. movement through the body over time.
   d. possible adverse reactions.

2. Which of the following factors may influence Ms. Snow's pharmacologic response to glyburide?
   a. absorption
   b. incidence of adverse reactions
   c. time of administration
   d. drug form used

3. Ms. Snow's primary nurse is unfamiliar with glyburide, so she reviews the literature about the drug before developing her teaching plan. She learns that glyburide's half-life is 10 hours. What does half-life mean?
   a. time required for the drug to be excreted
   b. time required for therapeutic response to occur
   c. time required for the blood drug concentration to decrease by half
   d. time required for drug to reach half of its therapeutic effect

Check your answers on page 1056.

CHAPTER 2

DRUG ADMINISTRATION

Administering drugs is one of the most important and most demanding nursing responsibilities. It's your responsibility to interpret and carry out the prescribed order and ensure its appropriateness for the particular patient. To ensure safe and effective drug therapy for your patients—and to protect yourself from liability for medication errors—you need to understand the legal implications of drug administration, your institution's policies and procedures on drug administration and its drug distribution system, administration routes, how to prepare for drug administration, and sources of medication errors.

LEGAL IMPLICATIONS

As a nurse, you face definite legal risks when administering drugs to patients. Understanding the basic legal principles involved in drug administration can help you minimize these risks.

In each state, a nurse practice act defines the legal scope of nursing practice in all areas, including drug dispensation, prescription, and administration. This scope varies among the states, with each state's board of nursing issuing its own rules and regulations. Generally, however, the nurse's role is limited to actually administering drugs to patients, with limited or no authority to prescribe or dispense them.

Other agencies and laws also regulate the use of drugs. State pharmacy practice acts and medical practice acts specify the responsibilities and liabilities of these two professions regarding drug prescription, preparation, dispensation, and administration. On a national level, the federal Food and Drug Administration (FDA) and Drug Enforcement Administration regulate the manufacture and use of drugs.

Basic to all state and federal drug regulations is the classification of drugs into four legal categories. *Over-the-counter* (OTC) drugs are those drugs available to the general public without a prescription; their use without the supervision of a health care professional has been determined to be relatively safe and their ingredients effective for the indications listed. *Prescription*, or *legend*, drugs are those drugs that can be dispensed and administered only on a doctor's order. *Controlled substances* are classified by the federal Controlled Substances Act of 1970 with respect to their physical or psychological abuse potential and accepted medical use. They also can be dispensed and administered only on a doctor's order.

GLOSSARY

Aerosol: a pressurized preparation that when activated releases a fine dispersion of liquid or solid materials in a gaseous medium.

Capsule: a solid dosage form containing one or more substances enclosed within a hard or soft gelatin shell.

Cream: a semisolid emulsion containing a drug suspension or solution in a water-soluble or fat-soluble base.

Drops: medicated oil or water intended to be dropped into the ears, eyes, nose, or mouth.

Elixir: a clear, sweetened, water-alcohol liquid containing flavoring substances and sometimes a medicinal agent.

Emulsion: an oil and water mixture in which one liquid is distributed as small globules throughout the body of a second liquid with which it cannot be mixed.

Enema: a liquid intended to be injected into the rectum.

Extended-release (timed-release, sustained-release): tablets or capsules specially formulated to more slowly release a drug, thereby producing a sustained duration of drug action.

Inhalation: drug droplets, vapor, or gas administered by the oral or nasal respiratory route via an aerosol or nebulizer.

Injection: a sterile, pyrogen-free preparation intended to be administered parenterally.

Lotion: a liquid suspension intended for external application to the skin.

Lozenges (troches): disk-shaped solid preparations intended to be slowly dissolved in the oral cavity for localized effects.

Ointment: a semisolid preparation intended for external application to the skin or mucous membranes.

Ophthalmic insert: a flexible, multilayered structure that permits a predetermined amount and rate of drug to be released into the eye.

Pellet (implant): a sterile, small, rod- or ovoid-shaped mass intended to be implanted under the skin for the purpose of providing the slow release of medication over an extended period of time.

Powder: a mixture of finely divided drugs or chemicals in dry form.

Solution: a liquid preparation containing soluble chemical substances usually dissolved in water (which, because of their ingredients or method of preparation, are not classified as another dosage form).

Spray: a liquid minutely divided or nebulized as by a jet of air or a stream.

Suppository: a solid dosage form intended for insertion into body orifices where it melts, softens, or dissolves and exerts its systemic or localized effects.

Suspension: a liquid preparation containing finely divided drug particles distributed somewhat uniformly throughout a vehicle in which the drug is only minimally soluble.

Syrup: a concentrated sugar solution in water that may contain a flavoring agent or drug.

(continued)

GLOSSARY *continued*

Tablet: a solid dosage form of varying weight, size, and shape that may be molded or compressed, and that contains a drug in a pure or diluted form. Enteric-coated tablets resist breakdown in the stomach, but not in the intestines, where the drug is absorbed.

Tincture: an alcohol or water-alcohol solution prepared from animal or vegetable material or from chemical substances.

Transcutaneous (transdermal) system: a solid preparation in which the drug is impregnated into an adhesive bandage or disk and from which the drug is released in predetermined amounts and rates; dosage form intended for systemic drug effects.

Finally, *investigational drugs* are those agents currently under FDA evaluation for approval for commercial release, based on their efficacy and safety. As such, their use requires an informed consent from the patient and typically involves extensive data collection regarding patient response.

POLICY CONSIDERATIONS

Beyond statutory requirements, nurses also must follow the policies and procedures for drug administration established by their individual institutions. Usually, such policies and procedures are formulated by the nursing and pharmacy departments and are subject to the approval of medical staff committees.

Specific policies and procedures will vary depending on applicable legal requirements and on the particular needs of the institution. But despite individual variations, all drug therapy-related policies and procedures should share a common goal: to minimize the potential for error, or to protect the patient from the administration of an inappropriate drug or the incorrect administration of an appropriate drug order. In a hospital setting, a doctor's order usually is required before dispensing and administering any drug, regardless of its legal category. Examples of other specific policies may include:

- the acceptance of doctor's verbal orders only in an emergency and the need to immediately document them
- standing orders to treat a particular disease or set of symptoms
- the use of automatic stop orders for certain drugs
- p.r.n. (Latin phrase that means "as the occasion arises") medication orders that allow the nurse to administer analgesics or laxatives as needed or to adjust the dose according to patient response
- stat orders for drugs that are to be administered immediately.

Institutional policies should also define who can receive medication orders and administer drugs, how to clarify unclear medication orders, when approved drugs may be prescribed for unapproved or unlabeled uses, and how to resolve conflicts about medication orders. All of the applicable legal statutes and guidelines should be listed in the institution's policies and procedures manual.

Drug distribution systems

To ensure a thorough knowledge of your institution's drug policies and procedures, you need to understand how drugs are dispensed in your institution. Today, most hospitals use some variation of one of these four basic drug distribution systems:
• floor stock system
• individual prescription order system
• centralized unit-dose system
• decentralized unit-dose system.

In the *floor stock system*, nearly all medications are stocked on the nursing unit. No patient-specific containers or individual-dose packaging are used. Only special drug products, such as chemotherapeutic drugs or diagnostic agents, are ordered from the pharmacy as needed.

In the *individual prescription order system*, all medications dispensed are labeled by the pharmacist for individual patients, much like a normal prescription vial from a retail pharmacy. Typically, a 5-day supply of a drug is dispensed at one time.

In a *centralized unit-dose system,* all orders are processed in the main pharmacy. Usually, duplicate patient medication bins are maintained in the pharmacy and exchanged at least once every 24 hours.

Because the centralized unit-dose system has often been associated with delays in the processing of orders, difficulty in accessing patient-specific information, and communication problems among the nursing, medical, and pharmacy staffs, *decentralized unit-dose systems* have been implemented in recent years. The decentralized system may involve the use of fixed pharmacy "satellites," located closer to the nursing units, or the placement of a mobile medication cart, staffed by a pharmacist, on the nursing unit. The decentralized unit-dose system incorporates the safeguards of a centralized unit-dose system with timely processing of medication orders, rapid access to patient-specific medication information, and improved communication among medical, nursing, and pharmacy staff members.

ADMINISTRATION ROUTES

Drugs may be administered by several different routes, as determined primarily by the intended site of action, the rapidity and duration of effect desired, and the chemical and physical properties of the drug itself. Routes of drug administration commonly used in nursing practice include the GI, parenteral, and dermatomucosal routes. Other routes of drug administration that may be used by the nurse include the ophthalmic, otic, nasal, respiratory, urethral, and vaginal routes. Additional methods of administration include intrathecal (instilling drugs directly into the CSF) and intra-articular (instilling a drug into a joint), as well as the use of special indwelling catheters such as the Hickman or Broviac catheter; these are used by the advanced nursing practitioner or doctor and are beyond the scope of this text.

GI routes of administration

The GI routes of administration may be further subdivided into oral, nasogastric and gastrostomy tube, and rectal administration.

Oral administration

Oral administration provides the most convenient and least expensive method of introducing medication into the body and is usually the route of choice for many drugs. Solid oral dosage forms include tablets, capsules, extended-release tablets or capsules, and enteric-coated tablets or capsules. Liquid dosage forms include syrups, elixirs, emulsions, and suspensions. See *Comparing drug forms.*

After ingestion, solid tablets and capsules disintegrate and dissolve in either the stomach or the small intestine. Because liquids do not undergo this transformation, they may be absorbed more rapidly and completely than tablets or capsules and reach therapeutic levels more rapidly.

Several other factors may influence oral drug absorption. The medication may adsorb to food in the stomach, slowing its passage into the small intestine and decreasing the rate (although not usually the extent) of absorption. Certain foods may hasten gastric emptying into the small intestine, speeding drug absorption; others, such as fatty foods, may slow gastric emptying and thus hinder drug absorption. In the stomach, polyvalent cations such as aluminum, calcium, and iron may combine with certain drugs (for example, tetracycline) and form nonabsorbable compounds, which will reduce drug effectiveness.

Because most drug absorption occurs in the small intestine, patients with intestinal abnormalities (for example, those who have undergone intestinal diversion procedures such as ileostomies and colostomies) may have trouble absorbing certain solid oral dosage forms. In such patients, disintegration and absorption of enteric-coated and extended-release tablets or capsules may be delayed and may not occur in the first part of the small intestine. In fact, these dosage forms may pass into ostomy bags intact. To ensure absorption, such patients should receive liquids or rapid-acting tablets. Consider that active medication from certain long-acting wax matrix tablets (Slow-K, Procan SR) may actually be "leached" from the tablet core, while the original matrix ("ghost") is excreted in the feces. This also occurs in patients with intact bowels.

Nasogastric and gastrostomy tube administration

The second route of drug administration using the GI tract is instillation of medication through a nasogastric (NG) or gastrostomy tube. Drugs administered through either type of gastric tube enter the stomach directly, thus bypassing the mouth and esophagus and the disintegration and dissolution processes that occur there. To administer a drug appropriately via an NG or a gastrostomy tube, the nurse must first reproduce the disintegration and dissolution processes by crushing a tablet and

(Text continues on page 28.)

COMPARING DRUG FORMS

DOSAGE FORM	DESCRIPTION	ADVANTAGES	DISADVANTAGES
Oral forms			
Tablet	Compressed or molded medication. May include one or more of these ingredients: • diluent (for example, dextrose) to ensure proper size and bulk • disintegrant (for example, starch) to speed disintegration process • coating	• Convenient and inexpensive • Protects gastric mucosa from irritation by medication • May be scored for easy breaking to divide a dose	• Variable absorption • May dissolve in the mouth
Enteric-coated tablet	Tablet with coating that resists breakdown from stomach acid	• Allows the tablet to pass through the stomach intact to dissolve in the small intestine • Produces less GI irritation than other tablets	• May be difficult for some patients to swallow • May pass undissolved
Coated tablet	Tablet with a hard coating	• Easier to swallow • Prevents the medication from dissolving in the mouth	• More expensive than plain tablets • May be difficult for some patients to swallow
Capsule	Small, soluble container, usually made of gelatin, enclosing a dose of medication	• Disintegrates in gastric fluids and is absorbed more rapidly than tablets	• Variable absorption
Extended-release tablet and capsule	Tablet or capsule containing particles of drug coated with substances that control release of the medication over a prolonged period of time	• Longer duration of medication effects • Requires fewer doses, promoting better patient compliance	• Variable absorption

(continued)

COMPARING DRUG FORMS *continued*

DOSAGE FORM	DESCRIPTION	ADVANTAGES	DISADVANTAGES
Oral forms *(continued)*			
Wax matrix extended-release tablet	Tablet in which the drug is embedded in a matrix that slowly breaks down during intestinal transit, releasing the medication in a sustained fashion	• Longer duration of medication effects • Requires fewer doses, promoting better patient compliance	• Variable absorption
Osmotic pump sustained-release tablet	Tablet covered with a semipermeable membrane that allows water to enter; in solution form, the drug leaves the tablet through a small hole in the membrane	• Longer duration of medication effects • Requires fewer doses, promoting better patient compliance	• Variable absorption
Sublingual and buccal tablet	Soft, compressed tablet combined with lactose (for rapid absorption) placed underneath the tongue (S.L.) or between the gum and cheek (buccal)	• Rapidly absorbed • Avoids some first-pass effects from stomach acids and foods	• May be chewed or swallowed mistakenly
Transmucosal tablet	Soft, compressed tablet combined with lactose placed between the upper lip and gum above the front teeth	• Longer-lasting effects than sublingual or buccal tablets	• May be swallowed mistakenly • Can produce mucosal irritation
Translingual spray	Medication applied by pressurized aerosol spray underneath the tongue	• Greater drug stability • Rapid drug absorption	• Patient may inhale instead of applying under the tongue • Flammable; patient should not smoke while using
Syrup	Liquid medication in a solution of sugar water to which various flavors can be added	• Disguises taste and aroma of medications, promoting patient compliance • Rapid drug absorption	• Pleasant taste may encourage overdose in children • High sugar content may influence glucose control in diabetic patients

COMPARING DRUG FORMS *continued*

DOSAGE FORM	DESCRIPTION	ADVANTAGES	DISADVANTAGES
Oral forms *(continued)*			
Elixir	Hydroalcoholic liquid flavored with volatile oils and slightly sweetened	• Rapid drug absorption	• Bad taste frequently causes poor compliance in children • Alcohol base may impair serum glucose control • Adverse reactions in alcoholics who are taking disulfiram (Antabuse)
Emulsion	Mixture of oil and water	• Increased palatability of oily liquids	• Variable ingestion and absorption
Suspension	Fine drug particles suspended in an aqueous vehicle	• Increased palatability • Ease of administration • Rapid drug absorption	• Must be shaken to ensure uniform dispersion of drug particles
Rectal forms			
Suppository	Solid medication in a firm base, such as cocoa butter, that melts at body temperature. May be molded in a variety of cylindrical shapes, usually about 1½″ (4 cm) long (smaller for infants and children)	• Provides a safe route if patient is vomiting, unconscious, or unable to swallow • Provides an effective route to treat vomiting • Doesn't irritate the patient's upper GI tract, as some oral medications do • Avoids destruction of medication by digestive enzymes in stomach and small intestine • Avoids biotransformation in liver because drugs absorbed from the lower rectum bypass the portal system	• May be uncomfortable and embarrassing for the patient • May result in irregular or incomplete drug absorption, depending on the patient's ability to retain the medication and whether feces are present in the rectum; because rectal absorption may be incomplete, rectal dosages of some medications may be larger than oral doses • May stimulate the patient's vagal nerve by stretching the anal sphincters; therefore, use the rectal route cautiously with cardiac patients

(continued)

COMPARING DRUG FORMS *continued*

DOSAGE FORM	DESCRIPTION	ADVANTAGES	DISADVANTAGES
Rectal forms *(continued)*			
Ointment	Semisolid medication that may be applied externally to the anus or internally to the rectum	• Same as for suppository	• Same as for suppository
Enema	Liquid given as either a *retention* enema (retained by the patient for at least 30 minutes or until absorbed) or a *nonretention* enema (retained by the patient for at least 10 minutes and then expelled) *Note:* Enemas given to clean the lower bowel usually aren't medicated	• Same as for suppository	• Same as for suppository
Parenteral forms			
Intradermal injection	Medication administered by injecting small amounts of solution, usually antigens, between the epidermal and dermal (skin) layers	• Convenient method to do skin tests • Less discomfort experienced than with other parenteral forms • Allows for multiple injections at one time	• Can only be used for drugs used in skin tests
Subcutaneous injection	Medication administered by injecting a substance under the skin into the layer of loose connective tissue	• Provides slow, sustained release of medication • Patient can learn self-administration • Causes only minimal tissue trauma and avoids damage to large blood vessels and nerves	• Cannot be used in patients with compromised perfusion, obesity, diseased tissue, burns, or dermatologic problems • Irritating drugs should not be administered by S.C. injection • No more than 2 ml of fluid can be injected at one site

COMPARING DRUG FORMS *continued*

DOSAGE FORM	DESCRIPTION	ADVANTAGES	DISADVANTAGES
Parenteral forms *(continued)*			
I.M. injection	Medication administered by injecting a solution into a muscle	• Provides rapid absorption of medication; onset of action usually within 10 to 15 minutes • I.M. injections of drugs that irritate subcutaneous tissues cause less pain than S.C. injections • Larger volume of fluid can be administered than by S.C. injection	• Blood flow to injection site affects absorption rate • Using an inappropriate injection site could result in permanent damage to the patient
Direct I.V. injection (I.V. bolus)	Medication administered by injecting into a vein to deliver rapidly	• Drug becomes effective immediately because it's injected directly into the patient's bloodstream • Blood levels more predictable than with other methods	• May cause speed shock • May irritate vein • Increases risk of complications: extravasation, systemic infection, and air embolism
Continuous I.V. drip (primary line infusion)	Medication administered by infusing into a vein to maintain delivery at a therapeutic level	• Less irritating than bolus injection • Requires less mixing and hanging than intermittent method • Easy to discontinue	• Can be dangerous if I.V. flow rate isn't carefully monitored • Many drugs too unstable for prolonged infusion • Increases risk of complications: extravasation, systemic infection, and air embolism • Mixing medications may cause incompatibility
Intermittent (additive set infusion) to administer drugs mixed with diluent	Medication infused intermittently or as a one-time dose	• Administration time longer than bolus injection and shorter than continuous I.V. drip therapy • Less likely to cause speed shock than bolus injection • Less irritating to veins than bolus injection	• Expensive • Increased risk of contamination by frequent port use • Mixing medications may cause incompatibility • Increases risks of complications: extravasation, systemic infection, and air embolism

(continued)

COMPARING DRUG FORMS *continued*

DOSAGE FORM	DESCRIPTION	ADVANTAGES	DISADVANTAGES
Dermatomucosal forms			
Powder	Inert chemical that may contain small particles of medication obtained by grinding a solid drug	• Faster relief from surface pain and itching than with systemic drugs • Less severe allergic reactions than with systemic drugs • Fewer adverse reactions than with systemic drugs • Comforting for the patient because he can witness the care	• Difficult to deliver in precise doses • May stain skin, clothing, furniture, or bed linen • Application procedure is time-consuming • Depending on the site, may be embarrassing to patient • Depending on the site, may be difficult for the patient to apply
Lotion	Suspension of insoluble powder in water or an emulsion without powder	• Same as for powder	• Same as for powder
Cream	Semisolid emulsion of oil and water	• Same as for powder	• Same as for powder
Ointment	Semisolid suspension of oil and water	• Same as for powder	• Same as for powder
Paste	Stiff mixture of powder and ointment	• Same as for powder	• Same as for powder

preparing a liquid form. When using an NG or gastrostomy tube, the nurse must know how the action of a medication changes when a tablet is crushed. A crushed tablet disintegrates immediately, and absorption from the GI tract occurs rapidly. These changes may not produce significant differences in blood levels and absorption rate if the tablet was designed for rapid disintegration and absorption. If, however, the tablet was designed for slow release and absorption, crushing can alter the drug's effect significantly.

In some cases, the nurse may consult the doctor about using a different form of the drug or a different route to achieve the intended effect.

Rectal administration

Rectal medications are available in various forms, including suppositories, creams, ointments, retention enemas, and rectal syringes. Because suppositories contain medication in a semisolid base, such as cocoa butter, that melts at body temperature, they must be refrigerated to prevent melting before use.

Rectal (P.R.) administration may be desirable for drugs that are rapidly degraded in the stomach or for drugs likely to cause gastric irritation. Drugs commonly administered P.R. include antipyretics, analgesics, antiemetics, bronchodilators, corticosteroids, and rectal evacuants.

P.R. administration can provide either local or systemic effects. Systemic absorption from this route may be unpredictable but usually is complete if the patient retains the medication long enough. The presence of feces in the rectum will decrease drug absorption. If the patient has diarrhea, the medication may be expelled before sufficient absorption has occurred. Rectal medications may exacerbate any local inflammatory conditions.

Parenteral administration

Parenteral drug administration can involve all routes other than the GI tract. The discussion in this chapter, however, concentrates on those medications given by injection. Nurses use the parenteral route to provide a rapid onset of action and to ensure high blood levels of the drug. The parenteral route also is used when the GI route would inactivate the drug, in unconscious patients, and in unstable or seriously ill patients who require precise administration and monitoring. Common administration techniques for parenteral drugs include intradermal, S.C., I.M., and I.V. administration.

Intradermal injections

Intradermal injection—injection into the dermis layer of the skin—is recommended to provide local drug effects or for allergy or anergy skin tests. Common sites of intradermal injection include the ventral forearm, the upper chest, and the shoulder blade. A short (⅝"), fine-gauge (26G or 27G) needle is used on a 1-ml syringe. Because absorption occurs in the capillaries of the dermis, which have a slower absorption rate than subcutaneous tissue or muscle, drug reactions are delayed. Reactions to intradermally injected drugs usually occur within 24 to 72 hours.

S.C. injections

Usually, S.C. injection—injection into the adipose tissues (fatty layer) beneath the skin—produces more sustained and slower absorption than I.M. injection. It also causes minimal tissue trauma and avoids damage to large blood vessels and nerves.

S.C. injection is undesirable for patients with compromised perfusion from conditions such as shock, edema, or occlusive peripheral vascular disease. It also is usually contraindicated in patients who are extremely obese or who have diseased tissue, dermatologic problems, or burns. Also, irritating drugs should not be administered S.C.; I.V. infusion may be more appropriate.

S.C. injection is appropriate in any part of the body where large nerves, large blood vessels, and bones are not near the surface. A short (½" to ⅝" [1.27 to 1.59 cm]) 25G to 27G needle is commonly used, and the maximum volume for injection is 2 ml. The most common sites for S.C.

injection include the outer aspects of the arms, the anterior thighs, the loose tissue of the lower abdomen just above the iliac crest, the buttocks, and the upper back.

I.M. injections

I.M. injection—injections into a muscle—is used to place medication deep into muscular tissue, where it is absorbed through many blood vessels. I.M. injection may be preferred in patients for whom I.V. access is difficult and in patients who are unable to swallow or are vomiting or unconscious. Because muscle tissue contains relatively fewer sensory nerve endings than most other tissues, irritating medications in volumes of up to 5 ml may be administered with less pain. Injectable formulations that should never be administered I.V. (such as oily solutions, suspensions, and other depot forms) commonly are administered by I.M. injection.

Absorption of drugs administered by I.M. injection depends on patient factors and on the properties of the drugs themselves. For example, drugs delivered by I.M. injection usually aren't well absorbed in patients with decreased peripheral perfusion resulting from disorders such as shock, edema, and occlusive peripheral vascular disease. For this reason, I.M. injections may be contraindicated in these patients. Certain drugs may crystallize after I.M. injection, resulting in delayed absorption. Such drugs, including diazepam (Valium), chlordiazepoxide (Librium), and phenytoin (Dilantin), are best administered I.V. if rapid effects are desired.

Although I.M. administration is inexpensive and generally safe, it does pose some special problems. This route may not be best for patients who are elderly, emaciated, or for some other reason do not have adequate muscle mass and for patients with altered coagulation states or thrombocytopenia or who are taking anticoagulants or antiplatelet drugs. I.M. injection may damage blood vessels, nerves, or bone if injected incorrectly. Inadvertent injection of drugs into fatty tissue in obese patients may cause sterile abscesses, draining lesions, low-grade fever, and pain. To prevent tissue damage and facilitate drug absorption, injections should be given into large muscle masses, such as the ventrogluteal, vastus lateralis, rectus femoris, dorsogluteal, and deltoid muscles.

I.V. injections

I.V. administration—injecting a medication directly into a vein—is another common parenteral route of administration. Many different drugs can be administered through I.V. infusion. Three types of I.V. infusion are used: direct (bolus), continuous, and intermittent. Bolus administration can quickly attain therapeutic drug concentrations, making it the method of choice in many emergency situations when rapid drug effect is desired; it also is used to deliver drugs that can't be diluted. The extremely rapid onset of drug effect provided by bolus administration is often a therapeutic advantage, but it also carries the risk of producing an immediate acute allergic reaction or anaphylaxis. Because of this risk, many drugs are inappropriate for bolus administration. Be sure to check with the pharmacist if you have any doubts about administering a drug as an I.V. bolus.

To sustain the desired action of a short-acting drug, continuous I.V. infusion can be administered at a rate calculated to maintain therapeutic serum levels of the drug. Intermittent I.V. infusion can be used to maintain therapeutic serum levels of longer-acting drugs.

Because many patients receive more than one drug simultaneously by I.V. infusion, ensuring the compatibility of different drugs in infusion containers and I.V. lines is essential. When evaluating I.V. drug compatibility, be sure to consider both physical and chemical incompatibilities. A physical incompatibility usually can be detected visually by the formation of a haze, color change, or precipitate in the solution. This problem usually results from differences in solubility among drugs. Infusion of physically incompatible drugs may cause precipitate formation, which can decrease or block the flow of I.V. fluid.

Chemical incompatibilities, which are more difficult to detect, may influence the action of one or more of the drugs administered. For example, administration of ticarcillin and gentamicin in combination causes inactivation of the gentamicin.

Dermatomucosal route

The dermal route, also known as the dermatomucosal route and more commonly the topical route, is generally used for local rather than systemic effects. One of several exceptions, nitroglycerin is given via the dermal route for its systemic rather than local effect.

Medication forms given via the dermal route include creams, lotions, ointments, powders, and patches. Patches contain a measured dose of medication that is delivered over an extended time. Medications in patch form include nitroglycerin (for angina pectoris), scopolamine (for motion sickness), clonidine (for hypertension), and estrogen (for menopausal symptoms).

Medication forms applied by the dermatomucosal route are absorbed through the epidermal layer into the dermis. The extent of absorption depends on the vascularity of and circulation in the region.

Other routes of drug administration

Other routes the nurse may use in the clinical setting include the ophthalmic, otic, nasal, respiratory, urethral, and vaginal routes.

Ophthalmic administration

Eye drops and ointments are applied directly to the eye for topical treatment of disease or as diagnostic aids. Ophthalmic agents include mydriatics (agents that dilate the pupil) and cycloplegics (agents that paralyze the accommodative muscle of the ciliary body of the eye), used primarily for intraocular examinations and refractions; miotics (agents used to treat glaucoma and to manage accommodative esotropia); drugs used to lower intraocular pressure; anesthetic agents used to relieve eye pain or discomfort, or so that instruments can be applied to measure intraocular pressure or remove foreign bodies; and anti-inflammatory and anti-infective agents, used to treat inflammation and infection.

If continuous release of certain ophthalmic drugs is indicated, an eye medication disk may be inserted in the conjunctival sac of the patient's lower eyelid. This small device consists of permeable inner and outer layers and a middle layer containing the medication. It can be worn continuously for up to 1 week and may be used with contact lenses.

Otic administration

Otic agents are instilled in the ear canal to treat infection, inflammation, and pain, and to soften cerumen (earwax). These drugs are categorized as anti-infective (single and compound), anti-inflammatory, local anesthetic, and ceruminolytic agents. Otic agents are administered via ear drops, ear irrigations, or ear wicks. Several combination products contain both anti-infective and anti-inflammatory agents.

Nasal administration

Medication can be applied topically to the nose in various forms, including liquid drops, sprays, and aerosols. The nurse administers these forms of medication by instillation or by an atomizer or nasal aerosol device, although the nasal aerosol device is now seldom used. The technique for its use resembles that for the atomizer and drop instillation methods. Nasal agents are primarily selected sympathomimetic amine decongestants used to provide immediate relief from nasal congestion and swollen mucous membranes when applied directly to the nasal mucosa.

Respiratory tract administration

Bronchodilators, corticosteroids, and antiallergy agents are commonly administered through oral or nasal inhalation. Hand-held metered-dose devices provide an inexpensive, safe, and convenient method for delivering medication systemically. These devices break up the medication into small particles that can reach the airways of the lungs when inhaled. The smaller the size of the particles and the deeper the patient inhales, the deeper the drug will reach into the lungs. Because only a small portion of the drug finds its way to the surface of the lung, inhalation usually causes fewer adverse reactions than oral administration.

An endotracheal tube can provide a valuable route of administration for some medications. Besides mucolytics, emergency drugs such as epinephrine, atropine, lidocaine, naloxone, and metaraminol can be delivered endotracheally and rapidly absorbed into systemic circulation via the alveoli. Delayed onset of drug action may occur in patients with conditions such as adult respiratory distress syndrome.

Drugs may be delivered directly to the throat through sprays, gargles, mouthwashes, and lozenges. Topical anesthetics are commonly administered in spray form for patients with pharyngitis or before a scheduled surgical procedure in the throat.

Urethral administration

Urethral drug administration may be used when local antibiotic or antifungal drug therapy is indicated for a lower GU tract condition. Such medication, in liquid form, is instilled into the urethra through a small-diameter urinary catheter under sterile conditions. The catheter then is removed or clamped so the medication can reach and bathe the bladder walls. How long the catheter remains clamped determines the duration of medication retention in the bladder. Occasionally an intracatheter with the needle removed may be inserted into the urethra for the instillation of liquid medication—for example, to treat epididymitis.

Urethral administration may be repeated several times a day for about a week or only performed once. The volume of medication can range from a few milliliters to almost a liter.

Vaginal administration
Vaginal medication, in suppositories, tablets, gels, creams, and ointments, is used to provide topical treatment of local infection and inflammation or for contraception. Suppositories are manufactured in a semisolid base, such as cocoa butter, that melts at body temperature in the vaginal mucosa. Medication then diffuses much like that from topical creams, gels, and ointments.

PREPARING FOR DRUG ADMINISTRATION
To ensure safe and effective drug therapy, you need a thorough understanding of the drug's pharmacokinetic and pharmacodynamic properties, as well as knowledge of correct administration techniques. Before administering any drug, you should be able to answer the following questions:
- What is the drug being used for?
- Is the dosage appropriate for this patient?
- Is the route of administration appropriate?
- What is the expected effect of the drug and how should this be monitored?
- What adverse reactions are common to this drug?
- How should any adverse reactions be managed?

For help, you can consult a variety of drug information sources, including the *American Hospital Formulary Service* (*AHFS*) and the *Physicians' Desk Reference* (*PDR*). Please note, however, that the *PDR* merely compiles the FDA-approved package inserts for the various drug products selected by the manufacturer and may or may not include a given drug's most up-to-date clinical information. Your institution's pharmacist and pharmacy department's drug information center may be the best source of updated information.

However, even when armed with all the necessary drug information, you are still vulnerable to medication errors. Such errors can result from problems or distraction at any point during drug prescription, dispensation, and administration. The following errors are most common: incorrectly transcribing a medication order onto a medication administration record (MAR), dispensing the wrong drug, administering the wrong dosage, using the wrong route of administration, and missing scheduled administration times. These errors may interfere with therapeutic effectiveness, produce adverse reactions, and, at worst, threaten the patient's life.

AVOIDING MEDICATION ERRORS
The following guidelines also will help you avoid medication errors.
- Utilize the classic safeguards, known as the five "rights" of medication administration (checking to be sure it's the right drug, dose, patient, time, and route before administration).

- Regardless of its legal classification, no drug—including OTC products and placebos—should be administered to a patient unless ordered by a doctor.
- Remember that verbal orders for drug therapy can be accepted only by a registered nurse, *only in emergencies,* and only with extreme care to ensure accuracy.
- If possible, avoid using a patient's own medications, the composition and condition of which may be unknown. If, however, they must be used, be sure to obtain a written doctor's order authorizing it, and have the drugs identified by a pharmacist before administering them.
- Store drugs and preparations meant for external use separate from internal medications. Make sure that such products are clearly labeled "for external use only."
- Store all controlled substances under a double-lock system, to limit access by unauthorized persons.
- When obtaining a drug from storage, check the drug name carefully. Pay particular attention to spelling—some dissimilar drugs have similar spellings. Consult a reliable reference if you are unsure about a drug name, and don't hesitate to ask another nurse or the pharmacist for verification.
- Always read the label to identify a drug. Don't rely on the color, shape, or shelf location of a container for identification.
- Check the drug's label against the doctor's order and the patient's MAR three times before administration: when obtaining the drug, when preparing the dose, and when returning the drug to storage or discarding its container.
- Wash your hands thoroughly before preparing or administering any medication.
- Prepare medications in a clean, distraction-free area.
- Never administer a medication that has been prepared by another nurse.
- Clearly label liquid doses drawn up in a syringe with the drug name, concentration, date and time drawn up, and your initials.
- Ensure the accuracy of your dosage calculations by having another nurse or a pharmacist double-check them.
- Administer a drug as close as possible to the scheduled administration time specified by the doctor's order and institution policy. Be especially punctual with drugs that must be maintained in adequate blood concentrations for optimal therapeutic effect, such as antibiotics, chemotherapeutic agents, and antimyasthenic drugs.
- Record the reason for any delayed or otherwise untimely administration in the nurses' notes and take other appropriate action, as defined by your institution's procedures.
- Before administering any drug, double-check the patient's identity by reading his wristband and addressing him by name.
- If the patient expresses concern about a drug you are about to administer, always take the time to double-check the drug and dosage information.

- If a patient refuses to take a medication, ask why. Often, your explanation of the drug's necessity and benefits will convince the patient to comply. If the patient still refuses, inform the patient care manager and doctor. Document the patient's noncompliance and your subsequent actions in the patient's chart.
- Never administer a drug that looks discolored, in which a precipitate has formed, or that otherwise appears abnormal. Instead, notify the pharmacist of your concern and have him evaluate the drug.
- Always check the expiration date before administering any drug. Return all expired drugs to the pharmacy for disposal.
- Never leave medications at the patient's bedside unless this is permitted by hospital policy and specifically authorized by a doctor's written order. If the patient is allowed to self-medicate, make sure that he can do so correctly, and monitor usage carefully.
- When administering a drug p.r.n., make sure that sufficient time has passed since the last dose.
- Provide privacy as needed when administering injections, suppositories, and enemas.
- Document all drug administration on the patient's chart.
- Always assess and record the patient's response after administering medications—especially after administering cardiac drugs and opioid analgesics.
- Discard used needles and syringes into proper disposal containers.
- Include any significant amounts of fluids used to deliver medications, such as I.V. piggyback fluid, in the patient's intake and output records, as applicable.

SELF-TEST

1. Timothy Jones, age 60, has osteoarthritis. His doctor has prescribed aspirin. On a follow-up visit, Mr. Jones complains of GI upset. The doctor then prescribes enteric-coated aspirin to reduce GI distress. Where do enteric-coated tablets dissolve?
   a. in the mouth
   b. in the stomach
   c. in the intestine
   d. in the rectum

2. Which of the following governing bodies regulates the nurse's legal responsibilities to administer drugs to hospital patients?
   a. nurse practice act in each state
   b. American Nurses' Association
   c. Food and Drug Administration
   d. state pharmacy practice act

3. Mr. Jones develops several complications after an MI and requires prolonged bed rest. His doctor has prescribed low-dose heparin to be administered subcutaneously to prevent thromboembolism. How many milliliters of solution may be administered per injection by the S.C. route?

    a. 1 ml

    b. 2 ml

    c. 3 ml

    d. 4 ml

Check your answers on page 1056.

CHAPTER 3

ADVERSE REACTIONS AND INTERACTIONS

An adverse reaction is any undesirable and unintended effect that follows administration of a drug. Types of adverse reactions include dose-related toxicity, side effects, and allergic and idiosyncratic reactions. Drug *toxicity* is usually caused by cumulative effect and buildup of excessive drug levels. Toxic effects may represent an exaggeration of the therapeutic effect. For example, guanethidine-induced norepinephrine depletion produces an antihypertensive effect; with larger doses, this same action often produces orthostatic hypotension, indicating drug toxicity.

A *side effect* is any pharmacologic but unintended action of a drug. For example, morphine given to relieve the pain of MI may also cause sedation as a side effect. Such sedation may be desirable in the patient with MI, but in an ambulatory patient, sedation could be hazardous, thereby qualifying as an adverse reaction.

An *allergic drug reaction* is an immunologically mediated adverse response requiring previous sensitization. It is usually unpredictable. An example is a penicillin rash.

An *idiosyncratic* drug reaction refers to an unusual and unpredictable response to a drug, such as chloramphenicol-induced aplastic anemia. Such a response may also take the form of extreme sensitivity to low doses of a drug or of insensitivity to high doses.

INCIDENCE OF ADVERSE REACTIONS
About 5% of patients who receive drug therapy experience serious adverse reactions. Nearly 20% of these involve new drugs, probably because less is known about their potential for adverse reactions. Many more patients experience minor, so-called insignificant side effects. Drug therapy causes life-threatening reactions in fewer than 1% of patients, but it accounts for up to 4% of hospitalizations. Clearly, the potential for causing adverse reactions is a major factor influencing the decision to prescribe drug therapy; the potential benefit to the patient should outweigh any risk of adverse effects.

EVALUATING THE RISKS AND BENEFITS
The following factors influence a decision to prescribe a drug that can produce serious adverse reactions:
• *Therapeutic index.* The standard measure of benefit to risk, this range between minimally effective and toxic plasma drug levels determines a drug's margin for safety. If a drug's therapeutic index is narrow, maintaining drug levels within the safe range is more difficult; therefore, the risk of adverse reactions is greater.

GLOSSARY

Adverse drug reaction: an undesirable and unintended effect ranging from mild to severe life-threatening hypersensitivity reactions.

Allergic drug reaction: an immunologically mediated adverse response requiring previous sensitization.

Anaphylaxis: a state of immediate hypersensitivity following sensitization to a foreign protein or drug.

Drug interaction: relationship between concurrently administered drugs or a reaction between a drug and a component of body fluids, food, or pharmaceutical preparations such as preservatives or binding agents used in drug formulations.

Idiosyncratic drug reaction: an unusual and unpredictable response to a drug.

Photodermatitis: a sunburnlike reaction that develops when a drug or its metabolite concentrates in the skin and absorbs ultraviolet light energy.

Serum sickness: a syndrome originally observed after a drug is administered, generally resulting in the occurrence in 8 to 12 days of an urticarial rash, edema, enlargement of lymph nodes, arthralgia, and fever.

Side effect: any pharmacologic but unintended action of a drug.

Toxicity: condition caused by excess drug in the body.

Urticaria: a skin condition characterized by the appearance of intensely itching wheals or welts with elevated, usually white, centers and a surrounding area of erythema; also known as hives.

- *The severity of the patient's condition.* A drug that has potential for serious adverse effects should not be prescribed for minor illness. For example, chloramphenicol, which can cause aplastic anemia, is not an appropriate treatment for an uncomplicated and ordinary respiratory infection. However, this drug may offer the best chance for recovery and thus be the drug of choice for life-threatening meningitis.
- *The severity of the adverse reaction.* For example, mouth dryness, a common reaction with decongestants (anticholinergics), is acceptable when it relieves a more distressing or dangerous condition.
- *The patient's ability to adjust to the adverse reaction.* For example, can the patient take the drug at bedtime to avoid orthostatic hypotension? Can he take a diuretic early in the day to avoid nocturia?

The patient's risk factors

For each patient who must receive drug therapy, you should consider these factors in light of the patient's individual risk factors, to help anticipate potential reactions and to detect them early enough to prevent major sequelae.

- To evaluate the risk of adverse reactions in a patient, you'll need to assess for the following factors.

- *Multiple drug therapy.* The incidence of adverse reactions is proportional to the number of drugs consumed. Because patients with chronic diseases and elderly patients with multiple impairments commonly need multiple drug therapy, they are at greater risk for adverse reactions.
- *A history of adverse drug reactions.* Patients with a history of sensitivity to medications or environmental allergens have an increased tendency to develop adverse drug reactions.
- *Pathologic factors.* Illness or systemic dysfunctions also increase the risk of adverse reactions. For example, hepatic or renal impairment causes accumulation of aminoglycoside antibiotics, such as gentamicin. Illness that causes fluid or electrolyte imbalance, such as vomiting or diarrhea, can cause sensitivity to drugs that require fluid and electrolyte balance for their action. For example, digitalis and antiarrhythmic agents are especially hazardous in patients with potassium imbalance.
- *Age.* Neonates have immature systems for drug metabolism and excretion, with potentially unstable homeostatic mechanisms. Elderly patients have diminished capacity to metabolize and excrete drugs, which makes them vulnerable to toxic drug accumulation.
- *Genetic predisposition.* Certain genetic characteristics can impair the biochemical pathways governing drug metabolism and increase the risk of adverse reactions. For example, in certain ethnic groups (Black Americans, Mediterranean Jews, and Chinese), congenital deficiency of the enzyme glucose-6-phosphate dehydrogenase (G6PD) increases the risk that certain oxidizing drugs, such as chloroquine and sulfacetamide, will cause hemolysis.
- *Sex.* Varying body fat and hormonal influences may affect drug therapy. However, sex-determined differences in drug effect generally appear to be of minor significance, except in pregnant women.

Dose-dependent responses: Predictable hazard
Even after careful assessment of risk factors, the patient is still at risk for severe reactions. Such reactions usually are dose-related; they may disappear rapidly if the drug is discontinued or its dosage reduced. Thus, dose-dependent toxicity is largely preventable.

DRUG ALLERGY AND SENSITIVITY
Allergic reactions account for about 6% of adverse drug reactions in hospitalized patients; of these patients, only about 5% have no history of drug allergy. A history of sensitivity most reliably indicates the potential for allergic reaction. But even with no such history, previous exposure usually increases the possibility of sensitization.

Cross-sensitivity
Drugs with similar chemical structures, such as penicillins and cephalosporins, may elicit a cross-sensitivity reaction. In patients known to be sensitive to either penicillin or cephalosporins, usually both are withheld or used with caution and prior skin testing.

In about 30% of adult patients with asthma and nasal polyps, aspirin produces an allergic reaction that may cause shortness of breath, severe urticaria, and anaphylaxis. Similar aspirin cross-sensitivity reactions occur in about 10% of those ingesting tartrazine (a yellow dye once used in the formulation of many drugs), in about 6% of those taking acetaminophen, and in most patients taking ibuprofen, indomethacin, naproxen, or other NSAIDs.

Common allergic reactions

The most common allergic reaction is a maculopapular rash. The most serious allergic reactions occur in patients in whom specific immunoglobulin E (IgE) antibodies for the drug have resulted from previous exposure. In such patients, drug ingestion causes rapid release of histamine, leukotrienes, and chemotactic factors that produce urticaria or even anaphylaxis.

A less acute systemic hypersensitivity reaction, *serum sickness* may develop within hours to weeks after the start of treatment with an antiserum. Its symptoms include urticaria, arthralgia, fever, arthritis, and adenopathy. Drugs associated with serum sickness include immune serums, cephalosporins, dextrans, hydralazine, penicillins, phenylbutazone, sulfonamides, and thiouracils.

Several types of skin disorders are also allergy-related:
- Cutaneous contact with some drugs causes *eczematous contact dermatitis,* an infiltration of T lymphocytes and mononuclear cells that leads to an inflammatory response and a transient rash. Neomycin, parabens, and topical antihistamines can cause such a reaction.
- Metronidazole, sulfonamides, penicillins, and phenolphthalein may cause *fixed drug eruptions* of the skin by unknown mechanisms. Typically, fixed eruptions produce a persistent, localized rash.
- Preceded by viruslike symptoms and characterized by vasculitis and severe, bullous lesions of the skin and mucous membranes, *erythema multiforme*, another hypersensitivity syndrome, and its life-threatening form, *Stevens-Johnson syndrome,* may follow use of barbiturates, codeine, or salicylates.
- *Photodermatitis* develops when a drug or its metabolite concentrates in the skin and absorbs ultraviolet light energy, causing a sunburnlike reaction. Drugs associated with this reaction include tetracyclines and phenothiazines, griseofulvin, nalidixic acid, sulfonamides, and thiazide diuretics.

Other types of allergy-based drug reactions include autoimmune reactions, hemolytic anemia, and drug fever:
- *Autoimmune reactions* are thought to develop when a drug, such as hydralazine or procainamide, causes nucleoprotein in the body to become antigenic, resulting in such conditions as systemic lupus erythematosus.
- *Hemolytic anemia* can result from the formation of immune complexes on RBCs. Drugs associated with hemolytic anemia include penicillins, phenothiazines, sulfonamides, methyldopa, and cisplatin.
- *Fever* may be associated with other symptoms of allergic drug reactions (for example, in serum sickness or vasculitis), but a sustained fever may be the *only* symptom of an allergic reaction. It usually subsides within

48 hours after discontinuation of the drug. Drugs that may produce drug fever include cephalosporins, penicillins, and other antibiotics; barbiturates; methyldopa; phenytoin; procainamide; and quinidine.

Management of allergic reactions

Potentially life-threatening allergic reactions require quick identification and immediate withdrawal of the drug. If your patient is receiving a commonly allergenic drug, be sure to double-check his drug and allergy history. Also, after administering such a drug, monitor the patient for signs of an allergic reaction for the first 15 minutes. When administering parenteral drugs (such as penicillin) in an outpatient setting, observe the patient for 30 to 60 minutes before discharge. Serious reactions may require airway maintenance and administration of epinephrine.

CARCINOGENIC AND TERATOGENIC REACTIONS

In the 1960s, the tragedy associated with thalidomide prompted close monitoring of drugs for potential to produce teratogenic and carcinogenic effects. Several drug groups have been implicated, including estrogens (childhood cancer), antihistamines (birth defects), tetracyclines (bone changes), and sulfonamides (jaundice). Because of the potential for teratogenicity, only the most necessary drugs are appropriate for use during the first trimester of pregnancy—the time of greatest risk to the developing fetus. Occupational exposure to toxic drugs is a source of similar concern. For example, health care workers should avoid handling cyclophosphamide, doxorubicin, vincristine, and other antineoplastic drugs during the first trimester of pregnancy. These drugs have been associated with fetal death. Before exposing themselves to toxic drugs, workers should review the guidelines for the safe handling of mutagenic compounds.

DRUG INTERACTIONS

A drug interaction occurs when a drug reacts with another drug or with any component of body fluids, foods, or pharmaceutical preparations (such as preservatives or binding agents).

Drug interactions may be intentional, producing a desirable or therapeutic effect, or unintentional, producing an undesirable, nontherapeutic, or possibly harmful effect. Most drug interactions are unintentional. Minor interactions may not influence therapy at all or may require only a change in dosage or schedule of administration. However, major interactions can hinder effective therapy or even be life-threatening.

The risk of a drug interaction increases with the number of drugs taken concomitantly. According to some sources, the average hospitalized patient receives 12 to 15 drugs; the chronically or critically ill patient easily could receive more. Drug interactions are sometimes mistaken for adverse drug reactions; reportedly, up to 25% of adverse reactions result from such interactions.

Classifying drug interactions into two broad categories—pharmacokinetic and pharmacodynamic interactions—can help clarify the subject. A *pharmacokinetic* interaction occurs when one drug changes the absorption, distribution, metabolism, or excretion of another drug. A *pharmaco-dynamic* interaction occurs when one drug changes the activity of another drug, producing additive or antagonistic effects.

Pharmacokinetic interactions

When a drug is prescribed, its absorption, distribution, metabolism, and excretion are expected to follow a predictable pattern. Interacting drugs can alter these patterns of activity through various mechanisms.

Altered absorption

Alteration in a drug's absorption pattern can produce a drug interaction from the following mechanisms: pH changes, complex formation, physical incompatibilities, or inactivation.

Any drug that alters the pH of the GI tract changes the absorption pattern for a drug taken later. For example, an antacid causes a patient's normally acidic gastric fluid to become more alkaline. As a result, any weakly alkaline drug that the patient subsequently ingests will remain non-ionized and be quickly absorbed. But a weakly acidic drug that is normally absorbed in the stomach is likely to become so highly ionized that it is poorly absorbed in the stomach.

Changes in gastric pH also can affect drug dissolution. If a patient takes an enteric-coated tablet shortly after taking an antacid, the alkaline environment in the stomach will dissolve the tablet's coating there instead of in the small intestine (as intended). This premature dissolution may cause gastric irritation—which the enteric coating was intended to prevent—and may lead to intensified drug effects from the unusually rapid absorption.

Another common interaction decreases absorption when certain antibiotics are taken with food or antacids. For example, the presence of food blocks penicillin absorption. The antibiotic tetracycline forms complexes with aluminum, calcium, and magnesium ions present in dairy products and antacids; such binding prevents the drug's passage into the bloodstream. Newer types of tetracyclines, such as doxycycline and minocycline, apparently do not form complexes with milk or food but do form complexes with the antacid aluminum hydroxide. Careful timing of doses can prevent such undesirable formation of complexes. Giving tetracycline 1 hour before an antacid usually allows enough time for drug absorption.

Physical or chemical incompatibility is another potential source of drug interactions. Combining incompatible drugs in a syringe may cause chemical complexes to form, which can inactivate the drug or prevent its absorption. For an overview of drug compatibility, see *Compatibility of drugs combined in a syringe*, pages 44 and 45. Physically incompatible drugs interact before they reach the site of action, usually interfering with the activity of one or both drugs. For example, exposing an aminoglycoside antibiotic (amikacin, gentamicin, tobramycin) to penicillins for a prolonged time inactivates the aminoglycoside. Mixing incompatible drugs can form precipitates or change a drug's color. Precipitate formation is especially dangerous for the patient if the solution is to be infused intravenously.

Some drug interactions enhance absorption. For example, giving a fat-soluble drug, such as griseofulvin, with fatty meals enhances its absorption. Similarly, giving vitamin C with iron supplements greatly increases iron absorption. Combining procaine and penicillin creates a complex that slows absorption of penicillin. This beneficial interaction sustains blood levels of penicillin for a longer time.

Altered distribution

After being absorbed and reaching the bloodstream, many drugs are bound to proteins in the plasma. And because only unbound drug can saturate the tissues and affect the body, the plasma proteins, mainly albumin (which binds acidic drugs) and alpha-lipoprotein (which binds alkaline drugs), in effect store the bound drug until more is needed. When two drugs bind to the same place on the same protein, they compete for binding sites, one displacing the other. This increases the amount of displaced drug that is free to act at its site of action. If a displaced drug normally is highly protein-bound (90% or more), its displacement can cause toxic overdose, particularly if the drug has a narrow therapeutic index. Phenytoin is one such drug. However, not all highly bound drugs pose a problem. Digitoxin, for instance, is highly bound, but no other drug displaces it significantly. Moreover, the fact that two drugs compete for the same proteins does not necessarily mean they can never be used together—but it does signal the need for careful monitoring when they are. Careful monitoring and compensatory dosage adjustment can make such combinations workable.

When an excess of free drug circulates, the body metabolizes and eliminates the extra molecules to bring the ratio of bound drug to free drug back to normal as soon as possible. The greater the drug's apparent volume of distribution, the more quickly compensation occurs.

Altered metabolism

Interactions that change a drug's pattern of metabolism involve either enzyme induction or enzyme inhibition.

In *enzyme induction,* a drug stimulates the production of the enzymes that metabolize it. If another drug is metabolized by the same enzyme system, a drug interaction may cause blood levels of either drug to fall suddenly to subtherapeutic levels. For example, barbiturates, such as phenobarbital, induce the production of the enzymes that inactivate phenytoin and warfarin. Therefore, in a patient stabilized on therapy with warfarin, the additional use of barbiturates may cause a sudden drop in warfarin blood levels and loss of anticoagulant effect.

(Text continues on page 46.)

COMPATIBILITY OF DRUGS COMBINED IN A SYRINGE

KEY
Y = compatible for at least 30 minutes
P = provisionally compatible; administer within 15 minutes
P(5) = provisionally compatible; administer within 5 minutes
N = not compatible
* = conflicting data

(A blank space indicates no available data.)

	atropine sulfate	benzquinamide HCl	butorphanol tartrate	chlorpromazine HCl	cimetidine HCl	codeine phosphate	dimenhydrinate	diphenhydramine HCl	droperidol	fentanyl citrate	glycopyrrolate	heparin Na	hydromorphone HCl	hydroxyzine HCl	meperidine HCl
atropine sulfate		Y	Y	Y	Y		P	P	P	P	Y	P(5)	Y	Y	Y
benzquinamide HCl	Y										Y			Y	Y
butorphanol tartrate	Y			Y	Y		N	Y	Y	Y				Y	P
chlorpromazine HCl	Y		Y		N		N	P	P	P	Y	N	Y	P	P
cimetidine HCl	Y		Y	N			Y	Y	Y	Y	Y	Y	Y	Y	Y
codeine phosphate											Y		Y		
dimenhydrinate	P		N	N				P	P	P	N	P(5)		N	P
diphenhydramine HCl	P		Y	P	Y	P			P	P	Y		Y	P	P
droperidol	P		Y	P	Y		P	P		P	Y	N		P	P
fentanyl citrate	P		Y	P	Y		P	P	P			P(5)	Y	Y	P
glycopyrrolate	Y	Y		Y	Y	Y	N	Y	Y				Y	Y	Y
heparin Na	P(5)		N	Y		P(5)		N	P(5)						N
hydromorphone HCl	Y		Y	Y			Y		Y	Y				Y	
hydroxyzine HCl	Y	Y	Y	P	Y	Y	N	P	P	Y	Y		Y		P
meperidine HCl	Y	Y	P	P	Y		P	P	P	P	Y	N		P	
metoclopramide HCl	P			P			P	Y	P	P		P(5)		P	P
midazolam HCl	Y	Y	Y	Y	Y		N	Y	Y	Y	Y		Y	Y	Y
morphine sulfate	P	Y	Y	P	Y		P	P	P	P	Y	N*		Y	N
nalbuphine HCl	Y			Y			Y						Y		
pentazocine lactate	P	Y	Y	P	Y		P	P	P	P	N	N	Y	Y	P
pentobarbital Na	P	N	N	N	N		N	N	N	N	N		Y	N	N
perphenazine	Y		Y	Y	Y		Y	Y	Y	Y					P
phenobarbital Na		N										P(5)			
prochlorperazine edisylate	P		Y	Y	Y		N	P	P	P	Y		N*	P	P
promazine HCl	P			P	Y		N	P	P	P	Y			P	P
promethazine HCl	P		Y	P	Y		N	P	P	P	Y	N	Y	P	Y
ranitidine HCl	Y			Y			Y	Y		Y	P		Y	N	Y
scopolamine HBr	P	Y	Y	P	Y		P	P	P	P	Y		Y	Y	P
secobarbital Na		N			N							N			
sodium bicarbonate												N			
thiethylperazine maleate			Y										Y		
thiopental Na		N			N		N	N				N			N

	metoclopramide HCl	midazolam HCl	morphine sulfate	nalbuphine HCl	pentazocine lactate	pentobarbital Na	perphenazine	phenobarbital Na	prochlorperazine edisylate	promazine HCl	promethazine HCl	ranitidine HCl	scopolamine HBr	secobarbital Na	sodium bicarbonate	thiethylperazine maleate	thiopental Na
atropine sulfate	P	Y	P	Y	P	P	Y		P	P	P	Y					
benzquinamide HCl		Y	Y		Y	N		N				Y	N				N
butorphanol tartrate		Y	Y		Y	N	Y		Y		Y		Y			Y	
chlorpromazine HCl	P	Y	P		P	N	Y		Y	P	P	Y	P				N
cimetidine HCl		Y	Y	Y	Y	N	Y		Y	Y	Y		Y	N			
codeine phosphate																	
dimenhydrinate	P	N	P		P	N	Y		N	N	N	Y	P				N
diphenhydramine HCl	Y	Y	P		P	N	Y		P	P	P	Y	P				N
droperidol	P	Y	P	Y	P	N	Y		P	P	P		P				
fentanyl citrate	P	Y	P		P	N	Y		P	P	P	Y	P				
glycopyrrolate		Y	Y		N	N			Y	Y	Y	Y	Y	N	N		N
heparin Na	P(5)		N*		N			P(5)		N							
hydromorphone HCl		Y			Y	Y			N*		Y	Y	Y	Y		Y	
hydroxyzine HCl	P	Y	Y	Y	Y	N			P	P	P	N	Y				
meperidine HCl	P	Y	N		P	N	P		P	P	Y	Y	P				N
metoclopramide HCl	■	Y	P		P		P		P	P	P	Y	P		N		N
midazolam HCl	Y	■	Y	Y		N	N		N	Y	Y	N	Y			Y	
morphine sulfate	P	Y	■		P	N*	Y		P*	P	P*	Y	P				N
nalbuphine HCl		Y		■		N			Y		Y	Y	Y			Y	
pentazocine lactate	P		P		■	N	Y		P	Y	Y	Y	P				
pentobarbital Na		N	N*	N	N	■	N		N	N	N		Y		Y		Y
perphenazine	P	N	Y		Y	N	■		Y			Y					
phenobarbital Na								■				N					
prochlorperazine edisylate	P	N	P*	Y	P	N	Y		■	P	P	Y	P				N
promazine HCl	P	Y	P		Y	N			P	■	P	P					
promethazine HCl	P	Y	P*	Y	Y	N			P	P	■	Y	P				N
ranitidine HCl	Y	N	Y	Y	Y		Y	N	Y	P	Y	■	Y			Y	
scopolamine HBr	P	Y	P	Y	P	Y			P		P	Y	■				Y
secobarbital Na														■			
sodium bicarbonate	N				Y										■		N
thiethylperazine maleate		Y		Y								Y				■	
thiopental Na			N			Y			N		N		Y		N		■

In *enzyme inhibition,* a drug decreases enzyme activity, significantly reducing another drug's metabolism and thereby usually prolonging its effects and leading to excessive drug accumulation unless dosage is reduced. For example, cimetidine interferes with the enzymes that influence the metabolism of warfarin, theophylline, and anticonvulsant drugs. Therefore, administration of cimetidine to a patient receiving one of these drugs can cause accumulation of the drug, excessive blood levels, and toxicity.

Altered excretion

Altering a drug's excretion pattern may produce a drug interaction by two mechanisms: pH changes or competition for elimination. The body removes drugs and their metabolites through excretion into waste fluids, mostly in urine or bile (excreted in feces); in smaller amounts in sweat, saliva, tears, respiratory gases, and breast milk. Drug excretion into breast milk, even in minute amounts, can significantly affect a breast-feeding infant.

The pH of an excretory fluid can change the drug's ionization. Depending on how urine pH levels change, a drug may be either reabsorbed or excreted to a greater extent than normal. For example, because salicylates and barbiturates are more ionized in alkaline media, alkalinization of urine is a common step in treating salicylate and barbiturate overdose.

Pharmacodynamic interactions

In this second category of drug interactions, one drug may alter the physiologic response to another drug with similar or opposite effects. Most commonly, such interactions are additive or antagonistic.

Additive interactions

In an *additive* interaction, two drugs with similar or complementary activity retain their full levels of effectiveness or toxicity. Their combined effects equal the sum of their individual effects. For example, aspirin taken with codeine produces additive pain relief, a beneficial interaction.

Occasionally, the concurrent administration of two drugs produces an exaggerated effect that exceeds the sum of the individual effects. This *synergistic* interaction, or *potentiation*, may be harmful, as in the increased drowsiness and respiratory depression that follow concurrent use of alcohol and narcotic analgesics. Or it may be useful, as in the enhanced effectiveness of gentamicin against some bacteria when it is administered with penicillin.

Antagonistic interactions

An *antagonistic* interaction may inhibit the activity of just one or both drugs. For example, the concurrent administration of propranolol and theophylline produces an undesirable antagonism. Propranolol may increase bronchial resistance or reduce the pharmacologic effect of theophylline. In rare exceptions, such antagonism can be useful. Because naloxone antagonizes the effects of opioid analgesics in the brain, it is used commonly to treat narcotic overdoses and to aid recovery from anesthesia. However, most antagonistic interactions result in ineffective or dangerous drug therapy.

Other interactions

Difficult to classify, some drug interactions occur through a common biochemical pathway, not through direct action. For example, a drug may alter serum electrolyte levels, which, in turn, can alter the effectiveness of a second drug. The classic example is the interaction of thiazide diuretics and digoxin. Thiazide diuretics, which are commonly used with digoxin to treat congestive heart failure, cause excessive potassium loss in the urine. If such loss leads to potassium deficiency (hypokalemia), digoxin toxicity can follow. But potassium excess also presents a risk for such a patient. If serum potassium levels rise too high, digoxin therapy will be less effective. In any patient, concurrent administration of digoxin and thiazide diuretics requires careful monitoring of potassium levels.

DRUG INTERACTIONS AND LIFE-STYLE

Anything that changes the chemical environment within the body can interact with a drug. Obvious problem areas include the careless use of OTC drugs, alcohol consumption, and the use of tobacco. Nutrition and exercise also can significantly influence drug therapy but are frequently overlooked.

Alcohol

A dangerous source of drug interaction, alcohol potentiates the CNS depression, lethargy, and coma associated with barbiturates, tranquilizers, antihistamines, and opiate analgesics. Furthermore, alcohol decreases the absorption of some drugs, such as thiamine and folic acid; induces liver enzyme metabolism of many drugs, including theophylline and diazepam; and increases the excretion of some nutrients, including potassium, magnesium, and zinc.

Probably the single most important drug interaction involving alcohol is the disulfiram (Antabuse) reaction. Disulfiram is administered to many recovering alcoholics to deter them from drinking. A patient who is taking disulfiram and ingests alcohol can expect to experience physical distress— flushing, headache, nausea, vomiting, and chest and abdominal pain. Several drugs can produce a disulfiram-like reaction in patients who drink alcohol. Such drugs include metronidazole, nitrofurantoin, and the sulfonylurea agents. Unfortunately, a severe disulfiram reaction can result in metabolic imbalance and may be fatal.

Tobacco

The use of tobacco can affect drug therapy as well. Whether smoked or chewed, tobacco releases chemicals that are potent inducers of liver enzyme activity. Such induction commonly affects theophylline metabolism. Long-term tobacco use may increase the amount of theophylline needed to achieve a therapeutic response. If the patient stops smoking, enzyme levels eventually return to nonsmoker levels, but this may take several months. Incidentally, marijuana induces the same theophylline-metabolizing enzymes.

OTC drugs

Many OTC drugs may interact with prescribed drug therapy or with one another. For example, OTC decongestants, such as pseudoephedrine, antagonize the action of antihypertensive drugs and potentiate the urine retention and dry mouth associated with anticholinergic drugs, such as propantheline. To prevent a potentially dangerous interaction, be sure to ask all patients about nonprescription drug use when they're taking prescription drugs.

Foods and nutrients

Taking medications with food can drastically affect drug absorption, but individual nutrients can interact with drugs in other ways as well.

- Many drugs (especially diuretics) may increase the excretion of nutrients, especially of minerals.
- The MAO inhibitors (isocarboxazid, pargyline, phenelzine, and tranylcypromine) and drugs that exhibit MAO inhibition (such as amphetamines, isoniazid, and procarbazine) decrease the metabolism of dopamine and of tyramine, which is found in many cheeses, red wines, beers, chicken livers, broad beans, avocados, bananas, and yeast extracts. This interaction can lead to life-threatening hypertension and CVA.
- Patients with hypertension should be discouraged from eating licorice. The flavoring source, glycyrrhiza, can cause sodium retention and can decrease the effectiveness of antihypertensive therapy.
- Consumption of high-protein and low-carbohydrate diets, diets high in cruciferous (cabbage family) vegetables, and charcoal-broiled foods, especially meats, induce liver enzyme activity and alter the metabolism of drugs such as theophylline.
- Charcoal-broiled meats may also decrease blood levels of phenytoin and warfarin through enzyme induction.

Exercise

Even exercise can lead to drug interactions, especially if before beginning an exercise program, the patient was stabilized on a drug regimen. Exercise most commonly affects patients with hypoglycemia and those requiring exogenous insulin. Because muscle tissue doesn't require insulin for glucose uptake, an active patient needs less insulin than a sedentary patient. A drastic change in activity level, such as from active outpatient to bedridden inpatient, may result in lost glucose control, requiring adjustment of insulin therapy.

PREVENTING DRUG INTERACTIONS

The first step in preventing drug interactions, history taking, gathers data that will identify patients at risk for dangerous or avoidable reactions.

Questions to ask during history taking

Begin by listing every drug the patient is taking or has taken during the previous 2 weeks. This list should include OTC as well as prescription medications. As you list the various medications, keep in mind those that commonly cause interactions—for example, MAO inhibitors, oral anticoagulants, cytotoxics, antihypertensives, and CNS depressants.

Ask specifically about vitamins and minerals, antacids, antidiarrheals, and laxatives. Is the patient taking any medication for allergies, cold or cough, or pain relief? Ask about whether the patient is taking anything to sleep at night or stay awake. Also, ask about a history of drug interactions.

Because food, caffeine, alcohol, and nicotine can affect drug therapy, gather detailed information about the patient's eating, drinking, and smoking habits. Keep in mind that people often minimize what they consider to be bad habits. By winning your patient's trust, you may be able to get him to reveal something significant about these habits.

Note any other factors that might increase the risk of a drug interaction—for example, age and body build. Elderly patients and infants are at increased risk, as are those who are extremely obese and those whose weight fluctuates dramatically.

From birth to death, the body's response to drugs constantly changes. In infants, drugs that the liver normally metabolizes may accumulate because infants' liver function is not fully developed. Also, proportions of body water and fat and serum protein levels differ between children and adults. Like infants and children, elderly patients also have altered body composition—for example, loss of muscle mass. They also are more likely to have impaired digestion, absorption, metabolism, or excretion. These age-related changes magnify the risk to elderly patients who require multiple drugs.

Ask the patient if he's being treated by more than one doctor. Does he have any other health problems—whether short-term or long-term, medical, dental, or psychological? For example, hepatic or renal dysfunction, which will delay a drug's metabolism and excretion, must be considered.

Reducing the risks

After identifying unnecessary drugs and, when possible, discontinuing their use, the doctor may identify the therapeutic equivalent (if any) for the interacting drug, which could be used in its place without incurring the interaction. (For example, can the infection be treated with a different, noninteracting antibiotic?)

If potentially interacting medications are the only or best choices for the patient, separating drug administration times or using different administration sites or routes may minimize drug interactions. For example, tetracycline and antacids won't interact if the tetracycline is administered 2 hours after the antacids, or if it is given intravenously instead of orally.

Before giving the patient any drug, evaluate the administration site for adequate absorption. For example, are the patient's mucous membranes too dry for sublingual medication? Is the injection site hard and knotty?

Also, keep in mind that some drugs cause the patient to lose or retain electrolytes and that others need certain electrolytes to act. Therefore, before you administer such drugs, be sure the patient's electrolyte status is normal.

Be aware

Remember: You're responsible for administering and evaluating the effectiveness of your patient's medications. So make sure that you are aware of the potential dangers and that you monitor for possible interactions diligently.

SELF-TEST

1. Florence Ellis, age 36, will receive cefuroxime (Ceftin) 250 mg P.O. b.i.d. for an upper respiratory infection. Several patient factors may predispose her to an adverse reaction to cefuroxime. Which of the following is a significant patient factor?
   a. multiple drug therapy
   b. drug dosage
   c. activity level
   d. dietary factors

2. The nurse observes Miss Ellis for an adverse drug reaction after administering cefuroxime. What is the most common allergic reaction?
   a. serum sickness
   b. urticaria
   c. anaphylaxis
   d. maculopapular rash

3. Miss Ellis also takes theophylline for asthma and phenytoin for a seizure disorder. Theophylline may interact with phenytoin by decreasing its therapeutic effects, thereby increasing the risk of seizure activity. This type of drug interaction is known as a(n):
   a. pharmacokinetic interaction.
   b. pharmacodynamic interaction.
   c. pharmacotherapeutic interaction.
   d. idiosyncratic interaction.

Check your answers on page 1056.

CHAPTER 4

DRUG THERAPY AND THE NURSING PROCESS

The nursing process guides nursing decisions about drug administration to ensure the patient's safety and meet medical and legal standards. This process, in five steps, provides thorough assessment, appropriate nursing diagnosis, effective planning, correct interventions, and constant evaluation. See *The nursing process and drug therapy*, page 53.

FIRST STEP: ASSESSMENT

During assessment, the nurse focuses on direct data collection by:
• obtaining a drug history from the patient, parent, spouse, or significant other
• reviewing the patient's previous medical history
• performing a physical examination
• obtaining relevant laboratory or diagnostic test results.

Drug history

Data collection begins at admission to the hospital or in an outpatient setting with specific questions about the patient's background, including allergies, medical history, medication history, habits, socioeconomic status, life-style and beliefs, sensory deficits, and clinical status. These aspects of the patient's background can significantly influence drug therapy.

Allergies

The patient's allergy profile includes the patient's reactions to both drugs and food. Information about allergic reactions to drugs must specify the drug, when the allergic reaction occurred, the situation and setting at the time of the reaction, a description of the reaction, and any contributing factors. Examples of contributing factors might include the concurrent use of stimulants, tobacco, alcohol, or illicit drugs, or a significant change in nutritional patterns. Asking the patient to describe his allergic reaction is especially important to help determine whether the patient actually reacts adversely to a drug or simply dislikes taking it.

Allergies to foods can also affect drug therapy. For example, allergies to shellfish can contraindicate use of drugs that contain iodine or are by-products of shellfish. Allergies to eggs are significant in patients who are to receive vaccines, which are commonly derived from chick embryos.

Medical history

In gathering the medical history, note any chronic diseases or disorders the patient may have and record the following information for each:
• date of diagnosis
• initial prescribed treatment
• current treatment
• the doctor in charge.

Careful attention to this part of the medical history can uncover one of the most important problems with drug therapy—conflicting and incompatible drug regimens. The patient who does not have a family doctor to oversee and coordinate all care may seek the care of several specialists who may prescribe drug treatment without knowing what other drugs the patient is taking. A carefully detailed medical history can uncover such problems. The nurse who identifies such conflicting or overlapping drug therapy must call it to the appropriate doctor's attention and then teach the patient about the importance of informing all caregivers about all drugs he is taking.

Medication history

The medication history should contain information about both prescription and OTC drugs. The patient's drug history should explore the following:
• the reason for using the drug
• the patient's knowledge of the appropriate dosage and schedule of administration
• the patient's knowledge about determining effectiveness of the drug (if appropriate), potential adverse reactions, what to do about adverse reactions, and when to contact the doctor
• route of administration
• the pattern of administration at home
• drug interactions with OTC drugs
• cognitive status.

Note any special monitoring the patient must perform, such as blood glucose monitoring before insulin administration or checking radial pulse rate before taking digoxin. Make sure the patient is performing such procedures correctly and that the results are within acceptable limits.

Discuss the effects of drug therapy with the patient and determine if new symptoms or unpredicted adverse reactions have developed. Noting the patient's pattern of administration may provide insight into why a particular drug regimen succeeds or fails.

OTC drugs

A comprehensive medication history should also list any OTC drugs the patient is taking. Many OTC drugs can inhibit or potentiate the effects of a prescribed drug. For example, aspirin potentiates the anticoagulant effects of warfarin.

OTC drugs include a wide range of products from common aspirin and nutritional supplements to various sprays and cleansing agents. The patient may not think of all of these products as drugs, so the nurse may have to suggest a general list of products to get an accurate response.

THE NURSING PROCESS AND DRUG THERAPY

Safe and effective drug therapy requires understanding of a drug's action as it applies to the individual patient. This chart relates patient factors and drug factors to each step of the nursing process. Considering each factor in sequence, as listed below, promotes the best individualized nursing care during drug therapy.

PATIENT FACTORS	DRUG FACTORS
Assessment	
• Physical assessment • Medical history • Current medical problems • Emotional state • Knowledge about condition and drugs • Environment • Allergies • Life-style: use of nicotine, caffeine, alcohol	• Completeness of drug order • Appropriateness of use • Appropriate drug route, dose, dosage form • Potential effect on laboratory findings • Food and drug interactions • Drug interactions • Contraindications • Institutional and unit policies for drug's administration
Diagnosis	
Patient problems, needs, strengths, weaknesses	Intended use and patient response
Planning	
Patient's scheduled activities, visitors, and other medications	Meals, patient need for p.r.n. medications, pharmacy schedule of delivery, and current supply
Interventions	
• Correct and accurate drug administration • Teaching and counseling • Comfort measures related to drug administration or adverse reactions • Observation for adverse reactions • Other care measures related to condition for which drug is used—for example, wound care for patient receiving antibiotics for wound infection • Recording of administration	• Accurate drug preparation • Safety measures related to drug action (such as side rails up with sedatives) • Storage
Evaluation	
• Cognitive abilities • Psychomotor abilities • Compliance factors	• Therapeutic effects • Nontherapeutic effects (toxic or other adverse effects) • Drug interactions

Dosage and frequency of use are just as important as the type of OTC product the patient is using. One tablet of aspirin taken once a day may have no effect on concomitant drug therapy; however, a higher dosage (such as that used for arthritis) could influence it profoundly.

Habits

Carefully consider dietary habits and the nontherapeutic use of drugs. Certain foods can directly affect the effectiveness of many drugs. For example, a person who is taking the anticoagulant warfarin (Coumadin) should not increase his intake of green leafy vegetables because they contain levels of vitamin K that can antagonize the drug's anticoagulant effect.

Nontherapeutic use of drugs can profoundly affect a patient's health and impair the effectiveness of drug therapy. Consider the possible use of alcohol, tobacco, caffeine, and illicit drugs, such as marijuana, cocaine, and heroin. For example, if the patient uses alcohol, note the frequency of use, the amount, and the type of alcohol consumed. Carefully document the intake of stimulants, such as caffeine, because they significantly affect a patient's cardiovascular status and nervous system. Record the type of stimulant (coffee, tea, soda, or chocolate), the frequency of intake, and the amount consumed.

For the patient who smokes, document the following information:
• the length of time the patient has smoked
• what the patient smokes (cigarettes, cigar, or pipe)
• how many cigarettes or cigars the patient smokes per day
• the brand of cigarettes or cigars the patient smokes or the brand of tobacco and how much he chews per day.

Defining the patient's use of illicit drugs may be difficult. However, the nurse who suspects such use should encourage the patient to discuss it honestly, emphasizing that these drugs have profound effects that may cause serious drug interactions. If the patient admits using illicit drugs, document the drug, the amount and frequency of use, and the route of administration.

Socioeconomic status

Note the patient's age, educational level, occupation, and insurance coverage. These factors may be significant to compliance and to an effective care plan. The patient's age, for example, can determine whom to include in the care plan (parents or other family members) and the level of information that is appropriate for teaching the patient.

Knowing the patient's educational background and occupation helps you select interventions at an appropriate level, plan a drug regimen that fits the patient's daily routine, and encourage compliance. Knowing the patient's insurance status may help you anticipate the need for financial assistance and counseling. Remember that noncompliance frequently results from inability to afford costly medications.

Life-style and beliefs

Support systems, marital status, childbearing status, attitudes toward health and health care, use of the health care system, and daily patterns of activities will affect the plan of care and patient compliance. For example, an 18-year-old single parent, who is a high-school dropout on medical assistance and has no family support, will probably require more teaching and support to gain a commitment to and compliance with drug therapy than a 40-year-old affluent professional, with a lot of family support, who can understand why she needs the drug and can readily pay for it.

Sensory deficits

Any sensory deficit can significantly alter an appropriate care plan. For example, impaired vision, paralysis of one or more extremities, loss of limb, or loss of sensation in an extremity can impair the patient's ability to administer a subcutaneous injection, break a scored tablet, or open a medication container. Color blindness may cause the patient difficulty in distinguishing between two medications. Hearing impairment can prevent him from receiving important patient instruction about a medication. Any sensory deficit requires careful consideration in any plan of prescribed drug therapy.

Clinical status

Two other factors can profoundly influence drug therapy: the patient's cognitive status and systemic effects of the prescribed drugs. A patient's intact cognitive abilities ensure that he can understand and implement the actions necessary for compliance. During the interview, note if the patient is alert and oriented, if he is able to interact appropriately with people, and if his conversation is appropriate. Consider whether the patient can think clearly and express his thoughts coherently. Finally, check both short-term and long-term memory because the patient needs both to follow a specified drug regimen. If such evaluation identifies a cognitive deficit, determine the probable cause, which can range from a transient drug-related effect to permanent neurologic impairment, and then determine whether or not the patient can carry out the prescribed drug regimen. If not, the nurse must find another way to ensure that the patient receives the prescribed therapy.

After completing the history, perform a physical examination to assess those body systems that may be affected by a particular drug the patient is taking or that may be prescribed. Every drug has a desired effect on a body system, but it may have also an undesired effect on another. For example, chemotherapeutic agents destroy cancerous cells, but they also affect normal cells and often cause the patient to experience hair loss, diarrhea, or nausea. Therefore, examine the patient for expected drug effects; also closely monitor the patient for potentially harmful adverse reactions.

SECOND STEP: FORMULATING A NURSING DIAGNOSIS

Using information gathered during assessment, define any potential or actual drug-related problems by formulating each in a relevant nursing diagnosis. The most common problem statements related to drug therapy are "Knowledge deficit," "Noncompliance," and "Alteration in health maintenance."

THIRD STEP: PLANNING

Nursing diagnoses provide the framework for planning interventions and outcome criteria (patient goals). Outcome criteria state the desired patient behaviors or responses that should result from nursing care. Outcome criteria should be measurable and objective, concise, realistic for the patient, and attainable by nursing management; they should express patient behavior in terms of expectations and specify a time frame. A typical outcome statement is "The patient verbalizes major adverse reactions related to his chemotherapy drugs prior to discharge."

FOURTH STEP: INTERVENTION

After developing the outcome criteria, the nurse determines the interventions needed to help the patient reach the desired behavior or goals. Drug-related interventions may focus on patient teaching, compliance, or effect of drug on health maintenance.

Appropriate interventions related to drug therapy will also include administration procedures and techniques, legal and ethical concerns, and any concerns related to special groups of patients (geriatric, pediatric, and pregnant or breast-feeding patients).

FIFTH STEP: EVALUATION

The final component of the nursing process, evaluation is a formal and systematic process for determining the effectiveness of nursing care. This process enables the nurse to determine whether outcome criteria were met and thereby make informed decisions about subsequent interventions. For example, if the patient experienced relief of headache within 1 hour after the nurse administered a p.r.n. analgesic, the outcome criterion was met. If the headache was the same or worse, the outcome criterion was not met and requires reassessment, which may require replanning or may yield new data that invalidate the nursing diagnosis or suggest new nursing interventions that are more specific or more acceptable to the patient. Such reassessment could lead to a higher dosage, a different analgesic, or a reevaluation of the cause of the headache.

Evaluation enables the nurse to design and implement a revised care plan, to continuously reevaluate outcome criteria, and to replan until each nursing diagnosis is resolved.

Documentation related to drug therapy

Although documentation is not a step in the nursing process, the nurse legally is required to document activities related to drug therapy, including the time of administration, the quantity administered, and the patient's reaction to the drug. To deliver the best possible patient care, the nurse also should record evaluation data. Because other nurses must be able to read the evaluation and implement appropriate nursing care, documentation must be clear, concise, and complete. It should begin with an evaluation of outcome criteria and proceed to a reassessment of specific interventions.

The format used to document the evaluation step in the nursing process can vary. The nurse may combine progress notes with flow sheets or add an evaluation column to the nursing care plan.

The nurse also must document each teaching session in the patient's chart so that other nurses and members of the health care team know what was covered, what patient learning resulted, and which areas need refinement or further instruction. The nurse must remember that the patient's education is the concern of the entire health care team, each member having a different area of expertise. To provide optimal patient education, the nurse must work closely with all other team members.

The chart is one method of sharing information. Other methods include informal health care team meetings, educational rounds, family conferences with the health care team, and discharge planning rounds. Above all, the patient's medical record must include complete documentation of all teaching efforts.

SELF-TEST

1. Patrick Lawson, age 30, is admitted to the hospital with pneumonia. The nurse takes a drug history that includes assessment of the patient's socioeconomic status. How would this information impact upon the patient's drug therapy?
   a. Age helps determine level of information that is appropriate for teaching about drug therapy.
   b. Beliefs about health care can influence types of drug interactions that may occur.
   c. Sensory deficits increase risk of adverse reactions.
   d. Smoking can enhance therapeutic action of some drugs.

2. When preparing a care plan for Mr. Lawson, the nurse writes several outcome criteria. Which of the following is written correctly?
   a. The patient adequately understands the need for antibiotic therapy.
   b. The patient states the importance of taking the antibiotic as prescribed.
   c. The patient knows he should take the antibiotic as prescribed.
   d. The patient believes he should take the antibiotic as prescribed.

3. Before Mr. Lawson is discharged, the nurse performs a thorough evaluation. What does the evaluation step of the nursing process determine?
   a. if the patient will recover
   b. if the outcome criteria have been met
   c. if the nurse has done a good job
   d. if the nursing diagnosis is correct

Check your answers on pages 1056 and 1057.

CHAPTER 5

AMEBICIDES AND TRICHOMONACIDES

chloroquine hydrochloride ✦ chloroquine phosphate
chloroquine sulphate ✦ iodoquinol ✦ emetine hydrochloride
metronidazole ✦ metronidazole hydrochloride ✦ paromomycin sulfate

OVERVIEW

- Amebicides and trichomonacides cure or control diseases caused by amebic or trichomonal infection, such as amebiasis, primary amebic meningoencephalitis, and trichomoniasis. Amebiasis, or amebic dysentery, is an intestinal disorder caused by the parasite *Entamoeba histolytica.* The condition is now being reported more often than it was in the past, particularly among homosexual males.
- Trichomoniasis is a relatively common vaginal infection caused by *Trichomonas vaginalis.* The infection spreads through sexual activity; infected males and about 70% of infected females are usually asymptomatic.

MAJOR USES

- Metronidazole is the drug of choice for amebic dysentery and trichomonal infections; it may also be useful in treating gram-negative anaerobic infections. Alternate drugs are usually administered in combination with at least one other drug and are not always efficacious.

MECHANISM OF ACTION

- Chloroquine is mainly an antimalarial (for further information about that use, see Chapter 8, Antimalarials). Its mechanism of amebicidal action is unknown, but it is useful in the treatment of extraintestinal amebiasis.
- Emetine kills *E. histolytica* by a mechanism related to the inhibition of protein synthesis.
- Iodoquinol is an iodine derivative with amebicidal activity in the intestinal lumen. Its mechanism of action is unknown.
- Metronidazole is a direct-acting trichomonacide and amebicide that works at both intestinal and extraintestinal sites.
- Paromomycin is an aminoglycoside antibiotic that acts as an amebicide in intestinal sites, effective in the presence or absence of bacteria. Its mechanism of action is unknown.

GLOSSARY

Amebicidal: pertaining to an agent that destroys amebae.
Anaerobe: microorganism that can live and grow only in the complete, or almost complete, absence of molecular oxygen.
Encephalitis: inflammation of the brain.
Infection: reactions of tissues to invading pathogenic microorganisms and the toxins these microorganisms generate.
Parasite: plant or animal that lives upon or within another living organism, at whose expense it obtains some advantage without return compensation.

ABSORPTION, DISTRIBUTION, METABOLISM, AND EXCRETION

Chloroquine is almost completely absorbed in the small intestine after oral administration. About 55% of the drug is bound to plasma proteins, and high concentrations are found in body tissues. It is excreted slowly in urine; small amounts are detectable after therapy is stopped—sometimes even years later.

Emetine is absorbed from parenteral sites, slowly detoxified by the liver, and excreted primarily by the kidneys. Detectable in urine 40 to 60 days after treatment, emetine concentrates in the liver, kidneys, and spleen.

Iodoquinol is poorly absorbed from the GI tract; most of it is eliminated in the stool.

Metronidazole is well absorbed after oral administration, primarily in the small intestine. Limited data suggest wide distribution, with significant concentration in abscesses, bile, CSF, and many tissues. From 60% to 70% is excreted unchanged in the urine; the remainder is metabolized in the liver.

Paromomycin is poorly absorbed from the GI tract after oral administration; almost all the drug is eliminated unchanged in the stool.

ONSET AND DURATION

Chloroquine: Daily doses of 50 mg result in peak blood levels of 125 mcg/ml within 2 to 4 hours; half-life is about 3 days. Onset of iodoquinol, emetine, and paromomycin is generally within 4 to 8 hours; effects can last 4 to 7 days. Single oral doses of 750 mg metronidazole cause peak blood levels of 10 to 15 mcg/ml within 2 to 4 hours; half-life is 6 to 12 hours.

ADVERSE REACTIONS

Amebicides and trichomonacides can exhibit significant but various adverse reactions, which may include the following:

CV reactions, including changes in ECG, CHF, pericarditis, myocarditis, precordial pain, hypotension, dyspnea, and edema, are associated with emetine. This drug may also cause severe nausea and vomiting with dizziness and headache. Neuromuscular reactions (muscle pain, tenderness, and stiffness), which usually precede severe reactions, can be used to monitor for toxicity.

CNS reactions, including dizziness, headache, vertigo, ataxia, neuritis, depression, syncope, peripheral neuropathy, and seizures, are associated with metronidazole.

GI reactions, including nausea, vomiting, taste dysfunction, and diarrhea, are the most common reactions to metronidazole.

Hematologic reactions, including agranulocytosis, aplastic anemia, hemolytic anemia, and thrombocytopenia. are associated with chloroquine.

Ophthalmic reactions, including blurred vision and retinal damage, are associated with chloroquine and iodoquinol.

Renal reactions, including polyuria, dysuria, incontinence and dark urine are associated with metronidazole, and nephrotoxicity is associated with paromomycin.

Serious toxicities may be prevented when using metronidazole if care is taken to avoid high dose and prolonged therapy. Seizures and peripheral neuropathy are the most serious, whereas dizziness, vertigo, ataxia, depression, headache, and syncope are of a less serious nature. The most common adverse effect of metronidazole is GI (nausea, vomiting, diarrhea, taste dysfunction).

The ingestion of alcohol while on metronidazole can increase adverse GI reactions. Other adverse effects of metronidazole can be polyuria, dysuria, incontinence, dark urine, vaginal dryness, and overgrowth of *Candida* organisms.

Paromomycin is an aminoglycoside antibiotic; with these drugs, nephrotoxicity and ototoxicity may occur because of drug absorption through damaged mucosa. Nausea, vomiting, other GI complaints, rash, and superinfection have also been reported.

PROTOTYPE: AMEBICIDES AND TRICHOMONACIDES

METRONIDAZOLE
(me troe ni' da zole)
Apo-Metronidazole†, Flagyl, Metizol, Metric 21, Metrogyl‡, Metrozine‡, Metryl, Neo-Metric†, Novonidazol†, PMS Metronidazole†, Protostat

METRONIDAZOLE HYDROCHLORIDE
Flagyl I.V., Flagyl I.V. RTU, Metro I.V., Novonidazol†
Classification: amebicide and trichomonacide
Pregnancy risk category B

How supplied
TABLETS: 200 mg‡, 250 mg, 400 mg‡, 500 mg
INJECTION: 500 mg/100 ml ready to use
POWDER FOR INJECTION: 500-mg single-dose vials

---

†Available in Canada only   ‡Available in Australia only

Indications and dosage
Amebic hepatic abscess
ADULTS: 500 to 750 mg P.O. t.i.d. for 5 to 10 days.
CHILDREN: 35 to 50 mg/kg daily (in three doses) for 10 days.

Intestinal amebiasis
ADULTS: 750 mg P.O. t.i.d. for 5 to 10 days.
CHILDREN: 35 to 50 mg/kg daily (in three doses) for 10 days. Follow this therapy with oral iodoquinol.

Trichomoniasis
ADULTS: 250 mg P.O. t.i.d. for 7 days or 2 g in single dose; 4 to 6 weeks should elapse between courses of therapy. In refractory cases, treatment may continue.

Bacterial infections caused by anaerobic microorganisms
ADULTS: Loading dose is 15 mg/kg I.V. infused over 1 hour (approximately 1 g for a 70-kg adult). Maintenance dose is 7.5 mg/kg I.V. or P.O. q 6 hours (approximately 500 mg for a 70-kg adult). The first maintenance dose should be administered 6 hours after the loading dose. Maximum dosage not to exceed 4 g daily.

Giardiasis
ADULTS: 250 mg P.O. t.i.d. for 5 days.
CHILDREN: 5 mg/kg P.O. t.i.d. for 5 days.

Prevention of postoperative infection in contaminated or potentially contaminated colorectal surgery
ADULTS: 15 mg/kg infused over 30 to 60 minutes and completed approximately 1 hour before surgery. Then, 7.5 mg/kg infused over 30 to 60 minutes at 6 and 12 hours after the initial dose.

Contraindications and precautions
Metronidazole is contraindicated in patients with known hypersensitivity to metronidazole or other nitroimidazole derivatives. It is also contraindicated during the first trimester of pregnancy.

Use cautiously in patients with a history of blood dyscrasia or CNS disorder, with retinal or visual field changes, with hepatic disease or in alcoholism, and with known hepatotoxic drugs.

Adverse reactions
BLOOD: transient leukopenia, neutropenia.
CNS: vertigo, headache, ataxia, incoordination, confusion, irritability, depression, restlessness, weakness, fatigue, drowsiness, insomnia, sensory neuropathy, paresthesia of extremities, psychic stimulation, neuromyopathy, **generalized seizures**, and peripheral neuropathy.
CV: ECG change (flattened T wave), edema (with I.V. preparation).
GI: abdominal cramping, stomatitis, *nausea*, vomiting, anorexia, diarrhea, constipation, proctitis, dry mouth.
GU: darkened urine, polyuria, dysuria, pyuria, incontinence, cystitis, decreased libido, dyspareunia, dryness of vagina and vulva, sense of pelvic pressure.

Italicized adverse reactions are common   Boldfaced adverse reactions are life-threatening

SKIN: pruritus, flushing.
LOCAL: thrombophlebitis after I.V. infusion.
OTHER: overgrowth of nonsusceptible organisms, especially *Candida* (glossitis, furry tongue); metallic taste; fever; gynecomastia.

Interactions

Alcohol: disulfiram-like reaction (nausea, vomiting, headache, cramps, flushing). Don't use together.
Barbiturates, phenytoin: diminished antimicrobial effect. Increased dosage may be required.
Cimetidine: decreased clearance of metronidazole. Monitor for adverse reactions.
Disulfiram: acute psychoses and confusional states. Don't use together.
Oral anticoagulants: prolonged prothrombin time.

Nursing considerations

Assessment

• Review the patient's history for a condition that contraindicates the use of metronidazole.
• Obtain a baseline assessment of the patient's infection, including appropriate specimen for culture and sensitivity, before therapy.
• Be alert for common adverse reactions.
• Evaluate the patient's and family's knowledge about metronidazole therapy.

Planning (Nursing Diagnoses)

Potential nursing diagnoses for the patient receiving metronidazole include:
• Potential for injury related to dosage regimen inadequate to alleviate infection.
• Alteration in nutrition: Less than body requirements related to anorexia, nausea, and vomiting.
• Knowledge deficit related to metronidazole therapy.

Implementation

Preparation and administration

—Metronidazole should be used only after *T. vaginalis* has been confirmed by wet smear or culture or after *E. histolytica* has been identified.
—Give oral form with meals to minimize GI distress.
—Follow package instructions carefully when mixing the I.V. solution.
—Don't refrigerate Flagyl I.V. RTU.
—The I.V. form should be administered only by slow infusion either as a continuous or intermittent infusion. Additives should not be introduced into solution. If used with a primary I.V. fluid system, discontinue the primary fluid during the infusion; do not give by I.V. push.
—Do not use equipment containing aluminum (for example, needles, cannulas) that would come in contact with the drug solution.
—Solution should be clear, pale yellow-green. Do not use cloudy or precipitated solutions.

Monitoring

—Monitor the effectiveness of therapy by regularly assessing for improvement of infectious process.
—Monitor the patient for adverse drug reactions.
—Monitor the patient's nutritional status, including body weight.
—Monitor the patient for signs of superinfection.
—Monitor the patient for drug interactions.
—Monitor diagnostic tests. Metronidazole may interfere with the chemical analyses of aminotransferase and triglyceride, leading to falsely decreased values. Rarely, it has been reported to flatten the T waves on ECG.
—Regularly reevaluate the patient's and family's knowledge about metronidazole therapy.

Intervention

—When treating amebiasis, record number and character of stools; send fecal specimens to laboratory promptly; infestation is detectable only in warm specimens.
—If the patient develops nausea or vomiting, obtain an order for an antiemetic.
—If the patient develops a superinfection, contact the doctor for appropriate treatment.
—Keep all health care team members advised of the patient's response to the drug.

Patient teaching

—Instruct the patient and family about metronidazole including the dosage, frequency, action, and adverse reactions.
—Explain disease process and rationale for therapy.
—Tell the patient to avoid alcohol or alcohol-containing medications during therapy and for at least 48 hours after therapy is completed.
—Tell the patient that drug may cause metallic taste and discolored (red-brown) urine.
—Tell patient to take tablets with meals to minimize GI distress and that tablets may be crushed to facilitate swallowing.
—Counsel the patient on need for medical follow-up after discharge.
—For the patient with amebiasis, explain that follow-up examinations of stool specimens are necessary for 3 months after treatment is discontinued, to ensure elimination of amebae. To help prevent reinfection, instruct the patient and family members in proper hygiene, including disposal of feces and hand washing after defecation; before handling, preparing, or eating food; and about the risks of eating raw food and the control of contamination by flies. Encourage other household members and suspected contacts to be tested and, if necessary, treated.
—For the patient with trichomoniasis, teach correct personal hygiene, including perineal care. Explain that the patient's asymptomatic sexual partner should be treated simultaneously to prevent reinfection; the patient should refrain from intercourse during therapy or have partner use condom.

— Tell the patient to notify the nurse or doctor if adverse reactions develop or questions arise about metronidazole therapy.

Evaluation

In the patient receiving metronidazole, appropriate evaluation statements include:
• Patient is free of infection.
• Patient maintains normal nutritional status.
• Patient and family state an understanding of metronidazole therapy.

SELECTED MAJOR DRUGS: AMEBICIDES AND TRICHOMONACIDES

DRUG, INDICATIONS, AND DOSAGES	SPECIAL PRECAUTIONS
chloroquine (Aralen) *Suppressive prophylaxis and treatment of acute attacks of malaria due to* Plasmodium vivax, P. malariae, P. ovale, *and susceptible strains of* P. falciparum — **Adults:** initially, 600 mg (base) P.O., then 300 mg at 6, 24, and 48 hours. Or 160 to 200 mg (base) I.M. initially; repeat in 6 hours if needed. Switch to oral therapy as soon as possible. **Children:** initially, 10 mg (base)/kg P.O., then 5 mg (base)/kg dose at 6, 24, and 48 hours (do not exceed adult dose). Or 5 mg (base)/kg I.M. initially; repeat in 6 hours if needed. Switch to oral therapy as soon as possible. *Malaria suppressive treatment —* **Adults and children:** 5 mg (base)/kg P.O. (not to exceed 300 mg) weekly on same day of the week (begin 2 weeks before entering endemic area and continue for 8 weeks after leaving). If treatment begins after exposure, double the initial dose (600 mg for adults, 10 mg/kg for children) in two divided doses 6 hours apart. *Extraintestinal amebiasis —* **Adults:** 160 to 200 mg (base) I.M. daily for no more than 12 days. As soon as possible, substitute 1 g (600 mg base) phosphate P.O. daily for 2 days; then 500 mg (300 mg base) daily for at least 2 to 3 weeks. Treatment is usually combined with an effective intestinal amebicide. **Children:** 10 mg/kg (base) for 2 to 3 weeks. Maximum is 300 mg daily. *Rheumatoid arthritis and lupus erythematosus —* **Adults:** 250 mg phosphate daily with evening meal.	• Contraindicated in patients with retinal or visual field changes or porphyria. • Use with extreme caution in patients with severe GI, neurologic, or blood disorders. • Drug concentrates in liver; use cautiously in patients with hepatic disease or alcoholism. • Use cautiously in patients with G6PD deficiency or psoriasis; drug may exacerbate these conditions.

(continued)

SELECTED MAJOR DRUGS: AMEBICIDES AND TRICHOMONACIDES
continued

DRUG, INDICATIONS, AND DOSAGES	SPECIAL PRECAUTIONS
emetine *Acute fulminating amebic dysentery—* **Adults:** 1 mg/kg daily up to 60 mg daily (one or two doses) deep S.C. or I.M. 3 to 5 days (only until symptoms are under control). Give another antiamebic drug simultaneously. **Children:** 1 mg/kg daily in two doses I.M. for up to 5 days. *Amebic hepatitis and abscess—* **Adults:** 60 mg daily (one or two doses) deep S.C. or I.M. for 10 days.	• Contraindicated in patients with cardiac or renal disease except with amebic abscess or hepatitis not controlled by chloroquine or metronidazole; in patients who have received emetine in previous 6 to 8 weeks; in children, except with severe dysentery unresponsive to other amebicides; and in patients with polyneuropathy or muscle disease. • Use cautiously and in reduced dosage in elderly, debilitated, or hypotensive patients or those about to undergo surgery.
iodoquinol (Diodoquin†, Moebiquin, Yodoxin) *Intestinal amebiasis—* **Adults:** 630 to 650 mg P.O. t.i.d. for 20 days. Total daily dosage should not exceed 2 g. **Children:** usual dosage is 30 to 40 mg/kg of body weight daily in two to three divided doses for 20 days. Additional courses of iodoquinol therapy should not be repeated before a resting interval of 2 to 3 weeks.	• Contraindicated in patients with known hypersensitivity to iodine or 8-hydroxyquinoline derivatives (iodoquinol causes hepatic damage in such patients) and in hepatic or renal disease or preexisting optic neuropathy. • Administer cautiously to patients with thyroid disease.
paromomycin (Humatin) *Intestinal amebiasis, acute and chronic—* **Adults:** 25 to 35 mg/kg daily P.O. in three doses for 5 to 10 days after meals. *Tapeworms (fish, beef, pork, dog)—* **Adults:** 1 g P.O. q 15 minutes for four doses. **Children:** 11 mg/kg P.O. q 15 minutes for four doses.	• Contraindicated in patients with impaired renal function or intestinal obstruction. • Use cautiously in patients with ulcerative bowel lesions to avoid inadvertent absorption and resulting renal toxicity. Poorly absorbed orally, but will accumulate with renal impairment or ulcerative lesions.

†Available in Canada only

SELF-TEST

1. Mary Ewing, age 31, has been complaining of perineal itching and a vaginal discharge. A culture of the discharge confirms *T. vaginalis*. Oral metronidazole is prescribed. She is told to take her medication:
   a. on an empty stomach at least 1 hour before or 2 hours after a meal.
   b. each morning at the same time for 10 days.
   c. three times daily with meals.
   d. until the vaginal discharge ceases.

2. While taking metronidazole, Ms. Ewing should observe for:
   a. furry tongue.
   b. interactions with other drugs she may be taking.
   c. tinnitus or reduction in hearing ability.
   d. bloody stools.

3. Ms. Ewing is sexually active but reports her partner is asymptomatic. She should:
   a. not worry about her partner unless he becomes symptomatic.
   b. discuss her infection with her partner and refrain from all sexual activity until she is free from her infection.
   c. have her partner treated simultaneously and use a condom throughout therapy.
   d. watch her partner for symptoms.

Check your answers on page 1057.

CHAPTER 6

ANTHELMINTICS

mebendazole ✦ niclosamide ✦ oxamniquine ✦ piperazine adipate
piperazine citrate ✦ praziquantel ✦ pyrantel embonate ✦ pyrantel pamoate
quinacrine hydrochloride ✦ thiabendazole

OVERVIEW
- Anthelmintics rid the body of helminths, or parasitic worms. Although helminthic infections are usually confined to the intestines, dissemination to the genitalia, peritoneum, and hematopoietic system may occur.

MAJOR USES
- Anthelmintics eradicate various helminths, including tapeworms, pinworms, hookworms, roundworms, and schistosomes.

MECHANISM OF ACTION
- Mebendazole appears to selectively and irreversibly inhibit uptake of glucose and other nutrients in susceptible helminths.
- Niclosamide inhibits the metabolic process of oxidative phosphorylation in tapeworms.
- Oxamniquine reduces the egg load of *Schistosoma mansoni*, but its exact mechanism of action is unknown.
- Piperazine and pyrantel block neuromuscular action, paralyzing the worm and causing its expulsion by normal peristalsis.
- Praziquantel causes a contraction of schistosomes by a specific effect on the permeability of the cell membrane.
- Quinacrine inhibits DNA metabolism.
- Mechanism of action of thiabendazole is unknown.

ABSORPTION, DISTRIBUTION, METABOLISM, AND EXCRETION
Mebendazole is poorly absorbed from the GI tract and mainly eliminated in the feces.

Niclosamide is not absorbed. Its action is solely in the GI tract.

Oxamniquine is well absorbed after oral administration. The drug is metabolized in the liver and excreted in the urine.

Piperazine is readily absorbed from the GI tract. Some piperazine is metabolized in the liver; the remainder is excreted unchanged in the urine.

Praziquantel is well absorbed in the GI tract, metabolized by the liver, and excreted in the urine.

GLOSSARY

Helminth: worm or wormlike parasite.
Parasite: plant or animal that lives upon or within another living organism, at whose expense it obtains some advantage without return compensation.
Schistosome: blood fluke that is a type of trematode parasite.

Pyrantel is poorly absorbed from the GI tract. It is metabolized primarily in the liver; the rest is eliminated unchanged in urine and feces. Rates of excretion vary greatly among patients.

Quinacrine is readily absorbed from the GI tract and is highly concentrated in the liver. Its metabolism and excretion are unknown.

Thiabendazole is rapidly absorbed from the GI tract; it is metabolized then excreted in the urine.

ONSET AND DURATION
Anthelmintics have a rapid onset and short duration of action.

ADVERSE REACTIONS
The most common adverse reactions are GI-related and include nausea, vomiting, abdominal pain, and anorexia. Other reactions include CNS effects (headache, dizziness, insomnia, drowsiness, and seizures) and dermatologic effects (various mild reactions to erythema multiforme).

PROTOTYPE: ANTHELMINTICS

PIPERAZINE ADIPATE
(pi′ per a zeen)
Entacyl†

PIPERAZINE CITRATE
Antepar, Bryrel, Pipril, Ta-Verm, Veriga†, Vermirex†, Vermizine
Classification: anthelmintic
Pregnancy risk category B

How supplied
adipate
ORAL SUSPENSION: 600 mg/5 ml
GRANULES: 2 g/packet
citrate
TABLETS: 250 mg
SYRUP: 500 mg/5 ml

---

†Available in Canada only

Indications and dosage
Pinworm
ADULTS AND CHILDREN: 65 mg/kg P.O. daily for 7 to 8 days. Maximum daily dosage is 2.5 g.

Roundworm
ADULTS: 3.5 g P.O. in single doses for 2 consecutive days.
CHILDREN: 75 mg/kg P.O. daily in single doses for 2 consecutive days. Maximum daily dosage is 3.5 g.

Contraindications and precautions
Piperazine is contraindicated in patients with known hypersensitivity to the drug; hepatic or renal impairment, or both; and seizure disorder. Use cautiously in severe malnutrition or anemia.

Because of potential neurotoxicity (especially in children), prolonged, repeated, and excessive treatment should be avoided. Because of the potential for severe toxicity in the infant, drug should not be used in women who are breast-feeding.

Adverse reactions
CNS: ataxia, tremor, choreiform movements, muscular weakness, myoclonus, hyporeflexia, paresthesia, **seizures**, sense of detachment, EEG abnormalities, memory defect, *headache*, vertigo.
EENT: nystagmus, blurred vision, paralytic strabismus, cataracts with visual impairment, lacrimation, difficulty in focusing, rhinorrhea.
GI: *nausea, vomiting, diarrhea, abdominal cramps.*
SKIN: urticaria, photodermatitis, **erythema multiforme**, purpura, eczematous skin reactions.
OTHER: arthralgia, fever, bronchospasm, **hemolytic anemia.**

Interactions
Chlorpromazine: exaggerated risk of extrapyramidal symptoms. Use with caution.
Pyrantel: possible pharmacologic antagonism. Don't administer together.

Nursing considerations
Assessment
• Review the patient's history for a condition that contraindicates the use of piperazine.
• Obtain a baseline assessment of the patient's infection, including appropriate specimens for culture and sensitivity, before therapy.
• Be alert for common adverse reactions.
• Evaluate the patient's and family's knowledge about piperazine therapy.

Planning (Nursing Diagnoses)
Potential nursing diagnoses for the patient receiving piperazine include:
• Altered health maintenance related to ineffectiveness of piperazine.
• Pain related to headache caused by piperazine.
• Knowledge deficit related to piperazine therapy.

Implementation

Preparation and administration

— Mix powder for oral suspension in 57 ml of water, milk, or fruit juice.
— Administer on an empty stomach because food may decrease the surface contact between the drug and parasite.
— Protect drug from light, air, and moisture.

Monitoring

— Monitor the effectiveness of therapy by regularly assessing for improvement of infectious process.
— Monitor the patient for adverse drug reactions.
— Monitor stools for worms. Absence of worms is the only confirmation of successful treatment.
— Monitor the patient for drug interactions.
— Monitor diagnostic test studies. Piperazine may cause EEG changes, particularly in children; it may also interfere with serum uric acid measurements, leading to falsely low values.
— Monitor the patient's compliance with piperazine therapy.
— Regularly reevaluate the patient's and family's knowledge about piperazine therapy.

Intervention

— If the patient develops headache, notify the doctor and obtain an order for an analgesic. Also report any other adverse reactions, obtain appropriate therapy, and provide appropriate supportive care.
— Ensure that all family members are treated; otherwise, pinworm and other nematode infections can recur.
— Keep all health care team members advised of the patient's response to the drug.

Patient teaching

— Instruct the patient and family about piperazine, including the dosage, frequency, action, and adverse reactions.
— Explain the disease process and rationale for therapy, including importance of compliance.
— Teach the patient and family about the need for good personal hygiene, especially proper hand-washing technique. To avoid reinfection, teach the patient to wash perianal area, to change undergarments and bedclothes daily, and to wash hands and clean fingernails before meals and after bowel movements.
— Explain that transmission can occur by direct or indirect transfer of ova by hands, food, or contaminated articles and that washing clothes in a household washing machine will destroy ova.
— Advise the patient to refrain from preparing food during infection.
— Inform the patient and family that no dietary restriction, laxatives, or enemas are necessary.
— Instruct the patient and family that the drug may be taken with food but that, for best effect, it should be taken on an empty stomach.

—Advise the patient and family to mix powder for oral suspension in 57 ml of water, milk, or fruit juice.

—Warn the patient and family not to exceed recommended dosage because of hazard of neurotoxicity at high doses.

—Tell the patient to notify the nurse or doctor if adverse reactions develop or questions arise about piperazine therapy.

Evaluation

In the patient receiving piperazine, appropriate evaluation statements include:

• Patient is free of infection and maintains normal health status.
• Patient is free of pain.
• Patient and family state an understanding of piperazine therapy.

SELECTED MAJOR DRUGS: ANTHELMINTICS

DRUG, INDICATIONS, AND DOSAGES	SPECIAL PRECAUTIONS
mebendazole (Vermox) *Pinworm—* **Adults and children over age 2:** 100 mg P.O. as a single dose. If infection persists 3 weeks later, repeat treatment. *Roundworm, whipworm, hookworm—* **Adults and children over age 2:** 100 mg P.O. b.i.d. for 3 days. If infection persists 3 weeks later, repeat treatment.	• Contraindicated in patients with known hypersensitivity to the drug. • Administer cautiously to patients with carcinogenesis, mutagenesis, and impairment of fertility; to pregnant and breast-feeding patients; and in pediatric use.
niclosamide (Niclocide, Yomesan‡) *Tapeworms (fish, beef, and pork)—* **Adults:** 4 tablets (2 g) chewed thoroughly as a single dose. **Children over 34 kg:** 3 tablets (1.5 g) chewed thoroughly as a single dose. **Children 11 to 34 kg:** 2 tablets (1 g) chewed thoroughly as a single dose. *Dwarf tapeworm—* **Adults:** 4 tablets chewed thoroughly as a single daily dose for 7 days. **Children over age 2** (over 34 kg): 3 tablets chewed thoroughly on the first day, then 2 tablets for the next 6 days. **Children over age 2** (11 to 34 kg): 2 tablets chewed thoroughly on the first day, then 1 tablet daily for the next 6 days.	• Contraindicated in patients with known hypersensitivity to the drug. • Administer cautiously to pregnant patients.
oxamniquine (Vansil) *Schistosomiasis caused by* Schistosoma mansoni, *western hemisphere strains—* **Adults and children** (more than 30 kg): 12 to 15 mg/kg given as a single oral dose. **Children under 30 kg:** 10 mg/kg P.O., followed by 10 mg/kg P.O. 2 to 8 hours later.	• Use cautiously in patients with a history of seizure disorders. Rarely, epileptiform seizures have been observed within the first few hours after ingestion. Patients with a history of seizures should be kept under medical supervision.

‡Available in Australia only

SELECTED MAJOR DRUGS: ANTHELMINTICS *continued*

DRUG, INDICATIONS, AND DOSAGES	SPECIAL PRECAUTIONS
praziquantel (Biltricide) *Schistosomiasis caused by* Schistosoma mekongi, S. japonicum, S. mansoni, *and* S. haematobium— **Adults and children ages 4 and over:** 20 mg/kg P.O. t.i.d. as a 1-day treatment. The interval between doses should be between 4 and 6 hours.	• Contraindicated in breast-feeding patients or in those with ocular cysticercosis or known hypersensitivity to the drug. • Administer cautiously to pregnant patients.
thiabendazole (Mintezol) *Systemic infection with pinworm, roundworm, threadworm, whipworm, cutaneous larva migrans, and trichinosis*— **Adults and children:** 25 mg P.O. b.i.d. Duration of therapy depends on infection: threadworm, 2 days; creeping eruption, 2 to 5 days; toxocariasis, 7 days; trichinosis, 2 to 4 days.	• Contraindicated in breast-feeding patients or in those with known hypersensitivity to the drug. • Administer cautiously to pregnant patients or to those with hepatic or renal dysfunction.

SELF-TEST

1. His school teacher noticed that Phillip, age 8, always looked undernourished and had a short attention span in class. She advised his mother to have him checked by his pediatrician. He was diagnosed as having a roundworm (ascariasis) infection for which piperazine was prescribed. Phillip's mother should be told that:
   a. he must be isolated from other family members until treatment is completed.
   b. he will need to take an oral suspension of the drug for at least 1 week to ensure that all the worms are gone.
   c. the drug should be taken on an empty stomach but may be mixed with fruit juice and taken at breakfast.
   d. headache and vertigo are common and no cause for concern.

2. Which of the following adverse reactions should the nurse tell Phillip's mother to watch for?
   a. nausea and vomiting
   b. hyperreflexia and tinnitus
   c. constipation
   d. tendencies to bleeding and infection

3. At follow-up examination, therapy will be considered successful if:
   a. Phillip's mother confirms that all of his clothing has been washed.
   b. Phillip and his mother have consistently followed the instructions related to good personal hygiene.
   c. no worms or fecal ova are found on examination of Phillip's stool after 3 weeks.
   d. no adverse reactions to the therapy have occurred and Phillip's mother reports that she saw worms in Phillip's stool after 2 days of treatment.

Check your answers on page 1057.

CHAPTER 7

ANTIFUNGALS

amphotericin B ✦ fluconazole ✦ flucytosine ✦ griseofulvin microsize
griseofulvin ultramicrosize ✦ ketoconazole ✦ miconazole ✦ nystatin

OVERVIEW

- Fungi resist most antibiotics at therapeutic levels; only the antifungals are currently effective against fungi. Amphotericin B has been the most widely used antifungal, although others have recently been developed.
- Much of the recent increase in systemic fungal infections is related to cancer chemotherapy's compromise of the immune system.

MAJOR USES

- Besides systemic fungal infections, antifungals are effective against meningitis, severe fungal infections caused by *Candida* and *Cryptococcus* organisms, and yeast infections.
- Amphotericin B is useful in the treatment of CNS, pulmonary, cardiac, renal, and other systemic fungal infections. It is effective against blastomycosis, histoplasmosis, cryptococcosis, candidiasis, sporotrichosis, aspergillosis, phycomycosis (mucormycosis), and coccidioidomycosis.
- Fluconazole is given orally or intravenously to treat various systemic fungal infections.
- Flucytosine is effective, usually in combination with amphotericin B, in the treatment of systemic candidiasis, cryptococcosis, and aspergillosis.
- Griseofulvin is used systemically in the treatment of tinea capitis and other tinea infections that do not respond to topical agents.
- Ketoconazole is given orally to treat a wide variety of systemic fungal infections previously susceptible only to parenteral agents.
- Miconazole is given intravenously to treat systemic coccidioidomycosis, candidiasis, cryptococcosis, and paracoccidioidomycosis. It is also used locally to treat vaginal fungal infections.
- Nystatin is used to treat oral, GI, and vaginal infections caused by *Candida albicans* and other *Candida* organisms. It is also used locally to treat vaginal infections. (See Chapter 84, Local Anti-Infectives.)

MECHANISM OF ACTION

- Amphotericin B and nystatin probably act by binding to sterols in the fungal cell membrane, altering cell permeability and allowing leakage of intracellular components. They may also inhibit glycolysis and protein synthesis.
- Fluconazole inhibits fungal P-450 cytochrome function, which causes weakening of the fungal cell wall.

GLOSSARY

Mycoses: diseases caused by fungi.
Sterol: monohydroxyl alcohol of high molecular weight commonly classified as a lipid.
Thrush: fungal infection characterized by whitish spots and shallow ulcers in the oral cavity, fever, and GI irritation; usually results from superinfection.

- Flucytosine appears to penetrate fungal cells, where it is converted to fluorouracil, a known metabolic antagonist. Flucytosine is incorporated into fungal RNA and causes defective protein synthesis.
- Griseofulvin arrests fungal cell activity by disrupting its mitotic spindle structure.
- Miconazole and ketoconazole inhibit purine transport and DNA, RNA, and protein synthesis; they also increase cell wall permeability, making the fungus more susceptible to osmotic pressure.

ABSORPTION, DISTRIBUTION, METABOLISM, AND EXCRETION

Amphotericin B is poorly absorbed from the GI tract; therefore, it is generally administered by I.V. infusion. It is 90% bound to plasma proteins; diffuses poorly into body cavities, eyes, and CSF; and is slowly excreted by the kidneys.

Fluconazole is well absorbed from the GI tract. The pharmacokinetics of the oral and injectable forms are similar. Approximately 80% of the dose is renally excreted and 11% is metabolized.

Flucytosine is rapidly absorbed from the GI tract, reaching peak levels in about 6 hours. About 90% is excreted unchanged in the urine. The drug is well distributed to all body tissues and to the CNS.

Griseofulvin, although almost completely absorbed through the duodenum in ultramicrosize formulation, is absorbed unpredictably in microsize formulation. Administration with a high-fat meal, however, may enhance absorption. The drug concentrates in skin, hair, nails, liver, fat, and skeletal muscles. The highest concentration is found in the outermost horny layer of the skin; the lowest, in the deep layers. Metabolized in the liver, griseofulvin is eliminated in urine, feces, and perspiration, mostly as inactive metabolite and unchanged drug.

Ketoconazole is well absorbed from the GI tract. The drug is extensively metabolized in the liver and excreted in the urine and bile.

Miconazole is poorly absorbed from the GI tract, rapidly metabolized in the liver, and excreted mainly as inactive metabolites. Miconazole penetrates joints but not the CNS.

Nystatin's oral absorption is negligible. The drug is not absorbed through intact skin or mucous membranes, and blood levels are not measurable at therapeutic doses. The drug is eliminated unchanged in the stool.

ONSET AND DURATION

Amphotericin B has an average peak blood level of 1 mcg/ml after I.V. infusion of 30 mg. Immediately after infusion, no more than 10% of the dose appears in blood; the half-life is 24 hours. Amphotericin B can be detected in blood and urine 4 weeks after therapy is discontinued.

Fluconazole steady-state drug concentrations are reached in 5 to 10 days if a loading dose isn't used. If a loading dose of twice the daily dose is used, this level can be reached in 2 days.

Flucytosine is well absorbed from the GI tract. It reaches peak blood levels of 30 to 45 mcg/ml within 6 hours of a single 2-g oral dose in patients with normal renal function. The dose must be altered, however, for patients with renal impairment. Flucytosine has a half-life of 6 hours and is eliminated unchanged, primarily in the urine.

Griseofulvin blood levels peak in 4 hours. It is undetectable in skin 2 days—and in blood 4 days—after drug is discontinued. Drug concentrations in skin are highest in warm climates.

Ketoconazole's peak blood level occurs within 1 to 2 hours after being administered with meals.

With I.V. infusion of 9 mg/kg, miconazole reaches blood levels of at least 1 mcg/ml, but the levels fall rapidly within 30 minutes. The half-life of miconazole is unchanged in patients with renal impairment.

Nystatin products vary in onset and duration.

ADVERSE REACTIONS

Adverse reactions occurring with antifungals may include GI effects (nausea, vomiting, diarrhea, and anorexia) and hematologic effects (anemia, leukopenia, thrombocytopenia, bone marrow suppression, and granulocytopenia). Other reactions include Stevens-Johnson syndrome, hepatotoxicity, cardiac arrhythmias, hypokalemia, azotemia, renal impairment, thrombophlebitis, fever, headache, dizziness, rash, photosensitivity, superinfection, gynecomastia, and pruritus.

Amphotericin B, the most effective antifungal, is associated with frequent adverse reactions in most organ systems. Among the most significant reactions are cardiac arrhythmias, hypokalemia, azotemia, permanent renal impairment, thrombophlebitis, fever, chills, anorexia, and nausea.

Fluconazole, comparatively free of adverse reactions, most commonly causes nausea and vomiting; rarely, hepatotoxicity and Stevens-Johnson syndrome.

Because flucytosine is usually used in combination with amphotericin B, its adverse effects may be difficult to identify. However, flucytosine causes anemia, leukopenia, thrombocytopenia, and bone marrow suppression as an extension of its pharmacologic action. It may also cause significant GI reactions (nausea, vomiting, and diarrhea).

Griseofulvin may also cause granulocytopenia that will require discontinuation of drug therapy. This drug's other adverse effects are less severe and include nausea, vomiting, headache, dizziness, diarrhea, rash, photosensitivity, and candidal overgrowth.

Ketoconazole may cause fatal hepatotoxicity indicated by elevated liver enzymes and by gynecomastia in males. It may also cause nausea, vomiting, itching, headache, and dizziness.

Miconazole may cause a transient decrease in serum sodium.

Nystatin is essentially free of adverse effects. However, high dosages may induce mild GI symptoms.

PROTOTYPE: ANTIFUNGALS

AMPHOTERICIN B

(am foe ter' i sin B)
Fungilin Oral‡, Fungizone
Classification: antifungal
Pregnancy risk category B

How supplied

TABLETS: 100 mg‡
ORAL SUSPENSION: 100 mg/ml‡
LOZENGES: 10 mg‡
INJECTION: 50-mg lyophilized cake

Indications and dosage

Systemic fungal infections (histoplasmosis, coccidioidomycosis, blastomycosis, cryptococcosis, disseminated moniliasis, aspergillosis, phycomycosis), meningitis

ADULTS: initially, 1 mg in 250 ml of dextrose 5% in water infused over 2 to 4 hours; or 0.25 mg/kg daily by slow infusion over 6 hours. Increase daily dosage gradually as patient tolerance develops to maximum of 1 mg/kg daily. Therapy must not exceed 1.5 mg/kg. If drug is discontinued for 1 week or more, administration must resume with initial dose and again increase gradually. For intrathecal injection, 25 mcg/0.1 ml diluted with 10 to 20 ml of CSF and administered by barbotage two or three times weekly. Initial dose should not exceed 100 mcg.

Candida albicans *infections involving the GI tract*

ADULTS: 100 mg P.O. q.i.d. for 2 weeks.

Oral and perioral candidal infections

ADULTS: 1 lozenge q.i.d. for 7 to 14 days. The lozenge should be sucked and allowed to dissolve slowly in the mouth.

Contraindications and precautions

Amphotericin B is contraindicated in patients with known hypersensitivity to the drug, unless no other therapy is effective. It should be used with caution in patients with mild to moderate renal function impairment, and in patients taking other nephrotoxic drugs.

Adverse reactions

BLOOD: normochromic, normocytic anemia.

CNS: *headache*, peripheral neuropathy; with intrathecal administration—peripheral nerve pain, paresthesia.

CV: hypotension, **arrhythmias, asystole.**

GI: *anorexia, weight loss, nausea, vomiting, dyspepsia, diarrhea, epigastric cramps.*

GU: *abnormal renal function with hypokalemia, azotemia, hyposthenuria, renal tubular acidosis, nephrocalcinosis*; with large doses—permanent renal impairment, anuria, oliguria.

LOCAL: *burning, stinging, irritation, tissue damage with extravasation, thrombophlebitis, pain at site of injection.*

OTHER: arthralgia, myalgia, muscle weakness secondary to hypokalemia, *fever, chills, malaise*, generalized pain.

Interactions

Other nephrotoxic antibiotics: may cause additive kidney toxicity. Administer very cautiously.

Nursing considerations

Assessment

• Review the patient's history for a condition that contraindicates the use of amphotericin B.
• Obtain a baseline assessment of patient's fungal infection before therapy.
• Be alert for common adverse reactions.
• Evaluate the patient's and family's knowledge about amphotericin B therapy.

Planning (Nursing Diagnoses)

Potential nursing diagnoses for the patient receiving amphotericin B include:
• Potential for injury related to ineffectiveness of amphotericin B to eradicate the infection.
• Altered health maintenance related to amphotericin B–induced adverse reactions.
• Knowledge deficit related to amphotericin B therapy.

Implementation

Preparation and administration

— Cultures and histologic and sensitivity testing must be completed and diagnosis confirmed before starting therapy in nonimmunocompromised patient.
— Prepare infusion as manufacturer directs, with strict aseptic technique, using only 10 ml of sterile water to reconstitute. To avoid precipitation, do not mix with solutions containing sodium chloride, other electrolytes, or bacteriostatic agents, such as benzyl alcohol.
— Lyophilized cake contains no preservatives. Do not use if solution contains a precipitate or other foreign particles. Store cake at 35.6° to 46.4° F (2° to 8° C). Protect drug from light and check expiration date.

—For I.V. infusion, use an in-line filter with a mean pore diameter larger than 1 micron.

—Infuse slowly; rapid infusion may cause CV collapse.

—Do not mix or piggyback antibiotics with amphotericin B infusion; the I.V. solution appears compatible with small amounts of heparin sodium, hydrocortisone sodium succinate, and methylprednisolone sodium succinate.

—Give in distal veins.

—Use topical products for folds of groin, neck, or armpit; avoid occlusive dressing with ointment and discontinue if signs of hypersensitivity develop. Topical products may stain skin or clothes.

—Store at room temperature. Solution is stable at room temperature and in indoor light for 24 hours or in refrigerator for 1 week.

Monitoring

—Monitor the effectiveness of therapy by regularly assessing for improvement of infectious process.

—Monitor I.V. site for discomfort or thrombosis.

—Monitor the patient for adverse drug reactions.

—Monitor vital signs every 30 minutes for at least 4 hours after start of I.V. infusion; fever may appear in 1 to 2 hours but should subside within 4 hours of discontinuing drug.

—Monitor intake and output and report changes in urine appearance or volume immediately; renal damage may be reversible if drug is stopped at earliest sign of dysfunction.

—Monitor potassium levels closely; monitor calcium and magnesium levels twice weekly; perform liver and renal function studies and CBC weekly.

—Monitor ECG for arrhythmias.

—Monitor the patient for drug interactions.

—Regularly reevaluate the patient's and family's knowledge about amphotericin B therapy.

Intervention

—Severity of some adverse reactions can be reduced by premedication with aspirin, acetaminophen, antihistamines, antiemetics, or small doses of corticosteroids; by addition of phosphate buffer to the solution; and by alternate-day dosing. If reactions are severe, drug may have to be discontinued for varying periods.

—If thrombosis occurs, alternate-day therapy may be prescribed.

—Obtain an order for an antiemetic or antidiarrheal agent as needed.

—Keep all health care team members advised of patient's response to the drug.

Patient teaching

—Instruct the patient and family about amphotericin B, including the dosage, frequency, action, and adverse reactions.

—Teach the patient signs and symptoms of hypersensitivity and other adverse reactions, especially those associated with I.V. therapy.

—Warn the patient that therapy may take several months; teach personal hygiene and other measures to prevent spread and recurrence of lesions.

—Urge the patient to adhere to regimen and to return as instructed for follow-up.

—Tell the patient that topical products may stain skin and clothing; cream or lotion may be removed from clothing with soap and water.

—Tell the patient to notify the nurse or doctor if adverse reactions develop or questions arise about amphotericin B therapy.

Evaluation

In the patient receiving amphotericin B, appropriate evaluation statements include:

• Patient's infection is alleviated.

• Patient does not experience serious adverse reactions associated with amphotericin B.

• Patient and family state an understanding of amphotericin B therapy.

SELECTED MAJOR DRUGS: ANTIFUNGALS

DRUG, INDICATIONS, AND DOSAGES

fluconazole (Diflucan)
Oropharyngeal candidiasis —
Adults: 200 mg P.O. or I.V. on the first day, followed by 100 mg daily. Therapy should continue for 2 weeks.
Esophageal candidiasis —
Adults: 200 mg P.O. or I.V. on the first day, followed by 100 mg daily. Higher doses (up to 400 mg daily) have been used, depending on the patient's condition and tolerance of treatment. Patients should receive the drug for at least 3 weeks and for 2 weeks after symptoms resolve.
Systemic candidiasis —
Adults: 400 mg P.O. or I.V. on the first day, followed by 200 mg daily. Treatment should continue for at least 4 weeks or for 2 weeks after symptoms resolve.
Cryptococcal meningitis —
Adults: 400 mg P.O. or I.V. on the first day, followed by 200 mg daily. Higher doses (up to 400 mg daily) may be used. Treatment should continue for 10 to 12 weeks after cultures of CSF are negative.
Suppression of relapse of cryptococcal meningitis in patients with AIDS —
Adults: 200 mg P.O. or I.V. daily.

SPECIAL PRECAUTIONS

• Contraindicated in patients with known hypersensitivity to the drug or any of its ingredients.

• Administer cautiously to pregnant or breast-feeding patients.

(continued)

SELECTED MAJOR DRUGS: ANTIFUNGALS *continued*

DRUG, INDICATIONS, AND DOSAGES	SPECIAL PRECAUTIONS
flucytosine (Ancobon) *Severe fungal infections caused by susceptible strains of* Candida *(including septicemia, endocarditis, urinary tract and pulmonary infections) and* Cryptococcus *(meningitis, pulmonary infection, and possible urinary tract infections)*— **Adults and children over 50 kg:** 50 to 150 mg/kg P.O. daily q 6 hours. **Adults and children under 50 kg:** 1.5 to 4.5 g/m² P.O. daily in four divided doses. Severe infections, such as meningitis, may require doses up to 250 mg/kg.	• Contraindicated in breast-feeding women or in patients with known hypersensitivity to the drug. • Administer with extreme caution to patients with impaired renal function or bone marrow depression. • Administer cautiously to pregnant women.
ketoconazole (Nizoral) *Systemic candidiasis, chronic mucocandidiasis, oral thrush, candiduria, coccidioidomycosis, histoplasmosis, chromomycosis, and paracoccidioidomycosis; severe cutaneous dermatophyte infections resistant to therapy with topical or oral griseofulvin*— **Adults and children over 40 kg:** initially, 200 mg P.O. daily as a single dose. Dosage may be increased to 400 mg daily in patients who don't respond to lower dosage. **Children under 20 kg:** 50 mg (¼ tablet) daily as a single dose. **Children 20 to 40 kg:** 100 mg (½ tablet) daily as a single dose.	• Contraindicated in breast-feeding women or in patients with known hypersensitivity to the drug. • Administer cautiously to pregnant patients. • Life-threatening ventricular arrhythmias have been reported in patients taking terfenadine (Seldane) with ketoconazole.
nystatin (Mycostatin, Nadostinet, Nilstat, Nystex) *GI infections*— **Adults:** 500,000 to 1 million units P.O. (oral tablets) t.i.d. *Oral, vaginal, and intestinal infections caused by* Candida albicans (Monilia) *and other* Candida *species*— **Adults:** 400,000 to 600,000 units P.O. (oral suspension) q.i.d. for oral candidiasis. **Children and infants over age 3 months:** 250,000 to 500,000 units P.O. (oral suspension) q.i.d. **Newborn and premature infants:** 100,000 units as oral suspension q.i.d. *Vaginal infections*— **Adults:** 100,000 units (vaginal tablets) inserted high into vagina daily or b.i.d. for 14 days.	• Contraindicated in patients with known hypersensitivity to the drug or any of its components.

†Available in Canada only

SELF-TEST

1. Anthony Kerry was admitted to the hospital for treatment of histoplasmosis. His doctor prescribed amphotericin B, 0.25 mg/kg I.V. daily. How should his nurse administer this drug?
   a. as a rapid infusion over 10 minutes
   b. by slow infusion over 6 hours
   c. divide the dose into four separate doses and administer each dose over 30 minutes 6 hours apart
   d. as a continuous infusion over 24 hours

2. Which electrolyte imbalance should the nurse monitor Mr. Kerry for?
   a. hypokalemia
   b. hyperkalemia
   c. hypocalcemia
   d. hypercalcemia

3. How often should the nurse take Mr. Kerry's vital signs after the start of the I.V. infusion?
   a. every 5 minutes for 1 hour
   b. every 10 minutes for 2 hours
   c. every 30 minutes for 4 hours
   d. every hour for 6 hours

Check your answers on page 1057.

CHAPTER 8

ANTIMALARIALS

chloroquine hydrochloride ◆ chloroquine sulphate
chloroquine phosphate ◆ hydroxychloroquine sulfate
mefloquine hydrochloride ◆ primaquine phosphate ◆ pyrimethamine
pyrimethamine with sulfadoxine ◆ quinine bisulfate ◆ quinine sulfate

OVERVIEW

- Quinine, the bitter alkaloid obtained from the bark of the cinchona tree; the 4-aminoquinoline derivatives (chloroquine and hydroxychloroquine); and related drugs are used in prophylaxis and treatment of malarial infections.
- In many areas of the world, malaria is a common infectious disease with a high mortality. Transmitted by the bite of the *Anopheles* mosquito, malaria is most commonly concentrated in Asia, Africa, and Latin America. In the United States, however, malarial infections are usually nonepidemic.

MAJOR USES

- Chloroquine, mefloquine, hydroxychloroquine, primaquine, and pyrimethamine suppress susceptible strains of *Plasmodium* (*P. vivax, P. malariae, P. ovale,* and *P. falciparum*).
- Chloroquine and hydroxychloroquine are also used in the treatment of systemic lupus erythematosus (SLE) and rheumatoid arthritis. Chloroquine is used in combination with emetine to treat amebic hepatic abscesses as well as certain fluke infections.
- Quinine is used to treat chloroquine-resistant malaria. The drug also is prescribed to relieve nocturnal leg cramps.
- Pyrimethamine is used in combination with sulfonamides to treat toxoplasmosis.

MECHANISM OF ACTION

- The 4-aminoquinoline compounds bind to, and alter the properties of, both microbial and mammalian DNA.
- Primaquine is a gametocidal drug that destroys exoerythrocytic forms and prevents delayed primary attack. Its precise mechanism of action is unknown.
- Pyrimethamine inhibits the enzyme dihydrofolate reductase, thereby impeding reduction of folic acid.
- Quinine's exact mechanism of action is unknown, but the drug is often referred to as a generalized protoplasmic poison.

GLOSSARY

Malaria: infectious febrile disease caused by protozoa transmitted by the bites of infected mosquitos; characterized by periodic attacks of chills, fever, and diaphoresis.
Prophylaxis: disease prevention.

* Mefloquine acts as a blood schizonticide; however, its exact mechanism of action is not known.

ABSORPTION, DISTRIBUTION, METABOLISM, AND EXCRETION

All antimalarials are rapidly absorbed from the GI tract. The 4-aminoquinoline compounds, bound to plasma proteins, achieve very high levels in the liver, spleen, kidneys, and lungs. They are metabolized in the liver and slowly excreted in the urine for months after treatment. Primaquine is rapidly metabolized in the liver. Only a small amount of unchanged drug is excreted in the urine; the rest is excreted as metabolite. Pyrimethamine is metabolized in the liver and excreted in the urine. Quinine, which is highly protein-bound, is excreted in the urine—mostly as inactive metabolite. Mefloquine is essentially all cleared hepatically and the drug is highly protein-bound.

ONSET AND DURATION

The 4-aminoquinolines and primaquine reach peak blood concentrations 6 hours after oral administration. Levels fall rapidly; only very small quantities are detectable after 24 hours. However, minute amounts may still be detectable in the urine months after therapy ends.

Pyrimethamine is eliminated slowly and has a half-life of 4 days. Therapeutic concentrations may remain in the blood for as long as 2 weeks.

Quinine achieves peak blood levels within 1 to 3 hours; only a negligible concentration can be measured 24 hours after therapy ends.

Mefloquine is absorbed within 30 minutes to 2 hours after oral administration and has a mean elimination half-life of 3 weeks.

ADVERSE REACTIONS

Chloroquine, hydroxychloroquine, and primaquine may cause agranulocytosis, aplastic anemia, thrombocytopenia, and, in patients with G6PD deficiency, hemolytic anemia. Visual reactions that range from the minor (blurred vision, difficulty in focusing) to the severe (optic disk atrophy, retinal degeneration). They also cause GI toxicities (anorexia, nausea, vomiting, and cramping), skin eruptions, and CNS toxicity (headache, fatigue, dizziness, and nightmares).

Mefloquine reactions most commonly include dizziness, myalgia, fever, nausea, headache, chills, diarrhea, fatigue, and tinnitus. Less common reactions include hair loss, bradycardia, pruritus, and seizures. These reactions are difficult to distinguish from the effects of malaria.

Pyrimethamine, with or without sulfadoxine, may produce various blood dyscrasia, such as agranulocytosis, aplastic anemia, leukopenia, thrombocytopenia, and pancytopenia. Seizures and CNS stimulation have occurred in acute overdose. Skin rashes may include Stevens-Johnson syndrome and toxic epidermal necrolysis.

Quinine is also known to produce significant hematologic toxicity (agranulocytosis, hemolytic anemia). CNS reactions include headache, syncope, delirium, and (with toxic doses) seizures. CV toxicity is associated with too-rapid I.V. administration or overdosage and includes hypotension and shock. Visual disturbances, impaired hearing, GI distress, and renal tubular damage have been noted but are usually mild.

PROTOTYPE: ANTIMALARIALS

CHLOROQUINE HYDROCHLORIDE
(klor′ oh kwin)
Aralen HCl, Chlorquin‡

CHLOROQUINE PHOSPHATE
Aralen Phosphate, Chlorquin‡

CHLOROQUINE SULPHATE
Nivaquine‡
Classification: antimalarial
Pregnancy risk category C

How supplied
hydrochloride
INJECTION: 50 mg/ml (40-mg/ml base)
phosphate
TABLETS: 250 mg (150-mg base), 500 mg (300-mg base)
sulphate
TABLETS: 200 mg (150-mg base)
SYRUP: 68 mg (50-mg base)/5 ml

Indications and dosage
Suppressive prophylaxis and treatment of acute attacks of malaria due to Plasmodium vivax, P. malariae, P. ovale, *and susceptible strains of* P. falciparum
ADULTS: initially, 600 mg (base) P.O., then 300 mg at 6, 24, and 48 hours. Or 160 to 200 mg (base) I.M. initially; repeat in 6 hours if needed. Switch to oral therapy as soon as possible.
CHILDREN: initially, 10 mg (base)/kg P.O., then 5 mg (base)/kg dose at 6, 24, and 48 hours (do not exceed adult dose). Or 5 mg (base)/kg I.M. initially; repeat in 6 hours if needed. Switch to oral therapy as soon as possible.

Malaria suppressive treatment
ADULTS AND CHILDREN: 5 mg (base)/kg P.O. (not to exceed 300 mg) weekly on same day of the week (begin 2 weeks before entering endemic area and continue for 8 weeks after leaving). If treatment begins after exposure, double the initial dose (600 mg for adults, 10 mg/kg for children) in 2 divided doses P.O. 6 hours apart.

Extraintestinal amebiasis
ADULTS: 160 to 200 mg hydrochloride (base) I.M. daily for no more than 12 days. As soon as possible, substitute 1 g (600 mg base) phosphate P.O. daily for 2 days; then 500 mg (300 mg base) daily for at least 2 to 3 weeks. Treatment is usually combined with an effective intestinal amebicide.
CHILDREN: 10 mg/kg of hydrochloride (base) for 2 to 3 weeks. Maximum is 300 mg daily.

Rheumatoid arthritis and SLE
ADULTS: 250 mg (phosphate) daily with evening meal.

Contraindications and precautions
Chloroquine is contraindicated in patients with known hypersensitivity to the drug or other 4-aminoquinoline compounds and in patients with retinal or visual field changes. However, the doctor may elect to use this drug after weighing possible benefits and risk to the patient. The drug should not be used during pregnancy or in patients with psoriasis or porphyria unless the benefit outweighs the potential hazard. Use cautiously in patients with hepatic disease, alcoholism, or G6PD deficiency and in those receiving other hepatotoxic drugs.

Adverse reactions
BLOOD: **agranulocytosis, aplastic anemia, hemolytic anemia,** thrombocytopenia.
CNS: mild and transient headache, neuromyopathy, psychic stimulation, fatigue, irritability, nightmares, **seizures**, dizziness.
CV: hypotension, ECG changes.
EENT: *visual disturbances* (blurred vision; difficulty in focusing; reversible corneal changes; generally irreversible, sometimes progressive or delayed retinal changes, such as narrowing of arterioles; macular lesions; pallor of optic disk; optic atrophy; patchy retinal pigmentation, often leading to blindness); ototoxicity (nerve deafness, vertigo, tinnitus).
GI: *anorexia, abdominal cramps,* diarrhea, nausea, vomiting.
SKIN: pruritus, lichen planus–like eruptions, skin and mucosal pigmentary changes, pleomorphic skin eruptions.

Interactions
Magnesium and aluminum salts, kaolin with pectin: Decreased GI absorption. Separate administration times.

Nursing considerations

Assessment
- Review the patient's history for a condition that contraindicates the use of chloroquine.
- Obtain a baseline assessment of the patient's infection before therapy.
- Be alert for common adverse reactions, especially visual disturbances.
- Evaluate the patient's and family's knowledge about chloroquine therapy.

Planning (Nursing Diagnoses)
Potential nursing diagnoses for the patient receiving chloroquine include:
- Potential for injury related to ineffective drug dosage.
- Sensory/perceptual alterations (visual) related to adverse reactions associated with chloroquine.
- Knowledge deficit related to chloroquine therapy.

Implementation

Preparation and administration
— Protect from light by storing in amber-colored containers.
— Tablets may be crushed and mixed with food or chocolate syrup for patients with difficulty swallowing, However, the drug has a bitter taste and patients may find the mixture unpleasant. The crushed tablets may be placed inside empty gelatin capsules which are easier to swallow.
— Prophylactic antimalarial therapy should begin 2 weeks before exposure and be continued for 6 to 8 weeks after leaving the endemic area.
— Administer with milk or meals to minimize GI distress.
— Administer at the same time of the same day each week.
— Missed doses should be taken as soon as possible. To avoid doubling doses in regimens requiring more than one dose per day, the patient should take missed dose within 1 hour of scheduled time or omit the dose.

Monitoring
— Monitor the effectiveness of therapy by regularly assessing for improvement of infectious process.
— Monitor the patient for adverse drug reactions.
— Monitor the patient's body weight for significant changes.
— Monitor for visual disturbances.
— Regularly monitor CBC and liver function studies during prolonged therapy. If severe blood disorder appears that is not attributable to disease under treatment, drug may need to be discontinued.
— Monitor the patient for drug interactions.
— Monitor diagnostic test results. Chloroquine may cause inversion or depression of the T wave or widening of the QRS complex on ECG. Rarely, it may cause decreased WBC, RBC, or platelet counts.
— Regularly reevaluate the patient's and family's knowledge about chloroquine therapy.

Intervention

— Notify the doctor of any significant weight changes. Drug dosage is calculated on the patient's weight.
— Institute safety measures if visual disturbances occur.
— Keep all health care team members advised of the patient's response to the drug.

Patient teaching

— Instruct the patient and family about chloroquine, including the dosage, frequency, action, and adverse reactions.
— Explain the disease process and rationale for therapy.
— To avoid exacerbated drug-induced dermatoses, warn the patient to avoid excessive exposure to sun.
— Review methods for reducing exposure to mosquitoes for the patient receiving this drug prophylactically.
— Caution the patient to avoid hazardous activities requiring alertness if dizziness or light-headedness occurs.
— Advise the patient to avoid alcohol while taking this drug.
— Tell the patient to keep drug out of children's reach. Fatalities have followed ingestion of as few as 3 or 4 tablets.
— Tell the patient to take drug immediately before or after meals on the same day each week to minimize gastric distress and to take missed doses as soon as possible.
— Advise the patient to have baseline and periodic ophthalmologic examinations. Tell the patient to report blurred vision, increased sensitivity to light, or muscle weakness. Check periodically for ocular muscle weakness after long-term use. Audiometric examinations are recommended before, during, and after therapy, especially long-term.
— Warn the woman of childbearing age who is traveling to an endemic area against becoming pregnant. Instruct her to continue contraceptive precautions for 2 months after the last dose of medication.
— Tell the patient to notify the nurse or doctor if adverse reactions develop or questions arise about chloroquine therapy.

Evaluation

In the patient receiving chloroquine, appropriate evaluation statements include:
• Patient is free of infection.
• Patient maintains normal vision throughout chloroquine therapy.
• Patient and family state an understanding of chloroquine therapy.

SELECTED MAJOR DRUGS: ANTIMALARIALS

DRUG, INDICATIONS, AND DOSAGES	SPECIAL PRECAUTIONS
mefloquine (Lariam) *Acute malarial infections caused by mefloquine-sensitive strains of* Plasmodium falciparum *or* P. vivax— **Adults:** 1,250 mg P.O. as a single dose. Patients with *P. vivax* infections should receive subsequent therapy with primaquine or other 8-aminoquinolines to avoid relapse after treatment of the initial infection. *Malaria prophylaxis—* **Adults:** 250 mg P.O. weekly for 4 weeks, then 250 mg every other week. Initiate prophylaxis 1 week before entering endemic area and continue prophylaxis for 4 weeks after returning from such areas. When returning to an area without malaria after a prolonged stay in an endemic area, prophylaxis ends after three doses.	• Contraindicated in patients with known hypersensitivity to mefloquine or related compounds. • Use cautiously in patients with cardiac disease.
primaquine *Radical cure of relapsing* Plasmodium vivax *malaria, eliminating symptoms and infection completely; prevention of relapse—* **Adults:** 15 mg (base) P.O. daily for 14 days. (26.3-mg tablet = 15 mg of base).	• Contraindicated in patients with lupus erythematosus and rheumatoid arthritis and in those taking bone marrow suppressants and potentially hemolytic drugs. • Use with a fast-acting antimalarial, such as chloroquine. Use full dose to reduce possibility of drug-resistant strains. • Administer cautiously to children and pregnant patients.
pyrimethamine (Daraprim) **pyrimethamine with sulfadoxine (Fansidar)** *Malaria prophylaxis and transmission control (pyrimethamine)—* **Adults and children over age 10:** 25 mg P.O. weekly. **Children ages 4 to 10:** 12.5 mg P.O. weekly. **Children under age 4:** 6.25 mg P.O. weekly. Continue in all age-groups at least 10 weeks after leaving endemic areas. *Acute attacks of malaria (pyrimethamine with sulfadoxine)—* **Adults:** 2 to 3 tablets as a single dose, either alone or in sequence with quinine or primaquine. **Children ages 9 to 14:** 2 tablets. **Children ages 4 to 8:** 1 tablet. **Children under age 4:** ½ tablet. *Malaria prophylaxis (pyrimethamine with sulfadoxine)—* **Adults:** 1 tablet weekly or 2 tablets q 2 weeks. **Children ages 9 to 14:** ¾ tablet weekly or 1½ tablets q 2 weeks. **Children ages 4 to 8:** ½ tablet weekly or 1 tablet q 2 weeks. **Children under age 4:** ¼ tablet weekly or ½ tablet q 2 weeks.	• Contraindicated in patients with chloroquine-resistant malaria. • Sulfadoxine, an ingredient in Fansidar, is a sulfonamide; therefore, this combination is contraindicated in porphyria. • Use cautiously in patients with impaired hepatic or renal function, severe allergy or bronchial asthma, or G6PD deficiency. Also, use cautiously in patients with seizure disorders; smaller doses may be needed. Additionally, use cautiously after treatment with chloroquine.

SELECTED MAJOR DRUGS: ANTIMALARIALS *continued*

DRUG, INDICATIONS, AND DOSAGES	SPECIAL PRECAUTIONS

pyrimethamine *(continued)*
Acute attacks of malaria (pyrimethamine) —
Not recommended alone in nonimmune persons; use
with faster-acting antimalarials, such as chloroquine, for
2 days to initiate transmission control and suppressive
cure.
Adults and children over age 15: 25 mg P.O. daily for 2
days.
Children under age 15: 12.5 mg P.O. daily for 2 days.
Toxoplasmosis (pyrimethamine) —
Adults: initially, 100 mg P.O., then 25 mg P.O. daily for
4 to 5 weeks; during same time, give 1 g sulfadiazine
P.O. q 6 hours.
Children: initially, 1 mg/kg P.O., then 0.25 mg/kg daily
for 4 to 5 weeks, along with 100 mg sulfadiazine/kg
P.O. daily in divided doses q 6 hours.

quinine (Quine, Strema)
Malaria due to Plasmodium falciparum *(chloroquine-re-sistant* —
Adults: 650 mg P.O. q 8 hours for 10 days, with 25 mg
pyrimethamine q 12 hours for 3 days, and with 500 mg
sulfadiazine q.i.d. for 5 days.
Nocturnal leg cramps —
Adults: 260 to 300 mg P.O. h.s. or after the evening
meal.

• Contraindicated in patients
with G6PD deficiency.
• Use cautiously in patients
with CV conditions.

SELF-TEST

1. Laura Dunn, age 35, is planning a 3-month tour of Southeast Asia. Because she knows that malaria is endemic in that part of the world,
she requested an antimalarial to prevent infection. Her nurse practitioner prescribed chloroquine. To prevent malaria, Ms. Dunn
should take the chloroquine weekly:
   a. from the time she arrives in Southeast Asia until she leaves that
   area.
   b. from 1 week before she leaves until 1 week after she returns.
   c. from 2 weeks before she leaves for Southeast Asia until she
   returns.
   d. from 2 weeks before she leaves for Southeast Asia to 8 weeks
   after leaving that area.

2. The nurse reviews Ms. Dunn's medication history for possible drug interactions. Which of the following OTC preparations should the nurse tell Ms. Dunn to avoid?
   a. aspirin
   b. acetaminophen
   c. antacids containing magnesium
   d. fat-soluble vitamins

3. Ms. Dunn will be traveling with two school-age children. The nurse should remind her:
   a. that children are not susceptible to malarial infection so no prophylactic treatment is required.
   b. that this medication is contraindicated in children.
   c. to keep this medication out of the reach of her children.
   d. that children should be treated only if they become infected.

Check your answers on pages 1057 and 1058.

CHAPTER 9

ANTITUBERCULARS

capreomycin sulfate ✦ cycloserine ✦ ethambutol hydrochloride
ethionamide ✦ isoniazid (INH) ✦ para-aminosalicylate sodium
pyrazinamide ✦ rifampin ✦ streptomycin sulfate

OVERVIEW

- Antituberculars combat different types of tuberculosis. This infection can attack any body organ but most commonly compromises the lungs.
- Once usually fatal, tuberculosis is now both controllable and curable. Becoming less prevalent in the United States, tuberculosis nevertheless remains a significant disease among alcoholics; in thickly populated, impoverished communities; on southwestern Indian reservations; and in parts of Asia, Africa, and Europe.

MAJOR USES

- Ethambutol, isoniazid, para-aminosalicylate sodium, rifampin, and streptomycin are the first-line drugs in the treatment of all forms of tuberculosis.
- Capreomycin, cycloserine, ethionamide, and pyrazinamide are second-line antitubercular, used in cases of drug resistance or in retreatment programs.
- Isoniazid is used prophylactically in susceptible persons exposed to tuberculosis.
- Rifampin is used prophylactically in meningococcal infections and *Haemophilus influenzae* meningitis. (It may be used with dapsone or sulfoxone in the initial management of lepromatous leprosy.)

MECHANISM OF ACTION

- Cycloserine inhibits cell-wall biosynthesis by inhibiting the utilization of amino acids (bacteriostatic).
- Ethambutol interferes with the synthesis of RNA, thus inhibiting protein metabolism (bacteriostatic).
- Isoniazid inhibits cell-wall biosynthesis by interfering with lipid and DNA synthesis (bactericidal).
- Para-aminosalicylate sodium inhibits the enzymes responsible for folic acid biosynthesis (bacteriostatic).
- Rifampin inhibits DNA-dependent RNA polymerase, thus impairing RNA synthesis (bactericidal).
- Streptomycin inhibits protein synthesis by binding to 30S ribosomal subunits (bactericidal).

GLOSSARY

Bactericidal: pertaining to an agent that destroys bacteria.
Bacteriostatic: pertaining to an agent that inhibits growth or multiplication of bacteria.
Meningitis: inflammation of the membranes that envelop in brain and spinal cord.
Resistance: natural ability of an organism to ward off deleterious effects of noxious agents, such as toxins, poisons, irritants, or pathogenic microorganisms.
Tuberculosis: infectious disease caused by a species of *Mycobacterium,* characterized by small rounded nodules in the tissues, as well as fever, emaciation, and night sweats.

• The mechanism of action of capreomycin (bactericidal), ethionamide (bacteriostatic), and pyrazinamide (bactericidal) is unknown.

ABSORPTION, DISTRIBUTION, METABOLISM, AND EXCRETION

Capreomycin is not significantly absorbed when given orally. Given I.M., it quickly reaches peak blood levels and is excreted in the urine essentially unchanged.

Cycloserine is rapidly absorbed when given orally. It is distributed throughout body fluids and tissues, including CSF. It is partially metabolized in the liver and excreted in the urine.

Ethambutol is well absorbed from the GI tract (75% to 80%). Distribution is unknown, but the drug is detoxified in the liver. Most is recovered unchanged from the urine and as much as 25% from the feces.

Ethionamide is rapidly absorbed when given orally and widely distributed; significant levels appear in CSF. Most of the drug is metabolized slowly in the liver and is subsequently excreted in the urine.

Isoniazid is readily absorbed when given orally or I.M., diffusing into all body fluids and tissues. About half the drug is metabolized in the liver and is excreted, together with unchanged drug (about 40%), in the urine.

Pyrazinamide is well absorbed from the GI tract. It is widely distributed, detoxified in the liver, and excreted in the urine.

Rifampin is well absorbed and widely distributed. Partially metabolized in the liver, rifampin is eliminated as both metabolite and unchanged drug in urine and feces.

Para-aminosalicylate sodium is readily absorbed from the GI tract, distributed throughout most body fluids and tissues, and excreted in the urine as both metabolite and free drug.

Streptomycin is well absorbed and widely distributed in most body tissues after I.M. injection. It is rapidly excreted, mostly unchanged, in the urine.

ONSET AND DURATION

Capreomycin reaches peak blood levels in 1 to 2 hours; duration is about 24 hours. Cycloserine reaches peak blood levels in 4 to 8 hours; duration is about 12 hours. Ethambutol reaches peak levels in 2 to 4 hours; duration is about 24 hours. Ethionamide produces peak levels in 3 hours; since it is metabolized slowly, blood levels are prolonged. Isoniazid reaches peak levels within 1 to 2 hours; levels decline to about 50% within either 50 minutes (rapid acetylators) or 3 hours (slow acetylators). Para-aminosalicylate sodium reaches peak levels within 1 hour; duration is about 10 to 12 hours. Pyrazinamide levels peak in 2 hours; duration is about 15 hours. Rifampin produces peak levels within 1½ to 4 hours; duration is 24 hours. Streptomycin's peak level occurs within 30 minutes to 2 hours; duration is about 8 to 12 hours.

ADVERSE REACTIONS

Adverse reactions to antituberculars occur primarily to the GI tract, peripheral nervous system, and hepatic system. GI reactions may include epigastric pain, nausea, vomiting, abdominal cramps, flatulence, anorexia, and diarrhea. Peripheral nervous system reactions may include peripheral neuritis, paresthesias (especially of the feet and hands), muscle twitching, dizziness, and ataxia. Hepatic effects may include liver dysfunction and hepatitis.

Other reactions may include visual disturbances, pruritus, joint pain, headache, muscle aches, psychoses and seizures, renal toxicity, hypersensitivity reactions, and red-orange discoloration of sweat, tears, saliva, urine, and feces. Hematologic reactions, including agranulocytosis, thrombocytopenia, and drug-induced lupus erythematosus, have also been reported.

PROTOTYPE: ANTITUBERCULARS

RIFAMPIN (RIFAMPICIN)
(rif′am pin)
Rifadin, Rifadin I.V., Rimactane, Rimycin‡, Rofact†
Classification: antitubercular
Pregnancy risk category C

How supplied
CAPSULES: 150 mg, 300 mg
KIT: 60 capsules, 300 mg
INJECTION: 600 mg

Indications and dosage
Primary treatment in pulmonary tuberculosis
ADULTS: 600 mg P.O. or I.V. daily as a single dose. Give P.O. dose 1 hour before or 2 hours after meals.

---

†Available in Canada only   ‡Available in Australia only

CHILDREN OVER AGE 5: 10 to 20 mg/kg P.O. or I.V. daily as a single dose. Give P.O. dose 1 hour before or 2 hours after a meal. Maximum dosage is 600 mg daily. Concomitant administration of other effective antituberculars is recommended.

Meningococcal carriers
ADULTS: 600 mg P.O. b.i.d. for 2 days.
CHILDREN AGES 1 TO 12: 10 mg/kg P.O. b.i.d. for 2 days, not to exceed 600 mg/dose.
INFANTS AGES 3 MONTHS TO 1 YEAR: 5 mg/kg P.O. b.i.d. for 2 days.

Prophylaxis of Haemophilus influenzae type b
ADULTS AND CHILDREN: 20 mg/kg P.O. daily for 4 days. Do not exceed 600 mg daily.

Contraindications and precautions
Rifampin is contraindicated in patients with known hypersensitivity to any of the rifamycins and in those with clinically active hepatitis. It should not be used to treat *Neisseria meningitidis* infections because of the risk of rapidly developing, resistant organisms. Use cautiously in patients with hepatic disease or in those receiving other hepatotoxic drugs.

Adverse reactions
BLOOD: thrombocytopenia, transient leukopenia, **hemolytic anemia.**
CNS: headache, fatigue, *drowsiness,* ataxia, dizziness, mental confusion, generalized numbness.
GI: epigastric distress, anorexia, *nausea, vomiting,* abdominal pain, diarrhea, flatulence, sore mouth and tongue.
METABOLIC: serious hepatotoxicity as well as transient abnormalities in liver function tests.
SKIN: pruritus, urticaria, *rash.*
OTHER: flulike syndrome, red-orange discoloration of body fluids, *fever.*

Interactions
Alcohol: may increase risk of hepatotoxicity.
Anticoagulants, corticosteroids, cyclosporine, cardiac glycoside preparations, quinidine, oral contraceptives, oral hypoglycemic agents (sulfonylurea), dapsone, narcotics, and analgesics: reduced drug activity. Avoid concomitant use.
Halothane: increased hepatotoxicity of both drugs. Avoid concomitant use.
Methadone, barbiturates, diazepam, verapamil, beta-adrenergic blockers, clofibrate, progestin, disopyramide, mexiletine, theophylline, chloramphenicol, and anticonvulsants: diminished drug effects. Monitor serum levels closely to detect subtherapeutic drug levels.
Oral contraceptives: impaired contraceptive effects. Patient should be advised to substitute nonhormonal methods of birth control.
Para-aminosalicylate sodium, ketoconazole: may interfere with absorption of rifampin. Give these drugs 8 to 12 hours apart.
Probenecid: may increase rifampin levels. Use together cautiously.

Nursing considerations

Assessment

• Review the patient's history for a condition that contraindicates the use of rifampin.
• Obtain a baseline assessment of the patient's infection before therapy.
• Be alert for common adverse reactions.
• Evaluate the patient's and family's knowledge about rifampin therapy.

Planning (Nursing Diagnoses)

Potential nursing diagnoses for the patient receiving rifampin include:
• Potential for injury related to dosage regimen inadequate to alleviate infection.
• Noncompliance (medication administration) related to prolonged therapy.
• Knowledge deficit related to rifampin therapy.

Implementation

Preparation and administration

— Obtain specimens for culture and sensitivity testing before first dose but do not delay therapy; repeat periodically to detect drug resistance.
— Give drug 1 hour before or 2 hours after meals for maximum absorption; capsule contents may be mixed with food or fluid to enhance swallowing.
— Increased liver enzyme activity inactivates certain drugs (especially warfarin, corticosteroids, and oral hypoglycemics), requiring dosage adjustments.
— Follow manufacturer's instructions for reconstitution of I.V. rifampin. Infuse within 3 hours.
— When administered during the last few weeks of pregnancy, rifampin can cause postnatal hemorrhage in the mother and infant, for which treatment with vitamin K may be indicated.

Monitoring

— Monitor the effectiveness of therapy by regularly assessing for improvement of the infectious process.
— Concomitant treatment with at least one other antitubercular is recommended.
— Monitor the patient for adverse drug reactions.
— Monitor for signs of hepatic impairment (anorexia, fatigue, malaise, jaundice, dark urine, and liver tenderness).
— Monitor hematologic, renal, and liver function studies and serum electrolytes.
— Monitor the patient for drug interactions.
— Monitor diagnostic studies.
— Rifampin alters standard serum folate and vitamin B_{12} assays. The drug's systemic effects may cause asymptomatic elevation of liver function tests (14%) and serum uric acid and may reduce vitamin D levels.

—Rifampin may cause temporary retention of sulfobromophthalein in the liver excretion test; it may also interfere with contrast material in gallbladder studies and urinalysis based on spectrophotometry.

—Monitor the patient's compliance with rifampin therapy. Therapy for tuberculosis should usually be continued for 6 to 9 months.

—Regularly reevaluate the patient's and family's knowledge about rifampin therapy.

Intervention

—If the patient develops an adverse reaction, notify the doctor and obtain an order for appropriate treatment. Provide supportive care as indicated.

—If the patient is unable to comply with treatment regimen, discuss reasons and offer suggestions to improve compliance (for example, clues patient can use to remind himself to take medication).

—Keep all health care team members advised of the patient's response to the drug.

Patient teaching

—Instruct the patient and family about rifampin, including the dosage, frequency, action, and adverse reactions.

—Explain the disease process and rationale for therapy.

—Tell the patient to take rifampin on an empty stomach, at least 1 hour before or 2 hours after a meal. If GI irritation occurs, the patient may need to take the drug with food.

—Urge the patient to comply with prescribed regimen, not to miss doses, not to double up on missed doses, and not to discontinue drug without checking with the doctor. Explain importance of follow-up appointments.

—Encourage the patient to report promptly to the doctor any flulike symptoms, weakness, sore throat, loss of appetite, unusual bruising, rash, itching, tea-colored urine, clay-colored stools, or yellow discoloration of eyes or skin.

—Explain that drug turns all body fluids a red-orange color; advise the patient of possible permanent stains on clothes and soft contact lenses.

—Advise oral contraceptive users to substitute other methods; rifampin inactivates such drugs and may alter menstrual patterns.

—Advise the patient to avoid alcoholic beverages while taking this drug because alcohol may increase the risk of hepatotoxicity.

—Warn the female patient that this drug is potentially teratogenic. Appropriate contraceptive measures should be taken while on this drug.

—Tell the patient to notify the nurse or doctor if adverse reactions develop or questions arise about rifampin therapy.

Evaluation

In the patient receiving rifampin, appropriate evaluation statements include:

• Patient is free of infection.

• Patient completes entire regimen of prescribed therapy.

• Patient and family state an understanding of rifampin therapy.

SELECTED MAJOR DRUGS: ANTITUBERCULARS

DRUG, INDICATIONS, AND DOSAGES

SPECIAL PRECAUTIONS

ethambutol (Etibi†‡, Myambutol)
Adjunctive treatment in pulmonary tuberculosis—
Adults and children over age 13: initial treatment for patients who have not received previous antitubercular therapy is 15 mg/kg P.O. daily as a single dose.
Retreatment: 25 mg/kg P.O. daily as a single dose for 60 days with at least one other antitubercular; then decrease to 15 mg/kg daily as a single dose.

• Contraindicated in patients with optic neuritis and in children under age 13.
• Use cautiously in patients with impaired renal function, cataracts, recurrent eye inflammations, gout, and diabetic retinopathy.

isoniazid (Laniazid, Nydrazid)
Primary treatment against actively growing tubercle bacilli—
Adults: 5 mg/kg P.O. or I.M. daily as a single dose, up to 300 mg daily, continued for 6 months to 2 years.
Infants and children: 10 to 20 mg/kg P.O. or I.M. daily as a single dose, up to 300 to 500 mg daily, continued for 18 months to 2 years. Concomitant administration of at least one other effective antitubercular is recommended.
Preventive therapy against tubercle bacilli of those closely exposed or those with positive skin tests whose chest X-rays and bacteriologic studies are consistent with nonprogressive tuberculous disease—
Adults: 300 mg P.O. daily as a single dose, continued for 1 year.
Infants and children: 10 mg/kg P.O. daily as a single dose, up to 300 mg daily, continued for 1 year.

• Contraindicated in patients with acute hepatic disease or isoniazid-associated hepatic damage.
• Use cautiously in patients with chronic non-isoniazid-associated hepatic disorders (especially those taking phenytoin), severe renal impairment, and chronic alcoholism and in elderly patients.

streptomycin
Streptococcal endocarditis—
Adults: 10 mg/kg I.M. (maximum 0.5 g) q 12 hours for 2 weeks with penicillin.
Primary and adjunctive treatment in tuberculosis—
Adults: with normal renal function, 1 g I.M. daily for 2 to 3 months, then 1 g 2 or 3 times a week. Inject deeply into upper outer quadrant of buttocks.
Children: with normal renal function, 20 mg/kg daily in divided doses injected deeply into large muscle mass. Give concurrently with other antituberculars, but not with capreomycin, and continue until sputum specimen becomes negative.
Patients with impaired renal function: initial dose is same as for those with normal renal function. Subsequent doses and frequency determined by renal function study results.
Enterococcal endocarditis—
Adults: 1 g I.M. q 12 hours for 2 weeks, then 500 mg I.M. q 12 hours for 4 weeks with penicillin.
Tularemia—
Adults: 1 to 2 g I.M. daily in divided doses injected deep into upper outer quadrant of buttocks. Continue until patient is afebrile for 5 to 7 days.

• Contraindicated in patients with labyrinthine disease.
• Use cautiously in elderly patients and in those with impaired renal function.

ANTITUBERCULAR COMBINATION

TRADE NAME AND CONTENT	SPECIAL CONSIDERATIONS
Rifamate rifampin 300 mg and isoniazid 150 mg	• The American Thoracic Society and Centers for Disease Control recommend rifampin 10 mg/kg (up to 600 mg daily) with isoniazid 5 mg/kg (up to 300 mg daily) for 6 months for the first 2 months with 15 to 30 mg/kg (up to 2 g) of pyrizinamide daily, • Combines rifampin and isoniazid into a single capsule; this may improve compliance by decreasing the number of medications that must be taken. • Monitor patients for common adverse reactions to rifampin (GI toxicity) and isoniazid (neurotoxicity). Remind patients to take daily pyridoxine (10 to 50 mg) to avoid neurotoxicity.

SELF-TEST

1. Robert Johnson, age 25, sought health care because of fever, night sweats, and a productive cough. He was admitted to the hospital for a workup of possible pulmonary tuberculosis. Mr. Johnson began treatment with rifampin 600 mg P.O. daily. The nurse should warn him that he may experience:
a. discoloration of teeth.
b. increased urine output.
c. red-orange urine.
d. increased sputum production.

2. Because Mr. Johnson's rifampin therapy will continue when he leaves the hospital, the nurse's discharge teaching should instruct him to:
a. report hearing loss immediately.
b. double up on the next dose if a dose is missed.
c. measure urine output daily.
d. take drug on an empty stomach.

3. Mr. Johnson asks how long drug treatment will continue. His nurse should reply that therapy for tuberculosis should usually continue for:
a. 4 to 6 weeks.
b. 4 to 6 months.
c. 6 to 9 weeks.
d. 6 to 9 months.

Check your answers on page 1058.

CHAPTER 10

AMINOGLYCOSIDES

━━━━━━━

amikacin sulfate ◆ gentamicin sulfate ◆ kanamycin sulfate
neomycin sulfate ◆ netilmicin sulfate ◆ streptomycin sulfate
tobramycin sulfate

───────

OVERVIEW

- Aminoglycosides are broad-spectrum antibiotics that act against both gram-positive and gram-negative bacteria as well as some strains of mycobacteria. Because of the risk of serious nephrotoxicity and ototoxicity (auditory and vestibular effects), their systemic use is generally reserved for infections caused by gram-negative organisms resistant to less toxic agents.

MAJOR USES

- Aminoglycosides combat serious bacterial infections and provide presurgical bacteriostatic and bactericidal action in the intestine.
- All aminoglycosides (except neomycin) may be used alone or in combination with penicillin to treat infections caused by group D streptococcus (enterococcus).
- Amikacin, gentamicin, kanamycin, netilmicin, and tobramycin may be used to treat serious infections caused by susceptible strains of *Escherichia coli, Klebsiella, Proteus, Enterobacter,* and *Pseudomonas aeruginosa.* They may also be used in combination with other antibiotics in serious infections when the organism has not been identified.
- Neomycin may be administered orally as adjunctive treatment in hepatic encephalopathy. It may also be used as an antimicrobial irrigating agent of the urinary tract.
- Neomycin and kanamycin may be used orally to promote bowel sterility before GI surgical procedures.

MECHANISM OF ACTION

- Aminoglycosides act directly on the ribosomes of susceptible organisms. By binding directly to the 30S ribosomal subunit, they inhibit protein synthesis. Generally, they are bactericidal in high concentrations and bacteriostatic in low concentrations.

ABSORPTION, DISTRIBUTION, METABOLISM, AND EXCRETION

Aminoglycosides are not well absorbed from the GI tract; therefore, they must be given parenterally for systemic effect. Given orally, they usually

GLOSSARY

Acid fast: organism that retains carbol-fuchsin stain after being decolorized with 95% ethyl alcohol and 3% hydrochloric acid—a unique characteristic of mycobacteria.

Antibiotic: substance, derived from cultures or semisynthetically produced, that inhibits growth of or kills other organisms, such as parasites.

Bacteria: group of single-cell organisms, usually possessing a rigid cell wall, dividing by binary fission and exhibiting either round, rod-like, or spiral form.

Mycobacteria: slender, gram-positive, acid-fast, rod-shaped microorganisms.

Ototoxicity: a destructive or poisonous effect upon the eighth cranial nerve or the organs of hearing and balance.

Superinfection: condition produced by the sudden overgrowth of resistant bacteria or fungi, which can occur in a patient on antibiotic therapy.

Toxicity: quality of being poisonous.

Trough levels: the lowest serum therapeutic concentration of a drug.

produce only a local effect (bowel sterilization). However, under certain conditions, substantial oral absorption may occur and lead to toxicity.

They are distributed uniformly to most body fluids and tissues; penetration into CSF, however, is inadequate. Since aminoglycosides accumulate in the kidneys, nephrotoxicity is possible. All aminoglycosides are rapidly excreted, mostly unchanged, in the urine by normal kidneys.

ONSET AND DURATION

Aminoglycoside blood levels peak within 30 minutes after I.V. infusion and within 60 minutes after I.M. injection. The half-life of all aminoglycosides is 2 to 4 hours but is significantly prolonged in patients with impaired renal function.

ADVERSE REACTIONS

Ototoxicity and nephrotoxicity are the most serious complications of aminoglycoside therapy. Ototoxicity involves both vestibular and auditory functions and usually is related to persistently high serum drug levels. Elderly patients and those with preexisting auditory loss are most susceptible, as are patients taking other potentially ototoxic drugs. In addition, tobramycin, gentamicin, and streptomycin primarily affect vestibular function; amikacin, kanamycin, netilmicin, and neomycin are primarily audiotoxic. Damage is reversible only if detected early and if drug is discontinued promptly.

Aminoglycosides may cause usually reversible nephrotoxicity. In order of increasing potential for nephrotoxicity, the drugs are streptomycin, tobramycin, kanamycin, amikacin, gentamicin, netilmicin, and neomycin.

The incidence of reported reactions ranges from 2% to 10%. The damage results in tubular necrosis. Mild proteinuria and granular cylindruria are early signs of declining renal function; elevated serum creatinine levels follow several days after the decline has begun. Nephrotoxicity usually begins on the fourth to seventh day of therapy and appears to be dose-related. At maximum risk are elderly patients, patients with hypovolemia or preexisting renal dysfunction, and those requiring extended therapy.

Neuromuscular blockade results in skeletal weakness and respiratory distress similar to that seen with the use of neuromuscular blocking agents, such as tubocurarine and succinylcholine. It is most likely to occur in patients receiving these blocking agents; in patients with preexisting neuromuscular disease such as myasthenia gravis; in those receiving general anesthetics; and in those with hypocalcemia.

Oral aminoglycoside therapy most often causes nausea, vomiting, and diarrhea. Less common adverse reactions include hypersensitivity effects (ranging from mild rashes, fever, and eosinophilia to fatal anaphylaxis); hematologic reactions include hemolytic anemia, transient neutropenia, leukopenia, and thrombocytopenia. Transient elevations of liver function values also occur.

Parenterally administered forms of aminoglycosides may cause local reactions: vein irritation, phlebitis, and sterile abscess.

PROTOTYPE: AMINOGLYCOSIDES

GENTAMICIN SULFATE
(jen ta mye' sin)
Cidomycin†‡, Garamycin, Gentafair, Jenamicin
Classification: aminoglycoside
Pregnancy risk category C

How supplied
INJECTION: 40 mg/ml (adult), 10 mg/ml (pediatric), 2 mg/ml (preservative-free for intrathecal use)

Indications and dosage
Serious infections caused by sensitive strains of Pseudomonas aeruginosa, Escherichia coli, Proteus, Klebsiella, Serratia, Enterobacter, Citrobacter, Staphylococcus
ADULTS WITH NORMAL RENAL FUNCTION: 3 mg/kg daily I.M. or I.V. infusion (in 50 to 200 ml of 0.9% sodium chloride solution or dextrose 5% in water infused over 30 minutes to 2 hours) in divided doses q 8 hours. May be given by direct I.V. push if necessary. For life-threatening infections, patient may receive up to 5 mg/kg daily in three or four divided doses.
CHILDREN WITH NORMAL RENAL FUNCTION: 2 to 2.5 mg/kg I.M. or I.V. infusion q 8 hours.
INFANTS AND NEONATES OVER AGE 1 WEEK WITH NORMAL RENAL FUNCTION: 2.5 mg/kg I.M. or I.V. infusion q 8 hours.

NEONATES UNDER AGE 1 WEEK: 2.5 mg/kg I.V. q 12 hours. For I.V. infusion, dilute in 0.9% sodium chloride solution or dextrose 5% in water and infuse over 30 minutes to 2 hours.

Meningitis
ADULTS: systemic therapy as above; may also use 4 to 8 mg intrathecally daily.
CHILDREN: systemic therapy as above; may also use 1 to 2 mg intrathecally daily.

Endocarditis prophylaxis for GI or GU procedure or surgery
ADULTS: 1.5 mg/kg I.M. or I.V. 30 to 60 minutes before procedure or surgery and q 8 hours after, for two doses. Given with aqueous penicillin G or ampicillin.
CHILDREN: 2.5 mg/kg I.M. or I.V. 30 to 60 minutes before procedure or surgery and q 8 hours after, for two doses. Given with aqueous penicillin G or ampicillin.
PATIENTS WITH IMPAIRED RENAL FUNCTION: initial dose is same as for those with normal renal function. Subsequent doses and frequency determined by renal function studies and serum concentrations of gentamicin.

Posthemodialysis to maintain therapeutic blood levels
ADULTS: 1 to 1.7 mg/kg I.M. or I.V. infusion after each dialysis.
CHILDREN: 2 mg/kg I.M. or I.V. infusion after each dialysis.

Contraindications and precautions
Gentamicin is contraindicated in patients with known hypersensitivity to the drug or other aminoglycosides. Safety for use in pregnancy has not been established. Use cautiously in patients with neuromuscular disorders, such as myasthenia gravis, and in elderly patients, neonates, infants, and those with impaired renal function.

Adverse reactions
CNS: headache, lethargy, neuromuscular blockade.
EENT: *ototoxicity* (tinnitus, vertigo, hearing loss).
GU: *nephrotoxicity* (cells or casts in the urine; oliguria; proteinuria; decreased creatinine clearance levels; increased BUN, nonprotein nitrogen, and serum creatinine levels).
OTHER: **hypersensitivity reactions, hepatic necrosis.**

Interactions
Cephalothin: increases nephrotoxicity. Use together cautiously.
Dimenhydrinate: may mask symptoms of ototoxicity. Use with caution.
General anesthetics, neuromuscular blocking agents: may potentiate neuromuscular blockade. Monitor patients closely.
I.V. loop diuretics (for example, furosemide): increase ototoxicity. Use together cautiously.
Other aminoglycosides, methoxyflurane, amphotericin B: increase ototoxicity and nephrotoxicity. Use together cautiously.
Parenteral penicillins (for example, carbenicillin and ticarcillin): gentamicin inactivation in vitro. Don't mix together in the same I.V. solution.

Nursing considerations
Assessment
• Review the patient's history for a condition that contraindicates the use of gentamicin.
• Obtain a baseline assessment of the patient's infection before therapy.
• Be alert for common adverse reactions.
• Evaluate the patient's and family's knowledge about gentamicin therapy.

Planning (Nursing Diagnoses)
Potential nursing diagnoses for patient receiving gentamicin include:
• Potential for injury related to dosage regimen inadequate to alleviate infection.
• Sensory/perceptual alterations (auditory) related to ototoxicity induced by gentamicin.
• Knowledge deficit related to gentamicin therapy.

Implementation
Preparation and administration
— Obtain specimen for culture and sensitivity tests before first dose. Therapy may begin pending test results.
— Weigh the patient and obtain baseline renal function studies before therapy begins.
— Ensure that the patient is well hydrated before therapy (unless contra-indicated) to decrease the risk of nephrotoxicity.
— Always consult manufacturer's directions for reconstitution, dilution, and storage. Check expiration dates.
— Administer I.M. dose deep into large muscle mass (gluteal or midlateral thigh); rotate injection sites to minimize tissue injury; do not inject more than 2 g of drug per injection site. Apply ice to injection site for pain.
— Refrigerate prepared I.V. aminoglycoside solution until use; infuse the drug over at least 30 minutes.
— Too-rapid I.V. administration may cause neuromuscular blockade. Infuse I.V. drug continuously or intermittently over 30 to 60 minutes for adults; 1 to 2 hours, for infants.
— Solutions should always be clear, colorless to pale yellow (in most cases, darkening indicates deterioration), and free of particles; do not give solutions containing precipitates or other foreign matter.
— Adequate dilution of I.V. solution and rotation of injection site every 48 hours help minimize local irritation; assess I.V. site frequently for infiltration or phlebitis. At end of infusion, flush line with 0.9% sodium chloride solution in water or dextrose 5% solution.
— Do not administer through heparinized I.V. line. If administering intermittent dose through heparin lock, flush with 0.9% sodium chloride solution before and after infusing gentamicin to provide a barrier between the gentamicin and the heparin used to keep the lock patent.
— Do not mix gentamicin in the same solution with extended-spectrum penicillins; drug may be inactivated.

— Administer gentamicin and an extended-spectrum penicillin or cephalosporin at least 2 hours apart to prevent a decrease in the drug level and half-life in a patient with normal renal function.

— Expect to adjust the dosage as prescribed when administering gentamicin to an elderly patient or one with renal impairment or receiving hemodialysis.

— Hemodialysis (8 hours) removes up to 50% of drug from blood. Do not administer before dialysis treatment.

— After loading dose, all further doses should be based on renal studies and serum levels of the drug. Draw blood for peak gentamicin level 1 hour after I.M. injection and 30 minutes to 1 hour after infusion ends; for trough levels, draw blood just before next dose. Do not collect blood in a heparinized tube because heparin is incompatible with aminoglycosides. Acceptable peak levels are 4 to 12 mcg/dl. Peak blood levels above 12 mcg/dl and trough levels above 2 mcg/dl may be associated with higher incidence of toxicity.

— Intrathecal form (without preservatives) should be used when intrathecal administration is indicated.

Monitoring

— Monitor the effectiveness of therapy by regularly assessing for improvement of infectious process.

— Monitor the patient for adverse drug reactions.

— Monitor renal function, including serum creatinine and BUN levels.

— Monitor intake and output, weight, urinalysis, and specific gravity.

— Monitor the patient's hearing and for signs of vestibular toxicity (dizziness, vertigo, nystagmus).

— Monitor for signs and symptoms of superinfection or new infection, especially of upper respiratory tract; oral candidiasis; vaginal discharge; or other signs of fungal overgrowth.

— Monitor respiratory rate and heart rate and rhythm, especially postoperatively, for signs of neuromuscular blockade.

— Monitor serum gentamicin level.

— Monitor the patient for drug interactions.

— Regularly reevaluate the patient's and family's knowledge about gentamicin therapy.

Intervention

— Notify the doctor of increased serum creatinine or BUN levels. Also report decreased intake and output, increased weight gain, increased casts in urine, and decreased specific gravity.

— Encourage the patient to maintain fluid intake of at least 2,000 ml/day (unless contraindicated).

— If ototoxicity is suspected, notify the doctor and prepare the patient for audiometric testing. Expect to discontinue gentamicin and initiate another type of antibiotic therapy. If the patient has signs of vestibular toxicity (dizziness), take safety precautions, such as supervising ambulation.

—Notify the doctor if patient's serum gentamicin peak or trough levels do not fall within the recommended range.

—Usual duration of therapy is 7 to 10 days. If no response in 3 to 5 days, therapy may be stopped and new specimens obtained for culture and sensitivity.

—After drawing blood specimen for determining serum gentamicin level, immediately place the blood sample on ice and transport it to the laboratory to prevent false changes of the gentamicin level.

—Keep all health care team members advised of the patient's response to the drug.

Patient teaching

—Instruct the patient and family about gentamicin, including the dosage, frequency, action, and adverse reactions.

—Instruct the patient to notify the doctor immediately if hearing changes occur.

—Instruct the patient to notify the doctor if other adverse reactions occur, if the infection does not improve, or if it worsens.

—Stress the importance of having blood tests done as instructed to monitor gentamicin level and renal function to determine the effectiveness of therapy or detect any increased risk of adverse drug reactions.

—Instruct the female patient to alert the doctor if pregnancy is suspected or confirmed during therapy.

—Emphasize the need to drink 1,500 to 2,000 ml of fluid each day, *not including* coffee, tea, or other caffeinated beverages.

—Tell the patient to notify the nurse or doctor if adverse reactions develop or questions arise about gentamicin therapy.

Evaluation

In the patient receiving gentamicin, appropriate evaluation statements include:

• Patient's serum gentamicin level remains in recommended dosage range.
• Patient is free of infection.
• Patient maintains normal auditory function.
• Patient and family state an understanding of gentamicin therapy.

SELECTED MAJOR DRUGS: AMINOGLYCOSIDES

DRUG, INDICATIONS, AND DOSAGES

SPECIAL PRECAUTIONS

amikacin (Amikin)
Serious infections caused by sensitive Pseudomonas aeruginosa, Escherichia coli, Proteus, Klebsiella, Serratia, Enterobacter, Acinetobacter, Providencia, Citrobacter, Staphylococcus —
Adults and children with normal renal function: 15 mg/ kg daily in divided doses q 8 to 12 hours by I.M. or I.V. infusion (in 100 to 200 ml dextrose 5% in water run in over 30 to 60 minutes). May be given by direct I.V. push if necessary.
Neonates with normal renal function: initially, 10 mg/ kg I.M. or I.V. infusion (in dextrose 5% in water run in over 1 to 2 hours), then 7.5 mg/kg I.M. or I.V. infusion q 12 hours.
Meningitis —
Adults: systemic therapy as above; may also use up to 20 mg intrathecally or intraventricularly daily.
Children: systemic therapy as above; may also use 1 to 2 mg intrathecally daily.
Uncomplicated urinary tract infections —
Adults: 250 mg I.M. or I.V. b.i.d.
Adults with impaired renal function: initially, 7.5 mg/ kg. Subsequent doses and frequency determined by blood amikacin levels and renal function studies.

• Contraindicated in patients with known hypersensitivity to amikacin; a history of hypersensitivity or serious toxic reactions to aminoglycosides may contraindicate the use of any other aminoglycosides because of the known cross-sensitivities of patients to drugs in this class.
• Use cautiously in elderly patients, in those with impaired renal function, and in neonates and infants.

kanamycin (Kantrex)
Serious infections caused by sensitive strains of Escherichia coli, Proteus, Enterobacter aerogenes, Klebsiella pneumoniae, Serratia marcescens, Acinetobacter —
Adults and children with normal renal function: 15 mg/ kg daily divided q 8 to 12 hours deep I.M. into upper outer quadrant of buttocks or I.V. infusion (diluted 500 mg/200 ml of 0.9% sodium chloride solution or dextrose 5% in water infused at 60 to 80 drops/minute). Maximum daily dosage is 1.5 g.
Neonates: 15 mg/kg I.M. or I.V. daily in divided doses q 12 hours.
Adjunctive treatment in hepatic coma —
Adults: 8 to 12 g P.O. daily in divided doses.
Preoperative bowel sterilization —
Adults: 1 g P.O. q 1 hour for four doses, then q 4 hours for four doses; or 1 g P.O. q 1 hour for four doses, then q 6 hours for 36 to 72 hours.
Intraperitoneal irrigation —
Adults: 500 mg in 20 ml sterile distilled water instilled via catheter into wound after patient is fully recovered from anesthesia and neuromuscular blocker effects.
Wound irrigation —
Adults: Up to 2.5 mg/ml in 0.9% sodium chloride solution irrigant.

• Oral use contraindicated in intestinal obstruction and treatment of systemic infection.
• Use cautiously in patients with impaired renal function and in elderly patients.

SELECTED MAJOR DRUGS: AMINOGLYCOSIDES *continued*

DRUG, INDICATIONS, AND DOSAGES	SPECIAL PRECAUTIONS

neomycin (Mycifradin, Neosulf‡)
Infectious diarrhea caused by enteropathogenic Escherichia coli —
Adults: 50 mg/kg P.O. daily in four divided doses for 2 to 3 days.
Children: 50 to 100 mg/kg P.O. daily in divided doses q 4 to 6 hours for 2 to 3 days.
Suppression of intestinal bacteria preoperatively —
Adults: 1 g P.O. q 1 hour for four doses, then 1 g q 4 hours for the balance of the 24 hours. A saline cathartic should precede therapy.
Children: 40 to 100 mg/kg P.O. daily in divided doses q 4 to 6 hours. First dose should be preceded by saline cathartic.
Adjunctive treatment in hepatic coma —
Adults: 1 to 3 g P.O. q.i.d. for 5 to 6 days; or 200 ml of 1% or 100 ml of 2% solution as enema retained for 20 to 60 minutes q 6 hours.

• Contraindicated in patients with intestinal obstruction.
• Use cautiously in patients with impaired renal function and ulcerative bowel lesions and in elderly patients.

netilmicin (Netromycin)
Serious infections caused by sensitive Pseudomonas aeruginosa, Escherichia coli, Proteus, Klebsiella, Serratia, Enterobacter, Citrobacter, Staphylococcus —
Adults and children over age 12: 3 to 6.5 mg/kg by I.M. injection or I.V. infusion daily. May be given q 12 hours to treat serious urinary tract infections and q 8 to 12 hours to treat serious systemic infections.
Infants and children ages 6 weeks to 12 years: 5.5 to 8 mg/kg by I.M. injection or I.V. infusion daily, given either as 1.8 to 2.7 mg/kg q 8 hours or as 2.7 to 4 mg/kg q 12 hours.
Neonates under age 6 weeks: 4 to 6.5 mg/kg by I.M. injection or I.V. infusion daily, given as 2 to 3 to 3.25 mg/kg q 12 hours.
Patients with impaired renal function: initial dose is the same as for patients with normal renal function. Subsequent doses and frequency are determined by renal function studies and serum concentration of netilmicin.

• Contraindicated in patients with known hypersensitivity to netilmicin or to any of the ingredients of the preparation.
• Use cautiously in patients with impaired renal function and in neonates, infants, and elderly patients.

streptomycin
Streptococcal endocarditis —
Adults: 10 mg/kg I.M. (maximum 0.5 g) q 12 hours for 2 weeks with penicillin.
Primary and adjunctive treatment in tuberculosis —
Adults: with normal renal function, 1 g I.M. daily for 2 to 3 months, then 1 g 2 or 3 times weekly. Inject deeply into upper outer quadrant of buttocks.
Children: with normal renal function, 20 mg/kg I.M. daily in divided doses injected deeply into large muscle mass. Give concurrently with other antituberculars, but *not* with capreomycin, and continue until sputum specimen becomes negative.

• Contraindicated in patients with labyrinthine disease.
• Use cautiously in patients with impaired renal function and in the elderly.

(continued)

‡Available in Australia only

SELECTED MAJOR DRUGS: AMINOGLYCOSIDES *continued*

DRUG, INDICATIONS, AND DOSAGES	SPECIAL PRECAUTIONS

streptomycin *(continued)*
Patients with impaired renal function: initial dose is same as for those with normal renal function. Subsequent doses and frequency determined by renal function study results.
Enterococcal endocarditis—
Adults: 1 g I.M. q 12 hours for 2 weeks, then 500 mg I.M. q 12 hours for 4 weeks with penicillin.
Tularemia—
Adults: 1 to 2 g I.M. daily in divided doses injected deep into upper outer quadrant of buttocks. Continue until patient is afebrile for 5 to 7 days.

tobramycin (Nebcin)
Serious infections caused by sensitive strains of Escherichia coli, Proteus, Klebsiella, Enterobacter, Serratia, Staphylococcus aureus, Pseudomonas, Citrobacter, Providencia—
Adults and children with normal renal function: 3 mg/kg I.M. or I.V. daily divided q 8 hours. Up to 5 mg/kg I.M. or I.V. daily in divided doses q 6 to 8 hours for life-threatening infections.
Neonates under age 1 week: up to 4 mg/kg I.M. or I.V. daily in divided doses q 12 hours. For I.V. use, dilute in 50 to 100 ml 0.9% sodium chloride solution or dextrose 5% in water for adults and in less volume for children. Infuse over 20 to 60 minutes.
Patients with impaired renal function: initial dose is same as for those with normal renal function. Subsequent doses and frequency determined by renal function study results and serum concentrations of tobramycin.

• Contraindicated in patients with known hypersensitivity to any aminoglycosides or serious toxic reactions to aminoglycosides because of known cross-sensitivities of patients to drugs in this class.
• Use cautiously in patients with impaired renal function and in elderly patients.

AMINOGLYCOSIDE COMBINATION

TRADE NAME AND CONTENT	SPECIAL CONSIDERATIONS
Neosporin GU Irrigant neomycin sulfate 40 mg and polymyxin B sulfate 200,000 units/ml	• Combines the effectiveness of neomycin sulfate, which is bactericidal against a wide range of gram-negative organisms (including *Proteus vulgaris*), and some gram-positive organisms with polymyxin B sulfate, which is effective against most gram-negative bacilli, including *Pseudomonas* infections. • Safety and effectiveness in patients with recent GU surgery have not been established. • Recommended maximum course of therapy is 10 days. • Although the risk of systemic absorption of the drug is small, monitor for nephrotoxicity and ototoxicity.

SELF-TEST

1. Stephanie Lynette, age 27, is admitted to the hospital with an infected prosthetic heart valve. She receives a loading dose of gentamicin 180 mg and then will continue treatment with gentamicin 80 mg I.V. q 8 hours. Which laboratory values should be monitored in this patient to assess for a predictable adverse reaction?
   a. CBC
   b. AST
   c. serum creatinine
   d. serum electrolytes

2. Besides monitoring for this adverse reaction, the nurse can help to prevent it by:
   a. changing the drug therapy to a less toxic drug.
   b. encouraging the patient to drink at least 2,000 ml of fluid daily.
   c. weighing the patient and monitoring blood pressure.
   d. having the patient sit on the side of the bed for a brief time before standing to walk.

3. Peak and trough levels of gentamicin are drawn around the third dose. Which of the following results indicate a therapeutic (peak) level of this drug?

a. 30 minutes after completing the infusion, the serum level is 8 mcg/dl

b. immediately before administration of the drug, the serum level is 4 mcg/dl

c. 60 minutes after completing the infusion, the serum level is 12 mcg/dl

d. immediately before administration of the drug, the serum level is 6 mcg/dl

Check your answers on page 1058.

CHAPTER 11

PENICILLINS

Natural penicillins
penicillin G benzathine ✦ penicillin G potassium ✦ penicillin G procaine
penicillin G sodium ✦ penicillin V ✦ penicillin V potassium

Penicillinase-resistant penicillins
cloxacillin sodium ✦ dicloxacillin sodium ✦ methicillin sodium
nafcillin sodium ✦ oxacillin sodium

Aminopenicillins
amoxicillin ✦ ampiciliin ✦ bacampicillin

Extended-spectrum penicillins
azlocillin sodium ✦ carbenicillin disodium ✦ carbenicillin indanyl sodium
mezlocillin sodium ✦ piperacillin sodium ✦ ticarcillin disodium

OVERVIEW

- More than 50 years after their discovery, penicillins remain the most popular class of antibiotic in clinical use. Chemical modifications of the original penicillin molecule have enhanced its activity against most gram-positive organisms.
- The penicillins are classified into four groups: natural penicillins, penicillinase-resistant penicillins, aminopenicillins, and extended-spectrum penicillins.

MAJOR USES

- Penicillins are highly effective against infections attributable to gram-positive cocci, such as *Streptococcus pneumoniae* and non-penicillinase-producing staphylococci; they are also effective against some gram-negative cocci, such as *Neisseria meningitidis* and *N. gonorrhoeae.* Penicillins are effective in varying degrees against *Bacillus anthracis, Bacteroides* species, *Clostridium perfringens, Treponema pallidum, Actinomyces,* and *Corynebacterium diphtheriae.* Penicillins are not effective against viruses, mycobacteria, yeasts, plasmodia, fungi, or rickettsiae.
- Amoxicillin and ampicillin are also active against strains of *Escherichia coli, Haemophilus influenzae, Proteus mirabilis,* and *Salmonella* and *Shigella* species.
- Azlocillin, carbenicillin, piperacillin, and ticarcillin have a broader activity than other penicillins against strains of *E. coli, Proteus* species, and *Pseudomonas aeruginosa.*

GLOSSARY

Anaphylaxis: life-threatening reaction of a person to a foreign protein or other substance.
Coccus: a spherical bacterial cell, usually slightly less than 1 micron in diameter.

- Cloxacillin, dicloxacillin, methicillin, nafcillin, and oxacillin are resistant to penicillinase and thus are extremely useful in the treatment of infections due to *Staphylococcus aureus*. They may be used prophylactically before orthopedic and cardiac surgery.

MECHANISM OF ACTION

- Penicillins are thought to be bactericidal against microorganisms by inhibiting cell wall synthesis during active multiplication. They are more effective against young, rapidly dividing organisms than against mature resting cells that are not in the process of cell-wall formation.
- Bacteria resist penicillin by producing penicillinases—enzymes that convert penicillin to inactive penicilloic acid. The penicillinase-resistant penicillins (cloxacillin, dicloxacillin, methicillin, nafcillin, and oxacillin) resist these enzymes.

ABSORPTION, DISTRIBUTION, METABOLISM, AND EXCRETION

Oral absorption occurs primarily in the duodenum; a small percentage of penicillin is absorbed in the stomach. Penicillins are widely distributed in body fluids and in such tissues as kidneys, liver, lungs, heart, spleen, skin, and intestine. Adequate penetration into CSF and the brain occurs only with meningeal inflammation.

Penicillins (except nafcillin) are excreted mostly unchanged in urine (nafcillin is extensively metabolized in the liver). Excretion is delayed in infants, elderly patients, and patients with impaired renal function.

Amoxicillin and bacampicillin are well absorbed orally and may be given with meals.

Ampicillin, cloxacillin, dicloxacillin, nafcillin, oxacillin, penicillin G, and penicillin V are all acid-labile, that is, broken down by gastric and duodenal acid. Therefore, they are best taken on an empty stomach 30 to 60 minutes before or 2 hours after meals. Parenteral administration results in higher but more transient blood levels.

Azlocillin, carbenicillin disodium, methicillin, mezlocillin, piperacillin, and ticarcillin are very poorly absorbed orally and should be reserved for parenteral use. Carbenicillin indanyl sodium is used to treat urinary tract infections.

Penicillin G benzathine is slowly absorbed from I.M. injection sites, and therapeutic levels for certain organisms (pneumococcus, *T. pallidum*) may be observed as long as 30 days after a dose.

Penicillin G procaine is more rapidly absorbed than penicillin G benzathine, but therapeutic levels may be observed as long as 24 hours after administration.

Carbenicillin indanyl sodium given orally reaches therapeutic levels only in the urine; therefore, it cannot be used for systemic infections.

ONSET AND DURATION

Peak blood levels for oral penicillins is usually reached within 1 to 2 hours. Because the half-lives of all penicillins are very short (30 to 60 minutes), frequent doses are necessary. Amoxicillin and bacampicillin, however, can be administered less frequently than the others.

After parenteral administration, ampicillin, azlocillin, carbenicillin, methicillin, mezlocillin, nafcillin, oxacillin, penicillin G, and piperacillin rapidly reach peak blood levels (immediately with I.V. infusion). The more insoluble procaine and benzathine salts of penicillin G are slowly absorbed from I.M. injections sites.

Duration of action is generally 3 to 6 hours in patients with normal renal function. In patients with impaired renal function, the drug may remain in the blood as long as 24 hours after administration.

ADVERSE REACTIONS

Penicillins, one of the most commonly used classes of antibiotics, exhibit some significant adverse effects. However, most patients receiving penicillins are relatively free of adverse reactions.

Hypersensitivity reactions can occur in 1% to 10% of patients receiving penicillins, with somewhat higher risk in patients with a history of other allergies. Allergic reactions include bronchospasm, laryngospasm, wheezing, urticaria, angioneurotic edema, and possibly vascular collapse and death. Myocarditis can also occur; it is not dose-related and can occur any time during therapy.

A maculopapular rash that is not due to penicillin allergy can occur with ampicillin (9%) and is more common in patients with concurrent viral illnesses (for example, virtually everyone with mononucleosis develops this rash after ampicillin therapy).

GI reactions are more common after oral use of penicillins but can occur with other administration routes. They can include sore mouth or tongue, furry tongue, nausea, vomiting, cramping, and mild diarrhea or more severe reactions, such as pseudomembranous colitis. Mild elevations of liver enzymes have been reported with semisynthetic penicillins (oxacillin and piperacillin) but rarely require discontinuation of the drug.

Interstitial nephritis has been reported with all penicillins but seems to occur most frequently with methicillin. If oliguria, proteinuria, and hematuria occur, the drug should be discontinued.

Higher dosage of penicillins, especially in patients with renal disease, have been associated with signs of CNS toxicity: lethargy, irritability, hallucinations, and seizures.

Electrolyte abnormalities can occur with high dosages of either sodium or potassium salts of penicillins. High dosages of the sodium salts can cause worsening of CHF; potassium salts can cause cardiac arrhythmias.

Various hematologic effects have been associated with penicillins: bone marrow depression, hemolysis, selected depression of blood cells (leukopenia, thrombocytopenia, anemia), eosinophilia, and prolongation of bleeding and prothrombin time. These reactions are reversible after discontinuation of the drug.

PROTOTYPE: NATURAL PENICILLINS

PENICILLIN G SODIUM (BENZYLPENICILLIN SODIUM)
(pen i sill′ in G)
Crystapen†
Classification: natural penicillin
Pregnancy risk category B

How supplied
INJECTION: 5 million units

Indications and dosage
Moderate to severe systemic infections
ADULTS: 1.2 to 24 million units I.M. or I.V. daily, divided into doses given q 4 hours.
CHILDREN: 25,000 to 300,000 units/kg I.M. or I.V. daily, divided into doses given q 4 hours.

Endocarditis prophylaxis for dental surgery
ADULTS: 2 million units I.V. or I.M. 30 minutes to 1 hour before procedure, then 1 million units 6 hours later.

Contraindications and precautions
Penicillin G sodium is contraindicated in patients with known hypersensitivity to any other penicillin or to cephalosporins.
Use cautiously in patients with renal impairment because it is excreted in urine: decreased dosage is required in patients with moderate to severe renal failure. Also use cautiously in patients with sodium restriction.

Adverse reactions
BLOOD: **hemolytic anemia**, leukopenia, thrombocytopenia.
CNS: neuropathy, **seizures**.
CV: **CHF** with high doses.
LOCAL: vein irritation, pain at injection site, thrombophlebitis.
OTHER: arthralgia, hypersensitivity (chills, fever, edema, maculopapular rash, **exfoliative dermatitis**, urticaria, **anaphylaxis**), overgrowth of non-susceptible organisms.

Interactions
Probenecid: increases blood levels of penicillin. Probenecid may be used for this purpose.

Boldfaced adverse reactions are life-threatening

Nursing considerations
Assessment
• Review the patient's history for a condition that contraindicates the use of penicillin G sodium.
• Obtain a baseline assessment of the patient's infection before therapy.
• Be alert for common adverse reactions.
• Evaluate the patient's and family's knowledge about penicillin G sodium therapy.

Planning (Nursing Diagnoses)
Potential nursing diagnoses for the patient receiving penicillin G sodium include:
• Potential for injury related to dosage regimen inadequate to alleviate infection.
• Impaired tissue integrity related to thrombophlebitis caused by I.V. administration.
• Knowledge deficit related to penicillin G sodium therapy.

Implementation
Preparation and administration
— Obtain specimen for culture and sensitivity tests before first dose. Therapy may begin pending test results.
— Before giving penicillin, ask the patient about previous allergic reactions to this drug. However, a negative history of penicillin allergy is no guarantee against a future allergic reaction.
— Administer I.M. dose deep into large muscle mass (gluteal or midlateral thigh); rotate injection sites to minimize tissue injury; do not inject more than 2 g of drug per injection site. Apply ice to injection site for pain.
— Do not add or mix other drugs with I.V. infusions—particularly aminoglycosides, which will be inactivated if mixed with penicillins; they are chemically and physically incompatible. If other drugs must be given I.V., temporarily stop infusion of primary drug.
— Infuse I.V. drug continuously or intermittently (over 30 minutes); intermittent I.V. infusion may be diluted in 50 to 100 ml sterile water, 0.9% sodium chloride solution, dextrose 5% in water, dextrose 5% in water and 0.45% sodium chloride solution, or lactated Ringer's solution.
— Solutions should always be clear, colorless to pale yellow, and free of particles; do not give solutions containing precipitates or other foreign matter.
— Give penicillin G sodium at least 1 hour before bacteriostatic antibiotics.
— Expect to alter dosage regimen of penicillin G sodium for a patient with reduced renal function. Because penicillins are dialyzable, patients undergoing hemodialysis may need dosage adjustments.

Monitoring

—Monitor the effectiveness of therapy by regularly assessing for improvement of infectious process.
—Monitor the patient for adverse drug reactions. Allergic reactions are the major adverse reactions to penicillin, especially with large doses, parenteral administration, or prolonged therapy. Keep in mind that the patient may become sensitized to penicillin through exposure.
—With large doses and prolonged therapy, bacterial or fungal superinfections may occur, especially in elderly, debilitated, or immunosuppressed patients. Close observation is essential.
—Monitor for decreased level of consciousness or seizures in a patient with decreased renal function who is receiving more than 20 million units of penicillin G sodium daily.
—Routinely monitor I.V. site.
—Monitor the patient for drug interactions.
—Monitor diagnostic test results: penicillin G sodium alters test results for urine and serum protein levels; it interferes with turbidimetric methods using sulfosalicylic acid, trichloracetic acid, acetic acid, and nitric acid. Penicillin G sodium alters urine glucose testing using copper sulfate; use reagent strip instead. Penicillin G sodium may cause falsely elevated results of urine specific gravity tests in patients with low urine output and dehydration and falsely elevated Norymberski and Zimmerman test results for 17-ketogenic steroids; it causes false-positive CSF protein test results and may cause positive Coombs' test results. Penicillin G sodium may falsely decrease serum aminoglycoside concentrations.
—Monitor for signs of renal failure or interstitial nephritis, such as fever, eosinophilia, hematuria, proteinuria, or pyuria, which usually occur 5 to 10 days after therapy begins in a patient receiving large parenteral doses of penicillin G sodium.
—Monitor for signs of hemolytic anemia, such as a positive Coombs' test. This reaction is most common when the patient is receiving high doses of I.V. penicillin G sodium (in excess of 10 million units/day in a uremic patient or 40 million units/day in a patient with normal renal function).
—Regularly reevaluate the patient's and family's knowledge about penicillin G sodium.

Intervention

—Discontinue the drug at once if the patient develops anaphylactic shock (exhibited by rapidly developing dyspnea and hypotension). Notify the doctor and prepare to administer immediate treatment, such as epinephrine, corticosteroids, antihistamines, and other resuscitative measures as indicated.
—The patient with a high blood level of this drug may have seizures. Institute seizure precautions.
—Change I.V. site every 48 hours.
—If the patient develops an adverse reaction, notify the doctor for appropriate treatment and provide supportive care as appropriate.

— Keep all health care team members advised of the patient's response to the drug.

Patient teaching

— Instruct the patient and family about penicillin G sodium, including the dosage, frequency, action, and adverse reactions.
— Explain disease process and rationale for therapy.
— Advise the patient who is allergic to penicillins to wear medical alert identification stating this information.
— Tell the patient to notify the nurse or doctor if adverse reactions develop or questions arise about penicillin G sodium therapy.

Evaluation

In the patient receiving penicillin G sodium, appropriate evaluation statements include:

• Patient is free of infection.
• Patient maintains good tissue integrity and exhibits no signs of thrombophlebitis.
• Patient and family state an understanding of penicillin G sodium therapy.

PROTOTYPE: PENICILLINASE-RESISTANT PENICILLINS

OXACILLIN SODIUM

(ox a sill' in)

Bactocill, Prostaphlin

Classification: penicillinase-resistant penicillin

Pregnancy risk category B

How supplied

CAPSULES: 250 mg, 500 mg
ORAL SOLUTION: 250 mg/5 ml (after reconstitution)
INJECTION: 250 mg, 500 mg, 1 g, 2 g, 4 g, 10 g
I.V. INFUSION: 1 g, 2 g, 4 g
PHARMACY BULK PACKAGE: 4 g, 10 g

Indications and dosage

Systemic infections caused by penicillinase-producing staphylococci

ADULTS: 2 to 4 g P.O. daily, divided into doses given q 6 hours; 2 to 12 g I.M. or I.V. daily, divided into doses given q 4 to 6 hours.
CHILDREN: 50 to 100 mg/kg P.O. daily, divided into doses given q 6 hours; 100 to 200 mg/kg I.M. or I.V. daily, divided into doses given q 4 to 6 hours.

Contraindications and precautions

Oxacillin is contraindicated in patients with known hypersensitivity to any other penicillin or to cephalosporins.

Adverse reactions

BLOOD: granulocytopenia, thrombocytopenia, eosinophilia, **hemolytic anemia,** transient neutropenia.

CNS: neuropathy, neuromuscular irritability, **seizures.**

GI: oral lesions.

GU: interstitial nephritis, transient hematuria, proteinuria.

HEPATIC: hepatitis, elevated enzymes.

LOCAL: thrombophlebitis.

OTHER: hypersensitivity (fever, chills, rash, urticaria, **anaphylaxis**), overgrowth of nonsusceptible organisms.

Interactions

Probenecid: increases blood levels of oxacillin and other penicillins. Probenecid may be used for this purpose.

Nursing considerations

Assessment

• Review the patient's history for a condition that contraindicates the use of oxacillin.

• Obtain a baseline assessment of the patient's infection before therapy.

• Be alert for common adverse reactions.

• Evaluate the patient's and family's knowledge about oxacillin therapy.

Planning (Nursing Diagnoses)

Potential nursing diagnoses for the patient receiving oxacillin include:

• Potential for injury related to ineffective drug dosage.

• Altered protection related to development of superinfection.

• Knowledge deficit related to oxacillin therapy.

Implementation

Preparation and administration

— Obtain specimen for culture and sensitivity tests before first dose. Therapy may begin pending test results.

— Before giving oxacillin, ask the patient about previous allergic reactions to penicillin. However, a negative history of penicillin allergy is no guarantee against a future allergic reaction.

— When given orally, drug may cause GI disturbances. Food may interfere with absorption, so give 1 to 2 hours before meals or 2 to 3 hours after.

— Give oral drug with water only; acid in fruit juice or carbonated beverage may inactivate drug.

— Give oral dose on empty stomach; food decreases absorption.

— When giving I.V., mix with dextrose 5% in water or 0.9% sodium chloride solution.

— Give I.V. intermittently to prevent vein irritation.

— Give oxacillin at least 1 hour before bacteriostatic antibiotics.

Monitoring

— Monitor the effectiveness of therapy by regularly assessing for improvement of infectious process.

— Monitor the patient for adverse drug reactions. Allergic reactions are the major adverse reactions to penicillin, especially with large doses, parenteral administration, or prolonged therapy. Keep in mind that the patient may become sensitized to penicillin through exposure.

— Monitor the patient for drug interactions.

— Monitor diagnostic test results. Oxacillin alters tests for urine and serum proteins; turbidimetric urine and serum proteins are often falsely positive or elevated in tests using sulfosalicylic acid or trichloroacetic acid. Oxacillin may cause transient reductions in RBC, WBC, and platelet counts. Elevations in liver function tests may indicate drug-induced hepatitis or cholestasis. Abnormal urinalysis results may indicate drug-induced interstitial nephritis. Oxacillin may falsely decrease serum aminoglycoside concentrations.

— Regularly reevaluate the patient's and family's knowledge about oxacillin therapy.

Intervention

— Discontinue the drug at once if the patient develops anaphylactic shock (exhibited by rapidly developing dyspnea and hypotension). Notify the doctor and prepare to administer immediate treatment, such as epinephrine, corticosteroids, antihistamines, and other resuscitative measures, as indicated.

— If giving the drug I.V., change site every 48 hours.

— If the patient develops an adverse reaction, notify the doctor for appropriate treatment and provide supportive care as appropriate.

— Notify the doctor if the patient develops a superinfection and provide supportive care as indicated.

— Keep all health care team members advised of the patient's response to the drug.

Patient teaching

— Instruct the patient and family about oxacillin, including the dosage, frequency, action, and adverse reactions.

— Explain the disease process and rationale for therapy.

— Tell the patient to take medication exactly as prescribed, even if he feels better. The entire quantity prescribed should be taken.

— Tell the patient to call the doctor if rash, fever, or chills develop. A rash is the most common allergic reaction.

— Explain the need to take oral preparations without food and to follow with water only because of acid content of fruit juice and carbonated beverages.

— Tell the patient to take oral penicillin 1 hour before or 2 hours after meals to ensure an optimal serum concentration.

— Advise the patient who is allergic to penicillins to wear medical alert identification stating this information.

— Tell the patient to notify the nurse or doctor if adverse reactions develop or questions arise about oxacillin therapy.

Evaluation
In the patient receiving oxacillin, appropriate evaluation statements include:
• Patient is free of infection.
• Patient exhibits no signs of superinfection.
• Patient and family state an understanding of oxacillin therapy.

PROTOTYPE: AMINOPENICILLINS

AMPICILLIN
(am pi sill' in)
Amcill, Ampicin†, Ampilean†, Apo-Ampi†, Novo Ampicillin†, Omnipen, Penbritin†, Principen

AMPICILLIN SODIUM
Ampicyn Injection‡, Omnipen-N, Polycillin-N, Totacillin-N

AMPICILLIN TRIHYDRATE
Amcill, Ampicyn Oral‡, D-Amp, Omnipen, Penamp-250, Penamp-500, Penbritin‡, Polycillin, Principen-250, Principen-500, Totacillin
Classification: aminopenicillin
Pregnancy risk category B

How supplied
CAPSULES: 250 mg, 500 mg
ORAL SUSPENSION: 100 mg/ml (pediatric drops), 125 mg/5 ml, 250 mg/5 ml, 500 mg/5 ml (after reconstitution)
INJECTION: 125 mg, 250 mg, 500 mg, 1 g, 2 g
INFUSION: 500 mg, 1 g, 2 g
PHARMACY BULK PACKAGE: 10-g vial

Indications and dosage
Systemic infections, acute and chronic urinary tract infections caused by susceptible strains of gram-positive and gram-negative organisms
ADULTS: 1 to 4 g P.O. daily, divided into doses given q 6 hours; or 2 to 12 g I.M. or I.V. daily, divided into doses given q 4 to 6 hours.
CHILDREN: 50 to 100 mg/kg P.O. daily, divided into doses given q 6 hours; or 100 to 200 mg/kg I.M. or I.V. daily, divided into doses given q 6 hours.

Meningitis
ADULTS: 8 to 14 g I.V. daily for 3 days, then I.M. divided q 3 to 4 hours.
CHILDREN: up to 300 mg/kg I.V. daily for 3 days, then I.M. divided q 4 hours.

Uncomplicated gonorrhea
ADULTS: 3.5 g P.O. with 1 g probenecid given as a single dose.

Contraindications and precautions

Ampicillin is contraindicated in patients with known hypersensitivity to any other penicillin or to cephalosporins. It should not be used in patients with infectious mononucleosis because many of these patients develop a rash during therapy. Use cautiously in patients with renal impairment because it is excreted in urine; decreased dosage is required in moderate to severe renal failure.

Adverse reactions

BLOOD: anemia, thrombocytopenia, thrombocytopenic purpura, eosinophilia, leukopenia.

GI: *nausea*, vomiting, diarrhea, glossitis, stomatitis.

LOCAL: pain at injection site, vein irritation, thrombophlebitis.

OTHER: hypersensitivity (erythematous maculopapular rash, urticaria, **anaphylaxis**), **overgrowth of nonsusceptible organisms**.

Interactions

Allopurinol: increased incidence of skin rash.

Probenecid: increases blood levels of ampicillin and other penicillins. Probenecid may be used for this purpose.

Nursing considerations

Assessment

• Review the patient's history for a condition that contraindicates the use of ampicillin.

• Obtain a baseline assessment of the patient's infection before therapy.

• Be alert for common adverse reactions.

• Evaluate the patient's and family's knowledge about ampicillin therapy.

Planning (Nursing Diagnoses)

Potential nursing diagnoses for the patient receiving ampicillin include:

• Altered health maintenance related to ineffectiveness of drug.

• Fluid volume deficit related to penicillin-induced adverse GI reactions.

• Knowledge deficit related to ampicillin therapy.

Implementation

Preparation and administration

—Obtain specimen for culture and sensitivity tests before first dose. Therapy may begin pending test results.

—Before giving ampicillin, ask the patient about any allergic reactions to penicillin. However, a negative history of penicillin allergy is no guarantee against a future allergic reaction.

—When given orally, drug may cause GI disturbances. Food may interfere with absorption, so give 1 to 2 hours before meals or 2 to 3 hours after.

—Dosage should be altered in the patient with impaired renal function.

—When giving I.V., mix with dextrose 5% in water or a saline solution. Don't mix with other drugs or solutions; they might be incompatible.

—Give I.V. intermittently to prevent vein irritation.

—Initial dilution in vial is stable for 1 hour. Follow manufacturer's direction for stability data when ampicillin is further diluted for I.V. infusion.

—In pediatric meningitis, may be given concurrently with parenteral chloramphenicol for 24 hours pending cultures.

—Give ampicillin at least 1 hour before bacteriostatic antibiotics.

Monitoring

—Monitor the effectiveness of therapy by regularly assessing for improvement of infectious process.

—Monitor the patient for adverse drug reactions. Allergic reactions are the major adverse reactions to penicillin, especially with large doses, parenteral administration, or prolonged therapy. Keep in mind that the patient may become sensitized to penicillin through exposure.

—With large doses or prolonged therapy, bacterial or fungal superinfections may occur, especially in elderly, debilitated, or immunosuppressed patients. Close observation is essential.

—Inspect the patient's skin routinely for rash.

—Monitor the patient for adverse GI reactions; if present, monitor the patient's hydration status.

—Monitor the patient for drug interactions.

—Monitor diagnostic test results. Ampicillin alters results of urine glucose tests that use copper sulfate (Benedict's test or Clinitest). Make urine glucose determinations with glucose enzymatic tests (Clinistix or Tes-Tape). Ampicillin may falsely decrease serum aminoglycoside concentrations.

—Regularly reevaluate the patient's and family's knowledge about ampicillin therapy.

Intervention

—Discontinue the drug at once if the patient develops anaphylactic shock (exhibited by rapidly developing dyspnea and hypotension). Notify the doctor and prepare to administer immediate treatment, such as epinephrine, corticosteroids, antihistamines, and other resuscitative measures, as indicated.

—If rash develops, notify the doctor and expect to discontinue the drug. If nausea, vomiting, diarrhea, or glossitis occurs, request a prescription for an antiemetic or antidiarrheal agent as needed. If the GI reactions are severe, expect the drug to be discontinued or replaced with a parenteral form.

—If the patient is receiving I.V. ampicillin, change I.V. site every 48 hours.

—If the patient develops an adverse reaction, notify the doctor for appropriate therapy and provide supportive care as appropriate.

—Keep all health care team members advised of the patient's response to the drug.

Patient teaching

—Instruct the patient and family about ampicillin, including the dosage, frequency, action, and adverse reactions.

—Explain the disease process and rationale for therapy.

—Tell the patient to take medication exactly as prescribed, even after he feels better. Entire quantity prescribed should be taken.

—Tell the patient to call the doctor if rash, fever, or chills develop. A rash is the most common allergic reaction.

—Warn the patient never to use leftover ampicillin for a new illness or to share it with family and friends.

—Advise the diabetic patient that urine glucose determinations may be false-positive with copper sulfate tests (Clinitest); glucose enzymatic tests (Clinistix, Tes-Tape) are not affected.

—Tell the patient to take oral penicillin 1 hour before or 2 hours after meals to ensure an optimal serum concentration.

—Advise the patient who is allergic to penicillin to wear medical alert identification stating this information.

—Tell the patient to notify the nurse or doctor if adverse reactions develop or questions arise about ampicillin therapy.

Evaluation

In the patient receiving ampicillin, appropriate evaluation statements include:

• Patient maintains normal health status and is free of infection.

• Patient does not develop dehydration during ampicillin therapy.

• Patient and family state an understanding of ampicillin therapy.

PROTOTYPE: EXTENDED-SPECTRUM PENICILLINS

TICARCILLIN DISODIUM
(tye kar sill′ in)
Ticar, Ticillin‡
Classification: extended-spectrum penicillin
Pregnancy risk category B

How supplied

INJECTION: 1 g, 3 g, 6 g
I.V. INFUSION: 3 g
PHARMACY BULK PACKAGE: 20 g, 30 g

Indications and dosage

Severe systemic infections caused by susceptible strains of gram-positive and especially gram-negative organisms (including Pseudomonas and Proteus)

ADULTS AND CHILDREN: 200 to 300 mg/kg I.V. or I.M. daily, divided into doses given q 4 to 6 hours.

‡Available in Australia only

Contraindications and precautions

Ticarcillin is contraindicated in patients with a history of allergic reaction to any of the penicillins. Before therapy, careful inquiry should be made about previous hypersensitivity reactions to penicillins and cephalosporins and other allergies.

Adverse reactions

BLOOD: leukopenia, neutropenia, eosinophilia, thrombocytopenia, **hemolytic anemia.**
CNS: **seizures**, neuromuscular excitability.
GI: *nausea*, diarrhea.
METABOLIC: hypokalemia.
LOCAL: pain at injection site, vein irritation, phlebitis.
OTHER: hypersensitivity (rash, pruritus, urticaria, chills, fever, edema, **anaphylaxis,**), overgrowth of nonsusceptible organisms.

Interactions

Aminoglycoside antibiotics (for example, gentamicin, tobramycin): chemically incompatible. Don't mix together in I.V.
Probenecid: increases blood levels of ticarcillin and other penicillins. Probenecid may be used for this purpose.

Nursing considerations

Assessment

• Review the patient's history for a condition that contraindicates the use of ticarcillin.
• Obtain a baseline assessment of the patient's infection before therapy.
• Be alert for common adverse reactions.
• Evaluate the patient's and family's knowledge about ticarcillin therapy.

Planning (Nursing Diagnoses)

Potential nursing diagnoses for the patient receiving ticarcillin include:
• Potential for injury related to dosage regimen inadequate to alleviate infection.
• Fluid volume excess related to administration of the drug.
• Knowledge deficit related to ticarcillin therapy.

Implementation

Preparation and administration

— Obtain specimen for culture and sensitivity tests before first dose. Therapy may begin pending test results.
— Before giving ticarcillin, ask the patient if he's had any allergic reactions to penicillin. However, a negative history of penicillin allergy is no guarantee against a future allergic reaction.
— Dosage should be decreased in the patient with impaired renal function.
— When giving I.V., mix with dextrose 5% in water or other suitable I.V. fluids.
— Give I.V. intermittently to prevent vein irritation.
— Administer deep I.M. into large muscle.
— Give ticarcillin at least 1 hour before bacteriostatic antibiotics.

—Ticarcillin is almost always used with another antibiotic, such as an aminoglycoside, in life-threatening situations.

—Because ticarcillin is dialyzable, the patient undergoing hemodialysis may need dosage adjustments.

Monitoring

—Monitor the effectiveness of therapy by regularly assessing for improvement of infectious process.

—Monitor the patient for adverse drug reactions.

—Monitor I.V. site routinely.

—With large doses and prolonged therapy, bacterial and fungal superinfections may occur, especially in elderly, debilitated, or immunosuppressed patients. Close observation is essential.

—Ticarcillin contains 5.2 mEq of sodium per gram of drug. Monitor serum electrolytes to prevent hypokalemia and hypernatremia.

—Monitor the patient's fluid balance (intake and output, weight).

—Monitor the patient for drug interactions.

—Monitor diagnostic test results. Ticarcillin alters tests for urine or serum proteins; it interferes with turbidimetric methods that use sulfosalicylic acid, trichloroacetic acid, acetic acid, or nitric acid. Ticarcillin may falsely decrease serum aminoglycoside concentrations. Systemic effects of ticarcillin may cause positive Coombs' test, hypokalemia, and hypernatremia and may prolong prothrombin times; it may also cause transient elevations in liver function studies and transient reductions in RBC, WBC, and platelet counts.

—Regularly reevaluate the patient's and family's knowledge about ticarcillin therapy.

Intervention

—If the patient develops signs of excess fluid volume (for example, edema, weight gain), notify the doctor.

—Change I.V. site every 48 hours.

—If the patient develops an adverse reaction, notify the doctor for appropriate treatment and provide supportive care as appropriate.

—Keep all health care team members advised of the patient's response to the drug.

Patient teaching

—Instruct the patient and family about ticarcillin, including the dosage, frequency, action, and adverse reactions.

—Explain the disease process and rationale for therapy.

—Advise the patient who is allergic to drug to wear medical alert identification stating this information.

—Tell the patient to notify the nurse or doctor if adverse reactions develop or questions arise about ticarcillin therapy.

Evaluation

In the patient receiving ticarcillin, evaluation statements may include:
• Patient is free of infection.
• Patient maintains normal fluid volume balance.
• Patient and family state an understanding of ticarcillin therapy.

SELECTED MAJOR DRUGS: PENICILLINS

DRUG, INDICATIONS, AND DOSAGES	SPECIAL PRECAUTIONS
azlocillin (Azlin, Securopen‡) *Serious infections caused by susceptible strains of gram-negative organisms, including* Pseudomonas aeruginosa— **Adults:** 200 to 350 mg/kg I.V. daily in four to six divided doses. Usual dose is 3 g q 4 hours (18 g daily). Maximum dosage is 24 g daily. May be administered by I.V. intermittent infusion or by direct slow I.V. injection. **Children with acute exacerbation of cystic fibrosis:** 75 mg/kg q 4 hours (450 mg/kg daily). Maximum dosage is 24 g daily. Azlocillin should not be used in neonates.	• Contraindicated in patients with known hypersensitivity reactions to any of the penicillins. • Use cautiously in patients hypersensitive to drugs, especially to cephalosporins (possible cross-allergenicity), and in bleeding tendencies, uremia, or hypokalemia.
bacampicillin (Penglobe†, Spectrobid) *Upper and lower respiratory tract infections due to streptococci, pneumococci, staphylococci, and* Haemophilus influenzae; *urinary tract infections due to* Escherichia coli, Proteus mirabilis, *and* Streptococcus faecalis; *skin infections due to streptococci and susceptible staphylococci*— **Adults and children weighing more than 25 kg:** 400 to 800 mg P.O. q 12 hours. *Gonorrhea*— **Adults:** Usual dosage 1.6 g and 1 g probenecid as a single dose. Not recommended for children under 25 kg.	• Contraindicated in patients with known hypersensitivity to any of the penicillins. • Use cautiously in patients with other drug allergies, especially to cephalosporins (possible cross-allergenicity), and in mononucleosis. This drug, like ampicillin, is linked to a high incidence of maculopapular rash.
carbenicillin disodium (Carbapen‡, Geopen, Pyopen) *Systemic infections caused by susceptible strains of gram-positive and especially gram-negative organisms (including* Proteus, Pseudomonas aeruginosa)— **Adults:** 30 to 40 g I.V. infusion daily, divided into doses given q 4 to 6 hours. **Children:** 300 to 500 mg/kg I.V. infusion daily, divided into doses given q 4 to 6 hours. *Urinary tract infections*— **Adults:** 200 mg/kg I.M. or I.V. infusion daily, divided into doses given q 4 to 6 hours. **Children:** 50 to 200 mg/kg I.M. or I.V. infusion daily, divided into doses given q 4 to 6 hours.	• Use cautiously in patients with other drug allergies, especially to cephalosporins (possible cross-allergenicity); in bleeding tendencies, uremia, and hypokalemia; and in patients on sodium-restricted diets; contains 4.7 mEq sodium/g.
carbenicillin indanyl sodium (Geocillin) *Urinary tract infection and prostatitis caused by susceptible strains of gram-negative organisms*— **Adults:** 382 to 764 mg P.O. q.i.d.	• Contraindicated in patients with known hypersensitivity to any of the penicillins. Not recommended for children. • Use cautiously in patients with other drug allergies, especially to cephalosporins (possible cross-allergenicity).

SELECTED MAJOR DRUGS: PENICILLINS *continued*

DRUG, INDICATIONS, AND DOSAGES	SPECIAL PRECAUTIONS
cloxacillin (Alclox‡, Cloxapen, Tegopen) *Systemic infections caused by penicillinase-producing staphylococci—* **Adults:** 2 to 4 g P.O. daily, divided into doses given q 6 hours. **Children:** 50 to 100 mg/kg P.O. daily, divided into doses given q 6 hours.	• Contraindicated in patients with known hypersensitivity to any of the penicillins.
dicloxacillin (Dycill, Dynapen, Pathocil) *Systemic infections caused by penicillinase-producing staphylococci—* **Adults:** 1 to 2 g P.O. daily, divided into doses given q 6 hours. **Children:** 25 to 50 mg/kg P.O. daily, divided into doses given q 6 hours.	• Contraindicated in patients with known hypersensitivity to any of the penicillins.
methicillin (Staphcillin) *Systemic infections caused by penicillinase-producing staphylococci—* **Adults:** 4 to 12 g I.M. or I.V. daily, divided into doses given q 4 to 6 hours. **Children:** 100 to 200 mg/kg I.M. or I.V. daily, divided into doses given q 4 to 6 hours.	• Same as cloxacillin.
mezlocillin (Mezlin) *Systemic infections caused by susceptible strains of gram-positive and especially gram-negative organisms (including* Proteus, Pseudomonas aeruginosa)— **Adults:** 200 to 300 mg/kg I.V. or I.M. daily in four to six divided doses. Usual dose is 3 g q 4 hours or 4 g q 6 hours. For very serious infections, up to 24 g daily may be administered. **Children up to age 12:** 50 mg/kg by I.V. infusion or direct I.V. injection q 4 hours.	• Contraindicated in patients with known hypersensitivity to any of the penicillins. • Use cautiously in patients with other drug allergies, especially to cephalosporins (possible cross-hypersensitivity), and in bleeding tendencies, uremia, and hypokalemia.
nafcillin (Nafcil, Nallpen, Unipen) *Systemic infections caused by penicillinase-producing staphylococci—* **Adults:** 2 to 4 g P.O. daily, divided into doses given q 6 hours; 2 to 12 g I.M. or I.V. daily, divided into doses given q 4 to 6 hours. **Children:** 50 to 100 mg/kg P.O. daily, divided into doses given q 4 to 6 hours; or 100 to 200 mg/kg I.M. or I.V. daily, divided into doses given q 4 to 6 hours.	• Contraindicated in patients with a history of allergic reaction to any of the penicillins. • Use cautiously in patients with other drug allergies, especially to cephalosporins (possible cross-allergenicity), and in GI distress.

(continued)

‡Available in Australia only

SELECTED MAJOR DRUGS: PENICILLINS *continued*

DRUG, INDICATIONS, AND DOSAGES	SPECIAL PRECAUTIONS
penicillin G benzathine (Bicillin-LA, Megacillin) *Congenital syphilis—* **Children under age 2:** 50,000 units/kg I.M. as a single dose. *Group A streptococcal upper respiratory infections—* **Adults:** 1.2 million units I.M. in a single injection. **Children over 27 kg:** 900,000 units I.M. in a single injection. **Children under 27 kg:** 300,000 to 600,000 units I.M. in a single injection. *Prophylaxis of poststreptococcal rheumatic fever—* **Adults and children:** 1.2 million units I.M. once a month or 600,000 units twice a month. *Syphilis of less than 1 year's duration—* **Adults:** 2.4 million units I.M. in a single dose. *Syphilis of more than 1 year's duration—* **Adults:** 2.4 million units I.M. weekly for three successive weeks.	• Contraindicated in patients with known hypersensitivity to any of the penicillins. • Use cautiously in patients with other drug allergies, especially to cephalosporins (possible cross-allergenicity).
penicillin G potassium (Pentids, Pfizerpen) *Moderate to severe systemic infections—* **Adults:** 1.6 to 3.2 million units P.O. daily in divided doses given q 6 hours (1 mg = 1,600 units); 1.2 to 24 million units I.M. or I.V. daily in divided doses q 4 hours. **Children:** 25,000 to 100,000 units/kg P.O. daily in divided doses q 6 hours; or 25,000 to 300,000 units/kg I.M. or I.V. daily in divided doses q 4 hours.	• Contraindicated in patients with known hypersensitivity to any of the penicillins. • Use cautiously in patients with other drug allergies, especially to cephalosporins (possible cross-allergenicity).
penicillin G procaine (Ayercillin†, Crysticillin AS, Wycillin) *Moderate to severe systemic infections—* **Adults:** 600,000 to 1.2 million unit I.M. daily as a single dose. **Children:** 300,000 units I.M. daily as a single dose. *Uncomplicated gonorrhea—* **Adults and children over age 12:** give 1 g probenecid; then 30 minutes later give 4.8 million units of penicillin G procaine I.M., divided into two injection sites. *Pneumococcal pneumonia—* **Adults and children over age 12:** 300,000 to 600,000 units I.M. daily q 6 to 12 hours.	• Contraindicated in patients with known hypersensitivity to any of the penicillins or to procaine. Use cautiously in patients with other drug allergies, especially to cephalosporins (possible cross-allergenicity).
penicillin V **penicillin V potassium (PVK‡, Veetids)** *Mild to moderate systemic infections—* **Adults:** 250 to 500 mg (400,000 to 800,000 units) P.O. q 6 hours. **Children:** 15 to 50 mg/kg (25,000 to 90,000 units/kg) P.O. daily, divided into doses given q 6 to 8 hours. *Endocarditis prophylaxis for dental surgery—* **Adults:** 2 g P.O. 30 to 60 minutes before procedure, then 1 g 6 hours after. **Children under 30 kg:** half of the adult dose.	• Contraindicated in patients with known hypersensitivity to any of the penicillins. • Use cautiously in patients with other drug allergies, especially to cephalosporins (possible cross-allergenicity), and in GI disturbances.

†Available in Canada only   ‡Available in Australia only

SELECTED MAJOR DRUGS: PENICILLINS *continued*

DRUG, INDICATIONS, AND DOSAGES

SPECIAL PRECAUTIONS

piperacillin (Pipracil, Pipril‡)
Systemic infections caused by susceptible strains of gram-positive and especially gram-negative organisms (including Proteus, Pseudomonas aeruginosa) —
Adults and children over age 12: 100 to 300 mg/kg I.V. or I.M. daily divided q 4 to 6 hours. Doses for children under age 12 are not established.
Prophylaxis of surgical infections —
Adults: 2 g I.V. 30 to 60 minutes before surgery. Depending on type of surgery, dose may be repeated during surgery and once or twice more after surgery.

• Contraindicated in patients with a history of allergic reactions to any of the penicillins.
• Use cautiously in patients hypersensitive to drugs, especially to cephalosporins (possible cross-hypersensitivity), and in bleeding tendencies, uremia, and hypokalemia.

‡Available in Australia only

SELF-TEST

1. Janice Kelly, age 27, is taking oral ampicillin for treatment of a bladder infection. She should:
  a. take with food to combat GI distress.
  b. take with milk or an antacid.
  c. take 1 hour before or 2 hours after a meal.
  d. open capsules and mix with orange juice if she has difficulty swallowing.

2. On the third day of ampicillin therapy, Ms. Kelly developed diarrhea. She should:
  a. stop taking the drug as this is an indication of toxicity.
  b. contact her health care provider about treatment of this diarrhea.
  c. ignore the diarrhea; it is a common adverse reaction that cannot be treated.
  d. drink plenty of fluid to compensate for the fluid lost in the diarrhea.

3. Jerry Lutz, age 65, has pneumonia. His doctor prescribed penicillin G sodium 3 million units I.V. q 4 hours. In taking a drug history from Mr. Lutz, it is especially important to assess for allergies to which of the following medications?
  a. aminoglycosides
  b. calcium channel blockers
  c. cephalosporins
  d. antituberculars

Check your answers on page 1058.

CHAPTER 12

CEPHALOSPORINS

First-generation cephalosporins
cefadroxil monohydrate ✦ cefazolin sodium ✦ cephalexin monohydrate
cephalothin sodium ✦ cephapirin sodium ✦ cephradine

Second-generation cephalosporins
cefaclor ✦ cefamandole nafate ✦ cefmetazole sodium ✦ cefonicid sodium
ceforanide ✦ cefotetan disodium ✦ cefoxitin sodium ✦ cefuroxime axetil
cefuroxime sodium

Third-generation cephalosporins
cefixime ✦ cefoperazone sodium ✦ cefotaxime sodium ✦ ceftazidime
ceftizoxime sodium ✦ ceftriaxone sodium ✦ moxalactam disodium

OVERVIEW
- Cephalosporins are beta-lactam antibiotics first isolated in 1948 from the fungus *Cephalosporium acremonium*. Their mechanism of action is similar to that of penicillins, but their antibacterial spectra differ. Over the past 15 years, intensive research and development has resulted in the availability of many newer cephalosporins, which are now classified by generations. Generations are differentiated in terms of individual antimicrobial activity.
- First-generation cephalosporins act like penicillins against gram-positive cocci and are also effective against some gram-negative organisms. Second-generation cephalosporins have increased activity against gram-negative organisms, including beta-lactamase-producing strains, but are less effective against gram-positive cocci than are first-generation drugs. Third-generation cephalosporins have a still broader spectrum of action, especially against gram-negative organisms, including some strains resistant to first- and second-generation drugs; some effectively attack *Pseudomonas*. However, they have less gram-positive activity than do first- and second-generation drugs. Moxalactam, an oxa-beta lactam, is chemically similar to third-generation cephalosporins and its antibacterial spectrum is similar to third-generation cephalosporins.
- The cephalosporins are classified into three groups: first-generation, second-generation, and third-generation cephalosporins.

MAJOR USES
- Parenteral cephalosporins are used to treat serious infections of the lungs, skin, soft tissue, bones, joints, urinary tract, blood (septicemia), abdomen, and heart (endocarditis).

GLOSSARY

Antimicrobial: substance used to treat infection with pathogenic microorganisms.
Bacillus: any rod-shaped, gram-positive, spore-forming microorganism.
Superinfection: condition produced by the sudden overgrowth of resistant bacteria or fungi, which can occur in a patient on antibiotic therapy.

- Third-generation cephalosporins (except moxalactam and cefoperazone) and the second-generation drug cefuroxime are used to treat CNS infections caused by susceptible strains of *Neisseria meningitidis, Haemophilus influenzae,* and *Streptococcus pneumoniae;* meningitis caused by *Escherichia coli* or *Klebsiella* can be treated by ceftriaxone, cefotaxime, or ceftizoxime.
- First-generation, and some second-generation, cephalosporins also can be given prophylactically to reduce postoperative infection after surgical procedures classified as contaminated or potentially contaminated; third-generation drugs are not usually indicated.
- Penicillinase-producing *N. gonorrhoeae* can be treated with cefoxitin, cefotaxime, ceftriaxone, ceftizoxime, or cefuroxime.
- Oral cephalosporins can be used to treat otitis media and infections of the respiratory tract, urinary tract, and skin and soft tissue; cefaclor is particularly effective against ampicillin-resistant middle ear infections caused by *H. influenzae.*

MECHANISM OF ACTION

- Cephalosporins are chemically and pharmacologically similar to penicillin; their structure contains a beta-lactam ring, a dihydrothiazine ring, and side chains, and they act by inhibiting bacterial cell wall synthesis, causing rapid cell lysis.
- The sites of action for cephalosporins are enzymes known as penicillin-binding proteins (PBPs). The affinity of certain cephalosporins for PBP in various microorganisms helps explain the differing spectra of activity in this class of antibiotics.
- Bacterial resistance to beta-lactam antibiotics is conferred most significantly by production of beta-lactamase enzymes (by both gram-negative and gram-positive bacteria) that destroy the beta-lactam ring and thus inactivate cephalosporins; decreased cell wall permeability and alteration in binding affinity to PBP also contribute to bacterial resistance.
- Cephalosporins are bactericidal; they act against many gram-positive and gram-negative bacteria and some anaerobic bacteria; they do not kill fungi or viruses.
- First-generation cephalosporins act against many gram-positive cocci, including penicillinase-producing *Staphylococcus aureus* and *S. epidermidis; Streptococcus pneumoniae,* group B streptococci, and

group A beta-hemolytic streptococci; susceptible gram-negative organisms include *Klebsiella pneumoniae, E. coli, Proteus mirabilis, and Shigella.*

- Second-generation cephalosporins are effective against all organisms attacked by first-generation drugs and have additional activity against *Branhamella catarrhalis, H. influenzae, Enterobacter, Citrobacter, Providencia, Acinetobacter, Serratia, and Neisseria; Bacteroides fragilis* is susceptible to cefotetan and cefoxitin.
- Third-generation cephalosporins are less active than first- and second-generation drugs against gram-positive bacteria but more active against gram-negative organisms, including those resistant to first- and second-generation drugs; they have the greatest stability against beta-lactamases produced by gram-negative bacteria. Susceptible gram-negative organisms include *E. coli, Klebsiella, Enterobacter, Providencia, Acinetobacter, Serratia, Proteus, Morganella,* and *Neisseria;* some third-generation drugs are active against *B. fragilis* and *Pseudomonas.*

ABSORPTION, DISTRIBUTION, METABOLISM, AND EXCRETION

Oral absorption of cephalosporins varies widely; many must be given parenterally. Most are distributed widely, the actual amount varying with individual drugs. CSF penetration by first- and second-generation drugs is minimal; third-generation drugs achieve much greater penetration. Cephalosporins cross the placenta. Degree of metabolism varies; some are not metabolized and others are extensively metabolized.

Cephalosporins are excreted primarily in urine, chiefly by renal tubular effects; elimination half-life ranges from 30 minutes to 10 hours in patients with normal renal function. (See *Pharmacokinetics of Cephalosporins*). Some drug is excreted in breast milk. Most cephalosporins can be removed by hemodialysis or peritoneal dialysis. Patients on dialysis may require dosage adjustment.

ONSET AND DURATION

Oral cephalosporins attain a peak concentration level within 1 to 2 hours after administration. After a 30-minute I.V. infusion, onset of action is rapid. Peak concentration usually is achieved within 1 hour. After I.V. administration of 1 g, the peak concentration is 50 to 100 mcg/ml for most cephalosporins. The higher concentration of cefazolin given I.V. or I.M. is a considerable advantage over other first-generation cephalosporins. After I.M. administration, the onset usually is delayed. The peak concentration achieved is about 50% of that achieved after I.V. administration.

The serum half-life of cephalosporins in adults with normal renal function ranges from 0.4 to 10.9 hours. Among first-generation cephalosporins, cefazolin has the longest half-life (2.2 hours), which allows an every-8-hour dosage schedule. Cefonicid is the longest-acting second-generation cephalosporin, with a serum half-life of nearly 6 hours and 90% to 98% of the drug bound to serum proteins. The drug normally is given once daily. In patients with renal impairment, the dosage and frequency of cefonicid administration depend on creatinine clearance. Among the

PHARMACOKINETICS OF CEPHALOSPORINS

DRUG (ROUTE)	ELIMINATION HALF-LIFE (hours)		SODIUM CONTENT (mEq/g)	CSF PENETRATION
	NORMAL RENAL FUNCTION	END-STAGE RENAL DISEASE		
cefaclor (oral)	0.5 to 1	3 to 5.5	Negligible	No
cefadroxil (oral)	1 to 2	20 to 25	Negligible	No
cefamandole (I.M., I.V.)	0.5 to 2	12 to 18	3.3	No
cefazolin (I.M., I.V.)	1.2 to 2.2	12 to 50	2.0	No
cefixime (oral)	3 to 4	11.5	Negligible	Unknown
cefmetazole (I.V.)	1.2	Unknown	49	Unknown
cefonicid (I.M., I.V.)	3.5 to 5.8	100	3.7	No
cefoperazone (I.M., I.V.)	1.5 to 2.5	3.4 to 7	1.5	Sometimes
ceforanide (I.M., I.V.)	2.5 to 3.5	5.5 to 25	Negligible	No
cefotaxime (I.M., I.V.)	1 to 1.5	11.5 to 56	2.2	Yes
cefotetan (I.M., I.V.)	2.8 to 4.6	13 to 35	3.5	No
cefoxitin (I.M., I.V.)	0.5 to 1	6.5 to 21.5	2.3	No
ceftazidime (I.M., I.V.)	1.5 to 2	35	2.3	Yes
ceftizoxime (I.M., I.V.)	1.5 to 2	30	2.6	Yes
ceftriaxone (I.M., I.V.)	5.5 to 11	15.7	3.6	Yes
cefuroxime (I.M., I.V.)	1 to 2	15 to 22	2.4	Yes

(continued)

PHARMACOKINETICS OF CEPHALOSPORINS *continued*

DRUG (ROUTE)	ELIMINATION HALF-LIFE (hours)		SODIUM CONTENT (mEq/g)	CSF PENETRATION
	NORMAL RENAL FUNCTION	END-STAGE RENAL DISEASE		
cephalexin (oral)	0.5 to 1	7.5 to 14	Negligible	No
cephalothin (I.M., I.V.)	0.5 to 1	19	2.8	No
cephapirin (I.M., I.V.)	0.5 to 1	1 to 1.5	2.4	No
cephradine (oral, I.M., I.V.)	0.5 to 2	8 to 15	6	No
moxalactam (I.M., I.V.)	2 to 3.5	5 to 10	3.8	Yes

third-generation cephalosporins, ceftriaxone displays the highest degree of plasma protein-binding (85% to 95%) and the longest serum half-life (up to 10.9 hours). Ceftriaxone usually is administered once daily. Dosage adjustments of ceftriaxone usually are unnecessary in patients with impaired renal or hepatic function. The remaining cephalosporins have a serum half-life of 0.5 to 4 hours and are administered at 4- to 12-hour intervals in patients with normal renal function.

ADVERSE REACTIONS

Many cephalosporins share a similar profile of adverse reactions. Hypersensitivity reactions range from mild rashes, fever, and eosinophilia to fatal anaphylaxis and are more common in patients with penicillin allergy. Hematologic reactions include positive direct and indirect antiglobulin (Coombs' test), thrombocytopenia or thrombocythemia, transient neutropenia, and reversible leukopenia. Adverse renal reactions may occur with any cephalosporin; they are most common in older patients, those with decreased renal function, and those taking other nephrotoxic drugs. GI reactions include nausea, vomiting, diarrhea, abdominal pain, glossitis, dyspepsia, and tenesmus; minimal elevation of liver function test results occurs occasionally. Local pain and irritation are common after I.M. injection; such reactions occur more often with higher doses and long-term therapy. Bacterial and fungal superinfection results from suppression of normal flora. Disulfiram-type reactions occur when cefamandole, cefoperazone, moxalactam, cefonicid, or cefotetan are administered within 48 to 72 hours of alcohol ingestion.

CEPHALEXIN MONOHYDRATE
(sef a lex′ in)
Ceporex†‡, Keflet, Keflex, Novolexin†

CEPHALEXIN HYDROCHLORIDE MONOHYDRATE
Keftab
Classification: first-generation cephalosporin
Pregnancy risk category B

How supplied
TABLETS: 250 mg, 500 mg, 1 g
CAPSULES: 500 mg, 1,250 mg
ORAL SUSPENSION: 100 mg/5 ml, 125 mg/5 ml, 250 mg/5 ml

Indications and dosage
Infections of respiratory or GU tract, skin and soft-tissue infections, bone and joint infections, and otitis media due to Escherichia coli *and other coliform bacteria, group A beta-hemolytic streptococci,* Haemophilus influenzae, Klebsiella, Proteus mirabilis, Streptococcus pneumoniae, *and* Staphylococcus
ADULTS: 250 mg to 1 g P.O. q 6 hours.
CHILDREN: 6 to 12 mg/kg P.O. q 6 hours. Maximum is 25 mg/kg q 6 hours.

Contraindications and precautions
Cephalexin is contraindicated in patients with known allergy to cephalosporins; should be given cautiously to penicillin-sensitive patients. Safety of this product for use during pregnancy has not been established. Use cautiously in markedly impaired renal function and in breast-feeding women. Safety in children has not been established.

Adverse reactions
BLOOD: transient neutropenia, eosinophilia, anemia.
CNS: dizziness, headache, malaise, paresthesia.
GI: pseudomembranous colitis, nausea, anorexia, vomiting, *diarrhea*, glossitis, *dyspepsia*, abdominal cramps, anal pruritus, tenesmus, oral candidiasis (thrush).
GU: genital pruritus and moniliasis, vaginitis.
SKIN: maculopapular and erythematous rashes, urticaria.
OTHER: hypersensitivity reactions (including rash, **anaphylaxis**), dyspnea.

Interactions
Probenecid: may increase blood levels of cephalosporins. Probenecid may be used for this purpose.

Nursing considerations

Assessment
- Review the patient's history for a condition that contraindicates the use of cephalexin.
- Obtain a baseline assessment of the patient's infection before therapy.
- Be alert for common adverse reactions.
- Evaluate the patient's and family's knowledge about cephalexin therapy.

Planning (Nursing Diagnoses)
Potential nursing diagnoses for the patient receiving cephalexin include:
- Potential for injury related to ineffectiveness of drug.
- Altered health maintenance related to an adverse drug reaction.
- Knowledge deficit related to cephalexin therapy.

Implementation

Preparation and administration
—Obtain specimen for culture and sensitivity tests before first dose. Therapy may begin pending test results.
—Preparation of oral suspension; add required amount of water to powder in two equal portions. Shake well after each addition. After mixing, store in refrigerator. Stable for 14 days without significant loss of potency. Keep tightly closed and shake well before using.
—Administer drug with food to prevent or minimize GI upset.
—To prevent toxic accumulation in the patient with impaired renal function, reduce dosage if creatinine clearance is below 40 ml/minute.
—Because cephalexin is dialyzable, the patient undergoing treatment with hemodialysis or peritoneal dialysis may require dosage adjustment.

Monitoring
—Monitor the effectiveness of therapy by regularly assessing for improvement of infectious process.
—Monitor the patient for adverse drug reactions.
—Monitor for signs of an allergic or anaphylactic reaction.
—With large doses or prolonged therapy, monitor for superinfection, especially in the high-risk patient.
—Monitor the patient for drug interactions.
—Monitor laboratory test results. A false-positive direct Coombs' test may occur in some patients, but only a few of these results indicate hemolytic anemia. Urine glucose determinations may be false-positive with copper sulfate tests (Clinitest); glucose enzymatic tests (Clinistix, Tes-Tape) are not affected.
—Regularly reevaluate the patient's and family's knowledge about cephalexin therapy.

Intervention
—Keep epinephrine on hand to treat anaphylaxis.
—If the patient develops an adverse reaction, notify the doctor for appropriate treatment and provide supportive care as indicated.

— Keep all health care team members advised of patient's response to the drug.

Patient teaching

— Instruct the patient and family about cephalexin, including the dosage, frequency, action, and adverse reactions.

— Explain the disease process and rationale for therapy.

— Tell the patient to take medication exactly as prescribed, even after he feels better.

— Tell the patient to take with food or milk to lessen GI discomfort.

— Advise the diabetic patient taking drug to test urine glucose levels with Tes-Tape or Clinistix (not Clinitest).

— Advise the patient using oral suspension to shake well before using. Store mixture in tightly closed container in refrigerator. Suspension is stable for 14 days without significant loss of potency.

— Tell the patient to notify the nurse or doctor if adverse reactions develop or questions arise about cephalexin therapy.

Evaluation

In the patient receiving cephalexin, appropriate evaluation statements include:

• Patient is free of infection.

• Patient maintains normal health maintenance status and has no adverse reactions to the drug.

• Patient and family state an understanding of cephalexin therapy.

PROTOTYPE: SECOND-GENERATION CEPHALOSPORINS

CEFACLOR
(sef′ a klor)
Ceclor
Classification: second-generation cephalosporin
Pregnancy risk category B

How supplied
CAPSULES: 250 mg, 500 mg
ORAL SUSPENSION: 125 mg/5 ml, 250 mg/5 ml

Indications and dosage
Infections of respiratory or urinary tracts, skin, and soft tissue; and otitis media due to Haemophilus influenzae, Streptococcus pneumoniae, Streptococcus pyogenes, Escherichia coli, Proteus mirabilis, Klebsiella species, *and* Staphylococcus

ADULTS: 250 to 500 mg P.O. q 8 hours. Total dose should not exceed 4 g daily.

CHILDREN: 20 mg/kg daily P.O. in divided doses q 8 hours. In more serious infections, 40 mg/kg daily is recommended, not to exceed 1 g daily.

Contraindications and precautions

Cefaclor is contraindicated in patients with known allergy to cephalosporins. Use cautiously in penicillin-sensitive patients; in those showing some form of allergy, particularly to drugs; in markedly impaired renal function; during pregnancy (use only if clearly needed); and in breast-feeding women. Safety in infants under age 1 month has not been established.

Adverse reactions

BLOOD: transient leukopenia, lymphocytosis, anemia, eosinophilia.
CNS: dizziness, headache, somnolence.
GI: *nausea*, vomiting, *diarrhea*, anorexia, pseudomembranous colitis.
GU: red and white cells in urine, vaginal moniliasis, vaginitis.
SKIN: *maculopapular rash*, dermatitis.
OTHER: hypersensitivity (including rash, **anaphylaxis**), fever, cholestatic jaundice.

Interactions

Probenecid: may inhibit excretion and increase blood levels of cefaclor.

Nursing considerations

Assessment

• Review the patient's history for a condition that contraindicates the use of cefaclor.
• Obtain a baseline assessment of the patient's infection before therapy.
• Be alert for common adverse reactions.
• Evaluate the patient's and family's knowledge about cefaclor therapy.

Planning (Nursing Diagnoses)

Potential nursing diagnoses for the patient receiving cefaclor include:
• Potential for injury related to dosage regimen inadequate to alleviate infection.
• Fluid volume deficit related to adverse GI reactions.
• Knowledge deficit related to cefaclor therapy.

Implementation

Preparation and administration

—Obtain specimen for culture and sensitivity tests before first dose. Therapy may begin pending test results.
—Administer the drug with food to prevent or minimize GI upset.
—If ordered, total daily dose of cefaclor may be administered twice daily rather than three times daily with similar therapeutic results.
—Reconstituted oral suspension is stable for 14 days if refrigerated.
—Because cefaclor is dialyzable, the patient who is receiving treatment with hemodialysis or peritoneal dialysis may require drug dosage adjustment.
—To prevent toxic accumulation, reduce dosage if the creatinine clearance is below 40 ml/minute.

Monitoring

— Monitor the effectiveness of therapy by regularly assessing for improvement of infectious process.
— Monitor the patient for adverse drug reactions. Monitor the patient's fluid volume (including intake and output).
— With large doses or prolonged therapy, monitor for superinfection, especially in the high-risk patient.
— Monitor for signs and symptoms of anaphylaxis.
— Monitor the patient for drug interactions.
— Monitor diagnostic test results. Cefaclor may cause false-positive Coombs' test results. Cefaclor also causes false-positive results in urine glucose tests utilizing copper sulfate (Benedict's test or Clinitest); use glucose enzymatic tests (Clinistix or Tes-Tape) instead. Cefaclor causes false elevations in serum or urine creatinine levels in tests using Jaffé reaction.
— Regularly reevaluate the patient's and family's knowledge about cefaclor therapy.

Intervention

— Keep epinephrine on hand to treat anaphylaxis.
— Obtain an order for an antiemetic or antidiarrheal agent if indicated.
— If the patient develops an adverse reaction, notify the doctor for appropriate treatment and provide supportive care as indicated.
— Keep all health care team members advised of patient's response to the drug.

Patient teaching

— Instruct the patient and family about cefaclor, including the dosage, frequency, action, and adverse reactions.
— Explain the disease process and rationale for therapy.
— Instruct the patient to complete the entire course of therapy, even if he's feeling better.
— Instruct the patient to take drug with food to prevent GI upset.
— Advise the diabetic patient taking drug to test urine glucose levels with Tes-Tape or Clinistix (not Clinitest).
— Tell the patient to store reconstituted suspension in refrigerator. Stable for 14 days if refrigerated. Shake well before using.
— Tell the patient to notify the nurse or doctor if adverse reactions develop or questions arise about cefaclor therapy.

Evaluation

In the patient receiving cefaclor, appropriate evaluation statements include:
• Patient is free of infection.
• Patient maintains normal fluid volume balance and experiences no adverse GI reactions.
• Patient and family state an understanding of cefaclor therapy.

CEFTAZIDIME
(sef tay′ zi deem)
Fortaz, Magnacef†, Tazicef, Tazidime
Classification: third-generation cephalosporin
Pregnancy risk category B

How supplied
INJECTION: 500 mg, 1 g, 2 g
INFUSION: 1 g, 2 g in 100-ml vials and bags
PHARMACY BULK PACKAGE: 6 g

Indications and dosage
Serious infections of the lower respiratory and urinary tracts, gynecologic infections, bacteremia, septicemia, intra-abdominal infections, CNS infections, and skin infections. Among susceptible microorganisms are streptococci, including Streptococcus pneumoniae *and* S. pyogenes; Staphylococcus aureus *(penicillinase- and non-penicillinase-producing);* Escherichia coli; Klebsiella; Proteus; Enterobacter; Haemophilus influenzae; Pseudomonas; *and some strains of* Bacteroides
ADULTS: 1 g I.V. or I.M. q 8 to 12 hours; up to 6 g daily in life-threatening infections.
CHILDREN AGES 1 MONTH TO 12 YEARS: 30 to 50 mg/kg I.V. q 8 hours.
NEONATES AGES 0 TO 4 WEEKS: 30 mg/kg I.V. q 12 hours.
　　Total daily dosage is the same for I.M. or I.V. administration and depends on susceptibility of organism and severity of infection. In the patient with impaired renal function, doses or frequency of administration must be modified according to degree of renal impairment, severity of infection, and susceptibility of organism.

Contraindications and precautions
Ceftazidime is contraindicated in patients with known hypersensitivity to the drug or other cephalosporins. Before therapy is instituted, careful inquiry should be made to determine whether the patient has had previous hypersensitivity reactions to ceftazidime or other cephalosporins, penicillins, or other drugs. Use cautiously in patients with some form of allergy, particularly to drugs; with type 1 hypersensitivity reactions to penicillin; and in those with a history of GI disease, particularly colitis. Use during pregnancy only if clearly needed and use cautiously in breast-feeding women.

Adverse reactions
BLOOD: eosinophilia, thrombocytosis, leukopenia.
CNS: headache, dizziness.
GI: pseudomembranous enterocolitis, *nausea*, vomiting, *diarrhea*, dysgeusia, abdominal cramps.
GU: genital pruritus and moniliasis.

---

†Available in Canada only
Italicized adverse reactions are common

HEPATIC: transient elevation in liver enzymes.

SKIN: maculopapular and erythematous rashes, urticaria.

LOCAL: at injection site—pain, induration, sterile abscesses, tissue slough- ing; phlebitis and thrombophlebitis with I.V. injection.

OTHER: hypersensitivity (including rash, **anaphylaxis**), dyspnea, elevated temperature.

Interactions

Sodium bicarbonate–containing solutions: make ceftazidime unstable. Don't mix together.

Nursing considerations

Assessment

- Review the patient's history for a condition that contraindicates the use of ceftazidime.
- Obtain a baseline assessment of the patient's infection before therapy.
- Be alert for common adverse reactions.
- Evaluate the patient's and family's knowledge about ceftazidime ther- apy.

Planning (Nursing Diagnoses)

Potential nursing diagnoses for the patient receiving ceftazidime include:
- Potential for injury related to dosage regimen inadequate to alleviate infection.
- Pain (injection site) related to I.V. or I.M. injection.
- Knowledge deficit related to ceftazidime therapy.

Implementation

Preparation and administration

— Obtain specimen for culture and sensitivity tests before first dose. Therapy may begin pending test results.

— The vials of ceftazidime are supplied under reduced pressure. When the antibiotic is dissolved, carbon dioxide is released and a positive pressure develops. Each brand of ceftazidime includes specific instruc- tions for reconstitution. Read and follow these instructions carefully.

— Because ceftazidime is hemodialyzable, the patient undergoing treat- ment with hemodialysis or peritoneal dialysis may require dosage adjustment.

— To prevent toxic accumulation, dosage reduction is necessary in the patient with a creatinine clearance below 50 ml/minute.

— For the patient on sodium restriction, note that ceftazidime contains 2.3 mEq of sodium per gram of drug.

— Ceftazidime powder for injection contains 118 mg sodium carbonate per gram of drug; ceftazidime is more water-soluble and is formed in situ upon reconstitution.

— Infuse I.V. ceftazidime over 30 minutes to prevent pain and irritation.

— Ceftazidime should be injected deep I.M. into a large muscle mass, such as gluteus or lateral aspect of thigh.

Monitoring

— Monitor the effectiveness of therapy by regularly assessing for improvement of infectious process.

— Monitor the patient for adverse drug reactions. Keep in mind that toxicity increases from the first to the third generation of cephalosporins.

— With large doses or prolonged therapy, monitor for superinfection, especially in the high–risk patient.

— If administering the drug I.V., monitor the I.V. site routinely for signs of thrombophlebitis, such as localized redness, swelling, and pain.

— Monitor the patient for drug interactions, such as those with sodium bicarbonate–containing solutions.

— Monitor diagnostic test results. Ceftazidime causes false-positive results in urine glucose tests using copper sulfate (Benedict's test or Clinitest); use glucose enzymatic test (Clinistix or Tes-Tape) instead. Ceftazidime also causes false elevations in urine creatinine levels in tests using Jaffé reaction. Ceftazidime may cause positive Coombs' test results and elevated liver function test results.

— Regularly reevaluate the patient's and family's knowledge about ceftazidime therapy.

Intervention

— Discontinue drug and notify the doctor if anaphylaxis occurs. Keep epinephrine readily available to treat anaphylaxis.

— Change I.V. site every 48 to 72 hours to prevent phlebitis. Manufacturer recommends discontinuing other I.V. solutions during I.V. administration of cephalosporins.

— If the patient develops an adverse reaction, notify the doctor for appropriate treatment and provide supportive care as indicated.

— Keep all health care team members advised of patient's response to the drug.

Patient teaching

— Instruct the patient and family about ceftazidime, including the dosage, frequency, action, and adverse reactions.

— Explain the disease process and rationale for therapy.

— Inform the patient that I.M. or I.V. administration may cause pain, inflammation, or tenderness at the injection site.

— Tell the patient to notify the nurse or doctor if adverse reactions develop or questions arise about ceftazidime therapy.

Evaluation

In the patient receiving ceftazidime, appropriate evaluation statements include:

• Patient is free of infection.
• Patient is free of pain at injection site.
• Patient and family state an understanding of ceftazidime therapy.

SELECTED MAJOR DRUGS: CEPHALOSPORINS

DRUG, INDICATIONS, AND DOSAGES	SPECIAL PRECAUTIONS

First-generation cephalosporins

cefadroxil (Duricef, Ultracef)
Urinary tract infections caused by Escherichia coli, Proteus mirabilis, *and* Klebsiella; *infections of skin and soft tissue; and streptococcal pharyngitis—*
Adults: 500 mg to 2 g P.O. daily, depending on the infection being treated. Usually given once daily or b.i.d.
Children: 30 mg/kg P.O. daily in two divided doses.

• Contraindicated in patients with hypersensitivity to other cephalosporins.
• Use cautiously in patients with impaired renal function and in those with a history of sensitivity to penicillins. Ask the patient if he's had any reaction to previous cephalosporin or penicillin therapy before administering first dose.

---

cefazolin (Ancel, Kefzol)
Serious infections of respiratory and GU tracts, skin and soft-tissue infections, bone and joint infections, septicemia, and endocarditis due to Escherichia coli, Enterobacteriaceae, *gonococci,* Haemophilus influenzae, Klebsiella, Proteus mirabilis, Staphylococcus aureus, Streptococcus pneumoniae, *and group A beta-hemolytic streptococci, and perioperative prophylaxis—*
Adults: 250 mg I.M. or I.V. q 8 hours to 1 g q 6 hours. Maximum is 12 g daily in life-threatening situations.
Children over age 1 month: 8 to 16 mg/kg I.M. or I.V. q 8 hours, or 6 to 12 mg/kg q 6 hours.
  Total daily dosage is same for I.M. or I.V. administration and depends on susceptibility of organism and severity of infection. In patients with impaired renal function, doses or frequency of administration must be modified according to degree of renal impairment, severity of infection, and susceptibility of organism. Should be injected deep I.M. into a large muscle mass, such as gluteus or lateral aspect of thigh.

• Contraindicated in patients with known allergies to cephalosporins.
• Use cautiously in patients with impaired renal function and in those with a history of sensitivity to penicillins. Ask the patient if he's ever had any reaction to cephalosporin or penicillin therapy before administering first dose.

---

cephalothin (Keflin)
Serious infections of respiratory, GU, or GI tract; skin and soft-tissue infections (including peritonitis); bone and joint infections; septicemia; and endocarditis due to Escherichia coli *and other coliform bacteria,* Enterobacteriaceae, *enterococci, gonococci, group A beta-hemolytic streptococci,* Haemophilus influenzae, Klebsiella, Proteus mirabilis, Salmonella, Staphylococcus aureus, Shigella, Streptococcus pneumoniae *and S.* viridans, *and staphylococci—*
Adults: 500 mg to 1 g I.M. or I.V. (or intraperitoneally) q 4 to 6 hours; in life-threatening infections, up to 2 g q 4 hours.
Children: 14 to 27 mg/kg I.V. q 4 hours, or 20 to 40 mg/kg q 6 hours; dose should be proportionately less in accordance with age, weight, and severity of infection.

• Use cautiously in patients with impaired renal function and in those with a history of sensitivity to penicillins. Ask the patient if he's had any reaction to previous cephalosporin or penicillin therapy before administering first dose.

(continued)

SELECTED MAJOR DRUGS: CEPHALOSPORINS *continued*

DRUG, INDICATIONS, AND DOSAGES

SPECIAL PRECAUTIONS

First-generation cephalosporins *(continued)*

cephalothin *(continued)*
Dosage schedule is determined by degree of renal impairment, severity of infection, and susceptibility of causative organism. Should be injected deep I.M. into a large muscle mass, such as gluteus or lateral aspect of thigh. I.V. route is preferable in severe or life-threatening infections.

cephapirin (Cefadyl)
Serious infections of respiratory, GU, or GI tract; skin and soft-tissue infections; bone and joint infections (including osteomyelitis); septicemia; endocarditis due to Streptococcus pneumoniae, Escherichia coli, *group A beta-hemolytic streptococci,* Haemophilus influenzae, Klebsiella, Proteus mirabilis, Staphylococcus aureus, *and* Streptococcus viridans—
Adults: 500 mg to 1 g I.V. or I.M. q 4 to 6 hours up to 12 g daily.
Children over age 3 months: 10 to 20 mg/kg I.V. or I.M. q 6 hours; dose depends on age, weight, and severity of infection.
Should be injected deep I.M. into a large muscle mass, such as gluteus or lateral aspect of thigh. Depending on causative organism and severity of infection, patients with reduced renal function may be treated adequately with a lower dose (7.5 to 15 mg/kg q 12 hours). Patients with severely reduced renal function and who are to be dialyzed should receive same dose just before dialysis and q 12 hours thereafter.

• Use cautiously in patients with impaired renal function and in those with a history of sensitivity to penicillins. Ask the patient if he's had any reaction to previous cephalosporin or penicillin therapy before administering first dose.

cephradine (Anspor, Velosef)
Serious infections of respiratory, GU, or GI tract; skin and soft-tissue infections; bone and joint infections; septicemia; endocarditis; and otitis media due to Escherichia coli *and other coliform bacteria, group A beta-hemolytic streptococci,* Haemophilus influenzae, Klebsiella, Proteus mirabilis, Staphylococcus aureus, Streptococcus pneumoniae *and* S. viridans, *and staphylococci*—
Adults: 500 mg to 1 g I.M. or I.V. b.i.d. to q.i.d.; do not exceed 8 g daily. Or 250 to 500 mg P.O. q 6 hours. Severe or chronic infections may require larger and/or more frequent doses (up to 1 g P.O. q 6 hours).
Children over age 1: 6 to 12 mg/kg P.O. q 6 hours. 12 to 25 mg/kg I.M. or I.V. q 6 hours.
Otitis media—19 to 25 mg/kg P.O. q 6 hours. Do not exceed 4 g daily.

• Contraindicated in patients with hypersensitivity to other cephalosporins.
• Use cautiously in patients with impaired renal function and in those with a history of sensitivity to penicillins. Ask the patient if he's had any reaction to previous cephalosporin or penicillin therapy before administering first dose.

SELECTED MAJOR DRUGS: CEPHALOSPORINS *continued*

DRUG, INDICATIONS, AND DOSAGES	SPECIAL PRECAUTIONS

First-generation cephalosporins *(continued)*

cephradine *(continued)*
All patients, regardless of age and weight: larger doses (up to 1 g q.i.d.) may be given for severe or chronic infections. Parenteral therapy may be followed by oral therapy. Injections should be given deep I.M. into a large muscle mass, such as gluteus or lateral aspect of thigh.

Second-generation cephalosporins

cefamandole (Mandol)
Serious infections of respiratory and GU tracts, skin and soft-tissue infections, bone and joint infections, septicemia, and peritonitis due to Escherichia coli *and other coliform bacteria,* Staphylococcus aureus *(penicillinase- and non-penicillinase-producing),* S. epidermidis, *group A beta-hemolytic streptococci,* Klebsiella, Haemophilus influenzae, Proteus mirabilis, *and* Enterobacter—
Adults: 500 mg to 1 g q 4 to 8 hours. If life-threatening infections, up to 2 g q 4 hours may be needed.
Infants and children: 50 to 100 mg/kg daily in equally divided doses q 4 to 8 hours. May be increased to total dose of 150 mg/kg daily (not to exceed maximum adult dose) for severe infections.
Total daily dosage is same for I.M. or I.V. administration and depends on susceptibility of organism and severity of infection. In patients with impaired renal function, doses or frequency of administration must be modified according to degree of renal impairment, severity of infection, and susceptibility of organism. Should be injected deep I.M. into a large muscle mass, such as gluteus or lateral aspect of thigh.

• Contraindicated in patients with hypersensitivity to other cephalosporins.
• Use cautiously in patients with impaired renal function and in those with a history of sensitivity to penicillins. Ask the patient if he's had any reaction to previous cephalosporin or penicillin therapy before administering first dose.

cefmetazole (Zefazone)
Lower respiratory tract infections caused by Streptococcus pneumoniae, Staphylococcus aureus *(penicillinase- and non-penicillinase-producing strains),* Escherichia coli, *and* Haemophilus influenzae *(non-penicillinase-producing strains); intra-abdominal infections caused by* E. coli *or* Bacteroides fragilis; *skin and skin structure infections caused by* S. aureus *(penicillinase- and non-penicillinase-producing strains),* S. epidermidis, Streptococcus pyogenes, S. agalactiae, E. coli, Proteus mirabilis, Klebsiella pneumoniae, *and* B. fragilis—
Adults: 2 g I.V. q 6 to 12 hours for 5 to 14 days.
Urinary tract infections caused by E. coli—
Adults: 2 g I.V. q 12 hours.

• Contraindicated in patients with hypersensitivity to cephalosporins. Ask the patient if he's had any reaction to previous cephalosporin or penicillin therapy before administering first dose.
• Administer cautiously to patients with renal impairment; to pregnant or breast-feeding women; to children; and to those at risk for carcinogenesis, mutagenesis, or impaired fertility.

(continued)

SELECTED MAJOR DRUGS: CEPHALOSPORINS *continued*

DRUG, INDICATIONS, AND DOSAGES	SPECIAL PRECAUTIONS

Second-generation cephalosporins *(continued)*

cefmetazole *(continued)*
Prophylaxis in patients undergoing vaginal hysterectomy—
Adults: 2 g I.V. 30 to 90 minutes before surgery as a single dose; or 1 g I.V. 30 to 90 minutes before surgery, repeated in 8 and 16 hours.
Prophylaxis in patients undergoing abdominal hysterectomy—
Adults: 1 g I.V. 30 to 90 minutes before surgery, repeated in 8 and 16 hours.
Prophylaxis in patients undergoing cesarean section—
Adults: 2 g I.V. as a single dose after clamping cord; or 1 g I.V. after clamping cord, repeated in 8 and 16 hours.
Prophylaxis in patients undergoing colorectal surgery—
Adults: 2 g I.V. as a single dose 30 to 90 minutes before surgery. Some clinicians follow with additional 2-g doses in 8 and 16 hours.
Prophylaxis in patients undergoing cholecystectomy (high risk)—
Adults: 1 g I.V. 30 to 90 minutes before surgery, repeated in 8 and 16 hours.

---

cefonicid (Monocid)
Serious infections of the lower respiratory and urinary tracts; skin and skin structure infections; septicemia; and bone and joint infections. Susceptible microorganisms include Streptococcus pneumoniae, S. pyogenes, Klebsiella pneumoniae, Escherichia coli, Haemophilus influenzae, Proteus mirabilis, Staphylococcus aureus, *and* S. epidermidis—
Adults: usual dosage is 1 g I.V. or I.M. q 24 hours; in life-threatening infections, 2 g q 24 hours.

Total daily dosage is same for I.M. or I.V. administration and depends on susceptibility of oragnism and severity of infection. In patients with impaired renal function, doses or frequency of administration must be modified according to degree of renal impairment, severity of infection, and susceptibility of organism. Should be injected deep I.M. into a large muscle mass, such as gluteus or lateral aspect of thigh.

• Contraindicated in patients with hypersensitivity to other cephalosporins.
• Use cautiously in patients with impaired renal function and in those with a history of sensitivity to penicillins. Ask the patient if he's had any reaction to previous cephalosporin or penicillin therapy before administering first dose.

---

ceforanide (Precef)
Serious infections of the lower respiratory and urinary tracts, skin and skin structure infections, endocarditis, septicemia, and bone and joint infections. Susceptible microorganisms include Streptococcus pneumoniae *and* S. pyogenes, Klebsiella pneumoniae, Escherichia coli, Haemophilus influenzae, Proteus mirabilis, *and* Staphylococcus aureus *and* S. epidermidis—

• Contraindicated in patients with hypersensitivity to other cephalosporins.
• Use cautiously in patients with impaired renal function and in those with a history of sensitivity to penicillins. Ask the patient if he's had a previous

SELECTED MAJOR DRUGS: CEPHALOSPORINS *continued*

DRUG, INDICATIONS, AND DOSAGES	SPECIAL PRECAUTIONS

Second-generation cephalosporins *(continued)*

ceforanide *(continued)*
Adults: 0.5 to 1 g I.V. or I.M. q 12 hours.
Children: 20 to 40 mg/kg daily in equally divided doses q 12 hours.
Prophylaxis in surgical infections—
Adults: 0.5 to 1 g I.M. or I.V. 1 hour before surgery.
   Total daily dosage is same for I.M. or I.V. administration and depends on susceptibility of organism and severity of infection. In patients with impaired renal function, doses or frequency of administration must be modified according to degree of renal impairment, severity of infection, and susceptibility of organism. Should be injected deep I.M. into a large muscle mass, such as gluteus or lateral aspect of thigh.

reaction to cephalosporin or penicillin therapy before administering first dose.

cefotetan (Cefotan)
Serious infections of the urinary and lower respiratory tracts; gynecologic, skin and skin structure, intra-abdominal, and bone and joint infections. Among susceptible microorganisms are streptococci, Staphylococcus aureus *(penicillinase- and non-penicillinase-producing) and* S. epidermidis, Escherichia coli, Klebsiella, Enterobacter, Proteus, Haemophilus influenzae, Neisseria gonorrhoeae, *and* Bacteroides, *including* B. fragilis—
Adults: 1 to 2 g I.V. or I.M. q 12 hours for 5 to 10 days. Up to 6 g daily in life-threatening infections.
   Total daily dosage is same for I.M. or I.V. administration and depends on susceptibility of organism and severity of infection. In patients with impaired renal function, doses or frequency of administration must be modified according ot degree of renal impairment, severity of infection, and susceptibility of organism. Should be injected deep I.M. into a large muscle mass, such as gluteus or lateral aspect of thigh.

• Contraindicated in patients with hypersensitivity to other cephalosporins.
• Use cautiously in patients with impaired renal status and in those with a history of sensitivity to penicillins. Ask the patient if he's had any reaction to previous cephalosporin or penicillin therapy before administering first dose.

cefoxitin (Mefoxin)
Serious infections of respiratory and GU tracts, skin and soft-tissue infections, bone and joint infections, bloodstream and intra-abdominal infections caused by Escherichia coli *and other coliform bacteria,* Staphylococcus aureus *(penicillinase- and non-penicillinase-producing) and* S. epidermidis, streptococci, Klebsiella, Haemophilus influenzae, *and* Bacteroides, *including* B. fragilis—
Adults: 1 to 2 g q 6 to 8 hours for uncomplicated forms of infection. Up to 12 g daily in life-threatening infections.
Children: 80 to 160 mg/kg daily in four to six equally divided doses.

• Contraindicated in patients with hypersensitivity to other cephalosporins.
• Use cautiously in patients with impaired renal status and in those with a history of sensitivity to penicillins. Ask the patient if he's had any reaction to previous cephalosporin or penicillin therapy before administering first dose.

(continued)

SELECTED MAJOR DRUGS: CEPHALOSPORINS *continued*

DRUG, INDICATIONS, AND DOSAGES	SPECIAL PRECAUTIONS

Second-generation cephalosporins *(continued)*

cefoxitin *(continued)*
Total daily dosage is same for I.M. or I.V. administration and depends on susceptibility of organism and severity of infection. In patients with impaired renal function, doses or frequency of administration must be modified according to degree of renal impairment, severity of infection, and susceptibility of organism. Should be injected deep I.M. into a large muscle mass, such as gluteus or lateral aspect of thigh.

cefuroxime axetil (Ceftin)
cefuroxime sodium (Kefurox, Zinacef)
Serious infections of the lower respiratory and urinary tracts, skin and skin structure infections, septicemia, meningitis, and gonorrhea. Among susceptible organisms are Streptococcus pneumoniae *and* S. pyogenes, Haemophilus influenzae, Klebsiella, Staphylococcus aureus, Escherichia coli, Enterobacter, *and* Neisseria gonorrhoeae —
Adults: usual dosage of (sodium) is 750 mg to 1.5 g I.M. or I.V. q 8 hours, usually for 5 to 10 days. For life-threatening infections and infections caused by less susceptible organisms, 1.5 g I.M. or I.V. q 6 hours; for bacterial meningitis, up to 3 g I.V. q 6 hours.
Alternatively, administer (axetil) 250 mg P.O. q 12 hours. For severe infections or less susceptible organisms, dosage may be increased to 500 mg P.O. q 12 hours.
Children and infants over age 3 months: 50 to 100 mg/kg daily (sodium) I.M. or I.V. Higher doses are administered when treating meningitis. Alternatively, give (axetil) 125 mg P.O. q 12 hours.
Uncomplicated urinary tract infections —
Adults: 125 to 250 mg P.O. q 12 hours.
Otitis media —
Children under age 2: 125 mg P.O. q 12 hours.
Children ages 2 and over: 250 mg P.O. q 12 hours.

• Contraindicated in patients with known hypersensitivity to other cephalosporins.
• Use cautiously in patients with impaired renal function and in those with a history of sensitivity to penicillins. Ask the patient if he's had any reaction to previous cephalosporin or penicillin therapy before administering first dose.

Third-generation cephalosporins

cefixime (Suprax)
Uncomplicated urinary tract infections caused by Escherichia coli *and* Proteus mirabilis; *otitis media caused by* Haemophilus influenzae *(beta-lactamase positive and negative strains),* Branhamella catarrhalis, *and* Streptococcus pyogenes; *pharyngitis and tonsillitis caused by* S. pyogenes; *acute bronchitis and acute exacerbations of chronic bronchitis caused by* S. pneumoniae *and* H. influenzae *(beta-lactamase positive and negative strains) —*

• Contraindicated in patients with hypersensitivity to other cephalosporins.
• Use cautiously and with reduced dosage in patients with renal dysfunction. Use cautiously in patients with a history of sensitivity to penicillins. Ask the patient if he's had any reaction to previous cephalospo-

SELECTED MAJOR DRUGS: CEPHALOSPORINS *continued*

DRUG, INDICATIONS, AND DOSAGES	SPECIAL PRECAUTIONS

Third-generation cephalosporins *(continued)*

cefixime *(continued)*
Adults: 400 mg P.O. daily as a single 400-mg tablet or 200 mg q 12 hours.
Children: 8 mg/kg oral suspension daily as a single dose or 4 mg/kg P.O. q 12 hours.
   Treat children over age 12 and those who weigh more than 50 kg with the recommended dose.

rin or penicillin therapy before administering first dose.

---

cefoperazone (Cefobid)
Serious infections of the respiratory tract; intra-abdominal, gynecologic, and skin infections; bacteremia; septicemia. Susceptible microorganisms include Streptococcus pneumoniae *and* S. pyogenes; Staphylococcus aureus *(penicillinase- and non-penicillinase-producing) and* S. epidermidis; enterococcus; Escherichia coli; Klebsiella; Haemophilus influenzae; Enterobacter; Citrobacter; Proteus; *some* Pseudomonas, *including* P. aeruginosa; *and* Bacteroides fragilis —
Adults: usual dosage is 1 to 2 g q 12 hours I.M. or I.V. In severe infections, or infections caused by less sensitive organisms, the total daily dosage or frequency may be increased up to 16 g daily in certain situations.
   No dosage adjustment is usually necessary in patients with renal impairment. However, doses of 4 g daily should be given very cautiously in patients with hepatic disease. Should be injected deep I.M. into a large muscle mass, such as gluteus or lateral aspect of the thigh.

• Contraindicated in patients with hypersensitivity to other cephalosporins.
• Use cautiously in patients with impaired renal function and in those with a history of sensitivity to penicillins. Ask the patient if he's had any reaction to previous cephalosporin or penicillin therapy before administering first dose.

---

cefotaxime (Claforan)
Serious infections of the lower respiratory and urinary tracts, CNS infections, gynecologic infections, bacteremia, septicemia, skin infections. Among susceptible microorganisms are streptococci, including Streptococcus pneumoniae *and* S. pyogenes; Staphylococcus aureus *(penicillinase- and non-penicillinase-producing) and* S. epidermidis; Escherichia coli; Klebsiella; Haemophilus influenzae; Enterobacter; Proteus; *and* Peptostreptococcus —
Adults: usual dose is 1 g I.V. or I.M. q 6 to 8 hours. Up to 12 g daily can be administered in life-threatening infections.
   Total daily dosage is same for I.M. or I.V. administration and depends on susceptibility of organism and severity of infection. In patients with impaired renal function, doses or frequency of administration must be modified according to degree of renal impairment, severity of infection, and susceptibility of organism. Should

• Contraindicated in patients with hypersensitivity to other cephalosporins.
• Use cautiously in patients with impaired renal function and in those with a history of sensitivity to penicillins. Ask the patient if he's had any reaction to previous cephalosporin or penicillin therapy before administering first dose.

(continued)

SELECTED MAJOR DRUGS: CEPHALOSPORINS *continued*

DRUG, INDICATIONS, AND DOSAGES	SPECIAL PRECAUTIONS

Third-generation cephalosporins *(continued)*

cefotaxime *(continued)*
be injected deep I.M. into a large muscle mass, such as
gluteus or lateral aspect of thigh.
Children age 1 month to 12 years: 50 to 180 mg/kg
I.M. or I.V. daily in four to six divided doses.
Neonates to age 1 week: 50 mg/kg I.V. q 12 hours.
Neonates ages 1 to 4 weeks: 50 mg/kg I.V. q 8 hours.

ceftizoxime (Cefizox)
*Serious infections of the lower respiratory and urinary
tracts, gynecologic infections, bacteremia, septicemia,
meningitis, intra-abdominal infections, bone and joint infections, and skin infections. Among susceptible microorganisms are streptococci, including* Streptococcus
pneumoniae *and* S. pyogenes; Staphylococcus aureus
(penicillinase- and non-penicillinase-producing) and S.
epidermidis; Escherichia coli; Klebsiella; Haemophilus influenzae; Enterobacter; Proteus; *some* Pseudomonas; *and*
Peptostreptococcus —
Adults: usual dosage is 1 to 2 g I.V. or I.M. q 8 to 12
hours. In life-threatening infections, up to 2 g q 4 hours.
   Total daily dosage is same for I.M. or I.V. administration and depends on susceptibility of organism and severity of infection. In patients with impaired renal
function, doses or frequency of administration must be
modified according to degree of renal impairment, severity of infection, and susceptibility of organism. Should
be injected deep I.M. into a large muscle mass, such as
gluteus or lateral aspect of thigh.

- Contraindicated in patients
with hypersensitivity to other
cephalosporins.
- Use cautiously in patients
with impaired renal function and
in those with a history of sensitivity to penicillins. Ask the patient if he's had any reaction to
previous cephalosporin or penicillin therapy before administering first dose.

ceftriaxone (Rocephin)
*Serious infections of the lower respiratory and urinary
tracts, gynecologic infections, bacteremia, septicemia,
intra-abdominal infections, skin infections, and Lyme
disease. Susceptible microorganisms are streptococci,
including* Streptococcus pneumoniae *and* S. pyogenes;
Staphylococcus aureus *(penicillinase- and non-penicillin-
ase-producing) and* S. epidermidis; Escherichia coli;
Klebsiella; Haemophilus influenzae; Neisseria meningitidis;
Enterobacter; Proteus; Pseudomonas; Peptostreptococcus, *and* Serratia marcescens —
Adults: 1 to 2 g I.M. or I.V. daily or in equally divided
doses. Total dose should not exceed 4 g daily.
Children: 50 to 75 mg/kg in divided doses q 12 hours.
Treatment of meningitis —
Adults and children: 100 mg/kg in divided doses q 12
hours. May give loading dose of 75 mg/kg.
   Total daily dose is same for I.M. or I.V. administration
and depends on susceptibility of organism and severity
of infection. Should be injected deep I.M. into a large
muscle mass, such as gluteus or lateral aspect of thigh.

- Contraindicated in patients
with hypersensitivity to other
cephalosporins.
- Administer cautiously to patients with a history of sensitivity to penicillins.

SELECTED MAJOR DRUGS: CEPHALOSPORINS *continued*

DRUG, INDICATIONS, AND DOSAGES	SPECIAL PRECAUTIONS

Third-generation cephalosporins *(continued)*

moxalactam (Moxam)
Serious infections of lower respiratory and urinary tract, CNS infections, intra-abdominal infections, gynecologic infections, bacteremia, septicemia, and skin infections. Susceptible microorganisms include Streptococcus pneumoniae *and* S. pyogenes; Staphylococcus aureus *(penicillinase- and non-penicillinase-producing) and* S. epidermidis; Escherichia coli; Klebsiella; Haemophilus influenzae; Enterobacter; Proteus; *some* Pseudomonas; *and* Peptostreptococcus —
Adults: usual dose is 2 to 6 g I.M. or I.V. daily in divided doses q 8 hours for 5 to 10 days, or up to 14 days. Up to 12 g daily may be needed in life-threatening infections or in infections due to less susceptible organisms.
Children: 50 mg/kg I.M. or I.V. q 6 to 8 hours.
Neonates: 50 mg/kg I.M. or I.V. q 8 to 12 hours.
  Total daily dosage is same for I.M. or I.V. administration and depends on susceptibility of organism and severity of infection. In patients with impaired renal function, doses or frequency of administration must be modified according to degree of impairment, severity of infection, and susceptibility of organism. Should be injected deep I.M. into the gluteus or lateral aspect of thigh.

• Contraindicated in patients with hypersensitivity to other cephalosporins.
• Use cautiously in patients with impaired renal function and in those with a history of sensitivity to penicillins. Before giving first dose, ask the patient if he's had any previous reaction to penicillins.

SELF-TEST

1. Joseph Essex, age 75, has undergone surgery to repair a fractured hip. Postoperative orders include ceftazidime 1 g I.V. q 8 hours. The nurse should infuse it:
  a. within 5 minutes.
  b. over 30 minutes.
  c. over 1 hour.
  d. over 2 hours.

2. Before administering the first dose, the nurse takes a drug history. She is especially concerned about any previous reactions to:
  a. penicillins.
  b. tetracyclines.
  c. aminoglycosides.
  d. sulfonamides.

3. On the second postoperative day, an oral cephalosporin, cephalexin, is substituted. The nurse should administer it:

a. q 8 hours to maintain a blood level.

b. at least 1 hour before or 2 hours after a meal.

c. until signs of infection are resolved.

d. with food or milk to minimize GI distress.

Check your answers on pages 1058 and 1059.

CHAPTER 13

TETRACYCLINES

demeclocycline hydrochloride ✦ doxycycline hyclate
minocycline hydrochloride ✦ oxytetracycline hydrochloride
tetracycline hydrochloride

OVERVIEW
- Tetracyclines are bacteriostatic antibiotics with broad activity against gram-positive and gram-negative bacteria, *Mycoplasma, Chlamydia,* and *Rickettsia.* Since chlortetracycline was first isolated in 1948, the pharmacologic and microbiologic effects of tetracyclines have been modified. However, because of widespread microbial resistance (for example, *Proteus* and *Pseudomonas* infection), tetracyclines are the drugs of choice in only a few clinical situations.

MAJOR USES
- Tetracyclines are used in prophylaxis and therapy of numerous bacterial diseases, especially of the mixed type, such as chronic bronchitis and peritonitis. They are drugs of choice in treatment of bubonic plague, brucellosis, cholera, mycoplasmosis, trachoma, lymphogranuloma venereum, and Rocky Mountain spotted fever. Tetracyclines are alternative therapeutic agents for syphilis, gonorrhea, anthrax, nocardiosis, and *Haemophilus influenzae* respiratory infections. Tetracyclines are effective against uncomplicated urinary tract infections from susceptible strains of *Escherichia coli, Klebsiella, Enterobacter,* and *Citrobacter* and in exacerbations of chronic bronchitis. Oral or topical tetracyclines are therapeutic against acne vulgaris.
- Minocycline is prophylactic in meningococcal infections when rifampin is contraindicated.
- Demeclocycline is a useful adjunct for treating SIADH.

MECHANISM OF ACTION
- Tetracyclines are thought to exert a bacteriostatic effect by binding to the 30S ribosomal subunit of microorganisms, thus inhibiting protein synthesis.

ABSORPTION, DISTRIBUTION, METABOLISM, AND EXCRETION
Most tetracyclines are readily absorbed (60% to 80%) after oral administration to fasting patients. Food, milk, or certain cations (including calcium, magnesium, zinc, and iron) may bind with tetracyclines in the GI tract and decrease their absorption.

GLOSSARY

Ribosome: one of the minute granules composed of nucleic acid, attached to the membranes of the endoplasmic reticulum of a cell where cellular protein synthesis occurs.

Thrush: fungal infection characterized by whitish spots and shallow ulcers in the oral cavity, fever, and GI irritation; usually results from superinfection.

Tetracyclines are widely distributed in most body fluids, including bile, sinus secretions, and synovial, pleural, and ascitic fluids. CSF levels vary, but the drugs tend to diffuse well when the meninges are inflamed; the drugs accumulate in bones, liver, spleen, and teeth.

Doxycycline and minocycline are partially metabolized by the liver; their elimination routes are unclear. The rest of the tetracyclines are eliminated unchanged in the feces (through the bile) and urine.

ONSET AND DURATION

Blood levels after oral administration peak in 2 to 4 hours. Blood levels of 1 to 3 mcg/ml persist for 6 or more hours. (Doxycycline and minocycline give the most prolonged blood levels.) Half-lives—hence blood levels—of all tetracyclines except doxycycline are prolonged in patients with severe renal impairment.

ADVERSE REACTIONS

Hepatic toxicity can result from high doses of tetracyclines or from use in patients with renal impairment; accumulation of drug in such patients may result in liver toxicity.

I.V. administration may produce rapid, high blood levels. Be sure to dilute the dose and give it slowly; phlebitis of the injected vein is common. Avoid extravasation.

Tetracyclines exhibit an antianabolic effect and may increase BUN levels. In patients with renal disease, reactions to tetracyclines (except doxycycline) can lead to worsening azotemia, hyperphosphatemia, and acidosis.

Photosensitivity reactions have been reported with all tetracyclines but appear to be more severe with demeclocycline and less frequent with minocycline.

Nephrogenic diabetes insipidus as manifested by polyuria, polydipsia, and weakness has occurred in patients treated with demeclocycline and is reversible upon discontinuation of the drug.

Transient light-headedness and vertigo can occur in patients taking minocycline.

Tetracyclines should be avoided during pregnancy and breast-feeding and in children unless the benefits outweigh the potential risks. Tetracyclines can affect both bone growth and tooth formation. Permanent discoloration of teeth in children under age 8 can occur. Animal studies have reported evidence of embryotoxicity.

Other adverse reactions may include nausea, vomiting, loose stools, hairy tongue, *Candida* overgrowth, skin pigmentation. Rarely, Stevens-Johnson syndrome (with minocycline) and pseudotumor cerebri may be seen; infants may display bulging fontanels.

PROTOTYPE: TETRACYCLINES

TETRACYCLINE HYDROCHLORIDE
(tet ra sye' kleen)

Achromycin, Achromycin V, Apo-Tetra†, Austramycin V‡, Bristacycline, Cyclopar, Hostacycline P‡, Kesso-Tetra, NorTet, Novotetra†, Panmycin**, Panmycin P‡, Robitet, Sarocycline, Sumycin, Tetracap, Tetracyn, Tetralan, Tetralean†

Classification: tetracycline
Pregnancy risk category D

How supplied
TABLETS: 250 mg, 500 mg
CAPSULES: 250 mg, 500 mg
ORAL SUSPENSION: 125 mg/5 ml
INJECTION: 100 mg, 250 mg, 500 mg

Indications and dosage
Infections caused by sensitive gram-negative and gram-positive organisms, trachoma, rickettsiae, Mycoplasma, and Chlamydia
ADULTS: 250 to 500 mg P.O. q 6 hours; or 250 to 500 mg I.V. q 8 to 12 hours.
CHILDREN OVER AGE 8: 25 to 50 mg/kg P.O. daily divided q 6 hours; or 10 to 20 mg/kg I.V. daily divided q 12 hours.

Uncomplicated urethral, endocervical, or rectal infection caused by Chlamydia trachomatis
ADULTS: 500 mg P.O. q.i.d. for at least 7 days.

Brucellosis
ADULTS: 500 mg P.O. q 6 hours for 3 weeks with streptomycin 1 g I.M. q 12 hours week 1 and daily week 2.
Gonorrhea in patients sensitive to penicillin
ADULTS: initially, 1.5 g P.O., then 500 mg q 6 hours for 7 days.

Syphilis in patients sensitive to penicillin
ADULTS: 30 to 40 g P.O. total in equally divided doses over 10 to 15 days.

Acne
ADULTS AND ADOLESCENTS: initially, 250 mg P.O. q 6 hours, then 125 to 500 mg P.O. daily or every other day.

---

†Available in Canada only   **May contain tartrazine   ‡Available in Australia only

Contraindications and precautions

Tetracycline is contraindicated in patients with known hypersensitivity to the drug or other tetracyclines. Avoid use cautiously during tooth development (last half of pregnancy, and children under age 8). Use cautiously in patients with renal or hepatic impairment.

Adverse reactions

BLOOD: neutropenia, eosinophilia.
CNS: dizziness, headache, **intracranial hypertension**.
CV: pericarditis.
EENT: sore throat, glossitis, dysphagia.
GI: anorexia, *epigastric distress*, *nausea*, vomiting, diarrhea, stomatitis, enterocolitis, inflammatory lesions in anogenital region.
HEPATIC: hepatotoxicity with large doses given I.V.
METABOLIC: increased BUN level.
SKIN: maculopapular and erythematous rashes, urticaria, photosensitivity, increased pigmentation.
LOCAL: irritation after I.M. injection, thrombophlebitis.

Interactions

Antacids (including sodium bicarbonate) and laxatives containing aluminum, magnesium, or calcium; food, milk, or other dairy products: decrease antibiotic absorption. Give tetracycline at least 1 hour before or 2 hours after any of the above.
Ferrous sulfate and other iron products, zinc: decrease antibiotic absorption. Give tetracycline 3 hours after or 2 hours before iron administration.
Lithium carbonate: may alter serum lithium levels.
Methoxyflurane: may cause severe nephrotoxicity with tetracycline. Avoid concomitant use.
Oral contraceptives: decreased contraceptive effectiveness and increased risk of breakthrough bleeding. Instruct patient to use a non-hormonal (such as barrier) form of contraception during tetracycline therapy.
Penicillin: interference with the bactericidal action of penicillin. Avoid giving tetracycline with penicillin.

Nursing considerations

Assessment

- Review the patient's history for a condition that contraindicates the use of tetracycline.
- Obtain a baseline assessment of the patient's infection before therapy.
- Be alert for common adverse reactions.
- Evaluate the patient's and family's knowledge about tetracycline therapy.

Planning (Nursing Diagnoses)

Potential nursing diagnoses for the patient receiving tetracycline include:
- Potential for injury related to dosage regimen inadequate to alleviate infection.
- Altered protection related to development of superinfection caused by tetracycline therapy.

• Knowledge deficit related to tetracycline therapy.

Implementation

Preparation and administration

— Obtain specimen for culture and sensitivity tests before first dose. Therapy may begin pending test results.

— Effectiveness is reduced when taken with milk or other dairy products, food, antacids, sodium bicarbonate, or iron products. Explain this to patient. Administer oral tetracycline to patient with a full glass of water on an empty stomach, at least 1 hour before meals or 2 hours afterward. Give at least 1 hour before bedtime to prevent esophagitis.

— Shake liquid preparation before administering.

— Monitor I.V. injection sites and rotate routinely to minimize local irritation. I.V. administration may cause severe phlebitis.

— Do not administer oral form within 1 to 3 hours of other medications.

— Check expiration date. Outdated or deteriorated tetracyclines have been associated with reversible nephrotoxicity (Fanconi's syndrome).

— Do not expose to light or heat.

— For I.V. use, reconstitute 100-mg and 250-mg powder for injection with 5 ml sterile water; 500 mg, with 10 ml. Further dilute in 100 to 1,000 ml volume of dextrose 5% in 0.9% sodium chloride solution. Refrigerate diluted solution for I.V. use and use within 24 hours.

— Do not mix tetracycline solution with any other I.V. additive.

— Tetracycline may be used as a pleural sclerosing agent in malignant pleural effusion. The drug is instilled through a chest tube by a doctor familiar with the technique.

Monitoring

— Monitor the effectiveness of therapy by regularly assessing for improvement of infectious process.

— Monitor the patient for adverse drug reactions.

— Monitor for signs and symptoms of superinfection.

— Watch for overgrowth of nonsusceptible organisms. Assess for signs of bacterial and fungal superinfections. Check the patient's tongue for signs of monilia infection (thrush).

— Observe the patient for diarrhea, which may result from local irrigation or superinfection.

— Monitor laboratory test results. Parenteral form may cause false-positive reading of urine glucose by copper sulfate test (Clinitest). All forms may cause false-positives by glucose enzymatic tests (Clinistix or Tes-Tape). Tetracycline may also cause false elevations in fluorometric tests for urinary catecholamines and may elevate BUN levels in the patient with decreased renal function.

— Monitor the patient for drug interactions.

— For the patient receiving I.V. therapy, monitor injection sites for local reactions.

— Regularly reevaluate the patient's and family's knowledge about tetracycline therapy.

Intervention

—If the patient develops a superinfection, or new infection, notify the doctor. Prepare to stop the drug and administer another antibiotic. If the patient develops oral thrush, provide good mouth care.

—If the patient develops diarrhea, nausea, or vomiting, request an anti-emetic or antidiarrheal agent, if needed. Expect to switch to a parenteral form of tetracycline or to a different antibiotic as prescribed.

—If the patient is unable to comply with therapy, discuss reasons and suggest possible methods to improve compliance (for example, clues patient may use to remind himself to take drug).

—For the patient receiving I.V. therapy, rotate site to minimize irritation.

—Keep all health care team members advised of the patient's response to the drug.

Patient teaching

—Instruct the patient and family about tetracycline, including the dosage, frequency, action, and adverse reactions.

—Explain the disease process and rationale for therapy.

—Advise the patient to avoid direct exposure to sunlight and ultraviolet light and to use a sunscreen with a sun protection factor (SPF) of 15 or higher to help prevent photosensitivity reactions. Remind the patient that photosensitivity persists after discontinuation of drug.

—Tell the patient to take oral tetracycline with a full glass of water (to facilitate passage to the stomach), 1 hour before or 2 hours after meals for maximum absorption, and not less than 1 hour before bedtime (to prevent irritation from esophageal reflux).

—Tell the patient *not* to take the drug with food, milk or other dairy products, antacids, sodium bicarbonate, or iron compounds, as it may interfere with absorption. Tell the patient to take antacids 3 hours after tetracycline.

—Emphasize importance of completing prescribed regimen exactly as ordered and keeping follow-up appointments.

—Tell the patient to check expiration dates and discard any outdated tetracycline as it may become toxic.

—Teach the patient to report signs of superinfection (furry overgrowth on tongue, vaginal itch or discharge, foul-smelling stool). Stress good oral hygiene.

—Advise the female patient taking an oral contraceptive to use an alternative means of contraception during tetracycline therapy and for 1 week after therapy is discontinued.

—Tell the patient to notify the nurse or doctor if adverse reactions develop or concerns or questions arise about tetracycline therapy.

Evaluation

In the patient receiving tetracycline, appropriate evaluation statements include:

• Patient is free of infection.

• Patient remains free of superinfection during tetracycline therapy.

• Patient and family state an understanding of tetracycline therapy.

SELECTED MAJOR DRUGS: TETRACYCLINES

DRUG, INDICATIONS, AND DOSAGES

demeclocycline (Declomycin, Ledermycin‡)
Infections caused by susceptible gram-negative and gram-positive organisms, trachoma, rickettsiae—
Adults: 150 mg P.O. q 6 hours or 300 mg P.O. q 12 hours.
Children over age 8: 6 to 12 mg/kg P.O. daily divided q 6 to 12 hours.
Gonorrhea—
Adults: initially, 600 mg P.O., then 300 mg P.O. q 12 hours for 4 days (total 3 g).
Uncomplicated urethral, endocervical, or rectal infection caused by Chlamydia trachomatis—
Adults: 300 mg P.O. q.i.d. for at least 7 days.
SIADH (a hyposmolar state)—
Adults: 600 to 1,200 mg P.O. daily in divided doses.

doxycycline (Vibramycin)
Infections caused by sensitive gram-negative and gram-positive organisms, trachoma, rickettsiae, Mycoplasma, Chlamydia, *and Lyme disease—*
Adults: 100 mg P.O. q 12 hours on first day, then 100 mg P.O. daily; or 200 mg I.V. on first day in one or two infusions, then 100 to 200 mg I.V. daily.
Children over age 8 (under 45 kg): 4.4 mg/kg P.O. or I.V. daily divided q 12 hours first day, then 2.2 to 4.4 mg/kg daily. For children over 45 kg, dosage is same as adults. Give I.V. infusion slowly (minimum 1 hour). Infusion must be completed within 12 hours (within 6 hours in lactated Ringer's solution or dextrose 5% in lactated Ringer's solution).
Gonorrhea in patients allergic to penicillin—
Adults: initially, 200 mg P.O., followed by 100 mg P.O. h.s. and 100 mg b.i.d. for 3 days; or 300 mg initially and repeat dose in 1 hour.
Primary or secondary syphilis in patients allergic to penicillin—
Adults: 300 mg P.O. daily in divided doses for 10 days.
Uncomplicated urethral, endocervical or rectal infections caused by Chlamydia trachomatis *or* Ureaplasma urealyticum—
Adults: 100 mg P.O. b.i.d. for at least 7 days.
To prevent "traveler's diarrhea" commonly caused by enterotoxigenic Escherichia coli—
Adults: 100 mg P.O. daily.

minocycline (Minocin)
Infections caused by sensitive gram-negative and gram-positive organisms, trachoma, amebiasis—
Adults: 200 mg I.V., then 100 mg I.V. q 12 hours. Do not exceed 400 mg daily. Or give 200 mg P.O. initially, then 100 mg P.O. q 12 hours. Some clinicians use 100 or 200 mg P.O. initially, followed by 50 mg q.i.d.

SPECIAL PRECAUTIONS

• Contraindicated in patients with known hypersensitivity to any of the tetracyclines.
• Use with extreme caution in patients with impaired renal or hepatic function. Use of these drugs during last half of pregnancy and in children under age 8 may cause permanent discoloration of teeth, enamel defects, and retardation of bone growth.

• Contraindicated in patients with known hypersensitivity to any of the tetracyclines.
• Use of these drugs during last half of pregnancy and in children under age 8 may cause permanent discoloration of teeth, enamel defects, and retardation of bone growth.

• Contraindicated in patients with known hypersensitivity to any of the tetracyclines.
• Use with extreme caution in patients with impaired renal or hepatic function. Use during last half of pregnancy and in chil-

(continued)

‡Available in Australia only

SELECTED MAJOR DRUGS: TETRACYCLINES *continued*

DRUG, INDICATIONS, AND DOSAGES

minocycline *(continued)*
Children over age 8: initially, 4 mg/kg P.O. or I.V., followed by 2 mg/kg q 12 hours. Give I.V. in 500- to 1,000-ml solution without calcium, and administer over 6 hours.
Gonorrhea in patients sensitive to penicillin—
Adults: initially, 200 mg P.O., then 100 mg q 12 hours for 4 days.
Syphilis in patients sensitive to penicillin—
Adults: initially, 200 mg P.O. then 100 mg q 12 hours for 10 to 15 days.
Meningococcal carrier state—
Adults: 100 mg P.O. q 12 hours for 5 days.
Uncomplicated urethral, endocervical, or rectal infection caused by Chlamydia trachomatis *or* Ureaplasma urealyticum—
Adults: 100 mg P.O. b.i.d. for at least 7 days.
Uncomplicated gonococcal urethritis in men—
Adults: 100 mg P.O. b.i.d. for 5 days.

oxytetracycline (Terramycin)
Infections caused by sensitive gram-negative and gram-positive organisms, trachoma, rickettsiae—
Adults: 250 mg P.O. q 6 hours; 100 mg I.M. q 8 to 12 hours; 250 mg I.M. as a single dose.
Children over age 8: 25 to 50 mg/kg P.O. daily in divided doses q 6 hours; 15 to 25 mg/kg I.M. daily in divided doses q 8 to 12 hours.
Brucellosis—
Adults: 500 mg P.O. q.i.d. for 3 weeks with streptomycin 1 g I.M. q 12 hours first week, once daily second week.
Syphilis in patients sensitive to penicillin—
Adults: 30 to 40 g P.O. divided equally over 10 to 15 days.
Gonorrhea in patients sensitive to penicillin—
Adults: initially, 1.5 g P.O., followed by 0.5 g q.i.d. for a total of 9 g.

SPECIAL PRECAUTIONS

dren under age 8 may cause permanent discoloration of teeth, enamel defects, and retardation of bone growth.

• Contraindicated in patients with epithelial herpes simplex keratitis, vaccinia, varicella, and many other viral diseases of the cornea and conjunctiva; mycobacterial infection of the eye; fungal diseases of ocular structures; or hypersensitivity to a compound of the medication.
• Use with extreme caution in patients with impaired renal or hepatic function. Use during last half of pregnancy and in children under age 8 may cause permanent discoloration of teeth, enamel defects, and retardation of bone growth.

SELF-TEST

1. Agnes Marshall, a 41-year-old university professor, will be traveling to the Middle East on a study tour. Her doctor prescribed tetracycline as prophylaxis for the organisms endemic in that area. In teaching Ms. Marshall about this medication, the nurse tells her:
   a. Take the drug with a full glass of water on an empty stomach to enhance absorption.
   b. Take the drug with food or an antacid to prevent esophagitis.
   c. Heat or light exposure does not affect the drug.
   d. A superinfection usually does not occur with this drug.

2. If Ms. Marshall were to become pregnant, this drug would be contraindicated during the last half of pregnancy because:

a. it is teratogenic.

b. it causes blurred vision.

c. it may cause permanent discoloration of her child's teeth.

d. pregnant women should not take any drugs.

3. Ms. Marshall is instructed to discard any leftover medication when
she returns because outdated tetracycline can cause which of the
following toxic reactions?

a. reversible nephrotoxicity

b. irreversible nephrotoxicity

c. hepatotoxicity

d. cardiomyotoxicity

Check your answers on page 1059.

CHAPTER 14

SULFONAMIDES

co-trimoxazole ✦ sulfadiazine ✦ sulfamethizole ✦ sulfamethoxazole
sulfapyridine ✦ sulfasalazine ✦ sulfisoxazole

OVERVIEW

- Sulfonamides were the first drugs to be used systemically for the treatment of bacterial infections in humans. First used clinically in the mid-1930s, sulfonamides significantly reduced incidence of morbidity and mortality of the treatable infectious diseases.

MAJOR USES

- Although increased microbial resistance in recent years has limited their utility, sulfonamides are still the drugs of choice for urinary tract infections, otitis media, conjunctivitis, toxoplasmosis, and trachoma.
- Co-trimoxazole is a primary prophylactic and therapeutic drug for acute and chronic urinary tract infections. It is therapeutic for bacterial prostatitis, shigellosis, otitis media, and *Pneumocystis carinii* pneumonia. It may also combat infections caused by organisms resistant to the simple sulfonamides (*Escherichia coli,* for example, which is resistant to sulfisoxazole).
- Sulfamethizole, sulfamethoxazole, and sulfisoxazole are useful in the treatment of cystitis and pyelonephritis caused by susceptible strains of *E. coli, Klebsiella, Staphylococcus aureus,* and *Proteus mirabilis.* Co-trimoxazole, sulfadiazine, sulfamethoxazole, and sulfisoxazole are also used in the treatment of chancroid, trachoma, and nocardiosis. They are effective against *Haemophilus influenzae* otitis media when combined with penicillin and against toxoplasmosis when combined with pyrimethamine.
- Sulfadiazine may be prophylactic for rheumatic heart disease in patients allergic to penicillin.
- Sulfapyridine is therapeutic for dermatitis herpetiformis.
- Sulfasalazine is useful in treating mild to moderate ulcerative colitis.

MECHANISM OF ACTION

- Sulfonamides have a broad spectrum of antibacterial action and are bacteriostatic. Chemically similar to PABA, these drugs competitively inhibit dihydropteroate synthetase, a bacterial enzyme responsible for incorporation of PABA into dihydrofolic acid (folic acid). This mechanism blocks folic acid synthesis. Therefore, nucleic acids—essential building blocks of the bacterial cell—cannot be synthesized. Bacteria are susceptible because they must synthesize their own folic acid.

GLOSSARY

Antibacterial: substance, derived from cultures or semisynthetically produced, that inhibits bacterial growth or kills bacteria.
Microbial: pertaining to minute living organisms capable of producing disease, including bacteria, protozoa, and fungi.
Spectrum: range of bacteria affected by an antibacterial.

ABSORPTION, DISTRIBUTION, METABOLISM, AND EXCRETION

Sulfonamides are rapidly and adequately absorbed from the GI tract, except for sulfasalazine, which is designed to produce a local effect in the bowel and is absorbed at a rate of only 10% to 15%. All sulfonamides are readily distributed throughout the body, largely metabolized in the liver, and excreted in the urine (excretion rate increases with alkaline urine).

ONSET AND DURATION

Peak blood levels of sulfonamides usually appear 2 to 8 hours after oral administration and within minutes after I.V. administration.

Co-trimoxazole and sulfamethoxazole have half-lives of 12 hours and may be administered twice daily. Sulfadiazine, sulfamethizole, sulfapyridine, and sulfisoxazole have half-lives of 4 to 6 hours and are usually administered four times daily. Sulfasalazine, usually administered several times daily, has a half-life of 4 to 10 hours.

ADVERSE REACTIONS

Hypersensitivity reactions are among the most severe adverse reactions to sulfonamides. Stevens-Johnson syndrome and Mucha-Habermann disease are two of the most serious. They are characterized by skin eruptions, epidermal necrolysis, urticaria, exfoliative dermatitis, anaphylactoid reactions, periorbital edema, conjunctival and scleral injection, arthralgia, eosinophilia, and sometimes decreased pulmonary function. Some reactions require immediate discontinuation of the drug.

Sulfonamides should be used cautiously in patients with decreased renal function because they can cause hematuria, crystalluria, proteinuria, nephrotic syndrome, oliguria, and anuria in normal patients.

Sulfonamides can cause agranulocytosis, anemia, leukopenia, and thrombocytopenia, as well as hemolytic anemia in patients with G6PD deficiency.

GI reactions include nausea, vomiting, diarrhea, impaired folic acid absorption and hepatitis. Headache, vertigo, tinnitus, peripheral neuropathy, seizures, ataxia, and hallucinations have also been reported in patients taking sulfonamides. Rare reactions include drug fever and a lupus erythematosus phenomenon.

CO-TRIMOXAZOLE
(SULFAMETHOXAZOLE-TRIMETHOPRIM)

(ko tri mox' a zol)

Apo-Sulfatrim†, Apo-Sulfatrim DS†, Bactrim*, Bactrim DS, Bactrim I.V. Infusion, Cotrim, Cotrim D.S., Novotrimel†, Novotrimel DS†, Protrin†, Protrin DF†, Resprim‡, Roubac†, Roubac DS†, Septra*, Septra DS, Septra I.V. Infusion, Septrin‡, SMZ-TMP, Sulfamethoprim, Sulfamethoprim DS, Sulmeprim, Trib‡, Uroplus DS, Uroplus SS

Classification: sulfonamide
Pregnancy risk category C (D if near term)

How supplied

TABLETS: trimethoprim 80 mg and sulfamethoxazole 400 mg; trimethoprim 160 mg and sulfamethoxazole 800 mg

ORAL SUSPENSION: trimethoprim 40 mg and sulfamethoxazole 200 mg/5 ml

INJECTION: trimethoprim 16 mg and sulfamethoxazole 80 mg/ml (5 ml/ampule)

Indications and dosage
Urinary tract infections and shigellosis

ADULTS: 160 mg trimethoprim/800 mg sulfamethoxazole (double strength tablet) P.O. q 12 hours for 10 to 14 days in urinary tract infections and for 5 days in shigellosis. For simple cystitis or acute urethral syndrome, may give one to three double strength tablets as a single dose. If indicated, give by I.V. infusion 8 to 10 mg/kg daily (based on trimethoprim component) in two to four divided doses q 6, 8, or 12 hours for up to 14 days.

CHILDREN: 8 mg/kg trimethoprim/40 mg/kg sulfamethoxazole P.O. daily in two divided doses q 12 hours (10 days for urinary tract infections; 5 days, for shigellosis).

Otitis media

CHILDREN: 8 mg/kg trimethoprim/40 mg/kg sulfamethoxazole P.O. daily in two divided doses q 12 hours for 10 days.

Pneumocystis carinii *pneumonitis*

ADULTS AND CHILDREN: 20 mg/kg trimethoprim/100 mg/kg sulfamethoxazole P.O. daily in equally divided doses q 6 hours for 14 days. If indicated, give by I.V. infusion 15 to 20 mg/kg daily (based on trimethoprim component) in three or four divided doses q 6 to 8 hours for up to 14 days.

Chronic bronchitis

ADULTS: 160 mg trimethoprim/800 mg sulfamethoxazole P.O. q 12 hours for 10 to 14 days. Not recommended for infants under age 2 months.

Contraindications and precautions

Co-trimoxazole is contraindicated in patients with known hypersensitivity to trimethoprim, sulfamethoxazole or other sulfonamides and in those with porphyria; in patients with documented megaloblastic anemia due to folate deficiency; in pregnancy at term; during breast-feeding; and in infants under age 2 months. Use cautiously in patients with impaired renal or hepatic function and in those with severe allergy, bronchial asthma, or G6PD deficiency.

Adverse reactions

BLOOD: **agranulocytosis**, aplastic anemia, megaloblastic anemia, thrombocytopenia, leukopenia, **hemolytic anemia.**
CNS: headache, mental depression, **seizures**, hallucinations.
GI: *nausea, vomiting, diarrhea*, abdominal pain, anorexia, stomatitis.
GU: toxic nephrosis with oliguria and anuria, crystalluria, hematuria.
HEPATIC: jaundice.
SKIN: **erythema multiforme (Stevens-Johnson syndrome), generalized skin eruption, epidermal necrolysis, exfoliative dermatitis**, photosensitivity, urticaria, pruritus.
OTHER: **hypersensitivity**, serum sickness, drug fever, **anaphylaxis.**

Interactions

Ammonium chloride, ascorbic acid: doses sufficient to acidify urine may cause precipitation of sulfonamide and crystalluria. Don't use together.
Oral anticoagulants: increased anticoagulant effect. Monitor closely for bleeding.
Oral contraceptives: decreased contraceptive effectiveness and increased risk of breakthrough bleeding. Instruct patient to use a nonhormonal form of contraception.
Oral hypoglycemic agents: increased hypoglycemic effect. Monitor closely for hypoglycemia; dosage adjustments may be necessary.

Nursing considerations

Assessment
• Review the patient's history for a condition that contraindicates the use of co-trimoxazole.
• Obtain a baseline assessment of the patient's infection before therapy.
• Be alert for common adverse reactions.
• Evaluate the patient's and family's knowledge about co-trimoxazole therapy.

Planning (Nursing Diagnoses)
Potential nursing diagnoses for the patient receiving co-trimoxazole include:
• Potential for injury related to dosage regimen inadequate to alleviate infection.
• Noncompliance (medication administration) related to prolonged therapy.
• Knowledge deficit related to co-trimoxazole therapy.

Italicized adverse reactions are common   Boldfaced adverse reactions are life-threatening

Implementation

Preparation and administration

—Obtain specimen for culture and sensitivity tests before first dose. Therapy may begin pending test results.

—Give oral drug with full glass (8 oz [240 ml]) of water at least 1 hour before or 2 hours after meals for maximum absorption.

—I.V. infusion must be diluted in dextrose 5% in water before administration. Don't mix with other drugs or solutions.

—I.V. infusion must be infused slowly over 60 to 90 minutes. Don't give by rapid infusion or bolus injection. Must be used within 2 hours of mixing. Do not refrigerate.

—Check solution carefully for precipitate before starting infusion. Do not use solution containing a precipitate.

—Shake oral suspension thoroughly before administering.

—This combination is often used in extremely ill, immunosuppressed patients when prescribed for treatment of *Pneumocystis carinii* pneumonia.

—Note that the "DS" or "DF" product means "double strength."

—Used effectively for treatment of chronic bacterial prostatitis.

—Used prophylactically for recurrent urinary tract infections in women and for "traveler's diarrhea."

Monitoring

—Monitor the effectiveness of therapy by regularly assessing for improvement of infectious process.

—Monitor the patient for adverse drug reactions.

—Monitor urine output and urine elimination pattern. Urine output should be at least 1,500 ml/day to ensure proper hydration. Inadequate urine output can lead to crystalluria or tubular deposits of the drug.

—Monitor the patient on long-term therapy for possible superinfection, especially the elderly or debilitated patient and the patient receiving immunosuppressant or radiation therapy.

—Monitor the patient for drug interactions.

—Monitor laboratory test results. Co-trimoxazole alters urine glucose test results using copper sulfate (Benedict's test or Clinitest). Co-trimoxazole may elevate liver function test results; it may decrease serum concentration levels of erythrocytes, platelets, or leukocytes.

—Regularly reevaluate the patient's and family's knowledge about co-trimoxazole therapy.

Intervention

—Force fluid intake. Patient's output should be at least 1,500 ml/day.

—Assess I.V. site for signs of phlebitis or infiltration. Change infusion site every 48 to 72 hours.

—Notify the doctor if the patient cannot consume adequate amounts of fluid or if the patient's urine elimination pattern changes for no apparent reason.

—If the patient develops an adverse reaction, notify the doctor for appropriate treatment and provide supportive care as indicated.
—If the patient is unable to comply with therapy, discuss reasons and suggest possible methods to improve compliance (for example, clues patient may use to remind himself to take medication).
—Keep all health care team members advised of the patient's response to the drug.

Patient teaching
—Instruct the patient and family about co-trimoxazole including the dosage, frequency, action, and adverse reactions.
—Explain the disease process and rationale for therapy.
—Tell the patient to take medication exactly as prescribed, even if he feels better, and to take entire amount prescribed.
—Advise the diabetic patient that drug may increase effects of oral hypoglycemic agents and not to monitor urine glucose levels with tests that use copper sulfate (such as Clinitest).
—Advise the patient to avoid exposure to direct sunlight because of risk of photosensitivity reaction.
—Tell the patient to take drug with a full glass of water and to drink at least four 8-oz glasses of fluid daily; explain that tablet may be crushed and swallowed with water.
—Tell the patient to notify the nurse or doctor if adverse reactions develop or questions arise about co-trimoxazole therapy.

Evaluation
In the patient receiving co-trimoxazole, appropriate evaluation statements include:
• Patient is free of infection.
• Patient completes entire prescribed therapy.
• Patient and family state an understanding of co-trimoxazole therapy.

PROTOTYPE: SULFONAMIDES

SULFISOXAZOLE
(SULFAFURAZOLE, SULPHAFURAZOLE)
(*sulf i sox′ a zole*)
Gantrisin, Novosoxazole†
Classification: sulfonamide
Pregnancy risk category B (D if near term)

How supplied
TABLETS: 500 mg
LIQUID: 500 mg/5 ml

Indications and dosage
Urinary tract and systemic infections
ADULTS: initially, 2 to 4 g P.O., then 1 to 2 g P.O. q.i.d.
CHILDREN OVER AGE 2 MONTHS: initially, 75 mg/kg P.O. daily or 2 g/m² P.O. daily in divided doses q 6 hours, then 150 mg/kg or 4 g/m² P.O. daily in divided doses q 6 hours.

Contraindications and precautions
Sulfisoxazole is contraindicated in patients with known hypersensitivity to sulfonamides and in those with porphyria; in infants under age 2 months (except for treatment of congenital toxoplasmosis); in pregnancy at term; and during breast-feeding. Use cautiously in patients with impaired renal or hepatic function and in those with severe allergy, bronchial asthma, or G6PD deficiency.

Adverse reactions
BLOOD: **agranulocytosis, aplastic anemia**, megaloblastic anemia, thrombocytopenia, leukopenia, **hemolytic anemia**.
CNS: headache, mental depression, seizures, hallucinations.
GI: *nausea*, vomiting, diarrhea, abdominal pain, anorexia, stomatitis.
GU: toxic nephrosis with oliguria and anuria, crystalluria, hematuria.
HEPATIC: jaundice.
SKIN: **erythema multiforme (Stevens-Johnson syndrome)**, generalized skin eruption, epidermal necrolysis, **exfoliative dermatitis**, photosensitivity, urticaria, pruritus.
OTHER: hypersensitivity, serum sickness, drug fever, **anaphylaxis**, bacterial and fungal superinfections.

Interactions
Ammonium chloride, ascorbic acid: doses sufficient to acidify urine may cause crystalluria and precipitation of sulfonamide. Don't use together.
Oral anticoagulants: increased anticoagulant effect. Monitor closely for bleeding; anticoagulant dosage may need to be changed.
Oral contraceptives: decreased contraceptive effectiveness and increased risk of breakthrough bleeding. Patient should use a nonhormonal form of contraception during therapy.
Oral hypoglycemic agents: increased hypoglycemic effect. Monitor closely for hypoglycemia; dosage adjustments may be necessary.
Folic acid, PABA-containing drugs: inhibit antibacterial action. Don't use together.

Nursing considerations
Assessment
• Review the patient's history for a condition that contraindicates the use of sulfisoxazole.
• Obtain a baseline assessment of the patient's infection before therapy.
• Be alert for common adverse reactions.
• Evaluate the patient's and family's knowledge about sulfisoxazole therapy.

Planning (Nursing Diagnoses)
Potential nursing diagnoses for the patient receiving sulfisoxazole include:
• Potential for injury related to ineffective drug dosage.
• Altered urinary elimination related to sulfonamide-induced crystalluria and tubular deposits of sulfonamide crystals.
• Knowledge deficit related to sulfisoxazole therapy.

Implementation
Preparation and administration
—Obtain results of culture and sensitivity tests before first dose, but therapy may begin before laboratory tests are complete; check test results periodically to assess drug efficacy. Monitor urine cultures, CBCs, prothrombin time, and urinalysis before and during therapy.
—Give oral dosage with full glass (8 oz [240 ml]) of water.
—Tablet may be crushed and swallowed with water to facilitate passage into stomach and maximum absorption.
—Always consult manufacturer's directions for reconstitution, dilution, and storage of drugs; check expiration dates.
—Give oral drug at least 1 hour before or 2 hours after meals for maximum absorption.
—Shake oral suspension well before administering to ensure correct dosage.
—When sulfisoxazole is given preoperatively, the patient should receive a low-residue diet and a minimal number of enemas and cathartics.
—Although often ordered, initial loading dose is not necessary.
—Sulfisoxazole-pyrimethamine combination is used in treating toxoplasmosis.

Monitoring
—Monitor the effectiveness of therapy by regularly assessing for improvement of infectious process.
—Monitor the patient for adverse drug reactions.
—Monitor continuously for possible hypersensitivity reactions or other untoward effects; patients with AIDS have a much higher incidence of adverse reactions.
—Monitor urine elimination pattern for such changes as an increase or decrease in amount voided, urinary frequency, or dysuria.
—Monitor fluid intake and output. The urine output should be at least 1,500 ml/day to ensure proper hydration. Inadequate urine output can lead to crystalluria or tubular deposits of the drug.
—Monitor the patient for drug interactions.
—Monitor urine cultures, CBCs, prothrombin times, and urinalyses before and during therapy. Also monitor other laboratory test results. Sulfisoxazole alters results of urine glucose tests using copper sulfate (Benedict's test or Clinitest). Sulfisoxazole may elevate liver function test results; it may decrease serum levels of erythrocytes, platelets, or leukocytes.

—Regularly reevaluate the patient's and family's knowledge about sulfisoxazole therapy.

Intervention

—Force fluid intake to 3,000 to 4,000 ml/day (the patient's output should be at least 1,500 ml/day).
—Notify the doctor if the patient cannot consume adequate amounts of fluid or if the patient's urine elimination pattern changes for no apparent reason. To aid in prevention of crystalluria, sodium bicarbonate may be administered to alkalinize urine.
—If the patient develops an adverse reaction, notify the doctor for appropriate treatment and provide supportive care as indicated.
—Keep all health care team members advised of the patient's response to the drug.

Patient teaching

—Instruct the patient and family about sulfisoxazole, including the dosage, frequency, action, and adverse reactions.
—Explain the disease process and rationale for therapy.
—Teach the patient to check expiration date of drug, how to store drugs, and to discard unused drug.
—Tell the patient to take medication exactly as prescribed, even if he feels better, and to take entire amount prescribed.
—Warn the patient to avoid direct sunlight and ultraviolet light to prevent photosensitivity reaction.
—Tell the patient to drink a full glass of water with each dose and to drink plenty of water throughout the day to prevent crystalluria. Monitor intake and output. Intake should be sufficient to produce output of 1,500 ml/day (between 3,000 and 4,000 ml/day for adults).
—Tell the patient to report early signs of blood dyscrasia (sore throat, fever, and pallor) immediately to doctor.
—Explain that tablet may be crushed and swallowed with water to ensure maximal absorption.
—Advise the diabetic patient that drug may increase effects of oral hypoglycemics and not to monitor urine glucose levels with tests that use copper sulfate (such as Clinitest).
—Tell the patient to notify the nurse or doctor if adverse reactions develop or questions arise about sulfisoxazole therapy.

Evaluation

In the patient receiving sulfisoxazole, appropriate evaluation statements include:
• Patient is free of infection.
• Patient maintains normal urinary output during sulfisoxazole therapy.
• Patient and family state an understanding of sulfisoxazole therapy.

SELECTED MAJOR DRUGS: SULFONAMIDES

DRUG, INDICATIONS, AND DOSAGES

SPECIAL PRECAUTIONS

sulfadiazine (Microsulfon)
Urinary tract infection—
Adults: initially, 2 to 4 g P.O., then 500 mg to 1 g P.O. q 6 hours.
Children: initially, 75 mg/kg or 2 g/m² P.O., then 150 mg/kg or 4 g/m² P.O. in four to six divided doses daily. Maximum dosage is 6 g daily.
Rheumatic fever prophylaxis, as an alternative to penicillin—
Children over 30 kg: 1 g P.O. daily.
Children under 30 kg: 500 mg P.O. daily.
Adjunctive treatment in toxoplasmosis—
Adults: 4 g P.O. in divided doses q 6 hours for 3 to 4 weeks, discontinued for 1 week; given with pyrimethamine 25 mg P.O. daily for 3 to 4 weeks.
Children: 100 mg/kg P.O. in divided doses q 6 hours for 3 to 4 weeks; given with pyrimethamine 2 mg/kg daily for 3 days, then 1 mg/kg daily for 3 to 4 weeks.

• Contraindicated in patients with porphyria and in infants under age 2 months (except in congenital toxoplasmosis).
• Use cautiously and in reduced doses in patients with impaired hepatic or renal function, bronchial asthma, history of multiple allergies, G6PD deficiency, and blood dyscrasia.

sulfamethizole
Urinary tract infections in the absence of obstructive uropathy or foreign bodies, when these infections are caused by susceptible strains of the following organisms: Escherichia coli, Klebsiella, Enterobacter, Staphylococcus aureus, Proteus mirabilis, *and* P. vulgaris—
Adults: 500 mg to 1 g 3 or 4 times daily.
Children and infants (over age 2 months): 30 to 45 mg/kg daily, divided into four doses.

• Contraindicated in patients with known hypersensitivity to sulfonamides; in infants under age 2 months; in pregnancy at term; and during breast-feeding because sulfonamides cross the placenta, are excreted in breast milk, and may cause kernicterus.
• Administer cautiously to patients with hepatic or renal impairment, severe allergy or bronchial asthma; and G6PD deficiency (in whom sulfonamides may cause hemolysis).

sulfamethoxazole (Gantanol)
Urinary tract and systemic infections—
Adults: initially, 2 g P.O., then 1 g P.O. b.i.d. up to t.i.d. for severe infections.
Children and infants over age 2 months: initially, 50 to 60 mg/kg P.O., then 25 to 30 mg/kg b.i.d. Maximum dosage should not exceed 75 mg/kg daily.
Lymphogranuloma venereum (genital, inguinal, or anorectal infection)—
Adults: 1 g P.O. daily for at least 2 weeks.

• Contraindicated in patients with porphyria and in infants under age 2 months (except in congenital toxoplasmosis).
• Use cautiously and in reduced dosages in patients with impaired hepatic or renal function and in patients with severe allergy or bronchial asthma, G6PD deficiency, and blood dyscrasia.

(continued)

SELECTED MAJOR DRUGS: SULFONAMIDES *continued*

DRUG, INDICATIONS, AND DOSAGES	SPECIAL PRECAUTIONS
sulfasalazine (Azulfidine) *Mild to moderate ulcerative colitis, adjunctive therapy in severe ulcerative colitis—* **Adults:** initially, 3 to 4 g P.O. daily in evenly divided doses; usual maintenance dosage is 1.5 to 2 g P.O. daily in divided doses q 6 hours. May need to start with 1 to 2 g initially, with a gradual increase in dosage to minimize adverse reactions. **Children over age 2:** initially, 40 to 60 mg/kg P.O. daily divided into three to six doses. May need to start at lower dose if GI intolerance occurs.	• Contraindicated in patients with porphyria and intestinal and urinary obstruction and in patients allergic to salicylates. • Use cautiously and in reduced dosages in impaired hepatic or renal function and in those with severe allergy, bronchial asthma, and G6PD deficiency.

COMPARING SULFONAMIDE COMBINATIONS

TRADE NAME AND CONTENT	SPECIAL CONSIDERATIONS
Azo Gantanol **Azo Sulfamethoxazole** **Uro Gantanol** sulfamethoxazole 500 mg and phenazopyridine hydrochloride 100 mg **Azo Gantrisin** **Azo Sulfisoxazole** sulfisoxazole 500 mg and phenazopyridine hydrochloride 100 mg	• Combine the bacteriostatic action of sulfamethoxazole or sulfisoxazole with the urinary tract analgesic phenazopyridine to treat urinary tract infections. • Treatment is usually limited to 2 days of therapy; if further antimicrobial therapy is necessary, the sulfonamide alone may be used. • Use cautiously in patients with impaired hepatic or renal function or with asthma or allergies. May cause hemolysis in patients with G6PD deficiency. • To avoid crystalluria, ensure adequate daily intake of fluids.

SELF-TEST

1. Ben Smythe, age 32, has an acute lower urinary tract infection. His doctor prescribes the sulfonamide, sulfisoxazole, for 10 days. How do sulfonamides produce their bacteriostatic effects?
   a. They inhibit cell wall synthesis.
   b. They inhibit folic acid production.
   c. They inhibit protein synthesis.
   d. They alter bacterial cell wall permeability.

2. Which of the following instructions should the nurse give Mr. Smythe about sulfisoxazole administration?

   a. Take the medication with meals to minimize adverse GI reactions.

   b. Take the medication with an antacid.

   c. Drink at least four 8-oz glasses of fluid daily.

   d. Limit fluid intake to 1,000 ml/day.

3. Co-trimoxazole P.O. has been prescribed for your patient's urinary tract infection. It is commonly administered every:

   a. 4 hours.

   b. 6 hours.

   c. 8 hours.

   d. 12 hours.

Check your answers on page 1059.

CHAPTER 15

QUINOLONES

cinoxacin ✦ ciprofloxacin ✦ nalidixic acid ✦ norfloxacin ✦ ofloxacin

OVERVIEW

• The quinolones are broad-spectrum, synthetic antibacterials. The fluoroquinolones have an altered structure that enhances their antimicrobial efficacy. This structural change increases potency against gram-negative organisms and broadens the spectrum of activity to cover grampositive organisms and pseudomonal strains. Both fluoroquinolones and quinolones are bactericidal.

MAJOR USES

• Quinolones are used for the treatment of infections caused by susceptible strains of microorganisms. Nalidixic acid, cinoxacin, and norfloxacin are approved for the treatment of urinary tract infections caused by susceptible microorganisms. Ciprofloxacin and ofloxacin achieve therapeutic levels in most tissues and fluids and are therefore indicated for urinary tract and systemic infections. Ofloxacin is also approved for use in prostatitis due to *Escherichia coli*. The broad range of activity covers susceptible organisms causing lower respiratory, skin and skin structure, bone and joint, and urinary tract infections and infectious diarrhea.

• Generally accepted, unlabeled uses for these drugs include the use of norfloxacin for the treatment of gonorrhea and endocervical gonococcal infection caused by *Neisseria gonorrhoeae*; ciprofloxacin, in patients with cystic fibrosis who have pulmonary exacerbations. Ciprofloxacin is possibly effective in the treatment of malignant external otitis. Fluoroquinolones may also be useful in treating bronchitis, pneumonia, selected types of osteomyelitis, as prophylaxis in urologic surgery, and for travelers' diarrhea.

MECHANISM OF ACTION

• These drugs achieve their bactericidal activity by interfering with DNA gyrase, an enzyme necessary for bacterial DNA production.

ABSORPTION, DISTRIBUTION, METABOLISM, AND EXCRETION

The quinolones are absorbed rapidly from the GI tract after oral administration. Food may delay absorption, but does not substantially affect overall absorption. Absorption also seems to be unaffected by age. Norfloxacin is least soluble at normal urinary pH. Quinolones are eliminated through metabolism, biliary excretion, and renal excretion. Elimi-

GLOSSARY

Microorganism: microscopic organism, including bacteria, spiral organisms, *Rickettsiae,* viruses, molds, yeasts, and protozoa.

nation is slowed with decreased renal function, including that in healthy elderly patients.

ONSET AND DURATION

Peak concentrations occur within 1 to 4 hours after an oral dose, depending on whether serum or urine concentrations are checked. Quinolones are usually administered b.i.d. to q.i.d., depending on the specific drug and the infection treated.

ADVERSE REACTIONS

Well tolerated by most patients, quinolones produce few adverse reactions. Any reactions that occur disappear with discontinuation of the drug. The most common reactions affect the GI tract and include nausea, vomiting, diarrhea, and abdominal pain; these reactions affect 2% to 10% of patients receiving quinolones. About 1% of patients develop CNS reactions, such as headache, drowsiness, seizures, visual disturbances, hallucinations, depression, and agitation. Ofloxacin may also cause insomnia and dizziness. Less common reactions affect the integumentary system.

In fewer than 1% of patients, quinolones produce hypersensitivity reactions that include urticaria, nonspecific rashes, pruritus, and edema. Other rare reactions include hematologic abnormalities, such as hemolytic anemia, that are associated with G6PD deficiency.

Because some quinolones have caused arthropathy in laboratory animals, they are generally contraindicated for use in children.

PROTOTYPE: QUINOLONES

CIPROFLOXACIN
(sip roe flox' a sin)
Cipro, Cipro I.V., Ciproxin‡
Classification: quinolone
Pregnancy risk category C

How supplied
TABLETS: 250 mg, 500 mg, 750 mg
INJECTION: 200 mg in 100 ml dextrose 5% in water, 400 mg in 200 ml dextrose 5% in water
VIALS: 200 mg/20 ml, 400 mg/40 ml

Indications and dosage
Mild to moderate urinary tract infections
ADULTS: 250 mg P.O. q 12 hours.

Severe or complicated urinary tract infections; mild to moderate bone and joint infections; mild to moderate respiratory tract infections; mild to moderate skin and skin structure infections; infectious diarrhea
ADULTS: 500 mg P.O. q 12 hours.

Severe or complicated bone or joint infections; severe respiratory tract infections; severe skin and skin structure infections
ADULTS: 750 mg P.O. q 12 hours.

Contraindications and precautions
Ciprofloxacin is contraindicated for use in patients with known hypersensitivity to the drug or other quinolones, in children, and in pregnant women. Use cautiously in CNS disorders, such as severe cerebral arteriosclerosis or seizure disorder, and in other patients who are at risk for seizures.

Adverse reactions
CNS: headache, restlessness, tremor, light-headedness, confusion, hallucinations, **seizures.**
GI: *nausea, diarrhea, vomiting, abdominal pain* or discomfort, oral candidiasis.
GU: crystalluria.
OTHER: *rash.*

Interactions
Iron or zinc supplements; antacids containing magnesium hydroxide or aluminum hydroxide: decreased ciprofloxacin absorption. Separate administration by at least 2 hours.
Probenecid: may elevate serum level of ciprofloxacin. Avoid concomitant use.
Theophylline: increased plasma theophylline concentrations and prolonged theophylline half-life. Monitor plasma theophylline levels closely.

Nursing considerations
Assessment
• Review the patient's history for a condition that contraindicates the use of ciprofloxacin.
• Obtain a baseline assessment of the patient's infection before therapy.
• Be alert for common adverse reactions.
• Evaluate the patient's and family's knowledge about ciprofloxacin therapy.

Planning (Nursing Diagnoses)
Potential nursing diagnoses for the patient receiving ciprofloxacin include:
• Potential for injury related to ineffectiveness of drug to alleviate infection.
• Noncompliance (medication administration) related to prolonged therapy.

• Knowledge deficit related to ciprofloxacin therapy.

Implementation

Preparation and administration

— Obtain specimen for culture and sensitivity tests before first dose. Therapy may begin pending test results.
— Administer drug 2 hours after a meal. Food does not affect absorption but may delay peak serum levels. Administer antacids, if prescribed, at least 2 hours after administering drug.
— Dosage adjustments may be necessary in the patient with renal dysfunction.
— Prolonged use may result in overgrowth of organisms that are resistant to ciprofloxacin.

Monitoring

— Monitor the effectiveness of therapy by regularly assessing for improvement of infectious process.
— Monitor the patient for adverse drug reactions.
— Monitor for seizures during therapy.
— Monitor the patient for drug interactions.
— Regularly reevaluate the patient's and family's knowledge about ciprofloxacin therapy.

Intervention

— Impose safety precautions if the patient experiences adverse CNS reactions.
— Take seizure precautions, such as padding bed rails, if needed. Notify the doctor if seizures occur.
— If the patient is unable to comply with therapy, discuss reasons and offer possible suggestions to improve compliance (for example, clues patient may use to remind himself to take medication).
— If the patient develops an adverse reaction, notify the doctor for appropriate treatment and provide supportive care.
— Keep all health care team members advised of the patient's response to the drug.

Patient teaching

— Instruct the patient and family about ciprofloxacin, including the dosage, frequency, action, and adverse reactions.
— Explain the disease process and rationale for therapy.
— May cause dizziness or light-headedness. Warn the patient to avoid hazardous tasks that require alertness, such as driving, until CNS effects of the drug are known.
— Advise the patient to drink plenty of fluids to reduce the risk of crystalluria.
— Tell the patient to take antacids, if prescribed, at least 2 hours after taking drug.
— Tell the patient to notify the nurse or doctor if adverse reactions develop or questions arise about ciprofloxacin therapy.

Evaluation

In the patient receiving ciprofloxacin, appropriate evaluation statements include:

• Patient is free of infection.

• Patient completes entire regimen as prescribed.

• Patient and family state an understanding of ciprofloxacin therapy.

SELECTED MAJOR DRUGS: QUINOLONES

DRUG, INDICATIONS, AND DOSAGES	SPECIAL PRECAUTIONS
cinoxacin (Cinobac) *Initial and recurrent urinary tract infections of* Escherichia coli, Klebsiella, Enterobacter, Proteus mirabilis, P. vulgaris, *and* P. morgani, Serratia, and Citrobacter— **Adults and children over age 12:** 1 g P.O. daily in two to four divided doses for 7 to 14 days. Not recommended for children under age 12.	• Contraindicated in patients with hypersensitivity to quinolones. • Administer cautiously to patients with impaired renal and hepatic function.
nalidixic acid (NegGram) *Acute and chronic urinary tract infections caused by susceptible gram-negative organisms* (Proteus, Klebsiella, Enterobacter, *and* Escherichia coli) — **Adults:** 1 g P.O. q.i.d. for 7 to 14 days; 2 g daily for long-term use. **Children over age 3 months:** 55 mg/kg P.O. daily divided q.i.d. for 7 to 14 days; 33 mg/kg daily for long-term use.	• Contraindicated in seizure disorders. • Use cautiously in patients with impaired hepatic or renal function or severe cerebral arteriosclerosis. Use very cautiously in prepubertal children; erosion of cartilage of immature animals has been reported.
norfloxacin (Noroxin) *Urinary tract infections caused by* E. coli, Klebsiella, Enterobacter, Proteus, Pseudomonas aeruginosa, Citrobacter, Staphylococcus aureus, *and* S. epidermidis), *and group D streptococci*— **Adults:** for uncomplicated infections, 400 mg P.O. b.i.d. for 7 to 10 days. For complicated infections, 400 mg b.i.d. for 10 to 21 days.	• Contraindicated in patients with hypersensitivity to quinolones.
ofloxacin (Floxin) *Lower respiratory tract infections caused by susceptible organisms*— **Adults:** 400 mg P.O. q 12 hours for 10 days. *Cervicitis or urethritis caused by* Chlamydia trachomatis *or* Neisseria gonorrhoeae— **Adults:** 300 mg P.O. q 12 hours for 7 days. *Acute, uncomplicated gonorrhea*— **Adults:** 400 mg P.O. as a single dose. *Mild-to-moderate skin and skin structure infections* (Haemophilus influenzae *or* Streptococcus pneumoniae) — **Adults:** 400 mg P.O. q 12 hours for 10 days. *Cystitis caused by* E. coli *or* Klebsiella pneumoniae— **Adults:** 200 mg P.O. q 12 hours for 3 days.	• Contraindicated in children and in breast-feeding women because drug has caused arthropathy or osteochondrosis in young animals. Breast milk concentrations are similar to those in plasma. Use during pregnancy only when benefits outweigh fetal risks. Also contraindicated in hypersensitivity to the drug or other quinolones. • Use cautiously in patients with a history of seizure disorders or other CNS diseases, such as cerebral arteriosclero-

SELECTED MAJOR DRUGS: QUINOLONES *continued*

DRUG, INDICATIONS, AND DOSAGES	SPECIAL PRECAUTIONS
ofloxacin *(continued)* *Urinary tract infections* Citrobacter diversus, Enterobacter aerogenes, Escherichia coli, Proteus mirabilis, *or* Pseudomonas aeruginosa) — **Adults:** 200 mg P.O. q 12 hours for 7 days. Complicated infections may require therapy for 10 days. *Prostatitis caused by* E. coli — **Adults:** 200 mg P.O. q 12 hours for 6 weeks. *Dosage adjustment for patients with renal failure —* If creatinine clearance is 10 to 50 ml/minute, decrease dosage interval to once q 24 hours; if < 10 ml/minute, give half the recommended dose q 24 hours.	sis. If the patient experiences excessive CNS stimulation (restlessness, tremor, confusion, hallucinations), discontinue medication and notify the doctor. Institute seizure precautions. • Because the drug is mainly eliminated by renal excretion, adjust dosage in patients with renal failure.

SELF-TEST

1. Diane Wilson, age 56, is a diabetic patient and seeks treatment for a recurrent urinary tract infection. Her doctor prescribed ciprofloxacin. Before administering ciprofloxacin to Mrs. Wilson, the nurse should obtain a complete medical history. Which of the following conditions require cautious administration of ciprofloxacin?
a. CV disease
b. CNS disorder
c. GI disorder
d. anemia

2. The nurse should monitor Mrs. Wilson for which of the following adverse drug reactions?
a. bronchospasm
b. tinnitus
c. seizures
d. constipation

3. Mrs. Wilson states that she takes an antacid when she experiences heartburn. When should Mrs. Wilson be instructed to take the antacid in relationship to the ciprofloxacin dose?
a. 2 hours after the ciprofloxacin dose
b. 2 hours before the ciprofloxacin dose
c. immediately after the ciprofloxacin dose
d. whenever the antacid is needed

Check your answers on page 1059.

CHAPTER 16

ANTIVIRALS

acyclovir sodium ◆ amantadine hydrochloride ◆ ganciclovir
ribavirin ◆ vidarabine monohydrate ◆ zidovudine

OVERVIEW

- Antivirals are used to treat various viral-induced infections. Acyclovir and zidovudine exert their effect by interfering with DNA synthesis and inhibiting viral replication, but the antiviral mechanism of action has not yet been established for many of these agents. Antivirals provide a range of alternatives for treating debilitating and life-threatening viral infections that were previously untreatable.
- Because of the wide range of potential adverse reactions, these drugs should be reserved for clearly diagnosed disease states that will respond to this level of therapy.

MAJOR USES

- Each of these agents is used for the treatment of a different viral infection.
- Acyclovir is used orally for the treatment of initial recurrent episodes of genital herpes. Treatment decisions are based on the severity of the disease, the patient's immune status, frequency and duration of episodes, and the degree of cutaneous or systemic involvement. It is also used for acute treatment of herpes zoster (shingles). The injectable form is used for the treatment of initial and recurrent mucosal and cutaneous infections caused by herpes simplex viruses (HSV) types 1 and 2; varicella zoster (chickenpox) infections in immunocompromised patients; herpes simplex encephalitis in patients over age 6 months; and severe initial episodes of genital herpes in patients who are not immunocompromised.
- Amantadine is used for prevention and treatment of respiratory tract illness caused by influenza A virus strains. It is especially indicated for use in patients who are considered high risk because of underlying CV, pulmonary, metabolic, neuromuscular, or immunodeficiency disease. Amantadine is also used for treatment of Parkinson's disease or parkinsonian syndrome and drug-induced extrapyramidal reactions.
- Ganciclovir is indicated for the treatment of CMV retinitis.
- Ribavirin is used as an aerosolized powder for the treatment of carefully selected hospitalized infants and young children with severe lower respiratory tract infections due to respiratory syncytial virus.
- Vidarabine, which has antiviral activity against HSV, is indicated in I.V. form for HSV, encephalitis, neonatal herpes simplex virus infections, and herpes zoster in immunosuppressed patients. An ophthalmic oint-

GLOSSARY

Virus: infectious agent characterized by a lack of independent metabolism and by an ability to replicate within living host cells only.

ment is available for the treatment of acute keratoconjunctivitis and recurrent epithelial keratitis due to HSV.
• Zidovudine, in oral form, is indicated for management of adults and children with AIDS who have evidence of impaired immunity before therapy; and for children over age 3 months who have human immunodeficiency virus– (HIV-) related symptoms or who are asymptomatic with abnormal laboratory values indicating significant HIV-related immunosuppression. The I.V. form is indicated for management of adults with symptomatic HIV infections (AIDS and advanced AIDS-related complex) who have a history of confirmed *Pneumocystis carinii* pneumonia or who are at high risk for this infection.

MECHANISM OF ACTION
• Acyclovir, ganciclovir, and zidovudine interfere with the synthesis and/or replication of viral DNA.
• The mechanism of action of amantadine is not completely understood. Its mode of action appears to be prevention of the release of infectious viral nucleic acid into the host cell and possible interference with viral penetration into the cells; this reaction appears to be virus specific for influenza A. Its antiparkinsonian action is thought to be mediated by the release of dopamine.
• Ribavirin has shown antiviral inhibitory activity but the mechanism of action is unknown; the mechanism of action of vidarabine has not yet been established.

ABSORPTION, DISTRIBUTION, METABOLISM, AND EXCRETION
Oral doses of acyclovir are slowly and incompletely absorbed from the GI tract. The drug is widely distributed in tissues and body fluids. The kidneys are the primary route of excretion.

Amantadine is readily absorbed, not metabolized, and excreted in the urine. The peak excretion rate is approximately 5 mg/hour. Renal clearance is reduced in otherwise healthy patients ages 65 and over. The dose for patients ages 65 and over is generally half the standard dose.

Ganciclovir is administered parenterally. In studies, the plasma level increased consistently over the duration of infusion, with the plasma half-life at 2.9 ± 1.3 hours, with normal renal function. The major route of elimination is through the kidney.

Ribavirin is available as an aerosolized powder and is absorbed systemically. The bioavailability of the drug is unknown. It has shown concentrations in respiratory tract secretions and RBCs.

Vidarabine is rapidly metabolized and promptly distributed into the tissues after I.V. administration. Systemic absorption is not expected to occur after ocular administration and/or swallowing of lacrimal secretions.

Zidovudine is rapidly absorbed from the GI tract after oral dosing; the rate of absorption of the syrup is greater than that of capsules. It is rapidly metabolized in the liver and excreted through the kidneys. The pharmacokinetics (absorption, distribution, metabolism, and excretion) are the same in adults and children over age 3.

ONSET AND DURATION

Peak concentrations of acyclovir are reached in 1.5 to 2 hours after oral administration. Duration and total body clearance depend on renal function. Maximum blood levels for amantadine are reached in approximately 4 hours. Peak urinary excretion rate approximates 15 hours. The plasma half-life for ganciclovir is 2.9 ± 1.3 hours with normal renal function. Accumulation of ribavirin in the RBCs after oral inhalation seems to plateau in about 4 days with an apparent half-life of 40 days. Vidarabine blood levels reflect the rate of infusion and show no accumulation over time. Excretion is primarily through the kidneys, and the drug may accumulate in patients with impaired renal function. Peak serum concentrations occur with zidovudine within 0.5 to 1.5 hours.

ADVERSE REACTIONS

Adverse reactions common to most of these agents include anorexia, chills, edema, nausea and vomiting, depression, diarrhea, confusion, dizziness, hallucinations, headache, and ataxia. Injectable agents can produce inflammation or phlebitis at injection site.

Acyclovir causes transient elevation of the serum creatinine or BUN levels; itching, rash, and hives; elevation of hepatic enzymes, encephalopathic changes (fatigue, lethargy, tremor, confusion, hallucinations, agitation, seizures, sore throat, or coma). The incidence of adverse reactions seems to increase with long-term and intermittent administration. Weakness and numbness have also been associated with long-term administration.

Amantadine most commonly causes nausea, dizziness, light-headedness, and insomnia; less frequently, it may cause depression, anxiety, irritability, hallucinations, confusion, anorexia, dry mouth, constipation, peripheral edema, orthostatic hypotension, and headache. Occasionally it causes CHF, psychosis, urine retention, dyspnea, fatigue, skin rash, vomiting, weakness, slurred speech, and visual disturbance. Rarely, seizures, leukopenia, neutropenia, eczematoid dermatitis, and oculogyric (involuntary movement of the eyes) episodes occur.

Ganciclovir is associated with granulocytopenia and thrombocytopenia. Granulocytopenia occurred in approximately 40% of patients, usually in the first or second week of treatment, but it may occur at any time during treatment. Thrombocytopenia is also common and may occur and may occur in up to 20% of patients. Adverse reactions include malaise, arrhythmia, hypertension, hypotension, abnormal thoughts or dreams, coma, nervousness, paresthesia, psychosis, somnolence, tremor, nausea, vomiting, anorexia, hemorrhage, abdominal pain, alopecia, pruritus, urticaria, increased serum creatinine level, inflammation, pain, phlebitis at the injection site, dyspnea, eosinophilia, retinal detachment in patients with CMV retinitis, and decreased blood glucose.

Ribavirin may cause worsening of respiratory status and deterioration of pulmonary function, bacterial pneumonia, pneumothorax, apnea, or ventilator dependence. It may also cause cardiac arrest, hypotension, digitalis toxicity, reticulocytosis, rash, and conjunctivitis.

Vidarabine may cause tremor, dizziness, headache, hallucinations, confusion, and psychosis, primarily in patients with impaired hepatic or renal function. Malaise and fatal metabolic encephalopathy have occurred. GI reactions include mild to moderate anorexia, nausea, vomiting, hematemesis, and diarrhea; liver function tests may be elevated. Hematologic reactions include decreased reticulocyte count, hemoglobin or hematocrit, WBC count, and platelet count. Other reactions may include weight loss, pruritus, rash, and pain at injection site. Ophthalmic use may cause lacrimation, foreign body sensation, burning, irritation, pain, photophobia, sensitivity, conjunctival injection, or superficial punctate keratitis.

Zidovudine most frequently causes hematologic toxicity, including granulocytopenia, severe anemia, and pancytopenia. Significant anemia most commonly occurred after 4 to 6 weeks of therapy and often required dose adjustment, discontinuation of drug, or blood transfusions.

PROTOTYPE: ANTIVIRALS

ZIDOVUDINE
(AZIDOTHYMIDINE, AZT)
(*zye doe' vue deen*)
Retrovir
Classification: antiviral
Pregnancy risk category C

How supplied
TABLETS: 100 mg
SYRUP: 50 mg/5 ml
INJECTION: 10 mg/ml

Indications and dosage
Patients with symptomatic human immunodeficiency virus (HIV) infection (AIDS or advanced AIDS-related complex [ARC]) who have a history of Pneumocystis carinii pneumonia or a CD4 lymphocyte count below 200 cells/mm^3
ADULTS: initially, 200 mg P.O. q 4 hours around the clock for 1 month, then 100 mg P.O. q 4 hours around the clock; or 1 to 2 mg/kg (infused over 1 hour) q 4 hours.
CHILDREN: dosage is individualized and will vary according to treatment protocol. Early studies have employed doses between 0.9 and 1.4

mg/kg/hour by continuous I.V. infusion; others have used 100 mg/m² I.V. or P.O. q 6 hours.

Asymptomatic HIV infection
ADULTS: 100 mg P.O. q 4 hours while awake (500 mg daily).

Postexposure prophylaxis (for example, after needle-stick injury)
ADULTS: dosage will vary according to study protocol, but most studies use 200 mg P.O. q 4 hours around the clock for 6 to 8 weeks. Some investigators attempt to initiate therapy within 1 hour of exposure.

Contraindications and precautions
Zidovudine is contraindicated in patients who have potentially life-threatening allergic reactions to any of the components of the formulations. Administer cautiously to patients who have bone marrow suppression, advanced symptomatic HIV disease, anemia, or granulocytopenia.

Adverse reactions
BLOOD: **severe bone marrow depression (resulting in anemia), granulocytopenia, thrombocytopenia.**
CNS: *headache*, agitation, restlessness, insomnia, confusion, anxiety.
GI: nausea, anorexia.
SKIN: rash, itching.
OTHER: myalgia.

Interactions
Acyclovir: possible lethargy and fatigue. Use together cautiously.
Co-trimoxazole, acetaminophen: may impair hepatic metabolism of zidovudine, increasing the drug's toxicity.
Other cytotoxic drugs: additive adverse effects on the bone marrow.
Pentamidine, dapsone, flucytosine, amphotericin B: increased risk of nephrotoxicity. Avoid concomitant use.
Probenecid: may decrease the renal clearance of zidovudine. Don't use together.

Nursing considerations
Assessment
• Review the patient's history for a condition that contraindicates the use of zidovudine.
• Obtain a baseline assessment of the patient's infection before therapy.
• Be alert for common adverse reactions.
• Evaluate the patient's and family's knowledge about zidovudine therapy.

Planning (Nursing Diagnoses)
Potential nursing diagnoses for the patient receiving zidovudine include:
• Potential for injury related to adverse drug reactions.
• Noncompliance (medication administration) related to prolonged therapy.
• Knowledge deficit related to zidovudine therapy.

Italicized adverse reactions are common   Boldfaced adverse reactions are life-threatening

Implementation

Preparation and administration

— Administer P.O. drug every 4 hours around the clock.

— For I.V. use, administer 1 to 2 mg/kg infused over 1 hour at a constant rate; administer every 4 hours around the clock (six times daily). Avoid rapid infusion or bolus injection.

— Do not give I.M.

— Patients should receive the I.V. infusion only until oral therapy can be administered.

— The I.V. dosing regimen equivalent to the oral administration of 100 mg every 4 hours is approximately 1 mg/kg I.V. every 4 hours.

— Dilute before administration. Remove the calculated dose from the vial; add to dextrose 5% injection to achieve a concentration that does not exceed 4 mg/ml.

— Admixture in biological or colloidal fluids (for example, blood products, protein solutions) is not recommended.

— After dilution, the solution is physically and chemically stable for 24 hours at room temperature and 48 hours if refrigerated at 35.6° to 46.4° F (2° to 8° C) to minimize the potential administration of a microbially contaminated solution. Store undiluted vials at 59° to 77° F (15° to 25° C) and protect from light.

— Health care workers who consider zidovudine prophylaxis after occupational exposure (needle-stick injury, for example) should understand that animal and human studies are insufficient to judge the drug's safety or efficacy. They should consider the potential toxicity of the drug, as well as the risk of acquiring HIV after occupational exposure. Some clinicians do not advocate such use of zidovudine.

Monitoring

— Monitor the patient for adverse drug reactions.

— Monitor blood studies (CBC and platelet count) for signs of anemia or granulocytopenia.

— Monitor the patient for drug interactions.

— Monitor for signs and symptoms of opportunistic infection (including pneumonia, meningitis, and sepsis).

— Regularly reevaluate the patient's and family's knowledge about zidovudine therapy.

Intervention

— If the patient develops significant anemia (hemoglobin level below 7.5 mg/dl or reduction by more than 25% of baseline value) and/or significant granulocytopenia (granulocyte count below 750/mm^3 or reduction by more than 50% of baseline value), notify the doctor; dose interruption may be necessary. For less significant anemia or granulocytopenia, a reduction in daily dose may be adequate. A blood transfusion may also be indicated.

— If the patient develops anemia, provide supportive care; for example, stagger the patient's activities to provide frequent rest periods.

—Keep all health care team members advised of patient's response to the drug.

—If signs of an opportunistic infection occurs, notify the doctor immediately.

—Administer a mild analgesic, as prescribed, if the patient experiences a headache. If the patient develops other adverse reactions, notify the doctor for appropriate treatment and provide supportive care as appropriate. For example, take safety precautions if the patient experiences adverse CNS reactions, such as dizziness; administer a mild sedative for insomnia as prescribed; or monitor hydration if the patient experiences nausea, vomiting, anorexia, or diarrhea. Obtain a prescription for an antiemetic or antidiarrheal agent if needed.

—If the patient is unable to comply with therapy, discuss reasons and offer possible suggestions to improve compliance (for example, clues patient can use to remind himself to take medication).

Patient teaching

—Instruct the patient and family about zidovudine, including the dosage, frequency, action, and adverse reactions.

—Explain the disease process and rationale for therapy.

—Drug does not cure HIV infection or AIDS but may reduce morbidity resulting from opportunistic infections and thus prolong the patient's life. However, the optimum duration of treatment, as well as the dosage for optimum effectiveness and minimum toxicity, is not yet known.

—Instruct the patient to take the drug every 4 hours around the clock, even though it means interrupting sleep. Suggest ways to avoid missing doses, such as the use of alarm clocks.

—Inform the patient that zidovudine does not reduce the risk of transmitting the virus to others through sexual contact or blood contamination.

—Caution the patient to avoid OTC medications or other drugs not medically approved to treat HIV infection without first checking with the doctor, pharmacist, or nurse.

—Inform the patient about the importance of follow-up medical visits to evaluate for adverse reactions and to monitor clinical status. Advise the patient that frequent (at least every 2 weeks) blood counts are strongly recommended.

—Advise the female patient that the manufacturer suggests that breast-feeding be discontinued during therapy with zidovudine.

—Warn the patient not to perform hazardous activities that require alertness if such adverse CNS reactions as dizziness occur.

—Tell the patient to store the drug at room temperature and to protect from light.

—Tell the patient to notify the nurse or doctor if adverse reactions develop or questions arise about zidovudine therapy.

—Zidovudine frequently causes a low RBC count by suppressing the bone marrow. Advise the patient that he may need blood transfusions during treatment with zidovudine.

Evaluation

In the patient receiving zidovudine, appropriate evaluation statements include:

• Patient exhibits no adverse reactions to zidovudine.

• Patient complies with prescribed therapy regimen.

• Patient and family state an understanding of zidovudine therapy.

SELECTED MAJOR DRUGS: ANTIVIRALS

DRUG, INDICATIONS, AND DOSAGES	SPECIAL PRECAUTIONS
acyclovir (Zovirax) *Initial and recurrent episodes of mucocutaneous herpes simplex virus (HSV-1 and HSV-2) infections in immuno-compromised patients; severe initial episodes of genital herpes in patients who are not immunocompromised—* **Adults and children over age 11:** 5 mg/kg given at a constant rate over a period of 1 hour by I.V. infusion q 8 hours for 7 days (5 days for genital herpes). **Children under age 12:** 250 mg/m^2 given at a constant rate over a period of 1 hour by I.V. infusion q 8 hours for 7 days (5 days for genital herpes). *Initial genital herpes—* **Adults:** 200 mg P.O. q 4 hours while awake (a total of 5 capsules daily). Treatment should continue for 10 days. *Intermittent therapy for recurrent genital herpes—* **Adults:** 200 mg P.O. q 4 hours while awake (a total of 5 capsules daily). Treatment should continue for 5 days. Initiate therapy at the first sign of recurrence. *Chronic suppressive therapy for recurrent genital herpes—* 200 mg P.O. t.i.d. for up to 6 months.	• Contraindicated in patients with known hypersensitivity to the drug. • Administer cautiously to patients with underlying neurologic abnormalities and to those with serious renal, hepatic, or electrolyte abnormalities or significant hypoxia; to patients with prior neurologic reactions to cytotoxic drugs or to those receiving concomitant intrathecal methotrexate or interferon.
ganciclovir (Cytovene) *CMV retinitis treatment of immunocompromised individuals, including patients with AIDS* **Adults:** induction treatment—initially, 5 mg/kg I.V. q 12 hours for 14 to 21 days (normal renal function); maintenance treatment—5 mg/kg I.V. once daily, for 7 days each week, or 6 mg/kg daily for 5 days each week.	• Contraindicated in patients with known hypersensitivity to ganciclovir or acyclovir. • Prepare ganciclovir solution cautiously because the solution is strongly alkaline. • Use cautiously in patients with renal impairment.
ribavirin (Virazole) *Treatment of hospitalized infants and young children infected by respiratory syncytial virus (RSV)—* **Infants and young children:** solution in concentration of 20 mg/ml delivered via the Viratek Small Particle Aerosol Generator (SPAG-2). Treatment is carried out for 12 to 18 hours daily for at least 3, and no more than 7, days.	• Contraindicated in women who are or may become pregnant during treatment with drug. Because the drug is administered by aerosol, nurses caring for patients taking ribavirin risk significant environmental exposure to the drug. Use caution. • Administer cautiously to patients with lower respiratory tract infection due to RSV; to those at risk for drug interac-

(continued)

SELECTED MAJOR DRUGS: ANTIVIRALS *continued*

DRUG, INDICATIONS, AND DOSAGES	SPECIAL PRECAUTIONS
ribavirin *(continued)*	tions, carcinogenesis, mutagenesis, and impairment of fertility; and to pregnant or breast-feeding patients.
vidarabine (Vira-A) *Herpes simplex virus encephalitis—* **Adults and children** (including neonates): 15 mg/kg I.V. daily for 10 days. Slowly infuse the total daily dose by I.V. infusion at a constant rate over 12- to 24-hour period. Avoid rapid or bolus injection.	• Contraindicated in patients who develop hypersensitivity reactions to the drug. • Administer cautiously to patients susceptible to fluid overload or cerebral edema; to patients with impaired renal or hepatic function; to those with herpes simplex encephalitis; and to neonates with herpes simplex infection.

SELF-TEST

1. Joyce Smith, age 30, is being treated for AIDS. To reduce opportunistic infections, her doctor prescribes zidovudine 200 mg P.O. q 4 hours. The nurse should instruct Mrs. Smith to:
  a. take the drug with meals.
  b. take the drug on an empty stomach.
  c. take the drug every 4 hours around the clock.
  d. take the drug every 4 hours except while sleeping.

2. Which adverse reaction should the nurse anticipate while Mrs. Smith is receiving zidovudine?
  a. severe bone marrow depression
  b. seizures
  c. renal dysfunction
  d. hypertension

3. Which of the following drugs is known to interact with zidovudine?
  a. penicillin
  b. acetaminophen
  c. atropine sulfate
  d. meprobamate

Check your answers on page 1059.

CHAPTER 17

ERYTHROMYCINS

erythromycin base ✦ erythromycin estolate ✦ erythromycin ethylsuccinate
erythromycin gluceptate ✦ erythromycin lactobionate
erythromycin stearate

OVERVIEW

- Erythromycins, which are macrolide antibacterials, contain a large macrocyclic lactone ring. They are used to treat various common infections. Because these highly effective drugs are considered one of the safest antibiotics, clinical indications for erythromycins continue to increase.

MAJOR USES

- Erythromycins are considered a drug of choice in the treatment of *Haemophilus influenzae*, *Entamoeba histolytica*, *Mycoplasma pneumoniae*, *Corynebacterium diphtheriae*, and *Bordetella pertussis.* They may be used as an alternate to penicillins or tetracycline in the treatment of *Streptococcus pneumoniae*, *S. viridans*, *Listeria monocytogenes*, *Staphylococcus aureus*, *Chlamydia trachomatis*, *Neisseria gonorrhoeae*, and *Treponema pallidum.*

MECHANISM OF ACTION

- Erythromycins are bacteriostatic antibacterials that inhibit bacterial protein synthesis by binding to ribosome's 50S subunit. They may be bactericidal in high concentrations or against highly susceptible organisms.

ABSORPTION, DISTRIBUTION, METABOLISM, AND EXCRETION

Because the base salt is acid-sensitive, it must be buffered or have enteric coating to prevent destruction by gastric acids. Acid salts and esters (estolate, ethylsuccinate, and stearate) are not affected by gastric acidity and therefore are well absorbed. Base and stearate preparations should be given on an empty stomach. Absorption of estolate and ethylsuccinate preparations is unaffected or possibly even enhanced by food. When administered topically, drug is absorbed minimally.

Erythromycin is distributed widely except to CSF, where it appears only in low concentrations. The drug crosses the placenta. About 80% of erythromycin base and 96% of erythromycin estolate are protein-bound.

Erythromycin is metabolized partially in the liver to inactive metabolites. It is excreted mainly unchanged in bile. Only small drug amounts (less than 5%) are excreted in urine; some drug is excreted in breast milk. In patients with normal renal function, plasma half-life is about 1½ hours.

Peritoneal hemodialysis does not remove drug.

ONSET AND DURATION
Peak serum concentration levels depend on several factors, including the chemical structure, coating, and number of doses of the drug and whether the patient is fasting. Enteric-coated erythromycin provides excellent bioavailability. The mean peak serum concentration occurs 2 to 4 hours after a single 250-mg dose in the fasting patient.

ADVERSE REACTIONS
Few adverse reactions are associated with erythromycin. Dose-related GI reactions (epigastric distress, nausea, vomiting, and diarrhea) are most common. Stomatitis, heartburn, anorexia, melena, and allergic reactions (rashes, fever, eosinophilia, and anaphylaxis) also can occur. Rarely, reversible sensorineural hearing loss can occur with I.V. erythromycin lactobionate, commonly in patients with renal failure who are receiving high doses of erythromycin. Venous irritation and thrombophlebitis can follow I.V. administration of erythromycin glucepate or lactobionate.

PROTOTYPE: ERYTHROMYCINS

ERYTHROMYCIN BASE
(er ith roe mye′ sin)
Apo-Erythro base†, EMU-V‡, E-Mycin, Eryc, Ery-Tab, Erythromid†, Ilotycin, Novorythro†, PCE Disperstabs, Robimycin

ERYTHROMYCIN ESTOLATE
Ilosone, Novorythro†

ERYTHROMYCIN ETHYLSUCCINATE
Apo-Erythro-ES†, E.E.S., EryPed, Erythrocin, Pediamycin, Wyamycin-E

ERYTHROMYCIN GLUCEPTATE
Ilotycin

ERYTHROMYCIN LACTOBIONATE
Erythrocin

ERYTHROMYCIN STEARATE
Apo-Erythro-S†, Erythrocin, Novorythro†, Wyamycin-S
Classification: erythromycin
Pregnancy risk category B

How supplied
base
TABLETS (ENTERIC-COATED): 250 mg, 300 mg, 500 mg
PELLETS (ENTERIC-COATED): 250 mg
ORAL SUSPENSION: 125 mg/5 ml, 200 mg/5 ml, 400 mg/5 ml

†Available in Canada only   ‡Available in Australia only

estolate
TABLETS: 250 mg, 500 mg
TABLETS (CHEWABLE): 125 mg, 250 mg
CAPSULES: 125 mg, 250 mg
ORAL SUSPENSION: 125 mg/5 ml, 250 mg/5 ml
DROPS: 100 mg/ml
ethylsuccinate
TABLETS (CHEWABLE): 200 mg, 400 mg
gluceptate
INJECTION: 250-mg, 500-mg, 1-g vials
lactobionate
INJECTION: 500-mg, 1-g vials
stearate
TABLETS (FILM-COATED): 250 mg, 500 mg

Indications and dosage

Acute pelvic inflammatory disease caused by Neisseria gonorrhoeae
WOMEN: 500 mg I.V. (gluceptate, lactobionate) q 6 hours for 3 days, then 250 mg (base, estolate, stearate) or 400 mg (ethylsuccinate) P.O. q 6 hours for 7 days.

Endocarditis prophylaxis for dental procedures in patients allergic to penicillin
ADULTS: 1 g (base, estolate, stearate) P.O. 1 hour before procedure, then 500 mg P.O. 6 hours later.

Intestinal amebiasis
ADULTS: 250 mg (base, estolate, stearate) P.O. q 6 hours for 10 to 14 days.
CHILDREN: 30 to 50 mg/kg (base, estolate, stearate) P.O. daily, divided q 6 hours for 10 to 14 days.

Mild to moderately severe respiratory tract, skin, and soft-tissue infections caused by sensitive group A beta-hemolytic streptococci, Streptococcus pneumoniae, Mycoplasma pneumoniae, Corynebacterium diphtheriae, Bordetella pertussis, Listeria monocytogenes
ADULTS: 250 to 500 mg (base, estolate, stearate) P.O. q 6 hours; or 400 to 800 mg (ethylsuccinate) P.O. q 6 hours; or 15 to 20 mg/kg I.V. daily as continuous infusion or divided q 6 hours.
CHILDREN: 30 mg/kg to 50 mg/kg (oral erythromycin salts) P.O. daily divided q 6 hours; or 15 to 20 mg/kg I.V. daily divided q 4 to 6 hours.

Syphilis
ADULTS: 500 mg (base, estolate, stearate) P.O. q.i.d. for 15 days.

Legionnaire's disease
ADULTS: 500 mg to 1 g (gluceptate) I.V. or (base) P.O. q 6 hours for 21 days.

Uncomplicated urethral, endocervical, or rectal infections in which tetracyclines are contraindicated
ADULTS: 500 mg (base) P.O. q.i.d. for at least 7 days.

Urogenital **Chlamydia trachomatis** *infections during pregnancy*
ADULTS: 500 mg (base) P.O. q.i.d. for at least 7 days or 250 mg (base) P.O. q.i.d. for at least 14 days.

Conjunctivitis caused by **C. trachomatis** *in neonates*
NEONATES: 50 mg/kg P.O. daily in four divided doses for at least 2 weeks.

Pneumonia of infancy due to **C. trachomatis**
INFANTS: 50 mg/kg P.O. daily in four divided doses for at least 3 weeks.

Contraindications and precautions
Erythromycin is contraindicated in patients with known hypersensitivity to the drug. Erythromycin estolate is contraindicated in patients with hepatic disease. Other erythromycin forms should be administered cautiously to patients with impaired hepatic function. Although safety for use in pregnancy has not been established, problems have not been reported.

Adverse reactions
EENT: hearing loss with high I.V. doses.
GI: *abdominal pain and cramping, nausea, vomiting, diarrhea.*
HEPATIC: cholestatic jaundice (with estolate).
SKIN: urticaria, rashes.
LOCAL: *venous irritation, thrombophlebitis* after I.V. injection.
OTHER: overgrowth of nonsusceptible bacteria or fungi; **anaphylaxis**; fever.

Interactions
Clindamycin, lincomycin: may be antagonistic. Don't use together.
Oral anticoagulants: increased anticoagulant effects. Monitor for bleeding problems; adjust dosage as ordered.
Theophylline: decreased erythromycin blood level and increased theophylline toxicity. Use together cautiously.

Nursing considerations
Assessment
• Review the patient's history for a condition that contraindicates the use of erythromycin.
• Obtain a baseline assessment of the patient's infection before therapy.
• Be alert for common adverse reactions.
• Evaluate the patient's and family's knowledge about erythromycin therapy.

Planning (Nursing Diagnoses)
Potential nursing diagnoses for the patient receiving erythromycin include:
• Potential for injury related to ineffective drug dosage.
• Noncompliance (medication administration) related to prolonged therapy.
• Knowledge deficit related to erythromycin therapy.

Italicized adverse reactions are common   Boldfaced adverse reactions are life-threatening

Implementation

Preparation and administration

— Obtain specimen for culture and sensitivity tests before first dose. Therapy may begin pending test results.

— For best absorption, administer oral drug form to the patient with a full glass of water 1 hour before or 2 hours after meals. If tablets are coated, they may be taken with meals. Do not administer drug with fruit juice. Advise the patient that chewable erythromycin tablets should not be swallowed whole.

— Coated forms of erythromycin are associated with lower incidence of GI problems and may be more tolerable to the patient.

— When administering suspension, be sure to note the concentration.

— Do not administer erythromycin stearate with food.

— Do not administer erythromycin by I.M. injection; the injection is painful and may cause abscess or local tissue necrosis.

— Administer I.V. dose over 60 minutes. Reconstitute according to manufacturer's directions and dilute each 250 mg in at least 100 ml 0.9% sodium chloride solution.

— Do not administer erythromycin lactobionate with other drugs because of chemical instability.

Monitoring

— Monitor the effectiveness of therapy by regularly assessing for improvement of the infectious process.

— Monitor the patient for adverse drug reactions.

— Erythromycin estolate may cause serious hepatotoxicity in adults (reversible cholestatic jaundice). Monitor hepatic function (increased levels of bilirubin, AST [SGOT], ALT [SGPT], and alkaline phosphatase may occur). Other erythromycin salts cause hepatotoxicity to a lesser degree. Patients who develop hepatotoxicity from estolate may react similarly to treatment with any erythromycin preparation.

— Monitor for signs and symptoms of superinfection. Drug may cause overgrowth of nonsusceptible bacteria or fungi.

— Monitor the patient for drug interactions.

— Observe the I.V. site for thrombophlebitis when administering erythromycin gluceptate or erythromycin lactobionate.

— If the patient is receiving erythromycin concomitantly with theophylline, monitor serum theophylline levels.

— If the patient is receiving erythromycin concomitantly with warfarin, monitor for prolonged prothrombin time and abnormal bleeding.

— Monitor laboratory tests. Erythromycin may interfere with fluorometric determination of urinary catecholamines. Liver function test results may become abnormal during erythromycin therapy (rare).

— Regularly reevaluate the patient's and family's knowledge about erythromycin therapy.

Intervention

—If adverse reactions occur (especially the signs and symptoms of cholestatic hepatitis), expect to discontinue the drug and administer another antibiotic.
—If the patient is unable to comply with therapy, discuss reasons and make possible suggestions to improve compliance (for example, clues patient may use to remind himself to take medication).
—If the patient develops an adverse reaction, notify the doctor for appropriate treatment and provide appropriate supportive care.
—Keep all health care team members advised of patient's response to the drug.

Patient teaching

—Instruct the patient and family about erythromycin including the dosage, frequency, action, and adverse reactions.
—Explain the disease process and rationale for therapy.
—Tell the patient to take medication for as long as prescribed, exactly as directed, and even after he feels better and to take entire amount prescribed.
—For best absorption, instruct the patient to take oral form with full glass of water 1 hour before or 2 hours after meals. (However, the patient receiving enteric-coated tablets may take them with meals.) Advise the patient not to take drug with fruit juice. If the patient is taking chewable tablets, instruct him not to swallow them whole.
—Teach the patient on long-term erythromycin therapy the importance of having routine liver function studies as prescribed.
—Instruct the patient receiving I.V. erythromycin lactobionate to notify the nurse if hearing changes occur.
—Tell the patient to notify the nurse or doctor if adverse reactions develop or questions arise about erythromycin therapy.

Evaluation

In the patient receiving erythromycin, appropriate evaluation statements include:
• Patient is free of infection.
• Patient completes prescribed therapy regimen.
• Patient and family state an understanding of erythromycin therapy.

SELF-TEST

1. Kate Conte, age 25, is being discharged with erythromycin to be taken 250 mg P.O. q 6 hours for treatment of pelvic inflammatory disease. The nurse should instruct Mrs. Conte to:
   a. take the drug with fruit juice.
   b. take the drug with water 1 hour before or 2 hours after meals.
   c. take the drug with milk.
   d. take the drug with an antacid.

2. After taking the drug for 6 days, Mrs. Conte develops oral thrush. This is probably a sign of which reaction?
   a. allergic reaction
   b. drug interaction
   c. superinfection
   d. erythromycin toxicity

3. When administering I.V. erythromycin, the nurse should be alert for:
   a. cholestatic hepatitis
   b. leukocytosis
   c. prolonged prothrombin time
   d. thrombophlebitis

Check your answers on pages 1059 and 1060.

CHAPTER 18

MISCELLANEOUS ANTI-INFECTIVES

amantadine hydrochloride ✦ aztreonam ✦ bacitracin zinc
chloramphenicol ✦ chloramphenicol palmitate
chloramphenicol sodium succinate ✦ clindamycin ✦ colistimethate sodium
colisten sulfate ✦ furazolidone ✦ imipenem/cilastatin sodium
lincomycin hydrochloride ✦ nitrofurantoin macrocrystals
nitrofurantoin microcrystals ✦ novobiocin ✦ pentamidine isethionate
polymyxin B sulfate ✦ spectinomycin hydrochloride ✦ trimethoprim
troleandomycin ✦ vancomycin hydrochloride

OVERVIEW

• These antibiotics provide a broad spectrum of activity against infecting agents through inhibition or destruction of susceptible microorganisms. Bacitracin, clindamycin, colistimethate, lincomycin, novobiocin, and polymyxin B sulfate, which have generally been replaced by newer, more effective, and less toxic agents, are primarily used when these newer agents are contraindicated or ineffective.

MAJOR USES

• Amantadine is a beta-lactam antibiotic used for prophylaxis and symptomatic treatment of respiratory tract illness caused by influenza A virus.
• Aztreonam is indicated for the treatment of complicated and uncomplicated urinary tract infections, lower respiratory infections, septicemia, skin and skin structure infections, bone and joint infections, intra-abdominal infections, and gynecologic infections caused by susceptible gram-negative aerobic bacteria.
• Bacitracin is used systemically to treat infants with pneumonia and empyema caused by susceptible staphylococci. In most cases, bacitracin has been replaced by newer agents with broader spectra of activities for such use. Oral bacitracin has been used effectively in a limited number of patients for the treatment of antibiotic-associated diarrhea and colitis, including pseudomembranous colitis caused by *Clostridium difficile*.

GLOSSARY

Antimicrobial: substance used to treat infection with pathogenic microorganisms.
Bacteremia: presence of bacteria in the blood.
Ototoxicity: exerting a destructive or poisonous effect upon the eighth cranial nerve or the organs of hearing and balance.
Resistance: natural ability of an organism to ward off deleterious effects of noxious agents, such as toxins, poisons, irritants, or pathogenic microorganisms.
Trough: the lowest serum therapeutic concentration of a drug.

- Chloramphenicol should be used only for the treatment of serious infections caused by susceptible bacteria, by *Rickettsia* when tetracyclines cannot be used, or by *Chlamydia* when potentially less toxic drugs are ineffective or contraindicated. Chloramphenicol is specifically indicated for the treatment of severe cases of typhoid fever caused by susceptible *Salmonella typhi*, in combination with I.M. or I.V. ampicillin for the initial treatment of meningitis caused by *Haemophilus influenzae* or for osteomyelitis, septic arthritis, cellulitis, epiglottiditis, septicemia, or other serious infections caused by this organism.
- Clindamycin is indicated for the treatment of serious respiratory tract infections, serious skin and soft-tissue infections, septicemia, intra-abdominal infections, and infections of the female pelvis and genital tract, caused by susceptible anaerobic bacteria. It is also used in acute hematogenous osteomyelitis caused by staphylococci, and as an adjunct to surgery in chronic bone and joint infections caused by susceptible organisms.
- Colistimethate is indicated for acute or chronic infections caused by susceptible strains of gram-negative bacteria when other more effective and less toxic agents are contraindicated or ineffective. It may be useful in the treatment of infections caused by *Pseudomonas aeruginosa*, especially urinary tract infections, which are resistant to aminoglycosides and extended-spectrum penicillins.
- Furazolidone is indicated for the specific and symptomatic treatment of diarrhea and enteritis caused by susceptible bacteria or protozoa. It may also be used for enteritis caused by *Giardia lamblia*; and as an adjunct to fluid and electrolyte replacement in the treatment of cholera.
- Imipenem/cilastatin sodium is indicated for serious infections caused by susceptible organisms, including lower respiratory tract, skin and skin structure, intra-abdominal, gynecologic, or bone and joint infections. It is also used to treat serious urinary tract infections, septicemia, or endocarditis caused by susceptible organisms.
- Lincomycin is indicated for serious respiratory tract and skin and soft-tissue infections caused by susceptible microorganisms when other more effective and less toxic agents are contraindicated or ineffective.

- Nitrofurantoin is used in the treatment of pyelonephritis, pyelitis, and cystitis caused by *Escherichia coli, Staphylococcus aureus,* enterococci, and certain strains of *Klebsiella, Proteus,* and *Citrobacter.*
- Novobiocin is indicated for infection caused by susceptible strains of *S. aureus* and *Proteus.*
- Pentamidine is indicated for *Pneumocystis carinii* pneumonia, which occurs primarily in immunocompromised patients. It is used in a solution for oral inhalation to prevent *P. carinii* pneumonia in patients at high risk for initial development or recurrence of this infection, primarily HIV-infected patients. It is also used for its antiprotozoal properties in the treatment and prophylaxis of susceptible organisms.
- Polymyxin B sulfate is used in treating susceptible microorganisms resistant to newer agents.
- Spectinomycin is used to treat uncomplicated gonorrhea caused by susceptible strains of *Neisseria gonorrhoeae.*
- Trimethoprim is available alone or in combination with sulfamethoxazole for the treatment of uncomplicated urinary tract infections due to susceptible microorganisms.
- Troleandomycin is used in the treatment of serious respiratory tract and skin and soft-tissue infections caused by susceptible microorganisms. It is rarely indicated because it is less effective than other agents.
- I.V. vancomycin is used to treat potentially life-threatening infections caused by susceptible organisms, primarily severe staphylococcal infections that cannot be treated with other effective, less toxic drugs. It has also been used alone successfully to treat endocarditis, osteomyelitis, pneumonia, septicemia, and soft-tissue infections caused by susceptible organisms, including methicillin-resistant strains. Oral vancomycin is generally considered the drug of choice for pseudomembranous colitis.

MECHANISM OF ACTION

- Amantadine appears to inhibit viral replication, but the exact mechanism of antiviral activity has not been fully defined.
- Aztreonam is bactericidal. Like other beta-lactam antibiotics, it inhibits mucopeptide synthesis in the bacterial cell wall.
- Bacitracin may be bactericidal or bacteriostatic in action, depending on the concentration of drug attained at the site of infection and the susceptibility of the infecting organism. It inhibits cell wall synthesis, preventing the incorporation of amino acids and nucleotides into the cell wall, and also damages the plasma membrane.
- Chloramphenicol may be bactericidal or bacteriostatic, depending on the concentration of drug attained at the site of infection and the susceptibility of the infecting organism. The drug inhibits protein synthesis.
- Clindamycin and lincomycin may be bacteriostatic or bactericidal, depending on the concentration of drug attained at the site of infection and the susceptibility of the infecting organism. These drugs appear to inhibit protein synthesis. Lincomycin is generally less active against susceptible organisms than clindamycin.
- Colistimethate is inactive until hydrolyzed to colistin. Colistin is usually bactericidal; it acts like a cationic detergent and binds to and damages

the bacterial cytoplasmic membrane of susceptible bacteria, causing leakage of essential intracellular metabolites and nucleosides.
- Furazolidone is bactericidal because it interferes with several bacterial enzyme systems.
- Imipenem/cilastatin sodium is bactericidal. Like other beta-lactam antibiotics, it inhibits mucopeptide synthesis in the bacterial cell wall.
- Nitrofurantoin is bactericidal or bacteriostatic, depending on microorganism and drug concentration. The drug inhibits bacterial enzyme systems.
- Novobiocin is bacteriostatic, apparently through interference with bacterial cell wall synthesis and inhibition of bacterial protein and nucleic acid synthesis. It also appears to affect the stability of the cell membrane by complexing with magnesium.
- Pentamidine's action is not well defined. It inhibits protein and nucleic acid synthesis in susceptible organisms, but the mechanism is unknown. It may also interfere with glucose utilization in susceptible organisms by inhibiting oxidative phosphorylation.
- Polymyxin B sulfate is bactericidal. It binds to phosphate groups in the lipids of bacterial cytoplasmic membrane and acts as a cationic detergent, altering the osmotic barrier of the membrane and causing leakage of essential metabolites.
- Spectinomycin is usually bacteriostatic and appears to inhibit protein synthesis in susceptible bacteria.
- Trimethoprim is slowly bactericidal. It inhibits bacterial thymidine synthesis.
- Troleandomycin may be bactericidal or bacteriostatic, depending on the concentration of the drug attained at the site of infection and the susceptibility of the infecting organism.
- Vancomycin is bactericidal and appears to inhibit protein synthesis.

ABSORPTION, DISTRIBUTION, METABOLISM, AND EXCRETION

Amantadine is well absorbed from the GI tract. Distribution in humans is not well reported. It is excreted unchanged in the urine by glomerular filtration and tubular secretion.

Aztreonam is poorly absorbed from the GI tract with a bioavailability of less than 1% after oral administration. The drug is rapidly and completely absorbed after I.M. and I.V. administration. Peak serum concentrations attained with an I.M. dose are slightly lower than with an equivalent I.V. dose. The drug is widely distributed into body tissues and fluids after I.M. or I.V. administration. Aztreonam is excreted principally in the urine as unchanged drug via both glomerular filtration and tubular secretion.

Bacitracin is not absorbed from the GI tract. It is rapidly and completely absorbed after I.M. injection.

Chloramphenicol is rapidly absorbed from the GI tract. I.V. absorption is variable. The drug is widely distributed into most body tissues and fluids with the highest concentrations found in the liver and kidneys.

Approximately 90% of an oral dose of clindamycin is rapidly absorbed from the GI tract. Serum concentrations increase predictably with increased dosage. The drug is distributed into many body tissues and fluids.

Colistin sulfate and colistimethate are not appreciably absorbed from the GI tract after oral administration. Colistimethate is well absorbed when administered by the I.M. and I.V. routes. Colistimethate and metabolites of the drug are excreted mainly via the kidneys by glomerular filtration.

Furazolidone is significantly absorbed after oral administration. It is rapidly and extensively metabolized, possibly in the intestine, and excreted in urine.

Imipenem/cilastatin sodium is not appreciably absorbed from the GI tract and therefore is given only parenterally. Imipenem is widely distributed. Imipenem, cilastatin, and their metabolites are excreted primarily in urine by both glomerular filtration and tubular excretion.

Lincomycin is rapidly absorbed from the GI tract; approximately 20% to 30% of an oral dose is absorbed. Food delays and decreases the extent of absorption. The I.M. dose is also well absorbed. The drug is distributed into many body tissues and fluids.

Nitrofurantoin is well absorbed from the GI tract. Drug absorption is enhanced when taken with food or when the macrocrystal form is used. Drug is 20% to 60% protein-bound; serum half-life is less than 30 minutes. Peak levels in the urine appear within 1 hour of dosing. Drug is partially metabolized in the liver; parent compound and metabolites are excreted in the urine.

Novobiocin is well absorbed from the GI tract. Food lowers peak serum concentrations. The drug diffuses into pleural, synovial, and ascitic fluid; it is excreted via the bile and feces. Approximately 3% is excreted in urine.

Pentamidine respiratory fluid concentrations are higher after oral inhalation than after I.V. administration. The drug appears to undergo limited absorption from the respiratory tract into systemic circulation. Distribution into body tissues and fluids has not been well defined but it appears to be rapidly and extensively distributed and/or bound to tissues. Little is known about the elimination of pentamidine in humans.

Polymyxin B sulfate is not absorbed from the GI tract, but is well absorbed intramuscularly. Reportedly, the serum half-life is 4.3 to 6 hours in adults. Approximately 60% of a dose is excreted unchanged into the urine by glomerular filtration; the fate of the remaining 40% is unknown.

Spectinomycin is not absorbed from the GI tract and is rapidly absorbed after I.M. administration. Distribution is not well defined.

Trimethoprim is readily and almost completely absorbed from the GI tract and is widely distributed into body tissues and fluids. It is metabolized in the liver and rapidly excreted in the urine via glomerular filtration and tubular secretion; small amounts are excreted in feces via biliary elimination.

Troleandomycin is rapidly but incompletely absorbed after oral administration. The metabolite is widely distributed into body tissues and fluids. The drug is excreted in urine and in feces via bile.

Vancomycin is usually not appreciably absorbed from the GI tract; however, limited data suggest that clinically significant serum concentrations may result after enteral or oral administration in some patients with colitis, particularly those with renal impairment. After I.V. administration, it is widely distributed in body tissues and diffuses readily into pericardial, pleural, ascitic, and synovial fluids. Oral doses are excreted primarily in the feces; absorbed drug is excreted primarily by glomerular filtration.

ONSET AND DURATION

Amantadine attains mean peak blood concentrations 1 to 4 hours after an oral dose. The elimination half-life has been reported as 9 to 37 hours, with an average of 24 hours. The long elimination half-life permits once daily dosage or two equally divided doses.

Aztreonam attains peak serum concentrations of a single oral dose in approximately 2 hours; serum concentrations were undetectable 8 hours after the dose.

Bacitracin attains the maximum serum concentration after a single I.M. dose and after 1 to 2 hours; detectable amounts are present in serum 6 to 8 hours after injection. The drug is widely distributed in all body organs and is present in ascitic and pleural fluids after I.M. injection. With I.M. injection, it is excreted slowly by glomerular filtration and appears in the urine within 24 hours. After oral administration, the drug is excreted in the feces. A considerable amount is thought to be either retained or destroyed in the body.

Chloramphenicol attains average peak plasma concentrations within 1 to 3 hours. After I.V. administration, plasma concentrations vary considerably. The plasma half-life is 1.5 to 4.1 hours. Excretion is through the kidney by glomerular filtration and tubular secretion.

Clindamycin attains peak serum concentrations after oral administration within 45 to 60 minutes. After I.M. administration, peak serum concentrations occur within 3 hours in adults and 1 hour in children. I.V. absorption is equally efficacious. The serum half-life is 2 to 3 hours in adults and children.

Colistimethate attains peak concentrations after I.M. administration within 2 hours and may be detectable 12 hours after the dose. After I.V. administration, peak serum concentrations are higher but decline more rapidly. The plasma half-life after I.M. or I.V. administration is reportedly 1.5 to 8 hours in adults.

Furazolidone is usually administered four times daily. Response should occur in 7 days; in 7 to 10 days, for giardiasis.

Imipenem/cilastatin sodium attains peak serum concentrations immediately after I.V. infusion of a single dose. Serum concentrations decline appreciably after 4 to 6 hours.

Lincomycin attains peak plasma concentrations after an oral dose within 2 to 4 hours; after I.M. administration, in 30 minutes. The plasma half-life is 4 to 6.4 hours. The drug is partially metabolized in the liver; both drug and metabolites are excreted in the urine, bile, and feces.

Nitrofurantoin's peak urine levels occur within 1 hour of dosing.

Novobiocin attains peak serum concentrations within 1 to 4 hours after oral administration. Serum concentrations may be detectable 24 hours after the dose.

Pentamidine attains peak plasma concentrations 1 to 14 days after initiation of therapy.

Polymyxin B sulfate attains peak serum concentrations within approximately 2 hours. Detectable amounts of the drug are present in the serum for up to 12 hours. The drug is widely distributed into body tissues.

Spectinomycin attains peak serum concentrations after I.M. administration within 1 hour. The plasma half-life is 1.2 to 2.8 hours.

Trimethoprim attains peak serum concentrations after oral administration in 1 to 4 hours. After multiple dose oral administration, steady-state peak serum concentrations are usually 50% greater than those obtained after single dose administration. Peak serum concentrations are reached after a 1-hour I.V. infusion. Steady-state peak concentrations are reached with every-8-hour I.V. dosing.

Troleandomycin attains peak serum concentrations of the metabolite within 2 hours; serum concentrations may be detectable 12 hours after the dose.

Vancomycin has been reported to have a serum elimination half-life of 4 to 6 hours.

ADVERSE REACTIONS

Amantadine most frequently causes nausea, dizziness, light-headedness, and insomnia. It may also cause CNS effects, dry mouth, constipation, ataxia, peripheral edema, livedo reticularis, orthostatic hypotension, headache, and dermatologic and hematologic reactions.

Aztreonam is generally well tolerated. GI reactions or rash have been reported in about 1% to 2% of the patients receiving the drug; hypotension, transient ECG changes, and CNS effects, in less than 1% of patients. Other reactions include hematologic effects; transient increases in hepatic and renal enzymes; local phlebitis or thrombophlebitis; and miscellaneous effects, including fever, chills, cold sweats, dyspnea, sneezing, nasal congestion, tinnitus, impaired hearing in one ear, diplopia, myalgia, vaginitis, vaginal candidiasis, and breast tenderness.

Bacitracin may cause renal tubular and glomerular necrosis, related to the total daily dose and the duration of therapy.

Chloramphenicol is known to cause two forms of bone marrow depression: a non-dose-related and irreversible type leads to aplastic anemia with a 50% or greater mortality rate, generally resulting from hemorrhage or infection. Bone marrow aplasia or hypoplasia may occur after a single dose but more often develops weeks or months after the drug has been discontinued. The second and more common type of bone marrow depression is dose-related and usually reversible upon discontinuation of the drug. Reversible bone marrow depression occurs regularly when chloramphenicol dosage in adults exceeds 4 g daily. Other adverse reactions include optic neuritis with long-term high-dose therapy, adverse GI effects, and hypersensitivity reactions. In neonates, it may cause a type of circulatory collapse known as gray syndrome. This syndrome has occurred in neonates born to mothers who received chloramphenicol during the final stages of pregnancy or labor, and in children as old as age 2.

Clindamycin most frequently causes a generalized morbilliform rash. Maculopapular rash, urticaria, pruritus, fever, hypotension, GI effects, and, rarely, polyarthritis and a few anaphylactoid reactions have also occurred. Thrombophlebitis, erythema, and pain and swelling have followed I.V. administration; cardiopulmonary arrest and hypotension have followed too-rapid I.V. administration of the drug.

Colistimethate may cause nephrotoxicity and neurotoxicity when the drug is used in higher-than-recommended dosages or in patients with impaired renal function. Transient CNS effects have occurred within the first 4 days of therapy; they disappear when the drug is discontinued. Neuromuscular blockage, which may result in respiratory arrest, has also occurred.

Furazolidone is known to cause allergic reactions, GI reactions, headache, malaise, disulfiram-like reactions, and mild reversible intravascular hemolysis in G6PD-deficient patients. Furazolidone should not be administered to neonates because they risk hemolytic anemia due to immature enzyme systems.

Imipenem/cilastatin sodium most commonly causes GI reactions, but CNS, hematologic, dermatologic, hepatic, and renal reactions have also been reported. Other adverse reactions are similar to those reported with other beta-lactam antibiotics.

Lincomycin may cause GI reactions with all routes of administration but may be severe enough to require discontinuation of the drug. Hypersensitivity reactions, localized irritation at injection site, and hepatic and hematologic changes have also occurred. Hypotension, syncope, and occasionally cardiac arrest have followed rapid I.V. administration.

Nitrofurantoin commonly causes adverse GI reactions, including anorexia, nausea, and vomiting (may be reduced by giving with food or milk or reducing dose). Pulmonary hypersensitivity reactions (including dyspnea, cough, or pulmonary infiltrates) may occur. Hepatitis, peripheral neuropathy, exfoliative dermatitis, and hemolytic anemia are severe reactions that rarely occur.

Novobiocin causes hepatic reactions, including jaundice. Dizziness, drowsiness, and light-headedness have also been reported.

Pentamidine most commonly causes nephrotoxicity or cough and bronchospasm. Fatalities due to severe hypotension, hypoglycemia, and cardiac arrhythmias have been reported.

Polymyxin B sulfate causes nephrotoxicity and neurotoxicity, which are more likely to occur with higher-than-recommended dosages or in patients with impaired renal function. Neuromuscular blockade, which may result in respiratory arrest, has occurred. Meningeal irritation may follow intrathecal administration. Anaphylactoid reactions have been reported rarely. Thrombophlebitis has been reported at I.V. injection sites.

Spectinomycin appears to have a low order of toxicity. The most frequent reaction is pain at the injection site. Other reactions include allergic reactions and decreases in hemoglobin and creatinine clearance.

Trimethoprim primarily causes dermatologic reactions—for example, rash occurs in 3% to 7% of patients. Other reactions include epigastric distress, nausea, vomiting, glossitis, hematologic changes, fever, and elevation of hepatic and renal enzymes.

Troleandomycin produces GI reactions and hypersensitivity reactions, including cholestatic hepatitis.

Vancomycin causes ototoxicity and nephrotoxicity, the most serious reactions to parenteral therapy; these effects have not been reported after oral therapy. Vancomycin is very irritating to tissue and causes necrosis when given I.M.; therefore, it must be administered I.V., with care to avoid extravasation. Pain and thrombophlebitis are common after I.V. administration; rapid I.V. administration has resulted in hypotension. Other reactions include hematologic effects, nausea, chills, fever, urticaria, macular rashes, a shocklike state, transient anaphylaxis, and, occasionally, vascular collapse. A throbbing pain in the neck and back muscles has been reported; it can usually be minimized or avoided by slower administration of the drug.

PROTOTYPE: MISCELLANEOUS ANTI-INFECTIVES

CHLORAMPHENICOL
(klor am fen′ i kole)
Chloromycetin, Novochlorocap†

CHLORAMPHENICOL PALMITATE
Chloromycetin Palmitate

CHLORAMPHENICOL SODIUM SUCCINATE
Chloromycetin, Pentamycetin†, Sodium Succinate
Classification: anti-infective
Pregnancy risk category C

How supplied
TABLETS: 250 mg, 500 mg
ORAL SUSPENSION: 150 mg/5 ml
INJECTION: 1-g, 10-g vials

Indications and dosage
Haemophilus influenzae *meningitis, acute* **Salmonella typhi** *infection, and meningitis, bacteremia, or other severe infections caused by sensitive* **Salmonella** *species,* **Rickettsia,** *lymphogranuloma, psittacosis, or various sensitive gram-negative organisms*
ADULTS AND CHILDREN: 50 to 100 mg/kg P.O. or I.V. daily in divided doses q 6 hours. Maximum dosage is 100 mg/kg daily.
PREMATURE INFANTS AND NEONATES AGES 2 WEEKS AND UNDER: 25 mg/kg P.O. or I.V. daily in divided doses q 6 hours. I.V. route must be used to treat meningitis.

---

†Available in Canada only

Contraindications and precautions
Chloramphenicol is contraindicated in patients with minor infections (such as influenza, throat infections, and colds) or as prophylaxis against infection. It is also contraindicated in patients with known hypersensitivity or a history of toxic reaction to the drug. Administer cautiously to pregnant patients at term or during labor; to premature and full-term infants, and to breast-feeding patients.

Adverse reactions
BLOOD: **aplastic anemia, hypoplastic anemia, granulocytopenia, thrombocytopenia.**
CNS: headache, mild depression, confusion, delirium, peripheral neuropathy with prolonged therapy.
EENT: optic neuritis (in patients with cystic fibrosis), glossitis, decreased visual acuity.
GI: nausea, vomiting, stomatitis, *diarrhea,* pseudomembranous colitis.
OTHER: infections caused by nonsusceptible organisms, hypersensitivity reaction (fever, rash, urticaria, **anaphylaxis**), jaundice, **gray syndrome** in neonates (abdominal distention, gray cyanosis, vasomotor collapse, respiratory distress, death within a few hours of onset of symptoms).

Interactions
Acetaminophen: elevates chloramphenicol levels. Monitor for chloramphenicol toxicity.
Chlorpropamide, dicumarol, phenobarbital, phenytoin, tolbutamide: blood levels of these agents may be increased by chloramphenicol. Monitor for toxicity.

Nursing considerations
Assessment
• Review the patient's history for a condition that contraindicates the use of chloramphenicol.
• Obtain a baseline assessment of the patient's infection before therapy.
• Be alert for common adverse reactions.
• Evaluate the patient's and family's knowledge about chloramphenicol therapy.

Planning (Nursing Diagnoses)
Potential nursing diagnoses for the patient receiving chloramphenicol include:
• Potential for injury related to inadequate dosage regimen.
• Altered protection related to chloramphenicol-induced aplastic anemia.
• Knowledge deficit related to chloramphenicol therapy.

Implementation
Preparation and administration
— Obtain specimen for culture and sensitivity tests before first dose. Therapy may begin pending test results. Chloramphenicol must not be used when less potentially dangerous agents will be effective.

—Give I.V. slowly over 1 minute.
—Reconstitute 1-g vial of powder for injection with 10 ml sterile water for injection. Concentration will be 100 mg/ml. Reconstituted solution is stable for 30 days at room temperature, but refrigeration is recommended. Do not use cloudy solutions.
—If administering drug concomitantly with penicillin, give penicillin 1 hour or more before chloramphenicol to avoid reduction in penicillin's bactericidal activity.
—Expect to decrease the chloramphenicol dosage as prescribed in a patient with serious hepatic dysfunction or renal failure or in a neonate to prevent bone marrow suppression, encephalitis, or gray syndrome.

Monitoring

—Monitor the effectiveness of therapy by regularly assessing for improvement of infectious process.
—Monitor the patient for adverse drug reactions.
—Observe the neonate for signs of gray syndrome. Observe the older patient for signs of toxicity (abdominal distention, vomiting, anorexia, tachypnea, cyanosis, green stools, lethargy, and an ashen color) if the serum concentration is above 40 mcg/ml. Observe the adult patient for evidence of encephalitis, such as decreased level of consciousness, headache, fever, seizures, and nuchal rigidity.
—Continue to observe the patient for signs and symptoms of aplastic anemia, such as anemia, infection, or bleeding, after chloramphenicol therapy has been discontinued.
—Monitor CBC, platelet counts, serum iron, and reticulocyte counts before and every 2 days during therapy.
—Monitor the patient for drug interactions.
—Monitor I.V. site daily for phlebitis and irritation.
—Monitor for evidence of superinfection by nonsusceptible organisms.
—Monitor plasma concentrations. Therapeutic plasma concentrations are 5 to 25 mcg/ml.
—Monitor diagnostic test results. Treatment with chloramphenicol will cause false-positive results on tests for urine glucose level using copper sulfate (Clinitest).
—Regularly reevaluate the patient's and family's knowledge about chloramphenicol therapy.

Intervention

—Discontinue drug immediately if anemia, reticulocytopenia, leukopenia, or thrombocytopenia develops and prepare to treat the patient's symptoms as indicated.
—If the patient's serum chloramphenicol concentration exceeds 25 mcg/ml, take bleeding precautions and infection-control measures because bone marrow suppression can occur.
—If the patient develops an adverse reaction, notify the doctor for appropriate treatment and provide supportive care as indicated.
—Keep all health care team members advised of the patient's response to the drug.

Patient teaching
—Instruct the patient and family about chloramphenicol, including the dosage, frequency, action, and adverse reactions.
—Explain the disease process and rationale for therapy.
—Tell the patient to take medication for as long as prescribed and exactly as directed, even after he feels better.
—Instruct the patient to take oral drug forms on an empty stomach 1 hour before or 2 hours after meals. (If patient develops adverse GI reactions, however, advise him to take drug with food.)
—Tell the patient to notify the nurse or doctor if adverse reactions develop or questions arise about chloramphenicol therapy.

Evaluation
In the patient receiving chloramphenicol, appropriate evaluation statements include:
• Patient is free of infection.
• Patient exhibits no adverse reactions to chloramphenicol therapy, including no signs of aplastic anemia.
• Patient and family state an understanding of chloramphenicol therapy.

PROTOTYPE: MISCELLANEOUS ANTI-INFECTIVES

CLINDAMYCIN HYDROCHLORIDE
(klin da mye′ sin)
Cleocin HCl, Dalacin C†‡

CLINDAMYCIN PALMITATE HYDROCHLORIDE
Cleocin Pediatric, Dalacin C Palmitate†‡

CLINDAMYCIN PHOSPHATE
Cleocin, Cleocin Phosphate, Dalacin C†‡, Dalacin C Phosphate
Classification: anti-infective
Pregnancy risk category C

How supplied
CAPSULES: 75 mg, 150 mg
ORAL SOLUTION: 75 mg/5 ml
INJECTION: 150 mg/ml

Indications and dosage
Infections caused by sensitive staphylococci, streptococci, pneumococci, Bacteroides, Fusobacterium, Clostridium perfringens, and other sensitive aerobic and anaerobic organisms
ADULTS: 150 to 450 mg P.O. q 6 hours; or 300 mg I.M. or I.V. q 6, 8, or 12 hours. Up to 2,700 mg I.M. or I.V. daily in divided doses q 6, 8, or 12 hours. May be used for severe infections.

CHILDREN OVER AGE 1 MONTH: 8 to 25 mg/kg P.O. daily, in divided doses q 6 to 8 hours; or 15 to 40 mg/kg I.M. or I.V. daily in divided doses q 6 hours.

Contraindications and precautions

Clindamycin is contraindicated in patients with known hypersensitivity to preparations containing clindamycin or lincomycin. Use cautiously in patients with a history of GI disease, particularly colitis; in atopic patients; in patients with very severe renal or hepatic disease; and in those receiving neuromuscular blocking agents.

Adverse reactions

BLOOD: transient leukopenia, eosinophilia, thrombocytopenia.

GI: *nausea*, vomiting, abdominal pain, *diarrhea,* pseudomembranous enterocolitis, esophagitis, flatulence, anorexia, bloody or tarry stools, dysphagia.

HEPATIC: elevated AST (SGOT), alkaline phosphatase, bilirubin.

SKIN: maculopapular rash, urticaria.

LOCAL: pain, induration, sterile abscess with I.M. injection; thrombophlebitis, erythema, and pain after I.V. administration.

OTHER: unpleasant or bitter taste, **anaphylaxis.**

Interactions

Erythromycin: antagonist that may block access of clindamycin to its site of action; don't use together.

Kaolin: decreased absorption of oral clindamycin. Separate administration times by at least 2 hours.

Neuromuscular blocking agents: clindamycin may potentiate neuromuscular blockade. Monitor for weakness or difficult breathing.

Nursing considerations

Assessment

• Review the patient's history for a condition that contraindicates the use of clindamycin.

• Obtain a baseline assessment of the patient's infection before therapy.

• Be alert for common adverse reactions.

• Evaluate the patient's and family's knowledge about clindamycin therapy.

Planning (Nursing Diagnoses)

Potential nursing diagnoses for the patient receiving clindamycin include:

• Potential for injury related to ineffective drug dosage.

• Potential fluid volume deficit related to adverse GI reactions.

• Knowledge deficit related to clindamycin therapy.

Implementation

Preparation and administration

—Obtain specimen for culture and sensitivity tests before first dose. Therapy may begin pending test results.

—Don't refrigerate reconstituted oral solution because it will thicken. Drug is stable for 2 weeks at room temperature.

Italicized adverse reactions are common   Boldfaced adverse reactions are life-threatening

—Give deep I.M. Rotate sites. Warn that I.M. injection may be painful. Doses greater than 600 mg/injection are not recommended.
—For I.V. infusion, dilute each 300 mg in 50 ml solution and give no faster than 30 mg/minute.

Monitoring

—Monitor the effectiveness of therapy by regularly assessing for improvement of infectious process.
—Monitor the patient for adverse drug reactions.
—Watch for superinfection (fever or other signs of new infection).
—If administering I.V., monitor site for signs of thrombophlebitis.
—If administering I.M., check injection site regularly for signs of irritation, such as induration and sterile abscess.
—Monitor the patient for drug interactions.
—Monitor hydration closely if the patient experiences GI upset, especially severe diarrhea.
—Monitor for signs of pseudomembranous colitis, such as mucus and blood in the stools.
—Monitor laboratory test results, especially renal, hepatic, and hematopoietic functions, during prolonged therapy. Liver function test results may become abnormal in some patients during clindamycin therapy. I.M. injection may cause creatinine phosphokinase level to rise because of muscle irritation.
—Regularly reevaluate the patient's and family's knowledge about clindamycin therapy.

Intervention

—If the patient develops GI upset, request an antiemetic or antidiarrheal, if needed.
—Don't give diphenoxylate compound (Lomotil) to treat drug-induced diarrhea. It may prolong and worsen diarrhea.
—If patient develops an adverse reaction, notify the doctor for appropriate treatment and provide supportive care as indicated.
—Keep all health care team members advised of the patient's response to the drug.

Patient teaching

—Instruct the patient and family about clindamycin, including the dosage, frequency, action, and adverse reactions.
—Explain the disease process and rationale for therapy.
—Instruct the patient to report adverse reactions, especially diarrhea, to the doctor. Warn the patient not to self-treat diarrhea.
—Advise the patient taking the capsule form to take with a full glass of water to prevent dysphagia.
—Instruct the patient to complete the entire course of therapy.
—Warn the patient receiving clindamycin I.M. that the injection may be painful.
—Instruct the patient receiving clindamycin I.V. to notify the nurse if discomfort is felt at the infusion site.

— Tell the patient to notify the nurse or doctor if adverse reactions develop or questions arise about clindamycin therapy.

Evaluation

In the patient receiving clindamycin, appropriate evaluation statements include:
• Patient is free of infection.
• Patient maintains normal fluid volume.
• Patient and family state an understanding of clindamycin therapy.

PROTOTYPE: MISCELLANEOUS ANTI-INFECTIVES

NITROFURANTOIN MACROCRYSTALS
Macrodantin

(nye troe fyoor an' toyn)

NITROFURANTOIN MICROCRYSTALS
Apo-Nitrofurantoin†, Furadantin, Furalan, Furan, Furanite, Macrodantin, Nephronex†, Nitrofan, Novofuran†

Classification: anti-infective
Pregnancy risk category B

How supplied

macrocrystals
CAPSULES: 25 mg, 50 mg, 100 mg
ORAL SUSPENSION: 25 mg/5 ml
microcrystals
TABLETS: 50 mg, 100 mg
CAPSULES: 50 mg, 100 mg
ORAL SUSPENSION: 25 mg/5 ml

Indications and dosage

***Pyelonephritis, pyelitis, and cystitis due to susceptible* Escherichia coli, Staphylococcus aureus, *enterococci; certain strains of* Klebsiella, Proteus, *and* Enterobacter**
ADULTS AND CHILDREN OVER AGE 12: 50 to 100 mg P.O. q.i.d. with milk or meals.
CHILDREN AGES 1 MONTH TO 12 YEARS: 5 to 7 mg/kg P.O. daily in divided doses q.i.d.

Long-term suppression therapy
ADULTS: 50 to 100 mg P.O. daily h.s.
CHILDREN: 1 to 2 mg/kg P.O. daily h.s.

Contraindications and precautions

Nitrofurantoin is contraindicated in patients with moderate to severe renal impairment, anuria, oliguria, or creatinine clearance under 40 ml/minute;

---

†Available in Canada only

in pregnant patients at term; in neonates; and in those with known hypersensitivity to the drug.

Adverse reactions

BLOOD: **hemolysis** in patients with G6PD deficiency (reversed after stopping drug), **agranulocytosis, thrombocytopenia.**
CNS: peripheral neuropathy, headache, dizziness, drowsiness, ascending polyneuropathy with high doses or renal impairment.
GI: *anorexia, nausea, vomiting, abdominal pain, diarrhea.*
HEPATIC: hepatitis.
SKIN: maculopapular, erythematous, or eczematous eruption; pruritus; urticaria; **exfoliative dermatitis; Stevens-Johnson syndrome.**
OTHER: **asthmatic attacks** in patients with history of asthma; **anaphylaxis;** hypersensitivity; transient alopecia; drug fever; overgrowth of nonsusceptible organisms in the urinary tract; pulmonary sensitivity reactions (cough, chest pains, fever, chills, dyspnea).

Interactions

Magnesium-containing antacids: decreased nitrofurantoin absorption. Separate administration times by 1 hour.
Nalidixic acid, norfloxacin: possible decreased effectiveness. Avoid using together.
Probenecid, sulfinpyrazone: increased blood levels and decreased urine levels. May result in increased toxicity and lack of therapeutic effect. Don't use together.

Nursing considerations

Assessment
• Review the patient's history for a condition that contraindicates the use of nitrofurantoin.
• Obtain a baseline assessment of the patient's infection before therapy.
• Be alert for common adverse reactions.
• Evaluate the patient's and family's knowledge about nitrofurantoin therapy.

Planning (Nursing Diagnoses)
Potential nursing diagnoses for the patient receiving nitrofurantoin include:
• Altered health maintenance related to the ineffectiveness of the drug.
• Noncompliance (medication administration) related to prolonged therapy.
• Knowledge deficit related to nitrofurantoin therapy.

Implementation
Preparation and administration
— Obtain specimen for culture and sensitivity tests before starting therapy and repeat as needed. Therapy may begin pending test results.
— Give with food or milk to minimize GI distress. Nitrofurantoin macrocrystals may be less irritating to the GI tract in some patients.

— Store in amber container. Keep away from metals other than stainless steel or aluminum to avoid precipitate formation.

— Continue treatment for 3 days after sterile urine specimens have been obtained.

— Give oral preparations 1 hour apart from magnesium-containing antacids. Oral suspension may be mixed with water, milk, fruit juice, and formulas.

— Dilute I.V. nitrofurantoin in 500 ml of I.V. solution before administering. Infuse at 50 to 60 drops/minute.

— For I.V. infusion, reconstitute in 20 ml of dextrose 5% solution or sterile water without preservatives.

Monitoring

— Monitor the effectiveness of therapy by regularly assessing for improvement of the infectious process.

— Monitor the patient for adverse drug reactions. Hypersensitivity may develop when used for long-term therapy.

— Monitor for superinfection. Use of nitrofurantoin may result in growth of nonsusceptible organisms, especially *Pseudomonas*.

— Monitor CBC regularly.

— Monitor intake and output carefully. May turn urine brown or rust-yellow.

— Monitor the patient for drug interactions.

— Monitor diagnostic test results. May cause false-positive results with urine sugar test using copper sulfate reduction method (Clinitest) but not with glucose enzymatic tests (Tes-Tape, Diastix, Clinistix).

— Regularly reevaluate the patient's and family's knowledge about nitrofurantoin therapy.

Intervention

— If the patient is unable to comply with therapy, discuss reasons and suggest possible methods to help improve compliance (for example, clues patient can use to remind himself to take medication).

— If the patient develops adverse reactions, notify the doctor for appropriate treatment and provide supportive care as indicated. If the patient displays adverse GI reactions during treatment with nitrofurantoin microcrystal formulation, discuss with doctor the possibility of changing the drug to nitrofurantoin macrocrystals, which are less likely to cause adverse GI reactions.

— Keep all health care team members advised of the patient's response to the drug.

Patient teaching

— Instruct the patient and family about nitrofurantoin, including the dosage, frequency, action, and adverse reactions.

— Explain disease process and rationale for therapy.

— Stress the importance of taking the drug for the prescribed length of time.

— Instruct the patient to take the drug with food or milk to minimize GI distress.
— Instruct the diabetic patient not to perform urine glucose determinations using copper sulfate (Clinitest) because false-positive results may occur during nitrofurantoin therapy.
— Warn the patient that drug may turn urine brown or rust-yellow.
— Warn the patient that oral suspension may temporarily discolor or stain teeth. To avoid this, suggest that the patient rinse his mouth with water after swallowing medication.
— Instruct the patient not to store drug in pillboxes made of stainless steel or aluminum.
— Tell the patient to notify the nurse or doctor if adverse reactions develop or questions arise about nitrofurantoin therapy.

Evaluation
In the patient receiving nitrofurantoin, appropriate evaluation statements include:
• Patient is free of infection.
• Patient completes entire therapy as prescribed.
• Patient and family state an understanding of nitrofurantoin therapy.

PROTOTYPE: MISCELLANEOUS ANTI-INFECTIVES

PENTAMIDINE ISETHIONATE
(pen tam' i deen)
NebuPent, Pentam 300
Classification: anti-infective
Pregnancy risk category C

How supplied
INJECTION: 300-mg vials
INHALATION: 300-mg vials

Indications and dosage
Pneumonia due to Pneumocystis carinii
ADULTS AND CHILDREN: 4 mg/kg I.V. or I.M. daily for 14 days.

Prevention of P. carinii pneumonia in high-risk individuals
ADULTS: 300 mg by inhalation (using a Respirgard II nebulizer) once q 4 weeks.

Contraindications and precautions
Pentamidine is contraindicated in patients with a history of an anaphylactic reaction to inhaled or parenteral pentamidine. Do not give to pregnant or breast-feeding women unless the potential benefits outweigh the unknown risks.

Once the diagnosis of *P. carinii* pneumonia has been firmly established, there are no absolute contraindications to the use of pentamidine. Use cautiously in patients with hypertension, hypotension, hypoglycemia, hyperglycemia, hypocalcemia, leukopenia, thrombocytopenia, anemia, and hepatic or renal dysfunction.

Adverse reactions
BLOOD: **leukopenia, thrombocytopenia**, anemia.
CNS: confusion, hallucinations.
CV: *hypotension*, tachycardia (parenteral form).
ENDOCRINE: **hypoglycemia,** hyperglycemia, hypocalcemia (parenteral form).
GI: nausea, anorexia, *metallic taste.*
GU: elevated serum creatinine, renal toxicity.
HEPATIC: elevated liver enzymes.
SKIN: rash, facial flushing, pruritus.
LOCAL: sterile abscess, pain or induration at injection site.
OTHER: fever, **anaphylaxis**, *coughing and bronchospasm* after aerosol form.

Interactions
Aminoglycosides, amphotericin B, cisplatin, vancomycin, zidovudine: increased risk of nephrotoxicity. Avoid concomitant use.

Nursing considerations
Assessment
• Review the patient's history for a condition that contraindicates the use of pentamidine.
• Obtain a baseline assessment of the patient's infection before therapy.
• Be alert for common adverse reactions.
• Evaluate the patient's and family's knowledge about pentamidine therapy.

Planning (Nursing Diagnoses)
Potential nursing diagnoses for the patient receiving pentamidine include:
• Potential for injury related to ineffective drug dosage.
• Noncompliance (medication administration) related to prolonged therapy.
• Knowledge deficit related to pentamidine therapy.

Implementation
Preparation and administration
—Make sure the patient has adequate fluid status before administering drug; dehydration may lead to hypotension and renal toxicity.
—Make sure the patient is lying down when he is receiving the drug because sudden, severe hypotension may develop. Monitor blood pressure during administration and several times thereafter until blood pressure is stable.
—To prepare drug for I.V. infusion, add 3 to 5 ml of sterile water for injection or dextrose 5% in water (D_5W) to 300-mg vial to yield 100 mg/ml or 60 mg/ml, respectively. Withdraw desired dose and dilute

further into 50 to 250 ml of D_5W; infuse over at least 60 minutes. Diluted solution remains stable for 5 days.

— To prepare drug for I.M. injection, add 3 ml of sterile water for injection to 300-mg vial to yield 100 mg/ml. Pain and induration occur universally with I.M. injection. Administer by deep I.M. injection.

— Dissolve nebulized pentamidine in sterile water and administer it via a Respirgard II nebulizer.

— When administering I.V., infuse over 60 minutes to minimize risk of hypotension.

— In the patient with AIDS, pentamidine may produce less severe adverse reactions than the alternative treatment with co-trimoxazole. Therefore, in some AIDS patients, pentamidine is considered the treatment of choice.

— Perform a respiratory assessment after administering nebulized pentamidine, particularly noting bronchospasm and cough.

Monitoring

— Monitor the effectiveness of therapy by regularly assessing for improvement of infectious process.

— Monitor the patient for adverse drug reactions.

— Monitor ECG during I.V. infusion.

— Monitor blood glucose, serum creatinine, and BUN levels daily. After parenteral administration, blood glucose levels may decrease initially; hypoglycemia may be severe in 5% to 10% of patients. This may be followed by hyperglycemia and insulin-dependent diabetes mellitus (which may be permanent).

— Monitor periodic electrolyte levels, CBC, platelet count, and liver function tests.

— Monitor the patient for drug interactions.

— Observe for signs and symptoms of hypoglycemia.

— Inspect the injection site periodically for signs of induration or sterile abscess when administering pentamidine I.M. Inspect the infusion site for evidence of phlebitis when administering pentamidine I.V.

— Monitor diagnostic test results: BUN, serum creatinine, AST (SGOT), and ALT (SGPT) levels may increase during pentamidine therapy.

— Regularly reevaluate the patient's and family's knowledge about pentamidine therapy.

Intervention

— Keep emergency drugs and equipment (including emergency airway, vasopressors, and I.V. fluids) on hand.

— If the patient is unable to comply with therapy, discuss reasons and suggest possible methods to improve compliance (for example, clues patient can use to help remind himself to take medication).

— If the patient develops an adverse reaction, notify the doctor for appropriate treatment and provide supportive care as indicated.

— Keep all health care team members advised of patient's response to the drug.

Patient teaching
— Instruct the patient and family about pentamidine, including the dosage, frequency, action, and adverse reactions.
— Explain disease process and rationale for therapy.
— Inform the patient that pain may occur at the injection site with I.M. administration of pentamidine.
— Advise the patient to alert the nurse or doctor if a cough or shortness of breath occur after inhalation therapy or if pruritus or skin changes occur with I.M. or I.V. therapy. Review the signs and symptoms of hyperglycemia or hypoglycemia with the patient.
— Tell the patient to notify the nurse or doctor if adverse reactions develop or questions arise about pentamidine therapy.

Evaluation
In the patient receiving pentamidine, appropriate evaluation statements include:
• Patient is free of infection.
• Patient completes prescribed therapy regimen.
• Patient and family state an understanding of pentamidine therapy.

PROTOTYPE: MISCELLANEOUS ANTI-INFECTIVES

VANCOMYCIN HYDROCHLORIDE
(van koe mye′ sin)
Vancocin
Classification: anti-infective
Pregnancy risk category C

How supplied
POWDER FOR ORAL SOLUTION: 1-g, 10-g bottles
POWDER FOR INJECTION: 500-mg, 1-g vials.

Indications and dosage
Severe staphylococcal infections when other antibiotics are ineffective or contraindicated
ADULTS: 500 mg I.V. q 6 hours, or 1 g q 12 hours.
CHILDREN: 44 mg/kg I.V. daily in divided doses q 6 hours.
NEONATES: 10 mg/kg I.V. daily in divided doses q 6 to 12 hours.

Antibiotic-associated pseudomembranous and staphylococcal enterocolitis
ADULTS: 125 to 500 mg P.O. q 6 hours for 7 to 10 days.
CHILDREN: 44 mg/kg P.O. daily in divided doses q 6 hours.

Endocarditis prophylaxis for dental procedures
ADULTS: 1 g I.V. slowly over 1 hour, starting 1 hour before procedure. No repeat dose is necessary.

Contraindications and precautions

Vancomycin is contraindicated in patients with known hypersensitivity to the drug. Administer cautiously to patients with renal insufficiency.

Adverse reactions

BLOOD: transient eosinophilia, leukopenia.
EENT: tinnitus, ototoxicity (deafness).
GI: *nausea.*
SKIN: "red-neck" syndrome with rapid I.V. infusion (maculopapular rash on face, neck, trunk, and extremities).
LOCAL: pain or thrombophlebitis with I.V. administration, necrosis.
OTHER: chills, fever, **anaphylaxis,** overgrowth of nonsusceptible organisms.

Interactions

Aminoglycosides, amphotericin B, cisplatin, pentamidine: increased risk of nephrotoxicity. Avoid concomitant use.

Nursing considerations

Assessment
• Review the patient's history for a condition that contraindicates the use of vancomycin.
• Obtain a baseline assessment of the patient's infection before therapy.
• Be alert for common adverse reactions.
• Evaluate the patient's and family's knowledge about vancomycin therapy.

Planning (Nursing Diagnoses)
Potential nursing diagnoses for the patient receiving vancomycin include:
• Altered health maintenance related to ineffectiveness of drug.
• Sensory-perceptual alterations (auditory) related to vancomycin-induced ototoxicity.
• Knowledge deficit related to vancomycin therapy.

Implementation
Preparation and administration
— Obtain culture and sensitivity tests before starting therapy (unless drug is being used for prophylaxis).
— To prepare drug for oral administration, reconstitute as directed in manufacturer's instructions. Reconstituted solution remains stable for 2 weeks when refrigerated.
— To prepare drug for I.V. injection, reconstitute 500-mg or 1-g vial with 10 ml of sterile water for injection to yield 50 mg/ml or 100 mg/ml, respectively. Withdraw desired dose and further dilute to 100 to 250 ml with 0.9% sodium chloride solution or 5% dextrose in water. Infuse over at least 60 minutes to avoid adverse reactions related to rapid infusion rate. Reconstituted solution remains stable for 96 hours when refrigerated.
— Do not give I.M. because drug is highly irritating.
— Assess the patient's renal status before beginning vancomycin therapy.

—Patients with impaired renal function may require dosage reduction. See dosage nomogram on package insert for initial dosage; monitor serum drug levels to titrate subsequent doses.

—Hemodialysis and peritoneal dialysis remove only minimal drug amounts. Patients receiving these treatments require usual dose only once every 5 to 7 days.

—Do not mix vancomycin with other drugs in the same I.V. solution.

Monitoring

—Monitor the effectiveness of therapy by regularly assessing for improvement of the infectious process.

—Monitor the patient for adverse drug reactions.

—Monitor carefully for "red-neck" syndrome. Stop infusion and notify the doctor promptly if you see this reaction.

—Monitor closely for signs of ototoxicity, especially in the patient with renal impairment or the patient receiving long-term high doses of I.V. vancomycin.

—Monitor vancomycin serum concentrations (peak and trough levels) and the serum creatinine level if the patient is receiving another ototoxic or nephrotoxic drug concurrently.

—Monitor I.V. infusion site for phlebitis and irritation.

—Monitor the patient for drug interactions.

—Monitor diagnostic test results. BUN and serum creatinine levels may increase and neutropenia and eosinophilia may occur during vancomycin therapy.

—Regularly reevaluate the patient's and family's knowledge about vancomycin therapy.

Intervention

—Withhold vancomycin and notify the doctor if tinnitus or hearing loss occurs. Expect to discontinue drug and initiate a different antibiotic as prescribed.

—If the patient develops maculopapular rash on face, neck, trunk, and upper extremities, slow infusion rate.

—If patient develops an adverse reaction, notify the doctor for appropriate treatment and provide supportive care as indicated.

—Keep all members of the health care team informed of the patient's response to the drug.

Patient teaching

—Instruct the patient and family about vancomycin, including the dosage, frequency, action, and adverse reactions.

—Explain the disease process and rationale for therapy.

—Tell the patient to take medication exactly as directed, even after he feels better, and to take entire amount prescribed. Treat staphylococcal endocarditis for at least 4 weeks.

—Tell the patient to report adverse reactions immediately, especially fullness or ringing in ears. Stop drug immediately if these occur.

— Advise the patient not to take antidiarrheals concomitantly with drug except under doctor's supervision.

— Tell the patient receiving I.V. drug to report pain at infusion site.

— Tell the patient to notify the nurse or doctor if adverse reactions develop or questions arise about vancomycin therapy.

Evaluation

In the patient receiving vancomycin, appropriate evaluation statements include:

• Patient is free of infection.

• Patient maintains normal hearing.

• Patient and family state an understanding of vancomycin therapy.

SELF-TEST

1. Debbie Golden, age 8, is receiving chloramphenicol for *Haemophilus influenzae* meningitis. Which adverse reaction limits chloramphenicol to treating serious infections only?

   a. ototoxicity

   b. drug-induced aplastic anemia

   c. nephrotoxicity

   d. bone marrow suppression

2. James Whyte, a diabetic patient, reports he tests his urine for glucose when he does not feel well. Which test produces a false-positive result for glucose during nitrofurantoin therapy?

   a. Clinistix

   b. Diastix

   c. Tes-Tape

   d. Clinitest

3. John Wright, age 52, has been receiving I.V. clindamycin for 3 days. He now complains of diarrhea. Which other signs should his nurse watch closely for?

   a. red, swollen oral mucous membranes

   b. bullae on the skin

   c. mucus and blood in the stools

   d. rash

Check your answers on page 1060.

CHAPTER 19

INOTROPIC AGENTS

Digitalis glycosides
deslanoside ✦ digitoxin ✦ digoxin

OVERVIEW

- Inotropic agents, primarily derivatives of digitalis, influence the force of myocardial contractility. The digitalis (or cardiac) glycosides, which are extracted from plants of the genus *Digitalis* or chemically synthesized, are used to treat CHF and tachyarrhythmias. All the digitalis glycosides act similarly on the CV system; however, they differ in extent of absorption, metabolism, and excretion.
- The range between therapeutic and toxic doses is extremely narrow. Toxicity may be due to altered absorption, serum electrolyte levels, renal or hepatic dysfunction, drug interactions, or other factors. The choice of digitalis glycoside and route of administration depend on the disorder and the desired onset of activity.

MAJOR USES

- Digitalis glycosides increase cardiac output in acute or chronic CHF. They control the rate of ventricular contraction in atrial flutter or fibrillation. They're also used to prevent or treat paroxysmal atrial tachycardia and angina associated with CHF.

MECHANISM OF ACTION

- Digitalis glycosides influence both mechanical and electrical activity of the heart. Their physiologic effects vary depending on drug concentration and cardiac status. Increasing the force of contraction may produce no significant effect on a normal heart; but, in the presence of CHF, it produces beneficial slowing of the heart rate according to the severity of compensatory tachycardia.
- The increased force of contraction (positive inotropic effect) is caused by increased calcium ion (Ca^{++}) availability to the contractile proteins actin and myosin. Increased Ca^{++} availability results from a complex series of interactions related to these drugs' ability to inhibit sodium-potassium adenosine triphosphatase (Na-K ATPase). This enzyme drives the "sodium pump," which exchanges intracellular sodium ions for extracellular potassium ions. In cardiac cells, a second exchange mechanism exchanges intracellular sodium for calcium in the presence of digitalis.

GLOSSARY

Afterload: pressure in the arteries leading from the ventricle that must be overcome for ejection to occur.
Contractility: capacity for shortening or contracting in response to a stimulus.
Diastole: period of ventricular dilation that occurs between the second and first heart sounds.
Inotropic: affecting the force of cardiac muscle contraction; a drug with a positive inotropic effect increases the strength of the muscle contraction.
Preload: blood volume in the ventricle at the end of diastole.
Stroke volume: blood output from the ventricle during systole, usually about 70 ml.
Systole: period of ventricular contraction that occurs between the first and second heart sounds.

- Digitalis glycosides also act on the CNS to decrease sympathetic activity and increase vagal activity. This increased vagal activity results in a slower firing rate of the sinoatrial (SA) node and slower conduction velocity through the atrioventricular (AV) node.

ABSORPTION, DISTRIBUTION, METABOLISM, AND EXCRETION

Deslanoside is given I.V. or I.M. only because absorption from the GI tract is erratic or incomplete. It is primarily excreted unchanged in the urine. It should be used with caution in patients with renal dysfunction.

Digitoxin is 90% to 100% absorbed after oral administration. Passing through the enterohepatic circulation, the drug is extensively metabolized in the liver to inactive metabolites and is excreted by the kidneys. Neither the drug nor its metabolites accumulate in the renal parenchyma when renal function is impaired, since biliary and fecal elimination increase.

Digoxin is 60% to 85% absorbed after oral administration (absorption varies with manufacturer). Although 80% is absorbed after I.M. administration, this route may cause pain and irritation at the injection site. Digoxin is excreted primarily unchanged in the urine. Use with caution in patients with renal dysfunction.

None of the digitalis glycosides is distributed to adipose tissues. In obese patients, dosage should be based on ideal body weight.

ONSET AND DURATION

The onset and duration of action of the digitalis glycosides vary. (See *Pharmacokinetics of Digitalis Glycosides*, page 224.)

ADVERSE REACTIONS

The adverse drug reactions associated with the digitalis glycosides fall into four groups: cardiac, neurologic, GI, and visual.

PHARMACOKINETICS OF DIGITALIS GLYCOSIDES

DRUG	ONSET	PEAK	HALF-LIFE	DURATION
deslanoside	10 to 30 minutes	1 to 2 hours	1½ days	2 to 5 days
digitoxin	30 to 120 minutes	4 to 12 hours	5 to 7 days	2 to 3 weeks
digoxin P.O.	15 to 30 minutes	2 to 6 hours	1½ days	2 to 3 days
digoxin I.V.	5 to 30 minutes	1 to 5 hours	1½ days	2 to 3 days

Cardiac reactions are usually caused by drug toxicity secondary to excessive blood levels. Digoxin levels above 2 mcg/liter or digitoxin levels above 35 mcg/liter may result in arrhythmias, most commonly premature ventricular contractions, AV node conduction block, paroxysmal supraventricular tachycardia, and bigeminy.

Neurologic reactions commonly associated with digitalis glycoside intoxication are headache, fatigue, depression, confusion, and insomnia. Less common reactions include psychosis, delirium, and neuralgia.

GI reactions include anorexia, nausea and vomiting and, less commonly, diarrhea and abdominal pain.

The most common visual reaction is blurred vision, but other signs of digitalis intoxication may include abnormal color vision, green and yellow halos, scotomata, and amblyopia.

PROTOTYPE: DIGITALIS GLYCOSIDES

DIGOXIN
(di jox'in)
Lanoxicaps, Lanoxin*, Novodigoxin†
Classification: digitalis glycoside
Pregnancy risk category C

How supplied
TABLETS: 0.125 mg, 0.25 mg, 0.5 mg
CAPSULES: 0.05 mg, 0.1 mg, 0.2 mg
ELIXIR: 0.05 mg/ml*
INJECTION: 0.05 mg/ml†, 0.1 mg/ml (pediatric), 0.25 mg/ml

---

*Liquid form contains alcohol   †Available in Canada only

Indications and dosage
CHF, paroxysmal supraventricular tachycardia, atrial fibrillation and flutter

ADULTS: loading dose is 0.5 to 1 mg I.V. or P.O. in divided doses over 24 hours; maintenance dosage is 0.125 to 0.5 mg I.V. or P.O. daily (average 0.25 mg). Larger doses are often needed for treatment of arrhythmias, depending on patient response. Smaller loading and maintenance doses should be given to patients with impaired renal function.

ADULTS OVER AGE 65: 0.125 mg P.O. daily as maintenance dose. Frail or underweight elderly patients may require only 0.0625 mg daily or 0.125 mg every other day.

CHILDREN OVER AGE 2: loading dose is 0.02 to 0.04 mg/kg P.O. divided q 8 hours over 24 hours; I.V. loading dose is 0.015 to 0.035 mg/kg; maintenance dosage is 0.012 mg/kg P.O. daily divided q 12 hours.

CHILDREN AGES 1 MONTH TO 2 YEARS: loading dose is 0.035 to 0.06 mg/kg P.O. in three divided doses over 24 hours, or 0.03 to 0.05 mg/kg I.V.; maintenance dosage is 0.01 to 0.02 mg/kg P.O. daily divided q 12 hours.

NEONATES: loading dose is 0.035 mg/kg P.O. divided q 8 hours over 24 hours, or 0.02 to 0.03 mg/kg I.V.; maintenance dosage is 0.01 mg/kg P.O. daily divided q 12 hours.

PREMATURE INFANTS: loading dose is 0.025 mg/kg I.V. in three divided doses over 24 hours; maintenance dosage is 0.01 mg/kg I.V. daily divided q 12 hours.

Contraindications and precautions

Digoxin is contraindicated in the presence of any digitalis-induced toxicity, ventricular fibrillation, or ventricular tachycardia unless caused by CHF. Use with extreme caution in elderly patients and in those with acute MI, incomplete AV block, sinus bradycardia, premature ventricular contractions, chronic constrictive pericarditis, idiopathic hypertrophic subaortic stenosis, renal insufficiency, severe pulmonary disease, or hypothyroidism. Dosage must be reduced in renal impairment.

Administering calcium salts to digitalized patients is contraindicated. Calcium affects cardiac contractility and excitability in much the same way as digitalis glycosides and may lead to serious arrhythmias in these patients.

Adverse reactions

The following signs of toxicity may occur with all digitalis glycosides:

CNS: fatigue, generalized muscle weakness, agitation, hallucinations, *headache,* malaise, dizziness, vertigo, stupor, paresthesia.

CV: increased severity of CHF, **arrhythmias** (most commonly conduction disturbances with or without AV block, premature ventricular contractions, and supraventricular arrhythmias), hypotension.

EENT: yellow-green halos around visual images, blurred vision, light flashes, photophobia, diplopia.

GI: *anorexia, nausea, vomiting, diarrhea.*

Note: Toxic effects on the heart may be life-threatening and require immediate attention.

Interactions

Amiloride: inhibits and increases digoxin excretion. Monitor for altered digoxin effect.

Amphotericin B, carbenicillin, ticarcillin, corticosteroids, and diuretics (including loop diuretics, chlorthalidone, metolazone, and thiazides): hypokalemia, predisposing patient to digitalis toxicity. Monitor serum potassium level.

Antacids, kaolin-pectin: decreased absorption of oral digoxin. Schedule doses as far as possible from oral digoxin administration.

Anticholinergics: may increase absorption of orally administered digoxin. Monitor blood levels and observe for toxicity.

Cholestyramine, colestipol, metoclopramide: decreased absorption of oral digoxin. Monitor for decreased effect and low blood levels of digoxin. Dosage may have to be increased.

Parenteral calcium, thiazides: hypercalcemia and hypomagnesemia, predisposing patient to digitalis toxicity. Monitor serum calcium and serum magnesium levels.

Quinidine, diltiazem, amiodarone, nifedipine, verapamil: increased digoxin blood levels. Monitor for toxicity.

Nursing considerations

Assessment

- Review the patient's history for a condition that contraindicates the use of digoxin and related compounds.
- Obtain a baseline assessment of the patient's heart rate and rhythm or degree of CHF present before therapy.
- Be alert for adverse reactions.
- Evaluate the patient's and family's knowledge about digoxin therapy.

Planning (Nursing Diagnoses)

Potential nursing diagnoses for the patient receiving digoxin include:
- Decreased cardiac output related to ineffectiveness of digoxin.
- Injury related to adverse CNS effects caused by potential digitalis toxicity.
- Fluid volume deficit related to potential digoxin-induced GI effects.
- Knowledge deficit related to digoxin therapy.

Implementation

Preparation and administration

— Obtain baseline data (heart rate and rhythm, blood pressure, and electrolyte levels) before giving first dose.
— Ask patient about recent use of digitalis glycosides (within the previous 2 to 3 weeks) before administering a loading dose.
— Withhold drug for 1 to 2 days before elective electrocardioversion. Adjust dosage after cardioversion.
— Don't substitute one brand for another.
— Always divide loading dose over first 24 hours unless clinical situation indicates otherwise.
— Infuse I.V. dose slowly over at least 5 minutes.

—Be aware that when changing from oral tablets or elixir to parenteral therapy or to liquid-filled capsules, the dosage is reduced by 20% to 25%. When changing from liquid-filled capsules to parenteral therapy, dosage is about equivalent because liquid-filled capsules are readily absorbed.

—Monitor hypothyroid patients carefully because they are very sensitive to digitalis glycosides; hyperthyroid patients may need larger doses.

—Be aware that, in obese patients, dosage should be based on ideal body weight.

Monitoring

—Monitor the effectiveness of therapy by taking an apical-radial pulse for a full minute before each dose, evaluating ECG when ordered, and regularly assessing patient's cardiopulmonary status for signs of improvement. Record and report to the doctor any significant changes (sudden increase or decrease in rate, pulse deficit, irregular beats, and particularly regularization of a previously irregular rhythm). Check blood pressure and obtain 12-lead ECG with these changes.

—Monitor the patient for adverse drug reactions.

—Dose is adjusted to the patient's clinical condition and is monitored by serum digoxin, calcium, potassium, and magnesium levels, and by ECG. Obtain blood for digoxin levels 8 hours after last oral dose. Therapeutic blood levels of digoxin range from 0.5 to 2 ng/ml.

—Regularly monitor for digitalis toxicity: nausea, vomiting, anorexia, visual disturbances, arrhythmias, and CNS reactions.

—Monitor the patient for drug interactions.

—Monitor the patient's cardiopulmonary status regularly for signs of recurring CHF (sudden weight gain, crackles in lung fields, S_3 heart sound, distended neck veins, peripheral edema).

—Regularly reevaluate the patient's and family's knowledge about digoxin therapy.

Intervention

—Excessive slowing of the pulse rate (60 beats/minute or less) may be a sign of digitalis toxicity. Withhold drug and notify doctor.

—Do not administer calcium salts to patients receiving digoxin; calcium affects cardiac contractility and excitability and may lead to serious arrhythmias.

—Institute safety precautions if CNS reactions occur.

—Obtain an order for an antiemetic or antidiarrheal agent if GI reactions occur. Also obtain a digoxin blood level to determine if symptoms are a result of toxicity. If so, expect to withhold dose.

—Keep all members of the health care team informed of the patient's response to the drug.

Patient teaching

—Inform the patient and family about digoxin, including the dosage, frequency, action, and adverse reactions.

—Teach the patient and family how to take a pulse before each dose.

—Stress the importance of notifying the doctor if digitalis toxicity is suspected because of visual disturbances, change in mental status, irregular pulse, or GI dysfunction.

—Encourage the patient to eat potassium-rich foods.

—Tell the patient that regular follow-up and periodic laboratory tests will be needed to evaluate the effectiveness of the drug.

—Tell the patient to notify the nurse or doctor if adverse reactions develop or questions arise about digoxin therapy.

Evaluation

In the patient receiving digoxin, appropriate evaluation statements include:

• Patient's ECG reveals correction of arrhythmia.

• Patient does not experience CNS reactions.

• Patient maintains adequate hydration.

• Patient and family state an understanding of digoxin therapy.

SELECTED MAJOR DRUGS: DIGITALIS GLYCOSIDES

DRUG, INDICATIONS, AND DOSAGES	SPECIAL PRECAUTIONS
deslanoside (Cedilanid-D) *CHF, paroxysmal atrial tachycardia, atrial fibrillation and flutter—* **Adults:** loading dose is 1.2 to 1.6 mg I.M. or slow I.V. in two divided doses over 24 hours; for maintenance, use another digitalis glycoside. Not recommended for children.	• Contraindicated in presence of any digitalis-induced toxicity, ventricular fibrillation, or ventricular tachycardia unless caused by CHF. • Administering calcium salts to digitalized patients is contraindicated. Calcium affects cardiac contractility and excitability in much the same way as digitalis glycosides and may lead to serious arrhythmias in such patients. • Use with extreme caution in elderly patients, and in those with acute MI, incomplete AV block, chronic constrictive pericarditis, idiopathic hypertrophic subaortic stenosis, renal insufficiency, severe pulmonary disease, or hypothyroidism. • Therapeutic drug levels have not been established.
digitoxin (Crystodigin) *CHF, paroxysmal atrial tachycardia, atrial fibrillation and flutter—* **Adults:** loading dose is 1.2 to 1.6 mg P.O. in divided doses over 24 hours; average maintenance dosage is 0.15 mg daily (range: 0.05 to 0.3 mg daily). **Children ages 2 to 12:** loading dose is 0.3 mg/kg or 0.75 mg/m² P.O. in divided doses over 24 hours; maintenance dosage is one-tenth of loading dose or 0.003 mg/kg or 0.075 mg/m² daily. Monitor closely for toxicity.	• Contraindicated in presence of any digitalis-induced toxicity, ventricular fibrillation, or ventricular tachycardia unless caused by CHF. • Administering calcium salts to digitalized patients is contraindicated. Calcium affects cardiac contractility and excitability in much the same way as digitalis glycosides and may lead to serious arrhythmias in such patients.

SELECTED MAJOR DRUGS: DIGITALIS GLYCOSIDES *continued*

DRUG, INDICATIONS, AND DOSAGES

digitoxin *(continued)*
Children ages 1 to 2: loading dose is 0.04 mg/kg
P.O. over 24 hours in divided doses; maintenance
dosage is 0.004 mg/kg daily. Monitor closely for
toxicity.
Infants ages 2 weeks to 1 year: loading dose is
0.045 mg/kg P.O. in divided doses over 24 hours;
maintenance dosage is 0.0045 mg/kg daily. Monitor
closely for toxicity.
Premature infants, neonates, severely ill older infants: loading dose is 0.022 mg/kg P.O. in divided
doses over 24 hours; maintenance dosage is 0.0022
mg/kg daily. Monitor closely for toxicity.

SPECIAL PRECAUTIONS

• Use with extreme caution in patients with acute MI, incomplete AV
block, chronic constrictive pericarditis, idiopathic hypertrophic subaortic
stenosis, severe pulmonary disease,
and hypothyroidism; and in elderly
patients.
• Therapeutic drug levels are 14 to
26 ng/ml.

SELF-TEST

Sara Rose, 57, is admitted to your unit with atrial fibrillation and ventricular arrhythmias. She has a history of coronary artery disease
and diabetes mellitus. Mrs. Rose is to receive a loading dose of
I.V. digoxin, a bolus of lidocaine I.V., and an I.V. lidocaine infusion.

1. For a patient Mrs. Rose's age, the usual loading dose of digoxin over a
24-hour period is:
 a. 0.125 mg I.V. q 8 hours.
 b. 0.5 mg/kg P.O. q 4 hours.
 c. 0.5 to 1 mg I.V. or P.O. in divided doses.
 d. 0.125 to 0.25 mg P.O. in divided doses.

2. Which of the following is not a common reaction to digoxin?
 a. nausea and vomiting
 b. hearing disturbances
 c. arrhythmias
 d. headache

3. Which of the following instructions should be given to Mrs. Rose
about digoxin administration?
 a. Stop the medication if the heart rate is stable.
 b. Monitor pulse rate daily.
 c. Notify the doctor if the heart rate is between 60 and 100
 beats/minute.
 d. Take only with milk.

4. Which of the following drugs will increase the digoxin concentration if given concurrently to Mrs. Rose while she is taking digoxin?
    a. nifedipine
    b. cholestyramine
    c. metoclopramide
    d. kaolin-pectin

5. How fast should the nurse administer I.V. digoxin?
    a. over 1 minute
    b. over 2 minutes
    c. over 5 minutes
    d. over 10 minutes

Check your answers on page 1060.

CHAPTER 20

ANTIARRHYTHMICS

Class I
moricizine hydrochloride

Class Ia
disopyramide phosphate ◆ procainamide hydrochloride
quinidine gluconate ◆ quinidine polygalacturonate ◆ quinidine sulfate

Class Ib
lidocaine hydrochloride ◆ mexiletine hydrochloride ◆ phenytoin
phenytoin sodium ◆ tocainide hydrochloride

Class Ic
flecainide acetate ◆ indecainide hydrochloride ◆ propafenone hydrochloride

Class II
acebutolol hydrochloride ◆ esmolol hydrochloride
propranolol hydrochloride

Class III
amiodarone hydrochloride ◆ bretylium tosylate

Class IV
verapamil hydrochloride

OVERVIEW

- Antiarrhythmics are used to prevent or treat atrial and ventricular arrhythmias, including those secondary to MI or digitalis toxicity.
- Bradycardia can be due to decreased generation of atrial impulses or to conduction of fewer atrial impulses to the ventricles. Similarly, ventricular tachycardia can develop from an increased number of impulses from either atrial or ventricular areas.
- As a group, the antiarrhythmics have a narrow therapeutic index (the toxic dose is not much greater than the therapeutic dose). Careful monitoring of therapy is imperative, since adverse reactions to these drugs are usually serious. Before therapy begins, underlying conditions such as electrolyte imbalances should be corrected.
- Synchronized cardioversion and electrical pacemakers are effective antiarrhythmic alternatives.

GLOSSARY

Arrhythmia: abnormal variation in cardiac conduction, rhythm, or rate.

Atrioventricular (AV) block: obstructed transmission of electrical impulses from the atria to the ventricles caused by AV node damage or depression.

Automaticity: ability to generate an electrical impulse independently.

Chronotropic: altering the rate of cardiac muscle contraction; a drug with a negative chronotropic effect slows the heart rate.

Conductivity: capacity of cells to conduct current.

Depolarization: neutralization of electrical polarity in cardiac cells caused by an influx of sodium ions.

Ectopy: generation of electrical impulses by cardiac cells outside the normal conduction pathways.

Excitability: readiness of a cell to respond to a stimulus.

Fibrillation: twitching movements of cardiac muscle resulting from so rapid a transmission of independent impulses that coordinated contractions cannot occur.

Proarrhythmia: arrhythmia that occurs when another already is present.

Reentry or circus movement: abnormal transmission of an electrical impulse around and around in cardiac muscle without stopping.

Refractory period: period of depolarization after excitation, during which cardiac muscle cannot respond to another normal cardiac impulse.

Repolarization: restoration of electrical polarity in cardiac cells caused by an outflow of potassium ions from the cells.

• The antiarrhythmic agents discussed in this chapter are classified into seven categories: Class I, Ia, Ib, Ic, II, III, and IV. These classifications are based upon the drugs' effects on the action potential of cardiac cells and their mechanisms of action. Although other drugs are used to treat certain arrhythmias (atropine, for example, is used to treat bradyarrhythmias), they are not included in this discussion. Among the Class Ib antiarrhythmics, phenytoin and phenytoin sodium are most often used to treat seizure disorders. (See Chapter 29, Anticonvulsants.)

MAJOR USES

• Antiarrhythmics are therapeutic for atrial and ventricular arrhythmias of various causes.

MECHANISM OF ACTION

• The most recently introduced Class I antiarrhythmic, moricizine, a potent anesthetic, produces its membrane-stabilizing effect by reducing the inward current carried by sodium ions.

- Class Ia antiarrhythmics (quinidine, procainamide, and disopyramide) block the transport of sodium ions, which results in a decreased conduction velocity and slow rate of repolarization.
- Class Ib antiarrhythmics (lidocaine, tocainide, and mexiletine) also block the transport of sodium ions, but cause almost no decrease in conduction velocity and increase the rate of repolarization.
- Class Ic antiarrhythmics (flecainide, indecainide, and propafenone) also block the transport of sodium ions. They cause a depression of conduction velocity but almost no decrease in repolarization rate.
- Class II antiarrhythmics (beta blockers) decrease conduction of impulses through the AV node and increase the effective refractory period. In addition to their beta blockade, Class II drugs also have reentry blocking effects similar to those of Class I. Acebutolol, esmolol, and propranolol are effective for supraventricular arrhythmias and, to a lesser extent, for ventricular arrhythmias.
- The Class III drug bretylium was originally used as an antihypertensive. It is an antiadrenergic agent whose action is mediated through the sympathetic division of the autonomic nervous system. Bretylium initially exerts short-lived adrenergic stimulatory effects (caused by release of norepinephrine) on the CV system. When norepinephrine is depleted, the adrenergic blocking actions predominate and orthostatic hypotension is common. Recent pharmacologic studies indicate that bretylium's action may be due to its large quaternary ammonium structure.
- Amiodarone, another Class III agent, produces its effect by prolonging the action potential and refractory period. It also produces noncompetitive alpha and beta inhibition.
- The calcium channel blocker, verapamil, a class IV antiarrhythmic, is used with digitalis to control the ventricular rate in chronic atrial flutter or fibrillation.

ABSORPTION, DISTRIBUTION, METABOLISM, AND EXCRETION

After oral administration, most antiarrhythmic drugs are well absorbed from the GI tract. Bretylium, however, is poorly absorbed and must be given parenterally.

All antiarrhythmics are widely distributed in body tissues and are metabolized primarily in the liver.

Procainamide is metabolized in the liver to an active metabolite, N-acetylprocainamide (NAPA), which accumulates in patients with impaired renal function. The other drugs are excreted partly as inactive metabolites and partly as unchanged drug by the kidneys.

Propranolol and lidocaine, although well absorbed when administered orally, enter the hepatic portal circulation immediately and are quickly metabolized in the first-pass effect. However, the first-pass effect may be nullified for propranolol by administering large oral doses (relative to parenteral doses). Therefore, propranolol is commonly used both orally and parenterally.

ONSET AND DURATION

See *Pharmacokinetics of Antiarrhythmics* for onset and duration of action of antiarrhythmics.

ADVERSE REACTIONS

Most Class I antiarrhythmics (Class I, Ia, Ib, or Ic) exhibit proarrhythmic effects. However, a large multicenter trial—the Cardiac Arrhythmia Suppression Trial (CAST)—investigating the effectiveness of antiarrhythmic medications found that two Class Ic agents, flecainide and encainide (which is no longer marketed), caused a higher incidence of mortality and nonfatal MI as compared to placebo. As a result of this finding, Class Ic agents are reserved for patients with life-threatening arrhythmias.

All patients taking antiarrhythmic drugs should be monitored for new or worsened arrhythmias. It may be particularly difficult to identify drug-induced arrhythmias because they may mimic the patient's underlying disorder.

Moricizine, a Class I agent, may also cause dizziness, headache, nausea, fatigue, and vomiting.

Class Ia antiarrhythmics commonly cause myocardial depression, diarrhea (a dose-limiting reaction with quinidine), dizziness, dry mouth, and blurred vision. Procainamide has been known to cause systemic lupus erythematosus (SLE) syndrome in some patients.

Class Ib antiarrhythmics are associated with neurologic reactions that are usually dose-limiting. Such reactions include confusion, dizziness, tremor, nystagmus, slurred speech, and seizures. Less often, Class Ib antiarrhythmics cause hypotension, myocardial depression, bradycardia, and heart block.

Class Ic antiarrhythmics are most commonly associated with bradycardia, dizziness (20% to 60%), tremor, and visual disturbances. Flecainide and propafenone have been associated with a metallic taste.

Class II antiarrhythmics, beta blockers, are commonly associated with nausea, dizziness, light-headedness, bradycardia, and fatigue. Less frequently, beta blockers are known to cause dry mouth, vomiting, hypotension, dyspnea, confusion, insomnia, rash, hyperglycemia, hypoglycemia, and impotence.

The Class III antiarrhythmic, amiodarone, may cause bradycardia, pneumonitis leading to fibrosis, photosensitivity, and pseudocyanosis. GI irritation commonly occurs with an amiodarone loading dose. Bretylium commonly causes orthostatic hypotension.

The Class IV antiarrhythmic, verapamil, most commonly causes constipation, hypotension, and bradycardia.

PHARMACOKINETICS OF ANTIARRHYTHMICS

GROUP	DRUG	ONSET (ORAL)	HALF-LIFE	DURATION	THERAPEUTIC BLOOD LEVELS
I	moricizine	2 hours	1½ to 3½ hours	10 to 24 hours	N/A
Ia	disopyramide	30 minutes	4 to 10 hours	6 to 7 hours	2 to 8 mcg/ml
	procainamide	30 minutes	2½ to 4½ hours	> 3 hours	4 to 8 mcg/ml
	quinidine	30 minutes	6 to 7 hours	6 to 8 hours	2 to 6 mcg/ml
Ib	lidocaine	(I.V.)	1 to 2 hours	15 minutes	1.5 to 6 mcg/ml
	mexiletine	< 3 hours	10 to 12 hours	variable	0.5 to 2 mcg/ml
	phenytoin	30 minutes to 1 hour	22 to 46 hours	24 hours	10 to 20 mcg/ml
	tocainide	< 3 hours	11 to 15 hours	variable	4 to 10 mcg/ml
Ic	flecainide	1 to 6 hours	12 to 27 hours	variable	0.2 to 1 mcg/ml
	propafenone	3.5 hours	2 to 10 hours	variable	0.06 to 1 mcg/ml
II	acebutolol	2 to 4 hours	3 to 4 hours	24 to 30 hours	unknown
	esmolol	(I.V.)	< 10 minutes	< 10 minutes	unknown
	propranolol	30 minutes	2 to 3 hours	3 to 5 hours	0.05 to 0.1 mcg/ml
III	amiodarone	1 to 3 weeks	25 to 100 days	variable	0.5 to 2.5 mcg/ml
	bretylium	(I.V.)	5 to 10 hours	6 to 8 hours	0.5 to 1.5 mcg/ml
IV	verapamil	30 minutes	3 to 7 hours	6 hours	0.08 to 0.3 mcg/ml

MORICIZINE HYDROCHLORIDE
(mor i' siz een)
Ethmozine
Classification: Class I antiarrhythmic
Pregnancy risk category B

How supplied
TABLETS: 200 mg, 250 mg, 300 mg

Indications and dosage
Life-threatening ventricular arrhythmias
ADULTS: individualized dosage is based on clinical response and patient tolerance. Therapy should begin in the hospital. Most patients respond to 600 to 900 mg P.O. daily, given in divided doses q 8 hours. Increase daily dosage q 3 days by 150 mg until the desired clinical effect is seen.

Patients with hepatic or renal function impairment
ADULTS: start therapy at 600 mg P.O. daily or less. Monitor closely and adjust dosage carefully.

Contraindications and precautions
Moricizine is contraindicated in patients with preexisting second- or third-degree AV block or right bundle branch block when associated with left hemiblock (bifascicular block) unless a pacemaker is present. It's also contraindicated in patients in cardiogenic shock and in those with known hypersensitivity to the drug.

Patients with hepatic or renal dysfunction will exhibit decreased moricizine clearance. Administer cautiously and monitor effects closely. Note ECG intervals before adjusting dosage. Administer with extreme care, if at all, to patients with severe hepatic insufficiency. Also use with extreme caution in patients with sick sinus syndrome; drug may cause sinus bradycardia or sinus arrest.

Note that the drug has been detected in breast milk. A decision should be made to discontinue breast-feeding or discontinue the drug, depending on the drug's potential benefit to the mother.

Adverse reactions
CNS: *dizziness, headache,* fatigue, anxiety, hypoesthesia, asthenia, nervousness, paresthesia, sleep disorders.
CV: **proarrhythmic events, ECG abnormalities** (including conduction defects, sinus pause, junctional rhythm, or AV block), **CHF**, palpitations, **sustained ventricular tachycardia,** chest pain, sinus bradycardia, **sinus arrest.**
EENT: blurred vision.
GI: *nausea,* vomiting, abdominal pain, dyspepsia, diarrhea, *dry mouth.*
GU: urine retention.
SKIN: rash.

Italicized adverse reactions are common   Boldfaced adverse reactions are life-threatening

OTHER: *dyspnea*, drug fever, sweating, musculoskeletal pain.

Interactions
Cimetidine: increased plasma levels and decreased clearance of moricizine. Begin moricizine therapy at low dosage (not more than 600 mg daily) and monitor plasma levels and therapeutic effect closely.
Propranolol, digoxin: additive prolongation of the PR interval. Monitor closely.
Theophylline: increased theophylline clearance and reduced plasma levels. Monitor plasma levels and therapeutic response; adjust theophylline dosage as needed.

Nursing considerations
Assessment
• Review the patient's history for a condition that contraindicates the use of moricizine.
• Obtain a baseline assessment of the patient's heart rate and rhythm before therapy.
• Be alert for common adverse reactions.
• Evaluate the patient's and family's knowledge about moricizine therapy.

Planning (Nursing Diagnoses)
Potential nursing diagnoses for the patient receiving moricizine include:
• Decreased cardiac output related to ineffectiveness of moricizine to correct arrhythmia.
• Altered protection related to moricizine-induced proarrhythmias.
• Fluid volume deficit related to potential moricizine-induced GI upset.
• Knowledge deficit related to moricizine therapy.

Implementation
Preparation and administration
—Be aware that the drug should be initially administered in the hospital with continuous ECG monitoring.
—Be aware that individual dosage is based on clinical response and patient tolerance.
—Correct electrolyte imbalances before administering drug, because hypokalemia, hyperkalemia, and hypomagnesemia may alter the drug's effects.
—Expect to administer reduced dosage to patients with hepatic or renal dysfunction.
—When substituting another antiarrhythmic, withdraw previous antiarrhythmic therapy for one to two half-lives of the drug before starting moricizine at recommended dosage. Patients who have shown a tendency to develop life-threatening arrhythmias after withdrawal of drug therapy should be hospitalized during withdrawal and adjustment to moricizine. Start moricizine therapy after:
    disopyramide, 6 to 12 hours after the last dose.
    mexiletine, 8 to 12 hours after the last dose.
    procainamide, 3 to 6 hours after the last dose.
    propafenone, 8 to 12 hours after the last dose.

quinidine, 6 to 12 hours after the last dose.

tocainide, 8 to 12 hours after the last dose.

—Be aware that the drug should be used only for patients with life-threatening ventricular arrhythmias.

Monitoring

—Monitor the effectiveness of moricizine therapy by continuous ECG recordings in a coronary care setting initially, followed by regular ECG assessments.

—Monitor the patient for proarrhythmic events and other ECG abnormalities throughout therapy.

—Monitor for electrolyte disturbances before and regularly throughout therapy.

—Monitor the patient for adverse drug reactions.

—Monitor for evidence of fluid volume deficit (dry skin, poor skin turgor, concentrated urine) if GI upset occurs.

—Monitor the patient for drug interactions.

—Regularly reevaluate the patient's and family's knowledge about moricizine therapy.

Intervention

—Notify the doctor immediately and obtain further administration guidelines if the patient develops a drug fever, proarrhythmias, or other ECG abnormalities.

—Keep emergency equipment nearby and be prepared to use other methods to treat arrhythmia if moricizine is ineffective or causes other life-threatening arrhythmias.

—Institute safety precautions if CNS reactions occur.

—Correct electrolyte imbalances as they arise throughout drug therapy.

—Administer a mild analgesic if a headache or musculoskeletal pain occurs.

—Assist the patient with daily activities if fatigue develops.

—Obtain an order for an antiemetic or antidiarrheal agent if needed. Ensure that patient maintains an adequate intake if GI upset occurs.

—Use measures to minimize CHF, such as fluid and sodium restriction, unless adverse GI effects are present.

—Keep all members of the health care team informed of the patient's response to the drug.

Patient teaching

—Inform the patient and family about moricizine, including the dosage, frequency, action, and adverse reactions.

—Inform breast-feeding mothers that because the drug is excreted in breast milk a decision will need to be made to discontinue breast-feeding or discontinue the drug.

—Warn the patient to avoid hazardous activities that require mental alertness until CNS effects are known.

—Stress importance of close follow-up care.

— Tell the patient to notify the nurse or doctor if adverse reactions develop or questions arise about moricizine therapy.

Evaluation

In the patient receiving moricizine, appropriate evaluation statements include:

• Patient's ventricular arrhythmia is abolished.
• Patient's ECG does not exhibit proarrhythmic activity.
• Patient maintains adequate hydration throughout therapy.
• Patient and family state an understanding of moricizine therapy.

PROTOTYPE: CLASS Ia ANTIARRHYTHMIC

PROCAINAMIDE HYDROCHLORIDE

(proe kane′a mide)

Procan SR, Promine, Pronestyl**, Pronestyl-SR, Rhythmin

Classification: Class Ia antiarrhythmic

Pregnancy risk category C

How supplied

TABLETS: 250 mg, 375 mg, 500 mg
TABLETS (SUSTAINED-RELEASE): 250 mg, 500 mg, 750 mg, 1,000 mg
CAPSULES: 250 mg, 375 mg, 500 mg
INJECTION: 100 mg/ml, 500 mg/ml

Indications and dosage

Premature ventricular contractions, ventricular tachycardia, atrial arrhythmias unresponsive to quinidine, paroxysmal atrial tachycardia

ADULTS: 100 mg slow I.V. push q 5 minutes, no faster than 25 to 50 mg/minute until arrhythmias disappear, adverse reactions develop, or 1 g has been given. (Usual effective dose is 500 to 600 mg.) When arrhythmias disappear, give continuous infusion of 2 to 6 mg/minute. If arrhythmias recur, repeat bolus as above and increase infusion rate; 0.5 to 1 g I.M. q 4 to 8 hours until oral therapy begins.

Loading dose for atrial fibrillation or paroxysmal atrial tachycardia

ADULTS: 1 to 1.25 g P.O. If arrhythmias persist after 1 hour, give additional 750 mg. If no change occurs, give 500 mg to 1 g P.O. q 2 hours until arrhythmias disappear or adverse reactions occur.

Loading dose for ventricular tachycardia

ADULTS: 1 g P.O. Maintenance dosage is 50 mg/kg daily in divided doses q 3 hours; average is 250 to 500 mg q 3 hours.

Note: Sustained-release tablet may be used for maintenance dosing when treating ventricular tachycardia, atrial fibrillation, or paroxysmal atrial tachycardia. Dose is 500 mg to 1 g q 6 hours.

**May contain tartrazine

Contraindications and precautions

Procainamide is contraindicated in patients with known hypersensitivity to procaine and related drugs; complete, second-, or third-degree heart block unassisted by electrical pacemaker; or myasthenia gravis. Use with caution in patients with CHF or other conduction disturbances, such as bundle branch block, sinus bradycardia, or digitalis glycoside intoxication, or hepatic or renal insufficiency.

Adverse reactions

BLOOD: **thrombocytopenia, neutropenia (especially with sustained-release forms), agranulocytosis, hemolytic anemia,** increased antinuclear antibodies (ANA) titer.

CNS: hallucinations, confusion, seizures, depression.

CV: severe hypotension, bradycardia, AV block, **ventricular fibrillation (after parenteral use).**

GI: *nausea,* vomiting, anorexia, diarrhea, bitter taste.

SKIN: maculopapular rash.

OTHER: fever, SLE syndrome (especially after prolonged administration), myalgia.

Interactions

Amiodarone: increased procainamide levels and possible drug toxicity. Monitor carefully for toxicity.

Anticholinergics: additive anticholinergic effects. Monitor carefully for toxicity.

Anticholinesterase agents: antagonized effect. Anticholinesterase dosage may need to be increased.

Cimetidine: may increase procainamide blood levels. Monitor for toxicity.

Neuromuscular blocking agents: increased skeletal muscle relaxant effects. Monitor patient closely.

Nursing considerations

Assessment

• Review the patient's history for a condition that contraindicates the use of procainamide and related compounds.

• Obtain a baseline assessment of the patient's heart rate and rhythm before therapy.

• Be alert for common adverse reactions.

• Evaluate the patient's and family's knowledge about procainamide therapy.

Planning (Nursing Diagnoses)

Potential nursing diagnoses for the patient receiving procainamide include:

• Decreased cardiac output related to ineffectiveness of drug or CV reactions to procainamide therapy.

• Altered protection related to procainamide-induced blood disorders.

• Fluid volume deficit related to potential procainamide-induced GI upset.

• Knowledge deficit related to procainamide therapy.

Implementation
Preparation and administration

—Procainamide solution for injection may become discolored. If so, check with pharmacy and prepare to discard.

—Note that the vials for I.V. injection contain 1 g of drug: 100 mg/ml (10 ml) or 500 mg/ml (2 ml).

—Patients receiving procainamide infusions must be attended at all times. Use an infusion pump to administer the infusion precisely.

—Follow administration guidelines closely. Do not administer too rapidly by the I.V. route, because hypotension can occur.

—Keep the patient supine for I.V. administration if hypotension occurs.

—Expect to decrease dosage in patients with hepatic and renal dysfunction, and give over 6 hours. Half-life of procainamide increases as much as threefold in these conditions.

—Be aware that patients with CHF have a lower volume of distribution and can be treated with lower dosage.

Monitoring

—Monitor the effectiveness of procainamide therapy by frequently assessing ECG recording.

—Monitor the patient for adverse drug reactions.

—Monitor the patient's serum electrolyte levels, especially potassium level. Hypokalemia predisposes patients to arrhythmias.

—Monitor blood pressure and ECG continuously during I.V. administration. Watch for prolonged QT and QRS intervals, heart block, and increased arrhythmias.

—Remember that elderly patients may be more likely to develop hypotension.

—Monitor CBC frequently during first 3 months of therapy, particularly in patients taking sustained-release dosage forms.

—Monitor the patient for drug interactions.

—Monitor the patient's hydration status if GI disturbances occur.

—Regularly reevaluate the patient's and family's knowledge about procainamide therapy.

Intervention

—If ECG disturbances occur, withhold the drug, obtain a rhythm strip, and notify the doctor immediately.

—Monitor the patient's serum creatinine levels because NAPA, an active metabolite, may accumulate when renal function is decreased. This may add to toxicity.

—After prolonged atrial fibrillation, restoration of normal rhythm may result in thromboembolism, due to dislodgment of thrombi from atrial wall. Be aware that anticoagulation is usually advised before restoration of normal sinus rhythm.

—Obtain an order for an antiemetic or antidiarrheal agent, as needed; maintain adequate fluid intake during GI upset to prevent dehydration.

—Maintain seizure precautions.

—Institute safety precautions if adverse CNS reactions occur.
—Keep all members of the health care team informed of the patient's response to the drug.

Patient teaching
—Inform the patient and family about procainamide, including the dosage, frequency, action, and adverse reactions.
—Stress importance of taking the drug exactly as prescribed. Patient may have to set an alarm clock for night doses.
—Reassure patients who are taking the extended-release form of procainamide that a wax matrix "ghost" from the tablet may be passed in the stool, and that the drug is completely absorbed before this occurs.
—Emphasize the importance of close follow-up care that includes frequent ECGs and blood tests.
—Warn the patient to avoid hazardous activities that require mental alertness until CNS effects of drug are known.
—Tell the patient how to handle troublesome GI reactions.
—Tell the patient to notify the nurse or doctor if adverse reactions develop or questions arise about procainamide therapy.

Evaluation
In the patient receiving procainamide, appropriate evaluation statements include:
• Patient's ECG reveals arrhythmia has been corrected.
• Patient's CBC remains normal throughout therapy.
• Patient does not develop a fluid volume deficit.
• Patient and family state an understanding of procainamide therapy.

PROTOTYPE: CLASS Ib ANTIARRHYTHMIC

LIDOCAINE HYDROCHLORIDE (LIGNOCAINE HYDROCHLORIDE)
(lye′doe kane)
LidoPen Auto-Injector, Xylocaine, Xylocard†‡
Classification: Class Ib antiarrhythmic
Pregnancy risk category B

How supplied
INJECTION (FOR DIRECT I.V. USE): 1% (10 mg/ml) in 5-ml, 10-ml syringes; 2% (20 mg/ml) in 5-ml vials, syringes, and ampules
INJECTION (FOR I.M. USE): 10% (100 mg/ml) in 3-ml automatic injection device or 5-ml ampules
INJECTION (FOR I.V. ADMIXTURES): 4% (40 mg/ml) in 25-ml, 50-ml vials and syringes; 10% (100 mg/ml) in 10-ml vials; 20% (200 mg/ml) in 5-ml, 10-ml vials and syringes
INFUSION (PREMIXED): 0.2% (2 mg/ml) in 500-ml vials; 0.4% (4 mg/ml) in 250-ml, 500-ml, 1,000-ml vials; 0.8% (8 mg/ml) in 250-ml, 500-ml vials

---

†Available in Canada only   ‡Available in Australia only

Indications and dosage
Ventricular arrhythmias caused by MI, cardiac manipulation, or digitalis glycosides; ventricular tachycardia
ADULTS: 50 to 100 mg (1 to 1.5 mg/kg) I.V. bolus at 25 to 50 mg/minute. Give half this amount to elderly patients or patients under 50 kg, and to those with CHF or hepatic disease. Repeat bolus q 3 to 5 minutes until arrhythmias subside or adverse reactions develop. Don't exceed 300-mg total bolus during a 1-hour period. Simultaneously, begin constant infusion of 1 to 4 mg/minute. If single bolus has been given, repeat smaller bolus 15 to 20 minutes after start of infusion to maintain therapeutic serum level. After 24 hours of continuous infusion, decrease rate by half, or as ordered.
I.M. administration—200 to 300 mg I.M. in deltoid muscle only.
CHILDREN: 1 mg/kg by I.V. bolus, followed by infusion of 30 mcg/kg/minute.

Contraindications and precautions
Lidocaine is contraindicated in patients with known hypersensitivity to related local anesthetics of the amide type, such as dibucaine. Do not use for ventricular escape beats. Atropine should be used instead. Use cautiously in patients with complete or second-degree heart block or sinus bradycardia. Also use cautiously in elderly patients and in those with CHF, with renal or hepatic disease, or those who weigh less than 110 lb (50 kg). Such patients need reduced dosage.

Adverse reactions
CNS: *confusion*, tremor, *lethargy, somnolence*, stupor, restlessness, slurred speech, euphoria, depression, light-headedness, paresthesia, muscle twitching, **seizures**.
CV: hypotension, bradycardia, **worsened arrhythmias**.
EENT: tinnitus, blurred or double vision.
OTHER: **anaphylaxis**, soreness at injection site, sensations of cold, diaphoresis.

Interactions
Cimetidine, beta blockers: decreased metabolism of lidocaine. Monitor for toxicity.
Phenytoin: additive cardiac depressant effects. Monitor carefully.

Nursing considerations
Assessment
- Review the patient's history for a condition that contraindicates the use of lidocaine and related compounds.
- Obtain a baseline assessment of the patient's heart rate and rhythm before therapy.
- Be alert for common adverse reactions.
- Evaluate the patient's and family's knowledge about lidocaine therapy.

Planning (Nursing Diagnoses)
Potential nursing diagnoses for the patient receiving lidocaine include:
- Decreased cardiac output related to ineffectiveness of lidocaine therapy.
- Altered thought processes related to lidocaine-induced confusion.

Italicized adverse reactions are common   Boldfaced adverse reactions are life-threatening

- Potential for injury related to lidocaine-induced seizures.
- Knowledge deficit related to lidocaine therapy.

Implementation

Preparation and administration

— Patients receiving lidocaine infusions must be attended at all times, and be on a cardiac monitor. Use an infusion pump to administer the infusion precisely. Do not exceed an infusion rate of 4 mg/minute, because a faster rate greatly increases risk of toxicity.
— A bolus dose not followed by infusion will have a short-lived effect. Do not use lidocaine with epinephrine (for local anesthesia) to treat arrhythmias.
— Patients over age 65 should initially receive half the recommended dosage.

Monitoring

— Monitor the effectiveness of lidocaine therapy by continuous ECG recordings.
— Closely monitor the patient for toxicity. In many severely ill patients, seizures may be the first sign of toxicity. However, severe reactions usually are preceded by somnolence, confusion, and paresthesias.
— Monitor the patient for adverse drug reactions.
— Monitor vital signs for hypotension or bradycardia.
— Monitor serum electrolyte, BUN, and creatinine levels. Also, monitor isoenzymes if using I.M. route. A patient who has received lidocaine I.M. will show a sevenfold increase in the serum creatine phosphokinase (CPK) level. Such CPK originates in the skeletal muscle, not the heart.
— Monitor serum lidocaine levels, if indicated. Normal therapeutic blood levels are 2 to 5 mcg/ml.
— Monitor the patient for drug interactions.

Intervention

— Notify the doctor promptly if abnormalities develop (changes in blood pressure and serum electrolyte, BUN, and creatinine levels).
— Discontinue the infusion and notify the doctor if arrhythmias worsen or ECG changes, such as widening QRS complex or substantially prolonged PR interval, are evident.
— If signs of toxicity (such as mental confusion, seizures, or somnolence) occur, stop administration at once and notify the doctor. Continued infusion could lead to seizures and coma. Give oxygen via nasal cannula, if not contraindicated.
— Keep emergency equipment nearby.
— Maintain seizure precautions.
— Institute safety precautions if the patient becomes confused and reorient patient as often as necessary until drug effect has worn off.
— Keep all members of the health care team informed of the patient's response to the drug.

Patient teaching
— Inform the patient and family about lidocaine, including method of administration, its action, and adverse reactions.
— Inform the patient that continuous ECG monitoring is required during lidocaine therapy.
— Tell the patient to notify the nurse or doctor if adverse reactions develop or questions arise about lidocaine therapy.

Evaluation
In the patient receiving lidocaine, appropriate evaluation statements include:
• Patient's ECG reveals correction of arrhythmia.
• Patient remains alert and oriented to person, place, and time throughout lidocaine therapy.
• Patient remains seizure-free.
• Patient and family state an understanding of lidocaine therapy.

PROTOTYPE: CLASS Ic ANTIARRHYTHMIC

FLECAINIDE ACETATE
(fle kay'nide)
Tambocor
Classification: Class Ic antiarrhythmic
Pregnancy risk category C

How supplied
TABLETS: 100 mg
INJECTION: 10 mg/ml‡

Indications and dosage
Life-threatening ventricular arrhythmias, such as sustained ventricular tachycardia
ADULTS: 100 mg P.O. q 12 hours. May be increased in increments of 50 mg b.i.d. q 4 days until efficacy is achieved. Maximum dosage is 400 mg daily for most patients.

Where available, flecainide may be given by I.V. injection. Dosage in adults is 2 mg/kg I.V. push over not less than 10 minutes; or dilute dose with dextrose 5% in water and administer as an infusion. Do not use any other solutions for infusion.

Initial dosage for patients with CHF is 50 mg q 12 hours.

Contraindications and precautions
Flecainide is contraindicated in patients with preexisting second- or third-degree AV block or right bundle branch block when associated with a left hemiblock, unless a pacemaker is present; it is also contraindicated in patients with cardiogenic shock. Use cautiously in patients with preexisting CHF, cardiomyopathy, severe renal or hepatic disease, prolonged QT interval, sick sinus syndrome, or blood dyscrasia.

‡Available in Australia only

Findings from the Cardiac Arrhythmia Suppression Trial (CAST) include a greater-than-twofold increase in the number of deaths and nonfatal cardiac arrest in patients treated with flecainide. Therefore, it should be used only to treat immediately life-threatening arrhythmias, such as sustained ventricular tachycardia.

Adverse reactions
CNS: *dizziness, headache, fatigue, tremor.*
CV: **new or worsened arrhythmias,** chest pain, **CHF, cardiac arrest.**
EENT: *blurred vision and other visual disturbances.*
GI: *nausea,* constipation, abdominal pain.
OTHER: *dyspnea,* edema, skin rash.

Interactions
Amiodarone, cimetidine: altered pharmacokinetics. Monitor for toxicity.
Digitalis glycosides: flecainide may increase plasma digoxin levels by 15% to 25%. Monitor for toxicity.
Propranolol: both flecainide and propranolol plasma levels increase by 20% to 30%. Monitor for toxicity.
Urine acidifying and alkalinizing agents: extremes of urine pH may substantially alter excretion of flecainide. Monitor blood levels closely.

Nursing considerations
Assessment
- Review the patient's history for a condition that contraindicates the use of flecainide and related compounds.
- Obtain a baseline assessment of the patient's heart rate and rhythm before therapy.
- Be alert for common adverse reactions.
- Evaluate the patient's and family's knowledge about flecainide therapy.

Planning (Nursing Diagnoses)
Potential nursing diagnoses for the patient receiving flecainide include:
- Decreased cardiac output related to ineffectiveness of flecainide therapy.
- Fluid volume excess related to flecainide therapy.
- Sensory/perceptual alterations (visual) related to flecainide-induced visual disturbances.
- Knowledge deficit related to flecainide therapy.

Implementation
Preparation and administration
— Flecainide can alter endocardial pacing thresholds. Determine pacing threshold 1 week before and after initiating therapy in patients with pacemakers.
— Correct hypokalemia or hyperkalemia before this drug is given, because both may alter the effect of flecainide.
— When administering flecainide orally, expect to increase dosage in increments of 50 mg b.i.d. every 4 days until efficacy is achieved or a maximum dosage of 400 mg daily is reached.
— When administering flecainide I.V. push, give over at least 10 minutes.

—When administering flecainide as an I.V. infusion, mix only with dextrose 5% in water.

—Most patients can be adequately maintained on an every-12-hour dosage schedule, but some need to receive flecainide every 8 hours. Monitor drug effects and consult with doctor about dosage schedule.

—Expect to administer I.V. lidocaine while awaiting full therapeutic effect of flecainide.

—Avoid loading doses, which may aggravate arrhythmias and are therefore not recommended.

—Twice-daily dosing for flecainide aids patient compliance.

Monitoring

—Monitor the effectiveness of flecainide therapy by continuous ECG monitoring initially; long-term oral administration requires regular ECG readings to monitor rhythm.

—Monitor the patient's vital signs, weight, and breath and heart sounds for evidence of CHF.

—Monitor the patient for adverse drug reactions.

—Normal therapeutic blood levels of flecainide range from 0.2 to 1 mcg/ml. Periodically monitor blood levels, especially in patients with renal failure or CHF. Incidence of adverse reactions increases when trough blood levels exceed 1 mcg/ml.

—Regularly monitor the patient's potassium level.

—Regularly monitor for visual disturbances.

—Monitor the patient for drug interactions.

—Regularly reevaluate the patient's and family's knowledge about flecainide therapy.

Intervention

—Withhold the drug and notify the doctor immediately if new or worsened arrhythmias occur.

—Know that full therapeutic effect of the drug may take 3 to 5 days.

—Institute measures to minimize CHF, such as fluid and sodium restriction, as needed.

—Institute safety precautions if CNS or visual reactions occur.

—Assist the patient with daily activities; schedule activities to promote adequate rest if fatigue occurs.

—Keep emergency equipment nearby.

—Keep all members of the health care team informed of the patient's response to the drug.

Patient teaching

—Inform the patient and family about flecainide, including the dosage, frequency, method of administration, action, and adverse reactions.

—Inform the patient that continuous ECG monitoring is needed initially to monitor drug effectiveness.

—Warn the patient against hazardous activities that require alertness or good vision if adverse CNS or visual reactions occur.

—Tell the patient to limit fluid and sodium intake to minimize CHF or fluid retention and to weigh himself daily. Emphasize that a sudden weight gain of 3 to 5 lb (1.4 to 2.3 kg) in 1 week should be reported to the doctor promptly.

—Tell the patient to notify the nurse or doctor if adverse reactions develop or questions arise about flecainide therapy.

Evaluation

In the patient receiving flecainide, appropriate evaluation statements include:

• Patient's ECG reveals arrhythmia has been corrected.
• Patient does not develop fluid retention.
• Patient states vision is unaffected by flecainide therapy.
• Patient and family state an understanding of flecainide therapy.

PROTOTYPE: CLASS II ANTIARRHYTHMIC

PROPRANOLOL HYDROCHLORIDE
(pro pran'oh lole)
Apo-Propranolol†, Deralin‡, Detensol†, Inderal, Inderal LA, Ipran, Novopranol†, PMS-Propranolol†
Classification: Class II antiarrhythmic
Pregnancy risk category C

How supplied

TABLETS: 10 mg, 20 mg, 40 mg, 60 mg, 80 mg, 90 mg
CAPSULES (SUSTAINED-RELEASE): 60 mg, 80 mg, 120 mg, 160 mg
ORAL SOLUTION: 4 mg/ml, 8 mg/ml; 80 mg/ml (concentrate)
INJECTION: 1 mg/ml

Indications and dosage

Management of angina pectoris

ADULTS: 10 to 20 mg P.O. t.i.d. or q.i.d., or 1 sustained-release capsule (80 mg) daily. Dosage may be increased at 7- to 10-day intervals. The average optimal dosage is 160 mg daily.

To reduce mortality after MI

ADULTS: 180 to 240 mg P.O. daily in divided doses. Usually administered t.i.d. to q.i.d.

Supraventricular, ventricular, and atrial arrhythmias; tachyarrhythmias caused by excessive catecholamine action during anesthesia, hyperthyroidism, and pheochromocytoma

ADULTS: 1 to 3 mg by slow I.V. push, not to exceed 1 mg/minute. After 3 mg have been given, another dose may be given in 2 minutes; subsequent doses, no sooner than q 4 hours. Drug may be given by direct injection or diluted in 50 ml dextrose 5% in water or 0.9% sodium chloride solution

---

and infused slowly. Usual maintenance dose is 10 to 80 mg P.O. t.i.d. to q.i.d.

Hypertension
ADULTS: initially, 80 mg P.O. daily in two to four divided doses or 1 sustained-release capsule daily. Increase at 3- to 7-day intervals to maximum daily dosage of 640 mg. Usual maintenance dosage is 160 to 480 mg daily.

Prevention of frequent, severe, uncontrollable, or disabling migraine or vascular headache
ADULTS: initially, 80 mg P.O. daily in divided doses or 1 sustained-release capsule daily. Usual maintenance dosage is 160 to 240 mg daily, divided t.i.d. or q.i.d.

Contraindications and precautions
Propranolol is contraindicated in patients with diabetes mellitus, asthma, or allergic rhinitis; during ethyl ether anesthesia; in patients with sinus bradycardia, second- or third-degree heart block, cardiogenic shock, or right ventricular failure secondary to pulmonary hypertension. Use cautiously in patients with CHF or respiratory disease and in patients taking other antihypertensive drugs.

Adverse reactions
CNS: *fatigue*, lethargy, *vivid dreams*, hallucinations.
CV: bradycardia, hypotension, **CHF**, peripheral vascular disease.
GI: nausea, vomiting, diarrhea.
METABOLIC: hypoglycemia without tachycardia.
SKIN: rash.
OTHER: increased airway resistance, fever, arthralgia.

Interactions
Aminophylline: antagonizes beta-blocking effects of propranolol. Use together cautiously.
Cimetidine: inhibits propranolol metabolism. Monitor for greater beta-blocking effect.
Digitalis glycosides, verapamil: excessive bradycardia and increased depressant effect on myocardium. Use together cautiously.
Epinephrine: severe vasoconstriction. Monitor blood pressure and observe patient carefully.
Insulin, oral antidiabetic agents: can alter requirements for these drugs in previously stabilized diabetics. Monitor for hypoglycemia.
Isoproterenol, glucagon: antagonize propranolol effect. May be used therapeutically and in emergencies. Monitor carefully.

Nursing considerations
Assessment
• Review the patient's history for a condition that contraindicates the use of propranolol or related compounds.
• Obtain a baseline assessment of the patient's heart rate and rhythm, anginal pain, blood pressure, or headache pattern before therapy.

- Be alert for common adverse reactions.
- Evaluate the patient's and family's knowledge about propranolol therapy.

Planning (Nursing Diagnoses)
Potential nursing diagnoses for the patient receiving propranolol include:
- Decreased cardiac output related to ineffectiveness of propranolol therapy.
- Fatigue related to adverse CNS reaction caused by propranolol.
- Impaired gas exchange related to propranolol-induced airway resistance.
- Fluid volume excess related to propranolol-induced CHF.
- Knowledge deficit related to propranolol therapy.

Implementation

Preparation and administration

— Double-check dose and route. I.V. doses are much smaller than oral doses.
— Food may increase the absorption of propranolol. Give consistently with meals.
— Compliance may be improved by administering this drug twice daily or by sustained-release capsule. Check with the patient's doctor.
— Elderly patients may experience enhanced adverse reactions. Dosage adjustment may be needed.

Monitoring

— Monitor the effectiveness of propranolol therapy by regularly evaluating the patient's ECG rate and pattern and blood pressure, especially during I.V. administration; if used for pain control, evaluate relief obtained by patient.
— Monitor the patient for adverse drug reactions.
— Monitor respiratory status, particularly for abnormal breath sounds and dyspnea suggestive of airway resistance.
— Monitor the patient for fluid retention that could lead to CHF.
— This drug masks common signs of shock and hypoglycemia. Monitor vital signs and blood glucose levels regularly.
— Monitor the patient's activity tolerance throughout propranolol therapy.
— Monitor the patient for drug interactions.
— Regularly reevaluate the patient's and family's knowledge about propranolol therapy.

Intervention

— If you detect extremes in pulse rates, withhold drug and call the doctor immediately.
— If the patient develops severe hypotension, notify the doctor, because a vasopressor may be indicated.
— After prolonged atrial fibrillation, restoration of normal sinus rhythm may cause thromboembolism due to dislodgment of thrombi from the atrial wall. Be aware that anticoagulation is often advised before restoration of normal atrial rhythm.

—Don't discontinue propranolol before surgery for pheochromocytoma. Before any surgical procedure, notify the anesthesiologist that the patient is receiving propranolol.

—Assist the patient with daily activities; schedule activities to promote adequate rest if fatigue occurs.

—Alert the doctor if dyspnea or abnormal breath sounds occur.

—Restrict the patient's fluid and sodium intake to minimize CHF.

—Have emergency drugs on hand to treat overdose. I.V. isoproterenol or atropine may be given; refractory cases may require a pacemaker. Glucagon is sometimes used.

—Keep all members of the health care team informed of the patient's response to the drug.

Patient teaching

—Inform the patient and family about propranolol, including the dosage, frequency, action, and adverse reactions.

—Teach the patient about his disease and therapy. Explain the importance of taking this drug as prescribed, even when he's feeling well.

—Tell outpatients not to discontinue this drug suddenly; abrupt discontinuation can exacerbate angina and MI.

—Teach the patient how to check pulse rate, and to do so before each dose.

—Tell the patient to schedule activities to allow adequate rest if fatigue becomes troublesome.

—Encourage the patient to restrict fluid and sodium intake to minimize CHF.

—Tell the patient to notify the nurse or doctor if adverse reactions develop or questions arise about propranolol therapy.

Evaluation

In the patient receiving propranolol, appropriate evaluation statements include:

• Patient's ECG reveals arrhythmia has been corrected.
• Patient is able to perform normal daily routine without fatigue.
• Patient's respiratory pattern and breath sounds are normal.
• Patient does not experience fluid retention.
• Patient and family state an understanding of propranolol therapy.

AMIODARONE HYDROCHLORIDE
(a mee'oh da rone)
Cordarone, Cordarone X‡
Classification: Class III antiarrhythmic
Pregnancy risk category C

How supplied
TABLETS: 100 mg†‡, 200 mg

Indications and dosage
Ventricular and supraventricular arrhythmias, including recurrent supraventricular tachycardia (Wolff-Parkinson-White syndrome), atrial fibrillation and flutter, and ventricular tachycardia refractory to other antiarrhythmics
ADULTS: loading dose is 800 to 1,600 mg P.O. daily for 1 to 3 weeks until initial therapeutic response occurs. Maintenance dosage is 200 to 600 mg P.O. daily.

Contraindications and precautions
Amiodarone is contraindicated in patients with preexisting sinus node dysfunction and bradycardia causing syncope or second- or third-degree heart block (except if patient has artificial pacemaker). Use cautiously in patients with preexisting bradycardia or sinus node disease, conduction disturbances, severely depressed ventricular function, and marked cardiomegaly. Use cautiously (if at all) in patients receiving Class I antiarrhythmics.

Adverse reactions
CNS: peripheral neuropathy, *extrapyramidal symptoms, headache, malaise, fatigue.*
CV: bradycardia, hypotension, **arrhythmias, CHF.**
EENT: corneal microdeposits, visual disturbances.
ENDOCRINE: hypothyroidism, hyperthyroidism, gynecomastia.
GI: *nausea, vomiting, constipation.*
HEPATIC: altered liver enzymes, hepatic dysfunction.
RESPIRATORY: **severe pulmonary toxicity** (pneumonitis/alveolitis).
SKIN: *photosensitivity,* blue-gray skin pigmentation.
OTHER: muscle weakness.

Interactions
Antiarrhythmic agents: use with amiodarone may induce torsades de pointes; amiodarone may reduce the hepatic or renal clearance of flecainide, procainamide, and quinidine. Monitor for adverse effects or toxicity.
Antihypertensives: increased hypotensive effect. Use together cautiously.
Beta blockers, calcium channel blockers: increased cardiac depressant effects; may potentiate slowing of sinus node and AV conduction. Use together cautiously.

Digitalis glycosides: increased serum digoxin levels. Monitor carefully for digitalis toxicity.

Phenytoin: phenytoin metabolism may be decreased. Monitor for phenytoin toxicity.

Warfarin: increased anticoagulant effect. Monitor patient closely.

Nursing considerations

Assessment

- Review the patient's history for the presence of a condition that contraindicates the use of amiodarone.
- Obtain a baseline assessment of the patient's heart rate and rhythm before therapy.
- Be alert for common adverse reactions.
- Evaluate the patient's and family's knowledge about amiodarone therapy.

Planning (Nursing Diagnoses)

Potential nursing diagnoses for the patient receiving amiodarone include:
- Decreased cardiac output related to ineffectiveness of amiodarone.
- Impaired gas exchange related to amiodarone-induced pulmonary toxicity.
- Fluid volume excess related to amiodarone-induced CHF.
- Potential fluid volume deficit related to amiodarone-induced nausea and vomiting.
- Knowledge deficit related to amiodarone therapy.

Implementation

Preparation and administration

— Divide oral loading dose into three equal doses and give with meals to decrease GI intolerance. Maintenance dosage may be given once daily, but may be divided into two doses taken with meals if GI intolerance occurs.

Monitoring

— Monitor the effectiveness of amiodarone therapy by regularly evaluating the patient's ECG. Monitor blood pressure and heart rate and rhythm frequently. Continuous ECG monitoring should be performed during initiation and alteration of dosage.

— Monitor the patient for adverse drug reactions.

— Closely monitor the patient who is receiving high doses, because adverse reactions are more prevalent at high doses. They are generally reversible after drug therapy is discontinued, but resolution of adverse reactions may take up to 4 months.

— Monitor carefully for pulmonary toxicity, which can be fatal. Incidence rises in patients receiving more than 400 mg/day.

— Monitor for symptoms of pneumonitis—exertional dyspnea, nonproductive cough, and pleuritic chest pain. Monitor pulmonary function tests and chest X-ray.

—Monitor hepatic and thyroid function tests. Monitor serum electrolyte levels, particularly potassium and magnesium levels.

—Monitor the patient for burning or tingling skin followed by erythema and possible skin blistering.

—Monitor closely for visual disturbances. These only occur in 2% to 3% of patients. However, most patients treated show corneal microdeposits on slit-lamp ophthalmologic examination. Onset of this effect occurs from 1 to 4 months after beginning amiodarone therapy.

—Monitor for signs of CHF—abnormal breath sounds, distended neck veins, dyspnea, and sudden weight gain.

—Monitor the patient's hydration status if adverse GI reactions occur.

—Monitor the patient for drug interactions.

—Regularly reevaluate the patient's and family's knowledge about amiodarone therapy.

Intervention

—Notify the doctor if arrhythmia persists despite amiodarone therapy.

—Institute safety precautions if CNS or visual disturbances occur.

—Obtain an order for a mild analgesic if the patient develops a headache.

—Schedule patient's activities to allow frequent rest periods if patient experiences fatigue.

—Obtain an order for an antiemetic if nausea and vomiting occur.

—Assist the patient with daily activities if muscle weakness occurs.

—To minimize corneal microdeposits, recommend instillation of methylcellulose ophthalmic solution during amiodarone therapy.

—Keep all members of the health care team informed of the patient's response to the drug.

Patient teaching

—Inform the patient and family about amiodarone, including dosage, frequency, action, and adverse reactions.

—Stress the importance of close follow-up and regular diagnostic studies to monitor drug action and assess for adverse reactions.

—Warn the patient that amiodarone may cause a blue-gray skin pigmentation.

—Advise the patient to use a sunscreen to prevent photosensitivity.

—Tell the patient to schedule activities to provide frequent rest periods if fatigue occurs.

—Teach the patient appropriate skin and foot care if peripheral neuropathy is present.

—Warn the patient to avoid hazardous activities that require manual dexterity or good vision if extrapyramidal symptoms or visual disturbances occur.

—Warn male patients about the possibility of gynecomastia.

—Tell the patient to limit fluid and sodium intake if fluid retention develops.

—Tell the patient to notify the nurse or doctor if adverse reactions develop or questions arise about amiodarone therapy.

Evaluation

In the patient receiving amiodarone, appropriate evaluation statements include:
* Patient's ECG reveals arrhythmia has been corrected.
* Patient's chest X-ray and pulmonary function studies remain normal throughout amiodarone therapy.
* Patient does not develop fluid retention.
* Patient maintains adequate hydration.
* Patient and family state an understanding of amiodarone therapy.

PROTOTYPE: CLASS IV ANTIARRHYTHMIC

VERAPAMIL HYDROCHLORIDE
(ver ap′a mill)
Calan, Calan SR, Cordilox Oral‡, Isoptin, Isoptin SR, Veradil‡
Classification: Class IV antiarrhythmic
Pregnancy risk category C

How supplied
TABLETS: 40 mg, 80 mg, 120 mg
TABLETS (SUSTAINED-RELEASE): 240 mg
INJECTION: 2.5 mg/ml in 2- and 4-ml vials, ampules, and syringes

Indications and dosage
Management of vasospastic (Prinzmetal's or variant) angina and classic chronic, stable angina pectoris; chronic atrial fibrillation
ADULTS: starting dose is 80 mg P.O. t.i.d. or q.i.d. Dosage may be increased at weekly intervals. Some patients may require up to 480 mg daily.

Supraventricular arrhythmias
ADULTS: 0.075 to 0.15 mg/kg (5 to 10 mg) I.V. push over 2 minutes with ECG and blood pressure monitoring. Repeat dose in 30 minutes if no response.
CHILDREN AGES 1 TO 15: 0.1 to 0.3 mg/kg as I.V. bolus over 2 minutes. Do not exceed 10 mg/dose. Repeat in 30 minutes if no response.
CHILDREN UNDER AGE 1: 0.1 to 0.2 mg/kg as I.V. bolus over 2 minutes with continuous ECG monitoring. Do not exceed 5 mg/dose. Dose can be repeated in 30 minutes if no response.

Migraine headache prophylaxis
ADULTS: 80 mg P.O. q.i.d.

Hypertension
ADULTS: 1 sustained-release tablet (240 mg) once daily in the morning. If response is not adequate, may give an additional half tablet in the evening or 1 tablet q 12 hours. Alternatively, may give 80 mg P.O. t.i.d. or q.i.d.

Contraindications and precautions

Verapamil is contraindicated in patients with advanced heart failure, AV block, severe left ventricular dysfunction, cardiogenic shock, sinus node disease, or severe hypotension. Use cautiously in patients with MI followed by coronary occlusion, sick sinus syndrome, impaired AV conduction, or heart failure with atrial tachyarrhythmia; and in patients with hepatic or renal disease.

Adverse reactions

CNS: *dizziness, headache, fatigue.*
CV: transient hypotension, **CHF**, bradycardia, AV block, **ventricular asystole**, peripheral edema.
GI: *constipation*, nausea (primarily from oral form).
HEPATIC: elevated liver enzymes.

Interactions

Carbamazepine, digitalis glycosides: verapamil may increase the serum levels of these drugs. Monitor patient for toxicity.
Lithium: verapamil may decrease serum lithium levels. Monitor patient closely.
Propranolol (and other beta blockers, including ophthalmic timolol), disopyramide: may cause heart failure. Use together cautiously.
Quinidine, antihypertensives: may result in hypotension. Monitor blood pressure.
Rifampin: may decrease oral bioavailability of verapamil. Monitor patient for lack of effect.

Nursing considerations

Assessment

- Review the patient's history for a condition that contraindicates the use of verapamil.
- Obtain a baseline assessment of the patient's heart rate and rhythm before therapy.
- Be alert for common adverse reactions.
- Evaluate the patient's and family's knowledge about verapamil therapy.

Planning (Nursing Diagnoses)

Potential nursing diagnoses for the patient receiving verapamil include:
- Decreased cardiac output related to ineffectiveness of drug to terminate arrhythmia.
- Decreased tissue perfusion (cerebral) related to verapamil-induced hypotension.
- Constipation related to adverse GI reactions to verapamil.
- Knowledge deficit related to verapamil therapy.

Implementation

Preparation and administration

— Patients with severely compromised cardiac function or those receiving beta blockers should receive lower doses of verapamil. Do not administer I.V. beta blockers at the same time as I.V. verapamil. Administer

I.V. doses over at least 3 minutes to minimize the risk of adverse reactions.

— Extended-release tablets should be taken on an empty stomach. Taking extended-release tablets with food may decrease rate and extent of absorption, but it allows smaller fluctuations of peak and trough blood levels.

Monitoring

— Monitor the effectiveness of verapamil therapy by monitoring patient's ECG regularly (if administered orally) or continuously (if administered I.V.), particularly the PR interval.
— Monitor the patient for adverse drug reactions.
— Monitor the patient's blood pressure for hypotension.
— Monitor liver function studies during prolonged treatment.
— Monitor bowel patterns for constipation.
— Monitor the patient for drug interactions.
— Regularly reevaluate the patient's and family's knowledge about verapamil therapy.

Intervention

— Notify the doctor if arrhythmia persists or patient develops signs of CHF, such as swelling of hands and feet, shortness of breath, or abnormal breath or heart sounds.
— Institute safety precautions if CNS reactions or hypotension occurs.
— Keep emergency equipment nearby and be prepared to treat arrhythmias such as AV block or ventricular asystole.
— Encourage the patient to increase fiber content of diet (if not contraindicated) to prevent constipation, or obtain an order for a laxative if constipation occurs.
— Assist the patient with daily activities if fatigue occurs.
— Obtain an order for a mild analgesic if a headache occurs.
— Keep all members of the health care team informed of the patient's response to the drug.

Patient teaching

— Inform the patient and family about verapamil, including the dosage, frequency, action, and adverse reactions.
— Explain to the patient that if verapamil is being used to terminate a supraventricular tachycardia, the doctor may instruct the patient to perform vagal maneuvers after receiving the drug.
— If the patient continues nitrate therapy during titration of oral verapamil dosage, urge continued compliance. Sublingual nitroglycerin, especially, may be taken as needed when anginal symptoms are acute.
— Warn the patient to avoid hazardous activities that require alertness if adverse CNS effects occur.
— Instruct patient to increase dietary fiber content and fluid (if not contraindicated) to prevent constipation.
— Tell the patient to notify the nurse or doctor if adverse reactions develop or questions arise about verapamil therapy.

Evaluation

In the patient receiving verapamil, appropriate evaluation statements include:

• Patient's ECG reveals arrhythmia has been corrected.
• Patient maintains adequate cerebral perfusion.
• Patient states bowel patterns are unchanged.
• Patient and family state an understanding of verapamil therapy.

SELECTED MAJOR DRUGS: ANTIARRHYTHMICS

DRUG, INDICATIONS, AND DOSAGES	SPECIAL PRECAUTIONS
Class Ia	
quinidine bisulfate (Biquin Durules‡) **quinidine gluconate (Duraquin, Quinaglute Dura-tabs)** **quinidine polygalacturonate (Cardioquin)** **quinidine sulfate (Apo-Quinidine, Quinora)** *Atrial flutter or fibrillation—* **Adults:** 200 mg (sulfate or equivalent base) P.O. q 2 to 3 hours for five to eight doses with subsequent daily increases until sinus rhythm is restored or toxic effects develop. Administer quinidine only after digitalization to avoid increasing AV conduction. Maximum dosage is 3 to 4 g daily. *Paroxysmal supraventricular tachycardia—* **Adults:** 400 to 600 mg (gluconate) I.M. q 2 to 3 hours until toxic reactions develop or arrhythmia subsides. *Premature atrial contractions, premature ventricular contractions (PVCs), paroxysmal AV junctional rhythm, paroxysmal atrial tachycardia, paroxysmal ventricular tachycardia, maintenance after cardioversion of atrial fibrillation or flutter—* **Adults:** test dose is 50 to 200 mg P.O., then monitor vital signs before beginning therapy. Give 200 to 400 mg (sulfate or equivalent base) P.O. q 4 to 6 hours; or initially, 600 mg (gluconate) I.M., then up to 400 mg q 2 hours p.r.n.; or 800 mg (gluconate) — 10 ml of the commercially available solution — added to 40 ml dextrose 5% in water, infused I.V. at 16 mg (1 ml)/minute. **Children:** test dose is 2 mg/kg; 3 to 6 mg/kg P.O. q 2 hours for five doses daily.	• Contraindicated in patients with digitalis toxicity when AV conduction is grossly impaired and in those with complete AV block with AV nodal or idioventricular pacemaker. • Use cautiously in patients with myasthenia gravis. Anticholinesterase drug doses may have to be increased.
disopyramide (Norpace, Rythmodan LA†) *PVCs (unifocal, multifocal, or coupled); ventricular tachycardia not severe enough to require electrocardioversion; to convert atrial fibrillation or flutter to normal sinus rhythm—* **Adults:** usual maintenance dosage 150 to 200 mg P.O. q 6 hours; for patients who weigh less than 50 kg (110 lb) or those with renal, hepatic, or cardiac impairment — 100 mg P.O. q 6 hours. May give sustained-release capsule q 12 hours. Recommended dosages in advanced renal insufficiency: creatinine clearance 15 to 40 ml/minute — 100 mg q 10 hours; creatinine clearance 5 to 15 ml/min-	• Contraindicated in patients with cardiogenic shock or second- or third-degree heart block with no pacemaker. • Use very cautiously, and avoid, if possible, in patients with CHF. Use cautiously in patients with underlying conduction abnormalities, urinary tract diseases (especially prostatic hypertrophy), hepatic or renal impairment, myasthenia gravis, or narrow-angle glaucoma. Adjust

SELECTED MAJOR DRUGS: ANTIARRHYTHMICS *continued*

DRUG, INDICATIONS, AND DOSAGES	SPECIAL PRECAUTIONS

Class Ia *(continued)*

disopyramide *(continued)*
ute — 100 mg q 20 hours; creatinine clearance 1 to 5 ml/minute — 100 mg q 30 hours.
Children ages 12 to 18: 6 to 15 mg/kg P.O. daily.
Children ages 4 to 12: 10 to 15 mg/kg P.O. daily.
Children ages 1 to 4: 10 to 20 mg/kg P.O. daily.
Children under age 1: 10 to 30 mg/kg P.O. daily.
All children's dosages should be divided into equal amounts and given q 6 hours.

dosage in renal insufficiency.

Class Ib

phenytoin (Dilantin)
phenytoin sodium (Dilantin Kapseals)
Ventricular arrhythmias unresponsive to lidocaine or pro-cainamide; supraventricular and ventricular arrhythmias induced by digitalis glycosides —
Adults: loading dose is 1 g P.O. divided over first 24 hours, followed by 500 mg daily for 2 days, then maintenance dose of 300 mg P.O. daily; 250 mg I.V. over 5 minutes until arrhythmias subside, adverse reactions develop, or 1 g has been given. Infusion rate should never exceed 50 mg/minute (slow I.V. push).
Alternate method — 100 mg I.V. q 15 minutes until adverse reactions develop, arrhythmias are controlled, or 1 g has been given. May also administer entire loading dose of 1 g I.V. slowly at 25 mg/minute. Can be diluted in 0.9% sodium chloride solution. I.M. dose not recommended because of pain and erratic absorption.
Children: 3 to 8 mg/kg P.O. or slow I.V. daily or 250 mg/ m² P.O. or I.V. daily given as single dose or in two divided doses.

• Contraindicated in patients with known hypersensitivity to phenytoin or other hydantoins.
• Use cautiously in patients with liver function impairment and in elderly or gravely ill patients.

tocainide (Tonocard)
Suppression of symptomatic ventricular arrhythmias, including frequent PVCs and ventricular tachycardia —
Adults: initially, 400 mg P.O. q 8 hours. Usual dosage is between 1,200 and 1,800 mg daily in three divided doses.

• Contraindicated in patients with known hypersensitivity to lidocaine or other amide-type local anesthetics and in patients with second- or third-degree AV block in the absence of a ventricular pacemaker.
• Use cautiously in patients with CHF or diminished cardiac reserve. Also use cautiously in patients with hepatic or renal impairment because these patients may often be treated effectively with a lower dose.

mexiletine (Mexitil)
Refractory ventricular arrhythmias, including ventricular tachycardia and PVCs —

• Contraindicated in patients with cardiogenic shock or pre-existing second- or third-degree

(continued)

SELECTED MAJOR DRUGS: ANTIARRHYTHMICS *continued*

DRUG, INDICATIONS, AND DOSAGES	SPECIAL PRECAUTIONS

Class Ib *(continued)*

mexiletine *(continued)*
Adults: 200 to 400 mg P.O. followed by 200 mg q 8 hours. May increase dose to 400 mg q 8 hours if satisfactory control is not obtained. Some patients may respond well to a q-12-hour schedule. May give up to 450 mg q 12 hours.
Where available, mexiletine may be given I.V. —
Adults: after a loading dose of 200 to 250 mg I.V. at a rate of 25 mg/minute, prepare an infusion solution of 250 mg mexiletine in 500 ml dextrose 5% in water (D_5W). Administer the first 120 ml (60 mg) over 1 hour. If clinical response is inadequate, give another bolus of 200 mg over 10 to 20 minutes. Maintenance dose is 0.5 mg/minute (1 ml/minute of prepared solution).

AV block (if pacemaker is not present).

Class Ic

indecainide (Decabid)
Life-threatening ventricular arrhythmias, such as sustained ventricular tachycardia —
Adults: initially, 50 mg P.O. q 12 hours. If necessary, increase the dosage to 75 mg q 12 hours,, but only after at least 4 days of treatment at initial dosage. After an additional 4 days, the dosage may be increased to 100 mg q 12 hours if necessary. Some patients may require higher dosages (up to 400 mg daily).
Patients with renal failure (creatinine clearance < 30 ml/minute, or serum creatinine of 3 mg/dl or more) should begin therapy at 50 mg P.O. daily. After at least 7 days of monitoring, dosage may be increased to 75 mg daily if necessary, but monitoring of trough blood levels should show that the plasma level is no higher than 900 mcg/liter. Further gradual increases may be made, to 50 mg b.i.d. or 100 mg daily, but only with close monitoring of renal function, clinical response, and trough blood levels.

• Contraindicated in patients with known hypersensitivity to the drug, in patients with cardiogenic shock, and in those with preexisting second- or third-degree AV block or bifascicular block (right bundle branch block associated with a left hemiblock) unless a pacemaker is present.
• Other Class Ic antiarrhythmics have been associated with a higher incidence of mortality and nonfatal cardiac arrest.
• Like other antiarrhythmic agents, indecainide can cause new or worsened arrhythmias ("proarrhythmic events"). Most occur during the first 2 weeks of therapy or when dosage is increased; they occur more frequently when total dosage exceeds 200 mg daily or when trough blood levels exceed 900 mcg/liter.

propafenone (Rythmol)
Suppression of life-threatening ventricular arrhythmias, such as episodic ventricular tachycardia —
Adults: initially, 150 mg P.O. q 8 hours. Dosage may be increased to 225 mg q 8 hours after 3 or 4 days; if necessary, increase dosage to 300 mg q 8 hours. Maximum daily dosage is 900 mg.

• Contraindicated in patients with severe or uncontrolled CHF; cardiogenic shock; SA, AV, or intraventricular disorders of impulse conduction; sinus node dysfunction in the absence of a pacemaker; severe bradycardia (50 beats/minute or less); marked hypotension; broncho-

SELECTED MAJOR DRUGS: ANTIARRHYTHMICS *continued*

DRUG, INDICATIONS, AND DOSAGES	SPECIAL PRECAUTIONS
Class Ic *(continued)*	

propafenone *(continued)*

spastic disorders; severe obstructive pulmonary disease; severe electrolyte imbalance; severe hepatic failure; and known hypersensitivity to the drug.
• Use cautiously in patients with CHF because propafenone can exert a negative inotropic effect on the heart, with other cardiac depressant drugs, and in hepatic or renal failure.

Class II

esmolol (Brevibloc)
Supraventricular tachycardia—
Adults: loading dose is 500 mcg/kg/minute by I.V. infusion over 1 minute, followed by a 4-minute maintenance infusion of 50 mcg/kg/minute. If adequate response does not occur within 5 minutes, repeat the loading dose followed by a maintenance infusion of 100 mcg/kg/minute for 4 minutes. Maximum maintenance infusion is 200 mcg/kg/minute.

• Contraindicated in patients with sinus bradycardia, second- or third-degree heart block, cardiogenic shock, or overt heart failure.
• Use cautiously in patients with impaired renal function, diabetes, or bronchospasm.
• Monitor continuous ECG and blood pressure during infusion. Up to 50% of all patients treated with esmolol develop hypotension. Monitor closely, especially if patient's pretreatment blood pressure was low.

Class III

bretylium (Bretylate†‡, Bretylol)
Ventricular fibrillation—
Adults: 5 mg/kg by I.V. push over 1 minute. If necessary, increase dose to 10 mg/kg and repeat q 15 to 30 minutes until 30 mg/kg have been given.
Children: safety and efficacy have not been established, but some clinicians use 2 to 5 mg/kg I.M. as a single dose, or 5 mg/kg I.V. followed by 10 mg/kg I.V. if fibrillation persists.
Other ventricular arrhythmias—
Adults: initially, 500 mg diluted to 50 ml with D_5W or 0.9% sodium chloride solution and infused I.V. over more than 8 minutes at 5 to 10 mg/kg. Dose may be repeated in 1 to 2 hours. Thereafter, repeat q 6 to 8 hours. For I.V. maintenance, infuse 1 to 2 mg/minute in diluted solution of 500 ml D_5W or 0.9% sodium chloride solution. For I.M. injection, give 5 to 10 mg/kg undiluted, repeated in 1 to 2 hours if needed. Thereafter, repeat q 6 to 8 hours.

• There are no contraindications to the use of bretylium in the treatment of ventricular fibrillation or life-threatening arrhythmias; however, patients with known hypersensitivity to corn or corn products should not receive the commercially available preparation mixed in D_5W.
• Use cautiously in patients with fixed cardiac output, aortic stenosis, and pulmonary hypertension to avoid severe and sudden drop in blood pressure.

†Available in Canada only   ‡Available in Australia only

SELF-TEST

1. Joseph Adams is admitted to the coronary care unit with a life-threatening ventricular arrhythmia. The doctor prescribes moricizine 300 mg P.O. q 8 hours. Which of the following ECG abnormalities would warrant extreme caution when moricizine is used?
   a. sick sinus syndrome
   b. atrial flutter
   c. frequent premature atrial contractions
   d. atrial fibrillation

2. Mr. Adams' ventricular arrhythmia was corrected. Before his discharge, his doctor prescribes procainamide 500 mg P.O. as a sustained-release tablet q 6 hours as maintenance therapy. What adverse reaction is especially associated with such use of procainamide?
   a. neutropenia
   b. hyperglycemia
   c. hypokalemia
   d. hypernatremia

3. Mary Jackson has had an acute massive MI and develops frequent premature ventricular contractions. Her doctor prescribed lidocaine 100 mg I.V. How should the nurse administer it?
   a. as a continuous I.V. infusion over 1 hour
   b. as a continuous I.V. infusion over 4 hours
   c. as an I.V. bolus at 25 to 50 mg/minute
   d. as an I.V. bolus over 10 minutes

4. Which of the following patients requires a reduced dosage of lidocaine?
   a. a patient with CHF
   b. a patient with diabetes mellitus
   c. a patient with COPD
   d. a patient with hypertension

5. In severely ill patients such as Mrs. Jackson, what may be the first sign of lidocaine toxicity?
   a. restlessness
   b. seizures
   c. syncope
   d. blurred vision

6. Mrs. Jackson developed a sustained ventricular tachycardia after lidocaine was discontinued. Her doctor ordered flecainide 100 mg P.O. q 12 hours to help treat the arrhythmia and to reinstate lidocaine therapy. What is the therapeutic serum level of flecainide?
   a. 0.1 to 0.2 mcg/ml
   b. 0.2 to 1 mcg/ml
   c. 1 to 2 mcg/ml
   d. 2 to 5 mcg/ml

7. Why should Mrs. Jackson receive both lidocaine and flecainide?
   a. Flecainide enhances the effect of lidocaine.
   b. Flecainide cannot be administered I.V; thus, lidocaine is given until flecainide has a chance to be absorbed.
   c. Full therapeutic effect of flecainide may take 3 to 5 days.
   d. Flecainide helps to prevent rapid metabolism of lidocaine.

8. Robert Jones developed tachyarrhythmia as a result of excessive catecholamine action during anesthesia for a cholecystectomy. His doctor prescribed propranolol 2 mg by slow I.V. push. How should the nurse interpret the word "slow"?
   a. Drug dosage should not exceed 0.25 mg/minute.
   b. Drug dosage should not exceed 0.5 mg/minute.
   c. Drug dosage should not exceed 1 mg/minute.
   d. Drug dosage should not exceed 2 mg/minute.

9. Jane Martin is hospitalized with CHF and has developed a ventricular tachycardia unresponsive to lidocaine. Her doctor prescribed amiodarone 5 mg/kg I.V. as a loading dose followed by an I.V. infusion of 10 mg/kg/day. Mrs. Martin is also taking digoxin 0.25 mg P.O. daily. Which of the following interactions may occur between amiodarone and digoxin?
   a. Amiodarone metabolism may be increased by digoxin, making amiodarone less effective.
   b. Amiodarone may potentiate the slowing of sinus node and AV conduction in the presence of digoxin.
   c. Amiodarone may increase serum digoxin levels and predispose patient to digitalis toxicity.
   d. Amiodarone may interfere with absorption of digoxin and cause it to be less effective.

10. During hospitalization for lung biopsy, Henry Woods developed a supraventricular tachycardia. His doctor prescribed verapamil 5 mg I.V. push over 2 minutes with continuous ECG and blood pressure monitoring. If this dose does not abolish Mr. Woods' arrhythmia, when can a repeat dose be given?
   a. 10 minutes
   b. 15 minutes
   c. 20 minutes
   d. 30 minutes

Check your answers on pages 1060 and 1061.

CHAPTER 21

ANTIANGINALS

Nitrates
amyl nitrite ◆ erythrityl tetranitrate ◆ isosorbide dinitrate ◆ nitroglycerin
pentaerythritol tetranitrate

Beta blockers
atenolol ◆ metoprolol tartrate ◆ nadolol ◆ propranolol hydrochloride

Calcium channel blockers
bepridil hydrochloride ◆ diltiazem hydrochloride ◆ nifedipine
verapamil hydrochloride

OVERVIEW

- Antianginals are used to treat angina pectoris, a syndrome of chest pain produced by an imbalance between myocardial oxygen demand and supply. Most antianginals treat this pain by reducing myocardial oxygen consumption. These drugs are effective in the treatment of classic effort-induced angina or angina that occurs at rest (Prinzmetal's, or variant, angina).
- Treatment with antianginals should be part of a general program designed to alleviate symptoms and reduce risk factors predisposing the patient to coronary artery disease.
- Antianginals are classified into three groups: nitrates, beta blockers, and calcium channel blockers.

MAJOR USES

- Sublingual nitroglycerin and sublingual or chewable isosorbide dinitrate are indicated for the relief of acute anginal episodes.
- Long-acting nitrates and topical, transdermal, transmucosal, and oral extended-release nitroglycerin products are used in the prophylaxis and long-term management of recurrent angina.
- I.V. nitroglycerin is used to treat unstable angina and CHF associated with MI.
- Nitrates are also used to reduce cardiac work load in patients with CHF.
- Beta blockers (atenolol, metoprolol, nadolol, and propranolol) are indicated for patients with moderate to severe angina. (See also Chapter 20, Antiarrhythmics, for additional discussion of beta blockers.)
- Calcium channel blockers are used to treat both classic, effort-induced angina and Prinzmetal's angina.

GLOSSARY

Angina pectoris: a paroxysmal thoracic pain caused most often by myocardial anoxia related to atherosclerosis of the coronary arteries.
Infarction: formation of a localized area of tissue necrosis caused by hypoxia resulting from inadequate blood flow to the area.
Ischemia: decreased blood supply to an area caused by vascular constriction or obstruction.

MECHANISM OF ACTION

- Nitrates (erythrityl tetranitrate, isosorbide dinitrate, nitroglycerin, pentaerythritol tetranitrate, and amyl nitrite) produce relief of angina by reducing the heart's oxygen demand. This reduction occurs because nitrates decrease left ventricular end-diastolic pressure (preload) and systemic vascular resistance (afterload). In addition, the nitrates increase blood flow through the collateral coronary vessels.
- Beta blockers (atenolol, metoprolol, nadolol, and propranolol) reduce the heart's oxygen demand by blocking catecholamine-induced increases in heart rate, blood pressure, and force of myocardial contraction.
- Calcium channel blockers (bepridil, diltiazem, nicardipine, nifedipine, and verapamil) reduce oxygen demand by inhibiting the influx of calcium through the muscle cell. This dilates the coronary arteries and decreases afterload.

ABSORPTION, DISTRIBUTION, METABOLISM, AND EXCRETION

Nitrates are well absorbed from all routes of administration, metabolized in the liver, and excreted mainly in the urine.

Beta blockers are absorbed in the GI tract. About 90% of a dose of propranolol is absorbed; only about 50% of an oral dose of the other beta blockers is absorbed. Atenolol, metoprolol, and propranolol are metabolized by the liver and excreted in the urine. Nadolol is excreted unchanged in the urine.

Calcium channel blockers are well absorbed in the GI tract, metabolized mainly in the liver, and excreted in the urine.

ONSET AND DURATION

Onset and duration of the nitrates depends on the drug used and the form and route of administration selected. (See *Pharmacokinetics of Nitrates,* page 266.)

Because they have a relatively slow onset of action after oral administration (30 minutes to 2 hours), beta-adrenergic blockers are most useful for the prophylaxis of anginal attacks.

PHARMACOKINETICS OF NITRATES

DRUG	FORM	ONSET	DURATION
erythrityl tetranitrate	chewable and S.L.	5 minutes	2 hours
	oral	30 minutes	3 to 4 hours
isosorbide dinitrate	chewable and S.L.	2 to 5 minutes	1 to 2 hours
	oral	15 to 30 minutes	4 to 6 hours
	oral, extended-release	1 hour	12 hours
nitroglycerin	I.V.	instantaneous	transient
	S.L.	3 minutes	10 to 30 minutes
	transmucosal	3 minutes	6 hours
	oral, extended-release	1 hour	8 to 12 hours
	topical ointment	30 to 60 minutes	4 to 6 hours
	transdermal	30 to 60 minutes	24 hours
pentaerythritol tetranitrate	oral	30 minutes	4 to 5 hours

Nifedipine begins to act in 10 minutes. Duration of action is approximately 4 hours. Verapamil, when administered I.V., has an onset of action of less than 5 minutes. The oral form begins to act within 1 to 2 hours. Duration of action is several hours.

ADVERSE REACTIONS

Adverse reactions commonly associated with nitrates include postural hypotension, headache due to vasodilation, reflex tachycardia, flushing, and rash. Intravenous preparations, in which ethanol is used to solubilize nitroglycerin, may cause ethanol intoxication.

Beta blockers most commonly cause bradycardia and hypotension, and possibly dizziness, shortness of breath, and fatigue. Bizarre or disturbing dreams are not uncommon, especially at the start of therapy.

Calcium channel blockers can cause bradycardia, dizziness, fatigue, hypotension, and constipation.

NITROGLYCERIN (GLYCERYL TRINITRATE)

(nye troe gli′ser in)

*Deponit, Klavikordal, Niong, Nitradisc‡, Nitro-Bid, Nitro-Bid IV,
Nitrocap, Nitrocap T.D., Nitrodisc, Nitro-Dur, Nitro-Dur II, Nitrogard,
Nitrogard SR, Nitrol, Nitrolate Ointment‡, Nitrolin, Nitrolingual, Nitrol
TSAR, Nitronet, Nitrong, Nitrong SR, Nitrospan, Nitrostat, Nitrostat IV,
NTS, Transderm-Nitro, Tridil*

Classification: nitrate
Pregnancy risk category C

How supplied

TABLETS (BUCCAL): 1 mg, 2 mg, 3 mg
TABLETS (SUBLINGUAL): 0.15 mg (gr 1/400), 0.3 mg (gr 1/200), 0.4 mg (gr
1/150), 0.6 mg (gr 1/100)
TABLETS (SUSTAINED-RELEASE): 2.6 mg, 6.5 mg, 9 mg
CAPSULES (SUSTAINED-RELEASE): 2.5 mg, 6.5 mg, 9 mg
SOLUTION FOR INFUSION: 0.5 mg/ml, 0.8 mg/ml in 10-ml ampules; 5 mg/ml
in 1-ml, 5-ml vials; 5 mg/ml in 10-ml vials and ampules
AEROSOL (TRANSLINGUAL): 0.4 mg/metered spray
TOPICAL: 2% ointment
TRANSDERMAL: 2.5 mg, 5 mg, 7.5 mg, 10 mg, 15 mg/24-hour systems

Indications and dosage

Prophylaxis against chronic anginal attacks
ADULTS: 2.5 mg sustained-release capsule P.O. q 8 to 12 hours. Alternatively, apply 2% ointment once daily. Start with ½" ointment, increasing
by ½" increments until headache occurs, then decreasing to previous dose.
Range of dosage with ointment is 2" to 5"; usual dose is 1" to 2".
Alternatively, transdermal disk or pad (Nitrodisc, Nitro-Dur, or Transderm-Nitro) may be applied to hairless site once daily.

**Relief of acute angina pectoris; to prevent or minimize anginal attacks
when taken immediately before stressful events**
ADULTS: 1 S.L. tablet (gr 1/400, 1/200, 1/150, 1/100) dissolved under the
tongue or in the buccal pouch immediately upon indication of anginal
attack. May repeat q 5 minutes for 15 minutes. Or, using Nitrolingual
spray, spray one or two doses into mouth, preferably onto or under the
tongue. May repeat q 3 to 5 minutes to a maximum of three doses within
a 15-minute period. Or, 1 to 3 mg (buccal tablet) q 3 to 5 hours during
waking hours.

**To control hypertension associated with surgery; to treat CHF
associated with MI; to relieve angina pectoris in acute situations; to
produce controlled hypotension during surgery**
ADULTS: initial I.V. infusion rate is 5 mcg/minute. May be increased by 5
mcg/minute q 3 to 5 minutes until a response is noted. If a 20 mcg/minute

‡Available in Australia only

rate doesn't produce a response, dosage may be increased by as much as 20 mcg/minute q 3 to 5 minutes.

Contraindications and precautions
Nitroglycerin is contraindicated in patients with known hypersensitivity to nitrates, head trauma, cerebral hemorrhage, hypertrophic cardiomyopathy, or severe anemia. Use cautiously in patients with hypotension.

Adverse reactions
CNS: *headache, sometimes with throbbing; dizziness;* weakness.
CV: orthostatic hypotension, *tachycardia,* flushing, palpitations, fainting.
GI: nausea, vomiting.
SKIN: cutaneous vasodilation.
LOCAL: *sublingual burning.*
OTHER: hypersensitivity reactions.

Interactions
Antihypertensives: possibly enhanced hypotensive effect. Monitor closely.

Nursing considerations
Assessment
• Review the patient's history for a condition that contraindicates the use of nitroglycerin and related compounds.
• Obtain a baseline assessment of the patient's angina or blood pressure (if used to control hypertension or produce controlled hypotension) before therapy.
• Be alert for common adverse reactions.
• Evaluate the patient's and family's knowledge about nitroglycerin therapy.

Planning (Nursing Diagnoses)
Potential nursing diagnoses for the patient receiving nitroglycerin include:
• Pain related to ineffectiveness of nitroglycerin.
• Potential for injury related to nitroglycerin-induced dizziness or orthostatic hypotension.
• Decreased cardiac output related to nitroglycerin-induced tachycardia.
• Knowledge deficit related to nitroglycerin therapy.

Implementation
Preparation and administration
— To apply ointment, spread uniform, thin layer on any hairless body area. Do not rub in. Cover with plastic film to aid absorption and to protect clothing. If using Tape-Surrounded Appli-Ruler (TSAR) system, keep the TSAR on skin to protect patient's clothing and to ensure that ointment remains in place.
— Be sure to remove all excess ointment from previous site before applying the next dose.
— Avoid getting ointment on fingers. (See *How to Apply Nitroglycerin Ointment.)*

HOW TO APPLY NITROGLYCERIN OINTMENT

The doctor has prescribed nitroglycerin as an ointment. In this form, nitroglycerin is continuously absorbed through the skin into the circulation; it's effective for about 4 hours.

To apply nitroglycerin, follow these instructions carefully:

1. Apply ointment to a hairless or shaved area of skin (chest, arm, thigh, abdomen, forehead, ankle, or back) to promote uniform absorption. Choose a new site each time you apply a new dose to prevent minor skin irritations. Remove any traces of ointment left from previous application.

2. Use the ruled applicator paper that comes with the ointment to measure your dose accurately.

3. Use the applicator paper to apply the ointment in a thin, uniform layer over an area of about 3″ to 6″ (7.5 to 15 cm). Leave the applicator paper on the site.

4. Cover the applicator paper with plastic wrap and secure it with tape. This will protect clothing and ensure maximum absorption.

Tell the patient to call the doctor immediately if headache, dizziness, fainting, or any redness or irritation occur. Such effects may require dosage adjustment.

— Transdermal dosage forms can be applied to any hairless part of the skin except distal parts of the arms or legs, because absorption will not be maximal at these sites.

— When terminating transdermal treatment of angina, gradually reduce the dosage and frequency of application over 4 to 6 weeks.

— The various brands of transdermal nitroglycerin can be interchanged to achieve the prescribed dose. Standardized labels specify the amount of nitroglycerin released over 24 hours.

— When administering sublingual tablets, place the tablet under the patient's tongue. Dose may be repeated every 10 to 15 minutes for a maximum of three doses. The patient who complains of tingling sensation with drug administration may try holding tablet in buccal pouch.

— Sublingual nitroglycerin tablets are still potent if they cause a burning sensation under the tongue. However, not all currently available preparations produce this sensation.

— When administering a buccal tablet, have the patient place the tablet between his lip and gum above the incisors or between his cheek and gum. Make sure the patient doesn't swallow or chew the tablet, as this will make it ineffective.

— Tolerance may develop rather quickly, especially with the long-acting forms of nitrates. To prevent tolerance, the patient should have a daily nitrate-free interval of 6 to 12 hours. Nitroglycerin patches should be applied in the morning and removed at bedtime. Sustained-release capsules should be taken morning, noon, and night as opposed to every 8 hours. Nitrate-free intervals help maintain responsiveness to the clinical effects of nitroglycerin.

— Nitroglycerin lingual spray should not be swallowed immediately after administering. Have the patient wait about 10 seconds or so before swallowing.

— Always administer I.V. nitroglycerin with an infusion pump and titrate the dose to desired patient response. Always mix in glass bottles and avoid use of I.V. filters because the drug binds to plastic. Regular polyvinyl chloride (PVC) tubing can bind up to 80% of the drug, requiring infusions of higher dosages. A special nonabsorbing (non-PVC) tubing is available from the manufacturer; patients receive more drug when these infusion sets are used. Always use the same type of infusion set when changing I.V. lines.

— Administer oral tablets on an empty stomach, either half an hour before or 1 to 2 hours after meals.

Monitoring

— Monitor the effectiveness of nitroglycerin therapy to prevent or relieve anginal pain by assessing patient's degree and frequency of pain.

— Monitor for headache, which may be throbbing but usually subsides in a few days as tolerance develops.

— Monitor blood pressure, heart rate, and intensity and duration of response to drug; ask the patient about palpitations.

— Closely monitor vital signs during infusion of nitroglycerin. Be particularly aware of blood pressure, especially if the drug is being used in a patient with an MI. Excessive hypotension may worsen the MI.

— Monitor the patient for drug interactions.

— Regularly reevaluate the patient's and family's knowledge about nitroglycerin therapy.

Intervention

— Alert the doctor immediately if nitroglycerin is ineffective; keep patient at rest during anginal attacks.

— Be sure to remove transdermal patch before defibrillation. Because the patch has an aluminum backing, the electric current may cause it to explode.

— Treat headache with aspirin or acetaminophen.

— Assist the patient to a sitting or standing position gradually to minimize effects of orthostatic hypotension.

— Maintain safety precautions during nitroglycerin therapy. Keep bed rails up and assist patient with activities such as walking if dizziness occurs (with long-acting forms of nitrates).

— Keep all members of the health care team informed of the patient's response to the drug.

Patient teaching

— Inform the patient and family about nitroglycerin, including the dosage, frequency, action, and adverse reactions.

— Tell the patient to take medication regularly, even long-term, as prescribed, and to keep it easily accessible at all times. Nitroglycerin is physiologically necessary but not habit-forming.

—Tell the patient that an additional dose may be taken before anticipated stress or at bedtime if angina is nocturnal.

—Teach the patient to take a sublingual tablet at the first sign of attack. Tell the patient that he should wet the tablet with saliva, place it under the tongue until completely absorbed, and sit down and rest. Dose may be repeated every 10 to 15 minutes for a maximum of three doses. If this provides no relief, the patient should call a doctor or go to a hospital emergency room. If the patient complains of a tingling sensation with drug placed sublingually, tell him to try holding the tablet in the buccal pouch.

—Tell the patient to place the buccal tablet between his lip and gum above the incisors, or between the cheek and gum. Tell the patient not to swallow or chew this tablet, because that will render it ineffective.

—Tell the patient to take the oral tablet on an empty stomach, either 30 minutes before or 1 to 2 hours after meals; to swallow oral tablets whole; and to chew chewable tablets thoroughly before swallowing.

—Teach the patient how to apply ointment or transdermal patch.

—Instruct patient to use caution when wearing a transdermal patch near a microwave oven. Leaking radiation may heat the patch's metallic backing and cause burns.

—If nitroglycerin lingual spray has been prescribed, instruct the patient how to use this device correctly. Remind the patient not to inhale the spray, but to release it onto or under the tongue.

—Tell the patient to store nitroglycerin sublingual tablets in their original container or another container specifically approved for this use; also tell the patient to store drug in cool, dark place in a tightly closed container. To ensure freshness, the patient should replace the supply of sublingual tablets every 3 months. Tell the patient to remove cotton from container, since it absorbs drug.

—Advise the patient not to carry bottle containing sublingual or buccal tablets close to body because body heat may accelerate the decomposition of the tablets. Patient should carry it in a jacket pocket or purse. Never store in a closed car or glove compartment.

—Inform the patient that headache usually subsides in a few days as tolerance develops; tell the patient to take a mild analgesic for headache relief until tolerance occurs.

—Nitroglycerin may cause orthostatic hypotension. Teach the patient how to minimize it: patient should change to upright position slowly, go up and down stairs carefully, and lie down at the first sign of dizziness.

—Tell the patient to notify the nurse or doctor if adverse reactions develop or questions arise about nitroglycerin therapy.

Evaluation

In the patient receiving nitroglycerin, appropriate evaluation statements include:

• Patient reports nitroglycerin relieves anginal pain.

- Patient does not experience injury as a result of dizziness or orthostatic hypotension.
- Patient maintains adequate cardiac output.
- Patient and family state an understanding of nitroglycerin therapy, including correct administration technique.

PROTOTYPE: BETA BLOCKERS

NADOLOL
(nay doe′ lole)
Corgard
Classification: beta blocker
Pregnancy risk category C

How supplied
TABLETS: 20 mg, 40 mg, 80 mg, 120 mg, 160 mg

Indications and dosage
Management of angina pectoris
ADULTS: initially, 40 mg P.O. daily. Dosage may be increased in 40- to 80-mg increments until optimal response occurs. Usual maintenance dosage range is 40 to 240 mg daily.

Hypertension
ADULTS: initially, 40 mg P.O. daily. Dosage may be increased in 40- to 80-mg increments until optimal response occurs. Usual maintenance dosage range is 40 to 320 mg daily. Doses of 640 mg may be necessary in rare cases.

Contraindications and precautions
Nadolol is contraindicated in patients with bronchial asthma, sinus bradycardia and second- or third-degree conduction block, and cardiogenic shock. Use cautiously in patients with heart failure, chronic bronchitis, renal or hepatic insufficiency, or emphysema.

Adverse reactions
CNS: fatigue, lethargy.
CV: *bradycardia*, hypotension, **CHF**, peripheral vascular disease.
GI: nausea, vomiting, diarrhea.
METABOLIC: hypoglycemia without tachycardia.
SKIN: rash.
OTHER: increased airway resistance, fever.

Interactions
Antihypertensives: enhanced antihypertensive effect. Use together cautiously.
Digitalis glycosides: excessive bradycardia and increased depressant effect on myocardium. Use together cautiously.

Epinephrine: severe vasoconstriction and reflex bradycardia. Monitor blood pressure and observe patient carefully.

Indomethacin: decreased antihypertensive effect. Monitor blood pressure and adjust dosage.

Insulin, oral antidiabetic agents (sulfonylureas): can alter dosage requirements in previously stabilized diabetics. Observe patient carefully.

Nursing considerations

Assessment

• Review the patient's history for a condition that contraindicates the use of nadolol and related compounds.
• Obtain a baseline assessment of the patient's anginal pain before therapy.
• Be alert for common adverse reactions.
• Evaluate the patient's and family's knowledge about nadolol therapy.

Planning (Nursing Diagnoses)

Potential nursing diagnoses for the patient receiving nadolol include:
• Pain related to ineffectiveness of nadolol therapy.
• Fluid volume excess related to nadolol-induced CHF.
• Altered tissue perfusion (cerebral) related to nadolol-induced bradycardia or hypotension.
• Knowledge deficit related to nadolol therapy.

Implementation

Preparation and administration

— Administer nadolol without regard to meals.
— Don't discontinue therapy abruptly; can exacerbate angina and MI. Expect to gradually reduce dosage over 1 to 2 weeks.

Monitoring

— Monitor the effectiveness of nadolol therapy by regularly evaluating the severity and frequency of the patient's anginal pain.
— Monitor elderly patients closely for enhanced adverse reactions.
— Monitor the patient for adverse drug reactions.
— Monitor vital signs regularly, because nadolol can mask common signs of shock.
— Check the patient's apical pulse for bradycardia before each dose.
— Regularly monitor the patient's thyroid studies and blood glucose levels, as nadolol can mask signs of hyperthyroidism and hypoglycemia.
— Monitor for signs of CHF (shortness of breath, abnormal heart and breath sounds, weight gain [reflecting edema], or changes in patient's skin color).
— Monitor the patient for drug interactions.
— Regularly reevaluate the patient's and family's knowledge about nadolol therapy.

Intervention
—If pulse is slower than 60 beats/minute, withhold drug and call the doctor.
—Consult the doctor if the patient does not experience pain relief.
—Institute measures to minimize CHF, such as limiting fluid and sodium intake.
—Maintain safety precautions if bradycardia and hypotension occur; assist the patient with daily activities to minimize energy expenditure.
—Keep all members of the health care team informed of the patient's response to the drug.

Patient teaching
—Inform the patient and family about nadolol, including the dosage, frequency, action, and adverse reactions.
—Teach the patient how to check pulse rate and to do so before taking drug; if rate is below 60 beats/minute, the patient should notify the doctor.
—Explain the importance of taking this drug as prescribed, even when feeling well.
—Tell outpatients not to discontinue nadolol suddenly, but to call the doctor if unpleasant adverse reactions occur.
—Teach the patient to restrict fluid and salt intake if fluid retention occurs.
—Teach the patient about disease and therapy.
—Tell the patient to notify the nurse or doctor if adverse reactions develop or questions arise about nadolol therapy.

Evaluation
In the patient receiving nadolol, appropriate evaluation statements include:
• Patient reports relief of anginal pain.
• Patient does not develop fluid retention leading to CHF.
• Patient maintains adequate cerebral tissue perfusion.
• Patient and family state an understanding of nadolol therapy.

PROTOTYPE: CALCIUM CHANNEL BLOCKERS

NIFEDIPINE
(nye fed'i peen)
Adalat, Adalat P.A.†, Procardia, Procardia XL
Classification: calcium channel blocker
Pregnancy risk category C

How supplied
TABLETS (SUSTAINED-RELEASE): 30 mg, 60 mg, 90 mg
CAPSULES: 10 mg, 20 mg

Indications and dosage
Management of vasospastic (Prinzmetal's or variant) angina and classic chronic stable angina pectoris; Raynaud's disease
ADULTS: starting dose is 10 mg P.O. t.i.d. Usual effective dosage range is 10 to 20 mg t.i.d. Some patients may require up to 30 mg q.i.d. Maximum daily dosage is 180 mg.

Hypertension
ADULTS: 30 or 60 mg P.O. (sustained-release form only) daily. Titrate over a 7- to 14-day period.

Contraindications and precautions
Nifedipine is contraindicated in patients with known hypersensitivity to the drug. Use cautiously in patients with CHF or hypotension. Also use cautiously in elderly patients because nifedipine's duration of action may be prolonged in such patients.

Adverse reactions
CNS: *dizziness, light-headedness*, flushing, *headache*, weakness, syncope.
CV: peripheral edema, hypotension, palpitations.
EENT: nasal congestion.
GI: *nausea, heartburn*, diarrhea.
METABOLIC: hypokalemia.
OTHER: muscle cramps, dyspnea.

Interactions
Cimetidine, ranitidine: decreased nifedipine metabolism. Monitor carefully for toxicity.
Propranolol (and other beta blockers): may cause hypotension and heart failure. Use together cautiously.

Nursing considerations
Assessment
• Review the patient's history for a condition that contraindicates the use of nifedipine and related compounds.
• Obtain a baseline assessment of the patient's angina before therapy.
• Be alert for common adverse reactions.
• Evaluate the patient's and family's knowledge about nifedipine therapy.

Planning (Nursing Diagnoses)
Potential nursing diagnoses for the patient receiving nifedipine include:
• Pain related to ineffectiveness of nifedipine therapy.
• Altered nutrition: Less than body requirements related to nifedipine-induced nausea and heartburn.
• Potential for injury related to nifedipine-induced dizziness or light-headedness.
• Knowledge deficit related to nifedipine therapy.

Implementation

Preparation and administration

— Protect capsules from direct light and moisture, and store at room temperature.

— No sublingual form of nifedipine is available. However, during an emergency the liquid in the oral capsule can be withdrawn by puncturing the capsule with a needle. The contents can then be instilled into the buccal pouch.

— Although a rebound effect hasn't been observed after withdrawal of the drug, expect dosage to be reduced slowly under a doctor's supervision.

Monitoring

— Monitor the effectiveness of nifedipine therapy by regularly assessing severity and frequency of pain.

— Monitor the patient for adverse drug reactions.

— Monitor blood pressure regularly, especially in patients who are also taking beta blockers or antihypertensives.

— Monitor serum potassium level regularly for hypokalemia.

— Continuous blood pressure and ECG monitoring is recommended if sublingual nifedipine is used to decrease blood pressure during hypertensive emergencies.

— Monitor the patient for drug interactions.

— Monitor the patient's nutritional intake and weight if the patient develops nausea or heartburn.

— Regularly monitor the patient for CNS reactions such as dizziness or light-headedness.

— Regularly reevaluate the patient's and family's knowledge about nifedipine therapy.

Intervention

— Consult the doctor if the patient does not obtain pain relief.

— Encourage small, frequent meals and a bland diet if nausea or heartburn occurs. If adverse GI reactions are severe or prolonged, obtain an order for an antiemetic.

— Institute safety precautions, such as assisting patient with ambulation, if CNS reactions occur.

— Keep all members of the health care team informed of the patient's response to the drug.

Patient teaching

— Inform the patient and family about nifedipine, including the dosage, frequency, action, and adverse reactions.

— If the patient is continuing nitrate therapy while drug dosage is being titrated, urge continued compliance. Sublingual nitroglycerin, especially, may be taken as needed when anginal symptoms are acute.

— Instruct the patient to swallow the capsule whole without breaking, crushing, or chewing it. Tell the patient that the sustained-release tablets should never be chewed, crushed, or broken.

—The patient may briefly develop anginal exacerbation when beginning drug therapy or when dosage is increased. Reassure him that this symptom is temporary.

—Tell the patient to notify a doctor if nifedipine does not relieve anginal pain.

—Advise the patient how to handle adverse GI reactions.

—Warn the patient to avoid hazardous activities that require mental alertness until CNS effects are known.

—Tell the patient to notify the nurse or doctor if adverse reactions develop or questions arise about nifedipine therapy.

Evaluation

In the patient receiving nifedipine, appropriate evaluation statements include:

• Patient reports relief of anginal pain.

• Patient maintains normal nutritional intake.

• Patient does not experience injury as a result of adverse CNS reactions to nifedipine.

• Patient and family state an understanding of nifedipine therapy.

SELECTED MAJOR DRUGS: ANTIANGINALS

DRUG, INDICATIONS, AND DOSAGES	SPECIAL PRECAUTIONS
Nitrates	
amyl nitrite *Relief of angina pectoris; relief of renal or gallbladder colic —* **Adults:** 1 glass ampule inhaler (0.2 to 0.3 ml) p.r.n.	• Contraindicated in patients with known hypersensitivity to nitrates and during an acute MI. • Use cautiously in patients with head injury, cerebral hemorrhage, hypotension, or glaucoma.
isosorbide dinitrate (Apo-ISDN†, Isordil) *Acute anginal attacks (sublingual and chewable tablets only); prophylaxis in situations likely to cause anginal attacks; chronic ischemic heart disease (by preload reduction) —* **Adults:** 2.5 to 10 mg S.L. for prompt relief of anginal pain, repeated q 5 to 10 minutes (maximum of three doses/30 minutes). For prophylaxis, 2.5 to 10 mg S.L. q 2 to 3 hours. Or 5 to 10 mg chewable form p.r.n. for acute attack or q 2 to 3 hours for prophylaxis but only after initial test dose of 5 mg to determine risk of severe hypotension. Or 5 to 30 mg P.O. q.i.d. for prophylaxis only (use smallest effective dose).	• Contraindicated in patients with known hypersensitivity to nitrates, head trauma, cerebral hemorrhage, or severe anemia. • Use cautiously in patients with hypotension. • Monitor blood pressure and intensity and duration of response to drug.

(continued)

†Available in Canada only

SELECTED MAJOR DRUGS: ANTIANGINALS *continued*

DRUG, INDICATIONS, AND DOSAGES	SPECIAL PRECAUTIONS

Nitrates *(continued)*

pentaerythritol tetranitrate (Peritrate)
Prophylaxis against angina pectoris—
Adults:10 to 20 mg P.O. q.i.d.; may be titrated upward
to 40 mg P.O. q.i.d. half an hour before or 1 hour after
meals and h.s.; or 80 mg sustained-release preparations
P.O. b.i.d.

• Contraindicated in patients
with head trauma, cerebral
hemorrhage, or severe anemia.
• Use cautiously in patients
with hypotension and glaucoma.

Beta-adrenergic blockers

atenolol (Noten‡, Tenormin)
Prophylaxis against angina pectoris—
Adults: 50 mg P.O. daily. May increase to 100 mg daily
after 7 days for optimal effect. May give as much as
200 mg daily.

• Contraindicated in patients
with sinus bradycardia and sec-
ond- or third-degree conduction
block, and cardiogenic shock.
• Use cautiously in patients
with cardiac failure.
• Similar to metoprolol, atenolol
is a cardioselective beta blocker.
Although atenolol can be used
in patients with bronchospastic
diseases such as asthma and
emphysema, the drug should
still be used cautiously in such
patients—especially when 100
mg are given. Twice-daily dosing may help minimize this risk.

metoprolol (Betaloc†‡, Lopressor)
Prophylaxis against angina pectoris—
Adults: 100 mg P.O. daily in divided doses. Gradually increase as needed and tolerated to a maximum of 400
mg daily.

• Use cautiously in patients
with heart failure, diabetes, respiratory or hepatic disease, or
in patients taking antihypertensives. Always check patient's
apical pulse rate before giving
this drug. If it's slower than 60
beats/minute, hold drug and call
doctor immediately.
• Although most patients with
asthma and bronchitis can take
this drug without fear of worsening their condition, doses over
100 mg daily should be used
cautiously.

propranolol (Apo-Propranolol†, Deralin‡, Inderal)
Management of angina pectoris—
Adults: 10 to 20 mg P.O. t.i.d. or q.i.d. or 1 sustained-
release capsule (80 mg) P.O. daily. Dosage may be increased at 7- to 10-day intervals. The average optimal
dosage is 160 mg daily.
To reduce mortality after MI—
Adults: 180 to 240 mg P.O. daily in divided doses. Usually administered t.i.d. to q.i.d.

• Contraindicated in patients
with diabetes mellitus, asthma,
or allergic rhinitis; during ethyl
ether anesthesia; with sinus
bradycardia and in second- or
third-degree heart block; in cardiogenic shock; and in right
ventricular failure secondary to
pulmonary hypertension.

---

†Available in Canada only   ‡Available in Australia only

SELECTED MAJOR DRUGS: ANTIANGINALS *continued*

DRUG, INDICATIONS, AND DOSAGES	SPECIAL PRECAUTIONS

Beta-adrenergic blockers *(continued)*

propranolol *(continued)*
Supraventricular, ventricular, and atrial arrhythmias; tachyarrhythmias caused by excessive catecholamine action during anesthesia, hyperthyroidism, and pheochromocytoma—
Adults: 1 to 3 mg I.V. diluted in 50 ml dextrose 5% in water or 0.9% sodium chloride solution infused slowly, not to exceed 1 mg/minute. After 3 mg have been infused, another dose may be given in 2 minutes; subsequent doses no sooner than q 4 hours. Usual maintenance dosage is 10 to 80 mg P.O.
Prevention of frequent, severe, uncontrollable, or disabling migraine or vascular headache—
Adults: initially, 80 mg P.O. daily in divided doses or 1 sustained-release capsule daily. Usual maintenance dosage is 160 to 240 mg daily, divided t.i.d. or q.i.d.

• Use cautiously in patients with CHF or respiratory disease, and in patients taking antihypertensive drugs.

Calcium channel blockers

bepridil (Vascor)
Chronic stable angina in patients intolerant of or unresponsive to other agents—
Adults: initially, 200 mg P.O. daily. After 10 days, increase dosage based on response. Maintenance dosage in most patients is 300 mg/day. Maximum daily dosage is 400 mg.

• Contraindicated in patients with known hypersensitivity to the drug.
• Not a first-line agent because of the risk of agranulocytosis.

diltiazem (Cardizem)
Management of vasospastic (Prinzmetal's or variant) angina and classic chronic stable angina pectoris—
Adults: 30 mg P.O. t.i.d. or q.i.d. before meals and h.s. Dosage may be gradually increased to a maximum of 360 mg/day in divided doses.
Hypertension—
Adults: 60 mg (sustained-release capsule) P.O. b.i.d. Titrate dosage to effect. Maximum recommended dosage is 360 mg/day.

• Contraindicated in patients with sick sinus syndrome, unless a functioning ventricular pacemaker is present; hypotension when systolic blood pressure is less than 90 mm Hg; and second- or third-degree AV block.
• Use cautiously in elderly patients because duration of action may be prolonged.

nicardipine (Cardene)
Management of angina pectoris; hypertension—
Adults: initially, 20 mg P.O. t.i.d. Increase as needed and tolerated. Usual dosage is 20 to 40 mg P.O. t.i.d.

• Contraindicated in patients with known hypersensitivity to nicardipine, and in advanced aortic stenosis.
• Use cautiously in patients with cardiac conduction disturbances, hypotension, and CHF.
• Some patients may experience increased frequency, severity, or duration of chest pain at beginning of therapy or during dos-

(continued)

SELECTED MAJOR DRUGS: ANTIANGINALS *continued*

DRUG, INDICATIONS, AND DOSAGES	SPECIAL PRECAUTIONS
Calcium channel blockers *(continued)*	

nicardipine *(continued)*

age adjustments. The mechanism for this adverse reaction is not known. Advise patient to report chest pain immediately.

verapamil (Calan, Isoptin)
Management of vasospastic (Prinzmetal's or variant) angina and classic chronic, stable angina pectoris —
Adults: starting dose is 80 mg P.O. t.i.d. or q.i.d. Dosage may be increased at weekly intervals. Some patients may require up to 480 mg daily.
Atrial arrhythmias —
Adults: 0.075 to 0.15 mg/kg (5 to 10 mg) I.V. push over 2 minutes with ECG and blood pressure monitoring. Repeat dose in 30 minutes if no response.
Children ages 1 to 15: 0.1 to 0.3 mg/kg as I.V. bolus over 2 minutes.
Children under age 1: 0.1 to 0.2 mg/kg as I.V. bolus over 2 minutes under continuous ECG monitoring. Dose can be repeated in 30 minutes if no response.
Migraine headache prophylaxis —
Adults: 80 mg P.O. q.i.d.
Hypertension —
Adults: 240 mg (sustained-release tablet) P.O. once daily in the morning. If response is not adequate, may give an additional half tablet in the evening or 1 tablet q 12 hours. Alternatively, may give 80-mg immediate-release tablet t.i.d. or q.i.d.

• Contraindicated in patients with advanced heart failure, AV block, severe left ventricular dysfunction, cardiogenic shock, sinus node disease, and severe hypotension.
• Use cautiously in elderly patients because duration of action may be prolonged; in MI followed by coronary occlusion, sick sinus syndrome, impaired AV conduction or heart failure with atrial tachyarrhythmias, and in hepatic or renal disease.

SELF-TEST

1. Timothy Parker, a 53-year-old accountant, is admitted to your unit for evaluation of the increasing frequency of his anginal attacks. He has a history of coronary artery disease and has been taking sublingual nitroglycerin and oral nifedipine at home. He reports that the pain is worse after meals and has increased from once a week to twice daily. The pain is usually relieved with rest and 1 nitroglycerin tablet S.L. When Mr. Parker develops anginal pain, the nurse administers an S.L. nitroglycerin tablet. Which of the following best explains the therapeutic action of nitroglycerin at this dose?
   a. increases the filling pressure (preload)
   b. causes vasoconstriction of the systemic arteriolar bed
   c. increases the systemic blood pressure
   d. decreases the myocardial oxygen consumption

2. Mr. Parker states that his pain is relieved but that he has a sudden pounding headache. The nurse is aware that the headache represents:
   a. a hypersensitivity reaction.
   b. a toxic adverse reaction.
   c. an expected adverse reaction.
   d. orthostatic hypotension.

3. Though there is no sublingual form of nifedipine, buccal administration can be accomplished by:
   a. crushing the capsule.
   b. puncturing the capsule with a needle.
   c. chewing the sustained-release tablet.
   d. dissolving the capsule in water.

4. The action of nadolol reflects:
   a. inhibition of calcium ion influx across cardiac and smooth muscle cells.
   b. reduction of the fast inward current carried by sodium ions.
   c. prolonging of the refractory period and action potential duration.
   d. blocking of the beta-adrenergic response.

Check your answers on page 1061.

CHAPTER 22

ANTIHYPERTENSIVES

Angiotensin converting enzyme (ACE) inhibitors
benazepril ◆ captopril ◆ enalapril maleate ◆ enalaprilat ◆ fosinopril
lisinopril ◆ ramipril

Beta-adrenergic blockers
acebutolol hydrochloride ◆ atenolol ◆ betaxolol hydrochloride
carteolol hydrochloride ◆ labetalol hydrochloride ◆ metoprolol tartrate
nadolol ◆ penbutolol sulfate ◆ pindolol ◆ propranolol hydrochloride
timolol maleate

Calcium channel blockers
diltiazem hydrochloride ◆ isradipine ◆ nicardipine hydrochloride
nifedipine ◆ verapamil hydrochloride

Alpha-adrenergic blockers
doxazosin ◆ phenoxybenzamine hydrochloride ◆ phentolamine mesylate
prazosin hydrochloride ◆ terazosin hydrochloride

Ganglionic blocking agents
mecamylamine hydrochloride ◆ trimethaphan camsylate

Centrally acting sympatholytics
clonidine hydrochloride ◆ guanabenz acetate ◆ guanfacine hydrochloride
methyldopa ◆ methyldopate hydrochloride

Vasodilators
diazoxide ◆ hydralazine hydrochloride ◆ minoxidil ◆ nitroprusside sodium

OVERVIEW

- Antihypertensives are used to lower blood pressure in patients whose diastolic blood pressure averages 90 to 95 mm Hg or more. To control blood pressure effectively with minimal adverse reactions, two or more antihypertensives—with different modes of action—may be needed.
- About 15% of adults are hypertensive. About half these people don't realize they're ill because they remain asymptomatic until complications occur. Untreated hypertension can lead to stroke and cardiac or renal disease.
- Hypertension is now one of the few chronic diseases for which effective therapy exists. However, treatment depends on accurate diagnosis.

GLOSSARY

Diastolic blood pressure: pressure exerted in the vessels when the ventricles are at rest.
Hypertension: systolic blood pressure of 160 mm Hg or higher and diastolic blood pressure of 95 mm Hg or higher on two or more occasions.
Orthostatic hypotension: decrease in blood pressure that occurs when a person stands erect; also called postural hypotension.
Peripheral vascular resistance: pressure that blood must overcome as it flows in a vessel.
Pulse pressure: difference between systolic and diastolic blood pressures, usually about 40 mm Hg.
Systolic blood pressure: pressure exerted in the vessels when the ventricles contract.

- Ensuring compliance with prescribed antihypertensive drug regimens is a major problem because, to the patient, the adverse reactions to the drugs may seem worse than the disease.
- Antihypertensives are classified into seven groups: ACE inhibitors, beta-adrenergic blockers, calcium channel blockers, alpha-adrenergic blockers, ganglionic blocking agents, centrally acting sympatholytics, and vasodilators. Calcium channel blockers are discussed in Chapter 21, Antianginals. Other drugs used for hypertension include diuretics (especially thiazides) and adrenergic neuron blocking agents (such as reserpine).

MAJOR USES

- Antihypertensives are used primarily to treat mild to severe essential hypertension (about 90% of all cases of hypertension). They can also be used to control hypertension in the 10% of patients who have secondary hypertension until a surgical cure can be obtained.
- Two alpha blockers—phenoxybenzamine and phentolamine—can be used to diagnose and manage pheochromocytoma until surgery, if feasible, can be performed.
- Some vasodilating antihypertensives can also be used in chronic refractory CHF to decrease the arterial resistance (afterload) that the heart must pump against. This decrease in arterial impedance causes an increase in cardiac output. Minoxidil, diazoxide, and hydralazine affect mainly the arterial bed, whereas prazosin and nitroprusside affect both the arterial and venous sides.
- A vasodilator affecting the arterial bed may be used alone or in combination with a nitrate to treat refractory CHF. Agents that affect both preload and afterload are used in combination with standard therapy for CHF (salt reduction, diuretics, and digoxin) to achieve maximal results.

MECHANISM OF ACTION

See *Actions of Antihypertensives* for a summary of the neuromuscular and enzymatic mechanisms of action of the major classes of antihypertensives.

ABSORPTION, DISTRIBUTION, METABOLISM, AND EXCRETION

Given orally, most antihypertensives are rapidly absorbed from the GI tract. Methyldopa, however, is erratically absorbed.

The extent of methyldopa absorption varies in patients from day to day but averages 50% of the administered dose. The drug's onset is delayed about 12 to 24 hours after an oral dose because methyldopa is biotransformed in the liver to the metabolite alpha-methylnorepinephrine, which produces the antihypertensive effect.

Captopril is well absorbed from the GI tract, distributed to most body tissues, and partially metabolized in the liver. Both metabolite and unchanged drug are excreted in the urine.

All antihypertensives are widely distributed in body tissues, and most are excreted predominantly through the kidneys. Prazosin, however, is eliminated through bile and feces.

Some patients acetylate (metabolize) hydralazine at a faster rate than others. Since acetylation inactivates the drug, rapid acetylators may require doses up to 60% larger than the usual dose to control their blood pressure.

ONSET AND DURATION

Actions of Antihypertensives describes the onset and duration of antihypertensives.

ADVERSE REACTIONS

The most common adverse reactions to ACE inhibitors include headache, tachycardia, dysgeusia, and orthostatic hypotension. Most of these dissipate after a few days to weeks of therapy. Other adverse reactions to these agents include allergic reactions, angioedema, proteinuria, hyperkalemia, and a persistent, nonproductive cough.

Many patients receiving beta-adrenergic blockers report fatigue, dizziness, or bradycardia, especially at the start of therapy. Some report bizarre dreams or nightmares, depression, or memory loss. Persons predisposed to airway difficulties (such as asthmatics) may experience increased airway resistance or bronchospasm with beta blocker therapy. Edema, CHF, persistent hypotension, or moderate to severe bradycardia can occur with excessive dosage.

Hypotension, bradycardia, and varying degrees of heart block may follow the use of a calcium channel blocker. Some patients report nausea or constipation. Headache, flushing, peripheral edema, or light-headedness may result from excessive peripheral vasodilation.

ACTIONS OF ANTIHYPERTENSIVES

DRUG	ROUTE	ONSET	DURATION	SITE AND MECHANISM OF ACTION
ACE inhibitors				
benazepril	P.O.	1 hour	24 hours	Blocks conversion of angiotensin I to angiotensin II by inhibiting ACE
captopril	P.O.	15 minutes	variable	Blocks conversion of angiotensin I to angiotensin II by inhibiting ACE
enalapril	P.O.	1 hour	24 hours	Blocks conversion of angiotensin I to angiotensin II by inhibiting ACE
enalaprilat	I.V.	15 minutes	6 hours	Blocks conversion of angiotensin I to angiotensin II by inhibiting ACE
fosinopril	P.O.	1 hour	24 hours	Blocks conversion of angiotensin I to angiotensin II by inhibiting ACE
lisinopril	P.O.	1 hour	24 hours	Blocks conversion of angiotensin I to angiotensin II by inhibiting ACE
ramipril	P.O.	1 to 2 hours	24 hours	Blocks conversion of angiotensin I to angiotensin II by inhibiting ACE
Beta-adrenergic blockers				
acebutolol	P.O.	variable	12 to 24 hours	Blocks beta$_1$ receptors
atenolol	P.O.	variable	24 to 36 hours	Blocks beta$_1$ receptors
betaxolol	P.O.	variable	24 to 36 hours	Blocks beta$_1$ receptors
carteolol	P.O.	variable	24 to 36 hours	Blocks beta$_1$ and beta$_2$ receptors
labetalol	P.O.	variable	12 to 24 hours	Blocks beta$_1$, beta$_2$, and alpha receptors
	I.V.	1 to 5 minutes	6 to 12 hours	Blocks beta$_1$, beta$_2$, and alpha receptors
metoprolol	P.O.	variable	12 to 24 hours	Blocks beta$_1$ receptors
	I.V.	1 to 5 minutes	4 to 6 hours	Blocks beta$_1$ receptors
nadolol	P.O.	variable	24 to 36 hours	Blocks beta$_1$ and beta$_2$ receptors

(continued)

ACTIONS OF ANTIHYPERTENSIVES *continued*

DRUG	ROUTE	ONSET	DURATION	SITE AND MECHANISM OF ACTION
Beta-adrenergic blockers *(continued)*				
penbutolol	P.O.	variable	24 to 36 hours	Blocks beta$_1$ and beta$_2$ receptors
pindolol	P.O.	variable	12 to 24 hours	Blocks beta$_1$ and beta$_2$ receptors
propranolol	P.O.	variable	12 to 24 hours	Blocks beta$_1$ and beta$_2$ receptors
	I.V.	1 to 5 minutes	4 to 6 hours	Blocks beta$_1$ and beta$_2$ receptors
timolol	P.O.	variable	12 to 24 hours	Blocks beta$_1$ and beta$_2$ receptors
Alpha-adrenergic blockers				
doxazosin	P.O.	2 to 6 hours	24 to 36 hours	Blocks postsynaptic alpha receptors
phenoxy-benzamine	P.O.	variable	variable	Irreversibly blocks both presynaptic and postsynaptic alpha receptors
phentol-amine	I.V.	immediate	30 minutes	Blocks both presynaptic and post-synaptic alpha receptors
prazosin	P.O.	1 to 3 hours	8 to 12 hours	Blocks postsynaptic alpha receptors
terazosin	P.O.	1 to 2 hours	12 to 24 hours	Blocks postsynaptic alpha receptors
Ganglionic blocking agents				
mecamyl-amine	P.O.	30 minutes to 2 hours	6 to 12 hours	Blocks parasympathetic and sympathetic neurotransmission at ganglia; hypotensive effects are primarily orthostatic
trimetha-phan	I.V.	immediate	10 to 30 minutes	Blocks parasympathetic and sympathetic neurotransmission at ganglia; also causes direct vasodilation and releases histamine

ACTIONS OF ANTIHYPERTENSIVES *continued*

DRUG	ROUTE	ONSET	DURATION	SITE AND MECHANISM OF ACTION
Centrally acting sympatholytics				
clonidine	P.O.	30 to 60 minutes	12 to 24 hours	May act as an agonist on inhibitory centers in the CNS, reducing sympathetic outflow
guanabenz	P.O.	1 hour	6 to 12 hours	May act as an agonist on inhibitory centers in the CNS, reducing sympathetic outflow
guanfacine	P.O.	variable	24 hours	May act as an agonist on inhibitory centers in the CNS, reducing sympathetic outflow
methyldopa	P.O.	2 hours	12 to 24 hours	Metabolized to alpha-methylnorepinephrine; may act as an agonist on inhibitory centers in the CNS, reducing sympathetic outflow; may also act as a false neurotransmitter
Vasodilators				
hydralazine	P.O.	45 minutes	6 to 8 hours	Alters calcium movement in vascular smooth muscle
	I.V.	10 to 20 minutes	2 to 4 hours	Alters calcium movement in vascular smooth muscle
minoxidil	P.O.	30 minutes	24 to 72 hours	Alters calcium movement in vascular smooth muscle

Alpha-adrenergic blockers can cause orthostatic hypotension. Doxazosin, prazosin, and terazosin can cause a syndrome referred to as the "first dose" effect: moderate to severe orthostatic hypotension and syncope at the start of therapy or following an increase in dosage. Other adverse reactions to the alpha blockers include tachycardia, nasal stuffiness, ocular congestion, or symptoms resembling a head cold.

The usefulness of the ganglionic blocking agents is limited by their adverse reactions. Orthostatic hypotension, sometimes severe, is a common problem. Other adverse reactions include GI disturbances, constipation, nausea, and vomiting.

Common adverse reactions to the centrally acting sympatholytics include dry mouth, drowsiness, constipation, and headache. Orthostatic hypotension, palpitations, and tachycardia may also occur.

Vasodilators can cause orthostatic hypotension, palpitations, and tachycardia. Less commonly they can cause other cardiac problems, including CHF, pleural or cardiac effusions, and ECG changes. Minoxidil has been associated with reversible hypertrichosis (elongation and thickening of fine body hair), and hydralazine may cause a systemic lupus erythematosus (SLE) syndrome, especially after prolonged high-dose therapy (more than 200 mg daily).

PROTOTYPE: ACE INHIBITORS

CAPTOPRIL
(kap' toe prill)
Capoten
Classification: ACE inhibitor
Pregnancy risk category C

How supplied
TABLETS: 12.5 mg, 25 mg, 50 mg, 100 mg

Indications and dosage
Hypertension
ADULTS: initially, 25 mg P.O. b.i.d. or t.i.d. If blood pressure isn't satisfactorily controlled in 1 to 2 weeks, dosage may be increased to 50 mg t.i.d. If not satisfactorily controlled after another 1 to 2 weeks, a diuretic should be added to regimen. If further blood pressure reduction is necessary, dosage may be raised to as high as 150 mg t.i.d. while continuing the diuretic. Maximum dosage is 450 mg daily. Daily dose may also be administered b.i.d.

CHF
ADULTS: initially, 6.25 to 12.5 mg P.O. t.i.d. May be gradually increased to 50 mg t.i.d. Maximum dosage is 450 mg daily.

Contraindications and precautions
Captopril is contraindicated in patients with known hypersensitivity to the drug or other ACE inhibitors. Use cautiously in patients with impaired renal function or serious autoimmune disease (particularly SLE), or in patients who have been exposed to other drugs known to affect WBC counts or immune response.

Adverse reactions
BLOOD: leukopenia, agranulocytosis, pancytopenia.
CNS: *headache,* dizziness, fainting.
CV: *tachycardia,* hypotension, angina pectoris, **CHF, pericarditis**, *orthostatic hypotension.*
EENT: *loss of taste (dysgeusia).*
GI: anorexia.
GU: proteinuria, nephrotic syndrome, membranous glomerulopathy, renal

---

Italicized adverse reactions are common　　　　　Boldfaced adverse reactions are life-threatening

failure (in patients with preexisting renal disease or those receiving high dosages), urinary frequency.

METABOLIC: hyperkalemia.

SKIN: urticarial rash, maculopapular rash, pruritus.

OTHER: fever, angioedema of face and extremities, transient increases in liver enzymes, persistent cough.

Interactions

Antacids: decreased captopril effect. Separate administration times.

Digitalis glycosides: may increase serum digoxin concentration by 15% to 30%. Monitor for signs of digoxin toxicity.

NSAIDs: may reduce antihypertensive effect. Monitor blood pressure.

Potassium supplements: increased risk of hyperkalemia. Avoid these supplements unless hypokalemic blood levels are confirmed.

Nursing considerations

Assessment

• Review the patient's history for a condition that contraindicates the use of captopril and related compounds.
• Obtain a baseline assessment of the patient's blood pressure before therapy.
• Be alert for common adverse reactions.
• Evaluate the patient's and family's knowledge about captopril therapy.

Planning (Nursing Diagnoses)

Potential nursing diagnoses for the patient receiving captopril include:
• Potential for injury related to ineffectiveness of captopril to lower blood pressure.
• Altered protection related to captopril-induced blood disorder or renal dysfunction.
• Knowledge deficit related to captopril therapy.

Implementation

Preparation and administration

— Administer 1 hour before meals because food in the GI tract may reduce absorption.
— Antacids decrease captopril effect; therefore, separate administration times.

Monitoring

— Monitor the effectiveness of captopril therapy by regularly assessing the patient's blood pressure and pulse rate before administration.
— Carefully monitor elderly patients because they may be more sensitive to the drug's hypotensive effect.
— Monitor the patient for adverse drug reactions.
— Monitor serum potassium level for hyperkalemia or hypokalemia.
— Monitor CBC, especially WBC and differential count, as well as signs of infection every 2 weeks for the first 3 months of therapy.
— Monitor renal function (BUN and creatinine clearance levels, urinalysis). Drug may further impair renal function.

—Monitor the patient for drug interactions.

—Regularly reevaluate the patient's and family's knowledge about captopril therapy.

Intervention

—Notify the doctor if urinalysis reveals proteinuria, elevated BUN or creatinine levels, or a low creatinine clearance.

—Hold dose and notify the doctor if the patient develops fever, sore throat, or leukopenia.

—Hold dose and notify the doctor if the patient develops hypotension or tachycardia.

—Institute safety precautions if CNS reactions develop.

—Protect the patient from exposure to other patients with infection.

—Limit the patient's fluid intake if CHF or renal dysfunction occurs.

—Keep all members of the health care team informed of the patient's response to the drug.

Patient teaching

—Instruct the patient and family about captopril, including the dosage, frequency, action, and adverse reactions.

—Instruct the patient not to take antacids at the same time as captopril.

—Tell the patient that periodic WBC with differential counts will be required during therapy.

—Advise the patient to report any signs of infection (fever, sore throat).

—Tell the patient that captopril may cause dizziness or fainting, especially at initiation of therapy. Patient should avoid sudden postural changes and should sit down immediately if he feels dizzy.

—Teach the patient about his disease.

—Explain the importance of taking this drug as prescribed, even when feeling well.

—Instruct the patient not to discontinue drug suddenly, but to call the doctor if unpleasant adverse reactions occur.

—Instruct the patient to check with the doctor or pharmacist before taking any OTC medications.

—Instruct the patient to take captopril 1 hour before meals.

—Tell the patient to notify the nurse or doctor if adverse reactions develop or questions arise about captopril therapy.

Evaluation

In the patient receiving captopril, appropriate evaluation statements include:

• Patient's blood pressure is within normal limits.

• Patient's WBC and differential counts and renal function studies are normal.

• Patient and family state an understanding of captopril therapy.

ATENOLOL
(a ten'oh lole)
Noten‡, Tenormin
Classification: beta-adrenergic blocker
Pregnancy risk category C

How supplied
TABLETS: 50 mg, 100 mg
INJECTION: 5 mg/10 ml

Indications and dosage
Hypertension
ADULTS: initially, 50 mg P.O. daily as a single dose. Dosage may be increased to 100 mg daily after 7 to 14 days. Dosages over 100 mg are unlikely to produce further benefit. Dosage adjustment is necessary in patients with creatinine clearance below 35 ml/minute/1.73 m².

Angina pectoris
ADULTS: 50 mg P.O. daily. May increase to 100 mg daily after 7 days for optimal effect. May give as much as 200 mg daily.

To reduce CV mortality and risk of reinfarction in patients with acute MI
ADULTS: 5 mg I.V. over 5 minutes, followed by another 5 mg I.V. 10 minutes later. After an additional 10 minutes, administer 50 mg P.O., followed by 50 mg P.O. in 12 hours. Thereafter, give 100 mg P.O. daily (as a single dose or 50 mg b.i.d.) for at least 7 days.

To reduce the incidence of supraventricular tachycardia in patients undergoing coronary artery bypass
ADULTS: 50 mg P.O. daily starting 3 days before surgery.

Contraindications and precautions
Atenolol is contraindicated in patients with sinus bradycardia and second- or third-degree conduction block, or cardiogenic shock. Use cautiously in patients with cardiac failure. Like metoprolol, atenolol is a cardioselective beta blocker. Although atenolol can be used in patients with bronchospastic diseases such as asthma and emphysema, the drug should still be used cautiously in such patients—especially when 100 mg are given.

Adverse reactions
CNS: *fatigue, dizziness,* lethargy.
CV: *bradycardia,* hypotension, **CHF,** peripheral vascular disease.
GI: nausea, vomiting, diarrhea.
SKIN: rash.
OTHER: fever.

‡Available in Australia only
Italicized adverse reactions are common   Boldfaced adverse reactions are life-threatening

Interactions

Antihypertensives: enhanced hypotensive effect. Use together cautiously.
Digitalis glycosides: excessive bradycardia and increased depressant effect on myocardium. Use together cautiously.
Indomethacin: decreased antihypertensive effect. Monitor blood pressure and adjust dosage.
Insulin, oral antidiabetic agents: can alter dosage requirements in previously stabilized diabetics. Observe patient carefully.

Nursing considerations

Assessment

- Review the patient's history for a condition that contraindicates the use of atenolol and related compounds.
- Obtain a baseline assessment of the patient's blood pressure before therapy.
- Be alert for common adverse reactions.
- Evaluate the patient's and family's knowledge about atenolol therapy.

Planning (Nursing Diagnoses)

Potential nursing diagnoses for the patient receiving atenolol include:
- Potential for injury related to ineffectiveness of atenolol to lower blood pressure.
- Decreased tissue perfusion (cerebral) related to atenolol-induced bradycardia and hypotension.
- Fluid volume excess related to potential for CHF caused by atenolol therapy.
- Knowledge deficit related to atenolol therapy.

Implementation

Preparation and administration

— I.V. doses may be mixed with 5% dextrose, sodium chloride injection, or dextrose and sodium chloride injection. The solution is stable for 48 hours after mixing.
— Administer I.V. dose over 5 minutes.
— Twice-daily dosing may help minimize risk of adverse reactions in patients with bronchospastic diseases.
— Dosage should be reduced if patient has renal insufficiency. Patients with a creatinine clearance of 15 to 35 ml/minute/1.73 m^2 should receive a maximum of 50 mg daily; if creatinine clearance is less than 15 ml/minute/1.73 m^2, the maximum dosage is 50 mg every other day. Hemodialysis patients should receive 50 mg after each dialysis session, but close supervision is mandatory because of the risk of marked decreases in blood pressure.

Monitoring

— Monitor the effectiveness of atenolol therapy by regularly checking the patient's blood pressure and pulse rate for bradycardia and hypotension before administration.
— Monitor ECG for arrhythmias such as heart block.

—Monitor the diabetic patient's blood glucose levels closely, because drug can alter dosage requirements for insulin and oral antidiabetic agents.

—Monitor for signs and symptoms of CHF (dyspnea on exertion, orthopnea, edema, jugular vein distension, crackles); drug has a cardiac depressant effect.

—Monitor creatinine clearance; dosage should be reduced if patient has renal insufficiency.

—Monitor the patient for drug interactions.

—Regularly reevaluate the patient's and family's knowledge about atenolol therapy.

Intervention

—Hold dose and notify the doctor if the patient develops apical rate below 60 beats/minute or second- or third-degree heart block, prolonged PR interval, or hypotension.

—Restrict the patient's fluid and sodium intake to minimize fluid retention.

—Institute safety measures if the patient becomes lethargic or develops peripheral vascular disease.

—Obtain an order for an antiemetic or antidiarrheal agent, as needed.

—Assist the patient with daily activities if fatigue, dyspnea, or bronchospasm occurs.

—Keep all members of the health care team informed of the patient's response to the drug.

Patient teaching

—Inform the patient and family about atenolol, including the dosage, frequency, action, and adverse reactions.

—Counsel your patient to take atenolol at a regular time every day. It can be dispensed in a 28-day calendar pack.

—Explain that the full antihypertensive effect may not appear for 1 or 2 weeks after initiating therapy.

—Instruct the patient not to discontinue the drug abruptly; can exacerbate angina and MI. Tell the patient that atenolol should be withdrawn gradually over a 2-week period.

—Teach the patient about his disease.

—Explain the importance of taking this drug as prescribed, even when feeling well.

—Instruct the patient to check with his doctor or pharmacist before taking any OTC medications.

—Tell the patient to limit fluid and sodium intake to minimize fluid retention.

—Warn the patient to avoid hazardous activities that require mental alertness if lethargy occurs.

—Teach the patient to prevent injury to lower extremities if peripheral vascular disease occurs.

—Tell the patient to notify the nurse or doctor if adverse reactions develop or questions arise about atenolol therapy.

Evaluation

In the patient receiving atenolol, appropriate evaluation statements include:
• Patient's blood pressure is within normal range.
• Patient remains mentally alert.
• Patient does not develop CHF.
• Patient and family state an understanding of atenolol therapy.

PROTOTYPE: ALPHA-ADRENERGIC BLOCKERS

PHENTOLAMINE MESYLATE

(fen' tole a meen)
Regitine, Rogitine†
Classification: alpha-adrenergic blocker
Pregnancy risk category C

How supplied

INJECTION: 5 mg/ml in 1-ml vials, 10 mg/ml‡

Indications and dosage

To aid in diagnosis of pheochromocytoma; to control or prevent hypertension before or during pheochromocytomectomy

ADULTS: for diagnosis, 5 mg I.V.; monitor blood pressure closely. Before surgical removal of tumor, give 2 to 5 mg I.M. or I.V. During surgery, patient may need small I.V. (1 mg) or I.M. (3 mg) doses.

CHILDREN: for diagnosis, 0.1 mg/kg or 3 mg/m² I.V. as single dose, with close blood pressure monitoring. Before surgery, give 1 mg I.V. or 3 mg I.M. During surgery, patient may need small I.V. doses (1 mg).

To treat extravasation

ADULTS AND CHILDREN: infiltrate area with 5 to 10 mg phentolamine in 10 ml 0.9% sodium chloride solution or give half the dosage through the infiltrated I.V. and the other half around the site. Must be done within 12 hours.

Contraindications and precautions

Phentolamine is contraindicated in patients with angina, coronary artery disease, and history of MI. Use cautiously in patients with gastritis or peptic ulcer and in those receiving other antihypertensives.

Adverse reactions

CNS: dizziness, weakness, *flushing.*
CV: *hypotension,* shock, arrhythmias, palpitations, tachycardia, angina pectoris.
GI: diarrhea, abdominal pain, nausea, vomiting, hyperperistalsis.
OTHER: *nasal stuffiness,* hypoglycemia.

---

†Available in Canada only   ‡Available in Australia only
Italicized adverse reactions are common.

Interactions

Antihypertensive agents: additive hypotensive effect. Use together cautiously.

Epinephrine: excessive hypotension. Don't use together.

Nursing considerations

Assessment

• Review the patient's history for a condition that contraindicates the use of phentolamine.
• Obtain a baseline assessment of the patient's blood pressure before therapy.
• Be alert for common adverse reactions.
• Evaluate the patient's and family's knowledge about phentolamine therapy.

Planning (Nursing Diagnoses)

Potential nursing diagnoses for the patient receiving phentolamine therapy include:
• Injury related to potential ineffectiveness of phentolamine therapy.
• Decreased cardiac output related to adverse CV reactions to phentolamine.
• Fluid volume deficit related to potential phentolamine-induced GI effects.
• Knowledge deficit related to phentolamine therapy.

Implementation

Preparation and administration

— When possible, do not give sedatives, analgesics, or narcotics for at least 24 hours before the phentolamine test. Rauwolfia alkaloids should be withdrawn at least 4 weeks before this test, which should not be performed until blood pressure returns to pretreatment levels.
— Administer I.V. dose slowly over several minutes.
— To treat extravasation, infiltrate affected area with phentolamine in 10 ml 0.9% sodium chloride solution, or give half the dosage through the infiltrated I.V. and the other half around the site.
— Do not administer epinephrine to treat phentolamine-induced hypotension, because it may cause an additional fall in blood pressure. Use norepinephrine instead.

Monitoring

— Monitor the effectiveness of phentolamine therapy by monitoring blood pressure constantly during administration. Test is positive for pheochromocytoma if I.V. test dose causes severe hypotension within 1 or 2 minutes; phentolamine has little effect on the blood pressure of a normal individual or patients with essential hypertension.
— Monitor the effectiveness of phentolamine to treat extravasation by inspecting area for signs of improvement.
— Monitor the patient for adverse drug reactions.
— Monitor ECG for arrhythmias.
— Monitor for dehydration if adverse GI reactions occur.

— Monitor blood glucose levels and observe for signs and symptoms of hypoglycemia.
— Monitor the patient for drug interactions.

Intervention

— Notify the doctor if the patient's blood pressure remains elevated despite phentolamine therapy.
— Keep emergency equipment nearby.
— Institute safety precautions if adverse CNS reactions occur.
— Notify the doctor if the patient experiences anginal pain and obtain orders for treatment.
— Obtain an order for an antiemetic or antidiarrheal agent as needed.
— Be prepared to treat hypoglycemia.
— Keep all members of the health care team informed of the patient's response to the drug.

Patient teaching

— Inform the patient and family about phentolamine, including the dosage, frequency, action, and adverse reactions.
— Inform the patient with an extravasation how phentolamine will be administered.
— Teach the patient about the phentolamine test for pheochromocytoma, if indicated.
— Tell the patient not to take sedatives or narcotics for at least 24 hours before a phentolamine test.
— Tell the patient to notify the nurse or doctor if adverse reactions develop or questions arise about phentolamine mesylate therapy.

Evaluation

In the patient receiving phentolamine, appropriate evaluation statements include:
• Patient's blood pressure is within normal limits.
• Patient maintains adequate cardiac output.
• Patient does not develop dehydration.
• Patient and family state an understanding of phentolamine therapy.

PROTOTYPE: GANGLIONIC BLOCKING AGENTS

TRIMETHAPHAN CAMSYLATE
(trye meth′a fan)
Arfonad
Classification: ganglionic blocking agent
Pregnancy risk category C

How supplied
INJECTION: 50 mg/ml in 10-ml ampules, 250 mg/vial‡

---

‡Available in Australia only

Indications and dosage
To lower blood pressure quickly in hypertensive emergencies; for controlled hypotension during surgery
ADULTS: 500 mg (10 ml) diluted in 500 ml dextrose 5% in water to yield concentration of 1 mg/ml I.V. Start I.V. drip at 1 to 2 mg/minute and titrate to achieve desired hypotensive response. Range is 0.3 to 6 mg/minute.

Contraindications and precautions
Trimethaphan is contraindicated in patients with anemia or respiratory insufficiency. Use cautiously in patients with arteriosclerosis; cardiac, hepatic, or renal disease; degenerative CNS disorders; Addison's disease; or diabetes. Also use cautiously in patients receiving glucocorticoids or other antihypertensives.

Adverse reactions
CNS: dilated pupils, *extreme weakness.*
CV: *severe orthostatic hypotension, tachycardia.*
GI: anorexia, *nausea, vomiting, dry mouth.*
GU: *urine retention.*
OTHER: respiratory depression.

Interactions
Anesthetics, antihypertensives, diuretics, procainamide: increased hypotensive effect. Monitor patient closely.
Tubocurarine, other neuromuscular blocking agents: additive muscle relaxant action. Monitor patient closely for adequate recovery of muscle strength before extubation.

Nursing considerations
Assessment
• Review the patient's history for a condition that contraindicates the use of trimethaphan and related compounds.
• Obtain a baseline assessment of the patient's blood pressure before therapy.
• Be alert for common adverse reactions.
• Evaluate the patient's and family's knowledge about trimethaphan.

Planning (Nursing Diagnoses)
Potential nursing diagnoses for the patient receiving trimethaphan include:
• Injury related to potential ineffectiveness of trimethaphan.
• Fluid volume deficit related to potential adverse GI reactions to trimethaphan.
• Activity intolerance related to potential trimethaphan-induced weakness.
• Knowledge deficit related to trimethaphan therapy.

Implementation
Preparation and administration
— Dose should be diluted in 5% dextrose in water. 500 mg (10 ml) yields a concentration of 1 mg/ml. Start I.V. drip at 1 to 2 mg/minute and titrate to achieve desired hypotensive response. Desired range is 0.3 to 6 mg/minute.

—Use continuous infusion pump to administer this drug slowly and precisely.

—The patient should be supine during drug administration. Elevate the head of the bed for maximal effect to avoid cerebral anoxia, but do not elevate it greater than 30 degrees.

—The patient should receive oxygen therapy during use of this drug.

—When used during surgery, this drug should be discontinued before wound closure to allow blood pressure to return to normal.

Monitoring

—Monitor the effectiveness of trimethaphan therapy by checking blood pressure continuously until it is stabilized at desired level, then every 5 minutes; monitor the patient for hypotension and tachycardia.

—Monitor the patient for adverse drug reactions.

—Monitor for respiratory distress, especially if large doses are used. Large doses have caused apnea and respiratory arrest.

—Monitor intake and output, because trimethaphan may reduce renal blood flow.

—Monitor the patient's hydration level if adverse GI reactions occur.

—Monitor muscle strength throughout drug therapy.

—Monitor infusion rate of the drug; normal rate is 0.3 to 6 mg/minute.

—Monitor the patient for urine retention throughout administration.

—Monitor the patient for drug interactions.

Intervention

—If extreme hypotension occurs, discontinue drug and notify doctor. Use phenylephrine or mephentermine to counteract hypotension.

—Be aware that anesthetics, diuretics, and procainamide may increase hypotensive effect.

—Assist the patient with all activities if weakness occurs, especially as drug may cause extreme weakness.

—Obtain an order for an antiemetic if nausea or vomiting occurs.

—Offer the patient frequent ice chips or sugarless candy to relieve dry mouth.

—Change the patient's position slowly because severe orthostatic hypotension is possible.

—Keep all members of the health care team informed of the patient's response to the drug.

Patient teaching

—Inform the patient and family about trimethaphan, including how it's administered, action, and adverse reactions.

—Tell the patient to notify the nurse or doctor if adverse reactions develop or questions arise about trimethaphan therapy.

Evaluation

In the patient receiving trimethaphan, appropriate evaluation statements include:

• Patient's blood pressure is within normal limits.

- Patient maintains adequate hydration throughout therapy.
- Patient is able to perform activities of daily living.
- Patient and family state an understanding of trimethaphan therapy.

PROTOTYPE: CENTRALLY ACTING SYMPATHOLYTICS

METHYLDOPA
(meth ill doe′pa)
Aldomet, Aldomet M‡, Apo-Methyldopa†, Dopamet†, Hydopa‡,
Novomedopa†

METHYLDOPATE HYDROCHLORIDE
(meth ill doe pate′)
Aldomet, Aldomet Ester Injection‡
Classification: centrally acting sympatholytic
Pregnancy risk category B

How supplied
methyldopa
TABLETS: 125 mg, 250 mg, 500 mg
ORAL SUSPENSION: 250 mg/5 ml
methyldopate hydrochloride
INJECTION: 250 mg/5 ml in 5-ml vials

Indications and dosage
For sustained mild to severe hypertension; should not be used for acute treatment of hypertensive emergencies
ADULTS: initially, 250 mg P.O. b.i.d. to t.i.d. in first 48 hours. Then increase as needed q 2 days. May give entire daily dosage in the evening or h.s. Dosage may need adjustment if other antihypertensives are added to or deleted from therapy. Maintenance dosage is 500 mg to 2 g daily in two to four divided doses. Maximum recommended daily dosage is 3 g. Alternatively, give 250 to 500 mg I.V. q 6 hours, diluted in dextrose 5% in water and administered over 30 to 60 minutes. Maximum dosage is 1 g q 6 hours. Switch to oral antihypertensives as soon as possible.
CHILDREN: initially, 10 mg/kg P.O. daily in two to three divided doses; or 20 to 40 mg/kg I.V. daily in four divided doses. Increase dose daily until desired response occurs. Maximum daily dose is 65 mg/kg, 2 g/m^2, or 3 g daily, whichever is least.

Contraindications and precautions
Methyldopa is contraindicated in patients with known hypersensitivity to the drug, in patients with active hepatic disease such as hepatitis or cirrhosis, and in those who developed hepatic dysfunction during previous therapy with methyldopa. Use cautiously in patients receiving other antihypertensives or MAO inhibitors and in patients with impaired hepatic function.

†Available in Canada only   ‡Available in Australia only

Methyldopa is frequently used to treat hypertension in pregnant women, apparently without ill effects to the fetus if the patient is closely monitored. Some clinicians recommend that therapy not begin between 16 and 20 weeks' gestation, if possible.

Adverse reactions

BLOOD: **hemolytic anemia, reversible granulocytopenia**, thrombocytopenia.

CNS: *sedation*, headache, asthenia, weakness, *dizziness, decreased mental acuity*, involuntary choreoathetotic movements, psychic disturbances, depression, nightmares.

CV: bradycardia, *orthostatic hypotension*, aggravated angina, myocarditis, edema, weight gain.

EENT: *dry mouth, nasal stuffiness.*

GI: diarrhea, pancreatitis.

HEPATIC: **hepatic necrosis.**

OTHER: gynecomastia, lactation, skin rash, drug-induced fever, impotence.

Interactions

Levodopa: additive hypotensive effects; possible increased adverse CNS reactions. Monitor carefully for toxicity.

MAO inhibitors, norepinephrine, phenothiazines, tricyclic antidepressants, amphetamines: possible hypertensive effects. Monitor carefully.

Tolbutamide: impaired tolbutamide metabolism and enhanced hypoglycemic effect. Monitor blood glucose levels.

Nursing considerations

Assessment
- Review the patient's history for a condition that contraindicates the use of methyldopa and related compounds.
- Obtain a baseline assessment of the patient's blood pressure before therapy.
- Be alert for common adverse reactions.
- Evaluate the patient's and family's knowledge about methyldopa therapy.

Planning (Nursing Diagnoses)
Potential nursing diagnoses for the patient receiving methyldopa include:
- Injury related to potential ineffectiveness of methyldopa to lower blood pressure.
- Altered body temperature related to potential drug fever induced by methyldopa.
- Altered oral mucous membrane related to dry mouth caused by methyldopa therapy.
- Decreased tissue perfusion (cerebral) related to methyldopa-induced hypotension.
- Knowledge deficit related to methyldopa therapy.

Implementation

Preparation and administration

— I.V. dose should be diluted in 5% dextrose in water and administered over 30 to 60 minutes.

— Administer once-daily dosages at bedtime to minimize CNS reactions.

Monitoring

— Monitor the effectiveness of therapy by checking blood pressure and pulse rate. When administering I.V., monitor blood pressure every 5 minutes during infusion.

— Monitor the patient's weight, intake and output, and evidence of edema because methyldopa may cause sodium and water retention.

— Monitor the patient's temperature for elevation.

— Monitor the patient for adverse drug reactions.

— Monitor CBC before and during therapy. Drug may cause hemolytic anemia.

— Monitor liver enzyme levels periodically, because methyldopa may cause hepatic necrosis.

— Monitor elderly patients carefully, because they are more likely to experience hypotension and sedation.

— Monitor for enhanced hypoglycemic effect in diabetic patients receiving tolbutamide.

— Check the patient's oral mucous membrane for dryness.

— Monitor the patient's mental status for adverse CNS reactions.

— Monitor the patient for drug interactions.

— Regularly reevaluate the patient's and family's knowledge about methyldopa therapy.

Intervention

— Hold dose and notify the doctor if the patient develops involuntary choreoathetoid (jerky) movements, hypotension, or bradycardia.

— After dialysis, monitor the patient for hypertension. Patient may need an extra dose of methyldopa.

— If the patient receives methyldopa for several months, positive reaction to direct Coombs' test indicates hemolytic anemia. If the patient requires a blood transfusion, make sure he gets direct and indirect Coombs' test to avoid cross-matching problems.

— Offer ice chips or sugarless chewing gum or hard candy if dry mouth occurs.

— Institute safety precautions if adverse CNS reactions occur.

— Restrict the patient's fluid and sodium intake to minimize fluid retention.

— Obtain an order for an antipyretic agent if drug-induced fever occurs.

— Keep all members of the health care team informed of the patient's response to the drug.

Patient teaching
— Inform the patient and family about methyldopa, including the dosage, frequency, action, and adverse reactions.
— Teach the patient about his disease.
— Explain the importance of taking drug as prescribed, even when feeling well.
— Instruct the patient not to stop taking this drug suddenly.
— Inform the patient that once-daily dosage given at bedtime will minimize daytime drowsiness.
— Instruct the patient to check with the doctor or pharmacist before taking OTC medications.
— Inform the patient that orthostatic hypotension can be minimized by rising slowly and avoiding sudden position changes. Instruct patient to sit down immediately if feeling dizzy.
— Tell the patient that dry mouth can be relieved with sugarless chewing gum, sour hard candy, or ice chips.
— Inform the patient that urine may turn dark in toilet bowls treated with bleach.
— Tell the patient to notify the nurse or doctor if adverse reactions develop or questions arise about methyldopa therapy.

Evaluation
In the patient receiving methyldopa, appropriate evaluation statements include:
• Patient's blood pressure is within normal limits.
• Patient's temperature remains normal throughout methyldopa therapy.
• Patient reports that measures to relieve dry mouth are effective.
• Patient does not experience light-headedness when changing position.
• Patient and family state an understanding of methyldopa therapy.

PROTOTYPE: VASODILATORS

HYDRALAZINE HYDROCHLORIDE
(hye dral' a zeen)
Alazine, Apresoline**, Novo-Hylazin†, Supres‡
Classification: vasodilator
Pregnancy risk category C

How supplied
TABLETS: 10 mg, 25 mg, 50 mg, 100 mg
INJECTION: 20 mg/ml in 1-ml ampules

Indications and dosage
Essential hypertension (alone or in combination with other antihypertensives); to reduce afterload in severe CHF (with nitrates)
ADULTS: initially, 10 mg P.O. q.i.d.; gradually increased to 50 mg q.i.d. Maximum recommended dosage is 200 mg daily, but some patients may

---
†Available in Canada only   **May contain tartrazine   ‡Available in Australia only

require 300 to 400 mg daily. Can be given b.i.d. for CHF.
CHILDREN: initially, 0.75 mg/kg P.O. daily in four divided doses (25 mg/m^2 daily). May increase gradually to 10 times this dosage, if necessary.

Severe essential hypertension (to lower blood pressure quickly)
ADULTS: 10 to 20 mg I.V. given slowly and repeated as necessary, generally q 4 to 6 hours; switch to oral antihypertensives as soon as possible. Or 20 to 40 mg I.M. repeated as necessary, generally q 4 to 6 hours; switch to oral antihypertensives as soon as possible.
CHILDREN: give slowly 1.7 to 3.5 mg/kg or 50 to 100 mg/m^2 I.V. daily in four to six divided doses. Or 1.7 to 3.5 mg/kg or 50 to 100 mg/m^2 I.M. daily in four to six divided doses. Switch to oral antihypertensives as soon as possible.

Contraindications and precautions
Hydralazine is contraindicated in patients with coronary artery disease or mitral valve disease following rheumatic fever and in patients with known hypersensitivity to the drug. Use cautiously in patients with cardiac disease, CVA, or severe renal impairment and in those taking other antihypertensives.

Adverse reactions
BLOOD: **neutropenia,** leukopenia.
CNS: peripheral neuritis, headache, dizziness.
CV: *orthostatic hypotension, tachycardia,* **arrhythmias**, angina, palpitations, sodium retention.
GI: nausea, vomiting, diarrhea, anorexia.
SKIN: rash.
OTHER: SLE-like syndrome (especially with high doses), weight gain.

Interactions
Diazoxide and other antihypertensive agents: may cause severe hypotension. Use together cautiously.

Nursing considerations
Assessment
- Review the patient's history for a condition that contraindicates the use of hydralazine and related compounds.
- Obtain a baseline assessment of the patient's blood pressure before therapy.
- Be alert for common adverse reactions.
- Evaluate the patient's and family's knowledge about hydralazine therapy.

Planning (Nursing Diagnoses)
Potential nursing diagnoses for the patient receiving hydralazine include:
- Injury related to potential ineffectiveness of hydralazine to control blood pressure.
- Fluid volume excess related to sodium retention associated with hydralazine.
- Knowledge deficit related to hydralazine therapy.

Implementation

Preparation and administration

— Give this drug with meals to increase absorption.
— Compliance may be improved by administering this drug b.i.d. Check with doctor.
— Inject I.V. drug as soon as possible after draining through needle into syringe; drug changes color after contact with metal.
— Remember that patients with renal impairment may respond to lower maintenance doses of hydralazine.
— When administering I.V., monitor blood pressure every 5 minutes until stable, then every 15 minutes; put patient in Trendelenburg's position if he is faint or dizzy. Too-rapid reduction in blood pressure can cause mental changes from cerebral ischemia.

Monitoring

— Monitor the effectiveness of hydralazine therapy by regularly monitoring the patient's blood pressure, pulse rate, and body weight.
— Monitor the patient closely for signs of SLE-like syndrome (sore throat, fever, muscle and joint aches, skin rash). Incidence is greatest in patients receiving more than 200 mg daily for prolonged periods.
— Monitor the patient for fluid retention (weight gain, distended neck veins, swollen ankles).
— Monitor the patient for adverse drug reactions.
— Monitor CBC, LE cell preparation, and antinuclear antibody titer determinations before therapy and periodically during long-term therapy.
— Monitor for postural hypotension.
— Monitor for hypersensitivity reaction; some preparations contain tartrazine, which may precipitate allergic reactions, especially in aspirin-sensitive patients.
— Monitor the patient's hydration status if adverse GI reactions occur.
— Monitor ECG for arrhythmias.
— Monitor the patient for drug interactions.
— Regularly reevaluate the patient's and family's knowledge about hydralazine therapy.

Intervention

— Alert doctor if blood pressure remains elevated.
— Remember that some clinicians combine hydralazine therapy with diuretics and beta-adrenergic blockers to decrease sodium retention and tachycardia and to prevent anginal attacks.
— Assist the patient with position changes to minimize orthostatic hypotension.
— Institute safety precautions if adverse CNS reactions occur.
— Obtain an order for an antiemetic or antidiarrheal agent as needed.
— Maintain sodium and fluid restriction diet to minimize sodium and fluid retention.

—Keep all members of the health care team informed of the patient's response to the drug.

Patient teaching

—Inform the patient and family about hydralazine, including the dosage, frequency, action, and adverse reactions.

—Teach the patient about his disease and therapy, and explain why he must take drug exactly as prescribed, even when feeling well; advise him never to discontinue drug suddenly because severe rebound hypertension may occur.

—Advise the patient to notify doctor of any unusual effects, especially symptoms of SLE (sore throat, fever, muscle and joint pain, and skin rash).

—Explain how to minimize impact of adverse reactions: to avoid performing hazardous tasks until tolerance develops to sedation, drowsiness, and other CNS reactions; to avoid sudden position changes, to minimize orthostatic hypotension; and to take drug with meals to enhance absorption and minimize gastric irritation.

—Reassure the patient that headaches and palpitations occurring 2 to 4 hours after initial dose usually subside spontaneously; if they do not, he should notify the doctor.

—Instruct the patient to weigh himself at least weekly, and advise him to notify the doctor if weight gain exceeds 5 lb (2.25 kg) per week.

—Warn the patient to check with doctor or pharmacist before taking OTC cold preparations and to avoid alcohol.

—Tell the patient to notify the nurse or doctor if adverse reactions develop or questions arise about hydralazine therapy.

Evaluation

In the patient receiving hydralazine, appropriate evaluation statements include:

• Patient's blood pressure is within normal limits during hydralazine therapy.

• Patient's water retention is kept to a minimum with fluid and sodium restriction while taking hydralazine.

• Patient and family state an understanding of hydralazine therapy.

SELECTED MAJOR DRUGS: ANTIHYPERTENSIVES

DRUG, INDICATIONS, AND DOSAGES	SPECIAL PRECAUTIONS

ACE inhibitors

enalapril (Vasotec)
enalaprilat (Vasotec I.V.)
Hypertension—
Adults: initially, 5 mg P.O. daily, then adjust according to response. Usual dosage range is 10 to 40 mg daily as a single dose or two divided doses. Alternatively give 1.25 mg by I.V. infusion over 5 minutes q 6 hours
To convert from I.V. therapy to oral therapy—
Adults: initially, 5 mg P.O. daily. Adjust dosage to response.
To convert from oral therapy to I.V. therapy—
Adults: 1.25 mg I.V. over 5 minutes q 6 hours. Higher doses have not demonstrated greater efficacy.

• Contraindicated in patients with known hypersensitivity to the drug.
• Use cautiously in patients with preexisting renal impairment, collagen disease, vascular disease, or immune disease.

---

lisinopril (Prinivil, Zestril)
Mild to severe hypertension—
Adults: initially, 10 mg P.O. daily. Most patients are well controlled on 20 to 40 mg daily as a single dose.

• Contraindicated in patients with known hypersensitivity to the drug and in patients with a history of angioedema related to previous treatment with an ACE inhibitor.
• Use cautiously in patients with impaired renal function or CHF, in hypertensive patients with unilateral or bilateral renal artery stenosis, or in pregnant or breast-feeding women.

---

ramipril (Altace)
Essential hypertension—
Adults: initially, 2.5 mg P.O. daily. Increase dosage p.r.n. based on patient tolerance and response. Maintenance dose is 2.5 to 20 mg daily as a single dose or in divided doses.

• Contraindicated in patients with known hypersensitivity to the drug and with a history of angioneurotic edema.
• Use cautiously in patients with renal insufficiency or diabetes mellitus, in patients receiving potassium supplements or potassium-sparing diuretics, and in those using potassium-containing sodium substitutes because such patients are at a higher risk for developing hyperkalemia.

Beta-adrenergic blockers

acebutolol (Monitan†, Sectral)
Hypertension—
Adults: 400 mg P.O. either as a single daily dose or divided b.i.d. Patients may receive as much as 1,200 mg daily.

• Contraindicated in patients with persistently severe bradycardia, second- and third-degree heart block, overt cardiac failure, or cardiogenic shock.

†Available in Canada only

SELECTED MAJOR DRUGS: ANTIHYPERTENSIVES *continued*

DRUG, INDICATIONS, AND DOSAGES	SPECIAL PRECAUTIONS

Beta-adrenergic blockers *(continued)*

acebutolol *(continued)*
Ventricular arrhythmias —
Adults: 400 mg P.O. daily divided b.i.d. Dosage is then increased to provide an adequate clinical response. Usual dosage is 600 to 1,200 mg daily.

• Use cautiously in patients with cardiac failure.

carteolol (Cartrol)
Hypertension —
Adults: initially, 2.5 mg P.O. as a single daily dose. Gradually increase dosage as required to 5 to 10 mg daily as a single dose.

• Contraindicated in patients with bronchial asthma, severe bradycardia, second- or third-degree heart block, cardiogenic shock, or uncontrolled CHF.
• Use cautiously in patients with CHF controlled by digitalis and diuretics because beta-adrenergic blockers do not block the inotropic effects of digitalis.

labetalol (Normodyne, Presolol‡, Trandate)
Hypertension —
Adults: 100 mg P.O. b.i.d. with or without a diuretic. Dose may be increased to 200 mg b.i.d. after 2 days. Further dosage increases may be made q 1 to 3 days until optimal response is reached. Usual maintenance dosage is 200 to 400 mg b.i.d.
For severe hypertension and hypertensive emergencies —
Adults: dilute 200 mg with 200 ml dextrose 5% In water (D_5W). Infuse at 2 mg/minute until satisfactory response is obtained. Then stop the infusion. May repeat q 6 to 8 hours. Alternatively, give 20 mg by slow I.V. injection over 2 minutes; repeat injections of 40 to 80 mg q 10 minutes p.r.n. until maximum dose of 300 mg is reached.

• Contraindicated in patients with bronchial asthma.
• Use cautiously in patients with CHF, hepatic failure, chronic bronchitis, emphysema, preexisting peripheral vascular disease, and pheochromocytoma.

metoprolol (Apo-Metoprolol†, Lopressor)
Hypertension; may be used alone or in combination with other antihypertensives —
Adults: initially, 50 mg P.O. b.i.d. or 100 mg P.O. daily. Maximum dosage is 200 to 400 mg daily in two to three divided doses. Not recommended for children.
Early intervention in acute MI —
Adults: three 5-mg I.V. bolus injections q 2 minutes. 15 minutes after last dose, start 50 mg P.O. q 6 hours for 48 hours.

• Contraindicated in patients with hypertension and angina and in MI.
• Use cautiously in patients with heart failure, diabetes, respiratory or hepatic disease, or in patients taking other antihypertensives. Always check patient's apical pulse rate before giving this drug. If slower than 60 beats/minute, hold drug and call doctor immediately.

nadolol (Corgard)
Hypertension —
Adults: initally, 40 mg P.O. daily. Dosage may be increased in 40- to 80-mg increments until optimal re-

• Contraindicated in patients with bronchial asthma, sinus bradycardia and second- or third-degree conduction block,

(continued)

†Available in Canada only   ‡Available in Australia only

SELECTED MAJOR DRUGS: ANTIHYPERTENSIVES *continued*

DRUG, INDICATIONS, AND DOSAGES	SPECIAL PRECAUTIONS
Beta-adrenergic blockers *(continued)*	

nadolol *(continued)*
sponse occurs. Usual maintenance dosage range is 40 to 320 mg daily. Doses of 640 mg may be necessary in rare cases.

• cardiogenic shock, or overt cardiac failure.
• Use cautiously in patients with impaired renal function and in pregnant and breast-feeding women.

---

penbutolol (Levatol)
Mild to moderate hypertension—
Adults: 20 mg P.O. daily. Usually given with other antihypertensives, such as thiazide diuretics.

• Contraindicated in patients allergic to penbutolol or other beta blockers. Also contraindicated in sinus bradycardia, cardiogenic shock, CHF, overt cardiac failure, and patients with second- or third-degree heart block. Beta-adrenergic blockers should be avoided in patients with pheochromocytoma unless alpha-adrenergic blockers are also used. They should also be avoided in patients with chronic airway disease, such as chronic bronchitis or emphysema.
• Use cautiously in patients with a history of CHF controlled by digitalis glycosides and diuretics.

---

pindolol (Barbloc‡, Visken)
Hypertension—
Adults: initially, 5 mg P.O. b.i.d. Dosage may be increased by 10 mg daily q 2 to 3 weeks up to a maximum of 60 mg daily.

• Contraindicated in patients with diabetes mellitus, asthma, and allergic rhinitis; during ethyl ether anesthesia; in sinus bradycardia and second- or third-degree heart block; in cardiogenic shock; and in right ventricular failure secondary to pulmonary hypertension.
• Use cautiously in patients with CHF or respiratory disease and in those taking other antihypertensives.

---

propranolol (Apo-Propranolol†, Deralin‡, Inderal)
Hypertension—
Adults: initially, 80 mg P.O. daily in two to four divided doses or the sustained-release form once daily. Increase at 3- to 7-day intervals to maximum daily dosage of 640 mg. Usual maintenance dose is 160 to 480 mg daily.

• Contraindicated in patients with cardiogenic shock, sinus bradycardia and second- or third-degree heart block, bronchial asthma, or CHF unless the failure is secondary to a tachyarrhythmia treatable with the drug.

---

†Available in Canada only   ‡Available in Australia only

SELECTED MAJOR DRUGS: ANTIHYPERTENSIVES *continued*

DRUG, INDICATIONS, AND DOSAGES	SPECIAL PRECAUTIONS
Beta-adrenergic blockers *(continued)*	
propranolol *(continued)*	• Use cautiously because of risk of carcinogenesis and in patients with impaired hepatic or renal function, in breast-feeding women, and in children. Use cautiously in patients receiving a beta blocker who are administered a calcium channel blocker, especially I.V. verapamil, because both agents may depress myocardial contractility or AV conduction.
timolol (Apo-Timol†, Blocadren) *Hypertension —* **Adults:** initially 10 mg P.O. b.i.d. Usual daily maintenance dosage is 20 to 40 mg. Maximum daily dosage is 60 mg. Drug is used either alone or in combination with diuretics. *MI (long-term prophylaxis in patients who have survived acute phase) —* **Adults:** 10 mg P.O. b.i.d.	• Contraindicated in patients with diabetes mellitus, asthma, allergic rhinitis; during ethyl ether anesthesia; and in sinus bradycardia and second- or third-degree heart block, cardiogenic shock, and right ventricular failure secondary to pulmonary hypertension. • Use cautiously in patients with CHF; hepatic, renal, or respiratory disease; and in those taking other antihypertensives.
Alpha-adrenergic blockers	
prazosin (Minipress) *For mild to moderate hypertension; used alone or in combination with a diuretic or other antihypertensive; also used to decrease afterload in severe chronic CHF —* **Adults:** oral test dose is 1 mg given at bedtime to prevent "first-dose" syncope. Initial dose is 1 mg P.O. t.i.d. Increase dosage slowly. Maximum daily dosage is 20 mg. Maintenance dosage is 3 to 20 mg daily in three divided doses. A few patients have required dosages larger than this (up to 40 mg daily). If other antihypertensives or diuretics are added to this regimen, decrease prazosin dosage to 1 to 2 mg t.i.d. and retitrate.	• Contraindicated in patients with known hypersensitivity to the drug. • Use cautiously in patients receiving other antihypertensives.
terazosin (Hytrin) *Hypertension —* **Adults:** initial dose is 1 mg P.O. h.s., gradually increased according to patient response. Usual dosage range is 1 to 5 mg daily. Maximum recommended dosage is 20 mg daily.	• Contraindicated in patients with known hypersensitivity to the drug. • Use cautiously in patients with orthostatic hypotension and in pregnant and breast-feeding women. *(continued)*

†Available in Canada only

SELECTED MAJOR DRUGS: ANTIHYPERTENSIVES *continued*

DRUG, INDICATIONS, AND DOSAGES	SPECIAL PRECAUTIONS

Ganglionic blocking agent

mecamylamine (Inversine)
Moderate to severe essential hypertension and uncompli-cated malignant hypertension—
Adults: initially, 2.5 mg P.O. b.i.d. Increase by 2.5 mg daily q 2 days. Average daily dose is 25 mg given in three divided doses. No dosing recommendations for children.

• Contraindicated in recent MI, uremia, or chronic pyelonephri-tis.
• Use cautiously in patients with lower urinary tract pathol-ogy, renal insufficiency, glau-coma, pyloric stenosis, coronary insufficiency, or in patients tak-ing other antihypertensives. Me-camylamine is usually reserved for moderate to severe hyper-tension that is refractory to other drugs.

Centrally acting sympatholytics

clonidine (Catapres, Dixarit†‡)
Essential, renal, and malignant hypertension—
Adults: initially, 0.1 mg P.O. b.i.d. Then increase by 0.1 to 0.2 mg daily on a weekly basis. Usual dosage range is 0.2 to 0.8 mg daily in divided doses; infrequently, dosages as high as 2.4 mg daily are given. No dosing recommendations for children.
Or apply transdermal patch to a hairless area of in-tact skin on the upper arm or torso q 7 days.
Prophylactic treatment of migraine; treatment of meno-pausal flushing—
Adults: 0.025 mg P.O. b.i.d. If there has been no remis-sion after 2 weeks, increase dosage to 0.05 mg b.i.d.
To suppress abstinence symptoms during narcotics withdrawal—
Adults: 0.1 mg P.O. t.i.d.

• There are no known contrain-dications.
• Use cautiously in patients with severe coronary insuffi-ciency, diabetes, MI, cerebrovas-cular disease, chronic renal failure or history of depression, and in those taking other anti-hypertensives.

guanabenz (Wytensin)
Hypertension—
Adults: initially, 4 mg P.O. b.i.d. Dosage may be in-creased in increments of 4 to 8 mg daily q 1 to 2 weeks. Maximum dosage is 32 mg b.i.d. To ensure ade-quate overnight blood pressure control, give last dose h.s.

• Contraindicated in patients with known hypersensitivity to the drug.
• Use cautiously in patients with vascular insufficiency, cor-onary insufficiency, recent MI, cerebrovascular disease, or se-vere hepatic or renal failure.

guanfacine (Tenex)
Mild to moderate hypertension—
Adults: initially, 0.5 to 1 mg P.O. daily h.s. Average dose is 1 to 3 mg daily.

• Contraindicated in patients with known hypersensitivity to the drug.
• Use cautiously in patients with severe coronary insuffi-ciency, recent MI, cerebrovascu-lar disease, or chronic renal or hepatic insufficiency.

SELECTED MAJOR DRUGS: ANTIHYPERTENSIVES *continued*

DRUG, INDICATIONS, AND DOSAGES	SPECIAL PRECAUTIONS

Vasodilators

diazoxide (Hyperstat)
Hypertensive crisis —
Adults and children: 1 to 3 mg/kg I.V. (up to a maximum of 150 mg) q 5 to 15 minutes until adequate response is seen. Repeat at intervals q 4 to 24 hours p.r.n., generally q 4 to 6 hours. Switch to oral antihypertensives as soon as possible. Alternatively, give 20 to 40 mg I.M., repeated as necessary, generally q 4 to 6 hours. Switch to oral antihypertensives as soon as possible.
Children: initially, 0.75 (25 mg/m^2) P.O. daily in four divided doses, increased gradually to 10 times this dosage, if necessary; or 1.7 to 3.5 mg/kg or 50 to 100 mg/m^2 given I.M. or slow I.V. daily in four to six divided doses.

• Contraindicated in treatment of compensatory hypertension, such as that associated with aortic coarctation or AV shunt, and in patients with known hypersensitivity to diazoxide, other thiazides, or other sulfonamide-derived drugs.
• Use cautiously in patients with impaired cerebral or cardiac function, diabetes or uremia and in those taking other antihypertensives.

minoxidil (Loniten, Minodyl)
Severe hypertension —
Adults: initially, 5 mg P.O. as a single dose. Effective dosage range is usually 10 to 40 mg daily. Maximum dosage is 100 mg daily.
Children under age 12: 0.2 mg/kg P.O. as a single daily dose. Effective dosage range usually is 0.25 to 1 mg/kg daily. Maximum dosage is 50 mg.

• Contraindicated in patients with pheochromocytoma.
• Use cautiously after MI, in patients with known hypersensitivity to the drug, in patients with renal failure or dialysis, in those receiving interacting drugs, and in those at risk for carcinogenesis, mutagenesis, and impairment of fertility and during pregnancy or breast-feeding.

nitroprusside (Nipride, Nitropress)
To lower blood pressure quickly in hypertensive emergencies; to control hypotension during anesthesia; to reduce preload and afterload in cardiac pump failure or cardiogenic shock; may be used with or without dopamine —
Adults: 50-mg vial diluted with 2 to 3 ml of D$_5$W I.V. and then added to 250, 500, or 1,000 ml D$_5$W. Infuse at 0.5 to 10 mcg/kg/minute. Average dose is 3 mcg/kg/minute. Maximum infusion rate is 10 mcg/kg/minute.
  Patients taking other antihypertensives along with nitroprusside are very sensitive to this drug. Adjust dosage accordingly.

• Use cautiously in patients with hypothyroidism or hepatic or renal disease or in patients receiving other antihypertensives. Keep patient supine when initiating or titrating nitroprusside therapy.

COMPARING ANTIHYPERTENSIVE COMBINATIONS

TRADE NAME AND CONTENT	SPECIAL CONSIDERATIONS
ACE inhibitors and diuretics	

Capozide 25/15
captopril 25 mg and hydrochlorothiazide 15 mg
Capozide 25/25
captopril 25 mg and hydrochlorothiazide 25 mg
Capozide 50/15
captopril 50 mg and hydrochlorothiazide 15 mg
Capozide 50/25
captopril 50 mg and hydrochlorothiazide 25 mg
Vaseretic
enalapril 10 mg and hydrochlorothiazide 25 mg
Prinizide
lisinopril 20 mg and hydrochlorothiazide 12.5 mg;
lisinopril 20 mg and hydrochlorothiazide 25 mg
Zestoretic
lisinopril 20 mg and hydrochlorothiazide 12.5 mg;
lisinopril 20 mg and hydrochlorothiazide 25 mg

• Combine the antihypertensive effectiveness of an ACE inhibitor (captopril, enalapril, or lisinopril) with the antihypertensive and diuretic actions of hydrochlorthiazide, a thiazide diuretic.
• Not intended for initial use in hypertensive patients. Dosage of the individual components should be titrated to maximal hypotensive effect before use of the fixed combination.

Beta-adrenergic blockers and diuretics

Lopressor HCT 50/25
metoprolol tartrate 50 mg and hydrochlorothiazide 25 mg
Lopressor HCT 100/25
metoprolol tartrate 100 mg and hydrochlorothiazide 25 mg
Corzide
nadolol 40 mg and bendroflumethiazide 15 mg
nadolol 80 mg and bendroflumethiazide 15 mg
Inderide 40/25
propranolol hydrochloride 40 mg and hydrochlorothiazide 25 mg
Inderide 80/25
propranolol hydrochloride 80 mg and hydrochlorothiazide 25 mg
Inderide LA 80/50
propranolol hydrochloride 80 mg and hydrochlorothiazide 50 mg
Normozide 100/25
labetalol hydrochloride 100 mg and hydrochlorothiazide 25 mg
Normozide 200/25
labetalol hydrochloride 200 mg and hydrochlorothiazide 25 mg
Normozide 300/25
labetalol hydrochloride 300 mg and hydrochlorothiazide 25 mg

• Combine the antihypertensive effectiveness of a beta-adrenergic blocker (labetalol, metoprolol, nadolol, or propranolol) with the antihypertensive and diuretic actions of a thiazide diuretic (bendroflumethiazide or hydrochlorothiazide).
• Not intended for initial use in hypertensive patients. Dosage of the individual components should be titrated to maximal hypotensive effect before use of the fixed combination.

COMPARING ANTIHYPERTENSIVE COMBINATIONS *continued*

TRADE NAME AND CONTENT	SPECIAL CONSIDERATIONS
Alpha-adrenergic blockers and diuretics	

Minizide 1 prazosin hydrochloride 1 mg and polythiazide 0.5 mg **Minizide 2** prazosin hydrochloride 2 mg and polythiazide 0.5 mg **Minizide 5** prazosin hydrochloride 5 mg and polythiazide 0.5 mg	• Combine the antihypertensive effectiveness of an alpha-adrenergic blocker (prazosin) with the antihypertensive and diuretic actions of a thiazide diuretic (polythiazide). • Not intended for initial use in hypertensive patients. Dosage of the individual components should be titrated to maximal hypotensive effect before use of the fixed combination.

Centrally acting sympatholytics and diuretics	

Combipres 0.1 clonidine hydrochloride 0.1 mg and chlorthalidone 15 mg **Combipres 0.2** clonidine hydrochloride 0.2 mg and chlorthalidone 15 mg **Aldochlor 150** methyldopa 250 mg and chlorothiazide 150 mg **Aldochlor 250** methyldopa 250 mg and chlorothiazide 250 mg **Aldoril 15** methyldopa 250 mg and hydrochlorothiazide 15 mg **Aldoril 25** methyldopa 250 mg and hydrochlorothiazide 25 mg	• Combine the antihypertensive effectiveness of a centrally acting sympatholytic (clonidine or methyldopa) with the antihypertensive and diuretic actions of a thiazide diuretic (hydrochlorothiazide) or a thiazide-like diuretic (chlorthalidone). • Not intended for initial use in hypertensive patients. Dosage of the individual components should be titrated to maximal hypotensive effect before use of the fixed combination.

Vasodilators and diuretics	

Apresazide 25/25 hydralazine hydrochloride 25 mg and hydrochlorothiazide 25 mg **Apresazide 50/50** hydralazine hydrochloride 50 mg and hydrochlorothiazide 50 mg **Apresazide 100/50** hydralazine hydrochloride 100 mg and hydrochlorothiazide 50 mg	• Combine the antihypertensive effectiveness of a vasodilator (hydralazine) with the antihypertensive and diuretic actions of a thiazide diuretic (hydrochlorothiazide). • Not intended for initial use in hypertensive patients. Dosage of the individual components should be titrated to maximal hypotensive effect before use of the fixed combination.

(continued)

COMPARING ANTIHYPERTENSIVE COMBINATIONS *continued*

TRADE NAME AND CONTENT	SPECIAL CONSIDERATIONS
Vasodilator, centrally acting adrenergic blocker, and diuretic	
Cam-Ap-Es, Cherapas, H-H-R, Ser-A-Gen, Seralazide, Ser-Ap-Es, Serpazide, Tri-Hydroserpine, Unipres hydralazine hydrochloride 25 mg, reserpine 0.1 mg, and hydrochlorothiazide 15 mg	• Combine the antihypertensive effectiveness of a vasodilator (hydralazine) and the antihypertensive effects of a centrally acting adrenergic blocker (reserpine) with the antihypertensive and diuretic actions of a thiazide diuretic (hydrochlorothiazide). • Not intended for initial use in hypertensive patients. Dosage of the individual components should be titrated to maximal hypotensive effect before use of the fixed combination.

SELF-TEST

1. Renata Porter, age 55, was admitted to the medical/surgical unit with uncontrolled hypertension (188/96 mm Hg) and acute CHF. She has a history of volatile blood pressure and has been treated with thiazides and prazosin without benefit. She has smoked one pack of cigarettes per day for 30 years. Currently Mrs. Porter is receiving atenolol 50 mg P.O. daily. Antihypertensives are used to lower blood pressure in a patient with:
   a. diastolic blood pressure that averages 90 to 95 mm Hg or more.
   b. diastolic blood pressure greater than 100 mm Hg.
   c. diastolic blood pressure that averages 85 to 90 mm Hg.
   d. diastolic blood pressure less than 85 mm Hg.

2. Atenolol is what type of antihypertensive drug?
   a. vasodilator
   b. beta-adrenergic blocker
   c. alpha blocker
   d. ACE inhibitor

3. What is the mechanism of action of atenolol?
   a. blocks beta stimulation, resulting in lessening work load on the heart
   b. vasodilates the arterial tree, lessening work load and blood pressure
   c. inhibits ACE, resulting in vasodilation
   d. decreases sympathetic outflow from the central vasomotor center

4. The doctor decided to change Mrs. Porter's antihypertensive agent to methyldopa 250 mg P.O. t.i.d. When can the nurse expect a dosage change if this dose of methyldopa does not reduce blood pressure?
  a. after 12 hours
  b. after 24 hours
  c. after 36 hours
  d. after 48 hours

5. If Mrs. Porter develops orthostatic hypotension, the nurse should:
  a. start I.V. fluids.
  b. start vasopressor agents.
  c. start oxygen therapy.
  d. assist with position changes.

6. Benjamin Taylor, age 82, has sinus bradycardia. After three follow-up visits to check his heart rate, he is diagnosed with mild hypertension. His doctor prescribed prazosin 1 mg t.i.d. When should the nurse administer the first dose to Mr. Taylor?
  a. in the morning when he awakens
  b. before a meal
  c. after a meal
  d. at bedtime

7. Mr. Taylor states that his sister who also has hypertension takes minoxidil. He asks why the doctor did not prescribe the same drug for him. The nurse should respond by explaining that:
  a. minoxidil is contraindicated in patients with sinus bradycardia.
  b. minoxidil is not used to treat mild hypertension.
  c. prazosin is more effective in controlling hypertension in the elderly.
  d. prazosin is not as effective in females because of a difference in metabolism.

8. Richard Bell is in the hospital for I.V. chemotherapy for lung cancer. During chemotherapy, the I.V. infiltrates and extravasation occurs. Which of the following antihypertensives will most likely be used to treat the extravasation?
  a. phentolamine mesylate
  b. reserpine
  c. methyldopa
  d. trimethaphan camsylate

9. Irma Peterson's blood pressure is elevated on a routine visit to her doctor. She has been taking captopril 25 mg P.O. t.i.d. for 6 months with good results. Before increasing her dosage, the doctor questions Mrs. Peterson about changes in her daily life and use of OTC medications that may be interfering with captopril's effect. Which OTC preparation should Mrs. Peterson take at a different time from her captopril to avoid such an interaction?

   a. multivitamin
   b. aspirin
   c. acetaminophen
   d. antacid

10. Glenn Sellers developed hypertensive crisis after eating some cheese while taking an MAO inhibitor for depression. He was brought to the emergency department and treated with trimethaphan. How should the nurse prepare this drug for administration?

   a. Dilute 500 mg of the drug in 500 ml dextrose 5% in water.
   b. Dilute 250 mg of the drug in 100 ml of 0.9% sodium chloride solution.
   c. Dilute 100 mg of the drug in 1,000 ml of dextrose 5% in water.
   d. Dilute 50 mg of the drug in 10 ml of 0.9% sodium chloride solution.

Check your answers on pages 1061 and 1062.

CHAPTER 23

VASODILATORS

cyclandelate ◆ dipyridamole ◆ ethaverine hydrochloride
isoxsuprine hydrochloride ◆ nylidrin hydrochloride
papaverine hydrochloride ◆ tolazoline hydrochloride

OVERVIEW

• Vasodilators have limited clinical value in patients with obstructive vascular disease, although they may be useful in patients with minimal organic involvement. Studies in healthy persons indicate that the peripheral vasodilators increase blood flow to vascular areas. Although we lack evidence of their vasodilating effect in diseased vascular areas, these drugs are still widely used. For additional information on vasodilators that are used to treat hypertension, see Chapter 22, Antihypertensives.

MAJOR USES

• Peripheral vasodilators are used to treat symptoms of peripheral vascular disease and vasospastic conditions as well as cerebrovascular disease.
• Dipyridamole (in combination with aspirin or warfarin) inhibits platelet aggregation to reduce risk of thrombus formation.
• Tolazoline is used to treat persistent pulmonary hypertension of the newborn (or persistent fetal circulation) when usual methods, such as mechanical ventilation or supplemental oxygen, are inadequate.

MECHANISM OF ACTION

• Some peripheral vasodilators directly relax smooth muscle. This effect may be due to the inhibition of phosphodiesterase, resulting in increased concentrations of cyclic adenosine monophosphate, which causes vasodilation.
• Other peripheral vasodilators have a different mechanism of action. Tolazoline is a direct vasodilator but also blocks alpha receptors; nylidrin also stimulates beta receptors. Although isoxsuprine originally was thought only to stimulate beta receptors, newer evidence indicates that it may also be a direct-acting peripheral vasodilator.
• Dipyridamole, originally classified as a coronary vasodilator, has no value in treating acute attacks of angina. In fact, evidence is lacking that its long-term use is beneficial in preventing chronic angina. It does, however, inhibit platelet adhesion and may be used in patients with prosthetic heart valves.

GLOSSARY

Vasoconstrictor: of or pertaining to a process, condition, or substance that causes the constriction of blood vessels.
Vasodilator: a nerve or agent that causes dilatation of blood vessels.
Vasomotor: of or pertaining to the nerves and muscles that control the caliber of the lumen of the blood vessels.

ABSORPTION, DISTRIBUTION, METABOLISM, AND EXCRETION

Vasodilators are well absorbed, widely distributed in body tissues, metabolized in the liver, and excreted mainly in the urine.

ONSET AND DURATION

Onset and duration of vasodilators depend on the drug used, form selected, and route of administration. Most of these drugs exhibit peak plasma levels within 1 to 4 hours of oral administration, and their effects last 3 to 6 hours. Nylidrin has the most rapid onset (about 10 minutes) and a short duration of action (about 2 hours).

ADVERSE REACTIONS

The most common adverse reactions to the vasodilators reflect the drugs' pharmacologic actions. Flushing, headache, hypotension, and tachycardia may be seen; orthostatic hypotension may be more common during the first few days of treatment.

GI disturbances, including vomiting, heartburn, and anorexia, may also occur. When tolazoline is used in neonates, many clinicians administer prophylactic antacids to prevent peptic ulcers.

Most patients tolerate these drugs well. If adverse reactions are troublesome, reduced dosage may be helpful.

PROTOTYPE: VASODILATORS

PAPAVERINE HYDROCHLORIDE

(pa pav' er een)

Cerespan, Genabid, Pavabid, Pavabid HP Capsulets, Pavabid Plateau Caps, Pavarine Spancaps, Pavasule, Pavatine, Pavatym, Paverolan Lanacaps

Classification: vasodilator
Pregnancy risk category C

How supplied

TABLETS: 30 mg, 60 mg, 100 mg, 150 mg, 200 mg, 300 mg
TABLETS (SUSTAINED-RELEASE): 200 mg

CAPSULES (SUSTAINED-RELEASE): 150 mg
INJECTION: 30 mg/ml in 2-ml and 10-ml ampules

Indications and dosage
Relief of cerebral and peripheral ischemia associated with arterial spasm and myocardial ischemia; treatment of smooth muscle spasm (coronary occlusion, angina pectoris, sequelae of peripheral and pulmonary embolism, certain cerebral angiospastic states) and visceral spasms (biliary, ureteral, or GI colic)
ADULTS: 60 to 300 mg P.O. one to five times daily, or 150- to 300-mg sustained-release preparation q 8 to 12 hours; 30 to 120 mg I.M. or I.V. q 3 hours, as indicated.

Contraindications and precautions
Papaverine is contraindicated for I.V. use in patients with Parkinson's disease or complete AV block. Use cautiously in patients with glaucoma.

Adverse reactions
CNS: *headache.*
CV: *increased heart rate*, increased blood pressure (with parenteral use), depressed AV and intraventricular conduction, hypotension, **arrhythmias.**
GI: *constipation,* nausea.
OTHER: sweating, flushing, malaise, increased depth of respiration, hepatic hypersensitivity reactions (with long-term use).

Interactions
Levodopa: papaverine may interfere with the therapeutic effects of levodopa in patients with Parkinson's disease. Monitor patient carefully.

Nursing considerations
Assessment
• Review the patient's history for a condition that contraindicates the use of papaverine.
• Obtain a baseline assessment of the patient's vascular status before therapy.
• Be alert for common adverse reactions.
• Evaluate the patient's and family's knowledge about papaverine therapy.

Planning (Nursing Diagnoses)
Potential nursing diagnoses for the patient receiving papaverine include:
• Decreased tissue perfusion (cerebral, peripheral areas) related to ineffectiveness of papaverine.
• Pain related to papaverine-induced headache.
• Potential for injury related to papaverine-induced hypertension.
• Knowledge deficit related to papaverine therapy.

Implementation
Preparation and administration
—Remember that papaverine is rarely used parenterally, except when immediate effect is desired.

—Give I.V. slowly (over 1 to 2 minutes) to avoid serious adverse reactions.

—Do not add lactated Ringer's injection to the injectable form because drug will precipitate.

Monitoring

—Monitor the effectiveness of papaverine therapy by assessing the patient's signs and symptoms.

—Monitor the patient for adverse drug reactions.

—Monitor the patient for drug-induced headache.

—Monitor blood pressure and heart rate and rhythm, especially in patients with cardiac disease.

—Monitor for adverse hepatic reactions in patients receiving long-term therapy.

—Monitor the patient for drug interactions.

—Regularly reevaluate the patient's and family's knowledge about papaverine therapy.

Intervention

—Withhold dose and notify the doctor immediately if changes in patient's health status occur.

—Obtain an order for a mild analgesic if patient experiences a headache.

—Keep all members of the health care team informed of the patient's response to the drug.

Patient teaching

—Inform the patient and family about papaverine, including the dosage, frequency, action, and adverse reactions.

—Tell patient to take the medication regularly; long-term therapy is required.

—Advise the patient to have blood pressure checked regularly and to notify the doctor promptly about signs and symptoms of hypertension (throbbing headache, visual changes).

—Tell the patient to take a mild analgesic for drug-induced headache.

—Encourage increased fluid and fiber intake (if not contraindicated) to prevent constipation.

—Tell the patient to notify the nurse or doctor if adverse reactions develop or questions arise about papaverine therapy.

Evaluation

In the patient receiving papaverine, appropriate evaluation statements include:

• Patient reports decrease or absence of signs and symptoms of vasoconstriction.

• Patient does not experience a headache.

• Patient's blood pressure remains normal throughout papaverine therapy.

• Patient and family state an understanding of papaverine therapy.

SELECTED MAJOR DRUGS: VASODILATORS

DRUG, INDICATIONS, AND DOSAGES	SPECIAL PRECAUTIONS
cyclandelate (Cyclan, Cyclospasmol) *Adjunct in intermittent claudication, arteriosclerosis obliterans, vasospasm and muscular ischemia associated with thrombophlebitis, nocturnal leg cramps, Raynaud's phenomenon, selected cases of ischemic cerebrovascular disease —* **Adults:** initially, 1.2 to 1.6 g P.O. daily, in divided doses before meals and h.s. For maintenance, decrease dosage by 200 mg daily to the lowest effective level. Maintenance dosage is usually 400 to 800 mg daily in two to four divided doses.	• There are no known contraindications. • Use with extreme caution in patients with severe obliterative coronary artery or cerebrovascular disease, because circulation to these diseased areas may be compromised by vasodilatory effects of the drug elsewhere (coronary steal syndrome). • Use cautiously in patients with glaucoma or hypotension.
dipyridamole (Apo-Dipyridamole†, Persantine 100‡, Persantine) *Inhibition of platelet adhesion in prosthetic heart valves, in combination with warfarin or aspirin —* **Adults:** 75 to 100 mg P.O. q.i.d. *Transient ischemic attack —* **Adults:** 400 to 800 mg P.O. daily in divided doses. *Diagnosis of coronary artery disease —* **Adults:** 0.142 mg/kg/minute for 4 minutes.	• Use cautiously in patients with hypotension and in those receiving anticoagulant therapy. • As a diagnostic agent, dipyridamole is given during thallium scan as an alternative to stress test.
isoxsuprine (Duvadilan‡, Vasodilan) *Adjunct for relief of symptoms associated with cerebrovascular insufficiency, peripheral vascular diseases (such as arteriosclerosis obliterans, thromboangiitis obliterans, Raynaud's disease) —* **Adults:** 10 to 20 mg P.O. t.i.d. or q.i.d.	• Contraindicated in immediate postpartum period and in patients with arterial bleeding. • Use with caution in patients with CV or cerebrovascular disease.
nylidrin (Arlidin, PMS Nylidrin†) *To increase blood supply in vasospastic disorders (arteriosclerosis obliterans, thromboangiitis obliterans, diabetic vascular disease, night leg cramps, Raynaud's phenomenon and disease, ischemic ulcer, frostbite, acrocyanosis, acroparesthesia, sequelae of thrombophlebitis) and in circulatory disturbances of the middle ear (primary cochlear ischemia, cochlear striae, vascular ischemia, macular or ampullar ischemia); other disturbances caused by labyrinth artery spasm or obstruction —* **Adults:** 3 to 12 mg P.O. t.i.d. or q.i.d.	• Contraindicated in patients with acute MI, paroxysmal tachycardia, angina pectoris, or thyrotoxicosis. • Use cautiously in patients with uncompensated heart disease or peptic ulcer.
tolazoline (Priscoline) *Persistent pulmonary hypertension in neonates —* **Neonates:** initially, 1 to 2 mg/kg I.V. over 10 minutes, followed by infusion of 1 to 2 mg/kg/hour. *Peripheral vasospastic disorders —* **Adults:** 10 to 50 mg I.M. or I.V. q.i.d.	• Contraindicated in patients with coronary artery disease or active peptic ulcer or after CVA. • Use cautiously in patients with a history of peptic ulcer disease, gastritis, or known or suspected mitral stenosis.

†Available in Canada only   ‡Available in Australia only

SELF-TEST

1. Reginald Smythe, age 68, is admitted to your unit with peripheral vascular disease. His admission orders include papaverine 300 mg P.O. b.i.d. Based on the nurse's knowledge of the usual adult dosage of this drug, the ordered dose is:
   a. within therapeutic dosage range.
   b. less than the usual dosage.
   c. greater than the usual dosage.
   d. within a toxic range.

2. A common adverse reaction to papaverine that may be observed in Mr. Smythe is:
   a. dry skin.
   b. headache.
   c. bradycardia.
   d. diarrhea.

3. The nurse reviews Mr. Smythe's medical history before administering the drug. Which of the following conditions requires cautious use of papaverine?
   a. hypertension
   b. asthma
   c. glaucoma
   d. diabetes mellitus

Check your answers on page 1061.

CHAPTER 24

ANTILIPEMICS

cholestyramine ◆ clofibrate ◆ colestipol hydrochloride
dextrothyroxine sodium ◆ gemfibrozil ◆ lovastatin ◆ niacin ◆ probucol

OVERVIEW

- Antilipemics can retard, and even arrest, atherosclerosis and its resultant complications. Atherosclerosis is associated with increased levels of certain blood lipids. Research thus far, however, has not been able to show a direct clinical relationship between lowered blood lipid levels and reduced incidence of atherosclerosis since other risk factors are reduced as well during the treatment period.
- Dietary restriction and physical exercise are essential in treating all hyperlipidemias. If strict dietary therapy does not effectively lower lipid levels after 2 or 3 months, drug therapy may be started.
- Hyperlipidemias may be primary or secondary to conditions such as hypothyroidism, hepatic disorders, renal failure, nephrosis, pancreatic insufficiency, malabsorption syndromes, and diabetes mellitus.
- Several types of antilipemics are currently in clinical use. The choice of drug depends on the type of hyperlipidemia. Excessive cholesterol levels can be treated with bile acid sequestrants (cholestyramine, colestipol) or cholesterol synthesis inhibitors (clofibrate, dextrothyroxine, gemfibrozil, lovastatin, niacin, probucol). Other antilipemics alter both cholesterol and triglyceride levels. (See *Effects of Antilipemics on Blood Lipids*, page 325.)

MAJOR USES

- Antilipemics counteract high concentrations of lipids in the blood. They do this by lowering levels of cholesterol or triglycerides or both, to different degrees.
- Reduction of serum lipid levels, particularly cholesterol levels, may reduce the risk of coronary artery disease and MI.

MECHANISM OF ACTION

- Both cholestyramine and colestipol combine with bile acid to form an insoluble compound that is excreted.
- Clofibrate—used when triglycerides are high and cholesterol levels are only moderately elevated—seems to inhibit biosynthesis of cholesterol at an early stage, but the exact mechanism is unknown.

GLOSSARY

Hyperlipoproteinemia: excess lipids in the blood.
Lipid: fatty substance in the blood.
Lipoprotein: combination of different lipids with proteins.

- Dextrothyroxine accelerates hepatic catabolism of cholesterol and increases bile secretion to lower cholesterol levels. The drug's serious adverse CV reactions restrict use to young patients with no history of coronary artery disease.
- Gemfibrozil inhibits peripheral lipolysis and also reduces triglyceride synthesis in the liver.
- Niacin, by an unknown mechanism, decreases synthesis of low-density lipoproteins and inhibits lipolysis in adipose tissue.
- Probucol inhibits cholesterol transport from the intestine and may also decrease cholesterol synthesis. The drug appears to be more effective in patients with mild cholesterol elevations than in those with severe hypercholesterolemia.
- Lovastatin acts by inhibiting the hepatic synthesis of cholesterol. It may also increase the number of low-density lipoprotein (LDL) receptors and enhance LDL catabolism.

ABSORPTION, DISTRIBUTION, METABOLISM, AND EXCRETION

Cholestyramine and colestipol are not appreciably absorbed from the GI tract. They are eliminated unchanged in the feces. Clofibrate and niacin are well absorbed from the GI tract; peak plasma levels of niacin occur less than 1 hour after an oral dose. Clofibrate is rapidly hydrolyzed to the active form of the drug, which is highly protein-bound. The active form of clofibrate is metabolized in the liver; 40% to 70% of the drug appears in the urine as metabolites. The plasma half-life of the active form of drug is about 15 hours. Niacin also undergoes hepatic metabolism; about 90% of the drug is excreted in the urine. Dextrothyroxine and probucol are poorly absorbed from the GI tract. Probucol is passed into the bile for elimination in the feces. Lovastatin is absorbed orally and is highly protein-bound. Lovastatin is metabolized in the liver; 10% of lovastatin is excreted in the urine and 83% in the feces. The absorption of lovastatin is greatly increased by administering it with food.

ONSET AND DURATION

Response to antilipemic therapy varies with adherence to drug and dietary regimens. Drug treatment is effective only when combined with an adequate dietary plan. For maximum benefit, blood cholesterol and triglyceride levels should be tested several times during the first few months of therapy and periodically thereafter. After administration of dietary or drug

EFFECTS OF ANTILIPEMICS ON BLOOD LIPIDS

DRUG	EFFECT ON CHOLESTEROL	EFFECT ON TRIGLYCERIDES
cholestyramine	◆	⊗ or ⌂
clofibrate	⌂	◆
colestipol	◆	⊗ or ⌂
dextrothyroxine	◆	⌂ or ⌂
gemfibrozil	⌂	◆
lovastatin	◆	◆
niacin	◆	⊗ or ⌂
probucol	⌂	⊗

KEY
⌂ = Mild decrease
◆ = Moderate decrease
⌂ = Mild increase
⊗ = No change

therapy, a new lipid steady-state level is reached in 4 weeks. Lipid levels should be rechecked at this time and the regimen changed, if necessary.

Clofibrate and probucol take up to 2 months to achieve maximum effect. Niacin's effect is transient; therefore, free fatty acid levels rebound between meals and at night. The bedtime dose is especially important to counteract the striking rise of free fatty acid levels during the nocturnal fast.

ADVERSE REACTIONS

The bile acid sequestrants cholestyramine and colestipol commonly cause constipation, bloating, nausea, flatulence, and an unpleasant taste. Clofibrate is associated with nausea, rash, weakness, and weight gain.

Nicotinic acid (niacin) most commonly causes cutaneous flushing, which may diminish over time or be relieved with prostaglandins. Niacin also causes headache, nausea, abdominal pain, rash, and exacerbation of ulcers. The sustained-release formulas may minimize flushing, but they increase GI discomfort.

Adverse reactions to lovastatin are usually GI related—diarrhea, constipation, and flatulence. This drug may also increase hepatic enzymes. Lovastatin has also caused rash, visual disturbances, and myositis in some patients.

The most common adverse reactions to gemfibrozil and probucol are diarrhea, flatulence, and abdominal pain. Gemfibrozil may also cause gallstones and elevate hepatic enzymes.

PROTOTYPE: BILE ACID SEQUESTRANTS

CHOLESTYRAMINE
(koe less'tir a meen)
Cholybar, Questran**
Classification: bile acid sequestrant
Pregnancy risk category C

How supplied
BAR: 4 g
POWDER: 378-g cans, 9-g single-dose packets. Each scoop of powder or single-dose packet contains 4 g of cholestyramine resin.

Indications and dosage
Primary hyperlipidemia, pruritus, and diarrhea due to excess bile acid; as adjunctive therapy for the reduction of elevated serum cholesterol in patients with primary hypercholesterolemia; and to reduce the risks of atherosclerotic coronary artery disease and MI
ADULTS: 4 g before meals and h.s., not to exceed 32 g daily. Each scoop or packet of Questran contains 4 g cholestyramine. Also available as Cholybar, a chewable candy bar (raspberry or caramel flavored) containing 4 g cholestyramine.
CHILDREN: 240 mg/kg daily P.O. in three divided doses with beverage or food. Safe dosage not established for children under age 6.

Contraindications and precautions
Cholestyramine is contraindicated in patients with complete biliary obstruction where bile is not secreted into the intestine and in those with known hypersensitivity to any of its components. Use cautiously in patients with hypothyroidism, diabetes mellitus, nephrotic syndrome, dysproteinemias, and obstructive liver disease.

Adverse reactions
GI: *constipation,* fecal impaction, hemorrhoids, *abdominal discomfort, flatulence, nausea,* vomiting, steatorrhea.
SKIN: rash; irritation of skin, tongue, and perianal area.
OTHER: vitamin A, D, E, and K deficiency from decreased absorption; hyperchloremic acidosis with long-term use or very high dosage.

Interactions
Acetaminophen, coumarin anticoagulants, beta-adrenergic blockers, corticosteroids, digitalis glycosides, fat-soluble vitamins (A, D, E, and K), iron preparations, thiazide diuretics, thyroid hormone: absorption may

---

**May contain tartrazine
Italicized adverse reactions are common

be substantially decreased by cholestyramine. Separate administration times by at least 2 hours.

Nursing considerations

Assessment
- Review the patient's history for a condition that contraindicates the use of cholestyramine and related compounds.
- Obtain a baseline assessment of the patient's serum triglyceride and cholesterol levels before therapy.
- Be alert for common adverse reactions.
- Evaluate the patient's and family's knowledge about cholestyramine therapy.

Planning (Nursing Diagnoses)
Potential nursing diagnoses for the patient receiving cholestyramine include:
- Potential for injury related to ineffectiveness of cholestyramine to lower blood lipid and cholesterol levels.
- Constipation related to adverse GI reactions.
- Altered nutrition: Less than body requirements related to decreased absorption of vitamins A, D, and K caused by cholestyramine therapy.
- Knowledge deficit related to cholestyramine therapy.

Implementation

Preparation and administration
— To mix powder, sprinkle on surface of preferred beverage or wet food. Let stand a few minutes, then stir to obtain uniform suspension. Mixing with carbonated beverages may result in excess foaming. Use large glass and mix slowly.
— Administer all other medications at least 1 hour before or 4 to 6 hours after cholestyramine to avoid blocking their absorption.
— Administer before meals and at bedtime.

Monitoring
— Monitor the effectiveness of cholestyramine therapy by checking the patient's serum cholesterol and triglyceride levels every 4 weeks.
— Monitor the patient for adverse drug reactions.
— Monitor the patient's bowel habits; drug may cause constipation.
— Monitor digitalis glycoside levels in patients receiving both medications concurrently. If cholestyramine therapy is discontinued, digitalis toxicity may result unless dosage is adjusted.
— Monitor for signs of vitamin deficiencies: A (visual disturbances, skin changes); D (alteration in calcium metabolism); and K (bleeding tendencies).
— Monitor the patient for drug interactions.
— Regularly reevaluate the patient's and family's knowledge about cholestyramine therapy.

Intervention
— If severe constipation develops, decrease dosage, add a stool softener, or discontinue drug.
— Keep all members of the health care team informed of the patient's response to the drug.

Patient teaching
— Inform the patient and family about cholestyramine, including the dosage, frequency, action, and adverse reactions.
— Teach the patient about the disease.
— Instruct the patient on all cardiac risk factors; in particular, counsel on weight control, stop-smoking programs, and exercise.
— Teach the patient about proper dietary management. Advise the patient to follow a diet low in saturated fats and high in fiber and vitamins A, D, and K.
— Teach the patient how to take the drug; instruct the patient to take before meals and at bedtime.
— Tell the patient to notify the nurse or doctor if adverse reactions develop or questions arise about cholestyramine therapy.

Evaluation
In the patient receiving cholestyramine, appropriate evaluation statements include:
• Patient's blood triglyceride and cholesterol levels are normal.
• Patient reports bowel habits are normal.
• Patient does not exhibit any signs or symptoms of vitamin A, D, or K deficiency.
• Patient and family state an understanding of cholestyramine therapy.

PROTOTYPE: CHOLESTEROL SYNTHESIS INHIBITORS

LOVASTATIN
(loe'va sta tin)
Mevacor
Classification: cholesterol synthesis inhibitor
Pregnancy risk category X

How supplied
TABLETS: 20 mg

Indications and dosage
Reduction of low-density lipoproteins and total cholesterol levels in patients with primary hypercholesterolemia (types IIa and IIb)
ADULTS: initially, 20 mg P.O. daily with the evening meal. For patients with severely elevated cholesterol levels (for example, over 300 mg/dl), the initial dose should be 40 mg. The recommended range is 20 to 80 mg in single or divided doses.

Contraindications and precautions

Lovastatin is contraindicated in patients with known hypersensitivity to the drug, active liver disease, unexplained persistent elevations of serum transaminases, or in pregnant and breast-feeding women.

Adverse reactions

CNS: *headache,* dizziness.
EENT: blurred vision, dysgeusia.
GI: *constipation, diarrhea, dyspepsia, flatus,* abdominal pain or cramps, heartburn, nausea.
METABOLIC: elevated serum transaminase levels, abnormal liver test results.
SKIN: rash, pruritus.
OTHER: peripheral neuropathy, muscle cramps, myalgia, myositis, **rhabdomyolysis**.

Interactions

Cholestyramine, clofibrate: enhanced lipid-reducing effects. Monitor carefully.
Immunosuppressive agents, gemfibrozil: possible increased risk of polymyositis and rhabdomyolysis. Maximum recommended lovastatin dosage is 80 mg daily; monitor patient closely.

Nursing considerations

Assessment

• Review the patient's history for a condition that contraindicates the use of lovastatin.
• Obtain a baseline assessment of the patient's serum lipoprotein and total cholesterol levels before therapy.
• Be alert for common adverse reactions.
• Evaluate the patient's and family's knowledge about lovastatin therapy.

Planning (Nursing Diagnoses)

Potential nursing diagnoses for the patient receiving lovastatin include:
• Potential for injury related to ineffectiveness of lovastatin to lower LDL and total cholesterol levels.
• Knowledge deficit related to lovastatin therapy.

Implementation

Preparation and administration
— Store tablets at room temperature in a light-resistant container.
— Administer with evening meal. Absorption is enhanced and biosynthesis is greater in the evening.

Monitoring
— Monitor the effectiveness of lovastatin therapy by regularly checking the patient's serum lipoprotein and total cholesterol levels.
— Regularly monitor serum transaminase levels and other liver function studies.
— Monitor the patient for adverse drug reactions.
— Monitor the patient for drug interactions.

Italicized adverse reactions are common   Boldfaced adverse reactions are life-threatening

—Regularly reevaluate the patient's and family's knowledge about lovastatin therapy.

Intervention

—Institute safety precautions if CNS reactions occur.
—Keep all members of the health care team informed of the patient's response to the drug.

Patient teaching

—Inform the patient and family about lovastatin, including the dosage, frequency, action, and adverse reactions.
—Teach the patient about his disease.
—Teach the patient proper dietary management (restricting total fat and cholesterol intake), weight control, and exercise. Explain their importance in controlling elevated serum lipids.
—Advise the patient to restrict alcohol intake, which can affect cholesterol profile.
—Instruct the patient to store drug at room temperature in a light-resistant container.
—Advise the patient to have regular eye examinations; lovastatin can cause blurred vision.
—Instruct the patient to take lovastatin with evening meal.
—Tell the patient to notify the nurse or doctor if adverse reactions develop or questions arise about lovastatin therapy.

Evaluation

In the patient receiving lovastatin, appropriate evaluation statements include:

• Patient's serum lipoprotein and total cholesterol levels are within normal limits.
• Patient and family state an understanding of lovastatin therapy.

SELECTED MAJOR DRUGS: ANTILIPEMICS

DRUG, INDICATIONS, AND DOSAGES	SPECIAL PRECAUTIONS
Bile sequestrants	
colestipol (Colestid) *Primary hypercholesterolemia and xanthomas—* **Adults:** 15 to 30 g P.O. daily in two to four divided doses.	• Contraindicated in patients with known hypersensitivity to any of its components. • Use cautiously in patients with diseases contributing to increased blood cholesterol, such as hypothyroidism, diabetes mellitus, nephrotic syndrome dysproteinemias or obstructive liver disease. • Consider that various drug interactions are possible with colestipol because it can bind drugs in the gut and alter their pharmacokinetics.

SELECTED MAJOR DRUGS: ANTILIPEMICS *continued*

DRUG, INDICATIONS, AND DOSAGES	SPECIAL PRECAUTIONS

Miscellaneous antilipemics

clofibrate (Arterioflexin‡, Atromid-S, Claripex†)
Hyperlipidemia and xanthoma tuberosum; type III hyperlipidemia that does not respond adequately to diet—
Adults: 2 g P.O. daily in four divided doses. Some patients may respond to lower doses as assessed by serum lipid monitoring.
　Should not be used in children.

• Contraindicated in patients with severe renal or hepatic disease.
• Use cautiously in patients with peptic ulcers and in those receiving anticoagulants.
• Drug should be used only with close monitoring of serum lipid levels. If no response occurs after 3 months, drug should be discontinued because there is a risk of cholelithiasis or cholecystitis.

dextrothyroxine (Choloxin)
Hyperlipidemia in euthyroid patients, especially when cholesterol and triglyceride levels are elevated—
Adults: initially, 1 to 2 mg P.O. daily, increased by 1 to 2 mg daily at monthly intervals to a total of 4 to 8 mg daily.
Children: initially, 0.05 mg/kg P.O. daily, increased by 0.05 mg/kg daily at monthly intervals to a total of 4 mg daily.

• Contraindicated in patients with hepatic or renal disease or iodism.
• Use cautiously in patients with history of cardiac disease, including arrhythmias, hypertension, or angina pectoris.

gemfibrozil (Lopid)
Type IV hyperlipidemia (hypertriglyceridemia) and severe hypercholesterolemia unresponsive to diet and other drugs—
Adults: 1,200 mg P.O. in two divided doses. Usual dosage range is 900 to 1,500 mg daily.

• Contraindicated in patients with hepatic or severe renal dysfunction, including primary biliary cirrhosis and preexisting gallbladder disease.
• Use only with close monitoring of serum lipid levels. If response is inadequate after 3 months of therapy, drug should be discontinued.

niacin
Adjunctive treatment of elevated cholesterol or triglycerides—
Adults: 1 to 2 g P.O. t.i.d. with meals. Maximum dosage is 8 g daily. Alternatively, give drug as sustained-release form—1 to 2 g P.O. daily or b.i.d.

• Contraindicated in patients with phenylketonuria, in pregnant or breast-feeding women, in patients with known hypersensitivity to any of the drug's ingredients, and in those receiving MAO inhibitors.
• Use cautiously (especially sustained-release form) in patients with peripheral vascular disease, hypotension, or bleeding.
• May cause liver damage; closely monitor liver enzyme levels.

probucol (Lorelco, Lurselle‡)
Primary hypercholesterolemia—
Adults: 500 mg P.O. b.i.d. with morning and evening meals. Do not exceed 1 g daily.
　Not recommended for children.

• Contraindicated in patients with arrhythmias. Drug should be stopped in any patient whose ECG shows prolonged QT interval. Monitor ECG periodically.
• Use cautiously in pregnant and breast-feeding women.

†Available in Canada only　‡Available in Australia only

SELF-TEST

1. Ed Gorman, age 36, underwent an uncomplicated coronary artery by-pass 4 days ago. His coronary risk profile includes positive family history, sedentary life-style, hypertension, ex-smoker, elevated cholesterol/triglycerides/low-density lipoprotein (LDL), and obesity. A 6-month trial period of nonpharmacologic therapy failed to lower his cholesterol/triglyceride/LDL levels. The doctor prescribed cholestyramine 4 g P.O. before meals and h.s. Which of the following is true regarding antilipemics?
   a. Antilipemics are indicated for total cholesterol greater than 300 mg/dl.
   b. Therapeutic response occurs in approximately 2 days.
   c. There are no known adverse reactions.
   d. Antilipemic therapy replaces dietary restrictions.

2. The nurse's teaching plan regarding Mr. Gorman's antilipemic therapy should include:
   a. need for yearly cholesterol checks.
   b. need to concurrently adhere to dietary restrictions.
   c. need to avoid aspirin products.
   d. need to be checked for colon cancer yearly.

3. Regina Smith has primary hypercholesterolemia, type IIa. Her doctor prescribed lovastatin 20 mg P.O. daily after a trial period of non-pharmacologic measures failed to reduce the cholesterol level. When should the nurse tell Mrs. Smith to take lovastatin?
   a. upon arising in the morning
   b. after a meal
   c. with the evening meal
   d. at bedtime

Check your answers on page 1062.

NONNARCOTIC ANALGESICS AND ANTIPYRETICS

Salicylates
aspirin ✦ choline magnesium trisalicylate ✦ choline salicylate
magnesium salicylate ✦ salsalate ✦ sodium salicylate
sodium thiosalicylate

Urinary tract analgesic
phenazopyridine hydrochloride

Nonsalicylates
acetaminophen ✦ methotrimeprazine hydrochloride

OVERVIEW

- Nonnarcotic analgesics and antipyretics are probably the most common drugs in medicine. Aspirin, most salicylate derivatives, and acetaminophen are available without a doctor's prescription. Salicylates or acetaminophen are combined with many other medications in varying amounts in many proprietary preparations that are available OTC. Urinary tract analgesics necessitate a doctor's prescription.
- Nonnarcotic analgesics and antipyretics are classified primarily into three groups: salicylates, urinary tract analgesics, and nonsalicylates.

MAJOR USES

- Salicylates relieve mild-to-moderate pain; alleviate inflammation of rheumatoid arthritis, osteoarthritis, and other conditions; and reduce fever.

  Aspirin also inhibits platelet aggregation, hindering coagulation. There is no evidence that aspirin is effective in reducing the incidence of transient ischemic attacks in women. Aspirin may prevent sunburn and relieve sunburn pain by preventing cells from manufacturing prostaglandins.
- Urinary tract analgesics ease the pain of frequent urination (burning and urgency) associated with cystitis, prostatitis, and urethritis. Once thought to have antiseptic properties, these agents are ineffective against microorganisms responsible for urinary tract infections.
- Among the nonsalicylates, acetaminophen relieves mild-to-moderate pain and fever. Methotrimeprazine alleviates moderate-to-severe pain.

GLOSSARY

Analgesic: a drug used to relieve pain.
Antipyretic: a drug used to reduce fever. Such drugs usually lower the thermodetection set point of the hypothalamic heat-regulating center, with resulting vasodilation and sweating. Antipyretic action is also referred to as an antifebrile, an antithermic, or a febrifuge.
Dysuria: discomfort or pain on urination, usually resulting from a bacterial infection or obstruction in the urinary tract.
Nonnarcotic analgesic: an analgesic drug that is not derived from an opioid source.
Prostaglandins: naturally occurring fatty acids abundant in cells that affect many different cellular functions including pain perception.
Salicylism: toxic effects that follow excessive ingestion of salicylic acid.

MECHANISM OF ACTION

- Salicylates produce analgesia by an ill-defined effect on the hypothalamus (central action) and by blocking generation of pain impulses (peripheral action). The peripheral action may involve inhibition of prostaglandin synthesis. Salicylates probably exert their anti-inflammatory effect by inhibiting prostaglandin synthesis; they may also inhibit the synthesis or action of other mediators of the inflammatory response. They relieve fever by acting on the hypothalamic heat-regulating center.
- The mechanism of action of the urinary tract analgesics is unknown.
- Among the nonsalicylates, acetaminophen produces analgesia by blocking generation of pain impulses. This action is probably due to inhibition of prostaglandin synthesis and possibly to inhibition of the synthesis or action of other substances that sensitize pain receptors to mechanical or chemical stimulation. It relieves fever by central action in the hypothalamic heat-regulating center. Methotrimeprazine is thought to suppress sensory impulses by acting on sites in the thalamus, hypothalamus, and reticular activating and limbic systems.

ABSORPTION, DISTRIBUTION, METABOLISM, AND EXCRETION

All oral and I.M. forms of nonnarcotic analgesics and antipyretics are well absorbed. The drugs are distributed in most body tissues and fluids, largely metabolized in the liver, and eliminated as inactive metabolites in urine and—through the bile—in feces. The urinary tract analgesics are eliminated as both inactive metabolites and unchanged drug.

ONSET AND DURATION

All of the nonnarcotic analgesics and antipyretics begin to act 30 to 60 minutes after oral administration and 15 to 30 minutes after I.M. injection. Peak blood levels are reached in 2 to 3 hours. Duration of action of these drugs is usually 4 to 6 hours.

ADVERSE REACTIONS

Adverse reactions to salicylates primarily involve the GI tract and commonly include dyspepsia, heartburn, epigastric distress, nausea, and abdominal pain. GI bleeding is possible and may range in severity from occult (common) to upper GI hemorrhage (rare). Salicylates can cause gastric mucosal damage varying from minor erythema to duodenal ulcers.

Aspirin is usually considered the salicylate that is most likely to cause adverse GI reactions. Such reactions typically occur in the first few days of therapy, often subside with continuous treatment, and can be minimized by administering the drug with food or milk, antacids, and always with at least 8 oz (240 ml) of fluid (usually water). Using enteric-coated forms of aspirin also reduces the incidence of adverse GI reactions.

In certain sensitive patients, usually those with rhinitis or nasal polyps and asthma (the aspirin triad), aspirin may induce bronchospasm with or without angioedema. This reaction is rare with other salicylates. Aspirin also causes adverse hematologic reactions. It irreversibly inhibits platelet aggregation—an effect that does not occur with other salicylates. Aspirin has been associated with increased preoperative and postoperative bleeding and after dental surgery. Adverse hematologic reactions have also been reported in neonates whose mothers ingested aspirin before delivery.

Chronic salicylate intoxication (salicylism) may occur with prolonged therapy at high doses. Manifestations include tinnitus, hearing loss, dimness of vision, headache, dizziness, mental confusion, lassitude, drowsiness, sweating, thirst, hyperventilation, tachycardia, hepatotoxicity, and adverse renal damage, but usual doses rarely cause significant adverse renal reactions. Acute aspirin overdosage produces manifestations similar to but more pronounced than those of chronic toxicity.

Adverse reactions to the urinary tract analgesic, phenazopyridine, occur occasionally and are usually mild. These reactions consist of headache, vertigo, rash, pruritus, and mild GI distress. Rarely, skin pigmentation, anemia, renal failure, jaundice, and hepatitis have occurred, usually associated with high doses or prolonged therapy. Phenazopyridine produces an orange-to-red color in the urine, which may stain fabric; contact lenses may also become stained.

Among the nonsalicylates, a therapeutic dosage of acetaminophen is associated with a relatively low incidence of adverse reactions. Allergic reactions include rash, urticaria, pruritus, laryngeal edema, and angioedema; anaphylactic reactions are rare.

Acetaminophen is often associated with acute toxicity, and the most serious complication is hepatic necrosis, which is potentially fatal. Liver damage becomes apparent 2 to 4 days after the ingestion and may be prevented if the antidote, acetylcysteine, is administered early. Other early signs of acetaminophen toxicity are nausea, vomiting, and abdominal pain. Methemoglobinemia may cause cyanosis, especially in children. CNS changes may include mental changes, stupor, confusion, agitation, and weakness. Severe toxicity may cause hypothermia, rapid shallow breathing, hypotension, and vascular collapse.

Common adverse reactions associated with methotrimeprazine include fainting, weakness, dizziness, orthostatic hypotension, and local reactions, such as pain, inflammation, and swelling at the injection site.

PROTOTYPE: SALICYLATES

ASPIRIN (ACETYLSALICYLIC ACID)
(as' pir in)

Ancasal†◊, Arthrinol†◊, ASA◊, Aspergum◊, Astrin†◊, Bex‡, Coryphen†◊, Easprin◊, Ecotrin◊, Empirin◊, Entrophen†◊, Measurin◊, Norwich Aspirin◊, Novasen†◊, Riphen-10†◊, Sal-Adult†◊, Sal-Infant†◊, Solprin‡, Supasa†◊, Triaphen-10†◊, Vincent's Powders‡, Winsprin Capsules‡, ZORprin◊

Classification: salicylate
Pregnancy risk category C (D in third trimester)

How supplied
TABLETS◊: 65 mg, 75 mg, 81 mg, 300 mg, 325 mg, 500 mg, 600 mg, 650 mg
TABLETS (CHEWABLE): 81 mg◊
TABLETS (ENTERIC-COATED): 325 mg◊, 500 mg◊, 650 mg◊, 975 mg
TABLETS (EXTENDED-RELEASE): 800 mg
TABLETS (TIMED-RELEASE): 650 mg◊
CAPSULES: 325 mg◊, 500 mg◊
POWDER: 500 mg
CHEWING GUM: 227.5 mg◊
SUPPOSITORIES: 60 to 120 mg◊

Indications and dosage
Arthritis
ADULTS: 2.6 to 5.4 g P.O. daily in divided doses.
CHILDREN: 90 to 130 mg/kg P.O. daily divided q 4 to 6 hours.

Mild pain
ADULTS: 325 to 650 mg P.O. or P.R. q 4 hours p.r.n.
CHILDREN: 65 to 100 mg/kg P.O. or P.R. daily divided q 4 to 6 hours p.r.n.

Fever
ADULTS: 325 to 650 mg P.O. or P.R. q 4 hours p.r.n.
CHILDREN: 40 to 80 mg/kg P.O. or P.R. daily divided q 6 hours p.r.n.

Thromboembolic disorders
ADULTS: 325 to 650 mg P.O. daily or b.i.d.

Transient ischemic attacks
MEN: 650 mg P.O. b.i.d. or 325 mg q.i.d.

To reduce the risk of heart attack in patients with previous MI or unstable angina
ADULTS: 325 mg P.O. daily.

Contraindications and precautions

Aspirin is contraindicated in patients with GI ulcer, GI bleeding, bleeding disorders, or known hypersensitivity to aspirin. Use cautiously in patients with hypoprothrombinemia and with vitamin K deficiency and in asthmatic patients with nasal polyps (may cause severe bronchospasm).

Because of epidemiologic association with Reye's syndrome, the Centers for Disease Control recommends that children or teenagers with chicken pox or influenza-like illness should not be given salicylates. Febrile, dehydrated children can develop toxicity rapidly. Elderly patients may be more susceptible to aspirin's toxic effects.

Adverse reactions

BLOOD: *prolonged bleeding time.*
EENT: *tinnitus and hearing loss.*
GI: *nausea, vomiting, GI distress, occult bleeding.*
HEPATIC: abnormal liver function studies, hepatitis.
SKIN: *rash*, bruising.
OTHER: **hypersensitivity manifested by anaphylaxis and/or asthma,** salicylism (with prolonged use).

Interactions

Ammonium chloride (and other urine acidifiers): increased blood levels of aspirin products. Monitor for aspirin toxicity.
Antacids in high doses (and other urine alkalinizers): decreased levels of aspirin products. Monitor for decreased aspirin effect.
Corticosteroids: enhance salicylate elimination and increase risk of GI bleeding. Monitor for decreased salicylate effect and for signs of GI bleeding.
Oral anticoagulants, heparin: increased risk of bleeding. Avoid using together if possible.
Oral hypoglycemic agents: increased hypoglycemic effect. Monitor glucose level.

Nursing considerations

Assessment

- Review the patient's history for a condition that contraindicates the use of aspirin.
- Obtain a baseline assessment of the patient's pain, temperature, or CV condition before therapy.
- Be alert for common adverse reactions.
- Evaluate the patient's and family's knowledge about aspirin therapy.

Planning (Nursing Diagnoses)

Potential nursing diagnoses for the patient receiving aspirin include:
- Pain related to ineffectiveness of aspirin therapy.
- Altered nutrition: Less than body requirements related to adverse GI reactions caused by salicylate therapy.

- Sensory/perceptual alteration (auditory) caused by chronic salicylate intoxication.

Implementation

Preparation and administration

— Give aspirin with food, milk, antacid, or large glass of water to reduce adverse GI reactions.

— For the patient who has difficulty swallowing, crush aspirin, combine it with soft food, or dissolve it in liquid. After mixing aspirin with a liquid, administer it immediately because the drug doesn't stay in solution. Don't crush enteric-coated aspirin.

— Remember that enteric-coated products are slowly absorbed and are not suitable for acute effects. They cause less GI bleeding and may be more suited for long-term therapy, such as arthritis therapy.

Monitoring

— Monitor the effectiveness of aspirin therapy regularly by reevaluating the patient's pain level or degree of fever or by questioning the patient about CV symptoms suggestive of ischemia.

— Therapeutic blood salicylate level in arthritis is 10 to 30 mg/dl. With chronic therapy, mild toxicity may occur at plasma levels of 20 mg/dl. Tinnitus may occur at plasma levels of 30 mg/dl and above, but this is not a reliable indicator of toxicity, especially in very young patients and those over age 60.

— Monitor the patient for adverse drug reactions.

— May cause an increase in serum levels of AST (SGOT), ALT (SGPT), alkaline phosphatase, and bilirubin.

— Question the patient regularly about any changes in nutritional intake caused by adverse GI reactions.

— Inspect the patient's skin regularly for bruising and question him regarding bleeding from gums, spontaneous epistaxis, or GI bleeding; test all emesis and stool for occult blood.

— Regularly question the patient about tinnitus or hearing changes.

— Monitor the patient for drug interactions.

— Regularly reevaluate the patient's and family's knowledge about aspirin therapy.

Intervention

— Hold dose and notify the doctor if the patient develops bleeding, salicylism (tinnitus, hearing loss), or adverse GI reactions.

— If possible, discontinue aspirin dosage 5 to 7 days before elective surgery.

— Keep all members of the health care team informed of the patient's response to the drug.

Patient teaching

— Instruct the patient and family about aspirin, including the dose, frequency, action, and adverse reactions.

— Advise the patient receiving prolonged treatment with large doses of aspirin to watch for petechiae, bleeding gums, and signs of GI bleeding

and to maintain adequate fluid intake. Encourage the use of a soft tooth brush.
— Because of the many possible drug interactions involving aspirin, warn the patient taking prescription drugs to check with the doctor or pharmacist before taking OTC combinations containing aspirin.
— Explain that concomitant use with alcohol, steroids, or other NSAIDs may increase the risk of GI bleeding.
— Explain that various OTC preparations contain aspirin and warn patient to read labels carefully to avoid overdosage.
— Instruct the patient to take aspirin with food or milk.
— Instruct the patient not to chew enteric-coated products.
— Emphasize safe storage of medications in the home. Teach the patient to keep drugs out of children's reach. Aspirin is a leading cause of poisoning in children. Encourage use of child-resistant containers in households that include children, even if only as occasional visitors.
— Tell the patient to inform the nurse or doctor if adverse reactions develop or questions arise about aspirin therapy.

Evaluation
In the patient receiving aspirin, appropriate evaluation statements include:
• Patient states aspirin has relieved pain.
• Patient's nutritional status is unaffected by adverse GI reactions.
• Patient exhibits no evidence of bleeding.
• Patient states hearing is unchanged.
• Patient and family state an understanding of aspirin therapy.

PROTOTYPE: URINARY TRACT ANALGESIC

PHENAZOPYRIDINE HYDROCHLORIDE
(fen az oh peer′ i deen)
Azo-Standard◊, Baridium◊, Di-Azo◊, Eridium◊, Geridium◊, Phenazo†,
Phenazodine◊, Pyrazodine◊, Pyridiate◊, Pyridin◊, Pyridium◊,
Pyronium†, Urodine◊, Urogesic◊, Viridium◊
Classification: urinary tract analgesic
Pregnancy risk category B

How supplied
TABLETS: 100 mg◊, 200 mg

Indications and dosage
Pain with urinary tract irritation or infection
ADULTS: 100 to 200 mg P.O. t.i.d.
CHILDREN: 100 mg P.O. t.i.d.

Contraindications and precautions
Phenazopyridine is contraindicated in renal and hepatic insufficiency.

---

†Available in Canada only   ◊ Available OTC

Adverse reactions

CNS: headache, vertigo.
GI: nausea.
SKIN: rash.

Interactions

None significant.

Nursing considerations

Assessment

- Review the patient's history for a condition that contraindicates the use of phenazopyridine.
- Obtain a baseline assessment of the patient's pain before therapy.
- Be alert for common adverse reactions.
- Evaluate the patient's and family's knowledge about phenazopyridine therapy.

Planning (Nursing Diagnoses)

Potential nursing diagnoses for the patient receiving phenazopyridine include:

- Pain related to ineffectiveness of phenazopyridine therapy.
- Injury related to phenazopyridine-induced vertigo.
- Knowledge deficit related to phenazopyridine therapy.

Implementation

Preparation and administration

— Administer phenazopyridine with meals to minimize GI distress.

Monitoring

— Monitor the effectiveness of phenazopyridine therapy regularly by questioning the patient about pain in the urinary tract.
— Monitor the patient for adverse drug reactions.

Intervention

— Notify the doctor if phenazopyridine does not relieve discomfort.
— Obtain urine samples for urinalysis and urine culture and sensitivity to detect infection as a source of the patient's dysuria.
— Use only as an analgesic.
— Use with an antibiotic to treat urinary tract infection.
— Discontinue drug if skin or sclera becomes yellow-tinged, which may indicate accumulation caused by impaired renal excretion.
— Use copper sulfate test (Clinitest) for accurate urine glucose test results; drug may alter glucose enzymatic (Clinistix or Tes-Tape) results.
— Institute safety measures, such as supervising patient activities and keeping bed rails up, if the patient develops vertigo.
— Keep all members of the health care team informed of the patient's response to the drug.

Patient teaching
—Instruct the patient and family about phenazopyridine, including the dose, frequency, action, and adverse reactions.

—Tell the patient the drug may be discontinued in 3 days if pain is relieved.

—Advise the diabetic patient to check urine with copper sulfate test for accurate urine glucose test results.

—Warn the patient that the drug colors urine red or orange and that it may stain fabrics.

—Caution the patient not to perform activities that require mental alertness or physical ability if vertigo occurs.

—Tell the patient to notify the nurse or doctor if adverse reactions develop or questions arise about phenazopyridine therapy.

Evaluation
In the patient receiving phenazopyridine, appropriate evaluation statements include:
• Patient states pain has been relieved.
• Patient does not experience injury if vertigo occurs.
• Patient and family state an understanding of phenazopyridine therapy.

PROTOTYPE: NONSALICYLATES

ACETAMINOPHEN (PARACETAMOL)
(a set a mee' noe fen)

Acephen◊, Aceta*◊, Ace-Tabs†◊, Acetaminophen Uniserts◊, Actamin◊, Actamin Extra◊, Anacin-3◊, Anacin-3 Maximum Strength◊, Anuphen◊, Apacet◊, Apacet Extra Strength◊, Apacet Oral Solution◊, APAP◊, Apo-Acetaminophen†◊, Atasol†◊, Atasol Forte†◊, Banesin◊, Campain†◊, Ceetamol‡, Children's Anacin-3◊, Children's Apacet◊, Children's Genapap◊, Children's Panadol◊, Children's Tylenol◊, Children's Ty-Pap◊, Children's Ty-Tab◊, Dapa◊, Datril◊, Datril Extra Strength◊, Dolanex*◊, Dymadon‡, Exdol†◊, Exdol Strong†◊, Genapap◊, Genebs◊, Genebs Extra Strength◊, Gentabs◊, Halenol◊, Infants' Anacin-3◊, Infants' Apacet◊, Infants' Tylenol◊, Infants' Ty-Pap◊, Junior Disprol‡, Liquiprin◊, Meda Cap◊, Meda Tab◊, Myapap◊, Neopap◊, Oraphen-PD◊, Panadol◊, Panadol Junior Strength Caplets◊, Panamax‡, Panex◊, Paraphen†◊, Parmol‡, Pedric*◊, Phenaphen◊, Robigesic†◊, Rounox†◊, Suppap◊, Tapanol◊, Tapanol Extra Strength◊, Tempra◊, Tenol◊, Ty Caplets◊, Ty Caps◊, Tylenol*◊, Tylenol Extra Strength◊, Ty Tab◊, Valadol*◊, Valorin◊

Classification: nonsalicylate
Pregnancy risk category B

How supplied
TABLETS: 160 mg◊, 325 mg◊, 500 mg◊, 650 mg◊
TABLETS (CHEWABLE): 80 mg◊

*Liquid form contains alcohol   †Available in Canada only   ‡Available in Australia only   ◊ Available OTC

CAPSULES: 325 mg◊, 500 mg◊
ORAL SOLUTION: 100 mg/ml◊
ORAL SUSPENSION: 120 mg/5 ml‡
ORAL LIQUID: 160 mg/5 ml◊, 500 mg/15 ml◊
ELIXIR: 120 mg/5 ml*◊, 160 mg/5 ml*◊, 320 mg/5 ml*◊
WAFERS: 120 mg◊
EFFERVESCENT GRANULES: 325 mg/capful◊
SUPPOSITORIES: 120 mg◊, 125 mg◊, 135 mg◊, 650 mg◊

Indications and dosage

Mild pain or fever
ADULTS AND CHILDREN OVER AGE 11: 325 to 650 mg P.O. or P.R. q 4 hours; or 1 g P.O. q.i.d. p.r.n. Maximum dosage should not exceed 4 g daily. Dosage for long-term therapy should not exceed 2.6 g daily.
CHILDREN AGE 11: 480 mg/dose.
CHILDREN AGES 9 TO 10: 400 mg/dose.
CHILDREN AGES 6 TO 8: 320 mg/dose.
CHILDREN AGES 4 TO 5: 240 mg/dose.
CHILDREN AGES 2 TO 3: 160 mg/dose.
CHILDREN AGES 12 TO 23 MONTHS: 120 mg/dose.
CHILDREN AGES 4 TO 11 MONTHS: 80 mg/dose.
CHILDREN UP TO AGE 3 MONTHS: 40 mg/dose.

Contraindications and precautions
Repeated use of acetaminophen is contraindicated in anemia or in renal or hepatic disease. Drug should not be used for self-medication of marked fever over 103.1° F (39.5° C), fever persisting longer than 3 days, or recurrent fever unless directed by doctor.

Adverse reactions
HEPATIC: **severe liver damage with toxic doses.**
SKIN: rash, urticaria.

Interactions
Diflunisal: increases acetaminophen blood levels. Don't use together.
Ethanol: increased risk of hepatic damage. Avoid concomitant use.
Warfarin: increased hypoprothrombinemic effect with chronic acetaminophen use. Monitor closely.

Nursing considerations

Assessment
• Review the patient's history for a condition that contraindicates the use of acetaminophen.
• Obtain a baseline assessment of the patient's pain or temperature before therapy.
• Be alert for common adverse reactions.
• Evaluate the patient's and family's knowledge about acetaminophen therapy.

---

*Liquid form contains alcohol ‡Available in Australia only ◊ Available OTC
Boldfaced adverse reactions are life-threatening

Planning (Nursing Diagnoses)

Potential nursing diagnoses for the patient receiving acetaminophen include:
- Pain related to ineffectiveness of acetaminophen.
- Potential for injury related to acetaminophen-induced liver damage with toxic doses.
- Knowledge deficit related to acetaminophen therapy.

Implementation

Preparation and administration

— Administer the liquid form for children and for all patients who have difficulty swallowing.

— Be aware that many OTC products contain acetaminophen and consider this when calculating total daily dosage.

Monitoring

— Monitor the effectiveness of acetaminophen therapy regularly by evaluating the degree of pain relief or the reduction of fever.

— Monitor the patient for adverse drug reactions.

— Monitor liver function studies regularly in the patient receiving large doses of the drug.

— Monitor closely for liver toxicity (change in mental status, jaundice) in the patient with known liver disease and in the high-risk patient, for example, one with a history of alcohol abuse.

— Monitor the patient for drug interactions.

— Regularly reevaluate the patient's and family's knowledge about acetaminophen therapy.

Intervention

— Hold drug and notify the doctor if the patient develops skin rash, urticaria, or any sign of liver damage (jaundice, change in mental status).

— Keep all members of the health care team informed of the patient's response to the drug.

Patient teaching

— Instruct the patient and family about acetaminophen, including the dosage, frequency, action, and adverse reactions.

— Warn the patient that high dosage or unsupervised chronic use can cause hepatic damage. Excessive ingestion of alcoholic beverages may increase the risk of hepatotoxicity.

— Advise the patient not to self-medicate for marked pain or fever (over 103.1° F), pain or fever that persists longer than 3 days, or recurrent fever unless directed by doctor.

— Tell the patient to notify the doctor if acetaminophen fails to relieve pain or fever.

— Tell the patient to notify the nurse or doctor if adverse reactions develop or questions arise about acetaminophen therapy.

Evaluation

In the patient receiving acetaminophen, appropriate evaluation statements include:

• Patient reports relief of pain or fever after acetaminophen use.
• Patient's liver function studies remain normal.
• Patient and family state an understanding of acetaminophen therapy.

SELECTED MAJOR DRUGS: NONNARCOTIC ANALGESICS AND ANTIPYRETICS

DRUG, INDICATIONS, AND DOSAGES	SPECIAL PRECAUTIONS
Salicylates	
choline salicylate (Arthropan) *Rheumatoid arthritis, osteoarthritis, minor pain or fever—* **Adults and children over age 12:** 1 teaspoonful (870 mg choline salicylate) P.O. q 3 to 4 hours p.r.n. If tolerated and needed, dosage may be increased to 2 teaspoonfuls. Do not exceed 6 teaspoonfuls daily. *Relief of pain from inflamed gums—* **Adults and children over age 2:** apply 1 cm of gel to affected area q 3 to 4 hours and h.s. p.r.n.	• Administer cautiously to patients with chronic renal failure, peptic ulcer disease, gastritis, and known allergy to salicylates.
magnesium salicylate (Doan's ◇, Mobidin ◇) *Arthritis—* **Adults:** 545 mg to 1.2 g P.O. t.i.d. or q.i.d. not to exceed 4 g daily. *Mild pain or fever—* **Adults:** 300 to 600 mg P.O. q 4 hours, not to exceed 3.5 g daily.	• Contraindicated in patients with severe chronic renal insufficiency because of risk of magnesium toxicity; with GI ulcer or bleeding; or with known hypersensitivity to aspirin. • Administer cautiously to patients with hypoprothrombinemia, vitamin K deficiency, and bleeding disorders.
Nonsalicylates	
methotrimeprazine (Levoprome, Nozinan†) *Postoperative analgesia—* **Adults and children over age 12:** initially, 2.5 to 7.5 mg I.M. q 4 to 6 hours, then adjust dose. *Preanesthetic medication—* **Adults and children over age 12:** 2 to 20 mg I.M. 45 minutes to 3 hours before surgery.	• Contraindicated in patients receiving concurrent antihypertensive drug therapy, including MAO inhibitors, and in patients with a history of seizure disorder; known hypersensitivity to phenothiazines; severe cardiac,

†Available in Canada only   ◇ Available OTC

SELECTED MAJOR DRUGS: NONNARCOTIC ANALGESICS AND
ANTIPYRETICS *continued*

DRUG, INDICATIONS, AND DOSAGES	SPECIAL PRECAUTIONS
Nonsalicylates *(continued)*	

methotrimeprazine *(continued)*
Sedation, analgesia—
Adults and children over age 12: 10 to 20 mg deep I.M. q 4 to 6 hours as required; or 6 to 25 mg P.O. daily in three divided doses with meals. For severe pain, dosage may be increased to 50 to 75 mg daily in two or three divided doses with meals.
Adults over age 65: 5 to 10 mg I.M. q 4 to 6 hours.
Psychosis—
Adults: 6 to 25 mg P.O. daily in three divided doses with meals. Dosage may be gradually increased p.r.n. and as tolerated to 50 to 74 mg P.O. daily in two or three divided doses.

hepatic, or renal disease; previous overdosage of CNS depressant; and coma.
• Administer cautiously to elderly or debilitated patients with cardiac disease or to any patients who may suffer serious consequences from a sudden drop in blood pressure, in asthmatic patients, or in patients with sulfite sensitivity.

COMPARING ANALGESIC COMBINATIONS

TRADE NAME AND CONTENT	SPECIAL CONSIDERATIONS
Salicylates	

Anacin Caplets ◇
Anacin Tablets ◇
aspirin 400 mg and
caffeine 32 mg
Anacin Maximum Strength ◇
aspirin 500 mg and
caffeine 32 mg
Cope ◇
aspirin 421 mg and
caffeine 32 mg

• Combine the analgesic and antipyretic actions of aspirin with caffeine. Considerable evidence exists that caffeine acts as a "coanalgesic"—it boosts the analgesic actions of both narcotic and nonnarcotic analgesics.
• Contraindicated in patients with peptic ulcers, known hypersensitivity to aspirin, or active bleeding.
• Use with extreme caution in patients with a history of peptic ulcer disease.

| **Urinary tract analgesics** | |

Pyridium Plus ◇
phenazopyridine hydrochloride 150 mg,
hyoscyamine hydrobromide 0.3 mg, and
butabarbital 15 mg

• Combines the analgesic effects of phenazopyridine with the antispasmotic action of hyoscyamine and the sedative effect of butabarbital.
• Contraindicated in patients with known hypersensitivity to any of the drug's components and in those with renal or hepatic insufficiency, bladder neck obstruction, glaucoma, and porphyria.

(continued)

◇ Available OTC

COMPARING ANALGESIC COMBINATIONS *continued*

TRADE NAME AND CONTENT	SPECIAL CONSIDERATIONS
Urinary tract analgesics *(continued)*	
Pyridium Plus *(continued)*	• Warn patients to avoid driving and other hazardous tasks that require alertness until CNS effects of the drug are known. • Emphasize that long-term use of butabarbital may result in drug dependence. • Tell patients that phenazopyridine may cause an orange-to-red color in urine, which may stain fabrics; contact lenses may also be stained.
Nonsalicylates	
Goody's Headache Powders ◊ acetaminophen 260 mg, aspirin 520 mg, and caffeine 32.5 mg/packet **Vanquish Caplets** ◊ acetaminophen 194 mg, aspirin 227 mg, and caffeine 33 mg **Excedrin Extra Strength** ◊ acetaminophen 250 mg, aspirin 250 mg, and caffeine 65 mg	• Combine the analgesic and antipyretic actions of acetaminophen and aspirin with caffeine, a suspected coanalgesic. • Contraindicated in patients with known hypersensitivity to any of the drug's components and in those with peptic ulcers and active bleeding. • Use with extreme caution in patients with a history of peptic ulcer disease. • Not intended for long-term use. Although some evidence exists that combining acetaminophen and aspirin may enhance the antipyretic actions of these agents, certain risks (hepatotoxicity, nephrotoxicity) are associated with long-term use.

◊ Available OTC

SELF-TEST

1. Mary Prokov has come to the emergency department complaining of ankle pain and swelling after falling down. The doctor diagnoses a sprained ankle, wraps her ankle with a woven elastic bandage, advises her to restrict activities, and prescribes aspirin 650 mg P.O. q 4 hours p.r.n. for pain. Before instructing Ms. Prokov about aspirin, the nurse reviews her medical history. Which of the following conditions would require cautious use of aspirin?
a. GI bleeding
b. vitamin K deficiency
c. hypertension
d. history of MI

2. How should the nurse teach Ms. Prokov to take the aspirin?
a. 1 hour before meals
b. 1 hour after meals
c. between meals or with water
d. with meals or milk

3. John Walker complains of frequency and painful urination. A routine urinalysis is normal. While waiting for the results of a urine culture and sensitivity test to rule out an infection, the doctor prescribed phenazopyridine 100 mg P.O. t.i.d. for Mr. Walker's dysuria. What adverse reactions should you instruct Mr. Walker to be alert for?
   a. drowsiness
   b. blurred vision
   c. vertigo
   d. diarrhea

4. Benny Saunders, age 4, has a middle ear infection. Besides an antibiotic, the doctor has prescribed acetaminophen for pain relief. What is the usual recommended dosage for a child Benny's age?
   a. 120 mg/dose
   b. 160 mg/dose
   c. 240 mg/dose
   d. 320 mg/dose

5. Which of the following drugs should not be used concurrently with acetaminophen?
   a. diflunisal
   b. Inderal
   c. phenytoin
   d. ibuprofen

Check your answers on page 1062.

CHAPTER 26

NONSTEROIDAL ANTI-INFLAMMATORY DRUGS

diclofenac sodium ✦ diflunisal ✦ etodolac ✦ fenoprofen calcium
flurbiprofen ✦ ibuprofen ✦ indomethacin ✦ indomethacin sodium trihydrate
ketoprofen ✦ ketorolac tromethamine ✦ meclofenamate sodium
mefenamic acid ✦ naproxen ✦ naproxen sodium ✦ oxyphenbutazone
phenylbutazone ✦ piroxicam ✦ sulindac ✦ tolmetin sodium

OVERVIEW
• Nonsteroidal anti-inflammatory drugs (NSAIDs) are useful alternatives
to the salicylates in the treatment of fever, pain, and inflammation. They
share many of the toxic effects of the salicylates as well. Most of these
drugs are used in the treatment of acute, painful musculoskeletal disorders or acute postoperative pain.

MAJOR USES
• NSAIDs are used to reduce inflammation associated with osteoarthritis,
rheumatoid arthritis, gout, and other conditions. Some are used to combat
dysmenorrhea and dental pain. Ketorolac is administered by I.M. injection for acute, short-term pain.

MECHANISM OF ACTION
• Although their exact mechanism of action is unknown, these drugs
probably inhibit prostaglandin synthesis.

ABSORPTION, DISTRIBUTION, METABOLISM, AND EXCRETION
• Oral forms of NSAIDs are well absorbed from the GI tract. Distributed
in most body tissues and fluids, these drugs are largely metabolized in
the liver. The inactive metabolites are eliminated in urine and—through
the bile—in feces.

GLOSSARY

Inflammation: the protective response of body tissues to irritation or injury. Inflammation may be acute or chronic; its cardinal signs are redness (rubor), heat (calor), swelling (tumor), and pain (dolor), accompanied by loss of function.

Reye's syndrome: a syndrome resulting from acute encephalopathy and fatty infiltration of the internal organs that may follow acute viral infections. It has been epidemiologically associated in children with administration of aspirin, other salicylates, and NSAIDs.

ONSET AND DURATION

- Onset of action after oral administration is within 30 to 60 minutes; after I.M. injection, within 15 to 30 minutes. Blood levels peak within 2 to 3 hours. Duration of action for most of the drugs is 4 to 6 hours. Optimal anti-inflammatory action develops only after 2 to 4 weeks of therapy.
- Naproxen and sulindac have a longer duration of action and are usually given twice daily.
- Piroxicam has the longest duration and should be given once daily.

ADVERSE REACTIONS

Adverse reactions to NSAIDs most frequently involve the GI tract and include epigastric distress, nausea, vomiting, occult blood in the stool, constipation, anorexia, diarrhea, and flatulence. Gastric or duodenal ulcers, GI bleeding, and perforation can occur at any time with or without warning symptoms in patients receiving chronic therapy with NSAIDs. The adverse GI reactions may be reduced by administering the NSAID with food or milk or, if severe, by the concomitant administration of misoprostol, a drug used to prevent NSAID-induced ulcers. Hepatitis and pancreatitis have also been associated with NSAIDs.

CNS effects commonly include dizziness, headache, and drowsiness. Light-headedness, nervousness, fatigue, malaise, anxiety, and mental confusion have also been reported. Indomethacin may aggravate depression or other psychiatric disturbances, seizure disorder, and parkinsonism. Rarely, aseptic meningitis has occurred with ibuprofen.

NSAIDs produce adverse renal reactions by reducing renal prostaglandin synthesis. Decreased renal function may cause fluid retention, which, in turn, may exacerbate CHF or hypertension. This effect is thought to be more common in elderly patients. Sulindac has the least renal effect because it is a prodrug that is not metabolized to its active form until it reaches its site of action and that is not activated by the kidneys. Like aspirin, NSAIDs produce an antiplatelet effect and may prolong bleeding time, which results in easy bruising. However, unlike aspirin, NSAIDs' antiplatelet effect is reversible when the NSAID is withdrawn. Rarely, other adverse hematologic reactions and blood dyscrasia have been reported.

Bronchospasm, difficult breathing, and anaphylactic reactions may result when patients sensitive to aspirin receive NSAIDs. Urticaria, other rashes, and pruritus are the most common dermatologic reactions. Visual disturbances; hearing disturbances, especially tinnitus; and alterations in taste perception may also occur.

PROTOTYPE: NONSTEROIDAL ANTI-INFLAMMATORY DRUGS

IBUPROFEN
(eye byoo proe' fen)

Aches-N-Pain◊, Advil◊, Amersol†, Apo-Ibuprofen†, Brufen‡, Cap-Profen◊, Genpril◊, Haltran◊, Ibuprin◊, Inflam‡, Medipren Caplets◊, Medipren Tablets◊, Midol 200◊, Motrin, Motrin IB◊, Novoprofen†, Nuprin◊, Pamprin-IB◊, Rafen‡, Rufen, Trendar◊

Classification: nonsteroidal anti-inflammatory drug
Pregnancy risk category B (D in third trimester)

How supplied
TABLETS: 200 mg◊, 300 mg, 400 mg, 600 mg, 800 mg
CAPLETS: 200 mg
ORAL SUSPENSION: 100 mg/5 ml

Indications and dosage
Mild to moderate pain, arthritis, primary dysmenorrhea, gout, postextraction dental pain
ADULTS: 200 to 800 mg P.O. t.i.d. or q.i.d. not to exceed 3.2 g daily.

Contraindications and precautions
Ibuprofen is contraindicated in asthmatic patients with nasal polyps. Use cautiously in GI disorders, angioedema, known hypersensitivity to other NSAIDs or salicylates (including aspirin), hepatic or renal disease, cardiac decompensation, known intrinsic coagulation defects, or a history of peptic ulcer disease.

Adverse reactions
BLOOD: prolonged bleeding time.
CNS: headache, drowsiness, dizziness, aseptic meningitis.
CV: peripheral edema.
EENT: visual disturbances, tinnitus.
GI: *epigastric distress*, nausea, occult blood loss, peptic ulceration.
GU: reversible renal failure.
HEPATIC: elevated enzymes.
SKIN: pruritus, rash, urticaria.
OTHER: **bronchospasm,** edema.

Interactions

Furosemide, thiazide diuretics: ibuprofen may decrease the effectiveness of diuretics. Monitor for decreased diuretic or antihypertensive effect.

Oral anticoagulants, lithium: ibuprofen may increase plasma levels or pharmacologic effects of these agents. Monitor for toxicity.

Nursing considerations

Assessment

• Review the patient's history for a condition that contraindicates the use of ibuprofen.
• Obtain a baseline assessment of the patient's pain before therapy.
• Be alert for common adverse reactions.
• Evaluate the patient's and family's knowledge about ibuprofen therapy.

Planning (Nursing Diagnoses)

Potential nursing diagnoses for the patient receiving ibuprofen include:
• Pain related to ineffectiveness of ibuprofen therapy.
• Potential for trauma related to drowsiness or dizziness caused by CNS reaction to ibuprofen.
• Impaired tissue integrity related to adverse GI reactions from ibuprofen administration.
• Knowledge deficit related to ibuprofen therapy.

Implementation

Preparation and administration

— Give with meals or milk to reduce adverse GI reactions.

Monitoring

— Regularly monitor the patient for relief of pain, keeping in mind that full therapeutic effects for arthritis may require as long as 2 to 4 weeks of therapy.
— Monitor the patient for adverse drug reactions.
— Test the patient's stool for occult blood.
— Regularly monitor the patient's renal and hepatic function in long-term therapy.
— Monitor the patient for fluid retention, especially if he is elderly.
— Monitor the patient for drug interactions.
— Regularly reevaluate the patient's and family's (if appropriate) knowledge about ibuprofen therapy.

Intervention

— Notify the doctor if the patient's pain is not relieved or if it worsens.
— If adverse CNS reactions occur, institute safety precautions, such as supervising ambulation and keeping the bed rails up.
— Hold dose and notify the doctor if the patient develops nausea, vomiting, or epigastric distress that is not relieved by taking drug with food or milk or if renal or hepatic abnormalities occur.
— Keep all members of the health care team informed of the patient's response to the drug.

Patient teaching
— Instruct the patient about ibuprofen, including the dosage, frequency, action, and adverse reactions.
— Tell the patient that the full therapeutic effect for arthritis may be delayed for 2 to 4 weeks. Explain that the analgesic effect occurs at low dosage levels, but the anti-inflammatory effect requires dosages above 400 mg q.i.d.
— Advise the patient to notify the doctor if pain persists or becomes worse.
— Instruct the patient not to exceed 1.2 g daily, nor to self-medicate for extended periods without consulting the doctor.
— Advise the patient to avoid driving and other hazardous activities that require mental alertness until CNS effects of the drug are known.
— Tell the patient to take the drug with food or milk.
— Because serious GI toxicity can occur at any time in chronic NSAID therapy, teach the patient signs and symptoms of GI bleeding. Tell the patient to report these to the doctor immediately.
— Concomitant use with aspirin, alcohol, or steroids may increase the risk of adverse GI reactions. Advise the patient to avoid aspirin and alcohol.
— Tell the patient to notify the nurse or doctor if adverse reactions develop or questions arise about ibuprofen therapy.

Evaluation
In the patient receiving ibuprofen, appropriate evaluation statements include:
• Patient states pain is relieved.
• Patient does not develop traumatic injuries as a result of adverse CNS reactions.
• Patient does not develop adverse GI reactions.
• Patient and family state an understanding of ibuprofen therapy.

SELECTED MAJOR DRUGS: NONSTEROIDAL ANTI-INFLAMMATORY DRUGS

DRUG, INDICATIONS, AND DOSAGES	SPECIAL PRECAUTIONS
diclofenac (Voltaren) *Ankylosing spondylitis —* **Adults:** 25 mg P.O. q.i.d. and h.s. *Osteoarthritis —* **Adults:** 50 mg P.O. b.i.d. or t.i.d., or 75 mg P.O. b.i.d. *Rheumatoid arthritis —* **Adults:** 75 to 100 mg P.O. b.i.d., or 50 to 100 mg P.R. (where available) h.s. as a substitute for the last oral dose of the day. Do not exceed 150 mg daily.	• Contraindicated in breast-feeding patients and in those with known hypersensitivity to the drug, with hepatic porphyria, and with aspirin- or NSAID-induced asthma, urticaria, or other allergic reactions. • Administer cautiously to patients with cardiac decompensation, hypertension, or other conditions that predispose to fluid retention.

SELECTED MAJOR DRUGS: NONSTEROIDAL ANTI-INFLAMMATORY DRUGS *continued*

DRUG, INDICATIONS. AND DOSAGES	SPECIAL PRECAUTIONS
diflunisal (Dolobid) *Mild to moderate musculoskeletal pain —* **Adults:** initially, 500 to 1,000 mg P.O., followed by 250 to 500 mg q 8 to 12 hours, not to exceed 1,500 mg daily. *Osteoarthritis —* **Adults:** 500 to 1,000 mg P.O. daily in two divided doses.	• Contraindicated in patients with known hypersensitivity to the drug or with diflunisal-induced acute asthmatic attacks, urticaria, or rhinitis. • Administer cautiously to pregnant or breast-feeding patients; to patients with compromised cardiac function; and to patients with reduced renal reserve, upper or lower GI disease, hypertension, or other conditions that predispose to fluid retention.
etodolac (Lodine) *Management of acute pain —* **Adults:** 200 to 400 mg P.O. q 6 to 8 hours, not to exceed 1.2 g daily. *Osteoarthritis —* **Adults:** 800 to 1,200 g P.O. daily in three or four divided doses. Smaller adults (< 132 lb [< 60 kg]) should receive a maximum of 20 mg/kg daily in divided doses.	• Contraindicated in patients with a history of allergy to other NSAIDs or aspirin. • Use cautiously in patients with a history of GI bleeding, renal dysfunction, or hepatic impairment.
fenoprofen (Nalfon) *Rheumatoid arthritis and osteoarthritis —* **Adults:** 300 to 600 mg P.O. q.i.d. Maximum dosage is 3.2 g daily. *Mild to moderate pain —* **Adults:** 200 mg P.O. q 4 to 6 hours p.r.n.	• Contraindicated in patients with known hypersensitivity, including aspirin or NSAID-induced asthma or urticaria. • Administer cautiously to elderly or debilitated patients and to those with impaired hepatic or renal function.
indomethacin (Indocin, Novomethacin†, Rheumatrin‡) *Moderate to severe arthritis, ankylosing spondylitis —* **Adults:** 25 mg P.O. or P.R. b.i.d. or t.i.d. With food or antacids, may increase dosage by 25 mg daily q 7 days up to 200 mg daily. Alternatively, may give sustained-release capsules (75 mg) — initially, 75 mg in the morning or h.s., followed, if necessary, by 75 mg b.i.d. *Acute gouty arthritis —* **Adults:** 50 mg P.O. t.i.d. Reduce dose as soon as possible, then stop. Sustained-release capsules shouldn't be used for this condition. *To close a hemodynamically significant patent ductus arteriosus in premature infants (I.V. form only) —* **Neonate under age 48 hours:** 0.2 mg/kg I.V., followed by two doses of 0.1/mg/kg at 12- to 24-hour intervals. **Neonate ages 2 to 7 days:** 0.2 mg/kg I.V., followed by two doses of 0.2 mg/kg at 12- to 24-hour intervals. **Neonates over 7 days:** 0.2 mg/kg I.V., followed by two doses 0.25 mg/kg at 12- to 24-hour intervals.	• Contraindicated in pregnant or breast-feeding patients and in those with known hypersensitivity to the drug, active or recurrent GI lesions, or aspirin- or NSAID-induced acute asthmatic attacks, urticaria, or rhinitis. Suppositories are contraindicated in patients with proctitis or recent rectal bleeding. • Administer cautiously to patients with reduced renal reserve, cardiac dysfunction, hypertension, or conditions that predispose to fluid retention or coagulation defects.

(continued)

SELECTED MAJOR DRUGS: NONSTEROIDAL ANTI-INFLAMMATORY DRUGS *continued*

DRUG, INDICATIONS. AND DOSAGES	SPECIAL PRECAUTIONS
ketoproten (Apo-Keto, Orudis) *Rheumatoid arthritis and osteoarthritis —* **Adults:** 150 to 300 mg P.O. in three or four divided doses. Usual dosage is 75 mg t.i.d. Maximum dosage is 300 mg daily. 　Alternatively, may use suppository where available — **Adults:** 100 mg P.R. b.i.d.; or 1 suppository h.s. (with oral ketoprofen during the day). *Mild to moderate pain, dysmenorrhea —* **Adults:** 25 to 50 mg P.O. q 6 to 8 hours p.r.n.	• Contraindicated in patients with aspirin- or NSAID-induced asthma, urticaria, or other allergic reactions. • Administer cautiously to patients with a history of peptic ulcer disease or renal dysfunction.
ketorolac (Toradol) *Short-term management of pain —* **Adults:** initially, give 30 or 60 mg I.M. as a loading dose, followed by half of the loading dose (15 or 30 mg) q 6 hours on a regular schedule or p.r.n. Subsequent dosage should be based on patient response. If pain returns before 6 hours, dosage may be increased by as much as 50% (up to 60 mg); if pain relief continues for 8 to 12 hours, increase interval between doses to q 8 to 12 hours or reduce dose. The recommended maximum dosage is 150 mg on the first day and 120 mg daily thereafter.	• Contraindicated in patients with known hypersensitivity to the drug or in those with the complete or partial syndrome of nasal polyps, angioedema, and bronchospastic reactivity to aspirin or NSAIDs. • Administer cautiously to patients with hepatic or renal impairment, cardiac disease, or hypertension.
meclofenamate (Meclofen, Meclomen) *Rheumatoid arthritis and osteoarthritis —* **Adults:** 200 to 400 mg P.O. daily in three or four equally divided doses. *Mild to moderate pain —* **Adults:** 50 to 100 mg P.O. q 4 to 6 hours. Maximum dosage is 400 mg daily.	• Contraindicated in patients with GI ulceration or inflammation. • Administer cautiously to patients with hepatic or renal disease, CV disease, blood dyscrasia, and diabetes mellitus; to asthmatic patients with nasal polyps; to patients with a history of peptic ulcer disease; or to elderly patients.
mefenamic acid (Ponstan†, Ponstel) *Mild to moderate pain, dysmenorrhea —* **Adults and children over age 14:** initially, 500 mg P.O., then 250 mg q 6 hours, p.r.n. Maximum therapy is 1 week.	• Contraindicated in patients with GI ulceration or with inflammation in patients in whom the potential exists for cross-sensitivity to aspirin or NSAID-inducing symptoms of bronchospasm, allergic rhinitis, or urticaria. • Administer cautiously to patients with hepatic or renal disease, CV disease, blood dyscrasia, and diabetes mellitus; to asthmatic patients with nasal polyps; and to patients with a history of peptic ulcer disease.

SELECTED MAJOR DRUGS: NONSTEROIDAL ANTI-INFLAMMATORY
DRUGS *continued*

DRUG, INDICATIONS. AND DOSAGES	SPECIAL PRECAUTIONS
naproxen (Apo-Naproxen†, Naprosyn, Naxen†‡) *Arthritis, primary dysmenorrhea —* **Adults:** 250 to 500 mg P.O. b.i.d. Alternatively, may use suppository where available — **Adults:** 500 mg P.R. h.s. with oral naproxen during the day. Maximum dosage is 1,250 mg daily.	• Contraindicated in breast-feeding or pregnant patients in the third trimester; in patients with known hypersensitivity to the drug or with aspirin-, other NSAID-, or analgesic-induced asthma, rhinitis, and nasal polyps. • Administer cautiously to patients with significantly impaired renal function, chronic alcoholic liver disease and other forms of cirrhosis, fluid retention, hypertension, or heart failure.
naproxen sodium (Anaprox, Apo-Napro-Na†) *Mild to moderate pain, primary dysmenorrhea —* **Adults:** 2 tablets (275 mg each tablet) P.O. to start, followed by 275 mg q 6 to 8 hours p.r.n. Maximum dosage should not exceed 1,375 mg daily.	• Contraindicated in breast-feeding or pregnant patients in the third trimester and in patients with known hypersensitivity to the drug or with aspirin-, other NSAID-, or analgesic-induced asthma, rhinitis, and nasal polyps. • Administer cautiously to patients with significantly impaired renal function, chronic alcoholic liver disease, and other forms of cirrhosis, fluid retention, hypertension, or heart failure.
phenylbutazone (Apo-Phenylbutazone, Butazolidin, Novobutazone†) *Pain, inflammation in arthritis, bursitis, acute superficial thrombophlebitis —* **Adults:** initially, 100 to 200 mg P.O. t.i.d. or q.i.d. Maximum dosage is 600 mg daily. When improvement is obtained, decrease dosage to 100 mg t.i.d. or q.i.d. *Acute, gouty arthritis —* **Adults:** initially, 400 mg P.O. as a single dose, then 100 mg q 4 hours for 4 days or until relief is obtained. *Note:* **Do not continue therapy for longer than 1 week.**	• Contraindicated in patients with known hypersensitivity to phenylbutazone or oxyphenbutazone and in those who have a bronchospastic reaction to aspirin or NSAIDs; in children under age 14; in senile patients; in patients with GI ulcer, blood dyscrasia, and thyroid disease; or in those receiving long-term anticoagulant therapy. • Administer cautiously to patients over age 60.
piroxicam (Apo-Piroxicam†, Feldene, Novopirocam†) *Osteoarthritis and rheumatoid arthritis —* **Adults:** 20 mg P.O. daily or divided if desired.	• Contraindicated in patients with known hypersensitivity to the drug or in those with aspirin- or NSAID-induced bronchospasm, nasal polyps, and angioedema.

(continued)

SELECTED MAJOR DRUGS: NONSTEROIDAL ANTI-INFLAMMATORY
DRUGS *continued*

DRUG, INDICATIONS, AND DOSAGES	SPECIAL PRECAUTIONS
piroxicam *(continued)*	• Use cautiously in elderly patients and in patients with angioedema, GI disorders, a history of renal or peptic ulcer disease, cardiac disease, or hypersensitivity to other NSAIDs.
sulindac (Apo-Sulin†, Clinoril) *Osteoarthritis, rheumatoid arthritis, ankylosing spondylitis—* **Adults:** initially, 150 mg P.O. b.i.d.; may increase to 200 mg P.O. b.i.d. *Acute subacromial bursitis or supraspinatus tendinitis, acute gouty arthritis—* **Adults:** 200 mg P.O. b.i.d. for 7 to 14 days. Dose may be reduced as symptoms subside.	• Contraindicated in patients with known hypersensitivity to the drug and in those with aspirin- or NSAID-induced acute asthmatic attacks, urticaria, or rhinitis. • Administer cautiously to patients with a history of ulcers and GI bleeding, renal dysfunction, compromised cardiac function, or hypertension or to those receiving oral anticoagulants or oral hypoglycemic agents.
tolmetin (Tolectin) *Rheumatoid arthritis, osteoarthritis, gout, dysmenorrhea, juvenile rheumatoid arthritis—* **Adults:** 400 mg P.O. t.i.d. or q.i.d. Maximum dose is 2 g daily. **Children ages 2 or over:** 15 to 30 mg/kg P.O. daily in divided doses.	• Contraindicated in breast-feeding patients or in those with known hypersensitivity to the drug or with aspirin- or NSAID-induced asthma, rhinitis, urticaria, or other symptoms of allergic or anaphylactic reactions. • Administer cautiously to pregnant patients or to those with compromised cardiac function, hypertension, or other conditions predisposing to fluid retention.

†Available in Canada only

SELF-TEST

1. Edward Thompson, age 77, has osteoarthritis, which causes pain in his hips and knees. The doctor prescribes ibuprofen 400 mg P.O. q.i.d. Which of the following nursing diagnoses might apply because Mr. Thompson is taking ibuprofen?
   a. constipation related to neuromuscular impairment
   b. altered urinary elimination related to urinary frequency
   c. potential for trauma related to drowsiness or dizziness
   d. potential for infection related to leukopenia.

2. Which adverse reaction associated with NSAIDs is Mr. Thompson at risk for developing because of his age?
   a. fluid retention
   b. orthostatic hypotension
   c. constipation
   d. thromboemboli

3. Which of the following instructions should the nurse include when teaching Mr. Thompson about ibuprofen therapy?
   a. Avoid the use of antacids.
   b. Take the drug with food or milk.
   c. Test urine daily for glucose.
   d. Wear medical alert identification.

Check your answers on pages 1062 and 1063.

CHAPTER 27

OPIOID ANALGESICS

Opioid agonists
alfentanil hydrochloride ✦ codeine phosphate ✦ codeine sulfate
fentanyl citrate ✦ hydrocodone bitartrate ✦ hydromorphone hydrochloride
levorphanol tartrate ✦ meperidine hydrochloride ✦ methadone hydrochloride
morphine hydrochloride ✦ morphine sulfate ✦ oxycodone hydrochloride
oxymorphone hydrochloride ✦ propoxyphene hydrochloride
propoxyphene napsylate ✦ sufentanil citrate

Opioid agonist-antagonists
buprenorphine hydrochloride ✦ butorphanol tartrate ✦ dezocine
nalbuphine hydrochloride ✦ pentazocine hydrochloride ✦ pentazocine lactate

OVERVIEW

- Opioid agonists relieve pain by acting at specific receptors in the brain and spinal cord. They can change a patient's perception of pain so that it's qualitatively less disturbing. Because use of these drugs may result in physical and psychological dependence, they should be reserved for treatment of severe pain unrelieved by nonnarcotic analgesics. Because they have a high potential for abuse, most of these drugs are classified as controlled substances (Schedule II) under the Controlled Substances Act of 1970.
- Opioid agonist-antagonists also act on specific pain receptors in the brain and spinal cord. Additionally, they block subsets of opiate receptors at these sites; they can precipitate a withdrawal syndrome in opioid-dependent persons. Several agents that have less potential for abuse are classified under controlled substance schedule IV (pentazocine) or schedule V (buprenorphine); others (butorphanol, dezocine, nalbuphine) are exempt from such control.
- The concern about addiction is generally unwarranted when narcotic analgesics are used for acute pain or in terminally ill patients. For patients with intractable (particularly cancer-related) pain, these drugs should be administered around the clock—not p.r.n. Such use of these drugs continually relieves pain and eases the patient's anxiety and anticipation of pain.
- Opioid analgesics are classified primarily into opioid agonists and opioid agonist-antagonists.

GLOSSARY

Competitive inhibition: displacement of an agent from an opiate receptor site by an antagonist.

Epidural block: loss of feeling or sensation produced by injecting an anesthetic agent between the vertebrae and beneath the ligaments into the space surrounding the dura.

Equianalgesic dose: amount of an analgesic drug that will produce the same level of pain relief as a standard agent used for comparison.

Opiate or narcotic: drug derived from opium or synthetically produced that alters pain perception, induces mental changes, promotes deep sleep, depresses respirations, constricts pupils, and decreases GI motility.

Neuroleptanesthesia: loss of feeling or sensation produced by using a narcotic, a neuroleptic, and nitrous oxide.

MAJOR USES

• Opioid agonists and opioid agonist-antagonists relieve moderate-to-severe pain and furnish preoperative sedation, alone or in combination with anxiolytics (such as diazepam and hydroxyzine).

MECHANISM OF ACTION

• Opioid agonists and opioid agonist-antagonists bind with opiate receptors at many sites in the CNS (brain, brain stem, and spinal cord), altering both perception of and emotional response to pain. The precise mechanism of action, however, is unknown.

ABSORPTION, DISTRIBUTION, METABOLISM, AND EXCRETION

Absorption of most opioid agonists and opioid agonist-antagonists is more effective after parenteral, than after oral, administration. However, hydrocodone and propoxyphene—available only in oral form—are well absorbed from the GI tract. Oxycodone, which is available in oral and rectal suppository forms, is also well absorbed from the GI tract after oral administration. Fentanyl is available in a transdermal form.

All opioid agonists and opioid agonist-antagonists are well distributed in body tissues, metabolized in the liver, and excreted in the urine.

ONSET AND DURATION

Onset of action for all analgesics is most rapid after I.V. administration (within 10 minutes). Onset is somewhat slower after I.M. injection (5 to 20 minutes) and is variable after oral administration.

Equianalgesic Doses of Opioid Agonist-Antagonists, page 360, and *Action of Opioid Analgesics,* page 361, list the duration time ranges for opioid agonists and opioid agonist-antagonists.

EQUIANALGESIC DOSES OF OPIOID AGONIST-ANTAGONISTS

The chart below compares equianalgesic doses of opioid agonist-antagonists.

	I.M. DOSE[1] (mg)	DURATION (hours)	ANTAGONIST ACTIVITY
buprenorphine	0.3	6	+ + + + +[2]
butorphanol	3	3 to 4	+ + + +
dezocine	10	2 to 4	+ +
nalbuphine	10	3 to 6	+ + +
pentazocine	30	3	+

[1]Compared to analgesic effect of 10 mg morphine I.M.
[2]Equipotent to naloxone.

ADVERSE REACTIONS

Opioid agonists and opioid agonist-antagonists cause respiratory depression, which may lead to apnea and respiratory arrest. Rapid I.V. administration of the drug increases the incidence of such respiratory depression. The narcotic antagonist, naloxone, reverses these respiratory depressant effects.

Adverse CNS reactions are common and include sedation, light-headedness, and dizziness. Euphoria, dysphoria, delirium, insomnia, agitation, anxiety, hallucinations, mental confusion, headache, tremor, and miosis are other adverse CNS reactions to the opioid analgesics. Fentanyl has been associated with chest wall rigidity and seizures. After prolonged use, the opioid analgesics may also cause both physical and psychological dependence, which results in withdrawal reactions.

Opioid agonists and opioid agonist-antagonists are commonly associated with nausea, vomiting, and constipation. They may cause biliary tract spasms (colic), with symptoms similar to an acute gallbladder attack, as well as diarrhea, cramps, abdominal pain, taste alterations, dry mouth, and anorexia.

Most opioid analgesics can cause bradycardia, which can be controlled with atropine. Meperidine and its analogs, however, may produce anticholinergic effects: tachycardia, palpitations, dry mouth, muscle tremor, flushing of the face and neck, faintness, hypertension, hypotension, orthostatic hypotension, and circulatory collapse.

ACTION OF OPIOID ANALGESICS

The chart below compares equianalgesic doses of opioid agonists.

DRUG	I.M. DOSE (mg)	DURATION (hours)	P.O. DOSE (mg)	DURATION (hours)	HALF-LIFE (hours)
alfentanil[1]	—	—	—	—	1.5
codeine	130	4 to 6	200[2]	4 to 6	2 to 4
fentanyl	0.1	1 to 2	—	—	3 to 4
hydrocodone	—	—	5 to 10	4 to 5	4
hydromorphone	1.5	4 to 5	7.5	4 to 6	2 to 3
levorphanol	2	4 to 5	4	4 to 7	12 to 16
meperidine	75	3 to 5	300	4 to 6	3 to 4
methadone	10	4 to 5	20	4 to 6	15 to 40
morphine	10	4 to 5	60	4 to 7	2
oxycodone	—	—	5 to 10	4 to 5	2 to 3
oxymorphone	1	4 to 6	5 (rectal)	4 to 6	2 to 3
propoxyphene	—	—	130 (HCl), 200 (napsylate)	4 to 6	6 to 12
sufentanil[2]	0.02	unknown	—	—	2 to 3

[1]Drug is usually used I.V. as an anesthetic adjunct.
[2]Analgesic (not antitussive) dose.

Allergic reactions may cause pruritus, urticaria or other rashes, laryngospasm and edema. Patients who are unable to take one opioid analgesic because of an allergic reaction, may be able to tolerate another drug of this class.

Opioid agonists may cause urine retention or hesitancy, most commonly in males with prostatic hypertrophy or those patients with urethral stricture. Decreased libido or potency may also occur.

MORPHINE HYDROCHLORIDE
(mor' feen)
Morphitec†, M.O.S.†, M.O.S.-S.R.†

MORPHINE SULFATE
Astramorph, Astramorph PF, Duramorph, Epimorph†, Morphine
H.P.†, MS Contin, MSIR, RMS Uniserts, Roxanol, Roxanol SR, Statex†
Classification: opioid agonist
Controlled substance schedule II
Pregnancy risk category B
(D for prolonged use or use of high doses at term)

How supplied
hydrochloride
TABLETS: 10 mg†, 20 mg†, 40 mg†, 60 mg†
ORAL SOLUTION†: 1 mg/ml, 5 mg/ml, 10 mg/ml, 20 mg/ml, 50 mg/ml
SYRUP: 1 mg/ml†, 5 mg/ml†
SUPPOSITORIES: 20 mg†, 30 mg†
sulfate
TABLETS: 15 mg, 30 mg
TABLETS (CONTROLLED-RELEASE): 30 mg, 60 mg
SOLUBLE TABLETS: 10 mg, 15 mg, 30 mg
ORAL SOLUTION: 10 mg/5 ml, 20 mg/5 ml, 20 mg/ml (concentrate)
SYRUP: 1 mg/ml, 5 mg/ml
INJECTION (WITH PRESERVATIVE): 1 mg/ml, 2 mg/ml, 3 mg/ml, 4 mg/ml, 5
mg/ml, 8 mg/ml, 10 mg/ml, 15 mg/ml
INJECTION (WITHOUT PRESERVATIVE): 500 mcg/ml, 1 mg/ml
SUPPOSITORIES: 5 mg, 10 mg, 20 mg, 30 mg

Indications and dosage
Severe pain
ADULTS: 4 to 15 mg S.C. or I.M.; or 30 to 60 mg P.O. or P.R. q 4 hours,
p.r.n. or around the clock. May be injected slow I.V. (over 4 to 5 minutes)
diluted in 4 to 5 ml water for injection. May also administer controlled-release tablets q 8 to 12 hours. As an epidural injection, 5 mg via an epidural
catheter q 24 hours.
CHILDREN: 0.1 to 0.2 mg/kg dose S.C. or I.M. q 4 hours. Maximum dosage
is 15 mg. In some situations, morphine may be administered by continuous
I.V. infusion or by intraspinal and intrathecal injection.

Contraindications and precautions
Use morphine with extreme caution in head injury, increased intracranial
pressure, seizures, asthma, COPD, alcoholism, prostatic hypertrophy,
severe hepatic or renal disease, acute abdominal conditions, hypothyroidism, Addison's disease, increased CSF pressure, urethral stricture, cardiac

arrhythmias, reduced blood volume, and toxic psychosis and in elderly or debilitated patients.

Adverse reactions

CNS: *sedation, somnolence, clouded sensorium,* euphoria, seizures with large doses, dizziness, nightmares (with long-acting oral forms).
CV: *hypotension,* bradycardia.
GI: *nausea,* vomiting, *constipation,* ileus.
GU: urine retention.
OTHER: respiratory depression, physical dependence, pruritus and skin flushing (with epidural administration).

Interactions

Alcohol, CNS depressants: additional effects. Use together cautiously.

Nursing considerations

Assessment
• Obtain a baseline assessment of the patient's pain before therapy.
• Be alert for common adverse reactions.
• Evaluate the patient's and family's knowledge about morphine therapy.

Planning (Nursing Diagnoses)
Potential nursing diagnoses for the patient receiving morphine include:
• Pain related to ineffectiveness or inadequate dosage of morphine.
• Altered thought processes related to CNS reactions induced by morphine.
• Decreased tissue perfusion (peripheral) related to morphine-induced hypotension.
• Ineffective breathing pattern related to morphine- induced respiratory depression.
• Knowledge deficit related to morphine therapy.

Implementation

Preparation and administration
— Oral solutions (sulfate) of various concentrations are available, as well as an concentrated oral solution (20 mg/ml). Be sure to note the strength you are administering.
— Do not crush or break controlled-release tablets.
— If S.L. administration is ordered, measure out oral solution with tuberculin syringe. Administer dose a few drops at a time to allow maximal S.L. absorption and to minimize swallowing.
— Rectal suppository available in 5-, 10-, 20-, and 30-mg dosages. Refrigeration is not necessary. Note that, in some patients, rectal and oral absorption may not be equivalent.
— Preservative-free preparations now available for epidural and intrathecal administration. Use of the epidural route is increasing.
— Around-the-clock administration is beneficial in severe, chronic pain.

Monitoring

—Monitor the effectiveness of morphine therapy after each dose by evaluating degree of pain relief.
—Monitor the patient for adverse drug reactions.
—Monitor respiratory status throughout morphine therapy noting any evidence of respiratory depression, such as decreased rate or depth of respiration.
—Monitor closely for respiratory depression up to 24 hours after epidural injection. Check respiratory rate and depth every 30 to 60 minutes for 24 hours.
—Regularly monitor blood pressure for hypotension and heart rate for bradycardia.
—Monitor bowel and bladder function daily for constipation or ileus or urine retention.
—Monitor the patient for drug interactions.
—Regularly reevaluate the patient's and family's knowledge about morphine therapy.

Intervention

—Notify the doctor and discuss increase of dosage or frequency if pain is not relieved.
—Hold dose and notify the doctor if he patient's respirations are below 12/minute or if significant hypotension occurs.
—Keep narcotic antagonist (naloxone) and resuscitative equipment available.
—Respiratory depression, hypotension, profound sedation, or coma may occur if used with general anesthetics, tranquilizers, sedatives, hypnotics, alcohol, tricyclic antidepressants, or MAO inhibitors. Morphine dose should be used with such drugs with extreme caution and at reduced dosage.
—Because adverse CNS reactions are possible, institute safety precautions, such as supervising ambulation and keeping bed rails up.
—If not contraindicated, obtain an order for a stool softener or other laxative and increase the patient's fluid and fiber intake to prevent or treat constipation, which can become severe during maintenance use of morphine.
—Maintain seizure precautions when administering large doses of morphine.
—If nausea and vomiting occur, obtain an order for an antiemetic.
—Be aware that morphine may worsen or mask gallbladder pain.
—Keep all members of the health care team informed of the patient's response to the drug.

Patient teaching

—Instruct the patient and family about morphine, including the dosage, frequency, action, and adverse reactions.
—Warn the ambulatory patient who is taking oral maintenance doses to avoid driving and other hazardous activities that require alertness.

—Teach the patient to remain in bed for 1 hour after I.M. injection and to obtain assistance before getting out of bed.

—When used postoperatively, encourage turning, coughing, and deep breathing and use of the incentive spirometer to avoid atelectasis.

—Suggest measures such as high-fiber diet and liberal fluid intake to prevent constipation in the patient on a maintenance regimen.

—Encourage the patient to ask for medication or to activate a patient-controlled analgesia (PCA) device before pain becomes severe.

—Warn the nonchronic patient about morphine's potential for dependence.

—Tell the patient to notify the nurse or doctor if adverse reactions develop or questions arise about morphine therapy.

Evaluation

In the patient receiving morphine, appropriate evaluation statements include:

• Patient reports relief of pain after administration of morphine.
• Patient remains alert and oriented.
• Patient's blood pressure is within the patient's normal range.
• Patient maintains normal respiratory rate and pattern after administration of morphine.
• Patient and family state an understanding of morphine therapy.

PROTOTYPE: OPIOID AGONIST-ANTAGONISTS

PENTAZOCINE HYDROCHLORIDE

(pen taz′ oh seen)

PENTAZOCINE LACTATE

Fortral, Talwin†, Talwin NX (contains naloxone hydrochloride 0.5 mg)
Classification: opioid agonist-antagonist
Controlled substance schedule IV
Pregnancy risk category B
(D for prolonged use or use of high doses at term)

How supplied

hydrochloride
TABLETS: 25 mg‡, 50 mg†‡
lactate
INJECTION: 30 mg/ml‡

Indications and dosage

Moderate to severe pain

ADULTS: 50 to 100 mg P.O. q 3 to 4 hours, p.r.n. or around the clock. Maximum oral dosage is 600 mg daily. Alternatively, may give 30 mg I.M., I.V., or S.C. q 3 to 4 hours, p.r.n. or around the clock. Maximum

---

†Available in Canada only   ‡Available in Australia only

parenteral dosage is 360 mg daily. Single doses above 30 mg I.V. or 60 mg I.M. or S.C. not recommended.

Contraindications and precautions

Pentazocine is contraindicated in emotional instability, drug abuse, head injury, and increased intracranial pressure. Use cautiously in hepatic or renal disease.

Adverse reactions

CNS: *sedation*, visual disturbances, *hallucinations*, drowsiness, *dizziness, light-headedness*, confusion, euphoria, headache, *psychotomimetic effects*.

GI: *nausea, vomiting*, dry mouth, constipation.

GU: *urine retention*.

LOCAL: induration, nodules, sloughing, and sclerosis of injection site.

OTHER: *respiratory depression*, physical and psychological dependence.

Interactions

Alcohol, CNS depressants: additive effects. Use together cautiously.

Narcotic analgesics: avoid concomitant use. Possible decreased analgesic effect.

Nursing considerations

Assessment

- Review the patient's history for a condition that contraindicates the use of pentazocine.
- Obtain a baseline assessment of the patient's pain before therapy.
- Be alert for common adverse reactions.
- Evaluate the patient's and family's knowledge about pentazocine.

Planning (Nursing Diagnoses)

Potential nursing diagnoses for the patient receiving pentazocine include:
- Pain related to ineffectiveness or inadequate dosage or frequency of pentazocine.
- Fluid volume deficit related to adverse GI reactions caused by pentazocine.
- Urinary retention related to potential adverse GU reactions caused by pentazocine.
- Ineffective breathing pattern related to pentazocine- induced respiratory depression.
- Knowledge deficit related to pentazocine therapy.

Implementation

Preparation and administration

—Before leaving the bedside, make sure the patient has swallowed the tablet.

Monitoring

—Monitor the effectiveness of pentazocine therapy by assessing the patient's degree of pain relief after each dose.

—Monitor the patient for adverse drug reactions.

Italicized adverse reactions are common

—If nausea or vomiting occurs, monitor the patient's fluid intake and evidence of dehydration.
—Monitor patient's rate and pattern of breathing for evidence of respiratory depression.
—Monitor the patient for drug interactions.
—Regularly reevaluate the patient's and family's knowledge about pentazocine therapy.

Intervention

—Notify the doctor if pain relief is not obtained.
—If nausea and vomiting prevents adequate oral intake, obtain an order for an antiemetic.
—Encourage the patient to void before administering dose; notify the doctor if urine retention is suspected and be prepared to catheterize the patient.
—Because the oral pentazocine preparation available in the United States contains the narcotic antagonist naloxone, this drug may precipitate abstinence syndrome in narcotic-dependent patients.
—Because of the potential for adverse CNS reactions, institute safety precautions, such as supervising ambulation.
—Hold drug and notify the doctor if the patient's respiratory rate declines.
—If not contraindicated, increase the patient's fluid and fiber intake to prevent constipation.
—Keep all members of the health care team informed of the patient's response to the drug.

Patient teaching

—Instruct the patient and family about pentazocine, including the dosage, frequency, action, and adverse reactions.
—Warn the patient about the drug's potential for causing physical or psychological dependence.
—Warn the patient to avoid driving and other hazardous activities that require mental alertness if adverse CNS reactions occur.
—Advise the patient to take precautions to prevent constipation.
—Alert the patient who is addicted to narcotics that U.S. preparation may precipitate abstinence syndrome.
—Encourage the patient to void before each dose and to withhold dose and notify the doctor if urine retention occurs.
—Tell the patient to notify the nurse or doctor if adverse reactions develop or questions arise about pentazocine therapy.

Evaluation

In the patient receiving pentazocine, appropriate evaluation statements include:
• Patient reports pain relief.
• Patient maintains adequate hydration.
• Patient reports no change in voiding pattern.
• Patient's respiratory rate and pattern remain normal.
• Patient and family state an understanding of pentazocine therapy.

SELECTED MAJOR DRUGS: OPIOID ANALGESICS

DRUG, INDICATIONS, AND DOSAGES	SPECIAL PRECAUTIONS

Opioid agonists

codeine phosphate (Paveralt)
Mild to moderate pain—
Adults: 15 to 60 mg P.O., S.C., or I.M. q 4 hours, p.r.n. or around the clock.
Children: 3 mg/kg P.O. daily divided q 4 hours, p.r.n. or around the clock.
Nonproductive cough—
Adults: 15 to 60 mg P.O., S.C., or I.M. q 4 hours, p.r.n. or around the clock.
Children: 3 mg/kg P.O. daily divided q 4 hours, p.r.n. or around the clock.
Adults: 10 to 20 mg P.O. q 4 to 6 hours. Maximum dosage is 120 mg daily.
Children ages 6 to 12: 5 to 10 mg P.O. q 4 to 6 hours. Maximum dosage is 60 mg daily.
Children ages 2 to 6: 2.5 to 5 mg P.O. q 4 hours. Do not exceed 30 mg daily.

• Administer with extreme caution to patients with head injury, increased intracranial pressure, increased CSF pressure, hepatic or renal disease, hypothyroidism, Addison's disease, acute alcoholism, seizures, severe CNS depression, asthma, COPD, respiratory depression, and shock and to elderly or debilitated patients.

codeine sulfate
Mild to moderate pain—
Adults: 15 to 60 mg P.O., S.C., or I.M. q 4 hours, p.r.n. or around the clock.
Children: 3 mg/kg P.O. daily divided q 4 hours, p.r.n. or around the clock.
Nonproductive cough—
Adults: 10 to 20 mg P.O. q 4 to 6 hours. Maximum dosage is 120 mg daily.
Children ages 6 to 12: 5 to 10 mg P.O. q 4 hours. Maximum dosage is 60 mg daily.
Children ages 2 to 6: 2.5 to 5 mg P.O. q 4 to 6 hours. Do not exceed 30 mg daily.

• Administer with extreme caution to patients with head injury, increased intracranial pressure, increased CSF pressure, hepatic or renal disease, hypothyroidism, Addison's disease, acute alcoholism, seizures, severe CNS depression, asthma, COPD, respiratory depression, and shock and to elderly or debilitated patients.

fentanyl citrate (Sublimaze)
Adjunct to general anesthetic—
Adults: 0.05 to 0.1 mg I.V. repeated q 2 to 3 minutes p.r.n. Dose should be reduced in elderly and high-risk patients.
Postoperatively for moderate to severe pain—
Adults: 0.05 to 0.1 mg I.M. q 1 to 2 hours p.r.n.
Preoperatively—
Adults: 0.05 to 0.1 mg I.M. 30 to 60 minutes before surgery.
Children ages 2 to 12: 1.7 to 3.3 mcg/kg I.M.

• Contraindicated in patients with known hypersensitivity to the drug.
• Administer cautiously to patients with head injury, increased CSF pressure, asthma, COPD, respiratory depression, and shock and to elderly or debilitated patients.

fentanyl transdermal system (Duragesic)
Management of chronic pain—
Adults: Highly individualized; most patients start therapy with the 25 mcg/hour system q 72 hours.

• Reserved for management of chronic pain.
• Alternate analgesics should be available for breakthrough pain, especially at the start of therapy.

SELECTED MAJOR DRUGS: OPIOID ANALGESICS *continued*

DRUG, INDICATIONS, AND DOSAGES	SPECIAL PRECAUTIONS

Opioid agonists *(continued)*

fentanyl transdermal system *(continued)*

• Serum levels drop slowly after the system is removed. Patients who are changing to another analgesic should wait for 18 hours before starting full doses of another opiate.

hydrocodone
Moderate to moderately severe pain—
Adults: 1 to 2 tablets q 4 to 6 hours p.r.n.

• Contraindicated in patients with known hypersensitivity or intolerance to the drug. When used in combination products that contain aspirin, the drug is contraindicated in patients with known hypersensitivity to aspirin; in patients with severe bleeding, disorders of coagulation or primary hemostasis, severe vitamin K deficiency, severe liver damage, anticoagulant therapy, peptic ulcer, or other serious GI lesions.
• Administer cautiously to elderly or debilitated patients and to those with severe impairment of hepatic or renal function, gallbladder disease or gallstones, respiratory impairment, cardiac arrhythmias, inflammatory disorders of the GI tract, hypothyroidism, Addison's disease, prostatic hypertrophy or urethral stricture, coagulation disorders, head injuries, or acute abdominal injury.

hydromorphone (Dilaudid)
Moderate to severe pain—
Adults: 1 to 6 mg P.O. q 4 to 6 hours, p.r.n. or around the clock; 2 to 4 mg I.M., S.C., or I.V. q 4 to 6 hours p.r.n. or q 6 to 8 hours around the clock (I.V. dose should be given over 3 to 5 minutes); or 3 mg P.R. (suppository) h.s., p.r.n. or q 6 to 8 hours around the clock.
Cough—
Adults: 1 mg P.O. q 3 to 4 hours.
Children ages 6 to 12: 0.5 mg P.O. q 3 to 4 hours p.r.n.

• Contraindicated in patients with known hypersensitivity to the drug; with an intracranial lesion associated with increased intracranial pressure; and whenever ventilatory function is depressed (COPD, cor pulmonale, emphysema, kyphoscoliosis, status asthmaticus).
• Administer cautiously to elderly or debilitated patients and to those with impaired renal or

(continued)

SELECTED MAJOR DRUGS: OPIOID ANALGESICS *continued*

DRUG, INDICATIONS, AND DOSAGES	SPECIAL PRECAUTIONS

Opioid agonists *(continued)*

hydromorphone *(continued)*

hepatic function, hypothyroidism, Addison's disease, prostatic hypertrophy, or urethral stricture.

levorphanol (Levo-Dromoran)
Moderate to severe pain—
Adults: 2 to 3 mg P.O. or S.C. q 6 to 8 hours, p.r.n. or around the clock.

• Contraindicated in patients with acute alcoholism, asthma, increased intracranial pressure, respiratory depression, and anorexia.
• Administer cautiously to patients with hepatic or renal disease, hypothyroidism, Addison's disease, seizures, head injury, severe CNS depression, brain tumor, COPD, and shock and to elderly or debilitated patients.

meperidine (Demerol)
Moderate to severe pain—
Adults: 50 to 150 mg P.O., I.M., or S.C. q 3 to 4 hours, p.r.n. or around the clock; or 15 to 35 mg/hour by continuous I.V. infusion.
Children: 1 to 1.8 mg/kg P.O., I.M., or S.C. q 4 to 6 hours. Maximum dosage is 100 mg q 4 hours, p.r.n. or around the clock.
Preoperatively—
Adults: 50 to 100 mg I.M. or S.C. 30 to 90 minutes before surgery.
Children: 1 to 2.2 mg/kg I.M. or S.C. 30 to 90 minutes before surgery.

• Contraindicated in patients with known hypersensitivity to the drug or in those who have recently received MAO inhibitors.
• Administer with extreme caution to patients receiving other CNS depressants; to those with head injury and increased intracranial pressure and asthma and other respiratory conditions; to pregnant and breast-feeding women; and to those susceptible to hypotension, such as postoperative patients who are volume-depleted or patients who have received phenothiazines or certain anesthetics.

methadone (Dolophine)
Severe pain—
Adults: 2.5 to 10 mg P.O., I.M., or S.C. q 6 to 8 hours, p.r.n. or around the clock.
Narcotic abstinence syndrome—
Adults: 15 to 40 mg P.O. daily (highly individualized). Maintenance dosage is 20 to 120 mg P.O. daily. Adjust dose as needed. Daily dosages over 120 mg require special state and federal approval.

• Contraindicated in patients with known hypersensitivity to the drug.
• Administer cautiously to elderly or debilitated patients, to patients with acute abdominal conditions, and to those with severe hepatic or renal impairment, hypothyroidism, Addison's disease, prostatic hypertrophy, urethral stricture, head injury, increased intracranial pressure, asthma, COPD, respiratory depression, and CNS depression.

SELECTED MAJOR DRUGS: OPIOID ANALGESICS *continued*

DRUG, INDICATIONS, AND DOSAGES	SPECIAL PRECAUTIONS

Opioid agonists *(continued)*

oxycodone (Endone‡, Roxicodone, Supeudol†)
Moderate to severe pain—
Adults: 1 to 2 tablets P.O. q 6 hours, p.r.n. or around the clock, or 5 mg (5 ml) of oral solution or tablets P.O. q 6 hours.
Adults: (Supeudol) 1 to 3 suppositories P.R. daily, p.r.n. or around the clock.

• Contraindicated in patients with known hypersensitivity to the drug.
• Administer with extreme caution in head injury, increased intracranial pressure, increased CSF pressure, seizures, asthma, COPD, alcoholism, prostatic hypertrophy, severe hepatic or renal disease, acute abdominal conditions, urethral stricture, hypothyroidism, Addison's disease, cardiac arrhythmias, reduced blood volume, and toxic psychosis and in elderly or debilitated patients.

oxymorphone (Nomorphan)
Moderate to severe pain—
Adults: 1 to 1.5 mg I.M. or S.C. q 4 to 6 hours, p.r.n. or around the clock; or 0.5 mg I.V. q 4 to 6 hours, p.r.n. or around the clock; or 2.5 to 5 mg P.R. q 4 to 6 hours, p.r.n. or around the clock.

• Contraindicated in patients with known hypersensitivity to the drug.
• Administer cautiously to elderly and debilitated patients; to those with known hypersensitivity to depressants, such as those with CV, pulmonary, or hepatic disease; and to those with hypothyroidism (myxedema), acute alcoholism, alcohol withdrawal syndrome, seizure disorders, asthma, and kyphoscoliosis.

propoxyphene hydrochloride (Darvon)
propoxyphene napsylate (Darvon-N)
Mild to moderate pain—
Adults: 65 mg (hydrochloride) P.O. q 4 hours p.r.n. Or 100 mg (napsylate) P.O. q 4 hours p.r.n.

• Contraindicated in patients with known hypersensitivity to propoxyphene, aspirin, or caffeine.
• Administer cautiously to patients with peptic ulcer or coagulation abnormalities and hepatic or renal impairment.

sufentanil (Sufenta)
Adjunct to general anesthetic—
Adults: 1 to 8 mcg/kg I.V. administered with nitrous oxide and oxygen.
Primary anesthetic—
Adults: 8 to 30 mcg/kg I.V. administered with 100% oxygen and a muscle relaxant.

• Contraindicated in patients with known hypersensitivity to the drug.
• Administer cautiously to patients with head injury, pulmonary disease, or decreased respiratory reserve.

(continued)

SELECTED MAJOR DRUGS: OPIOID ANALGESICS *continued*

DRUG, INDICATIONS, AND DOSAGES	SPECIAL PRECAUTIONS
Opioid agonist-antagonists	

buprenorphine (Buprenex)
Moderate to severe pain—
Adults: 0.3 mg I.M. or slow I.V. q 6 hours, p.r.n. or around the clock. May administer up to 0.6 mg/dose if necessary.

• Contraindicated in patients with known hypersensitivity to the drug.
• Administer cautiously to elderly or debilitated patients and to those with severe hepatic, pulmonary, or renal impairment; myxedema or hypothyroidism; Addison's disease; CNS depression or coma; toxic psychoses; prostatic hypertrophy or urethral stricture; acute alcoholism; alcohol withdrawal syndrome; or kyphoscoliosis.

butorphanol (Stadol)
Moderate to severe pain—
Adults: 1 to 4 mg I.M. q 3 to 4 hours, p.r.n. or around the clock; or 0.5 to 2 mg I.V. q 3 to 4 hours, p.r.n. or around the clock.

• Contraindicated in patients with known hypersensitivity to the drug.
• Administer cautiously in patients with head injury, increased intracranial pressure, acute MI, ventricular dysfunction, coronary insufficiency, respiratory disease or depression, and renal or hepatic dysfunction.

dezocine (Dalgan)
Moderate to severe pain—
Adults: 5 to 20 mg I.M. q 3 to 6 hours p.r.n.; or 2.5 to 10 mg I.V. q 2 to 4 hours p.r.n.

• Contraindicated in patients with known hypersensitivity to the drug.
• Administer cautiously to patients with head injury, increased intracranial pressure, respiratory depression, COPD, hepatic or renal disease, and biliary surgery; to those who are taking CNS depressants; to those who are using alcohol; to pregnant women; and to geriatric patients.

nalbuphine (Nubain)
Moderate to severe pain—
Adults: 10 to 20 mg S.C., I.M., or I.V. q 3 to 6 hours, p.r.n. or around the clock. Maximum dosage is 160 mg daily.

• Contraindicated in patients with known hypersensitivity to the drug.
• Administer cautiously to patients with impaired renal or hepatic function, MI, biliary tract surgery, impaired respiration (for example, from other medication, uremia, asthma, severe infection, cyanosis, or respiratory obstructions).

COMPARING OPIOID ANALGESIC COMBINATIONS

TRADE NAME AND CONTENT	SPECIAL CONSIDERATIONS
Darvocet-N 50 propoxyphene napsylate 50 mg and acetaminophen 325 mg **Darvocet-N 100, Propacet 100** propoxyphene napsylate 100 mg and acetaminophen 650 mg **Darvon-N with A.S.A.** propoxyphene napsylate 100 mg and aspirin 325 mg **Darvon Compound-65, Bexophene** propoxyphene hydrochloride 65 mg and aspirin 389 mg, caffeine 32.4 mg **Dolene-AP-65, Genagesic, Wygesic** propoxyphene hydrochloride 65 mg and acetaminophen 650 mg	• Darvocet-N combines the analgesic activity of propoxyphene and the antipyretic analgesic activity of acetaminophen. This combination produces greater analgesia than that produced by administration of either propoxyphene or acetaminophen alone. • Contraindicated in patients with known hypersensitivity to any component of the drug and in those who are vulnerable to accidents or addiction. • Administer cautiously to patients taking tranquilizers or antidepressants and to those who drink alcohol in excess because excessive dosage of propoxyphene, either alone or in combination with other CNS depressants including alcohol, is a known cause of drug-related deaths. • Tell patients not to exceed the recommended dose and to limit their intake of alcohol. • The propoxyphene portion of this drug may produce psychological dependence and, less commonly, physical dependence and tolerance if taken in higher-than-recommended doses over long periods of time. • Caution patients that drug may impair the mental and physical abilities necessary for safe performance of hazardous tasks. • Expect a reduction of daily dosage in patients with hepatic or renal adverse reactions. • Monitor patients for common adverse reactions, such as dizziness, sedation, nausea, and vomiting. Such reactions may be alleviated if the patient lies down.
Tylenol with Codeine No. 1 codeine phosphate 7.5 mg and acetaminophen 300 mg **Tylenol with Codeine No. 2** codeine phosphate 15 mg and acetaminophen 300 mg **Tylenol with Codeine No. 3** **Papadeine No. 3** codeine phosphate 30 mg and acetaminophen 300 mg **Tylenol with Codeine No. 4** codeine phosphate 60 mg and acetaminophen 300 mg	• Tylenol with Codeine combines the analgesic effect of a centrally acting opiate analgesic (codeine) with a nonopiate analgesic (acetaminophen). • Contraindicated in patients with known hypersensitivity to any component of the drug. • Administer cautiously to elderly and debilitated patients and to those with severe impairment of hepatic or renal function, hyperthyroidism, Addison's disease, and prostatic hypertrophy or urethral stricture. • Be aware that this drug may obscure the clinical course of patients with head injuries or acute abdominal conditions.

(continued)

COMPARING OPIOID ANALGESIC COMBINATIONS *continued*

TRADE NAME AND CONTENT	SPECIAL CONSIDERATIONS
Tylenol with Codeine Elixir codeine phosphate 120 mg/5 ml and acetaminophen 120 mg/5 ml **Phenaphen with Codeine No. 2** codeine phosphate 15 mg and acetaminophen 325 mg **Phenaphen with Codeine No. 3** **Aceta with Codeine** codeine phosphate 30 mg and acetaminophen 325 mg **Phenaphen with Codeine No. 4** codeine phosphate 60 mg and acetaminophen 325 mg	• Safe use of this drug has not been established in children under age 3. Monitor patients closely for adverse reactions such as light-headedness, dizziness, sedation, shortness of breath, nausea, and vomiting. These effects are more prominent in ambulatory than nonambulatory patients; some of these effects may be alleviated if the patient lies down. • Be aware that this drug may also cause allergic rash, euphoria, dysphoria, constipation, abdominal pain, and pruritus. At higher dosage, codeine may cause respiratory depression. • Tylenol with Codeine tablets are Schedule III controlled substances; Tylenol with Codeine Elixir is a Schedule V controlled substance. Codeine in the combination can produce psychic or physical dependence with repeated administration.

SELF-TEST

1. John Pedro has just had a subtotal gastrectomy. His doctor has prescribed morphine 10 mg I.M. q 4 hours p.r.n. for incisional pain. Select the most critical nursing assessment to be done before administering morphine to Mr. Pedro.
   a. Palpate urinary bladder for distention.
   b. Auscultate abdomen for bowel sounds.
   c. Count respiratory rate and assess depth.
   d. Inspect skin for rash.

2. Before administering the first dose of morphine, the nurse also reviews Mr. Pedro's medical history. Which of the following conditions would require extreme caution when administering morphine? Explain why.
   a. hyperthyroidism
   b. alcoholism
   c. hypertension
   d. leukemia

3. Mr. Pedro asks how soon he can begin to experience pain relief after morphine is administered I.M. The nurse should respond by telling him the onset of action of morphine is:
   a. within 20 minutes.
   b. 20 to 30 minutes.
   c. 30 to 45 minutes.
   d. 45 to 60 minutes.

4. The nurse should tell Mr. Pedro to report which of the following adverse reactions?
   a. nervousness
   b. headache
   c. hematuria
   d. urine retention

Check your answers on page 1063.

CHAPTER 28

SEDATIVE-HYPNOTICS

Barbiturates
amobarbital ✦ amobarbital sodium ✦ aprobarbital ✦ butabarbital
butabarbital sodium ✦ mephobarbital ✦ pentobarbital
pentobarbital sodium ✦ phenobarbital ✦ phenobarbital sodium
secobarbital sodium

Benzodiazepines
estazolam ✦ flurazepam hydrochloride ✦ quazepam ✦ temazepam
triazolam

Miscellaneous agents
acetylcarbromal ✦ chloral hydrate ✦ ethchlorvynol ✦ glutethimide
methotrimeprazine hydrochloride ✦ methyprylon
paraldehyde

OVERVIEW

• Most of the drugs in this chapter are barbiturates (amobarbital, aprobarbital, butabarbital, mephobarbital, pentobarbital, phenobarbital, and secobarbital). Until recently, these agents were used extensively as nighttime sedative-hypnotics to induce sleep. However, because of the high risk of barbiturate toxicity and dependence, most doctors no longer regard barbiturates as the drugs of choice for this indication and they are rarely used.

• Benzodiazepines (estazolam, flurazepam, quazepam, temazepam, and triazolam) are more desirable for nighttime sedation because they are as therapeutically effective as the barbiturates and have a much greater therapeutic index (margin between toxic and therapeutic doses). The other drugs in this chapter (except paraldehyde) more closely resemble the barbiturates in their potential to cause toxicity and drug dependence.

• Sedative-hypnotics are classified primarily into three groups: barbiturates, benzodiazepines, and miscellaneous agents.

MAJOR USES

• Sedative-hypnotics are used to treat insomnia, induce sleep before operative or test procedures, and provide sedation and relief of anxiety.

• Mephobarbital and paraldehyde alleviate alcohol withdrawal syndrome.

• Phenobarbital controls acute psychotic agitation.

GLOSSARY

Hypersomnia: disorder of excessive somnolence, such as narcolepsy (sleep attacks).

Hypnotic: agent that induces sleep.

Insomnia: inability to sleep; abnormal wakefulness.

Non–rapid eye movement (NREM) sleep: first four stages of sleep, which progress from light to deep sleep and are characterized by NREM.

Parasomnia: dysfunction associated with sleep, sleep stages, or partial arousals.

Rapid eye movement (REM) sleep: fifth and last stage of sleep characterized by REMs. REM sleep is essential for physiologic and mental restoration.

Sedative: agent that allays excitement and produces drowsiness.

Serotonin: neurotransmitter secreted by the rapheal nuclei that inhibits pain pathways and helps control an individual's mood; it may induce sleep.

MECHANISM OF ACTION

- Although their mechanism of action is not completely defined, most sedative-hypnotics probably interfere with transmission of impulses from the thalamus to the cortex of the brain.
- Benzodiazepines act on the limbic system, thalamus, and hypothalamus of the CNS to produce hypnotic effects.

ABSORPTION, DISTRIBUTION, METABOLISM, AND EXCRETION

Barbiturates are well absorbed from all administration routes; the sodium salts are absorbed more rapidly than the acids. They are distributed to all tissues and body fluids, with high concentrations in the brain and liver. Barbiturates are metabolized slowly in the liver. Both metabolites and unchanged drug are excreted in urine. Trace amounts are also eliminated in feces and perspiration.

Chloral hydrate is well absorbed from the GI tract after oral or rectal administration. It is rapidly reduced and distributed to all tissues. Both the unchanged drug and active metabolites are detected in CSF, umbilical-cord blood, fetal blood, and amniotic fluid. Chloral hydrate is metabolized in the liver and RBCs. It is eliminated primarily in urine and partially in feces through the bile.

Ethchlorvynol is rapidly absorbed from the GI tract after oral administration. Both the unchanged drug and metabolites are detected in the liver, kidneys, spleen, brain, bile, and CSF. The drug is metabolized primarily in the liver and excreted in urine.

Ethinamate is well absorbed from the GI tract. Although it is rapidly destroyed in the tissues, its pattern of distribution is unknown. The liver is not significantly involved in the drug's metabolism. Small amounts are excreted in the urine.

Benzodiazepines are well absorbed from the GI tract after oral administration. Distributed to all tissues and metabolized in the liver, they're eliminated primarily in urine.

Glutethimide is absorbed irregularly from the GI tract after oral administration. The unchanged drug and active metabolites are detected in the liver, kidneys, brain, and bile. The drug is metabolized in the liver and eliminated in both urine and feces.

Acetylcarbromal is a ureide derivative. It is metabolized to urea and releases bromine, which acts as a CNS depressant. This metabolism occurs in the liver; bromine is excreted in the urine. Because of the risk of bromide toxicity, acetylcarbromal is now rarely used.

Methotrimeprazine is rapidly absorbed after I.M. injection. It is well distributed to body tissues, including the CSF, metabolized in the liver, and eliminated slowly in urine and feces.

Methyprylon's absorption and distribution are not well known. The drug is metabolized in the liver. Some of its metabolites are secreted in the bile and reabsorbed; the rest are excreted in urine.

Paraldehyde is rapidly absorbed from either the GI tract or muscles, depending on the route of administration. Although its distribution is not well known, the drug is metabolized in the liver and excreted in urine and through the lungs. Significant quantities are exhaled unchanged, emitting a characteristic odor.

ONSET AND DURATION

Onset and Duration of Sedative-Hypnotics summarizes onset and duration of these agents.

ADVERSE REACTIONS

Benzodiazepines usually produce adverse reactions that are extensions of their pharmacologic effects. These include the CNS effects of drowsiness, ataxia, fatigue, confusion, weakness, headache, dizziness, vertigo, and syncope. Patients with hepatic or renal dysfunction, elderly or debilitated patients, and children are more likely to develop these adverse reactions and should receive a lower initial dosage. All patients, but especially the elderly, may have increased daytime sedation or other prolonged adverse CNS reactions from taking a benzodiazepine for sleep. This effect is potentiated if the benzodiazepine is taken every night because serum levels will increase, reflecting accumulation. Other CNS reactions include euphoria, nightmares, and hallucinations with benzodiazepine use. Psychological and physical dependence occur and may result in withdrawal symptoms. Rare paradoxical reactions produce an acute hyperexcited state with anxiety, hallucinations, insomnia, or rage and require discontinuation of the drug. Triazolam has been associated with paradoxical reactions and with anterograde amnesia.

ONSET AND DURATION OF SEDATIVE-HYPNOTICS

ONSET AND DURATION	DRUGS P.O./I.M.	DRUGS I.V.
Ultra short-acting: few minutes' onset; short-term duration (less than 1 hour)	None	amobarbital ethchlorvynol pentobarbital phenobarbital secobarbital
Short-acting: 10 to 15 minutes' onset; 3 hours' or less duration	acetylcarbromal paraldehyde pentobarbital secobarbital	
Intermediate-acting: 10 to 30 minutes' onset; 3 to 6 hours' duration	amobarbital aprobarbital butabarbital chloral hydrate ethchlorvynol methotrimeprazine temazepam triazolam	
Long-acting: 30 to 60 minutes' onset; 6 or more hours' duration	estazolam flurazepam glutethimide mephobarbital methyprylon phenobarbital quazepam	

GI reactions include constipation, dry mouth, taste alterations, anorexia, nausea, vomiting, and abdominal discomfort. Hiccups have also been reported. Respiratory depression may occur, but is usually associated with an overdose or an interaction with another respiratory depressant agent. Rare reactions include tachycardia, palpitations, and hypotension; rashes, urticaria and flushing; and urinary incontinence or urine retention.

Drowsiness, lethargy, vertigo, headache, and CNS depression are common with barbiturates and other sedative-hypnotics. After hypnotic doses, a hangover effect, subtle distortion of mood, and impairment of judgment or motor skills may continue for many hours. After a decrease in dosage or discontinuation of sedative-hypnotics used for hypnosis, rebound insomnia or increased dreaming or nightmares may occur. Barbiturates cause hyperalgesia in subhypnotic doses. Hypersensitivity reactions (rash, fever, serum sickness) are not common and are more likely to occur in patients with a history of asthma or allergies to other drugs; reactions include urticaria, rash, angioedema, and Stevens-Johnson syndrome. Barbiturates can cause paradoxical excitement at low doses, confusion in elderly patients, and hyperactivity in children. High fever, severe headache, stomatitis, conjunctivitis, or rhinitis may precede skin eruptions. Because of the potential for fatal consequences, discontinue barbiturates if dermatologic reactions occur.

Withdrawal symptoms may occur after as little as 2 weeks of uninterrupted therapy. Symptoms of abstinence usually occur within 8 to 12 hours after the last dose but may be delayed up to 5 days. They include weakness, anxiety, nausea, vomiting, insomnia, hallucinations, and possibly seizures.

PROTOTYPE: BARBITURATES

SECOBARBITAL SODIUM
(see koe bar' bi tal)
Novosecobarb†, Seconal Sodium
Classification: barbiturate
Controlled substance schedule II
Pregnancy risk category D

How supplied
TABLETS: 100 mg
CAPSULES: 50 mg, 100 mg
INJECTION: 50 mg/ml
RECTAL INJECTION: 50 mg/ml

Indications and dosage
Sedation, preoperatively
ADULTS: 200 to 300 mg P.O. 1 to 2 hours before surgery.
CHILDREN: 50 to 100 mg P.O. or 4 to 5 mg/kg P.R. 1 to 2 hours before surgery.

Insomnia
ADULTS: 100 to 200 mg P.O. or I.M.
CHILDREN: 3 to 5 mg/kg I.M., not to exceed 100 mg, with no more than 5 ml injected in any one site or 4 to 5 mg/kg P.R.

Acute tetanus seizure
ADULTS AND CHILDREN: 5.5 mg/kg I.M. or slow I.V., repeated q 3 to 4 hours, if needed; I.V. injection rate not to exceed 50 mg/15 seconds.

Acute psychotic agitation
ADULTS: initially, 50 mg/minute I.V. up to 250 mg I.V.; additional doses given cautiously after 5 minutes if desired response is not obtained. Not to exceed 500 mg total.

Status epilepticus
ADULTS AND CHILDREN: 250 to 350 mg I.M. or I.V.

Contraindications and precautions
Secobarbital is contraindicated in uncontrolled severe pain, respiratory disease with dyspnea or obstruction, known hypersensitivity to barbitu-

rates, previous addiction to sedatives, or porphyria. Use cautiously in hepatic or renal impairment and in pregnant women with toxemia or a history of bleeding.

Adverse reactions

CNS: *drowsiness, lethargy, hangover,* paradoxical excitement in elderly patients.
GI: nausea, vomiting.
SKIN: rash, urticaria.
OTHER: **Stevens-Johnson syndrome**, angioedema, exacerbation of porphyria.

Interactions

Alcohol or other CNS depressants, including narcotic analgesics: excessive CNS and respiratory depression. Use together cautiously.
Griseofulvin: decreased absorption of griseofulvin. Avoid concomitant use.
MAO inhibitors: inhibit metabolism of barbiturates; may cause prolonged CNS depression. Reduce barbiturate dosage during concomitant use.
Oral anticoagulants, estrogens and oral contraceptives, doxycycline, corticosteroids: secobarbital sodium may enhance the metabolism of these drugs. Monitor for decreased effect.
Rifampin: may decrease barbiturate levels. Monitor for decreased effect.

Nursing considerations

Assessment
- Review the patient's history for a condition that contraindicates the use of secobarbital.
- Obtain a baseline assessment of sleeping patterns before therapy.
- Be alert for common adverse reactions., especially CNS reactions such as drowsiness, lethargy, or hangover.
- Evaluate the patient's and family's knowledge about secobarbital.

Planning (Nursing Diagnoses)
Potential nursing diagnoses for the patient receiving secobarbital include:
- Sleep pattern disturbance related to ineffectiveness of secobarbital.
- Activity intolerance related to adverse CNS reactions caused by secobarbital.
- Knowledge deficit related to secobarbital therapy.

Implementation

Preparation and administration
— Use injectable solution within 30 minutes after opening container to minimize deterioration. Don't use cloudy solution.
— Secobarbital injection is compatible with Ringer's injection and 0.9% sodium chloride solution. Don't mix with acidic solutions, such as lactated Ringer's injection, because it is not compatible; a precipitate may form.
— To reconstitute, rotate ampule. Do not shake.

— I.V. injection should be reserved for emergency treatment and should be given under close supervision. Be prepared to give artificial respiration.

— Give I.M. injection deeply. Superficial injection may cause pain, sterile abscess, and sloughing.

— Expect to reduce dosage during labor because barbiturates potentiate the effects of opiates.

— Before leaving the bedside, make sure the patient has swallowed tablet or capsule.

Monitoring

— Regularly monitor the effectiveness of secobarbital sodium by evaluating the patient's ability to sleep after administration.

— Monitor the patient for adverse drug reactions.

— Monitor the patient's mental status and activity level after the patient awakens for evidence of adverse CNS reactions.

— Monitor the elderly patient's response to the drug as these patients are more sensitive to the drug's adverse CNS reactions.

— Monitor for signs of barbiturate toxicity: coma, pupillary constriction, cyanosis, clammy skin, and hypotension. Overdose can be fatal.

— Monitor the neonate's respiratory status closely if the mother received drug during labor because excessive dosage may cause respiratory depression in the neonate.

— Monitor the patient for drug interactions.

— Regularly reevaluate the patient's and family's knowledge about secobarbital therapy.

Intervention

— After administration, institute safety precautions: keep the patient on bed rest, keep bed rails up, and supervise or assist ambulations.

— Withhold the drug if barbiturate toxicity is suspected.

— Do not discontinue the drug abruptly if the patient has been using it for an extended period. The drug may cause dependence and severe withdrawal symptoms. Withdraw barbiturates gradually.

— Take precautions to prevent hoarding or self-overdosing, especially by the patient who is depressed or suicidal or has a history of drug abuse.

— Consult with the patient's doctor to obtain an analgesic order if the patient has pain. Barbiturates have no analgesic effect and may cause restlessness or delirium in presence of pain.

— Keep all members of the health care team informed of the patient's response to the drug.

Patient teaching

— Instruct the patient and family about secobarbital, including the dosage, frequency, action, and adverse reactions.

— Morning "hangover" is common after hypnotic dose. Encourage the patient to report "hangover" or feeling oversedated so the doctor can be consulted for change of dose or drug.

—Explain that hypnotic drugs suppress rapid eye movement (REM) sleep. When drug is discontinued, the patient may experience increased dreaming.
—Instruct the patient to remain in bed after taking drug and to call for assistance to use the bathroom.
—Warn the patient that drug may cause physical dependence.
—Warn the patient to avoid hazardous activities that require mental alertness if adverse CNS reactions are present after awakening.
—Advise the patient to avoid alcoholic beverages during therapy with secobarbital because it may cause excessive CNS depression.
—Tell the patient to notify the nurse or doctor if adverse reactions develop or questions arise about secobarbital therapy.

Evaluation

In the patient receiving secobarbital, appropriate evaluation statements include:
• Patient states drug was effective in inducing sleep.
• Patient can perform usual daily activities.
• Patient and family state an understanding of secobarbital therapy.

PROTOTYPE: BENZODIAZEPINES

FLURAZEPAM HYDROCHLORIDE
(flure az′ e pam)
Apo-Flurazepam†, Dalmane, Durapam, Novoflupam†, Som-Pam†
Classification: benzodiazepine
Controlled substance schedule IV
Pregnancy risk category D

How supplied
CAPSULES: 15 mg, 30 mg

Indications and dosage
Insomnia
ADULTS: 15 to 30 mg P.O. h.s. May repeat dose once.
ADULTS OVER AGE 65: 15 mg P.O. h.s.

Contraindications and precautions
Flurazepam is contraindicated in patients with known hypersensitivity to the drug. Use with caution in patients with impaired hepatic or renal function, mental depression, suicidal tendencies, or history of drug abuse.

Adverse reactions
BLOOD: **leukopenia**, granulocytopenia.
CNS: *daytime sedation, dizziness, drowsiness, disturbed coordination,* lethargy, confusion, *headache.*
GI: nausea, vomiting, heartburn.
METABOLIC: elevated liver enzymes.

---

† Available in Canada only
Italicized adverse reactions are common   Boldfaced adverse reactions are life-threatening

Interactions

Alcohol or other CNS depressants, including narcotic analgesics: excessive CNS depression. Use together cautiously.

Cimetidine: increased sedation. Monitor carefully.

Nursing considerations

Assessment

• Review the patient's history for any condition that contraindicates the use of flurazepam.

• Obtain a baseline assessment of the patient's sleeping patterns before therapy.

• Be alert for common adverse reactions.

• Evaluate the patient's and family's knowledge about flurazepam therapy.

Planning (Nursing Diagnoses)

Potential nursing diagnoses for the patient receiving flurazepam include:

• Sleep pattern disturbance related to ineffectiveness of flurazepam.

• Pain related to flurazepam-induced headache.

• Potential for injury related to drug-induced CNS effects.

• Knowledge deficit related to flurazepam therapy.

Implementation

Preparation and administration

—Before leaving the bedside, make sure the patient has swallowed capsule.

Monitoring

—Regularly monitor the effectiveness of flurazepam by evaluating the patient's ability to sleep after administration. Be aware that drug is more effective on second, third, and fourth nights of use.

—Monitor the patient for adverse drug reactions.

—Monitor the patient's mental status and activity tolerance after awakening for adverse CNS reactions. Remember that elderly patients are more sensitive to the drug's adverse CNS effects.

—Monitor the patient for evidence of dependency during prolonged use.

—Regularly monitor the patient's CBC and liver enzymes for abnormalities.

—Monitor the patient for drug interactions.

—Regularly reevaluate the patient's and family's knowledge about flurazepam therapy.

Intervention

—After dosing, institute safety precautions: keep patient on bed rest, keep bed rails up, and supervise or assist ambulations.

—Take precautions to prevent hoarding or self-overdosing, especially by the patients who is depressed, suicidal, or drug-dependent or who has a history of drug abuse.

—Obtain an analgesic order if the patient experiences a headache after administration of the drug.

—If the patient develops chronic insomnia, attempt to use non-pharmacologic methods to induce sleep to avoid physical dependence.

—Monitor and assist the patient with daytime activities if adverse CNS reactions occur.

—Keep all members of the health care team informed of the patient's response to the drug.

Patient teaching

—Instruct the patient and family about flurazepam, including the dosage, frequency, action, and adverse reactions.

—Explain to the patient that drug is more effective on second, third, and fourth nights of use because active metabolite accumulates. Encourage the patient to continue drug if it doesn't work the first night.

—Instruct the patient to remain in bed after taking drug and to call for assistance to use bathroom.

—Warn the patient to avoid driving and other hazardous activities that require mental alertness if adverse CNS reactions are present after awakening.

—Advise the patient to avoid alcoholic beverages during therapy with flurazepam because they may cause excessive CNS depression.

—Tell the patient that long term use may cause dependency; encourage the patient to induce sleep with nonpharmacologic measures.

—Tell the patient to take a mild analgesic, if not contraindicated, for flurazepam-induced headaches.

—Tell the patient to notify the nurse or doctor if adverse reactions develop or questions arise about therapy.

Evaluation

In the patient receiving flurazepam, appropriate evaluation statements include:

• Patient states drug was effective in inducing sleep.
• Patient states pain is relieved.
• Patient does not experience injury as a result of CNS effects of the drug.
• Patient and family state an understanding of flurazepam therapy.

PROTOTYPE: MISCELLANEOUS SEDATIVE-HYPNOTICS

CHLORAL HYDRATE
(klor′ al hi′ drate)
Aquachloral Supprettes, Noctec, Novochlorhydrate†
Classification: sedative-hypnotic
Controlled substance schedule IV
Pregnancy risk category C

How supplied
CAPSULES: 250 mg, 500 mg

SYRUP: 250 mg/5 ml, 500 mg/5 ml
SUPPOSITORIES: 325 mg, 500 mg, 648 mg

Indications and dosage

Sedation
ADULTS: 250 mg P.O. or P.R. t.i.d. after meals.
CHILDREN: 8 mg/kg P.O. t.i.d. Maximum dosage is 500 mg t.i.d.

Insomnia
ADULTS: 500 mg to 1 g P.O. or P.R. 15 to 30 minutes before bedtime.
CHILDREN: 50 mg/kg P.O. as a single dose. Maximum dosage is 1 g daily.

Premedication for EEG
CHILDREN: 25 mg/kg P.O. as a single dose. Maximum dosage is 1 g daily.

Contraindications and precautions
Chloral hydrate is contraindicated in marked hepatic or renal impairment
and hypersensitivity to chloral hydrate or trichloroethanol. Oral administration is contraindicated in gastric disorders. Use cautiously in patients
with severe cardiac disease, mental depression, and suicidal tendencies.

Adverse reactions
BLOOD: eosinophilia.
CNS: *hangover, drowsiness,* nightmares, dizziness, ataxia, paradoxical
excitement.
GI: *nausea,* vomiting, diarrhea, flatulence.
SKIN: **hypersensitivity reactions**.

Interactions
Alcohol and other CNS depressants, including narcotic analgesics: ex-
cessive CNS depression or vasodilation reaction. Use together cautiously.
Furosemide I.V.: sweating, flushes, variable blood pressure, and uneasi-
ness. Use together cautiously or use a different hypnotic drug.
Oral anticoagulants: increased risk of bleeding. Monitor patient closely.

Nursing considerations

Assessment
• Review the patient's history for a condition that contraindicates the use
of chloral hydrate.
• Obtain a baseline assessment of patient's sleeping patterns before ther-
apy.
• Be alert for common adverse reactions.
• Evaluate the patient's and family's knowledge about chloral hydrate
therapy.

Planning (Nursing Diagnoses)
Potential nursing diagnoses for the patient receiving chloral hydrate in-
clude:
• Sleep pattern disturbance related to ineffectiveness of chloral hydrate.
• Fluid volume deficit related to potential chloral hydrate–induced adverse
GI reactions (nausea, vomiting, diarrhea).
• Knowledge deficit related to chloral hydrate therapy.

Implementation

Preparation and administration

— Dilute syrup with adequate fluid (4 oz glass water, fruit juice, or ginger ale) or administer with 8 oz of liquid to minimize unpleasant taste and stomach irritation. Administer after meals.
— Store drug in dark container; store suppositories in refrigerator.
— Before leaving the bedside, make sure the patient has swallowed oral medication.

Monitoring

— Monitor the effectiveness of chloral hydrate by evaluating the patient's ability to sleep after administration.
— Monitor the patient for adverse drug reactions.
— Monitor the patient's mental status and activity level after patient awakens for evidence of adverse CNS effects.
— Monitor the patient's fluid intake and watch for evidence of dehydration if adverse GI reactions occur.
— Monitor the patient for drug interactions.
— Regularly reevaluate the patient's and family's knowledge about chloral hydrate therapy.

Intervention

— After dosing, institute safety precautions: keep patient on bed rest, keep bed rails up, and supervise or assist ambulations.
— Notify the doctor if adverse GI reactions occur and obtain an antiemetic order as needed. Encourage the patient to sip water or ice chips frequently until adverse GI reactions disappear; expect the doctor to discontinue chloral hydrate if adverse GI reactions are severe.
— When interpreting test results, be aware that high dosage may raise BUN level and may interfere with fluorometric tests for urine catecholamines and Reddy-Jenkins-Thorn test for urine 17-hydroxycorticosteroids. Do not administer drug for 48 hours before fluorometric test.
— Take precautions to prevent hoarding or self-overdosing by the patient who is depressed, suicidal, or drug-dependent or who has a history of drug abuse.
— Keep all members of the health care team informed of the patient's response to the drug.

Patient teaching

— Instruct the patient and family about chloral hydrate, including dosage, frequency, action, and adverse reactions.
— Instruct the patient to remain in bed after taking the drug and to call for assistance to use the bathroom.
— Explain to the patient that morning "hangover" can occur after drug administration. Encourage the patient to report such effects or feelings of oversedation so the doctor can be consulted to adjust or change drug.
— Warn the patient to avoid hazardous activities that require mental alertness if adverse CNS reactions occur after awakening.

— Advise the patient to avoid alcoholic beverages during chloral hydrate therapy because this combination may cause excessive CNS depression.

— Tell the patient to notify the nurse or doctor if adverse reactions develop or questions arise about chloral hydrate therapy.

Evaluation

In the patient receiving chloral hydrate, appropriate evaluation statements include:

• Patient states drug was effective in inducing sleep.
• Patient maintains adequate hydration.
• Patient and family state an understanding of chloral hydrate therapy.

SELECTED MAJOR DRUGS: SEDATIVE-HYPNOTICS

DRUG, INDICATIONS, AND DOSAGES	SPECIAL PRECAUTIONS
Barbiturates	
amobarbital (Amytal) **amobarbital sodium (Amytal Sodium)** *Sedation—* **Adults:** usually 30 to 50 mg P.O. b.i.d. or t.i.d. but may range from 15 to 120 mg b.i.d. to q.i.d. **Children:** 3 to 6 mg/kg P.O. daily in four equally divided doses. *Insomnia—* **Adults:** 65 to 200 mg P.O. or deep I.M. h.s.; I.M. injection not to exceed 5 ml in any one site. Maximum dosage is 500 mg daily. **Children:** 3 to 5 mg/kg deep I.M. h.s.; I.M. injection not to exceed 5 ml in any one site. *Preanesthetic sedation—* **Adults and children:** 200 mg P.O. or I.M. 1 to 2 hours before surgery. *Manic reactions, as an adjunct in psychotherapy, anticonvulsant—* **Adults and children over age 6:** 65 to 500 mg slow I.V.; rate not to exceed 100 mg/minute. Maximum dosage is 1 g. **Children under age 6:** 3 to 5 mg/kg slow I.V. or I.M.	• Contraindicated in patients with known hypersensitivity to barbiturates, uncontrolled severe pain, respiratory disease with dyspnea or obstruction, previous addiction to sedatives, or porphyria. • Use cautiously in patients with hepatic or renal impairment.
aprobarbital (Alurate) *Sedation—* **Adults:** 15 to 40 mg P.O. t.i.d. or q.i.d.; usual dose is 40 mg t.i.d. *Insomnia—* **Adults:** 40 to 160 mg P.O. h.s.	• Contraindicated in patients with known hypersensitivity to barbiturates, uncontrolled severe pain, respiratory disease with dyspnea or obstruction, previous addiction to sedatives, or porphyria. • Use cautiously in patients with hepatic or renal impairment and in elderly patients.

SELECTED MAJOR DRUGS: SEDATIVE-HYPNOTICS *continued*

DRUG, INDICATIONS, AND DOSAGES	SPECIAL PRECAUTIONS

Barbiturates *(continued)*

butabarbital sodium (Barbased, Butalan, Buticaps, Butisol)
Sedation—
Adults: 15 to 30 mg P.O. t.i.d. or q.i.d.
Children: 6 mg/kg P.O. divided t.i.d. Dosage range is 7.5 to 30 mg P.O. t.i.d.
Preoperatively—
Adults: 50 to 100 mg P.O. 60 to 90 minutes before surgery.
Insomnia—
Adults: 50 to 100 mg P.O. h.s.

• Contraindicated in patients with known hypersensitivity to barbiturates, uncontrolled severe pain, respiratory disease with dyspnea or obstruction, previous addiction to sedatives, or porphyria.
• Use cautiously in patients with hepatic or renal impairment.

pentobarbital (Nembutal)
pentobarbital sodium (Nembutal Sodium)
Sedation—
Adults: 20 to 40 mg P.O. b.i.d., t.i.d., or q.i.d.
Children: 6 mg/kg P.O. daily in divided doses.
Insomnia—
Adults: 100 to 200 mg P.O. h.s. or 150 to 200 mg deep I.M.; initially, 100 mg I.V., then additional doses up to 500 mg; or 120 to 200 mg P.R.
Children: 3 to 5 mg/kg I.M. Maximum dosage is 100 mg. Rectal dosages are ages 2 months to 1 year, 30 mg; ages 1 to 4, 30 to 60 mg; ages 5 to 12, 60 mg; ages 12 to 14, 60 to 120 mg.
Preanesthetic medication—
Adults: 150 to 200 mg I.M. or P.O. in two divided doses.

• Contraindicated in patients with emotional instability and with a history of drug abuse, head injury, or increased intracranial pressure.
• Use cautiously in patients with hepatic and renal disease. These patients may overreact to customary doses.

phenobarbital (Barbita, Luminal†)
phenobarbital sodium (Luminal†)
Sedation—
Adults: 30 to 120 mg P.O. daily in two or three divided doses.
Children: 6 mg/kg P.O. divided t.i.d.
Insomnia—
Adults: 100 to 320 mg P.O. or I.M.
Children: 3 to 6 mg/kg.
Preoperative sedation—
Adults: 100 to 200 mg I.M. 60 to 90 minutes before surgery.
Children: 16 to 100 mg I.M. 60 to 90 minutes before surgery.

• Contraindicated in patients with known hypersensitivity to barbiturates, porphyria, hepatic dysfunction, respiratory disease with dyspnea or obstruction, and nephritis and in breast-feeding women.
• Use cautiously in hyperthyroidism, diabetes mellitus, and anemia and in elderly or debilitated patients.

(continued)

†Available in Canada only

SELECTED MAJOR DRUGS: SEDATIVE-HYPNOTICS *continued*

DRUG, INDICATIONS, AND DOSAGES	SPECIAL PRECAUTIONS
Benzodiazepines	
estazolam (ProSom) *Insomnia* — **Adults:** 1 mg P.O. h.s. Some patients may require 2 mg.	• Contraindicated in patients with known hypersensitivity to the drug or other benzodiazepines, in pregnant women, and in patients with suspected or established sleep apnea.
quazepam (Doral) *Insomnia* — **Adults:** 15 mg P.O. h.s. Some patients may respond to lower doses. Decrease dosage in elderly patients to 7.5 mg P.O. h.s. after 2 days of therapy.	• Contraindicated in patients with known hypersensitivity to the drug or other benzodiazepines, in pregnant women, and in patients with suspected or established sleep apnea.
temazepam (Restoril) *Insomnia* — **Adults:** 15 to 30 mg P.O. h.s. **Adults over age 65:** 15 mg P.O. h.s.	• Use cautiously in patients with impaired hepatic or renal function, mental depression, suicidal tendencies, and a history of drug abuse. Use caution and low end-of-dosage range for elderly or debilitated patients.
triazolam (Halcion) *Insomnia* — **Adults:** 0.125 to 0.25 mg P.O. h.s. **Adults over age 65:** 0.125 mg P.O. h.s.; increase to 0.25 mg P.O. h.s. p.r.n.	• Use cautiously in patients with impaired hepatic or renal function, mental depression, suicidal tendencies, or a history of drug abuse.
Miscellaneous agents	
acetylcarbromal (Paxarel) *Anxiety states* — **Adults:** 250 to 300 mg P.O. b.i.d. or t.i.d.	• Acts by releasing bromine in the serum; therefore, contraindicated in patients with known hypersensitivity to bromides.
ethchlorvynol (Placidyl) *Sedation* — **Adults:** 100 to 200 mg P.O. b.i.d. or t.i.d. *Insomnia* — **Adults:** 500 mg to 1 g P.O. h.s. May repeat 100 to 200 mg if awakened in early morning.	• Contraindicated in patients with uncontrolled pain and porphyria. • Use cautiously in patients with hepatic or renal impairment and in patients with mental depression with suicidal tendencies, in elderly or debilitated patients, and if patient has previously overreacted to barbiturates or alcohol.

SELECTED MAJOR DRUGS: SEDATIVE-HYPNOTICS *continued*

DRUG, INDICATIONS, AND DOSAGES	SPECIAL PRECAUTIONS

Miscellaneous agents *(continued)*

glutethimide (Doriden)
Insomnia —
Adults: 250 to 500 mg P.O. h.s. May be repeated, but not less than 4 hours before intended awakening. Total dosage should not exceed 1 g daily.

• Contraindicated in patients with uncontrolled pain, severe renal impairment, or porphyria.
• Use cautiously in patients with mental depression, suicidal tendencies, a history of drug abuse, prostatic hypertrophy, stenosing peptic ulcer, pyloroduodenal or bladder-neck obstruction, narrow-angle glaucoma, and cardiac arrhythmias.

methotrimeprazine (Levoprome, Nozinan†)
Postoperative analgesia —
Adults and children over age 12: 2.5 to 7.5 mg I.M. q 4 to 6 hours, then adjust dose.
Preanesthetic medication —
Adults and children over age 12: 2 to 20 mg I.M. 45 minutes to 3 hours before surgery.
Sedation, analgesia —
Adults and children over age 12: 10 to 20 mg deep I.M. q 4 to 6 hours as required; or 6 to 25 mg P.O. daily in three divided doses with meals. For severe pain, dosage may be increased to 50 to 75 mg daily in two or three divided doses with meals.
Adults over age 65: 5 to 10 mg I.M. q 4 to 6 hours.
Psychosis —
Adults: 6 to 25 mg P.O. daily in three divided doses with meals. Dosage may be gradually increased p.r.n. and as tolerated to 50 to 75 mg P.O. daily in two or three divided doses.

• Contraindicated in patients receiving concurrent antihypertensive drug therapy, including MAO inhibitors, and in those with a history of seizure disorder; known hypersensitivity to phenothiazines; severe cardiac, hepatic, or renal disease; previous overdose of CNS depressant; or coma.
• Use with extreme caution in elderly or debilitated patients with cardiac disease or in patients who may suffer serious consequences from a sudden drop in blood pressure. Because the injectable form contains sulfites, use cautiously in asthmatic patients or in patients with sulfite sensitivity.

methyprylon (Noludar)
Insomnia —
Adults: 200 to 400 mg P.O. 15 minutes before bedtime.
Children over age 3 months: 50 mg P.O. h.s., increased to 200 mg if necessary. Maximum dosage is 400 mg daily.

• Use with extreme caution in head injury, increased intracranial pressure, seizures, asthma, COPD, alcoholism, increased CSF pressure, acute abdominal conditions, prostatic hypertrophy, severe hepatic or renal disease, urethral stricture, CNS depression, respiratory depression, hypothyroidism, Addison's disease, cardiac arrhythmias, reduced blood volume, and toxic psychosis and in elderly or debilitated patients.

†Available in Canada only

SELF-TEST

1. Tim O'Connor, age 76, is in skeletal traction for the treatment of a femoral fracture. His doctor has ordered secobarbital 100 mg P.O. h.s. p.r.n. When the nurse offers his bedtime dose, Mr. O'Connor tells her, "I'll take it after I finish watching the ball game on TV. Please leave it here by my glass of water." The nurse should tell Mr. O'Connor she will:
   a. leave the medication and come back in 30 minutes to see if he has taken it.
   b. phone his doctor to obtain an order permitting compliance with this request.
   c. return with the medication when the ball game is over.
   d. withhold the medication for tonight.

2. After administering secobarbital to Mr. O'Connor, the nurse should observe him for which of the following adverse reactions?
   a. paradoxical excitement
   b. bronchospasms
   c. abdominal cramps
   d. headache

3. May Smith is recovering from an abdominal hysterectomy. She requests a sleeping pill the second night postoperatively because of insomnia. The nurse obtains an order for chloral hydrate 500 mg P.O. h.s. p.r.n. Before administering the drug, she reviews Ms. Smith's medical history. Which of the following conditions contraindicates the use of this drug?
   a. peptic ulcer disease
   b. hepatic impairment
   c. mental depression
   d. asthma

4. Barbara Tyler, a 68-year-old retired teacher, was admitted yesterday with pneumonia. She received flurazepam last night. This morning she tells the nurse she believes the drug was not helpful because she did not experience a restful sleep. The nurse should then:
   a. consult with the doctor about the possibility of increasing the drug dose.
   b. tell the patient she'll ask the doctor to change to another bedtime sedative.
   c. explain that this drug becomes more effective after the first dose.
   d. encourage the patient to ask for the drug earlier in the evening.

5. What is the usual dosage for an adult over age 65?
   a. 5 mg
   b. 15 mg
   c. 30 mg
   d. 45 mg

Check your answers on page 1063.

CHAPTER 29

ANTICONVULSANTS

Barbiturate derivatives
mephobarbital ✦ phenobarbital ✦ phenobarbital sodium ✦ primidone

Benzodiazepine derivatives
clonazepam ✦ diazepam

Hydantoin derivatives
ethotoin ✦ mephenytoin ✦ phenacemide ✦ phenytoin

Miscellaneous agents
acetazolamide ✦ carbamazepine ✦ divalproex sodium ✦ ethosuximide
methsuximide ✦ paramethadione ✦ phensuximide ✦ trimethadione
valproate sodium ✦ valproic acid

OVERVIEW

- Each anticonvulsant is used to treat specific seizure disorders. Frequently, these drugs are used in combination for complex or mixed-seizure disorders. For specific indications in seizures, see *Use of Anticonvulsants in Seizure Disorders,* page 395. Seizures may be of unknown origin (idiopathic) or secondary to some organic or acquired condition. When their etiology is known, therapy is often aimed at the underlying cause as well.
- Anticonvulsants are classified primarily into four groups: barbiturate derivatives, benzodiazepine derivatives, hydantoin derivatives, and miscellaneous agents (including succinimide and oxazolinedione derivatives).

MAJOR USES

- Anticonvulsants prevent or reduce the frequency or severity of seizures in idiopathic seizure disorder or seizures secondary to drugs, hypoglycemia, hypomagnesemia, meningitis, eclampsia, encephalitis, alcohol withdrawal syndrome, or traumatic brain injury.

MECHANISM OF ACTION

- Barbiturate derivatives depress monosynaptic and polysynaptic transmission in the CNS and increase the threshold for seizure activity in the motor cortex.

GLOSSARY

Absence seizure: generalized seizure characterized by an abrupt loss of consciousness or unawareness with staring; formerly called petit mal seizure.

Atonic seizure: generalized seizure accompanied by akinesia and usually loss of consciousness.

Clonic seizure: generalized seizure characterized by rhythmic contraction and relaxation of muscles, loss of consciousness, and marked autonomic signs and symptoms.

Electroencephalogram: graphic recording of electrical currents produced in the brain.

Epilepsy: disorder characterized by one or more of the following signs and symptoms: paroxysmally recurring impairment or loss of consciousness, involuntary excess or cessation of muscle movements, psychic or sensory disturbances, and derangement of the autonomic nervous system. Also called seizure disorder.

Generalized seizure: bilaterally symmetrical, violent, involuntary contractions of voluntary muscles involving loss of consciousness; more specifically classified as absence, myoclonic, clonic, tonic, tonic-clonic, or atonic seizure.

Myoclonic seizure: generalized seizure characterized by bilaterally symmetrical, involuntary lightning jerks of voluntary muscles lasting from seconds to minutes; consciousness is maintained.

Partial seizure: focal or local violent, involuntary contractions of voluntary muscles; more specifically classified as simple or complex.

Relaxant: agent that reduces or lessens muscle tension.

Rigidity: abnormal muscle stiffness or inflexibility.

Status epilepticus: series of rapidly repeated seizures without periods of consciousness separating them.

Tonic-clonic seizure: generalized seizure characterized by contraction of all skeletal muscles in rhythmic alternating tonic and clonic patterns, followed by depression of all central functions; formerly known as grand mal seizure.

Tonic seizure: generalized seizure characterized by an abrupt increase in muscle tone, resulting in contraction, loss of consciousness, and marked autonomic signs and symptoms.

- Benzodiazepine derivatives appear to act on the limbic system, thalamus, and hypothalamus to produce anticonvulsant effects. Both benzodiazepines and barbiturates are also used as sedative-hypnotics (see Chapter 28, Sedative-Hypnotics).

- Hydantoin derivatives and carbamazepine stabilize neuronal membranes and limit seizure activity by either increasing efflux or decreasing influx of sodium ions across cell membranes in the motor cortex during generation of nerve impulses.

USE OF ANTICONVULSANTS IN SEIZURE DISORDERS

DRUG	GENERAL-IZED TONIC-CLONIC	ABSENCE	MYO-CLONIC	MIXED	COMPLEX PARTIAL	STATUS EPILEPTI-CUS
Barbiturate derivatives						
mephobarbital	✔	✔				
phenobarbital	✔	✔	✔	✔	✔	
primidone	✔				✔	
Benzodiazepine derivatives						
clonazepam		✔	✔			
diazepam						✔
Hydantoin derivatives						
ethotoin	✔				✔	
mephenytoin	✔				✔	
phenacemide				✔	✔	
phenytoin	✔				✔	✔
Miscellaneous agents						
acetazolamide		✔				
carbamazepine	✔			✔	✔	
ethosuximide		✔				
methsuximide		✔				
paramethadione		✔				
phensuximide		✔				
trimethadione		✔				
valproic acid and its derivatives		✔				

Note: Magnesium sulfate and paraldehyde are not included in this list since they are used to control nonepileptic seizures.

- Miscellaneous agents exert their effects by various mechanisms. Acetazolamide may inhibit carbonic anhydrase in the CNS and decrease abnormal paroxysmal or excessive neuronal discharge. (For discussion of diuretic use of acetazolamide, see Chapter 61, Diuretics.)
- Oxazolidinedione derivatives raise the threshold for cortical seizures but do not modify seizure patterns. They decrease projection of focal activity and reduce both repetitive spinal-cord transmission and spike-and-wave patterns of absence seizures.
- Succinimide derivatives raise the seizure threshold. They reduce the paroxysmal spike-and-wave pattern of absence seizures by depressing nerve transmission in the motor cortex.
- Valproic acid may increase brain levels of gamma-aminobutyric acid, which transmits inhibitory nerve impulses in the CNS.

ABSORPTION, DISTRIBUTION, METABOLISM, AND EXCRETION

Anticonvulsants are generally well absorbed from the GI tract and widely distributed in the tissues, including the CNS. They're metabolized by the liver and excreted by the kidneys.

Because barbiturate derivatives induce microsomal enzymes in the liver, they may accelerate metabolism of other anticonvulsant drugs given concurrently.

ONSET AND DURATION

Onset and duration of action vary with each drug and from patient to patient. When parenteral preparations are used for acute episodes (for example, status epilepticus or eclampsia), onset is immediate.

Most anticonvulsants have half-lives of several hours to days, and they may require days or even weeks of therapy to achieve steady-state blood concentrations.

ADVERSE REACTIONS

Adverse reactions to barbiturate derivatives most commonly reflect CNS depression and may include drowsiness, the most common reaction, lethargy, vertigo, headache, and confusion. In patients with severe pain, in elderly patients, or in children, they may cause paradoxical excitement. Because barbiturate derivatives produce hyperalgesia, they should be used cautiously in patients with severe untreated or chronic pain. Long-term use is associated with the development of tolerance and dependence. When hypnotic doses of barbiturate derivatives are discontinued, the patient may experience increased dreams or nightmares; when barbiturate derivatives used to control seizures are abruptly withdrawn or dosage is reduced, seizure activity may rebound. Headache and fever have been reported with chronic use of phenobarbital. Other reactions to barbiturate derivatives may include respiratory depression leading to apnea and circulatory collapse, laryngospasm, and bronchospasm. Bradycardia, hypotension, and syncope may occur, especially after rapid I.V. administration. GI reactions include constipation or diarrhea, nausea, vomiting, and epigastric pain. Allergic reactions most frequently associated with phenobarbital, and mephobarbital result in skin rashes, urticaria, angioedema, fever, and serum sickness; rarely, erythema multiforme or Stevens-Johnson syndrome may occur.

Benzodiazepine derivatives usually produce adverse reactions that include the CNS effects of drowsiness, ataxia, fatigue, confusion, weakness, headache, dizziness, vertigo, and syncope. These reactions are most likely to occur in patients with hepatic or renal dysfunction and in children or elderly or debilitated patients; such patients should receive lower initial doses of these drugs. All patients who take a benzodiazepine as a sleeping aid, especially those who are elderly, may have increased daytime sedation or other prolonged adverse CNS reactions. This effect is intensified if the benzodiazepine is taken for prolonged periods because serum levels of the medication will increase. Prolonged use of benzodiazepines with a long half-life, such as diazepam, clorazepate, or chlordiazepoxide, has been associated with increased incidence of falls in elderly patients. Other adverse CNS reactions include euphoria, nightmares, and hallucinations. Psychological and physical dependence occur with long-term use and may result in withdrawal symptoms. Rarely, paradoxical reactions produce an acute hyperexcited state with anxiety, hallucinations, insomnia, or rage; such reactions require discontinuation of the drug. Triazolam has been associated with paradoxical reactions and anterograde amnesia.

Adverse GI reactions include constipation, dry mouth, taste alterations, anorexia, nausea, vomiting, and abdominal discomfort. Hiccups have also been reported. Respiratory depression may occur but is usually associated with overdosage or an interaction with another respiratory depressant. Other adverse reactions are rare. They include CV effects (tachycardia, palpitations, and hypotension), dermatologic reactions (rashes, urticaria, and flushing), and urinary incontinence or urine retention.

Hydantoin derivatives frequently produce adverse reactions that vary widely and may have serious consequences. Most patients tolerate the hydantoin derivatives when blood concentrations are maintained in the therapeutic range. Adverse reactions may subside during chronic therapy.

Adverse CNS reactions are the most common and are usually dose-related. Ataxia, slurred speech, mental confusion, dizziness, insomnia, nervousness, twitching, drowsiness, and headache are possible. Nystagmus is dose-related and may be one of the first symptoms of toxicity. Diplopia and blurred vision may also occur.

GI reactions are common but usually consist of nausea, vomiting, diarrhea, or constipation. These reactions may be minimized by administration of the drug with meals. Gingival hyperplasia, especially in children, is frequently associated with phenytoin and may be severe enough to require surgical intervention. Meticulous oral hygiene may reduce the incidence of gingival hyperplasia.

CV reactions usually follow I.V. administration of phenytoin and may include hypotension (if the drug is administered too rapidly), ventricular fibrillation, and CV collapse. These reactions are more common in patients who are elderly and gravely ill.

Dermatologic reactions include scarlatiniform or morbilliform rashes; bullous, exfoliative, or purpuric dermatitis; Stevens-Johnson syndrome; lupus erythematosus; hirsutism; toxic epidermal necrolysis, and photosensitivity. Many of these reactions may be fatal. Coarsening of the facial features, enlargement of the lips, and Peyronie's disease may be the result of long-term use of hydantoin derivatives.

Hydantoin derivatives have also been associated with hepatitis and liver damage and with severe hematologic reactions: thrombocytopenia, leukopenia, granulocytopenia, agranulocytosis, and pancytopenia. Anemia may also occur and usually responds to folic acid therapy.

Among the miscellaneous anticonvulsants, valproic acid has been associated with hepatic failure. This reaction is more common when the drug is used in high doses or in combination with other anticonvulsants, especially in children under age 2. Baseline hepatic function tests and periodic monitoring of liver function tests are recommended.

Most anticonvulsants, including succinimide derivatives (ethosuximide, methsuximide, and phensuximide), carbamazepine, and oxazolidinedione derivatives (paramethadione and trimethadione), have been associated with aplastic anemia or agranulocytosis. The overall risk of these disorders is low, but undiagnosed bone marrow suppression can be fatal. Therefore, patients should receive a thorough hematologic evaluation before therapy and periodic blood studies during therapy.

Acetazolamide may cause metabolic acidosis or hypokalemia.

Other adverse reactions include dizziness, drowsiness, unsteadiness, nausea, and vomiting. These adverse reactions can be minimized by starting therapy at a low dosage and gradually increasing as needed and tolerated.

Oxazolidinedione derivatives (paramethadione and trimethadione) were once the drugs of choice for absence seizures but are now used only when the seizures are refractory to other anticonvulsants. They are of no use in generalized tonic-clonic seizures and may actually precipitate new seizures or increase the frequency of preexisting generalized tonic-clonic seizures.

PHENOBARBITAL (PHENOBARBITONE)
(fee noe bar' bi tal)
Barbita, Gardenal†, Luminal†, Solfoton

PHENOBARBITAL SODIUM (PHENOBARBITONE SODIUM)
Luminal Sodium†
Classification: barbiturate derivative
Controlled substance schedule IV
Pregnancy risk category D

How supplied
TABLETS: 8 mg, 15 mg, 16 mg, 30 mg, 32 mg, 60 mg, 65 mg, 100 mg
CAPSULES: 16 mg
ORAL SOLUTION: 15 mg/5 ml, 20 mg/5 ml
ELIXIR: 20 mg/5 ml
INJECTION: 30 mg/ml, 60 mg/ml, 65 mg/ml, 130 mg/ml
POWDER FOR INJECTION: 120 mg/ampule

Indications and dosage
All forms of seizure disorder, febrile seizures in children
ADULTS: 100 to 200 mg P.O. daily divided t.i.d. or given as a single dosage h.s.
CHILDREN: 4 to 6 mg/kg P.O. daily usually divided q 12 hours. It can, however, be administered once daily usually h.s.

Status epilepticus
ADULTS: 10 mg/kg as I.V. infusion no faster than 50 mg/minute. May give up to 20 mg/kg total. Administer in acute care or emergency area only.
CHILDREN: 5 to 10 mg/kg I.V. May repeat q 10 to 15 minutes up to a total of 20 mg/kg I.V. Injection rate should not exceed 50 mg/minute.

Sedation
ADULTS: 30 to 120 mg P.O. daily in two or three divided doses.
CHILDREN: 6 mg/kg P.O. divided t.i.d.

Insomnia
ADULTS: 100 to 320 mg P.O. or I.M.
CHILDREN: 3 to 6 mg/kg P.O.

Preoperative sedation
ADULTS: 100 to 200 mg I.M. 60 to 90 minutes before surgery.
CHILDREN: 16 to 100 mg I.M. 60 to 90 minutes before surgery.

Hyperbilirubinemia
NEONATES: 7 mg/kg P.O. daily from first to fifth day of life; or 5 mg/kg daily I.M. on first day, repeated P.O. on second to seventh days.

Chronic cholestasis
ADULTS: 90 to 180 mg P.O. daily in two or three divided doses.

---

†Available in Canada only

CHILDREN UNDER AGE 12: 3 to 12 mg/kg P.O. daily in two or three divided doses.

Contraindications and precautions
Phenobarbital is contraindicated in barbiturate hypersensitivity, porphyria, hepatic dysfunction, respiratory disease with dyspnea or obstruction, and nephritis and in lactating women. Use cautiously in hyperthyroidism, diabetes mellitus, and anemia and in elderly or debilitated patients.

Adverse reactions
CNS: *drowsiness, lethargy, hangover,* paradoxical excitement in elderly patients.
GI: nausea, vomiting.
SKIN: rash, **Stevens-Johnson syndrome,** urticaria.
LOCAL: pain, swelling, thrombophlebitis, necrosis, nerve injury.
OTHER: angioedema, **respiratory depression** (with overdose).

Interactions
Alcohol and other CNS depressants, including narcotic analgesics: excessive CNS depression. Use cautiously.
Diazepam: increased effects of both drugs. Use together.
Griseofulvin: decreased absorption of griseofulvin. Monitor for decreased effectiveness.
MAO inhibitors: potentiated barbiturate effect. Monitor for increased CNS and respiratory depression.
Oral anticoagulants, estrogens and oral contraceptives, doxycycline, corticosteroids: may enhance the metabolism of these drugs. Monitor for decreased effect.
Primidone: increased phenobarbital blood levels. Monitor for excessive phenobarbital blood levels.
Rifampin: may decrease barbiturate levels. Monitor for decreased effect.
Valproic acid: increased phenobarbital levels. Monitor for toxicity.

Nursing considerations
Assessment
- Review the patient's history for a condition that contraindicates the use of phenobarbital.
- Obtain a baseline assessment of the patient's seizure activity, including type, frequency, and presence of aura before therapy.
- Be alert for common adverse reactions.
- Evaluate the patient's and family's knowledge about phenobarbital therapy.

Planning (Nursing Diagnoses)
Potential nursing diagnoses for the patient receiving phenobarbital include:
- Potential for trauma related to uncontrolled seizure activity caused by ineffectiveness of current phenobarbital regime.
- Noncompliance related to need for long-term use of phenobarbital anticonvulsant therapy.

Italicized adverse reactions are common   Boldfaced adverse reactions are life-threatening

• Knowledge deficit related to phenobarbital therapy.

Implementation

Preparation and administration

— Do not use injectable solution if it contains a precipitate.
— Do not mix parenteral form with acidic solutions such as tetracyclines, metaraminol, or methyldopate hydrochloride; precipitation may result. Check with pharmacist before mixing.
— Give I.M. injection deeply. Superficial injection may cause pain, sterile abscess, and tissue sloughing.
— I.V. injection should be reserved for emergency treatment and should be given slowly under close supervision. When administering I.V., do not give more than 60 mg/minute. Have resuscitative equipment readily available.

Monitoring

— Monitor the effectiveness of phenobarbital therapy regularly by assessing seizure activity.
— Monitor the patient for adverse drug reactions.
— Monitor the patient for drug interactions.
— Closely monitor the patient's respiratory rate and depth when administering phenobarbital I.V.
— Monitor for therapeutic blood levels, for example, 15 to 40 mcg/ml for phenobarbital.
— Monitor for signs of barbiturate toxicity: coma, asthmatic breathing, depressed respiratory function, cyanosis, clammy skin, and hypotension.
— Regularly reevaluate the patient's and family's knowledge about phenobarbital therapy.

Intervention

— Maintain seizure precautions; full therapeutic effect of phenobarbital is delayed 2 to 3 weeks, unless loading dose is used.
— Notify the doctor if seizure activity persists despite phenobarbital therapy.
— Withhold dose and notify the doctor if barbiturate toxicity is suspected, then expect to have the patient's barbiturate level determined; if confirmed, anticipate giving a different anticonvulsant.
— Consider and try to prevent potential for noncompliance that may result from the patient's health belief system or life-style.
— If drowsiness or lethargy occurs, institute safety precautions, such as supervising activities.
— Obtain an order for an antiemetic if nausea or vomiting occurs.
— Keep all members of the health care team informed of the patient's response to the drug.

Patient teaching

— Instruct the patient and family about phenobarbital, including the dosage, frequency, action, and adverse reactions.

— Warn the patient to avoid driving and other activities that require alertness and good psychomotor coordination until CNS effects of the drug are known.
— Warn the patient not to discontinue drug abruptly and to call the doctor immediately if adverse reactions develop or if seizure activity occurs.
— Make sure the patient is aware that phenobarbital is available in different milligram strengths. Tell the patient to check with pharmacist if a refill looks different from previous supply.
— Stress the importance of compliance with the prescribed regimen.
— Tell the patient that phenobarbital may interact with different medications; the patient should alert all prescribing doctors that he is taking phenobarbital.
— Advise the patient to carry or wear medical alert identification indicating a seizure disorder and phenobarbital use.
— Warn the patient to avoid alcohol because it may cause excessive CNS depression when used concomitantly with phenobarbital.
— Tell the patient to notify the nurse or doctor if adverse reactions develop or questions arise about phenobarbital therapy.

Evaluation
In the patient receiving phenobarbital, appropriate evaluation statements include:
• Patient is free of seizure activity.
• Patient's barbiturate blood level is within therapeutic range.
• Patient and family state an understanding of phenobarbital therapy.

PROTOTYPE: BENZODIAZEPINE DERIVATIVES

DIAZEPAM
(dye az′ e pam)

Diazemuls†, Apo-Diazepam†, Diazepam Intensol, E-Pam†, Meval†, Novodipam†, Q-Pam, Rival†, Valium, Valrelease, Vazepam, Vivol†, Zetran

Classification: benzodiazepine derivative
Controlled substance schedule IV
Pregnancy risk category D

How supplied
TABLETS: 2 mg, 5 mg, 10 mg
CAPSULES (EXTENDED-RELEASE): 15 mg
ORAL SOLUTION: 5 mg/5 ml, 5 mg/ml
INJECTION: 5 mg/ml
STERILE EMULSION FOR INJECTION: 5 mg/ml†

Indications and dosage

Tension, anxiety, adjunct in seizure disorders or skeletal muscle spasm

ADULTS: 2 to 10 mg P.O. t.i.d. or q.i.d.; or 15 to 30 mg (extended-release capsule) once daily.

CHILDREN OVER AGE 6 MONTHS: 1 to 2.5 mg P.O. t.i.d. or q.i.d.

Tension, anxiety, muscle spasm, endoscopic procedures, seizures

ADULTS: initially, 5 to 10 mg I.V., up to 30 mg in 1 hour or possibly more for cardioversion or status epilepticus, depending on response.

CHILDREN AGES 5 AND OLDER: 1 mg I.V. or I.M. slowly q 2 to 5 minutes to maximum of 10 mg. Repeat q 2 to 4 hours.

CHILDREN AGES 30 DAYS TO 5 YEARS: 0.2 to 0.5 mg I.V. or I.M. slowly q 2 to 5 minutes to maximum of 5 mg. Repeat q 2 to 4 hours.

Tetanic muscle spasms

CHILDREN OVER AGE 5: 5 to 10 mg I.M. or I.V. q 3 to 4 hours p.r.n.

INFANTS OVER AGE 30 DAYS: 1 to 2 mg I.M. or I.V. q 3 to 4 hours p.r.n.

Status epilepticus

ADULTS: 5 to 20 mg by slow I.V. push 2 to 5 mg/minute; may repeat q 5 to 10 minutes up to maximum total dose of 60 mg. Use 2 to 5 mg in elderly or debilitated patients. May repeat therapy in 20 to 30 minutes with caution if seizures recur.

CHILDREN: 0.1 to 0.3 mg/kg by slow I.V. push (1 mg/minute over 3 minutes). May repeat q 15 minutes for two doses. Maximum single dose in children under age 5 is 5 mg; in children over age 5, 10 mg.

Contraindications and precautions

Diazepam is contraindicated in shock, coma, acute alcohol intoxication, acute narrow-angle glaucoma, psychoses, and myasthenia gravis; in oral form, for children under age 6 months. Use with caution in blood dyscrasia, hepatic or renal damage, depression, and open-angle glaucoma; in elderly and debilitated patients; and in those with limited pulmonary reserve.

Adverse reactions

CNS: *drowsiness, lethargy, hangover, ataxia,* fainting, slurred speech, tremor.

CV: transient hypotension, bradycardia, **cardiovascular collapse.**

EENT: diplopia, blurred vision, nystagmus.

GI: nausea, vomiting, abdominal discomfort.

SKIN: rash, urticaria.

LOCAL: desquamation, *pain, phlebitis at injection site (with I.V. use).*

OTHER: **respiratory depression.**

Interactions

Alcohol, other CNS depressants: increased CNS depression. Avoid concomitant use.

Cimetidine: increased sedation. Monitor carefully.

Phenobarbital: increased effects of both drugs. Use together cautiously.

Nursing considerations

Assessment

• Review the patient's history for a condition that contraindicates the use of diazepam.
• Obtain a rapid assessment of status epilepticus before therapy.
• Be alert for common adverse reactions.
• Evaluate the patient's and family's knowledge about I.V. diazepam therapy for the treatment of status epilepticus after the patient's condition has stabilized.

Planning (Nursing Diagnoses)

Potential nursing diagnoses for the patient receiving diazepam include:
• Potential for injury related to potential for recurring seizures.
• Ineffective breathing pattern related to the depressive effect of diazepam on the respiratory system.
• Impaired tissue integrity related to phlebitis at the I.V. site.
• Knowledge deficit related to I.V. diazepam therapy used to treat status epilepticus.

Implementation

Preparation and administration

—Do not mix injectable form with other drugs because diazepam is incompatible with most drugs.
—Considerable controversy surrounds the use of diluted diazepam solutions for continuous I.V. infusion because of its low aqueous solubility. Under certain conditions, it may be compatible with 0.9% sodium chloride solution or Ringer's lactate injection, but the diluted solution may not be stable. Consult hospital pharmacy for further information.
—Avoid extravasation. Do not inject into small veins.
—Give I.V. slowly at rate not exceeding 5 mg/minute. When injecting I.V., administer directly into the vein. If this is not possible, inject slowly through the infusion tubing as close as possible to the vein insertion site.
—I.V. route is more reliable; I.M. administration is not recommended because absorption is variable and injection is painful (because the solution is highly alkaline).
—Do not store diazepam in plastic syringes.
—Dosage should be reduced in elderly or debilitated patients because they may be more susceptible to the adverse CNS effects of the drug.

Monitoring

—Monitor the effectiveness of I.V. diazepam therapy to abolish seizure activity after each dose.
—Monitor respirations every 5 to 15 minutes and before each repeated I.V. dose.
—Monitor the patient for adverse drug reactions.
—Frequently inspect I.V. site for phlebitis.
—Monitor the patient for drug interactions.

Intervention

—Maintain seizure precautions; seizures may recur within 20 to 30 minutes of initial control because of redistribution of the drug.
—Keep emergency equipment and oxygen at the patient's bedside.
—Determine if status epilepticus resulted from noncompliance and take corrective measures as indicated.
—Institute safety precautions because of CNS effects until the effect of diazepam has worn off.
—Change I.V. site if phlebitis occurs.
—Remember that naloxone does not reverse the respiratory depression produced by diazepam.
—Keep all members of the health care team informed of the patient's response to the drug.

Patient teaching

—Inform the patient and family about the use of diazepam to treat status epilepticus. Include the action and adverse reactions.
—Warn the patient to avoid driving and other hazardous activities that require alertness and good psychomotor coordination until CNS effects of the drug have worn off.
—Stress the importance of adhering to the prescribed drug regimen.
—Tell the patient to notify the nurse or doctor if adverse reactions develop or questions arise about diazepam therapy.

Evaluation

In the patient receiving I.V. diazepam, appropriate evaluation statements include:
• Patient is free of seizure activity.
• Patient maintains adequate respiratory function.
• Patient does not develop phlebitis at the I.V. site.
• Patient and family state an understanding of diazepam therapy in the treatment of status epilepticus.

PHENYTOIN
(fen' i toyn)
Dilantin, Dilantin Infatabs, Dilantin-30 Pediatric, Dilantin-125

PHENYTOIN SODIUM
Dilantin

PHENYTOIN SODIUM (EXTENDED)
Dilantin Kapseals

PHENYTOIN SODIUM (PROMPT)
Diphenylan
Classification: hydantoin derivative
Pregnancy risk category D

How supplied

phenytoin
TABLETS CHEWABLE: 50 mg
ORAL SUSPENSION: 30 mg/5 ml, 125 mg/5 ml
phenytoin sodium
CAPSULES: 30 mg (27.6-mg base), 100 mg (92-mg base)
INJECTION: 50 mg/ml (46-mg base)
phenytoin sodium (extended)
CAPSULES: 30 mg (27.6 mg-base), 100 mg (92-mg base)
phenytoin sodium (prompt)
CAPSULES: 30 mg (27.6 mg-base), 100 mg (92-mg base)

Indications and dosage
Generalized tonic-clonic seizures, status epilepticus, nonepileptic seizures (post–head trauma, Reye's syndrome)
ADULTS: loading dose is 900 mg to 1.5 g I.V. at 50 mg/minute or P.O. divided t.i.d., then start maintenance dosage of 300 mg P.O. daily (extended only) or divided t.i.d. (extended or prompt).
CHILDREN: loading dose is 15 mg/kg I.V. at 50 mg/minute or P.O. divided q 8 to 12 hours, then start maintenance dosage of 5 to 7 mg/kg P.O. or I.V. daily divided q 12 hours.

If the patient has not received phenytoin previously or has no detectable blood level, use loading dose
ADULTS: 900 mg to 1.5 g I.V. divided t.i.d. at 50 mg/minute. Do not exceed 500 mg each dose.
CHILDREN: 15 mg/kg I.V. at 50 mg/minute.

If the patient has been receiving phenytoin but has missed one or more doses and has subtherapeutic levels
ADULTS: 100 to 300 mg I.V. at 50 mg/minute.
CHILDREN: 5 to 7 mg/kg I.V. at 50 mg/minute. May repeat lower dose in 30 minutes if needed.

Neuritic pain (migraine, trigeminal neuralgia, Bell's palsy)
ADULTS: 200 to 400 mg P.O. daily.

Ventricular arrhythmias unresponsive to lidocaine or procainamide; supraventricular and ventricular arrhythmias induced by digitalis glycosides
ADULTS: loading dose is 1 g P.O. divided over first 24 hours, followed by 500 mg daily for 2 days, then maintenance dosage of 300 mg P.O. daily; or 250 mg I.V. over 5 minutes; repeat dosage as needed until arrhythmias subside, adverse reactions develop, or 1 g has been given. Infusion rate should never exceed 50 mg/minute (slow I.V. push).
Alternate method: 100 mg I.V. q 15 minutes until adverse reactions develop, arrhythmias are controlled, or 1 g has been given. May also administer entire loading dose of 1 g I.V. slowly at 25 mg/minute. Can be diluted in 0.9% sodium chloride solution. I.M. dose not recommended because of pain and erratic absorption.
CHILDREN: 3 to 8 mg/kg P.O. or slow I.V. daily or 250 mg/m² daily given as a single dose or in two divided doses.

Contraindications and precautions
Phenytoin is contraindicated in phenacemide or hydantoin hypersensitivity, bradycardia, SA and AV block, or Stokes-Adams syndrome. Use cautiously in hepatic or renal dysfunction, hypotension, myocardial insufficiency and respiratory depression; in elderly or debilitated patients; and in those receiving other hydantoin derivatives.

Adverse reactions
BLOOD: **thrombocytopenia, leukopenia, agranulocytosis, pancytopenia,** macrocytosis, megaloblastic anemia.
CNS: *ataxia,* slurred speech, *drowsiness,* confusion, *dizziness,* insomnia, nervousness, twitching, headache.
CV: hypotension, **ventricular fibrillation.**
EENT: nystagmus, diplopia, *blurred vision.*
GI: *nausea,* vomiting, gingival hyperplasia (especially children).
HEPATIC: toxic hepatitis.
SKIN: scarlatiniform or morbilliform rash; **bullous, exfoliative, or purpuric dermatitis; Stevens-Johnson syndrome;** lupus erythematosus; hirsutism; **toxic epidermal necrolysis;** photosensitivity.
LOCAL: pain, necrosis, and inflammation at injection site; purple glove syndrome.
OTHER: periarteritis nodosa, lymphadenopathy, hyperglycemia, osteomalacia, hypertrichosis.

Interactions

Alcohol, dexamethasone, folic acid: decreased phenytoin activity. Monitor closely.

Oral anticoagulants, antihistamines, amiodarone, chloramphenicol, cimetidine, cycloserine, diazepam, diazoxide, disulfiram, influenza vaccine, isoniazid, phenylbutazone, salicylates, sulfamethizole, valproic acid: increased phenytoin activity. Monitor for toxicity.

Oral tube feedings with Osmolite or Isocal: may interfere with absorption of oral phenytoin. Schedule feedings as far as possible from drug administration.

Nursing considerations

Assessment

• Review the patient's history for a condition that contraindicates the use of phenytoin.
• Obtain a baseline assessment of seizure activity before therapy.
• Be alert for common adverse reactions.
• Evaluate the patient's and family's knowledge about phenytoin therapy.

Planning (Nursing Diagnoses)

Potential nursing diagnoses for the patient receiving phenytoin include:
• Potential for injury related to ineffectiveness of phenytoin to control seizure activity.
• Fluid volume deficit related to adverse GI reactions caused by phenytoin.
• Sensory/perceptual alterations (visual) related to phenytoin-induced diplopia.
• Knowledge deficit related to phenytoin therapy.

Implementation

Preparation and administration

—Be aware that this drug was formerly known as diphenylhydantoin (DPH).
—Phenytoin sodium (extended) is the only form that can be given once daily. Patients should be stabilized on the prompt formulation before switching to the extended form.
—Oral suspension is available as 30 mg/5 ml or 125 mg/5 ml. Read label carefully.
—Shake oral suspension well before each dose. Use solid forms (tablets or capsules) if possible.
—Give divided doses with or after meals to minimize GI reactions.
—Elderly patients may require lower dosages because they tend to metabolize phenytoin slowly.
—Use only clear solution for parenteral injection. Slight yellow color is acceptable. Don't refrigerate.
—Avoid administering I.V. push phenytoin injections into veins in the back of the hand. Inject into larger veins to avoid discoloration known as purple glove syndrome.
—Don't mix drug with dextrose 5% in water because it will precipitate. Clear I.V. tubing first with 0.9% sodium chloride solution. Never use

cloudy solution. May mix with 0.9% sodium chloride solution if necessary to give as an infusion. Administer infusion over 30 to 60 minutes when possible. Infusion must begin within 1 hour after preparation and should run through an in-line filter. Discard 4 hours after preparation. Preferably, administer slowly (50 mg/minute) as an I.V. bolus.

— Do not give I.M. unless dosage adjustments are made. Drug may precipitate at injection site, cause pain, and be erratically absorbed.

Monitoring

— Monitor the effectiveness of phenytoin by evaluating the patient's seizure activity.

— Monitor phenytoin blood levels regularly. Therapeutic blood level of phenytoin is 10 to 20 mcg/ml.

— Monitor the patient for adverse drug reactions.

— Monitor for visual disturbances, such as blurred vision or diplopia.

— Monitor the patient's fluid intake if nausea or vomiting occurs; assess the patient for dehydration.

— Monitor the patient for drug interactions.

— Monitor CBC and serum calcium levels every 6 months, and periodically monitor blood glucose levels and hepatic function.

— Phenytoin requirements usually increase during pregnancy. Monitor serum levels closely and assess for seizures.

— Phenytoin levels may be decreased in mononucleosis. Monitor for increased seizure activity.

— Regularly reevaluate the patient's and family's knowledge about phenytoin therapy.

Intervention

— Don't withdraw drug suddenly. Call the doctor immediately if adverse reactions develop.

— Drug should be discontinued if rash appears. If rash is scarlet or measles-like, drug may be resumed after rash clears; it should not be resumed if rash is exfoliative, purpuric, or bullous. If rash reappears, drug should be discontinued.

— Folic acid and vitamin B_{12} may be prescribed if megaloblastic anemia is evident.

— Maintain seizure precautions.

— If adverse CNS reactions or visual disturbances occur, institute safety measures, such as assisting patient with ambulation and keeping bed rails up.

— If nausea and vomiting occur, obtain an order for an antiemetic. Offer the patient sips of water or ice chips frequently; provide bland diet during GI upset.

— Schedule oral tube feedings containing Osmolite or Isocal as far as possible from drug administration.

— Keep all members of the health care team informed of the patient's response to the drug.

Patient teaching
— Instruct the patient and family about phenytoin, including the dosage, frequency, action, and adverse reactions.
— Warn the patient to avoid driving and other hazardous activities that require alertness and good psychomotor coordination until CNS effects of the drug are known.
— Tell the patient to carry identification stating that he's taking phenytoin.
— Stress importance of good oral hygiene and regular dental examinations. Gingivectomy may be necessary periodically if dental hygiene is poor.
— Advise the patient not to change brands or dosage forms once stabilized on therapy.
— Inform the patient that heavy use of alcoholic beverages may diminish benefits of drug.
— Tell the patient to take oral phenytoin with or after meals to minimize adverse GI reactions.
— Tell the patient to notify the doctor if nausea or vomiting occurs and to take frequent sips of fluid or ice chips to maintain hydration.
— Stress importance of compliance.
— Advise the patient to withhold the drug and notify the doctor at once if skin rash appears.
— Inform the patient that phenytoin may color the urine pink, red, or reddish brown but that this effect is harmless.
— Tell the patient to notify the nurse or doctor if other adverse reactions develop or questions arise about phenytoin therapy.

Evaluation
In the patient receiving phenytoin, appropriate evaluation statements include:
• Patient is free of seizure activity.
• Patient maintains adequate hydration.
• Patient states vision is unaffected by phenytoin therapy.
• Patient and family state an understanding of phenytoin therapy.

PROTOTYPE: SUCCINIMIDE DERIVATIVES

ETHOSUXIMIDE
(eth oh sux′ i mide)
Zarontin
Classification: succinimide derivative
Pregnancy risk category C

How supplied
CAPSULES: 250 mg
SYRUP: 250 mg/5 ml

Indications and dosage

Absence seizures

ADULTS AND CHILDREN OVER AGE 6: initially, 250 mg P.O. b.i.d. May increase by 250 mg q 4 to 7 days up to 1.5 g daily.

CHILDREN AGES 3 TO 6: 250 mg P.O. daily or 125 mg P.O. b.i.d. May increase by 250 mg q 4 to 7 days up to 1.5 g daily.

Contraindications and precautions

Ethosuximide is contraindicated in hypersensitivity to succinimide derivatives. Use cautiously in hepatic or renal disease.

Adverse reactions

BLOOD: **leukopenia, eosinophilia, agranulocytosis, pancytopenia, aplastic anemia.**

CNS: *drowsiness,* headache, *fatigue, dizziness,* ataxia, irritability, hiccups, euphoria, lethargy.

EENT: myopia.

GI: *nausea,* vomiting, diarrhea, gum hypertrophy, weight loss, cramps, tongue swelling, anorexia, epigastric and abdominal pain.

GU: vaginal bleeding.

SKIN: urticaria, pruritic and erythematous rashes, hirsutism.

Interactions

None significant.

Nursing considerations

Assessment

• Review the patient's history for a condition that contraindicates the use of ethosuximide.

• Obtain a baseline assessment of patient's seizure activity before therapy.

• Be alert for common adverse reactions.

• Evaluate the patient's and family's knowledge about ethosuximide therapy.

Planning (Nursing Diagnoses)

Potential nursing diagnoses for the patient receiving ethosuximide include:

• Potential for injury related to ineffectiveness of ethosuximide to control seizure activity.

• Altered protection related to ethosuximide-induced blood disorders.

• Knowledge deficit related to ethosuximide therapy.

Implementation

Preparation and administration

— Administer drug with food to minimize GI distress.

Monitoring

— Monitor the effectiveness of therapy by regularly assessing seizure activity.

— Monitor CBC every 3 months and monitor for dermatologic reactions, joint pain, unexplained fever, or unusual bruising or bleeding (which may signal hematologic or other severe adverse reactions).

—Monitor serum blood levels; therapeutic levels range between 40 and 80 mcg/ml.
—Monitor the patient for adverse drug reactions.
—Monitor for increased frequency of generalized tonic-clonic seizures. Drug may increase frequency of such seizures when used alone in patients who have mixed types of seizures.
—Regularly reevaluate the patient's and family's knowledge about ethosuximide therapy.

Intervention

—Never withdraw drug suddenly. Abrupt withdrawal may precipitate absence seizures. Call the doctor immediately if adverse reactions develop.
—Be aware that drug may cause a positive direct Coombs' test.
—Institute safety precautions if the patient develops adverse CNS reactions.
—If blood disorders occur, provide supportive measures, such as assisting the anemic patient with activities and providing frequent rest periods.
—Obtain an order for an antiemetic or antidiarrheal agent if indicated.

Patient teaching

—Instruct the patient and family about ethosuximide, including the dose, frequency, action, and adverse reactions.
—Tell the patient to take drug with food or milk to prevent GI distress, to avoid use with alcoholic beverages, and to avoid driving and other hazardous tasks that require alertness if drug causes drowsiness, dizziness, or blurred vision.
—Warn the patient not to discontinue drug abruptly; this may cause seizures.
—Encourage the patient to wear medical alert identification indicating seizure disorder and ethosuximide use.
—Tell the patient to report the following reactions to the doctor: skin rash, joint pain, fever, sore throat, or unusual bleeding or bruising.
—Tell the patient to consult the doctor promptly if pregnancy is suspected.
—Advise the parents to protect pediatric syrup from freezing.
—Tell the patient to notify the nurse or doctor if adverse reactions develop or questions arise about ethosuximide therapy.

Evaluation

In the patient receiving ethosuximide, appropriate evaluation statements include:
• Patient is free of seizures.
• Patient's CBC is normal.
• Patient and family state an understanding of ethosuximide therapy.

VALPROATE SODIUM
(val proe' ate)
Depakene Syrup, Epilim‡, Myproic Acid Syrup

VALPROIC ACID
(val proe' ik acid)
Dalpro, Depakene, Myproic Acid

DIVALPROEX SODIUM
(dye val' proe ex)
Depakote, Epival†, Valcote‡
Classification: miscellaneous anticonvulsant
Pregnancy risk category D

How supplied
valproate sodium
SYRUP: 250 mg/ml‡, 250 mg/5 ml
valproic acid
TABLETS (ENTERIC-COATED): 200 mg‡, 500 mg‡
CRUSHABLE TABLETS: 100 mg‡
CAPSULES: 250 mg
SYRUP: 200 mg/5 ml‡, 250 mg/5 ml
divalproex sodium
TABLETS (ENTERIC-COATED): 125 mg, 250 mg, 500 mg

Indications and dosage
Simple and complex absence seizures, mixed seizure types (including absence seizures), generalized tonic-clonic seizures
ADULTS AND CHILDREN: initially, 15 mg/kg P.O. daily divided b.i.d. or t.i.d.; then may increase by 5 to 10 mg/kg daily at weekly intervals up to maximum of 60 mg/kg daily divided b.i.d. or t.i.d.

Contraindications and precautions
Valproic acid and its derivatives are contraindicated in hepatic dysfunction. Use cautiously in children under age 2; in children with congenital metabolic disorders or mental retardation; in patients with organic brain disease; and in those who are taking multiple anticonvulsants.

Adverse reactions
Because this drug is usually used concomitantly with other anticonvulsants, adverse reactions may not be caused by valproic acid or its derivatives alone.
BLOOD: **inhibited platelet aggregation, thrombocytopenia, increased bleeding time.**

---

†Available in Canada only   ‡Available in Australia only
Boldfaced adverse reactions are life-threatening

CNS: *sedation,* emotional upset, depression, psychosis, aggression, hyper-activity, behavioral deterioration, muscle weakness, tremor.
EENT: stomatitis.
GI: *nausea, vomiting,* indigestion, *diarrhea, abdominal cramps,* constipa-tion, increased appetite and weight gain, anorexia, pancreatitis. (*Note:* lower incidence of GI effects with divalproex.)
HEPATIC: elevated enzymes, **toxic hepatitis.**
METABOLIC: elevated serum ammonia.
OTHER: alopecia.

Interactions
Antacids, aspirin: may cause valproic acid toxicity. Use together cau-tiously and monitor blood levels.
Phenobarbital: increased phenobarbital levels. Monitor for toxicity.
Phenytoin: increased or decreased phenytoin levels. Monitor closely.

Nursing considerations
Assessment
• Review the patient's history for a condition that contraindicates the use of valproic acid or its derivatives.
• Obtain a baseline assessment of patient's seizure activities before ther-apy.
• Be alert for common adverse reactions.
• Evaluate the patient's and family's knowledge about drug therapy.

Planning (Nursing Diagnoses)
Potential nursing diagnoses for the patient receiving valproic acid or its derivatives include:
• Potential for injury related to ineffectiveness of valproic acid or its derivatives.
• Altered protection related to drug-induced bleeding.
• Activity intolerance related to drug-induced sedation.
• Knowledge deficit related to drug therapy.

Implementation
Preparation and administration
— Give drug with food or milk to reduce adverse GI reactions. Advise against chewing capsules, which causes irritation of mouth and throat.
— Available as pleasant-tasting red syrup. Keep out of reach of children.
— Syrup is more rapidly absorbed. Peak effect is reached within 15 minutes.
— Syrup shouldn't be mixed with carbonated beverages because it may be irritating to mouth and throat.
— Don't administer syrup to the patient who needs sodium restriction. Consult the doctor to provide alternate drug form.

Monitoring
— Regularly monitor the effectiveness of therapy by evaluating seizure activity.
— Monitor degree of sedation.

—Monitor the patient for adverse drug reactions.

—Regularly monitor liver function studies, platelet count, prothrombin time, and pancreatic enzyme levels.

—Monitor for nonspecific symptoms, such as malaise, fever, and lethargy, which may precede serious or fatal hepatotoxicity.

—Monitor for bleeding tendencies, such as easy bruising and spontaneous epistaxis.

—Monitor ketosis-prone diabetic patients for clinical signs of ketosis. Drug may produce false-positive results for urine ketones.

—Monitor the patient for drug interactions.

—Regularly reevaluate the patient's and family's knowledge about drug therapy.

Intervention

—Maintain seizure precautions.

—Institute safety precautions until sedative effects of the drug is known; assist the patient with activities as needed.

—Institute bleeding precautions. Advise the patient to use an electric shaver and soft toothbrush, and to avoid cuts and bruises.

—Expect dosage reduction if the patient develops tremor.

—Keep all members of the health care team informed of the patient's response to the drug.

Patient teaching

—Instruct the patient and family about the drug, including the dosage, frequency, action, and adverse reactions.

—Warn the patient to avoid driving and other hazardous activities that require alertness and good psychomotor coordination until CNS effects of the drug are known.

—Instruct the patient to take bleeding precautions.

—Warn the patient not to discontinue the drug suddenly.

—Inform the diabetic patient that drug may produce false positive test results for ketones in urine.

—Stress importance of follow-up care and periodic diagnostic tests.

—Tell the patient to report nonspecific symptoms, such as malaise, fever, lethargy, and bleeding, immediately.

—Advise the patient to take drug with food or milk to reduce adverse GI reactions. Warn against chewing capsules or mixing syrup with carbonated beverages.

—Tell the patient to notify the nurse or doctor if adverse reactions develop or questions arise about therapy.

Evaluation

In the patient receiving valproic acid or its derivatives, appropriate evaluation statements include:

• Patient is free of seizure activity.

• Patient does not experience bleeding throughout valproic acid therapy.

• Patient's daily activity needs are met.

• Patient and family state an understanding of drug therapy.

CARBAMAZEPINE
(kar ba maz′ e peen)

Apo-Carbamazepine†, Epitol, Mazepine†, Tegretol, Tegretol CR†, Teril‡

Classification: miscellaneous anticonvulsant
Pregnancy risk category C

How supplied
TABLETS: 200 mg
TABLETS (CHEWABLE): 100 mg
ORAL SUSPENSION: 100 mg/5 ml

Indications and dosage
Generalized tonic-clonic and complex-partial seizures, mixed seizure patterns
ADULTS AND CHILDREN OVER AGE 12: initially, 200 mg P.O. b.i.d. May increase by 200 mg daily in divided doses at 6- to 8-hour intervals. Adjust to minimum effective level when control achieved.
CHILDREN UNDER AGE 12: 10 to 20 mg/kg P.O. daily in two to four divided doses.

Trigeminal neuralgia
ADULTS: initially, 100 mg P.O. b.i.d. with meals. Increase by 100 mg q 12 hours until pain is relieved. Don't exceed 1.2 g daily. Maintenance dose is 200 to 400 mg P.O. b.i.d.

Contraindications and precautions
Carbamazepine is contraindicated in bone marrow suppression and hypersensitivity to carbamazepine or tricyclic antidepressants. Use cautiously in cardiac, renal, or hepatic damage and increased intraocular pressure.

Also use cautiously in children with mixed seizure disorders because these children may experience an increased incidence of seizures (usually atypical absence or generalized seizures).

Adverse reactions
BLOOD: **aplastic anemia, agranulocytosis,** eosinophilia, leukocytosis, thrombocytopenia.
CNS: *dizziness,* vertigo, *drowsiness,* fatigue, ataxia, worsening of seizures.
CV: **CHF,** hypertension, hypotension, aggravation of coronary artery disease.
EENT: conjunctivitis, dry pharynx, blurred vision, diplopia, nystagmus.
GI: *nausea,* vomiting, abdominal pain, diarrhea, anorexia, stomatitis, glossitis, dry mouth.
GU: urinary frequency, urine retention, impotence, albuminuria, glycosuria, elevated BUN level.
HEPATIC: abnormal liver function tests, hepatitis.
METABOLIC: water intoxication.

SKIN: rash, urticaria, **erythema multiforme, Stevens-Johnson syndrome.**
OTHER: diaphoresis, fever, chills, pulmonary hypersensitivity.

Interactions

Phenytoin, primidone, phenobarbital, nicotinic acid: may decrease carbamazepine levels. Monitor for decreased effect.
Phenytoin, warfarin, doxycycline, theophylline, haloperidol: carbamazepine may decrease blood levels of these drugs. Monitor for decreased effect.
Propoxyphene, troleandomycin, erythromycin, isoniazid, verapamil: may increase carbamazepine blood levels. Use cautiously.

Nursing considerations

Assessment

- Review the patient's history for a condition that contraindicates the use of carbamazepine.
- Obtain a baseline assessment of seizure activity before therapy.
- Be alert for common adverse reactions.
- Evaluate the patient's and family's knowledge about carbamazepine therapy.

Planning (Nursing Diagnoses)

Potential nursing diagnoses for the patient receiving carbamazepine include:
- Potential for injury related to ineffectiveness of carbamazepine.
- Altered protection related to carbamazepine-induced blood disorders.
- Altered oral mucous membrane related to carbamazepine-induced stomatitis.
- Knowledge deficit related to carbamazepine therapy.

Implementation

Preparation and administration
—Administer drug in divided doses, when possible, to maintain consistent blood levels.
—Administer with food to minimize GI distress.

Monitoring
—Monitor the effectiveness of carbamazepine therapy by evaluating seizure activity.
—Monitor therapeutic blood levels closely. Ask patient when last dose of medication was taken to approximately evaluate blood levels. Therapeutic levels of carbamazepine are 3 to 9 mcg/ml.
—Monitor the patient for adverse drug reactions.
—Obtain baseline determinations of urinalysis, BUN, liver function, CBC, platelet and reticulocyte counts, and serum iron levels. Monitor periodically during therapy.
—Monitor for mild-to-moderate dizziness and drowsiness at start of therapy. Effect usually disappears within 3 to 4 days.

—Monitor for signs of anorexia or subtle appetite changes, which may indicate excessive blood levels.

—Monitor for stomatitis (red, painful ulcerations in oral cavity) throughout therapy.

—Monitor for signs of anemia (pallor, fatigue), infection (fever, chills, drainage), or bleeding (easy bruising, spontaneous epistaxis).

—Monitor the patient for drug interactions.

—Regularly reevaluate the patient's and family's knowledge about carbamazepine therapy.

Intervention

—Never discontinue the drug suddenly when treating seizures or status epilepticus. Notify the doctor immediately if adverse reactions occur.

—If anemia occurs, assist the patient with activities, schedule activities to allow frequent rest periods. Expect to administer additional agents to treat anemia.

—If the patient's WBC counts are low, institute infection control measures. Advise the patient to get adequate rest, maintain adequate hydration, and avoid exposure to colds and other infections.

—If the patient exhibits bleeding tendencies, institute bleeding precautions. Advise the patient to use an electric shaver and to avoid cuts and bruises.

—Advise meticulous oral hygiene for the patient with stomatitis; encourage a bland diet and obtain an order for a local anesthetic to ease mouth discomfort.

—Maintain seizure precautions.

—If CNS reactions occur, institute safety precautions.

—Keep all members of the health care team informed of the patient's response to the drug.

Patient teaching

—Instruct the patient and family about carbamazepine, including the dosage, frequency, action, and adverse reactions.

—Warn the patient to avoid driving and other hazardous activities that require alertness and good psychomotor coordination until CNS effects of the drug are known.

—Advise the patient to have periodic eye examinations.

—Tell the patient to notify the doctor immediately if fever, sore throat, mouth ulcers, or easy bruising or bleeding occur. Instruct the patient about appropriate protective measures.

—Tell the patient how to manage stomatitis.

—Instruct the patient to take the drug with food to minimize GI discomfort.

—Stress importance of compliance.

—Explain the importance of follow-up care, including periodic diagnostic studies.

—Reassure the patient that dizziness and drowsiness usually disappear after 3 to 4 days of therapy.

— Tell the patient to notify the nurse or doctor if adverse reactions develop or questions arise about carbamazepine therapy.

Evaluation

In the patient receiving carbamazepine, appropriate evaluation statements include:
• Patient remains free of seizure activity.
• Patient's CBC remains normal.
• Patient does not exhibit signs of stomatitis.
• Patient and family state an understanding of carbamazepine therapy.

SELECTED MAJOR DRUGS: ANTICONVULSANTS

DRUG, INDICATIONS, AND DOSAGES	SPECIAL PRECAUTIONS
Barbiturate derivatives	
mephobarbital (Mebaral) *Generalized tonic-clonic or absence seizures —* **Adults:** 400 to 600 mg P.O. daily or in divided doses. **Children:** 6 to 12 mg/kg P.O. daily divided q 6 to 8 hours (smaller doses are given initially and increased over 4 to 5 days p.r.n.).	• Contraindicated in patients with known hypersensitivity to barbiturates and in those with porphyria or respiratory disease with dyspnea or obstruction. • Use cautiously in patients with hepatic, renal, cardiac, or respiratory function impairment; myasthenia gravis; and myxedema.
primidone (Apo-Primidone†, Myidone, Mysoline, Sertan†) *Generalized tonic-clonic seizures, complex-partial seizures —* **Adults and children over age 8:** 250 mg P.O. daily. Increase by 250 mg weekly, up to maximum of 2 g daily, divided q.i.d. **Children under age 8:** 125 mg P.O. daily. Increased by 125 mg weekly, up to maximum of 1 g daily divided q.i.d.	• Contraindicated in patients with known hypersensitivity to phenobarbital and with porphyria.
Benzodiazepine derivatives	
clonazepam (Klonopin, Rivotril) *Absence and atypical absence seizures; akinetic and myoclonic seizures —* **Adults:** initial dosage should not exceed 1.5 mg P.O. daily in three divided doses. May be increased by 0.5 to 1 mg q 3 days until seizures are controlled. Maximum recommended dosage is 20 mg daily. **Children up to age 10 or 30 kg:** 0.01 to 0.03 mg/kg P.O. daily (not to exceed 0.05 mg/kg daily) divided q 8 hours. Increase dosage by 0.25 to 0.5 mg q third day to a maximum maintenance dosage of 0.1 to 0.2 mg/kg daily. *Status epilepticus (if parenteral form is available) —* **Adults:** 1 mg by slow I.V. infusion. **Children:** 0.5 mg by slow I.V. infusion.	• Contraindicated in patients with known hypersensitivity to the drug, significant liver disease, and acute narrow-angle glaucoma and in pregnant and breast-feeding women. • Administer cautiously to patients with impaired renal function and chronic respiratory disease.

(continued)

SELECTED MAJOR DRUGS: ANTICONVULSANTS *continued*

| DRUG, INDICATIONS, AND DOSAGES | SPECIAL PRECAUTIONS |

Hydantoin derivatives

ethotoin (Peganone)
Generalized tonic-clonic or complex-partial seizures —
Adults: initially, 250 mg P.O. q.i.d. after meals. May increase slowly over several days to 3 g daily divided q.i.d.
Children: initially, 250 mg P.O. b.i.d. May increase up to 250 mg P.O. q.i.d.

• Contraindicated in patients with hepatic abnormalities, hematologic disorders, or known hypersensitivity to hydantoin derivatives.
• Administer cautiously to patients receiving other hydantoin derivatives.

mephenytoin (Mesantoin)
Generalized tonic-clonic or complex-partial seizures —
Adults: 50 to 100 mg P.O. daily. May increase by 50 to 100 mg weekly up to 200 mg P.O. t.i.d.
Children: initially, 50 to 100 mg P.O. daily or 100 to 450 mg/m² P.O. daily in three divided doses. Dosage must be adjusted individually.

• Contraindicated in patients with known hypersensitivity to hydantoin derivatives.
• Administer cautiously to patients with liver diseases, blood dyscrasia, and skin and mucous membrane manifestations.

phenacemide (Phenurone)
Refractory, complex-partial, generalized tonic-clonic, absence, and atypical absence seizures —
Adults: 500 mg P.O. t.i.d. May increase by 500 mg weekly, up to 5 g daily, p.r.n.
Children ages 5 to 10: 250 mg P.O. t.i.d. May increase by 250 mg weekly, up to 1.5 g daily, p.r.n.

• Contraindicated in patients with preexisting personality disturbances or in those receiving satisfactory seizure control with other anticonvulsants.
• Administer cautiously to patients with hepatic dysfunction or history of allergy and when a hydantoin derivative is used concomitantly.

Miscellaneous agents

acetazolamide (Apo-Acetazolamide†, Diamox)
Myoclonic, refractory generalized tonic-clonic or absence, or mixed seizures —
Adults: 375 mg P.O., I.M., or I.V. daily up to 250 mg q.i.d. Alternatively, use sustained-release form 250 to 500 mg P.O. daily or b.i.d. When used with other anticonvulsants, initial dosage is usually 250 mg daily.
Children: 8 to 30 mg/kg P.O. daily divided t.i.d. or q.i.d. Maximum dosage is 1.5 g daily, or 300 to 900 mg/m² daily.
Narrow-angle glaucoma —
Adults: 250 mg q 4 hours; or 250 mg P.O., I.M., or I.V. b.i.d. for short-term therapy.
Edema in CHF —
Adults: 250 to 375 mg P.O., I.M., or I.V. daily in morning.
Children: 5 mg/kg daily in morning.
Open-angle glaucoma —
Adults: 250 mg daily to 1 g P.O., I.M., or I.V. divided q.i.d.
Prevention or amelioration of acute mountain sickness —
Adults: 250 mg P.O. q 8 to 12 hours.

• Contraindicated in patients in long-term therapy for chronic noncongestive narrow-angle glaucoma and in those with hyponatremia or hypokalemia, renal or hepatic disease or dysfunction, adrenal gland failure, or hyperchloremic acidosis.
• Administer cautiously to patients with respiratory acidosis, emphysema, and chronic pulmonary disease and in those receiving other diuretics.

SELECTED MAJOR DRUGS: ANTICONVULSANTS *continued*

DRUG, INDICATIONS, AND DOSAGES	SPECIAL PRECAUTIONS
Miscellaneous agents	

methsuximide (Celontin) *Refractory absence seizures—* **Adults and children:** initially, 300 mg P.O. daily. May increase by 300 mg weekly. Maximum daily dosage is 1.2 g in divided doses.	• Contraindicated in patients with known hypersensitivity to succinimide derivatives. • Administer cautiously to patients with hepatic or renal dysfunction.
paramethadione (Paradione) *Refractory absence seizures—* **Adults:** initially, 300 mg P.O. t.i.d. May increase by 300 mg weekly, up to 600 mg q.i.d., if needed. **Children over age 6:** 0.9 g P.O. daily in divided doses t.i.d. or q.i.d. **Children ages 2 to 6:** 0.6 g P.O. daily in divided doses t.i.d. or q.i.d. **Children under age 2:** 0.3 g P.O. daily in divided doses b.i.d.	• Contraindicated in patients with known hypersensitivity to the drug, renal and hepatic dysfunction, or severe blood dyscrasia. • Administer cautiously to patients with retinal or optic nerve diseases.
phensuximide (Milontin) *Absence seizures—* **Adults and children:** 500 mg to 1 g P.O. b.i.d. to t.i.d.	• Contraindicated in patients with known hypersensitivity to succinimide derivatives. • Administer cautiously to patients with hepatic or renal dysfunction.
trimethadione (Tridione) *Refractory absence seizures—* **Adults and children over age 13:** initially, 300 mg P.O. t.i.d. May increase by 300 mg weekly up to 600 mg P.O. q.i.d. **Children:** 13 mg/kg P.O. t.i.d. or 335 mg/m² P.O. t.i.d.; alternatively— **Children under age 2:** 100 mg P.O. t.i.d. **Children ages 2 to 6:** 200 mg P.O. t.i.d. **Children ages 6 to 13:** 300 mg P.O. t.i.d.	• Contraindicated in patients with known hypersensitivity to the drug and to paramethadione and in those with severe blood dyscrasia or hepatic dysfunction. • Administer cautiously to patients with retinal and optic nerve diseases.

ANTICONVULSANT COMBINATION

TRADE NAME AND CONTENT	SPECIAL CONSIDERATION
Dilantin with phenobarbital phenytoin 100 mg and phenobarbital 16 mg, phenytoin 100 mg and phenobarbital 32 mg	• Fixed combination drug is usually used only after patient's dosage is titrated to therapeutic levels with individual drugs.

SELF-TEST

1. Pat Kosta has been admitted with generalized tonic-clonic seizures. The nurse prepares to administer a dose of phenytoin 900 mg as an I.V. bolus. What is the minimum injection time for this bolus of medication?
   a. 10 minutes
   b. 18 minutes
   c. 20 minutes
   d. 40 minutes

2. Ms. Kosta has an I.V. of dextrose 5% in water (D_5W). To administer a bolus dose of I.V. phenytoin, the nurse should:
   a. stop the D_5W and inject the Dilantin into the lowest port on the I.V. line.
   b. flush the line with 0.9% sodium chloride solution before and after the Dilantin.
   c. insert a p.r.n. device (heparin lock) to use for injecting the Dilantin.
   d. request a change of I.V. fluid orders from D_5W to dextrose in lactated Ringer's solution.

3. When teaching Ms. Kosta about the self-care needed during maintenance phenytoin therapy, the nurse should explain that, because of possible adverse effects of this drug, Ms. Kosta should schedule regular examinations by a/an:
   a. dentist.
   b. otologist.
   c. cardiologist.
   d. gynecologist.

4. Suzie Ames takes phenobarbital 50 mg P.O. t.i.d. for seizure control. Ms. Ames informed the nurse that she is pregnant and plans to breast-feed her infant. What information should Ms. Ames' nurse give her?
   a. Phenobarbital is contraindicated during pregnancy.
   b. Phenobarbital is contraindicated during breast-feeding.
   c. The dosage of phenobarbital must be increased during pregnancy.
   d. The dosing interval of phenobarbital must be spaced evenly throughout 24 hours when breast-feeding.

5. Joe Batts' doctor prescribed carbamazepine 200 mg P.O. b.i.d. for a seizure disorder. Which of the following instructions should the nurse give Mr. Batts?
   a. Dosing interval will be decreased to once daily when seizure control is attained.
   b. Antacids interfere with the absorption of the drug and should be avoided.
   c. The drug can be taken with food to minimize GI reactions.
   d. The drug may cause constipation; therefore, patient should increase his fiber and fluid intake.

6. Mr. Batt's doctor could have prescribed valproic acid as an alternative anticonvulsant. Which of the following conditions would contraindicate the use of valproic acid?
  a. renal dysfunction
  b. cardiac dysfunction
  c. respiratory dysfunction
  d. hepatic dysfunction

7. John Saunders develops seizures after a head injury. One month after discharge he returns to the hospital with status epilepticus. The physician prescribed diazepam 10 mg slow I.V. push 5 mg/minute. How soon can another dose of diazepam be given if seizures continue?
  a. 1 to 2 minutes
  b. 2 to 3 minutes
  c. 3 to 5 minutes
  d. 5 to 10 minutes

Check your answers on pages 1063 and 1064.

CHAPTER 30

ANTIDEPRESSANTS

Monoamine oxidase inhibitors
isocarboxazid ✦ phenelzine sulfate ✦ tranylcypromine sulfate

Tricyclic antidepressants
amitriptyline hydrochloride ✦ amoxapine ✦ clomipramine hydrochloride
desipramine hydrochloride ✦ doxepin hydrochloride
imipramine hydrochloride ✦ nortriptyline hydrochloride
protriptyline hydrochloride ✦ trimipramine maleate

Miscellaneous agents
bupropion hydrochloride ✦ fluoxetine hydrochloride
maprotiline hydrochloride ✦ trazodone hydrochloride

OVERVIEW

- Tricyclic antidepressants (TCAs) are the drugs of choice for most types of depression. Since their introduction in the late 1950s, TCAs have totally supplanted amphetamines and other psychomotor stimulants for this indication. This change has occurred because of their effectiveness and relative safety.
- Monoamine oxidase inhibitors (MAO inhibitors, or MAOIs) are another class of antidepressants. These can cause more serious adverse reactions than the TCAs; thus, they are generally omitted until two TCAs have been tried unsuccessfully. Despite the official warning against the combined use of a TCA and an MAO inhibitor, reports have documented the success of such combination therapy.
- Fluoxetine is the most recent antidepressant to become available. It differs chemically from both the TCAs and MAO inhibitors.
- Bupropion, maprotiline, and trazodone are also chemically different but share similar activity and adverse reaction profiles.
- The antidepressants are classified primarily into three groups: MAO inhibitors, TCAs, and miscellaneous agents.

MAJOR USES

- All antidepressants are used to treat psychotic and neurotic endogenous depression and to prevent recurrent depression.
- Imipramine is used to treat enuresis in children and adolescents.
- MAO inhibitors may be effective in closely supervised patients who are unresponsive to other antidepressant therapy for severe reactive or endogenous depression.

GLOSSARY

Affective disorder: mood disturbance in the presence of an elated or depressive state.
Antidepressant: agent that prevents or relieves depression.
Antimanic: agent that prevents or diminishes mania.
Bipolar disorder: mood disorder in which manic and depressive episodes occur. Formerly known as manic-depressive disorder.
Depression: emotional dejection characterized by an absence of cheerfulness and hope disproportionate to circumstances.
Mania: mood disorder characterized by an expansive emotional state, elation, hyperirritability, over-talkativeness, a flight of ideas, and increased motor activity.
Monoamine oxidase (MAO): enzyme in the nerve endings that breaks down catecholamines.

MECHANISM OF ACTION

• Endogenous depression may be caused by a lack of biogenic amines (norepinephrine, dopamine, and serotonin) within certain areas of the CNS. Antidepressants act to increase the availability of these neurotransmitters to their receptor sites.

• TCAs, bupropion, and trazodone are thought to increase the action of norepinephrine or serotonin, or both, in the CNS by blocking the reuptake of norepinephrine or serotonin by the presynaptic neurons. This prolongs the action of these neurotransmitters in the synapse.

• MAO inhibitors block MAO (which helps metabolize neurotransmitters within the neuron), causing buildup of certain neurotransmitters, including norepinephrine.

• Fluoxetine is believed to inhibit serotonin reuptake from the synaptic cleft.

ABSORPTION, DISTRIBUTION, METABOLISM, AND EXCRETION

TCAs have rapid and uniformly good absorption after oral administration. MAO inhibitors are rapidly and uniformly absorbed after oral administration, metabolized by the liver, and excreted by the kidneys, usually within 24 hours. Although the half-lives of these drugs are short, their pharmacologic effects are long-lasting because the drugs permanently inactivate enzymes.

All antidepressants are widely distributed to body tissues. TCAs, bupropion, fluoxetine, and trazodone are metabolized in the liver and excreted by the kidneys as inactive metabolites. Most of the drugs and metabolites are excreted within 72 hours.

ONSET AND DURATION

Of the MAO inhibitors, isocarboxazid and phenelzine have a very slow onset that may not occur for several weeks or months. Effects may persist for up to 3 weeks after therapy is stopped. Tranylcypromine has a more rapid onset of action (usually several days), and MAO activity is restored 3 to 5 days after the drug is discontinued.

TCAs and trazodone produce sedative effects within a few hours after oral administration. Also, anticholinergic adverse effects occur soon after therapy begins, except for trazodone, which causes fewer anticholinergic effects. Antidepressant effects occur 7 to 14 days after onset of therapy because of the slow effect on the brain's neurotransmitter metabolism. The claim that some of the newer TCAs (amoxapine and trimipramine) supply a more rapid onset of action is not well substantiated.

ADVERSE REACTIONS

See *Comparing Adverse Reactions to Antidepressants* for comparative severity of anticholinergic, sedative, and hypotensive reactions. MAO inhibitors' most serious adverse reactions involve blood pressure. Hypotensive reactions appear to follow gradual accumulation of false neurotransmitters (phenylethylamines) in adrenergic nerve terminals; normal breakdown of these agents is also inhibited by MAO. Severe hypertension also may result from interaction with drugs with sympathomimetic activity, such as pseudoephedrine, phenylephrine, and phenylpropanolamine, other false neurotransmitters, and other drugs with vasoconstrictive effects. Ingestion of food or beverages containing tyramine may provoke hypertensive crisis—a rapid and severe increase in blood pressure. Hypertensive crisis is attributed to displacement of norepinephrine by false neurotransmitters; prodromal symptoms include severe occipital headache, tachycardia, sweating, and visual disturbances.

All MAO inhibitors cause adverse CNS reactions, including restlessness, hyperexcitability, insomnia, and headache. Over time, tolerance develops to most adverse reactions.

TCAs frequently cause sedation and anticholinergic effects. Other less frequent adverse CNS reactions include dizziness, weakness, headache, and mental confusion (more marked in elderly patients). Numbness, tingling, paresthesia of the extremities, incoordination, and tremor may occur. Extrapyramidal symptoms may occur in patients taking TCAs; tardive dyskinesia and neuroleptic malignant syndrome has been reported with amoxapine. The TCAs may also lower the seizure threshold and allow seizures to develop in predisposed individuals. Excitation, anxiety, nervousness, vivid dreams, and decreased libido have also been reported.

Anticholinergic reactions include GI effects: dry mouth, constipation, paralytic ileus, abdominal cramping, and effects on the urinary tract: urine retention, delayed micturition, and dilation of the urinary tract may occur, especially in patients with preexisting conditions, such as prostatic hypertrophy. The anticholinergic reactions may produce blurred vision, disturbances of accommodation, increased intraocular pressure, and mydriasis. Another possible anticholinergic effect is hyperthermia.

COMPARING ADVERSE REACTIONS TO ANTIDEPRESSANTS

DRUG	USUAL ADULT DOSAGE	ANTICHOLINERGIC EFFECTS	SEDATIVE EFFECTS	HYPOTENSIVE EFFECTS
Tricyclic antidepressants				
amitriptyline	50 to 100 mg daily	HIGH	HIGH	MODERATE
amoxapine	150 to 300 mg daily	LOW	MODERATE	LOW
desipramine	50 to 150 mg daily	LOW	LOW	MODERATE
doxepin	50 to 150 mg daily	MODERATE	HIGH	HIGH
imipramine	50 to 150 mg daily	MODERATE	MODERATE	HIGH
nortriptyline	50 to 100 mg daily	MODERATE	MODERATE	LOW
protriptyline	10 to 40 mg daily	LOW	LOW	MODERATE
trimipramine	50 to 150 mg daily	MODERATE	MODERATE	MODERATE
Monoamine oxidase inhibitors				
isocarboxazid	10 to 30 mg daily	LOW	LOW	MODERATE
phenelzine	60 to 90 mg daily	LOW	MODERATE	MODERATE
tranylcypromine	10 to 30 mg daily	LOW	NONE	MODERATE
Miscellaneous agents				
bupropion	300 to 450 mg daily	NONE	NONE	LOW
fluoxetine	20 to 80 mg daily	VERY LOW	LOW	LOW
maprotiline	50 to 150 mg daily	LOW	MODERATE	LOW
trazodone	150 to 300 mg daily	NONE	HIGH	MODERATE

The TCAs may produce adverse CV reactions. Orthostatic hypotension may occur and may cause syncope and falls in the elderly. Tachycardia, palpitations, cardiac arrhythmias, and heart block may occur and may precipitate MI, stroke, or CHF. TCA therapy has also been associated with sudden death.

Rarely, TCAs have been associated with bone marrow depression, hepatic dysfunction, and sensitivity reactions. These drugs have also been reported to cause weight gain and, occasionally, weight loss. Decreased libido, impotence, testicular swelling, breast engorgement, and galactorrhea in females and gynecomastia in males have also been reported.

Among the miscellaneous antidepressants, fluoxetine or trazodone commonly cause anxiety, headache, nervousness, and insomnia; less often, sedation, tremor, dizziness, fatigue, diminished concentration, abnormal dreams, and agitation. GI reactions commonly include nausea, diarrhea, dry mouth, anorexia, and dyspepsia. Nausea is usually mild and subsides after a few weeks of therapy.

Bupropion is associated with seizures in about 0.4% of patients taking doses up to 450 mg daily, an incidence that may be four times greater than that of other antidepressants. The incidence of seizures rises with increasing dosage. It may also be associated with a history of seizures, head trauma, concomitant medication that lowers the seizure threshold, or CNS tumor.

PROTOTYPE: MONOAMINE OXIDASE INHIBITORS

TRANYLCYPROMINE SULFATE
(tran ill sip′ roe meen)
Parnate
Classification: monoamine oxidase inhibitor
Pregnancy risk category C

How supplied
TABLETS: 10 mg

Indications and dosage
Depression
ADULTS: 10 mg P.O. b.i.d. Increase to maximum of 30 mg daily, if necessary, after 2 weeks. Not recommended for children under age 16.

Contraindications and precautions
Tranylcypromine is contraindicated in severe hepatic or renal impairment; CHF; pheochromocytoma, hypertension, or CV or cerebrovascular disease; in severe or frequent headaches; in patients taking antihypertensive

drugs or diuretics; in elderly or debilitated patients; in patients for whom close supervision is not possible; and in hyperactive, agitated, or schizophrenic patients. Drug is also contraindicated with foods containing tryptophan or tyramine and during therapy with other MAO inhibitors (phenelzine, isocarboxazid) or within 7 days of such therapy and within 7 days of elective surgery requiring general anesthetic, cocaine, or local anesthetic containing sympathomimetic vasoconstrictors. Use cautiously with antiparkinsonian drugs and spinal anesthetics; in renal disease, diabetes, seizure disorder, and hyperthyroidism and in patients at risk for suicide.

Adverse reactions
CNS: *dizziness*, vertigo, headache, overactivity, hyperreflexia, tremor, muscle twitching, mania, jitters, confusion, memory impairment, fatigue.
CV: *orthostatic hypotension,* arrhythmias, paradoxical hypertension.
EENT: blurred vision.
GI: dry mouth, *anorexia*, nausea, diarrhea, constipation, abdominal pain.
GU: impotence.
SKIN: rash.
OTHER: peripheral edema, sweating, weight changes, chills, altered libido.

Interactions
Alcohol, barbiturates, and other sedatives; narcotics; dextromethorphan; TCAs: increased drug effects. Use with caution and in reduced dosage.
Amphetamines, antihistamines, ephedrine, levodopa, meperidine, metaraminol, methotrimeprazine, methylphenidate, phenylephrine, phenylpropanolamine: pressor effects of these drugs are enhanced by tranylcypromine. Use together cautiously.
Insulin, oral hypoglycemic agents: tranylcypromine may alter requirements of antidiabetic medications. Monitor blood glucose and adjust dosage as ordered.

Nursing considerations
Assessment
• Review the patient's history for a condition that contraindicates the use of tranylcypromine.
• Obtain a baseline assessment of the patient's degree of depression before therapy.
• Be alert for common adverse reactions.
• Evaluate the patient's and family's knowledge about tranylcypromine therapy.

Planning (Nursing Diagnoses)
Potential nursing diagnoses for the patient receiving tranylcypromine include:
• Altered thought processes related to ineffectiveness of tranylcypromine therapy.
• Potential for injury related to tranylcypromine induced dizziness or orthostatic hypotension.
• Altered nutrition: Less than body requirements related to tranylcypromine-induced anorexia.
• Knowledge deficit related to tranylcypromine therapy.

Implementation

Preparation and administration

— Ask the patient about recent ingestion of tyramine-rich foods before administering drug.

— Administer the drug at bedtime when possible to minimize discomfort from CNS and anticholinergic reactions.

— Be aware that drug is used only when TCA or electroconvulsive therapy is ineffective or contraindicated.

— Dosage is usually reduced to maintenance level as soon as possible.

Monitoring

— Regularly monitor effectiveness by asking about patient's feelings and by observing behavior.

— Monitor the patient for adverse drug reactions.

— Monitor nutritional status and weight if anorexia occurs.

— Obtain baseline blood pressure readings, CBC, and liver function tests before beginning therapy and monitor throughout treatment.

— Monitor for suicidal tendencies.

— Monitor the patient for drug interactions.

— Monitor blood pressure for paradoxical hypertension.

— Regularly reevaluate the patient's and family's knowledge about tranylcypromine therapy.

Intervention

— Confer with doctor if patient does not respond to drug.

— If adverse CNS reactions occur, institute safety measures, such as assisting with activities.

— Advise the patient to change positions slowly to minimize orthostatic hypotension.

— If the patient develops symptoms of overdose (palpitations, severe hypotension, or frequent headaches), hold dose and notify the doctor.

— Do not withdraw drug abruptly.

— Have phentolamine (Regitine) available to combat severe hypertension.

— If anorexia develops, encourage the patient to eat highly nutritious foods and more frequent smaller meals.

— Tell the patient to expect delay of 2 weeks or more before noticeable effect. Full effect may take 4 weeks or more.

— Instruct the patient to continue precautions for 7 days after discontinuing the drug because of residual effects.

— Keep all members of the health care team informed of the patient's response to the drug.

Patient teaching

— Instruct the patient and family about tranylcypromine, including the dosage, frequency, action, and adverse reactions.

— MAO inhibitors are most often reported to cause hypertensive crisis with high-tyramine ingestion; warn the patient to avoid foods high in

tyramine or tryptophan (aged cheese, Chianti wine, beer, avocados, chicken livers, chocolate, bananas, soy sauce, meat tenderizers, salami, bologna) and self-medication with OTC cold, hay fever, or weight-loss preparations. (Give patient a list of foods to avoid when taking MAO inhibitors.)
— Tell the patient to avoid combining with alcohol or other CNS depressants.
— Advise the patient how to overcome anorexia.
— Warn the patient to avoid driving and other hazardous activities that require mental alertness if adverse CNS reactions occur.
— Tell the diabetic patient to monitor blood glucose level closely as drug may alter levels.
— Tell the patient to notify the nurse or doctor if adverse reactions develop or questions arise about tranylcypromine therapy.

Evaluation
In the patient receiving tranylcypromine, appropriate evaluation statements include:
• Patient reports improved feelings about himself and life.
• Patient is not injured as a result of adverse CNS reactions.
• Patient maintains adequate nutritional intake.
• Patient and family state an understanding of tranylcypromine therapy.

PROTOTYPE: TRICYCLIC ANTIDEPRESSANTS

AMITRIPTYLINE HYDROCHLORIDE
(a mee trip' ti leen)
Amitril, Apo-Amitriptyline†, Elavil, Emitrip, Endep, Enovil, Laroxyl‡,
Levate†, Meravil†, Novotriptyn†
Classification: tricyclic antidepressant
Pregnancy risk category D

How supplied
TABLETS: 10 mg, 25 mg, 50 mg, 75 mg, 100 mg, 150 mg
INJECTION: 10 mg/ml

Indications and dosage
Depression
ADULTS: 50 to 100 mg P.O. h.s., increasing to 200 mg daily; maximum dosage is 300 mg daily if needed; or 20 to 30 I.M. q.i.d. Alternatively, the entire dosage can be given h.s.
ELDERLY PATIENTS AND ADOLESCENTS: 30 mg P.O. daily in divided doses. May be increased to 150 mg.

Contraindications and precautions
Amitriptyline is contraindicated during the acute recovery phase of MI, in patients with a history of seizure disorders, and in those with prostatic

hypertrophy. Use cautiously in patients who are at risk for suicide; in patients with urine retention, narrow-angle glaucoma, increased intraocular pressure, CV disease, impaired hepatic function, or hyperthyroidism; and in those receiving thyroid medications, electroconvulsive therapy, or elective surgery.

Adverse reactions

CNS: *drowsiness, dizziness*, excitation, tremor, weakness, confusion, headache, nervousness.

CV: *orthostatic hypotension, tachycardia*, **ECG changes**, hypertension.

EENT: *blurred vision*, tinnitus, mydriasis.

GI: *dry mouth, constipation*, nausea, vomiting, anorexia, paralytic ileus.

GU: *urine retention.*

SKIN: rash, urticaria.

OTHER: *sweating,* allergy.

AFTER ABRUPT WITHDRAWAL OF LONG-TERM THERAPY: nausea, headache, malaise. (Does not indicate addiction.)

Interactions

Barbiturates: decrease TCA blood levels. Monitor for decreased antidepressant effect.

Cimetidine, methylphenidate: increases TCA blood levels. Monitor for enhanced antidepressant effect.

Epinephrine, norepinephrine: increase hypertensive effect. Use with caution.

MAO inhibitors: may cause severe excitation, hyperpyrexia, or seizures, usually with high dosage. Use together cautiously.

Nursing considerations

Assessment

• Review the patient's history for a condition that contraindicates the use of amitriptyline.

• Obtain a baseline assessment of the patient's depression before therapy.

• Be alert for common adverse reactions.

• Evaluate the patient's and family's knowledge about amitriptyline therapy.

Planning (Nursing Diagnoses)

Potential nursing diagnoses for the patient receiving amitriptyline include:

• Altered thought processes related to ineffectiveness of amitriptyline therapy.

• Constipation related to anticholinergic effects of amitriptyline.

• Altered health maintenance related to cardiovascular reactions to amitriptyline.

• Potential for injury related to adverse CNS reactions to amitriptyline.

• Knowledge deficit related to amitriptyline therapy.

Implementation

Preparation and administration

— Whenever possible, patient should take full dose at bedtime.

—Expect reduced dosage in elderly or debilitated patients and adolescents.

Monitoring

—Monitor effectiveness by asking the patient about degree of depression and by evaluating the patient's behavior.
—Monitor the patient for adverse drug reactions.
—Monitor blood pressure for alterations, heart rate for tachycardia, and ECG for changes.
—Watch for signs of oversedation, especially in the elderly patient.
—Monitor bowel patterns for constipation.
—Monitor for suicidal tendencies.
—Monitor the patient for drug interactions.
—Regularly reevaluate the patient's and family's knowledge about amitriptyline therapy.

Intervention

—Discuss alternative therapy or changes in regimen with doctor if drug is ineffective.
—Institute safety precautions if adverse CNS reactions occur.
—Do not withdraw drug abruptly.
—If psychotic signs increase, dosage should be reduced. Allow minimum supply of tablets to lessen suicide risk.
—Dry mouth may be relieved with sugarless hard candy or gum. Saliva substitutes may be necessary.
—If not contraindicated, increase the patient's fluid and fiber intake to prevent constipation; if needed, obtain an order for a laxative.
—Assist the patient in changing positions slowly to minimize orthostatic hypotension.
—Keep all members of the health care team informed of the patient's response to the drug.

Patient teaching

—Instruct the patient and family about amitriptyline, including the dosage, frequency, action, and adverse reactions.
—Teach the patient to increase fluids to lessen constipation. Suggest stool softener or high-fiber diet, if needed.
—Warn the patient to avoid driving and other hazardous activities that require alertness and good psychomotor coordination until CNS effects of the drug are known. Tell the patient that drowsiness and dizziness usually subside after first few weeks. Inform the patient that drug has strong sedative effects. Warn against combining with alcohol or other CNS depressants.
—Tell the patient to expect delay of 2 weeks or more before noticeable effect. Full effect may take 4 weeks or more. Encourage the patient to continue to take medication until it achieves its full therapeutic effect.
—Advise the patient not to take any other drugs (prescription or OTC) without first consulting the doctor.

— Warn the patient about the possibility of morning orthostatic hypotension. Instruct the patient to rise slowly and to sit for several minutes before standing up.
— Tell the patient to notify the nurse or doctor if adverse reactions develop or questions arise about amitriptyline therapy.

Evaluation
In the patient receiving amitriptyline, appropriate evaluation statements include:
• Patient reports improvement of depression.
• Patient reports regular bowel habits.
• Patient's vital signs and ECG are normal.
• Patient does not experience injury from adverse CNS reactions.
• Patient and family state an understanding of amitriptyline therapy.

PROTOTYPE: MISCELLANEOUS ANTIDEPRESSANTS

FLUOXETINE HYDROCHLORIDE
(floo ox′ e teen)
Prozac
Classification: miscellaneous antidepressant
Pregnancy risk category B

How supplied
PULVULES: 20 mg

Indications and dosage
Short-term management of depressive illness
ADULTS: initially, 20 mg P.O. in the morning; dosage increased according to patient response. May be given b.i.d. in the morning and at noon. Maximum dosage is 80 mg daily.

Contraindications and precautions
Fluoxetine is contraindicated in patients with known hypersensitivity to the drug and in patients who have received MAO inhibitors within 14 days of starting therapy. Fluoxetine should be used with close monitoring and psychiatric evaluation. The possibility of a suicide attempt is inherent in depressed patients. Because patients may experience significant weight loss while taking this drug, use cautiously in underweight individuals.

In early clinical trials, about 4% of patients developed a rash while taking fluoxetine. Some of these patients developed further systemic symptoms, including fever, leukocytosis, and arthralgia. Drug should be discontinued if a rash develops during therapy.

Adverse reactions
CNS: *nervousness, anxiety, insomnia, headache, drowsiness, tremor, dizziness,* abnormal dreams.
CV: palpitations, flushing, bradycardia, arrhythmias.

Italicized adverse reactions are common

EENT: flulike syndrome, nasal congestion, upper respiratory infection, pharyngitis, cough, sinusitis, visual disturbances, tinnitus, respiratory distress.

GI: *nausea, diarrhea,* dry mouth, *anorexia,* dyspepsia, constipation, abdominal pain, vomiting, taste change, flatulence, increased appetite.

GU: sexual dysfunction, urine retention.

SKIN: *rash.*

OTHER: muscle pain, *weight loss,* rash, pruritus, urticaria, asthenia, edema, lymphadenopathy, *excessive sweating.*

Interactions

Diazepam: half-life may be prolonged. Drugs highly bound to plasma proteins (warfarin, digitoxin) can displace drug and cause toxic effects.

Nursing considerations

Assessment
- Obtain a baseline assessment of patient's depression before therapy.
- Be alert for common adverse reactions.
- Evaluate the patient's and family's knowledge about fluoxetine therapy.

Planning (Nursing Diagnoses)
Potential nursing diagnoses for the patient receiving fluoxetine include:
- Altered thought processes related to ineffectiveness or inadequate fluoxetine therapy.
- Sleep pattern disturbance related to fluoxetine-induced insomnia.
- Diarrhea related to fluoxetine effects on the GI tract.
- Knowledge deficit related to fluoxetine therapy.

Implementation

Preparation and administration
— Expect reduced dosage or longer intervals between doses in elderly or debilitated patients and in patients with renal or hepatic dysfunction.
— Make sure the patient has swallowed the medication after each dose.
— To prevent insomnia, avoid administering the drug in the evening.

Monitoring
— Monitor effectiveness by asking the patient about feelings of depression and by evaluating the patient's behavior.
— Monitor the patient for adverse drug reactions.
— Monitor sleep patterns for evidence of insomnia.
— Monitor changes in bowel patterns, especially for diarrhea.
— Monitor the patient for drug interactions.
— Monitor for skin changes suggestive of allergy: rash, pruritus, or urticaria.
— Regularly reevaluate the patient's and family's knowledge about fluoxetine therapy.

Intervention
— Discuss with doctor alternative therapies or change in fluoxetine regimen if drug is ineffective.

—Help the patient use nonpharmacologic measures to combat insomnia. For example, recommend relaxation techniques, reading before going to bed, and listening to soothing music.

—If needed, obtain an order for an antidiarrheal agent.

—If adverse CNS reactions occur, institute safety precautions, such as supervising patient's activities.

—If infection occurs, provide fluids and opportunities to rest as well as use of prescribed medications to treat fever, aches and pains, and signs and symptoms of infection.

—Ask the patient to void before dosing to avoid urine retention.

—Weigh the patient regularly to monitor for weight loss resulting from adverse GI reactions.

—Keep all members of the health care team informed of the patient's response to the drug.

Patient teaching

—Instruct the patient and family about the fluoxetine, including the dosage, frequency, action, and adverse reactions.

—Tell the patient that fluoxetine and its active metabolite have a long elimination half-life. Clinical effects of dosage changes may not be evident for weeks; full antidepressant effects may not appear for 4 or more weeks of treatment.

—Because fluoxetine commonly causes nervousness and insomnia, tell the patient to avoid taking the drug in the evening to prevent sleep disturbances. Also teach the patient use of nonpharmacologic measures to induce sleep if insomnia occurs.

—Drug may cause dizziness or drowsiness in some patients; therefore, warn the patient to avoid driving and other hazardous activities that require alertness until CNS effects of the drug are known.

—Tell the patient to rest, drink adequate fluids, and to notify the doctor if an infection occurs.

—Advise the patient to weigh himself daily and report sudden weight gains (greater than 3 to 5 lb [1.4 to 2.3 kg]), which suggests edema, or weight losses (greater than 5 lb), which suggests adverse GI reactions.

—Inform the patient that fluoxetine can cause sexual dysfunction.

—Tell the patient to notify the nurse or doctor if adverse reactions develop or questions arise about fluoxetine therapy.

Evaluation

In the patient receiving fluoxetine, appropriate evaluation statements include:

• Patient reports feeling renewed interest in life.
• Patient reports ability to sleep at night.
• Patient does not experience diarrhea.
• Patient and family state an understanding of fluoxetine therapy.

SELECTED MAJOR DRUGS: ANTIDEPRESSANTS

DRUG, INDICATIONS, AND DOSAGES	SPECIAL PRECAUTIONS

Monoamine oxidase inhibitors

isocarboxazid (Marplan)
Depression—
Adults: 30 mg P.O. daily in divided doses. Reduce to 10 to 20 mg daily when condition improves. Not recommended for children under age 11.

• Contraindicated in patients with known hypersensitivity to the drug; in elderly or debilitated patients; and in those with severe hepatic or renal impairment; CHF; pheochromocytoma; hypertension; CV or cerebrovascular disease; or severe or frequent headaches. Also contraindicated within 10 days of elective surgery requiring general anesthesia, cocaine, or a local anesthetic containing sympathomimetic vasoconstrictors and with concurrent use of other MAO inhibitors, buspirone, clomipramine, CNS depressants, sympathomimetic drugs, high-tryptophan foods, high-tyramine foods, or excessive amounts of caffeine.
• Administer cautiously to hyperactive, agitated, schizophrenic, or suicidal patients; to patients with diabetes mellitus or seizure disorder; or to those taking antihypertensive drugs, including thiazide diuretics. Also administer cautiously to pregnant or breast-feeding patients.

phenelzine (Nardil)
Depression—
Adults: 45 mg P.O. daily in divided doses, increasing rapidly to 60 mg daily. Then dosage can usually be reduced to 15 mg daily. Maximum is 90 mg daily.

• Contraindicated in patients with known hypersensitivity to the drug, pheochromocytoma, CHF, a history of liver disease or abnormal liver function tests, hypertension, and CV or cerebrovascular disease; with foods containing tryptophan or tyramine; during therapy with other MAO inhibitors (including isocarboxazid and tranylcypromine) or within 10 days of such therapy; within 10 days of elective surgery requiring general anesthetic, cocaine, or local anesthetic containing sympathomimetic vasoconstrictors; and in hyperactive, agitated, or schizophrenic patients.
• Administer cautiously with antihypertensive drugs containing thiazide diuretics, with spinal anesthetics, and to patients with diabetes mellitus or at risk for suicide.

Tricyclic antidepressants

amoxapine (Asendin)
Depression—
Adults: initially, 50 mg P.O. t.i.d. Maximum dosage is 600 mg in hospitalized patients.

• Contraindicated in patients during acute recovery phase of MI, with a history of seizure disorder, and with prostatic hypertrophy.

(continued)

SELECTED MAJOR DRUGS: ANTIDEPRESSANTS *continued*

DRUG, INDICATIONS, AND DOSAGES	SPECIAL PRECAUTIONS
Tricyclic antidepressants *(continued)*	

amoxapine *(continued)*

- Administer cautiously to patients who are at risk for suicide; to patients with urine retention, narrow-angle glaucoma, increased intraocular pressure, CV disease, impaired hepatic function, or hyperthyroidism; and to those receiving thyroid medications, electroconvulsive therapy, or elective surgery.

desipramine (Norpramin, Pertofrane)
Depression—
Adults: 75 to 150 mg P.O. daily in divided doses, increasing to maximum of 300 mg daily.
Elderly patients and adolescents: 25 to 50 mg P.O. daily, increasing gradually to maximum of 100 mg daily.

- Contraindicated in patients receiving MAO inhibitors and in hyperpyretic crises, severe seizures, and the acute recovery phase of MI.
- Administer cautiously to patients with CV disease, urine retention, glaucoma, thyroid disease, and seizure disorders; to pregnant and breast-feeding women; to children; and with alcohol.

doxepin (Adapin, Deptran‡, Sinequan, Triadapin‡)
Depression—
Adults: initially, 50 to 75 mg P.O. daily in divided doses, to maximum of 300 mg daily. Alternatively, entire dosage may be given h.s.

- Contraindicated in patients with known hypersensitivity to the drug, glaucoma, or urine retention.
- Administer cautiously to pregnant and breast-feeding women, children under age 12, patients taking MAO inhibitors, and those at risk for suicide.

imipramine (Apo-Imipramine†, Imiprin‡, Janimine, Tofranil)
Depression—
Adults: 75 to 100 mg P.O. or I.M. daily in divided doses, with 25- to 50-mg increments up to 200 mg. Maximum dosage is 300 mg daily. Alternatively, the entire dosage may be given h.s.
Children ages 6 and over: 25 mg P.O. 1 hour before bedtime. If no response within 1 week, increase to 50 mg if the child is under age 12 and to 75 mg for children ages 12 and over; not to exceed 2.5 mg/kg daily in either case.

- Contraindicated in patients during acute recovery phase of MI and in those with a history of seizure disorder.
- Administer cautiously to patients with CV disease, prostatic hypertrophy, urine retention, narrow-angle glaucoma or increased intraocular pressure, thyroid disease, blood dyscrasia, or impaired hepatic function; in patients who are at risk for suicide; and in those receiving electroconvulsive therapy, thyroid medication, or elective surgery.

maprotiline (Ludiomil)
Depression—
Adults: initially, 75 mg P.O. daily for patients with mild to moderate depression. Dosage may be increased as required to a dose of 150 mg daily. Maximum dosage is 225 mg in patients who are not hospitalized. More severely depressed, hospitalized patients may receive up to 300 mg daily.

- Contraindicated in patients with known hypersensitivity to the drug and in those with seizure disorder; concomitantly with MAO inhibitors; or during the acute recovery phase of MI.
- Administer cautiously to patients with a history of MI, with CV disease, and at risk for suicide; with narrow-angle glaucoma, thyroid disease, blood dyscrasia, and impaired hepatic function; and to those receiving electroconvulsive therapy or elective surgery.

SELECTED MAJOR DRUGS: ANTIDEPRESSANTS *continued*

DRUG, INDICATIONS, AND DOSAGES	SPECIAL PRECAUTIONS
Tricyclic antidepressants *(continued)*	
nortriptyline (Aventyl, Pamelor) *Depression—* **Adults:** 25 mg P.O. t.i.d. or q.i.d., gradually increasing to a maximum of 150 mg daily. Alternatively, entire dose may be given h.s.	• Contraindicated in patients with known hypersensitivity to the drug; in use with MAO inhibitors; and during the acute recovery phase of MI. • Administer cautiously to patients with CV disease, urine retention, glaucoma, thyroid disease, impaired hepatic function, or blood dyscrasia; to patients who are at risk for suicide; or to those receiving electroconvulsive therapy, thyroid medication, or elective surgery.
trimipramine (Surmontil) *Depression—* **Adults:** 75 mg P.O. daily in divided doses, increased to 200 mg daily. Dosages over 300 mg daily not recommended. *Enuresis—* **Children over age 6:** initially, 25 mg P.O. 1 hour before bedtime; if no response, increase to 50 mg in children under age 12, and to 75 mg in children over age 12.	• Contraindicated in patients with known hypersensitivity to the drug, in use with MAO inhibitors and tricyclic compounds, during the acute recovery phase of MI, in patients with prostatic hypertrophy, in patients with a history of seizure disorder, in those at risk for suicide, and in those receiving electroconvulsive therapy, thyroid medication, or elective surgery. • Administer cautiously to patients with CV disease, urine retention, narrow-angle glaucoma or increased intraocular pressure, thyroid disease, blood dyscrasia, or impaired hepatic function.
Miscellaneous agents	
bupropion (Wellbutrin) *Depression—* **Adults:** 100 mg P.O. b.i.d. If necessary, dosage is increased after 3 days to the usual dose of 100 mg t.i.d. If there is no response after several weeks of therapy, dosage may be increased to 150 mg t.i.d.	• Contraindicated in patients who are allergic to the drug; who have taken MAO inhibitors within previous 14 days; and who have seizure disorders. About 0.4% of patients treated at doses up to 450 mg daily experience seizures; incidence rises tenfold if dosage is increased to 600 mg daily. Also contraindicated in patients with a history of bulimia or anorexia nervosa because of higher incidence of seizures in these patients. Patients who experience seizures often have predisposing factors (history of head trauma, prior seizure, or CNS tumors) or may be taking a drug that lowers the seizure threshold.
trazodone (Desyrel, Trazon, Trialodine) *Depression—* **Adults:** initially, 150 mg P.O. daily in divided doses, which can be increased by 50 mg daily q 3 to 4 days. Average dosage ranges from 150 to 400 mg daily. Maximum dosage is 600 mg daily.	• Contraindicated in patients with known hypersensitivity to the drug, in patients during the acute recovery phase of MI, and in those receiving electroconvulsive therapy.

SELF-TEST

1. Alison Cote is hospitalized for the treatment of acute bronchitis. She is on long-term drug therapy with tranylcypromine (Parnate) for endogenous depression. You are helping her to select her menu. All of the following foods are choices for lunch. Which would you remind her to *avoid*?
   a. hamburger
   b. tuna salad
   c. baked chicken
   d. grilled cheese sandwich

2. You would schedule Ms. Cote's maintenance dose of tranylcypromine to be given:
   a. ½ hour before breakfast.
   b. 1 hour after breakfast.
   c. with supper.
   d. at bedtime.

3. Betty Shapiro started taking amitriptyline (Elavil) 1 week ago for treatment of endogenous depression. On her return visit to the mental health clinic, she complains that she feels no better than before she started on amitriptyline. The nurse would:
   a. encourage her to continue the medication since it can take up to 4 weeks to be effective.
   b. consult with the doctor about the possibility of changing to a more effective medication.
   c. teach her to take the medication 2 hours before a meal to enhance absorption.
   d. suggest she increase her intake of chocolate and cheese because these foods improve the drug's metabolism.

4. Susan Little, age 67, is severely depressed after the recent death of her spouse of 40 years. Her doctor prescribed fluoxetine 20 mg P.O. daily to be taken in the morning. Subsequent dosage will be increased in two follow-up visits. What is the maximum dosage Ms. Little should receive?
   a. 40 mg
   b. 60 mg
   c. 80 mg
   d. 100 mg

5. How should Ms. Little's age influence the dosage prescribed to treat her depression?
   a. Higher than normal dosages may be required.
   b. Lower than normal dosages may be required.
   c. More frequent dosing throughout the day may be required.
   d. A night-time dose may be required.

Check your answers on page 1064.

CHAPTER 31

ANXIOLYTICS

Antihistamines
hydroxyzine hydrochloride ✦ hydroxyzine pamoate

Benzodiazepines
alprazolam ✦ chlordiazepoxide hydrochloride ✦ clorazepate dipotassium
diazepam ✦ halazepam ✦ lorazepam ✦ oxazepam ✦ prazepam

OVERVIEW
- Anxiolytics, also known as antianxiety agents, reduce anxiety without inducing sleep; they are indicated for patients suffering from various neuroses or mild depression. Most anxiolytics have muscle-relaxant and anticonvulsant properties. They produce a dose-dependent, nonspecific depression of the CNS and closely resemble sedative-hypnotics, such as benzodiazepines, in pharmacologic properties.
- Anxiolytics are classified primarily into two groups: antihistamines and benzodiazepines.

MAJOR USES
- Anxiolytics are used to treat anxiety, relax skeletal muscles, prevent and treat alcohol withdrawal symptoms and seizures (especially chlordiazepoxide, diazepam, and lorazepam), treat status epilepticus (especially I.V. diazepam), and supply premedication for I.V. general anesthetic for short procedures (especially diazepam and lorazepam). For information about anticonvulsant use of clonazepam and diazepam, see Chapter 29, Anticonvulsants.

MECHANISM OF ACTION
- Benzodiazepines (alprazolam, chlordiazepoxide, clorazepate, diazepam, halazepam, lorazepam, oxazepam, and prazepam) appear to depress the CNS at the limbic and subcortical levels of the brain, with sedative skeletal muscle relaxant and anticonvulsant effects. They can produce physical and psychological dependence.
- The mechanisms of action of the other anxiolytics are still unclear.

ABSORPTION, DISTRIBUTION, METABOLISM, AND EXCRETION
Hydroxyzine is well absorbed orally, distributed to most body tissues, metabolized in the liver, and eliminated in both the urine and feces.

GLOSSARY

Anxiety: feeling of apprehension, uncertainty, and fear.
Anxiety disorder: primary medical condition or disorder secondary to another medical or social problem; may be nonphobic (such as a generalized anxiety, obsessive-compulsive, or panic disorder) or phobic (such as a fear of crowds or heights).

Benzodiazepines are very well absorbed when given orally. Well distributed to body tissues and fluids, they're all metabolized in the GI tract and the liver to either active or inactive metabolites. These metabolites are then excreted by the kidneys. Alprazolam, the first of a new type of benzodiazepine, is more rapidly metabolized and excreted than most of the other benzodiazepines and has a lower incidence of lethargy than other drugs in this class. Absorption of chlordiazepoxide and diazepam after I.M. injection is variable, painful, and unpredictable. After I.M. injection, lorazepam absorption is much more dependable and less painful than that of diazepam and chlordiazepoxide.

ONSET AND DURATION

Hydroxyzine acts within 15 to 20 minutes and its effect lasts 4 to 6 hours. All benzodiazepines have a fairly prompt onset of action (1 to 2 hours); diazepam has the fastest (about 1 hour). Generally, those agents that are changed into active (long-acting) metabolites have longer duration of action (up to 24 hours) than those that are not changed. The long therapeutic half-lives of the active metabolites permit once-daily dosing when steady-state levels are reached. Alprazolam, lorazepam, and oxazepam, which have shorter half-lives, must be given two to four times daily.

ADVERSE REACTIONS

At therapeutic dosage levels, most antihistamines are likely to cause drowsiness and impaired motor function during initial therapy. Also, their anticholinergic action usually causes dry mouth and throat, blurred vision, and constipation. Antihistamines that are also phenothiazines, such as promethazine, may cause other adverse reactions, including cholestatic jaundice (thought to be a hypersensitivity reaction), and may predispose patients to photosensitivity; patients taking such drugs should avoid prolonged exposure to sunlight.

Toxic doses elicit a combination of CNS depression and excitation as well as atropine-like symptoms, including sedation, reduced mental alertness, apnea, CV collapse, hallucinations, tremor, seizures, dry mouth, flushed skin, and fixed, dilated pupils. Toxic effects reverse when medication is discontinued. Used appropriately and in correct dosages, antihistamines are safe for prolonged use.

Benzodiazepines usually produce adverse reactions that include CNS effects, such as drowsiness, ataxia, fatigue, confusion, weakness, headache, dizziness, vertigo, and syncope. These reactions are most likely to occur in patients with hepatic or renal dysfunction and in children or elderly or debilitated patients; such patients should receive lower initial doses of these drugs. All patients who take a benzodiazepine as a sleeping aid, especially those who are elderly, may have increased daytime sedation or other prolonged adverse CNS reactions. This effect is intensified if the benzodiazepine is taken for prolonged periods because serum levels of the drug will increase. Prolonged use of benzodiazepines with a long half-life, such as diazepam, clorazepate, or chlordiazepoxide, has been associated with increased incidence of falls in elderly patients.

Other adverse CNS reactions associated with benzodiazepines include anterograde amnesia, euphoria, nightmares, and hallucinations. Psychological and physical dependence occur with long-term use and may result in withdrawal symptoms. Rarely, paradoxical reactions produce an acute hyperexcited state with anxiety, hallucinations, insomnia, or rage; such reactions require discontinuation of the drug.

GI reactions include constipation, dry mouth, taste alterations, anorexia, nausea, vomiting, and abdominal discomfort. Hiccups have also been reported. Respiratory depression may occur but is usually associated with overdosage or an interaction with another respiratory depressant. Other adverse reactions are rare but may include CV effects (tachycardia, palpitations, and hypotension), dermatologic reactions (rashes, urticaria, and flushing), and urinary incontinence or urine retention.

PROTOTYPE: ANTIHISTAMINES

HYDROXYZINE HYDROCHLORIDE (HYDROXYZINE EMBONATE)
(hye drox′ i zeen)
Anxanil, Apo-Hydroxyzine†, Atarax*, Atozine, Durrax, E-Vista, Hydroxacen, Hyzine-50, Multipax†, Novohydroxyzin†, Quiess, Vistacon-50, Vistaject, Vistaquel 50, Vistaril, Vistazine 50

HYDROXYZINE PAMOATE
Hy-Pam, Vamate, Vistaril
Classification: piperazine antihistamine
Pregnancy risk category C

How supplied
hydrochloride
TABLETS: 10 mg, 25 mg, 50 mg, 100 mg
CAPSULES: 10 mg†‡, 25 mg†‡, 50 mg†‡
SYRUP: 10 mg/5 ml
INJECTION: 25 mg/ml, 50 mg/ml
pamoate
CAPSULES: 25 mg, 50 mg, 100 mg
ORAL SUSPENSION: 25 mg/5 ml

Indications and dosage

Anxiety and tension
ADULTS: 25 to 100 mg P.O. t.i.d. or q.i.d.

Anxiety, tension, hyperkinesia
CHILDREN AGES 6 AND OVER: 50 to 100 mg P.O. daily in divided doses.
CHILDREN UNDER AGE 6: 50 mg P.O. daily in divided doses.

Preoperative and postoperative adjunctive therapy
ADULTS: 25 to 100 mg I.M. q 4 to 6 hours.
CHILDREN: 1.1 mg/kg I.M. q 4 to 6 hours.

Rashes, pruritus
ADULTS: 25 mg P.O. t.i.d. or q.i.d.
CHILDREN AGES 6 AND OVER: 50 to 100 mg P.O. daily in divided doses.
CHILDREN UNDER AGE 6: 50 mg P.O. daily in divided doses.

Contraindications and precautions
Hydroxyzine is contraindicated in patients with known hypersensitivity to the drug and in those in shock or comatose states.

Adverse reactions
CNS: *drowsiness*, involuntary motor activity.
GI: *dry mouth.*
LOCAL: marked discomfort at site of I.M. injection.

Interactions
Alcohol, other CNS depressants: increased CNS depression. Avoid concomitant use.

Nursing considerations

Assessment
- Review the patient's history for a condition that contraindicates the use of hydroxyzine.
- Obtain a baseline assessment of the patient's anxiety level before therapy.
- Be alert for common adverse reactions.
- Evaluate the patient's and family's knowledge about hydroxyzine therapy.

Planning (Nursing Diagnoses)
Potential nursing diagnoses for the patient receiving hydroxyzine include:
- Anxiety related to ineffectiveness of hydroxyzine.
- Activity intolerance related to hydroxyzine-induced drowsiness.
- Altered oral mucous membrane related to hydroxyzine-induced dry mouth.
- Knowledge deficit related to hydroxyzine therapy.

Implementation

Preparation and administration
——Parenteral form (hydrochloride) for I.M. use only (Z-track injection is preferred). Never administer I.V.

Italicized adverse reactions are common

—Aspirate injection carefully to prevent inadvertent intravascular injection. Inject deep into a large muscle.

—Dosage should be reduced in elderly or debilitated patients.

Monitoring

—Regularly monitor effectiveness by asking the patient about feelings of anxiety and by observing the patient's behavior.

—Monitor the patient for adverse drug reactions.

—Monitor degree of dry mouth.

—Monitor for excessive sedation due to potentiation with other CNS drugs.

—Monitor the patient for drug interactions.

—Regularly reevaluate the patient's and family's knowledge about hydroxyzine therapy.

Intervention

—If drowsiness or involuntary motor activity occurs, institute safety precautions, such as supervising ambulation.

—Provide frequent sips of water or ice chips for dry mouth.

—Provide encouragement for other supportive measures such as counseling and problem identification with a health professional.

—Keep all members of the health care team informed of the patient's response to the drug.

Patient teaching

—Instruct the patient and family about hydroxyzine, including the dosage, frequency, action, and adverse reactions.

—Warn the patient to avoid driving and other hazardous activities that require alertness and good psychomotor coordination until CNS effects of the drug are known.

—Warn the patient not to combine drug with alcohol or other CNS depressants.

—Alert the patient to expect some marked discomfort at the injection site.

—Suggest sugarless hard candy, ice chips, or gum to relieve dry mouth.

—Tell the patient to notify the nurse or doctor if adverse reactions develop or questions arise about hydroxyzine therapy.

Evaluation

In the patient receiving hydroxyzine, appropriate evaluation statements include:

• Patient states he is less anxious.

• Patient is able to maintain normal daily activities.

• Patient states that use of sugarless candy, ice chips, or gum relieves the discomfort of dry mouth.

• Patient and family state an understanding of hydroxyzine therapy.

ALPRAZOLAM
(al pray′ zoe lam)
Xanax
Classification: benzodiazepine
Controlled substance schedule IV
Pregnancy risk category D

How supplied
TABLETS: 0.25 mg, 0.5 mg, 1 mg

Indications and dosage
Anxiety and tension
ADULTS: usual starting dose is 0.25 to 0.5 mg P.O. t.i.d. Maximum total dosage is 4 mg daily in divided doses. In elderly or debilitated patients, usual starting dose is 0.25 mg b.i.d. or t.i.d.

Contraindications and precautions
Alprazolam is contraindicated in patients with known hypersensitivity to the drug or other benzodiazepines and in those with acute narrow-angle glaucoma, psychoses, or anxiety-free psychiatric disorders. Reduce dosage in elderly or debilitated patients because they may be more susceptible to adverse CNS reactions.

Adverse reactions
CNS: *drowsiness, light-headedness, headache,* confusion, hostility.
CV: transient hypotension, tachycardia.
EENT: dry mouth.
GI: nausea, vomiting, constipation, discomfort.

Interactions
Alcohol, other CNS depressants: increased CNS depression. Avoid concomitant use.
Cimetidine: increased sedation. Monitor carefully.
Tricyclic antidepressants (TCAs): increased plasma levels of TCAs. Monitor for toxicity.

Nursing considerations
Assessment
• Review the patient's history for a condition that contraindicates the use of alprazolam.
• Obtain a baseline assessment of the patient's anxiety level before therapy.
• Be alert for common adverse reactions.
• Evaluate the patient's and family's knowledge about alprazolam therapy.

Planning (Nursing Diagnoses)

Potential nursing diagnoses for the patient receiving alprazolam include:
• Anxiety related to ineffectiveness of alprazolam.
• Potential for injury related to alprazolam-induced CNS reactions.
• Knowledge deficit related to alprazolam therapy.

Implementation

Preparation and administration

—When administering alprazolam, make sure the patient has swallowed the tablets before leaving the bedside.
—Expect to administer lower dosage at longer intervals in elderly or debilitated patients.

Monitoring

—Regularly monitor the effectiveness of alprazolam therapy by asking the patient about feelings of anxiety and by evaluating the patient's behavior.
—Monitor the patient for adverse drug reactions.
—Monitor vital signs for hypotension or tachycardia.
—Monitor bowel patterns to detect constipation before it becomes severe.
—Monitor the patient for drug interactions.
—Regularly reevaluate the patient's and family's knowledge about alprazolam therapy.

Intervention

—Provide encouragement and support with other measures prescribed to augment alprazolam therapy, such as counseling and problem identification with professionals.
—If drowsiness, light-headedness, or confusion occurs, institute safety measures, such as supervising patient activities. Reorient patient as needed and ensure a safe environment.
—Provide frequent sips of water or ice chips for dry mouth.
—If not contraindicated, increase the patient's fluid intake and dietary fiber to prevent constipation.
—Be aware that drug should not be prescribed for everyday stress or for long-term use (more than 4 months).
—Do not withdraw drug abruptly. Abuse or addiction is possible and withdrawal symptoms may occur.
—Keep all members of the health care team informed of the patient's response to the drug.

Patient teaching

—Instruct the patient and family about alprazolam, including the dosage, frequency, action, and adverse reactions.
—Warn the patient not to combine drug with alcohol or other CNS depressants and also to avoid driving and other hazardous activities that require alertness and psychomotor coordination until adverse CNS effects of the drug are known.
—Caution the patient against giving medication to others.

— Warn the patient to take this drug only as directed and not to discontinue drug without the doctor's approval. Inform the patient of the drug's potential for dependence if taken longer than directed.

— Recommend sugarless chewing gum or hard candy or ice chips to relieve dry mouth.

— Tell the patient to increase fluid and fiber intake to prevent constipation.

— Tell the patient to notify the nurse or doctor if adverse reactions develop or questions arise about alprazolam therapy.

Evaluation

In the patient receiving alprazolam, appropriate evaluation statements include:

• Patient states he is less anxious.

• Patient does not experience injury as a result of adverse CNS reactions.

• Patient and family state an understanding of alprazolam therapy.

SELECTED MAJOR DRUGS: ANXIOLYTICS

DRUG, INDICATIONS, AND DOSAGES	SPECIAL PRECAUTIONS
Benzodiazepines	
chlordiazepoxide (Libritabs) **chlordiazepoxide hydrochloride (Apo-Chlordiazepoxide†, Librium, Mitran)** *Mild to moderate anxiety and tension—* **Adults:** 5 to 10 mg P.O. t.i.d. or q.i.d. **Children over age 6:** 5 mg P.O. b.i.d. to q.i.d. Maximum dosage is 10 mg P.O. b.i.d. to t.i.d. *Severe anxiety and tension—* **Adults:** 20 to 25 mg P.O. t.i.d. or q.i.d. *Withdrawal symptoms of acute alcoholism—* **Adults:** 50 to 100 mg P.O., I.M., or I.V. Maximum dosage is 300 mg daily. *Preoperative apprehension and anxiety—* **Adults:** 5 to 10 mg P.O. t.i.d. or q.i.d. on day preceding surgery; or 50 to 100 mg I.M. 1 hour before surgery.	• Contraindicated in patients with known hypersensitivity to the drug. • Administer cautiously to patients with mental depression, psychiatric disturbances, blood dyscrasia, porphyria, or hepatic or renal disease and to those undergoing anticoagulant therapy.
clorazepate (Tranxene) *Acute alcohol withdrawal syndrome—* **Adults:** Day 1—initially, 30 mg P.O., followed by 30 to 60 mg P.O. in divided doses; Day 2—45 to 90 mg P.O. in divided doses; Day 3—22.5 to 45 mg P.O. in divided doses; Day 4—15 to 30 mg P.O. in divided doses. Gradually reduce daily dosage to 7.5 to 15 mg. *Anxiety—* **Adults:** 15 to 60 mg P.O. daily. *As an adjunct in seizure disorder—* **Adults and children over age 12:** maximum recommended initial dosage is 7.5 mg P.O. t.i.d. Dosage increases should be no greater than 7.5 mg weekly. Maximum daily dosage should not exceed 90 mg daily.	• Contraindicated in patients with known hypersensitivity to the drug and in those with acute narrow-angle glaucoma. • Administer cautiously to patients with hepatic or renal damage.

†Available in Canada only

SELECTED MAJOR DRUGS: ANXIOLYTICS *continued*

DRUG, INDICATIONS, AND DOSAGES	SPECIAL PRECAUTIONS

Benzodiazepines *(continued)*

clorazepate *(continued)*
Children ages 9 to 12: maximum recommended initial dosage is 7.5 mg P.O. b.i.d. Dosage increases should be no greater than 7.5 mg weekly. Maximum dosage should not exceed 60 mg daily.

---

diazepam (Apo-Diazepam†, Novodiazepam†, Valium)
Tension, anxiety, adjunct in seizure disorders, or skeletal muscle spasm—
Adults: 2 to 10 mg P.O. t.i.d. or q.i.d. or 15 to 30 mg (extended-release capsule) daily.
Children over age 6 months: 1 to 2.5 mg P.O. t.i.d. or q.i.d.
Tension, anxiety, muscle spasm, endoscopic procedures, seizures—
Adults: initially, 5 to 10 mg I.V. up to 30 mg in 1 hour or possibly more for cardioversion or status epilepticus, depending on response.
Children ages 5 and over: 1 mg I.V. or I.M. slowly q 2 to 5 minutes to maximum of 10 mg. Repeat q 2 to 4 hours.
Children ages 30 days to 5 years: 0.2 to 0.5 mg I.V. or I.M. slowly q 2 to 5 minutes to maximum of 5 mg. Repeat q 2 to 4 hours.

• Contraindicated in patients with shock, coma, acute alcohol intoxication, acute narrow-angle glaucoma, psychoses, or myasthenia gravis and in oral form for children under age 6 months.
• Use cautiously in patients with blood dyscrasia, hepatic or renal damage, depression, and open-angle glaucoma; in elderly and debilitated patients; and in those with limited pulmonary reserve.

---

halazepam (Paxipam)
Relief of anxiety and tension—
Adults: usual dose is 20 to 40 mg P.O. t.i.d. or q.i.d. Optimal daily dosage is generally 80 to 160 mg. Daily dosages up to 600 mg have been given. In elderly or debilitated patients, initial dosage is 20 mg daily or b.i.d.

• Contraindicated in patients with acute narrow-angle glaucoma, psychoses, or anxiety-free psychiatric disorders.
• Administer cautiously to patients with hepatorenal impairment.

---

lorazepam (Apo-Lorazepam†, Ativan)
Anxiety, tension, agitation, irritability, especially in anxiety neuroses or organic (especially GI or CV) disorders—
Adults: 2 to 6 mg P.O. daily in divided doses. Maximum dosage is 10 mg daily.
Insomnia—
Adults: 2 to 4 mg P.O. h.s.
Premedication before operative procedure—
Adults: 0.05 mg/kg I.M. or I.V., not to exceed 4 mg.

• Contraindicated in patients with known hypersensitivity to benzodiazepines or their vehicles (polyethylene glycol, propylene glycol, and benzyl alcohol) and in those with acute narrow-angle glaucoma.
• Administer cautiously to patients with organic brain syndrome, myasthenia gravis, and renal or hepatic impairment.

(continued)

SELECTED MAJOR DRUGS: ANXIOLYTICS *continued*

DRUG, INDICATIONS, AND DOSAGES	SPECIAL PRECAUTIONS
Benzodiazepines *(continued)*	
oxazepam (Apo-Oxazepam†, Novoxapam†, Serax) *Alcohol withdrawal syndrome —* **Adults:** 15 to 30 mg P.O. t.i.d. or q.i.d. *Severe anxiety —* **Adults:** 15 to 30 mg P.O. t.i.d. or q.i.d. *Tension, mild to moderate anxiety —* **Adults:** 10 to 15 mg P.O. t.i.d. or q.i.d.	• Contraindicated in patients with known hypersensitivity to oxazepam and in psychoses. • Administer cautiously to patients with a history of seizure disorder, drug allergies, blood dyscrasia, renal disease, and depression.
prazepam (Centrax) *Anxiety —* **Adults:** 30 mg P.O. in divided doses. Range 20 to 60 mg daily. May be administered as single daily dose h.s.; start with 20 mg.	• Contraindicated in patients with acute narrow-angle glaucoma, psychoses, or anxiety-free psychiatric disorders. • Administer cautiously to patients with renal or hepatic impairment.

†Available in Canada only

SELF-TEST

1. Paul Hernandez, age 72, has acute anxiety. His doctor orders alprazolam 25 mg P.O. q.i.d. The nurse should:
   a. follow the order promptly because acute anxiety can be life-threatening.
   b. question the order because it exceeds the safe dosage and frequency.
   c. refuse to give the drug because it is contraindicated in elderly patients.
   d. institute seizure precautions after administering the first dose.

2. Mr. Hernandez will be taking alprazolam at home. Which of the following instructions are appropriate regarding safe use of this drug?
   a. Stop the medication if it makes you sleepy.
   b. Do not drink any alcohol while taking this medication.
   c. Stay out of the sun when taking this medication.
   d. Call your doctor if you develop dry mouth.

3. Mary Smith is hospitalized for treatment of acute anxiety. Her doctor prescribed an initial dose of hydroxyzine 25 mg parenterally, followed by a P.O. dose of 25 mg t.i.d. How should the nurse administer the injection?
   a. direct I.V. push
   b. I.M. using Z-track technique
   c. inject into a small muscle to limit discomfort
   d. subcutaneously into the deltoid muscle

4. How should the patient's age influence hydroxyzine therapy?
   a. Dosage should be increased in children.
   b. Dosage should be decreased in elderly patients.
   c. Frequency of administration should be increased in elderly patients.
   d. Frequency of administration should be decreased in elderly patients.

5. Mrs. Smith's nurse should monitor for which of the following adverse reactions?
   a. nausea and vomiting
   b. orthostatic hypotension and cardiac arrhythmias
   c. bronchospasms and shortness of breath
   d. drowsiness and involuntary motor activity

Check your answers on pages 1064 and 1065.

CHAPTER 32

ANTIPSYCHOTIC AGENTS

Phenothiazines
acetophenazine maleate ◆ chlorpromazine hydrochloride
fluphenazine decanoate ◆ fluphenazine enanthate
fluphenazine hydrochloride ◆ mesoridazine besylate ◆ perphenazine
prochlorperazine ◆ prochlorperazine edisylate ◆ prochlorperazine maleate
prochlorperazine mesylate ◆ promazine ◆ thioridazine
thioridazine hydrochloride ◆ trifluoperazine

Nonphenothiazines
chlorprothixene ◆ clozapine ◆ haloperidol ◆ haloperidol decanoate
haloperidol lactate ◆ loxapine hydrochloride ◆ loxapine succinate
thiothixene ◆ thiothixene hydrochloride

OVERVIEW

- Antipsychotic agents (also called neuroleptic agents) are used to help control the symptoms of psychoses and may help patients become more receptive to psychotherapy. These agents modify thought disorders, blunted affect (deadened emotions and apathy), and abnormal behaviors associated with psychomotor and mental retardation. They lessen symptoms of paranoia, agitation, hallucinations, delusions, and autistic behavior.
- Because antipsychotic agents cause many and potentially severe adverse reactions, they should be reserved for severe mental illness. For milder disturbances, anxiolytics, such as benzodiazepines, are safer and probably more effective.
- Because antipsychotic agents do not control the causes of psychoses, symptoms may recur after the drugs are discontinued.
- Antipsychotic agents are classified primarily into phenothiazines and nonphenothiazines.

MAJOR USES

- Antipsychotic agents may be used to treat symptoms of acute and chronic psychoses, especially those attended by increased psychomotor activity (including schizophrenia and the manic phase of bipolar disorders).
- Haloperidol and thioridazine are more commonly used than other antipsychotic agents to control agitation in organic brain syndrome.
- Chlorpromazine and certain other phenothiazines may also be used as antiemetics, antihistamines, and antipruritics.

GLOSSARY

Antipsychotic: agent that prevents or diminishes psychosis.
Drug holiday: discontinuation of an antipsychotic agent for 4 or more weeks to detect tardive dyskinesia, which may be masked by the drug's effects.
Dystonia: disordered muscle tone; a common adverse reaction to antipsychotic agents.
Euphoria: exaggerated sense of well-being.
Phobia: persistent, abnormal dread or fear.
Pseudoparkinsonism: state resembling Parkinson's disease; characterized by muscle rigidity, tremor, shuffling gait, drooling, and decreased arm swing and associative movements when walking; a common adverse reaction to antipsychotic agents.
Psychosis: mental disorder characterized by loss of contact with reality and derangement of personality.
Tardive dyskinesia: neurologic syndrome characterized by abnormal muscle movement, particularly around the mouth (such as smacking, rhythmic darting of the tongue, and constant chewing movements), and slow, aimless involuntary movements of the arms and legs; a common adverse reaction to antipsychotic agents.

MECHANISM OF ACTION

- As antipsychotic agents, these drugs block postsynaptic dopamine receptors in the brain.
- As antiemetics, they block dopamine receptors in the medullary chemoreceptor trigger zone.

ABSORPTION, DISTRIBUTION, METABOLISM, AND EXCRETION

Although absorption after oral administration of these agents is efficient (faster with liquid concentrate than with tablets), it varies markedly among patients. Absorption after I.M. administration is usually more complete (about one-half the oral dose produces equal effect).

Antipsychotic agents are widely distributed to body tissues, and highest concentrations of unchanged drug occur in the brain. Metabolites predominate in the lungs, liver, kidneys, and spleen.

All antipsychotics are metabolized in the liver; the metabolites are eliminated in the urine and—through the bile—in the feces.

ONSET AND DURATION

Onset of action is 2 to 6 hours for most drugs given orally and I.M., although haloperidol's onset (administered I.M.) is much shorter (20 to 30 minutes). Although symptoms may diminish with the first few doses, maximal effect may require weeks or months to develop.

Long half-lives generally permit once-daily dosing (usually at bedtime). Divided doses are sometimes necessary for drugs causing significant hypotension (for example, thioridazine and chlorpromazine). Administering large doses of antipsychotics at the beginning of drug therapy (rapid neuroleptization) is sometimes ordered. Drugs such as haloperidol and thiothixene are then given hourly until symptoms abate.

ADVERSE REACTIONS

Antipsychotic agents, both phenothiazines and nonphenothiazines, may produce extrapyramidal symptoms (dystonic movements, torticollis, oculogyric crisis, parkinsonian symptoms) from akathisia during early treatment to tardive dyskinesia after long-term use. In most patients, such symptoms can be relieved by dosage reduction or treatment with diphenhydramine, trihexyphenidyl, or benztropine mesylate. Dystonia usually occurs during initial therapy or at increased dosage in children and young adults; parkinsonian symptoms and tardive dyskinesia more often affect older patients, especially women.

Neuroleptic malignant syndrome, resembling severe parkinsonism, may occur (most often in young men taking fluphenazine). The signs and symptoms include rapid onset of hyperthermia, muscular hyperreflexia, marked extrapyramidal and autonomic dysfunction, arrhythmias, and sweating. Although rare, this condition carries a 10% mortality rate and requires immediate treatment, including cooling blankets, a skeletal muscle relaxant (such as dantrolene), and supportive measures.

A significant risk of agranulocytosis and seizures is associated with clozapine. Patients receiving clozapine therapy require close monitoring for flulike symptoms or any symptoms suggestive of infection. Recommended monitoring includes weekly WBC and differential counts; to ensure compliance, no more than a 7-day supply of this drug should be given to the patient. Therapy should be interrupted if the total WBC count falls below $3,000/mm^3$ or the granulocyte count falls below $1,500/mm^3$. At any sign of infection, the patient should have appropriate cultures performed and an antibiotic prescribed.

Other adverse reactions are similar to those with the tricyclic antidepressants. They include varying sedative and anticholinergic effects, orthostatic hypotension with reflex tachycardia, fainting and dizziness, and arrhythmias; GI reactions, such as, nausea, vomiting, abdominal pain, and gastric irritation; ocular and visual changes; skin eruptions; and photosensitivity (See *Comparing Adverse Reactions to Phenothiazines* for comparative incidence of sedative, extrapyramidal, hypotensive, and anticholinergic effects.) Allergic reactions are usually marked by elevations of liver enzymes progressing to obstructive jaundice.

Generally, mesoridazine and thioridazine have the most pronounced CV effects; prochlorperazine has the least. Because of the rapid absorption, parenteral administration is more often associated with CV effects.

COMPARING ADVERSE REACTIONS TO PHENOTHIAZINES

The chart below indicates the relative potential of phenothiazines and nonphenothiazines to produce specific adverse reactions.

DRUG	SEDATIVE EFFECTS	EXTRA-PYRAMIDAL EFFECTS	HYPOTENSIVE EFFECTS	ANTICHOLIN-ERGIC EFFECTS
Phenothiazines				
acetophenazine	Moderate	Moderate	Low	Moderate
chlorpromazine	High	Moderate	High	High
fluphenazine	Low	High	Low	Low
mesoridazine	High	Low	Moderate	Moderate
perphenazine	Moderate	Moderate	Low	Low
prochlorperazine	Moderate	High	Low	Moderate
promazine	Moderate	Moderate	Moderate	High
thioridazine	High	Low	Moderate	Very high
trifluoperazine	Low	High	Low	Low
Nonphenothiazines				
chlorprothixene	High	Moderate	Moderate	Moderate
clozapine	High	Low	Low	Low
haloperidol	Low	Very high	Low	Very low
loxapine	Low	Moderate	Low	Low
thiothixene	Low	Moderate	Moderate	Low

PROTOTYPE: PHENOTHIAZINES

CHLORPROMAZINE HYDROCHLORIDE
(klor pro′ mah zeen)
Clorpromanyl†*, Largactil‡*, Novochlorpromazine†*, Ormazine, Thorazine
Classification: phenothiazine
Pregnancy risk category C

How supplied
TABLETS: 10 mg, 25 mg, 50 mg, 100 mg, 200 mg
CAPSULES (SUSTAINED-RELEASE): 30 mg, 75 mg, 150 mg, 200 mg, 300 mg
SYRUP: 10 mg/5 ml
ORAL CONCENTRATE: 30 mg/ml, 100 mg/ml

*Liquid form contains alcohol   †Available in Canada only   ‡Available in Australia only

SUPPOSITORIES: 25 mg, 100 mg
INJECTION: 25 mg/ml

Indications and dosage

Psychosis
ADULTS: 30 to 75 mg P.O. daily in two to four divided doses. Dosage may be increased twice weekly by 20 to 50 mg until symptoms are controlled. Most patients respond to 200 mg daily, but doses up to 800 mg may be necessary.
CHILDREN: 0.25 mg/kg P.O. q 4 to 6 hours; or 0.25 mg/kg I.M. q 6 to 8 hours. Maximum dosage is 40 mg in children under age 5 and 75 mg in children ages 5 to 12.

Acute management of psychosis in severely agitated patients
ADULTS: 25 mg I.M.; may be repeated with 25 to 50 mg in 1 hour. May be gradually increased over several days to a maximum of 400 mg q 4 to 6 hours.

Nausea and vomiting
ADULTS: 10 to 25 mg P.O. or I.M. q 4 to 6 hours p.r.n.;
or 50 to 100 mg P.R. q 6 to 8 hours p.r.n.
CHILDREN AND INFANTS: 0.25 mg/kg P.O. q 4 to 6 hours; or 0.25 mg/kg I.M. q 6 to 8 hours; or 0.5 mg/kg P.R. q 6 to 8 hours.

Intractable hiccups
ADULTS: 25 to 50 mg P.O. or I.M. t.i.d. or q.i.d.

Contraindications and precautions
Chlorpromazine is contraindicated in patients with known hypersensitivity to phenothiazines and related compounds, including allergic reactions involving hepatic function; in patients with blood dyscrasia and bone marrow depression because chlorpromazine may induce agranulocytosis; in patients with disorders accompanied by coma, brain damage, or CNS depression because of additive CNS depressant effects. Drug is contraindicated in patients with circulatory collapse or cerebrovascular disease because of the potential for hypotensive or adverse cardiac effects and for use with adrenergic blocking agents or spinal or epidural anesthetics because of the alpha blocking potential.

Use chlorpromazine cautiously in patients with cardiac disease (arrhythmias, CHF, angina pectoris, valvular disease or heart block), encephalitis, Reye's syndrome, head injury, respiratory disease, seizure disorders, glaucoma, prostatic hyperplasia, urine retention, hepatic or renal dysfunction, Parkinson's disease, pheochromocytoma, or hypocalcemia.

Adverse reactions
BLOOD: transient leukopenia, **agranulocytosis.**
CNS: **sedation, pseudoparkinsonism, drowsiness, dizziness, headache, insomnia, exacerbation of psychotic symptoms,** *extrapyramidal symptoms including tardive dyskinesia (dose-related, with long-term therapy),* **neuroleptic malignant syndrome.**
CV: *orthostatic hypotension*, tachycardia, fainting, arrhythmias, ECG

---

changes, increased anginal pain (after I.M. injection).

EENT: *blurred vision,* ocular changes.

GI: *dry mouth, constipation.*

GU: *urine retention,* dark urine, menstrual irregularities, gynecomastia, inhibited ejaculation.

HEPATIC: cholestatic jaundice, abnormal liver function test.

SKIN: *mild photosensitivity,* dermal allergic reactions

LOCAL: *pain at I.M. injection site, sterile abscess.*

OTHER: increased appetite, weight gain, hyperprolactinemia.

Interactions

Alcohol, other CNS depressants: increased CNS depression. Avoid concomitant use.

Antacids: inhibits absorption of oral chlorpromazine. Separate antacid and chlorpromazine by at least 2 hours.

Anticholinergics (including antidepressants and antiparkinsonian agents): increased anticholinergic activity, aggravated parkinsonian symptoms. Use with caution.

Barbiturates: may decrease chlorpromazine effect. Monitor closely.

Beta blockers: may inhibit chlorpromazine metabolism, increasing plasma levels and toxicity. Use together with caution.

Bromocriptine: antagonizes bromocriptine's inhibition of prolactin secretion. Avoid using together.

Centrally acting antihypertensive agents: decreased antihypertensive effect. Monitor patient carefully.

Lithium: may cause severe neurotoxicity with encephalitis-like syndrome and decreased therapeutic effects. Avoid using together.

Oral anticoagulants: decreased anticoagulant effect. Monitor closely.

Nursing considerations

Assessment

- Review the patient's history for a condition that contraindicates the use of chlorpromazine and related compounds.
- Obtain baseline assessment of patient's mental status, including psychotic symptoms, before therapy.
- Be alert for common adverse reactions.
- As appropriate, evaluate the patient's and family's knowledge about chlorpromazine therapy.

Planning (Nursing Diagnoses)

Potential nursing diagnoses for the patient receiving chlorpromazine include:

- Impaired physical mobility related to potential for extrapyramidal symptoms.
- Constipation related to potential adverse GI reactions to chlorpromazine.
- Urinary retention related to potential adverse GU reactions.
- Knowledge deficit related to chlorpromazine therapy.

Implementation

Preparation and administration

— Sustained-release preparations should not be crushed but rather swallowed whole.
— Because oral formulations may cause stomach upset, administer food or milk.
— Dilute the concentrate in 2 to 4 oz of liquid, preferably water, carbonated drinks, fruit juice, tomato juice, milk, puddings or applesauce.
— Shake the syrup before administration.
— Store suppositories in a cool place.
— Avoid skin contact with the injectable or liquid form because it may cause a rash.

Monitoring

— Regularly observe the patient's behavior and notice if psychotic symptoms have been relieved or diminished.
— Observe the patient for adverse reactions, such as extrapyramidal or other CNS symptoms, cholinergic effects (blurred vision, dry mouth, constipation, urine retention), or allergic reactions.
— Monitor weekly bilirubin tests during the first month of therapy; regular blood tests (CBC and liver function), and ophthalmic tests during prolonged use.
— Observe the patient for orthostatic hypotension, especially after parenteral administration; monitor ECG for changes.
— Check and record blood pressure before and after I.M. administration.
— Monitor the patient for drug interactions.
— Monitor elderly patients carefully because they are more likely to develop adverse reactions, particularly tardive dyskinesia.
— Regularly reevaluate the patient's and family's knowledge about chlorpromazine therapy.

Intervention

— Hold dose and notify the doctor if the patient develops jaundice, symptoms of blood dyscrasia (fever, sore throat, infection, cellulitis, weakness), or severe adverse reactions.
— Steady-state serum level is reached in 4 to 7 days.
— Keep the patient supine for 1 hour after I.M. administration. Then assist patient to get up slowly to avoid orthostatic hypotension.
— Do not discontinue drug abruptly unless required by severe adverse reactions.
— Assist the patient with ambulation and daily activities if extrapyramidal symptoms occur. Notify the doctor and expect possible dosage adjustment.
— Expect to treat acute dystonic reactions with I.V. diphenhydramine (Benadryl).
— Increase the patient's fluid and fiber intake–if not contraindicated–to prevent constipation. If necessary, request doctor's order for a laxative.

—Before administering chlorpromazine, ask the patient to void. If urine retention occurs, notify he doctor and prepare to perform catheterization.

—Keep all members of the health care team informed of the patient's response to the drug.

Patient teaching

—Inform the patient about chlorpromazine, including the dosage, frequency, action, and adverse reactions.

—Tell the patient to avoid exposure to the sun and to use a sunscreen when going outdoors to prevent photosensitivity reactions. (*Note:* Sun lamps and tanning beds may cause burning of the skin or skin discoloration.)

—Warn the patient that a pink-brown coloration of urine may be observed but that this effect is harmless.

—Tell the patient to take the drug exactly as prescribed and not to take double doses to compensate for missed ones.

—Tell the patient not to stop taking the drug suddenly.

—Explain that many drug interactions are possible. Patient should seek medical approval before taking any OTC medication.

—Encourage the patient to report difficulty urinating, sore throat, dizziness, or fainting.

—Advise the patient to increase fluid and fiber in the diet, if appropriate.

—Tell the patient to avoid driving and other hazardous activities that require alertness until the effect of the drug is established. Excessive sedative effects tend to subside after several weeks.

—Explain which fluids are appropriate for diluting the concentrate and show the dropper technique for measuring dose. Warn the patient not to spill liquid preparation on skin because rash and irritation may occur.

—Tell the patient that sugarless hard candy or chewing gum or ice chips can alleviate dry mouth.

Evaluation

In the patient receiving chlorpromazine, appropriate evaluation statements include:
• Patient demonstrates a decrease in psychotic behavior.
• Patient maintains physical mobility.
• Patient states bowel patterns are unchanged.
• Patient voids without difficulty.
• Patient and family state an understanding of chlorpromazine therapy.

HALOPERIDOL
(ha loe per′ i dole)
Apo-Haloperidol†, Haldol**, Haloperon, Novoperidol†, Peridol†

HALOPERIDOL DECANOATE
Haldol Decanoate, Haldol LA†

HALOPERIDOL LACTATE
Haldol
Classification: nonphenothiazine
Pregnancy risk category C

How supplied
haloperidol
TABLETS: 0.5 mg, 1 mg, 2 mg, 5 mg, 10 mg, 20 mg
haloperidol decanoate
INJECTION: 50 mg/ml
haloperidol lactate
ORAL CONCENTRATE: 2 mg/ml
INJECTION: 5 mg/ml

Indications and dosage
Psychotic disorders
ADULTS: dosage varies for each patient. Initial range is 0.5 to 5 mg P.O.
b.i.d. or t.i.d.; or 2 to 5 mg I.M. q 4 to 8 hours, increasing rapidly if
necessary for prompt control. Maximum dosage is 100 mg P.O. daily.
Doses over 100 mg have been used for patients with severely resistant
conditions.

Chronic psychotic patients who require prolonged therapy
ADULTS: 50 to 100 mg I.M. (decanoate) q 4 weeks.

*Control of tics, vocal utterances in Gilles de la Tourette's syndrome,
agitation in elderly patients with senile dementia*
ADULTS: 0.5 to 2 mg P.O. b.i.d. or t.i.d., increasing p.r.n.

Contraindications and precautions
Haloperidol is contraindicated in parkinsonism, coma, or CNS depression.
Use with caution in elderly or debilitated patients; in severe CV disorders,
allergies, glaucoma, urine retention; and with anticonvulsant, anticoagulant, antiparkinsonian, or lithium medications.

Adverse reactions
BLOOD: transient leukopenia and leukocytosis.
CNS: *high incidence of severe extrapyramidal reactions, tardive dyskine-
sia;* low incidence of sedation.
CV: low incidence with therapeutic dosages.
EENT: blurred vision, dry mouth.

---

†Available in Canada only   **May contain tartrazine
Italicized adverse reactions are common

GU: urine retention, menstrual irregularities, gynecomastia.

SKIN: rash.

OTHER: rarely, **neuroleptic malignant syndrome** (fever, tachycardia, tachypnea, profuse diaphoresis).

Interactions

Alcohol, other CNS depressants: increased CNS depression. Avoid concomitant use.

Lithium: lethargy and confusion with high doses, Observe patient.

Methyldopa: possible symptoms of dementia. Observe patient.

Nursing considerations

Assessment

• Review the patient's history for a condition that contraindicates the use of haloperidol.

• Obtain a baseline assessment of the patient's mental status, including psychotic symptoms, before therapy.

• Be alert for common adverse reactions.

• Evaluate the patient's (if appropriate) and family's knowledge about haloperidol therapy.

Planning (Nursing Diagnoses)

Potential nursing diagnoses for the patient receiving chlorpromazine include:

• Impaired thought processes related to ineffectiveness of therapy.

• Impaired physical mobility related to potential for extrapyramidal effects.

• Altered oral mucus membrane related to haloperidol-induced dry mouth.

• Sensory/perceptual alterations (visual) related to potential blurred vision.

• Knowledge deficit related to haloperidol therapy.

Implementation

Preparation and administration

— When changing from tablets to decanoate injection, patient should receive 10 to 15 times the oral dose once a month (maximum 100 mg).

— Don't administer the decanoate form I.V.

— Protect medication from light. Slight yellowing of injection or concentrate is common and does not affect potency. Discard markedly discolored solutions.

— Dose of 2 mg is therapeutic equivalent of 100 mg of chlorpromazine.

— Elderly patients usually require lower initial dosage and more gradual dosage titration.

Monitoring

— Monitor the effectiveness of haloperidol by regularly observing the patient's behavior and noting if psychotic symptoms have abated or diminished.

— Monitor the patient for adverse drug reactions, especially extrapyramidal and anticholinergic effects (blurred vision, dry mouth, constipation, urine retention), and tardive dyskinesia, during prolonged therapy.

—Monitor the patient for drug interactions.

Intervention

—Do not withdraw drug abruptly unless required by severe adverse reactions.

—Assist the patient with ambulation and daily activities if extrapyramidal symptoms occur. Notify doctor of symptoms and expect to implement change of drug or dosage.

—Expect to treat dystonic reactions with I.V. diphenhydramine.

—Institute safety precautions if the patient develops blurred vision.

—Keep all members of the health care team informed of the patient's response to the drug.

Patient teaching

—Inform the patient and family about haloperidol, including the dosage, frequency, action, and adverse reactions.

—Tell the patient to take drug exactly as prescribed and not to double doses to compensate for missed ones.

—Warn the patient to avoid alcohol and other CNS depressants during haloperidol therapy because their combined use causes excessive CNS depression.

—Advise the patient to avoid driving and other hazardous activities that require alertness or normal vision until full effect of the drug is known.

—Recommend sugarless hard candy or chewing gum or ice chips to relieve dry mouth.

Evaluation

In the patient receiving haloperidol, appropriate evaluation statements include:

• Patient demonstrates decreased psychotic behavior.
• Patient maintains physical mobility.
• Patient states that dry mouth is relieved.
• Patient's vision remains unchanged.
• Patient and family state an understanding of haloperidol therapy.

SELECTED MAJOR DRUGS: ANTIPSYCHOTIC AGENTS

DRUG, INDICATIONS, AND DOSAGE	SPECIAL PRECAUTIONS

Phenothiazines

fluphenazine decanoate (Prolixin Decanoate)
fluphenazine enanthate (Prolixin Enanthate)
fluphenazine hydrochloride (Prolixin)
Psychotic disorders—
Adults: initially, 0.5 to 10 mg (hydrochloride) P.O. daily in divided doses q 6 to 8 hours; may increase cautiously to 20 mg. Higher doses (50 to 100 mg) have been given. Maintenance dosage is 1 to 5 mg P.O. daily. I.M. doses are 1/3 to 1/2 oral doses.
Adults and children over age 12: 12.5 to 25 mg of long-acting esters (decanoate and enanthate) I.M. or S.C. q 1 to 6 weeks. Maintenance dosage is 12 to 100 mg p.r.n.
Adults over age 65: 1 to 2.5 mg (hydrochloride) daily.
Children: 0.25 to 3.5 mg (hydrochloride) P.O. daily in divided doses q 4 to 6 hours; or 1/3 to 1/2 of oral dose I.M.; maximum dosage is 10 mg daily.

• Use parenteral form cautiously in asthmatic patients and in patients allergic to sulfites.
• High incidence of extrapyramidal reactions.

---

mesoridazine (Serentil)
Alcoholism—
Adults and children over age 12: 25 mg P.O. b.i.d. up to maximum of 200 mg daily.
Behavioral problems with chronic brain syndrome—
Adults and children over age 12: 25 mg P.O. t.i.d. up to maximum of 300 mg daily.
Psychoneurotic manifestations (anxiety)—
Adults and children over age 12: 10 mg P.O. t.i.d. up to maximum of 150 mg daily.
Schizophrenia—
Adults and children over age 12: initially, 50 mg P.O. t.i.d. or 25 mg I.M. repeated in 30 to 60 minutes p.r.n.

• Contraindicated in acutely ill or dehydrated children.
• High incidence of sedation.

---

perphenazine (Trilafon)
Hospitalized psychiatric patients—
Adults: initially, 8 to 16 mg P.O. b.i.d., t.i.d., or q.i.d., increasing to 64 mg daily.
Children over age 12: 6 to 12 mg P.O. daily, divided.
Mental disturbances, acute alcoholism, nausea, vomiting, hiccups—
Adults and children over age 12: 5 to 10 mg I.M. p.r.n. Maximum is 15 mg daily in ambulatory patients; 30 mg daily, in hospitalized patients.

• Use cautiously in patients exposed to extreme heat or cold (including antipyretic therapy).

---

thioridazine (Mellaril)
Psychosis—
Adults: initially, 25 to 100 mg P.O. t.i.d., with gradual increments up to 800 mg daily in divided doses, if needed. Dosage varies.
Adults over age 65: initial dose, 25 mg P.O. t.i.d.
Depressive neurosis, alcohol withdrawal, dementia in geriatric patients, behavioral problems in children—

• Use cautiously in patients exposed to extreme heat or cold (including antipyretic therapy), in those with suspected brain tumor or intestinal obstruction, and in acutely ill or dehydrated children.
• Very high incidence of anti-

(continued)

SELECTED MAJOR DRUGS: ANTIPSYCHOTIC AGENTS *continued*

DRUG, INDICATIONS, AND DOSAGE	SPECIAL PRECAUTIONS

Phenothiazines *(continued)*

thioridazine *(continued)*
Adults: initially, 25 mg P.O. t.i.d. Maintenance dosage is 20 to 200 mg daily.
Children over age 2: 0.5 to 3 mg/kg P.O. daily, divided.

cholinergic reactions.

trifluoperazine (Stelazine)
Anxiety states —
Adults: 1 to 2 mg P.O. b.i.d.
Schizophrenia and other psychotic disorders —
Adults: *outpatients —*1 to 2 mg P.O. b.i.d., up to 4 mg daily; *hospitalized patients —*2 to 5 mg P.O. b.i.d.; may gradually increase to 40 mg daily. 1 to 2 mg I.M. q 4 to 6 hours p.r.n.
Children ages 6 to 12: *hospitalized or under close supervision —*1 mg P.O. daily or b.i.d.; may increase gradually to 15 mg daily.

• Use cautiously in patients with suspected brain tumor or intestinal obstruction and in acutely ill or dehydrated children.

Nonphenothiazines

chlorprothixene (Taractan)
Psychotic disorders —
Adults: initially, 10 mg P.O. t.i.d. or q.i.d. Increase gradually to maximum of 600 mg daily.
Children over age 6: 10 to 25 mg P.O. t.i.d. or q.i.d.
Agitation of severe neurosis, depression, schizophrenia —
Adults: 25 to 50 mg P.O. or I.M. t.i.d. or q.i.d. Increase p.r.n. to maximum of 600 mg.

• Use cautiously in patients with suspected brain tumor or intestinal obstruction and in acutely ill or dehydrated children.
• High incidence of sedation.

clozapine (Clozaril)
Severe schizophrenia unresponsive to other therapies —
Adults: initially, 25 mg P.O. q.i.d. or b.i.d., titrated upward at 25 to 50 mg daily (if tolerated) to a daily dosage of 300 to 450 mg by the end of 2 weeks. Individual dosage is based on clinical response, patient tolerance, and adverse reactions. Subsequent dosage should not be increased more than once or twice weekly, and should not exceed 100 mg. Many patients respond to doses of 300 to 600 mg daily, but some may require as much as 900 mg daily. Do not exceed 900 mg daily.

• Contraindicated with history of clozapine-induced agranulocytosis or severe granulocytopenia; in patients with WBC counts below 3,500/mm³; with other bone marrow suppressant drugs; with myelosuppressive disorders; and with severe CNS depression or coma.
• Weekly WBC count determination required during therapy.
• High incidence of sedation.

thiothixene (Navane)
Acute agitation —
Adults: 4 mg I.M. b.i.d. to q.i.d. Maximum dosage is 30 mg daily I.M. Change to P.O. as soon as possible.
Mild to moderate psychosis —
Adults: initially, 2 mg P.O. t.i.d. May increase gradually to 15 mg daily.
Severe psychosis —
Adults: initially, 5 mg P.O. b.i.d. May increase gradually to 15 to 30 mg daily. Maximum recommended daily dosage is 60 mg. Not recommended in children under age 12.

• Contraindicated in patients with seizures, circulatory collapse, coma, CNS depression, blood dyscrasia, or bone marrow suppression and with use of spinal or epidural anesthetic or adrenergic blockers.
• Use cautiously in patients exposed to extreme heat or cold (including antipyretic therapy) or excessive sunlight.

SELF-TEST

1. Peter Korbin is on a maintenance regimen of chlorpromazine for treatment of psychosis. This drug produces its therapeutic effects by:
   a. blocking the brain's postsynaptic dopamine receptors.
   b inhibiting the medullary chemoreceptor zone.
   c. stabilizing neuronal membranes in the hypothalamus.
   d. stimulating the production of endorphins.

2. Which of the following diagnostic studies should be done regularly because Mr. Korbin is receiving chlorpromazine?
   a. serum electrolytes
   b. CSF analysis
   c. urine culture
   d. liver function studies

3 Which of the following dose-related adverse reactions should the nurse watch for during long-term therapy?
   a tardive dyskinesia
   b diarrhea
   c. weight loss
   d. hypertension

4. Mary Smith is being treated for schizophrenia with haloperidol 4 mg P.O. b.i.d. What is the maximum daily dosage Ms. Smith could safely receive?
   a. 12 mg
   b. 24 mg
   c. 50 mg
   d. 100 mg

5. Which rare but potentially fatal adverse reaction could Ms. Smith develop as a result of haloperidol therapy?
   a. neuroleptic malignant syndrome
   b. malignant hypertension
   c. ventricular tachycardia
   d. severe respiratory depression

Check your answers on page 1065.

CHAPTER 33

ANTIMANIC AGENTS

lithium carbonate ◆ lithium citrate

OVERVIEW

- Lithium salts have been used throughout the world for more than 20 years to combat bipolar disorders (also known as manic-depressive illness). In the United States, however, lithium has been used only since 1970. (Many deaths occurred during the 1940s when lithium was improperly used as a sodium substitute.)
- Under proper supervision, lithium may prevent up to 80% of manic and depressive episodes. Episodes that occur during lithium therapy are usually less severe and shorter than those that might occur without such therapy. Close monitoring to maintain therapeutic lithium blood levels allows safe use of this drug. However, lithium's toxic level is very close to its therapeutic level.
- Consistent dietary sodium and fluid intake are necessary every day to help prevent toxicity. Conditions that may cause excess sodium and water loss (such as sweating or diarrhea) may require supplemental fluid or sodium administration.
- This chapter describes the major uses, mechanisms of action, and adverse reactions of lithium salts.

MAJOR USES

- Lithium salts are used to treat acute manic or hypomanic episodes of manic-depressive disorders and to prevent their recurrence. They are also used investigationally to stimulate WBC count production in patients receiving antineoplastic drugs.

MECHANISM OF ACTION

- Lithium alters chemical transmitters in the CNS, possibly by interfering with ionic pump mechanisms in brain cells. Its exact mechanism of action in mania, however, is unknown.

ABSORPTION, DISTRIBUTION, METABOLISM, AND EXCRETION

Lithium is readily absorbed orally. It is distributed to body tissues, with highest concentrations in the kidneys and lowest concentrations in brain tissue. The drug is almost entirely excreted through the kidneys as unchanged lithium ions. Lithium has a relatively narrow therapeutic window: effective antimanic activity is exhibited with plasma levels of 0.6 to 1.2 mEq/liter; toxicity usually occurs when levels exceed 1.5 mEq/liter.

ONSET AND DURATION
Blood levels of lithium peak within 2 to 4 hours. The antimanic action is delayed for 5 to 10 days.

ADVERSE REACTIONS
Lithium produces various CNS reactions; most commonly, these include lethargy, fatigue, muscle weakness, headache, mental confusion, and hand tremor, which occur in up to 50% of patients.

Restlessness, stupor, blackouts, coma, seizures, exacerbation of psychotic symptoms, and hyperexcitability may also occur.

GI reactions are also common at the start of therapy but tend to be mild and reversible. These reactions include nausea, vomiting, bloating, anorexia, diarrhea, or abdominal pain and may signal lithium toxicity. Weight gain may be seen in 25% of patients.

Polyuria and polydypsia may develop in up to 50% of patients; polyuria may cause dry mouth. A diabetes insipidus–like syndrome has been observed. Serum electrolyte abnormalities are possible.

Hypothyroidism may require thyroid supplementation. Cardiac arrhythmias, bradycardia, and other reversible changes may occur. Lithium toxicity parallels serum concentration and produces the same reactions already listed in greater severity. Symptoms are usually amplifications of the adverse reactions.

PROTOTYPE: ANTIMANIC AGENTS

LITHIUM CARBONATE
(lith' ee um)
Camcolit‡, Carbolith†, Duralith†, Eskalith, Eskalith CR, Lithane**, Lithicarb‡, Lithizine†, Lithobid, Lithonate, Lithotabs, Priadel‡

LITHIUM CITRATE
Cibalith-S*

Classification: antimanic agent
Pregnancy risk category D

How supplied
TABLETS: 250 mg‡, 300 mg (300 mg = 8.12 mEq lithium)
TABLETS (SUSTAINED-RELEASE): 300 mg, 400 mg‡, 450 mg
CAPSULES: 300 mg
SYRUP (SUGARLESS): 300 mg/5 ml*

Indications and dosage
Prevention or control of mania
ADULTS: 300 to 600 mg P.O. up to q.i.d., increasing on the basis of blood levels to achieve optimal dosage. Recommended therapeutic lithium blood levels: 1 to 1.5 mEq/liter, for acute mania, 0.6 to 1.2 mEq/liter for maintenance therapy, and 2 mEq/liter as maximum.

Note: 5 ml lithium citrate (liquid) contains 8 mEq lithium equal to 300 mg lithium carbonate.

Contraindications and precautions

Lithium is contraindicated if therapy cannot be closely monitored. Use cautiously with haloperidol, other antipsychotics, neuromuscular blocking agents, and diuretics; in elderly or debilitated persons; and in thyroid disease, seizure disorder, renal or CV disease, brain damage, severe debilitation or dehydration, and sodium depletion.

Adverse reactions

BLOOD: leukocytosis of 14,000 to 18,000 (reversible).

CNS: *tremor,* drowsiness, headache, confusion, *restlessness,* dizziness, psychomotor retardation, stupor, lethargy, coma, blackouts, **epileptiform seizures,** EEG changes, worsened organic brain syndrome, impaired speech, ataxia, muscle weakness, incoordination, hyperexcitability.

CV: reversible ECG changes, **arrhythmias,** hypotension, **peripheral circulatory collapse,** allergic vasculitis, ankle and wrist edema.

EENT: tinnitus, impaired vision.

GI: *nausea,* vomiting, anorexia, diarrhea, *dry mouth, thirst, metallic taste.*

GU: polyuria, glycosuria, incontinence, renal toxicity with long-term use.

METABOLIC: transient hyperglycemia, goiter, hypothyroidism (lowered T_3, T_4, and protein-bound iodine, but elevated ^{131}I uptake), hyponatremia.

SKIN: pruritus, rash, diminished or lost sensation, drying and thinning of hair.

Interactions

Aminophylline, sodium bicarbonate, and sodium chloride: ingestion of these salts increases lithium excretion. Avoid salt loads and monitor lithium levels.

Carbamazepine, probenecid, indomethacin, methyldopa, and piroxicam: increased effect of lithium. Monitor for lithium toxicity.

Diuretics: increased reabsorption of lithium by kidneys, with possible toxic effect. Use with extreme caution and monitor lithium and electrolyte levels (especially sodium).

Haloperidol and thioridazine: encephalopathic syndrome (lethargy, tremor, extrapyramidal symptoms). Watch for syndrome and stop drug if it occurs.

Thyroid hormones: lithium may induce hypothyroidism. Monitor for increased need for thyroid supplements.

Nursing considerations

Assessment

- Assess the patient's situation to determine if therapy can be closely monitored. Use of lithium is contraindicated if therapy cannot be closely monitored.
- Obtain a baseline assessment of the patient's behavior before therapy.
- Be alert for common adverse reactions.
- Evaluate the patient's and family's knowledge about lithium therapy.

Planning (Nursing Diagnoses)

Potential nursing diagnoses for the patient receiving lithium include:
• Altered thought processes related to ineffectiveness of lithium.
• Fatigue related to adverse CNS reactions induced by lithium therapy.
• Potential for trauma related to drowsiness, ataxia, and/or confusion caused by lithium therapy.
• Noncompliance with lithium therapy related to lack of insight secondary to mania.
• Knowledge deficit related to lithium therapy.

Implementation

Preparation and administration

— Administer with plenty of water and after meals to minimize GI upset.
— Before leaving the bedside, make sure the patient has swallowed medication.
— Make sure the patient can have regular checks of lithium blood levels as this is crucial to the safe use of the drug. If regular follow-up is doubtful, confer with doctor before administering the drug.

Monitoring

— Regularly monitor the effectiveness of lithium therapy by observing the patient's behavior.
— Monitor the patient for adverse drug reactions.
— Monitor WBC count for leukocytosis, serum sodium level for hyponatremia, blood glucose level for hyperglycemia, thyroid function studies for results suggestive of hypothyroidism, and renal function studies suggestive of renal toxicity.
— Monitor ECG for changes or arrhythmias and blood pressure for hypotension.
— Monitor the patient's intake and output for thirst, polyuria, or oliguria suggestive of renal toxicity with long-term use and urine specific gravity for diabetes insipidus syndrome.
— Monitor mental status and level of consciousness throughout lithium therapy.
— Monitor for wrist or ankle edema, skin rash, change in skin sensation, and drying or thinning of hair.
— Monitor the patient for drug interactions.
— Monitor lithium blood levels 8 to 12 hours after first dose, usually before morning dose, two or three times weekly first month, then weekly to monthly on maintenance. When blood levels of lithium are below 1.5 mEq/liter, adverse reactions usually remain mild.
— Regularly reevaluate the patient's and family's knowledge about lithium therapy.

Intervention

— Notify the doctor if the patient's behavior does not improve in 1 to 3 weeks or if it worsens.
— Withhold drug if lithium toxicity is suspected (diarrhea, vomiting, drowsiness, muscular weakness, ataxia) and notify the doctor promptly.

— Adjust fluid and sodium ingestion to compensate if excessive loss occurs through protracted sweating or diarrhea. Under normal conditions, patients should have fluid intake of 2,500 to 3,000 ml daily and a balanced diet with adequate sodium intake.

— Have outpatient follow-up of thyroid and renal functions every 6 to 12 months.

— If adverse CNS reactions occur, institute safety precautions, such as supervising ambulation.

— Assist the patient with activities of daily living, space activities throughout the day, and provide rest periods as the patient's degree of fatigue dictates.

— Identify a responsible family member or friend to oversee the patient's compliance with drug therapy.

— Institute seizure precautions as needed.

— Keep all members of the health care team informed of the patient's response to the drug.

Patient teaching

— Instruct the patient and family about lithium, including the dosage, frequency, action, and adverse reactions.

— Warn the patient and family to watch for signs of toxicity (diarrhea, vomiting, drowsiness, muscular weakness, ataxia) and to expect transient nausea, polyuria, thirst, and discomfort during first few days. Tell the patient to withhold one dose and call the doctor if toxic symptoms appear but not to discontinue drug abruptly.

— Tell the patient to expect lag of 1 to 3 weeks before drug's beneficial effects are noticed.

— Explain that lithium has a narrow therapeutic margin of safety. A blood level that is even slightly too high can be dangerous.

— Instruct the patient to carry an identification card (available from pharmacy) with toxicity and emergency information.

— Warn the ambulatory patient to avoid driving and other hazardous activities that require alertness and good psychomotor coordination until CNS effects of the drug are known.

— Tell the patient not to switch brands of lithium or to take other drugs (prescription or OTC) without doctor's guidance.

— Stress the importance of compliance to lithium therapy.

— Tell the patient to take frequent rest periods and space activities throughout the day if fatigue becomes a problem.

— Explain the importance of having laboratory and other diagnostic studies done when ordered.

— Tell the patient to take the drug with plenty of water and after meals to minimize GI upset.

— Advise the patient to increase fluid and sodium intake if excessive fluid loss occurs.

— Tell the patient to notify the nurse or doctor if adverse reactions develop or questions arise about lithium therapy.

Evaluation

In the patient receiving lithium, appropriate evaluation statements include:

• Patient exhibits improved behavior and thought processes.
• Patient experiences minimal fatigue.
• Patient does not experience trauma with adverse CNS reactions.
• Patient is compliant with drug regimen.
• Patient and family state an understanding of lithium therapy.

SELF-TEST

1. Ellen Johnson has a manic-depressive disorder for which the doctor prescribed lithium 300 mg P.O. b.i.d. How is lithium excreted by the body?
   a. feces
   b. bile
   c. urine
   d. liver metabolism

2. The nurse must monitor Mrs. Johnson's therapeutic lithium blood levels closely. When is toxicity most likely to occur?
   a. when levels exceed 0.5 mEq/liter
   b. when levels exceed 0.8 mEq/liter
   c. when levels exceed 1.2 mEq/liter
   d. when levels exceed 1.5 mEq/liter

3. Which endocrine reaction should the nurse watch for?
   a. diabetes mellitus
   b. diabetes insipidus–like syndrome
   c. hyperthyroidism
   d. Addison's disease

4. Which of the following nursing diagnoses would be appropriate for patients like Mrs. Johnson receiving lithium?
   a. constipation
   b. urine retention
   c. fatigue
   d. ineffective thermoregulation

5. Because Mrs. Johnson has difficulty swallowing the tablets, the nurse requests the syrup form. How many ml of syrup would provide 300 mg of lithium?
   a. 2 ml
   b. 3 ml
   c. 5 ml
   d. 10 ml

Check your answers on page 1065.

CHAPTER 34

CEREBRAL STIMULANTS

amphetamine sulfate ✦ benzphetamine hydrochloride
caffeine ✦ caffeine, citrated ✦ caffeine and sodium benzoate
dextroamphetamine sulfate ✦ diethylpropion hydrochloride
fenfluramine hydrochloride ✦ mazindol ✦ methamphetamine hydrochloride
methylphenidate hydrochloride ✦ pemoline ✦ phendimetrazine tartrate
phenmetrazine hydrochloride ✦ phentermine hydrochloride

OVERVIEW

- Amphetamines are the prototypes for CNS stimulants. They are the first agents to have been used as appetite suppressants (anorexigenics). Recently, however, the FDA proposed that weight reduction in obesity be deleted as an approved indication for these drugs. Their use as anorexigenics should be limited to short-term weight control only as prescribed by a doctor.
- Amphetamines, or "uppers" in street language, are common drugs of abuse. Also included in this class are isomers of amphetamines (amphetamine-like drugs that are also used for weight control), but they have less potential for abuse because their euphoric effects aren't as great.
- All of the agents discussed in this chapter, except caffeine, are officially listed by the Drug Enforcement Administration as controlled substances.

MAJOR USES

- Amphetamines and amphetamine-like drugs may suppress appetite, promote weight reduction in exogenous obesity, and supply short-term adjunctive therapy for weight control and dieting. Dextroamphetamine and methylphenidate are used as therapeutic adjuncts in attention deficit hyperactivity disorder (ADHD).
- Dextroamphetamine, amphetamine sulfate, and methylphenidate are used to treat narcolepsy.

MECHANISM OF ACTION

- Amphetamines and amphetamine-like drugs, caffeine, methylphenidate, and pemoline are sympathomimetics whose main sites of activity appear to be the cerebral cortex and the reticular activating system. They probably promote nerve impulse transmission by releasing stored norepinephrine from nerve terminals in the brain. In children with ADHD, amphetamines may have a paradoxical calming effect that is probably related to the actions of the drug on CNS neurotransmitters. The mech-

GLOSSARY

Analeptic: drug used to stimulate the CNS; restorative agent.
Anorexiant: agent that produces a decrease in appetite; also called anorexigenic agent.
Hyperkinesis: abnormally increased motor function or activity; also called hyperactivity.

anism by which amphetamines produce mental and behavioral effects in children, however, has not been established.
• Fenfluramine, an amphetamine congener, differs structurally from amphetamines. Its exact mechanism of action has not been defined.

ABSORPTION, DISTRIBUTION, METABOLISM, AND EXCRETION

Cerebral stimulants are readily absorbed from the GI tract. They are well distributed to most body tissues, with high concentrations in the brain and CSF. Fenfluramine is rapidly absorbed and widely distributed in almost all body tissues. Elimination is more rapid when urine is acidic.

Amphetamines and amphetamine-like drugs are excreted by the kidneys, largely unchanged, in about 3 hours. They are excreted more readily in acidic urine than they are in alkaline urine.

Caffeine and methylphenidate are partially metabolized by the liver and excreted by the kidneys. Pemoline probably undergoes the greatest metabolic change of these drugs, with more than 50% being metabolized to an active metabolite before being excreted by the kidneys.

ONSET AND DURATION

Onset is usually within 1 to 2 hours. Duration is from 4 to 10 hours, with most drugs requiring multiple doses for continued anorexigenic effect. Some are longer-acting (6 to 12 hours).

ADVERSE REACTIONS

Adverse reactions to the cerebral stimulants are commonly extensions of their pharmacologic activity on the CNS. They include nervousness, insomnia, irritability, dizziness, headache, overstimulation, and dysphoria. These drugs' peripheral activity, particularly on the CV system, may cause tachycardia, palpitations, and hypertension or hypotension. GI reactions include anorexia with weight loss, dry mouth, nausea, vomiting, diarrhea or constipation, and metallic taste. Physical or psychological dependence is possible with prolonged use. Because fenfluramine differs pharmacologically from amphetamines, it produces signs of CNS depression such as drowsiness.

AMPHETAMINE SULFATE
(am fet' a meen)
Classification: amphetamine
Controlled substance schedule II
Pregnancy risk category C

How supplied
TABLETS: 5 mg, 10 mg
CAPSULES: 5 mg, 10 mg

Indications and dosage
Attention deficit hyperactivity disorder (ADHD)
CHILDREN AGES 6 AND OVER: 5 mg P.O. daily, with 5-mg increments weekly, p.r.n.
CHILDREN AGES 3 TO 5: 2.5 mg P.O. daily, with 2.5-mg increments weekly, p.r.n.

Narcolepsy
ADULTS: 5 to 60 mg P.O. daily in divided doses.
CHILDREN OVER AGE 12: 10 mg P.O. daily, with 10-mg increments weekly, p.r.n.
CHILDREN AGES 6 TO 12: 5 mg P.O. daily, with 5-mg increments weekly, p.r.n.

Short-term adjunct in exogenous obesity
ADULTS: 1 10- or 15-mg long-acting capsule daily; or 2, if needed, up to 30 mg daily; or 5 to 30 mg daily in divided doses 30 to 60 minutes before meals. Not recommended for children under age 12.

Contraindications and precautions
Amphetamine sulfate is contraindicated in symptomatic CV diseases, hyperthyroidism, nephritis, angina pectoris, moderate to severe hypertension, parkinsonism due to arteriosclerosis, certain types of glaucoma, advanced arteriosclerosis, and agitated states or in patients with a history of drug abuse. Use cautiously in diabetes mellitus and in elderly, debilitated, or hyperexcitable patients. Also use cautiously in children with Gilles de la Tourette's syndrome.

Not recommended for first-line treatment of obesity. Use as an anorexigenic agent is prohibited in some states. Use as an analeptic is usually discouraged, because CNS stimulation superimposed on CNS depression can lead to neuronal instability and seizures. Drug should not be used to combat fatigue.

Adverse reactions
CNS: *restlessness*, tremor, *hyperactivity, talkativeness, insomnia,* irritability, dizziness, headache, chills, overstimulation, dysphoria.
CV: *tachycardia, palpitations,* hypertension, hypotension.
GI: nausea, vomiting, cramps, dry mouth, diarrhea, constipation, metallic

---
Italicized adverse reactions are common

taste, *anorexia, weight loss.*
OTHER: urticaria, impotence, altered libido.

Interactions

Ammonium chloride, ascorbic acid: acidifies urine and speeds up excretion. Observe for decreased amphetamine effect.
Antacids, sodium bicarbonate, acetazolamide: increased renal reabsorption. Monitor for enhanced effect.
MAO inhibitors: severe hypertension; possible hypertensive crisis. Don't use together.

Nursing considerations

Assessment

- Review the patient's history for a condition that contraindicates the use of amphetamine sulfate.
- Obtain a baseline assessment of the patient's condition (ADHD, narcolepsy, or exogenous obesity) before therapy.
- Be alert for common adverse reactions.
- Evaluate the patient's and family's knowledge about amphetamine sulfate therapy.

Planning (Nursing Diagnoses)

Potential nursing diagnoses for the patient receiving amphetamine sulfate include:

- Activity intolerance related to ineffectiveness or inadequate dosage of amphetamine sulfate.
- Sleep pattern disturbance related to amphetamine sulfate–induced insomnia.
- Decreased cardiac output related to adverse CV effects of amphetamine sulfate.
- Knowledge deficit related to amphetamine sulfate therapy.

Implementation

Preparation and administration

— Administer drug at least 6 hours before bedtime to avoid interference with sleep.
— When used for obesity, administer drug 30 to 60 minutes before meals.
— Avoid prolonged administration because physical dependency may occur, especially in patients with a history of drug addiction. After prolonged use, reduce dosage gradually to prevent acute rebound depression.

Monitoring

— Monitor the effectiveness of amphetamine sulfate therapy regularly by observing the patient's behavior or assessing the patient's weight.
— Monitor the patient for adverse drug reactions.
— Monitor vital signs for evidence of tachycardia or blood pressure changes; question the patient regularly about palpitations.
— Monitor sleeping pattern and bowel habits for changes.

— Monitor blood glucose levels in diabetic patients because drug may alter daily insulin needs.

— Monitor the patient for drug interactions.

— Regularly reevaluate the patient's and family's knowledge about amphetamine sulfate therapy.

Intervention

— Provide frequent rest periods and assistance with activities as needed; fatigue may result as drug effects wear off.

— Institute safety precautions by making environment safe and providing supervision of patient's activities.

— Suggest nonpharmacologic measures to overcome insomnia.

— When used for obesity, make sure the patient is also on a weight-reduction program. Do calorie counts, if necessary.

— Keep all members of the health care team informed of the patient's response to the drug.

Patient teaching

— Instruct the patient and family about amphetamine sulfate, including the dosage, frequency, action, and adverse reactions.

— Warn the patient to avoid activities that require alertness or good psychomotor coordination until CNS effects of the drug are known.

— Tell the patient to avoid beverages containing caffeine, which increase the stimulant effects of amphetamines and related amines.

— Have the patient report signs of excessive stimulation.

— Instruct the patient about calorie restriction if drug is used to lower weight.

— Tell the patient to weigh himself weekly in the same clothes at the same time of day to evaluate effectiveness in obesity therapy.

— Inform the patient that drug may cause impotence or altered libido.

— Tell the diabetic patient to monitor blood glucose levels closely.

— Teach the patient how to take the drug to minimize insomnia and enhance effectiveness.

— Tell the patient that, when tolerance to anorexigenic effect develops, dosage should not be increased, but drug discontinued. Patient should call the doctor to report decreased effectiveness of drug. Warn the patient against stopping drug abruptly.

— Tell the patient to notify the nurse or doctor if adverse reactions develop or questions arise about amphetamine sulfate therapy.

Evaluation

In the patient receiving amphetamine sulfate, appropriate evaluation statements include:

• Patient demonstrates clinical improvement.

• Patient is able to sleep without difficulty.

• Patient's cardiac output does not diminish.

• Patient and family state an understanding of amphetamine sulfate therapy.

SELECTED MAJOR DRUGS: CEREBRAL STIMULANTS

DRUG, INDICATIONS, AND DOSAGES	SPECIAL PRECAUTIONS
diethylpropion (Propiont, Tenuate, Tepanil) *Short-term adjunct in exogenous obesity—* **Adults:** 25 mg P.O. before meals t.i.d.; or 75 mg controlled-release tablet P.O. in midmorning.	• Contraindicated in patients with known hypersensitivity or idiosyncrasy to sympathomimetic amines and in those with advanced arteriosclerosis, hyperthyroidism, glaucoma, severe hypertension, agitation, a history of drug abuse, and during or within 14 days after administration of MAO inhibitors because hypertensive crises may result. • Administer cautiously to patients with hypertension or symptomatic CV disease, including arrhythmias; to patients with seizure disorder; to patients with diabetes mellitus; and to those in hyperexcitability states.
fenfluramine (Ponderalt, Pondimin) *Short-term adjunct in exogenous obesity—* **Adults:** initially, 20 mg P.O. t.i.d. before meals. Maximum dosage is 40 mg t.i.d. Adjust dosage according to patient's response.	• Contraindicated in patients with known hypersensitivity to sympathomimetic amines and in those with glaucoma, symptomatic CV disease, alcoholism, or a history of drug abuse. • Administer cautiously to patients with hypertension, a history of mental depression, and diabetes mellitus.
mazindol (Mazanor, Sanorex) *Short-term adjunct in exogenous obesity—* **Adults:** 1 mg P.O. t.i.d. 1 hour before meals, or 2 mg daily 1 hour before lunch. Use lowest effective dosage.	• Contraindicated in patients with known hypersensitivity or idiosyncrasy to mazindol and in those with glaucoma, agitation, a history of drug abuse, and during or within 14 days after administration of MAO inhibitors. • Administer cautiously to patients with diabetes mellitus, hypertension, and hyperexcitability states.
methylphenidate (Ritalin) *Attention deficit hyperactivity disorder (ADHD)—* **Children ages 6 and over:** initially, 5 to 10 mg P.O. daily before breakfast and lunch, with 5- to 10-mg increments weekly p.r.n., up to 60 mg daily.	• Contraindicated in patients with known hypersensitivity to the drug and in those with marked anxiety, tension, and agitation; glaucoma; and motor

(continued)

SELECTED MAJOR DRUGS: CEREBRAL STIMULANTS *continued*

DRUG, INDICATIONS, AND DOSAGES	SPECIAL PRECAUTIONS
methylphenidate *(continued)* *Narcolepsy—* **Adults:** 10 mg P.O. b.i.d. or t.i.d. ½ hour before meals. Dosage varies with patient needs. Dosage range is 5 to 10 mg daily.	tics or a family history of Gilles de la Tourette's syndrome. • Administer cautiously to elderly, debilitated, or hyperexcitable patients and to those with a history of CV disease, diabetes, or seizures.
pemoline (Cylert) *Attention deficit hyperactivity disorder (ADHD)—* **Children ages 6 and older:** initially, 37.5 mg P.O. in the morning. Daily dose can be raised by 18.75 mg weekly. Effective dosage range is 56.25 to 75 mg daily; maximum dosage is 112.5 mg daily.	• Contraindicated in patients with known hypersensitivity or idiosyncrasy to the drug and in those with impaired hepatic function. • Administer cautiously to patients with impaired renal function or a history of Gilles de la Tourette's syndrome.
phenmetrazine (Preludin) *Short-term adjunct in exogenous obesity—* **Adults:** 25 mg P.O. b.i.d. or t.i.d. 1 hour before meals, up to 75 mg daily; or single 50- to 75-mg extended-release tablet daily in midmorning.	• Contraindicated in patients with known hypersensitivity to the drug or idiosyncrasy to sympathomimetic amines and in those with advanced arteriosclerosis, symptomatic CV disease, moderate to severe hypertension, hyperthyroidism, glaucoma, agitation, and a history of drug abuse; concomitant use of CNS stimulants; and during or within 14 days after administration of MAO inhibitors. • Administer cautiously to patients in hyperexcitability states.
phentermine (Fastin, Ionamin) *Short-term adjunct in exogenous obesity—* **Adults:** 8 mg P.O. t.i.d. ½ hour before meals; or 15 to 30 mg daily before breakfast.	• Contraindicated in patients with known hypersensitivity or idiosyncrasy to the drug and in those with advanced arteriosclerosis, symptomatic CV disease, moderate to severe hypertension, hyperthyroidism, glaucoma, agitation, and drug abuse and during or within 14 days after administration of MAO inhibitors. • Administer cautiously to patients in hyperexcitability states or with a history of drug addiction.

COMPARING CEREBRAL STIMULANT COMBINATIONS

TRADE NAME AND CONTENT	SPECIAL CONSIDERATIONS
Biphetamine 12½ dextroamphetamine sulfate 6.25 mg and amphetamine sulfate 6.25 mg **Biphetamine 20** dextroamphetamine sulfate 10 mg and amphetamine sulfate 10 mg	• Combines the actions of two amphetamine derivatives, dextroamphetamine and amphetamine sulfate. • Contraindicated in patients with a history of drug abuse. • Use cautiously in patients with CV disorders or diabetes mellitus.

SELF-TEST

1. John Cole is taking amphetamine sulfate for short-term treatment of exogenous obesity. Which of the following self-care measures should the nurse teach Mr. Cole?
   a. Take this medication before meals and at bedtime.
   b. Avoid coffee, tea, and carbonated beverages containing caffeine.
   c. Stop taking the medication if you notice your hands are shaky.
   d. You can increase your food intake now that you are on this drug.

2. Which OTC preparation should Mr. Cole avoid?
   a. antacids
   b. aspirin
   c. acetaminophen
   d. complex B vitamins

3. Mr. Cole is also an insulin-dependent diabetic patient. How may amphetamine sulfate therapy affect Mr. Cole's diabetic treatment?
   a. He will need more calories to cover his insulin requirements; thus, weight loss will be slower.
   b. He may need to alter his daily insulin dosage because amphetamine sulfate causes weight loss.
   c. He will need to avoid using a reagent strip to test his urine glucose level because a false-positive result may occur.
   d. He will need to exercise more to keep blood glucose levels under control because amphetamine sulfate therapy may cause hyperglycemia.

Check your answers on pages 1065 and 1066.

CHAPTER 35

ANTIPARKINSONIAN AGENTS

Dopaminergic agents
amantadine hydrochloride ✦ bromocriptine mesylate ✦ carbidopa-levodopa
levodopa ✦ pergolide mesylate ✦ selegiline hydrochloride

Miscellaneous agents
benztropine mesylate ✦ biperiden hydrochloride
diphenhydramine hydrochloride ✦ orphenadrine hydrochloride
procyclidine hydrochloride ✦ trihexyphenidyl hydrochloride

OVERVIEW

- Parkinsonism is a syndrome characterized by disordered movement, including akinesia, tremor at rest, rigidity, and loss of postural reflexes. These effects have been linked to the destruction, degeneration, or depletion of dopamine within the basal ganglia of the brain.
- Within the basal ganglia, dopamine-containing (dopaminergic) neurons act as inhibitory modulators to acetylcholine-containing (cholinergic) neurons. When their inhibitory action is withdrawn, either from destruction of the neurons (for example, in idiopathic parkinsonism) or by blocking central dopamine receptors (for example, by the use of certain drugs, such as the antipsychotic agents), the unopposed cholinergic excitation produces parkinsonian symptoms.
- Idiopathic Parkinson's disease, characterized by degenerative changes within the basal ganglia, is responsible for about 85% of all cases of parkinsonian syndrome. The remaining 15% results from drugs, head trauma, encephalitis, arteriosclerosis, or other neurologic disorders.
- Antiparkinsonian agents are classified primarily into two groups: dopaminergic agents and miscellaneous agents.

MAJOR USES

- Drugs used in the treatment of parkinsonism act to restore the delicate balance of cholinergic and dopaminergic actions within the basal ganglia. Anticholinergic drugs are usually used to treat drug-induced parkinsonism and may also be particularly useful in idiopathic parkinsonism associated with symptoms of excessive cholinergic activity, such as seborrhea, drooling, and excessive sweating. Anticholinergics are commonly used early after the diagnosis of the disease.

GLOSSARY

Dopamine: neurotransmitter produced by the decarboxylation of dopa, an intermediate product in norepinephrine synthesis.
Dopaminergic: stimulated, activated, or transmitted by dopamine.
Dyskinesia: impaired power of voluntary movement resulting in fragmentary or incomplete movements.
Hyperkinesis: abnormally increased motor function or activity; also called hyperactivity.
Parkinson's disease: disorder characterized by muscular rigidity, immobile facies, tremor that disappears upon volitional movement, and loss of associated autonomic movement and salivation.
Rigidity: abnormal muscle stiffness or inflexibility.
Tremor: involuntary trembling or quivering.

- Amantadine, an antiviral agent, has also been used to treat parkinsonism. However, its effectiveness is limited. Many patients show no improvement after 6 months of therapy.
- Levodopa, carbidopa-levodopa, bromocriptine, pergolide, and selegiline, which enhance dopaminergic transmission, are more effective than anticholinergics or amantadine. Some clinicians will use the less effective agents until the disease progresses; others may use combinations of all of these drugs to restore normal motor activity.

MECHANISM OF ACTION

- Drugs with anticholinergic properties block the excessive cholinergic input into the basal ganglia. The antihistamines diphenhydramine and orphenadrine are useful in the treatment of parkinsonism because they exert substantial anticholinergic effects. Other anticholinergics include trihexyphenidyl, procyclidine, biperiden, and benztropine.
- Because dopamine does not cross the blood-brain barrier, it is not useful in treating parkinsonism. However, levodopa, a metabolic precursor to dopamine, enters the CNS and is converted to dopamine within the surviving dopaminergic neurons of the basal ganglia.
- Levodopa increases central dopaminergic activity; the peripheral decarboxylase inhibitor carbidopa enhances the amount of levodopa that reaches the brain by preventing the breakdown of levodopa in peripheral tissues.
- Bromocriptine and pergolide directly stimulate dopamine receptors within the basal ganglia. Pergolide is used as an adjunct to carbidopa-levodopa therapy.
- Selegiline, a selective MAO type B inhibitor, enhances central dopaminergic transmission by preventing the breakdown of dopamine in the CNS. It is usually reserved for patients who no longer respond to carbidopa-levodopa therapy.

ABSORPTION, DISTRIBUTION, METABOLISM, AND EXCRETION

Detailed pharmacokinetic information for each of the anticholinergic agents is not available. However, most of these drugs appear to be well absorbed after oral administration, and their effectiveness does not appear to be altered by food. They readily enter the CNS and act within the basal ganglia. Most of these drugs, except trihexyphenidyl, are metabolized by the liver. They are excreted as metabolites and unchanged drug, except for trihexyphenidyl, which is excreted unchanged.

The antihistamines diphenhydramine and orphenadrine are also well absorbed and readily enter the CNS. Both are extensively metabolized by the liver and excreted in the urine as metabolites.

Among the dopaminergic agents, levodopa is absorbed by an active transport process within the small intestine. Because levodopa competes with dietary amino acids for absorption, the presence of food in the GI tract will decrease blood levels of the drug. Large amounts of the drug are metabolized peripherally (either within the lumen of the stomach or the liver or in peripheral tissues) to dopamine or other compounds; these metabolites are excreted in the urine. Because it cannot cross the blood-brain barrier, peripherally produced dopamine cannot reach the CNS. Carbidopa, a peripheral decarboxylase inhibitor, has no antiparkinsonian activity. However, by preventing its metabolic conversion into dopamine, it increases the amount of levodopa that is available for entry into the CNS. In the CNS, levodopa is taken up by dopaminergic neurons where it is converted into dopamine, which is stored in storage granules until it is released by a nerve impulse. After activating its receptors, dopamine is returned to storage in the dopaminergic neurons.

Other dopaminergic agents are well absorbed by the GI tract and readily enter the CNS. Bromocriptine and pergolide are highly bound (90% to 95%) to plasma proteins. Most of these drugs are extensively metabolized in the liver and excreted by the kidneys. Bromocriptine is primarily excreted in the feces. Selegiline is metabolized to amphetamine, methamphetamine, and n-desmethyldeprenyl; all of these metabolites appear in the urine.

ONSET AND DURATION

For most anticholinergic agents, onset of action occurs within 1 hour, peak levels occur in 2 to 4 hours, and duration of action is up to 6 hours. Benztropine's effects may last up to 24 hours.

The action of levodopa is highly variable among patients. Onset and peak blood levels are usually seen within 1 hour of dosing. The drug's effects may last up to 5 hours; half-life is about 1 hour but may be prolonged to 2 hours when combined with carbidopa. A sustained-release formulation of carbidopa-levodopa is less bioavailable (70% to 75%) but is designed to release its contents over 4 to 6 hours. With this formulation, the time to peak concentration is prolonged (up to 2 hours), but peak plasma levels are only about 35% of those that follow immediate release of levodopa.

The action of other dopaminergic agents is not well defined. Amantadine exhibits peak levels in 1 to 4 hours and has a long half-life (24 hours). Bromocriptine exhibits onset within 90 minutes and peak levels within 2 hours; its half-life is 6 hours and duration of action is 3 to 5 hours. Pergolide has a rapid onset (15 to 30 minutes) with peak levels within 1 to 3 hours. Selegiline achieves peak levels within 2 hours.

ADVERSE REACTIONS

Most anticholinergic adverse reactions reflect an extension of their pharmacologic effects and commonly include dry mouth, palpitations or tachycardia, constipation, and urine retention. Less common reactions may include blurred vision, confusion, restlessness, agitation, insomnia, dyspnea, decreased sweating, nausea, and vomiting.

Adverse reactions to levodopa or carbidopa are usually dose-related and commonly include nausea, vomiting, anorexia, and orthostatic hypotension. At higher dosages, CV reactions may include palpitations, tachycardia, arrhythmias, or flushing. Confusion, irritability, or hallucinations may also occur. Levodopa may lose its effectiveness over time; it may become ineffective gradually or erratically, causing sharp fluctuations between mobility and immobility. This problem, called the on-off phenomenon, is a common cause of falls in elderly patients taking the drug for idiopathic parkinsonism.

Amantadine is usually well tolerated. However, prolonged use may cause livedo reticularis, characterized by diffuse mottled reddening of the skin, usually confined to the lower extremities. Amantadine has also been associated with confusion, edema, anorexia, nausea, and constipation.

Bromocriptine commonly causes orthostatic hypotension, especially at the start of therapy. It may also cause palpitation, arrhythmias, and exacerbations of angina, edema, flushing, and GI reactions (including nausea and vomiting).

Pergolide can cause hallucinations, confusion, dyskinesia, nausea, and constipation. It has also been associated with flulike symptoms and orthostatic hypotension.

Selegiline is usually well tolerated at normal dosage range. However, because it is an MAO inhibitor, higher-than-recommended dosages may cause hypotension, palpitations, and acute hypertensive crisis after ingestion of tyramine-containing foods or administration of some sympathomimetic agents.

PROTOTYPE: DOPAMINERGIC AGENTS

LEVODOPA
(lee voe doe' pa)
Dopar, Larodopa, Levopa,
Classification: dopaminergic agent
Pregnancy risk category C

How supplied
TABLETS: 100 mg, 250 mg, 500 mg
CAPSULES: 100 mg, 250 mg, 500 mg

Indications and dosage
Idiopathic parkinsonism, postencephalitic parkinsonism, and symptomatic parkinsonism after carbon monoxide or manganese intoxication; or in association with cerebral arteriosclerosis
ADULTS AND CHILDREN OVER AGE 12: initially, 0.5 to 1 g P.O. daily, given b.i.d., t.i.d., or q.i.d. with food; increase by no more than 0.75 g daily q 3 to 7 days until usual maximum of 8 g is reached. Carefully adjust dosage to individual requirements, tolerance, and response. Higher dosage requires close supervision.

Contraindications and precautions
Levodopa is contraindicated in patients with narrow-angle glaucoma, melanoma, or undiagnosed skin lesions. Use cautiously in CV, renal, hepatic, and pulmonary disorders; peptic ulcer; psychiatric illness, MI with residual arrhythmias; bronchial asthma; emphysema; and endocrine disease.

Adverse reactions
BLOOD: **hemolytic anemia,** leukopenia.
CNS: aggressive behavior; choreiform, dystonic, and dyskinetic movements; involuntary grimacing; head movements; myoclonic body jerks; ataxia; *tremor; muscle twitching;* bradykinetic episode; psychiatric disturbances; memory loss; *mood changes; nervousness; anxiety; disturbing dreams;* euphoria; malaise; fatigue; severe depression; **suicidal tendencies;** dementia; delirium; hallucinations (may necessitate reduction or withdrawal of drug).
CV: *orthostatic hypotension,* cardiac irregularities, flushing, hypertension, phlebitis.
EENT: blepharospasm, *blurred vision,* diplopia, mydriasis or miosis, widening of palpebral fissures, activation of latent Horner's syndrome, oculogyric crises, nasal discharge.
GI: *nausea, vomiting, anorexia,* weight loss (may occur at start of therapy), constipation, flatulence, diarrhea, epigastric pain, hiccups, sialorrhea, dry mouth, bitter taste.
GU: urinary frequency or incontinence, urine retention, darkened urine, excessive and inappropriate sexual behavior, priapism.

Italicized adverse reactions are common   Boldfaced adverse reactions are life-threatening

HEPATIC: hepatotoxicity.

OTHER: dark perspiration, hyperventilation.

Interactions

Antacids: increased absorption of levodopa. Avoid concomitant use.

Antihypertensives: additive hypotensive effect. Monitor patient closely.

High-protein foods: decreased absorption of levodopa. Avoid concomitant use.

Metoclopramide: accelerated gastric emptying of levodopa. Avoid concomitant use.

Papaverine, phenothiazines and other antipsychotics, phenytoin: decreased levodopa effect. Monitor closely.

Pyridoxine: reduced efficacy of levodopa. Examine vitamin preparations and nutritional supplements for content of vitamin B_6 (pyridoxine).

Sympathomimetics: increased risk of cardiac arrhythmias. Monitor closely.

Nursing considerations

Assessment

- Review the patient's history for a condition that contraindicates the use of levodopa.
- Obtain a baseline assessment of the patient's parkinsonism signs and symptoms before therapy.
- Be alert for common adverse reactions.
- Evaluate the patient's and family's knowledge about levodopa therapy.

Planning (Nursing Diagnoses)

Potential nursing diagnoses for the patient receiving levodopa include:

- Impaired physical mobility related to ineffectiveness of levodopa to control parkinsonian syndrome.
- Altered thought processes related to levodopa-induced CNS reactions.
- Fluid volume deficit related to potential adverse GI reactions.
- Knowledge deficit related to levodopa therapy.

Implementation

Preparation and administration

— Adjust dosage according to patient's response and tolerance.

— Crush pills and mix with applesauce or baby food fruits for patients who have difficulty swallowing pills.

— Withdraw MAO inhibitors at least 2 weeks before levodopa therapy.

— Administer with food to prevent GI discomfort.

— If therapy is interrupted for a long time, dosage should be adjusted gradually to previous level.

— Patient who must undergo surgery should continue levodopa as long as oral intake is permitted, generally 6 to 24 hours before surgery. After surgery, administer drug as soon as patient is able to take oral medication.

— Protect levodopa from heat, light, and moisture. If preparation darkens, it has lost potency and should be discarded.

Monitoring

— Monitor the effectiveness of therapy by regularly checking the patient's body movements for signs of improvement; therapeutic response usually follows each dose and disappears within 5 hours but varies considerably.
— Carefully monitor the patient who is also receiving an antihypertensive and a hypoglycemic agent.
— Monitor for signs of overdose; muscle twitching and blepharospasm (twitching of eyelids) may be early signs of drug overdosage; report them to the doctor immediately.
— Monitor the patient for adverse drug reactions.
— Monitor the patient on long-term therapy for diabetes and acromegaly; repeat blood tests and liver and kidney function studies periodically.
— Monitor dietary intake of protein because high-protein foods can decrease levodopa absorption.
— Monitor for abnormal body movements, for example, dystonic, choreiform, and dyskinetic movements.
— Monitor vital signs closely, especially during dosage adjustment.
— Monitor for dehydration if adverse GI reactions occur.
— Monitor the patient for drug interactions.
— Regularly reevaluate the patient's and family's knowledge about levodopa therapy.

Intervention

— Withhold dose and notify the doctor if significant changes in mental status occur. Reduced dosage or discontinuation of levodopa may be necessary.
— Institute safety precautions.
— A doctor-supervised period of drug discontinuance (called a drug holiday) may reestablish the effectiveness of a lower dosage regimen.
— Evaluate test results carefully: Coombs' test occasionally becomes positive during extended use. Expect uric acid elevations with colorimetric method but not with uricase method. Alkaline phosphatase, AST (SGOT), ALT (SGPT), lactate dehydrogenase, bilirubin, BUN, and protein-bound iodine levels show transient elevations in patients receiving levodopa; WBC counts, hemoglobin, and hematocrit show occasional reduction.
— Assist the patient with daily activities as needed.
— Obtain an order for an antiemetic if needed.
— Keep all members of the health care team informed of the patient's response to the drug.

Patient teaching

— Instruct the patient and family about levodopa, including the dosage, frequency, action, and adverse reactions.
— Warn the patient of possible dizziness and orthostatic hypotension, especially at start of therapy. The patient should change position slowly

and dangle legs before getting out of bed. Inform the patient that elastic stockings may control this adverse reaction.

— Advise the patient and family that multivitamin preparations, fortified cereals, and certain OTC medications may contain pyridoxine (vitamin B_6), which can reverse the effects of levodopa.

— Warn the patient and family not to increase dosage without the doctor's orders (they may be tempted to do this as disease symptoms of parkinsonism progress).

— Instruct the family to notify the doctor if they notice changes in the patient's behavior or mental status.

— Advise the patient to avoid driving and other hazardous activities that require mental alertness until adverse CNS reactions are known.

— Instruct the patient to take levodopa with food.

— Tell the patient to notify the nurse or doctor if adverse reactions develop or questions arise about levodopa therapy.

Evaluation
In the patient receiving levodopa, appropriate evaluation statements include:
• Patient exhibits reduced severity of parkinsonism symptoms.
• Patient remains mentally alert throughout levodopa therapy.
• Patient does not develop dehydration.
• Patient and family state an understanding of levodopa therapy.

PROTOTYPE: MISCELLANEOUS ANTIPARKINSONIAN AGENTS

BENZTROPINE MESYLATE
(benz′ troe peen)
Apo-Benztropine†, Bensylate†, Cogentin, PMS Benztropine†
Classification: anticholinergic agent
Pregnancy risk category C

How supplied
TABLETS: 0.5 mg, 1 mg, 2 mg
INJECTION: 1 mg/ml in 2-ml ampules

Indications and dosage
Acute dystonic reaction
ADULTS: 1 to 2 mg I.V. or I.M., followed by 1 to 2 mg P.O. b.i.d. to prevent recurrence.

Parkinsonism
ADULTS: 0.5 to 6 mg P.O. daily. Initial dose is 0.5 mg to 1 mg. Increase by 0.5 mg q 5 to 6 days. Adjust dosage to meet individual requirements. Usual maintenance dose is 1 to 2 mg daily.

Contraindications and precautions

Benztropine is contraindicated in narrow-angle glaucoma. Use cautiously in prostatic hypertrophy and tendency to tachycardia and in elderly or debilitated patients. Drug produces atropine-like adverse reactions and may aggravate tardive dyskinesia.

Adverse reactions

CNS: disorientation, restlessness, irritability, incoherence, hallucinations, headache, *sedation,* depression, muscular weakness.
CV: palpitations, tachycardia, paradoxical bradycardia.
EENT: dilated pupils, blurred vision, photophobia, difficulty swallowing.
GI: *constipation, dry mouth,* nausea, vomiting, epigastric distress.
GU: urinary hesitancy, urine retention.
SKIN: warming, dry skin, flushing.

Some adverse reactions may be due to pending atropine-like toxicity and are dose-related.

Interactions

Amantadine, phenothiazines, tricyclic antidepressants (TCAs): additive anticholinergic adverse reactions, such as confusion and hallucinations. Reduce dosage before administering amantadine.

Nursing considerations

Assessment

- Review the patient's history for a condition that contraindicates the use of benztropine.
- Obtain a baseline assessment of the patient's parkinsonism signs and symptoms before therapy.
- Be alert for common adverse reactions.
- Evaluate the patient's and family's knowledge about benztropine therapy.

Planning (Nursing Diagnoses)

Potential nursing diagnoses for the patient receiving benztropine include:
- Impaired physical mobility related to ineffectiveness of benztropine to control parkinsonism signs and symptoms.
- Constipation related to benztropine's adverse effect on the GI tract.
- Altered oral mucous membrane related to dry mouth caused by benztropine.
- Knowledge deficit related to benztropine therapy.

Implementation

Preparation and administration
—To help prevent GI distress, administer after meals.
—Never discontinue this drug abruptly. Dosage must be reduced gradually.

Monitoring
—Monitor the effectiveness of therapy by regularly checking the patient's body movements for signs of improvement; full effect of drug may take 2 to 3 days.

— Monitor the patient for adverse drug reactions.

— Monitor for intermittent constipation, distention, and abdominal pain, which may signal onset of paralytic ileus.

— Monitor vital signs carefully. Watch closely for adverse reactions, especially in elderly or debilitated patients.

— Regularly check the patient's oral mucous membranes for dryness.

— Monitor the patient's mental status and behavior closely.

— Monitor the patient's GU status for urinary hesitancy or urine retention.

— Monitor the patient for drug interactions.

— Regularly reevaluate the patient's and family's knowledge about benztropine therapy.

Intervention

— Notify the doctor if the patient develops serious adverse reactions that may require dosage reduction.

— Provide a high-fiber diet to prevent constipation; obtain an order for a laxative if needed.

— Give the patient fluids, ice chips, or sugarless gum or hard candy to relieve dry mouth.

— Assist the patient with activities as needed.

— Institute safety precautions.

— Encourage the patient to void before each dose.

— Keep all members of the health care team informed of the patient's response to the drug.

Patient teaching

— Instruct the patient and family about benztropine, including the dosage, frequency, action, and adverse reactions.

— Warn the patient to avoid driving and other hazardous activities that require alertness until CNS effects of the drug are known.

— Explain that drug may take 2 to 3 days to exert full effect.

— Advise the patient to report signs of urinary hesitancy or urine retention.

— Advise the patient to limit activities during hot weather because drug-induced anhydrosis may result in hyperthermia.

— Tell the patient to take the drug after meals to minimize GI discomfort.

— Warn the patient not to discontinue drug abruptly.

— Tell the patient how to manage troublesome adverse reactions such as constipation and dry mouth.

— Tell the patient to notify the nurse or doctor if adverse reactions develop or questions arise about benztropine therapy.

Evaluation

In the patient receiving benztropine, appropriate evaluation statements include:

• Patient exhibits reduced severity of parkinsonism symptoms.

• Patient reports normal bowel patterns.

• Patient reports relief of dry mouth.

• Patient and family state an understanding of benztropine therapy.

SELECTED MAJOR DRUGS: ANTIPARKINSONIAN AGENTS

DRUG, INDICATIONS, AND DOSAGES	SPECIAL PRECAUTIONS

Dopaminergic agents

bromocriptine (Parlodel)
Parkinson's disease —
Adults: 1.25 mg P.O. b.i.d. with meals. Dosage may be increased q 14 to 28 days, up to 100 mg daily.
Amenorrhea and galactorhea associated with hyperprolactinemia; female infertility —
Women: 1.25 to 2.5 mg P.O. daily. Increase dosage by 2.5 mg daily at 3- to 7-day intervals until desired effect is achieved. Safety and efficacy of doses greater than 100 mg daily have not been established.
Prevention of postpartum lactation —
Women: 2.5 mg P.O. b.i.d. with meals for 14 days. Treatment may be extended for up to 21 days, if necessary.
Acromegaly —
Adults: 1.25 to 2.5 mg P.O. for 3 days. An additional 1.25 to 2.5 mg may be added q 3 to 7 days until patient receives therapeutic benefit.

• Contraindicated in patients with known hypersensitivity to ergot derivatives.
• Use cautiously in patients with preexisting psychiatric disorders.

carbidopa-levodopa (Sinemet)
Idiopathic Parkinson's disease, postencephalitic parkinsonism, and symptomatic parkinsonism resulting from carbon monoxide or manganese intoxication —
Adults: 3 to 6 tablets of 25 mg carbidopa/250 mg levodopa daily in divided doses. Do not exceed 8 tablets daily. Optimum daily dosage must be determined by careful titration for each patient.

• Contraindicated in patients with narrow-angle glaucoma, melanoma, or undiagnosed skin lesions.
• Use cautiously in patients with CV, renal, hepatic, and pulmonary disorders; a history of peptic ulcer; and psychiatric illness, MI with residual arrhythmias, bronchial asthma, emphysema, and endocrine disease.

pergolide (Permax)
Adjunct therapy with levodopa and carbidopa-levodopa in management of symptoms associated with Parkinson's disease —
Adults: initially 0.05 mg P.O. daily for 2 days, increased by 0.1 to 0.15 mg daily q third day for 12 days, then increased by 0.25 mg daily q third day until a therapeutic dosage is reached.

• Contraindicated in patients with known hypersensitivity to the drug.
• Administer cautiously to patients with residual arrhythmias after MI; to patients with a history of peptic ulcer disease, psychosis, or seizure disorders; or to those experiencing hallucinations, confusion, or dyskinesia.
• Advise female patients to notify the doctor of pregnancy or breast-feeding.

selegiline (Eldepryl)
Adjunctive treatment to carbadopa-levodopa in the management of the symptoms associated with Parkinson's disease —

• Contraindicated in patients with known hypersensitivity to the drug.

SELECTED MAJOR DRUGS: ANTIPARKINSONIAN AGENTS *continued*

DRUG, INDICATIONS, AND DOSAGES	SPECIAL PRECAUTIONS

Dopaminergic agents *(continued)*

selegiline *(continued)*
Adults: 10 mg P.O. daily, taken as 5 mg at breakfast and 5 mg at lunch. After 2 or 3 days of therapy, begin gradual decrease of carbidopa-levodopa dosage.

Miscellaneous agents

biperiden (Akineton)
Extrapyramidal disorders—
Adults: 2 to 6 mg P.O. daily, b.i.d., or t.i.d., depending on severity. Usual dose is 2 mg daily, or 2 mg I.M. or I.V. q ½ hour, not to exceed four doses or 8 mg total daily.
Parkinsonism—
Adults: 2 mg P.O. t.i.d. to q.i.d. Some patients may require as much as 16 mg daily.

• Use cautiously in patients with prostatism, cardiac arrhythmias, narrow-angle glaucoma, and seizure disorders.

procyclidine (Kemadrin, Procyclid†)
Parkinsonism, muscle ridigity—
Adults: initially, 2 to 2.5 mg P.O. t.i.d. after meals. Increase gradually as needed. Usual dosage range is 20 to 30 mg daily, but some patients may require up to 60 mg daily.
   Also used to relieve extrapyramidal dysfunction that accompanies treatment with phenothiazines and rauwolfia derivatives. Also controls excessive salivation from neuroleptic medications.

• Contraindicated in patients with narrow-angle glaucoma.
• Use cautiously in patients with tachycardia, hypotension, urine retention, and prostatic hypertrophy.

trihexyphenidyl (Aparkane†, Artane, Trihexane)
Drug-induced parkinsonism—
Adults: 1 mg P.O. on first day, 2 mg on second day, then increase by 2 mg q 3 to 5 days until total of 6 to 10 mg is given daily. Usually given t.i.d. with meals and, if needed, q.i.d. (last dose should be before bedtime) or extended-release form b.i.d. Postencephalitic parkinsonism may require total daily dosage of 12 to 15 mg daily.

• Use cautiously in patients with narrow-angle glaucoma; cardiac, hepatic, or renal disorders; hypertension; obstructive disease of the GI and GU tracts; and possible prostatic hypertrophy; in patients over age 60; and in those with arteriosclerosis or a history of drug hypersensitivities.
• Adverse reactions are usually mild and transient.

†Available in Canada only

SELF-TEST

1. Janet Walker has idiopathic parkinsonism and takes levodopa 2 g P.O. q.i.d. Which of the following adverse reactions may require reduced dosage or withdrawal of the drug?
   a. seizures
   b. hallucinations
   c. urinary tract infection
   d. endocarditis

2. At routine follow-up, Mrs. Walker mentions that she has had indigestion several times over the past few weeks and has taken an antacid to relieve it. Which drug interaction occurs with levodopa and antacids?
   a. Antacids increase the absorption of levodopa.
   b. Antacids decrease the absorption of levodopa.
   c. Antacids decrease the efficacy of levodopa.
   d. Antacids increase the efficacy of levodopa.

3. Donald Brown's doctor prescribes benztropine P.O. for parkinsonism. What is the usual initial adult dosage for Mr. Brown's condition?
   a. 0.5 to 1 mg
   b. 1 to 1.5 mg
   c. 1.5 to 2 mg
   d. 2 to 3 mg

Check your answers on page 1066.

CHAPTER 36

CHOLINERGICS

Cholinesterase inhibitors
ambenonium chloride ✦ edrophonium chloride ✦ neostigmine bromide
neostigmine methylsulfate ✦ physostigmine salicylate
pyridostigmine bromide

Parasympathomimetic agent (cholinergic agonist)
bethanechol chloride

OVERVIEW

- When stimulated, parasympathetic nerves release acetylcholine from their nerve endings. Acetylcholine binds to specific sites (muscarinic receptors) in the tissue innervated by the parasympathetic nerve. This interaction starts the mechanisms that result in a typical parasympathetic response.
- The parasympathetic division of the autonomic nervous system innervates various body organs and systems and acts on the heart, GI tract, urinary bladder, and respiratory tract. The parasympathetic division works in concert with its sympathetic counterpart to provide continuous control of body functions that occur without conscious thought (for example, digestion, respiration, and maintenance of blood pressure).
- Cholinergics (also called parasympathomimetic agents) mimic the action of acetylcholine in that they produce parasympathetic responses. They are not organ-specific. When bethanechol, for example, is administered to treat postoperative urine retention, it is distributed throughout the body, and other organs innervated by the parasympathetic system are activated. Thus, these drugs can produce a therapeutic effect at one location (for example, by preventing urine retention in the bladder) and annoying adverse reactions at another (for example, by causing excess production of saliva by the salivary glands).

  Drug therapy can influence autonomic processes in one of two ways: it can mimic acetylcholine at muscarinic receptor sites (by administration of parasympathomimetic agents) or it can inhibit the breakdown of acetylcholine at these sites, prolonging its action (by administration of cholinesterase inhibitors).

GLOSSARY

Acetylcholine: an acetic acid ester of choline, normally present in the body. It is a neurotransmitter at the neuromuscular junction, in sympathetic and parasympathetic ganglia, and at parasympathetic nerve endings.

Autonomic nervous system: portion of the nervous system that controls the involuntary visceral functions of the body.

Cholinergic: stimulated, activated, or transmitted by acetylcholine or a similar substance.

Muscarinic receptor: receptor located in effector cells that is stimulated by acetylcholine, muscarine, or a similar substance.

Neurotransmitter: chemical substance secreted by the neuron at the synapse that acts on receptor proteins in the membrane of the adjacent neuron or muscle to stimulate, inhibit, or modify its activity.

Parasympathetic nervous system: cholinergic division of the autonomic nervous system.

Parasympathomimetic: agent that produces effects similar to those from stimulation of the parasympathetic nerves; also called cholinergic or muscarinic.

Nerves that innervate skeletal muscle also release acetylcholine when stimulated. The released acetylcholine binds to specific sites in skeletal muscle, triggering contraction. Disordered release of acetylcholine from these nerves or impaired binding with skeletal muscle leads to profound muscle weakness (myasthenia gravis). Cholinesterase inhibitors (for example, neostigmine) improve muscular performance in patients with this disease.

- Cholinergics are classified primarily into the cholinesterase inhibitors and the parasympathomimetic agents.

MAJOR USES

- Ambenonium, neostigmine, and pyridostigmine are used to treat symptoms of myasthenia gravis.
- Edrophonium and neostigmine aid differential diagnosis of myasthenia gravis.
- Neostigmine is used to prevent and treat postoperative urine retention.
- Neostigmine and pyridostigmine reverse the effect of neuromuscular blocking agents used in surgery.
- Physostigmine is an antidote in anticholinergic poisoning, such as poisoning caused by tricyclic antidepressants (TCAs). However, because of the risk of adverse reactions, it is not commonly used.
- Bethanechol is used to prevent and treat postoperative urine retention, postoperative gastric atony and retention, abdominal distention, and megacolon.

MECHANISM OF ACTION

- Ambenonium, edrophonium, neostigmine, physostigmine, and pyridostigmine inhibit the destruction of acetylcholine released from the parasympathetic nerves. Acetylcholine accumulates, promoting increased stimulation of the receptor.
- Bethanechol directly binds to muscarinic receptors, mimicking the action of acetylcholine.

ABSORPTION, DISTRIBUTION, METABOLISM, AND EXCRETION

All cholinergics except physostigmine are poorly absorbed orally. They are widely distributed to organs innervated by the parasympathetic nervous system, metabolized in the liver, and excreted by the kidneys as water-soluble metabolites.

Physostigmine, the only cholinergic that effectively crosses the blood-brain barrier, is useful for TCA and anticholinergic poisoning.

ONSET AND DURATION

Ambenonium's onset and duration are variable. The drug's effects on skeletal muscle usually last 4 to 8 hours. Edrophonium's onset after I.V. injection occurs within 30 to 60 seconds; therapeutic activity lasts 5 to 10 minutes. When the drug is given I.M., onset occurs in 2 to 10 minutes and its duration of action is 5 to 30 minutes. Neostigmine has an onset of action on the GI tract 2 to 4 hours after oral administration, 10 to 30 minutes after I.M. injection. Duration of action on skeletal muscle after I.M. injection is 2½ to 4 hours. Physostigmine's onset occurs in 3 to 8 minutes after parenteral administration; its duration of action is 30 minutes to 5 hours. Pyridostigmine's action on skeletal muscle begins within 30 to 45 minutes when the drug is given orally. Its action persists 3 to 6 hours. After I.M. injection, onset occurs within 15 minutes. After I.V. infusion, onset occurs in 2 to 5 minutes; its duration of action is 2 to 3 hours.

Bethanechol has an onset between 60 and 90 minutes (occasionally as soon as 30 minutes) after oral administration. Therapeutic effects persist for about 1 hour. After S.C. injection, onset occurs within 5 to 15 minutes and action peaks in 15 to 30 minutes. Therapeutic effects wane thereafter and disappear after 2 hours.

ADVERSE REACTIONS

Stimulation of the parasympathetic nervous system can occur either directly by parasympathomimetics acting on cholinergic receptors or indirectly, by cholinesterase inhibitors causing a buildup of acetylcholine. The resulting adverse reactions include sweating, GI disturbances (nausea, diarrhea, abdominal cramping), cardiac problems (bradycardia, hypotension, and arrhythmias), and respiratory difficulties (increased airway secretions).

Cholinesterase inhibitors promote the action of acetylcholine at all of its effector sites, including the neuromuscular junction, autonomic ganglia, and CNS. Cholinesterase inhibitors can cause parasympathetic adverse reactions. In high dosages, these drugs can cause neuromuscular blockade, which can lead to weakness, difficulty breathing, and ptosis. These symptoms are similar to those of myasthenia gravis and those in patients receiving cholinesterase inhibitors as drug therapy. Differentiating between advancing disease and excessive drug dosage requires a specific diagnostic test.

Some cholinergics produce CNS reactions, including headache, confusion, nervousness, and, with high dosages, seizures. Visual reactions include problems of accommodation, miosis, excessive lacrimation, and diplopia.

PROTOTYPE: CHOLINESTERASE INHIBITORS

NEOSTIGMINE BROMIDE
(nee oh stig' meen)
Prostigmin Bromide

NEOSTIGMINE METHYLSULFATE
Prostigmin
Classification: cholinesterase inhibitor
Pregnancy risk category C

How supplied
bromide
TABLETS: 15 mg
methylsulfate
INJECTION: 0.25 mg/ml, 0.5 mg/ml, 1 mg/ml

Indications and dosage
Antidote for nondepolarizing neuromuscular blocking agents
ADULTS: 0.5 to 2 mg I.V. slowly. Repeat p.r.n. to a total of 5 mg. Give 0.6 to 1.2 mg atropine sulfate I.V. before antidote dose.

Postoperative abdominal distention and bladder atony
ADULTS: 0.5 to 1 mg I.M. or S.C. q 4 to 6 hours.

Postoperative ileus
ADULTS: 0.25 to 1 mg I.M. or S.C. q 4 to 6 hours.

Diagnosis of myasthenia gravis
ADULTS: 0.022 mg/kg I.M. 30 minutes after 0.011 mg/kg atropine sulfate.

Treatment of myasthenia gravis
ADULTS: 15 to 30 mg P.O. t.i.d. (range is 15 to 375 mg daily); or 0.5 to 2 mg I.M. or I.V. q 1 to 3 hours. Dosage must be individualized, depending on response and tolerance of adverse reactions. Therapy may be required day and night.
CHILDREN: 7.5 to 15 mg P.O. t.i.d. to q.i.d.
Note: 1:1,000 solution of injectable solution contains 1 mg/ml; 1:2,000 solution, 0.5 mg/ml.

Contraindications and precautions

Neostigmine is contraindicated in patients with known hypersensitivity to cholinergics or bromide, mechanical obstruction of the intestine or urinary tract, bradycardia, or hypotension. Use with extreme caution in bronchial asthma. Use cautiously in seizure disorder, recent coronary occlusion, peritonitis, vagotonia, hyperthyroidism, cardiac arrhythmias, and peptic ulcer.

Adverse reactions

CNS: dizziness, muscle weakness, mental confusion, jitters, sweating, respiratory depression.
CV: bradycardia, hypotension.
EENT: miosis.
GI: *nausea, vomiting, diarrhea, abdominal cramps,* excessive salivation.
GU: urinary frequency.
SKIN: rash (bromide).
OTHER: **bronchospasm, bronchoconstriction,** *muscle cramps.*

Interactions

Atropine, cholinergic blockers, procainamide, aminoglycosides, quinidine: may block cholinergic effect on muscle. Observe for lack of drug effect.

Nursing considerations

Assessment

- Review the patient's history for a condition that contraindicates the use of neostigmine.
- Obtain a baseline assessment of the patient's underlying condition before initiating neostigmine therapy.
- Be alert for common adverse reactions.
- Evaluate the patient's and family's knowledge about neostigmine therapy.

Planning (Nursing Diagnoses)

Potential nursing diagnoses for the patient receiving neostigmine include:
- Impaired physical mobility related to the ineffectiveness of neostigmine in treatment of myasthenia gravis.
- Diarrhea related to adverse GI effect of neostigmine.
- Pain related to neostigmine-induced abdominal or muscle cramps.
- Knowledge deficit related to neostigmine therapy.

Implementation

Preparation and administration
—Make sure that all other cholinergics have been discontinued before administering this drug.
—In myasthenia gravis, schedule the dose before periods of fatigue. For example, if patient has dysphagia, schedule dose 30 minutes before each meal.
—Adverse GI reactions may be reduced by taking drug with milk or food.

Italicized adverse reactions are common   Boldfaced adverse reactions are life-threatening

—Hospitalized patient with chronic myasthenia gravis may request bed-side supply of tablets for self-administration. This will enable patient to take each dose precisely as ordered. Seek approval for self-medication program according to hospital policy, but continue to oversee medication.

—Be prepared to administer I.M. neostigmine instead of edrophonium to diagnose myasthenia gravis; may be preferable to edrophonium when limb weakness is the only symptom.

Monitoring

—Monitor the effectiveness of therapy by regularly assessing signs and symptoms of the underlying disorder for evidence of relief or diminished severity; patients may develop resistance to this drug.

—Monitor the patient for adverse drug reactions.

—Monitor vital signs frequently; check respirations carefully.

—Monitor and document the patient's response after each dose because it is difficult to determine optimum dosage.

—Monitor closely for improvement in strength, vision, and ptosis 45 to 60 minutes after each dose.

—Monitor for diarrhea and other adverse GI reactions; if present, monitor hydration status.

—Monitor for abdominal or muscle cramping.

—Monitor the patient for drug interactions.

—Regularly reevaluate the patient's and family's knowledge about neostigmine therapy.

Intervention

—Have atropine injection readily available and be prepared to give as ordered to reverse toxicity; provide respiratory support as needed.

—Use to prevent abdominal distention and GI distress may require insertion of a rectal tube to help passage of gas.

—Report severe muscle weakness to doctor, who will determine if it reflects drug-induced toxicity or exacerbation of myasthenia gravis. Test dose of edrophonium I.V. will worsen drug-induced weakness but will temporarily relieve weakness caused by disease.

—Obtain an order for an antidiarrheal or antiemetic as needed.

—Consult with the doctor to manage abdominal or muscle cramping.

—Keep all members of the health care team informed of the patient's response to the drug.

Patient teaching

—Instruct the patient and family about neostigmine, including the dosage, frequency, action, and adverse reactions.

—Instruct the patient about underlying disease condition requiring treatment with neostigmine.

—Tell the patient how to handle troublesome GI reactions and abdominal or muscle cramping.

— Tell the patient to notify the nurse or doctor if adverse reactions develop or questions arise about neostigmine therapy.

Evaluation
In the patient receiving neostigmine, appropriate evaluation statements include:
• Patient is able to perform activities of daily living without assistance.
• Patient's bowel patterns are unaffected by neostigmine therapy.
• Patient does not experience abdominal or muscle cramping.

PROTOTYPE: PARASYMPATHOMIMETIC AGENTS

BETHANECHOL CHLORIDE
(be than' e kole)
Duvoid, Urabeth, Urecholine, Urocarb Liquid‡, Urocarb Tablets‡
Classification: parasympathomimetic agent
Pregnancy risk category C

How supplied
TABLETS: 5 mg, 10 mg, 25 mg, 50 mg
LIQUID: 1 mg/5 ml‡
INJECTION: 5 mg/ml

Indications and dosage
Acute postoperative and postpartum nonobstructive (functional) urine retention, neurogenic atony of urinary bladder with retention, abdominal distention, megacolon, or reflux esophagitis caused by low esophageal sphincter pressure
ADULTS: 10 to 30 mg P.O. b.i.d. to q.i.d. Or 2.5 to 10 mg S.C. Never give I.M. or I.V. When used for urine retention, some patients may require 50 to 100 mg P.O./dose. Use such doses with extreme caution.
   Test dose is 2.5 mg S.C., repeated at 15- to 30-minute intervals to total of four doses to determine the minimal effective dose; then use minimal effective dose q 6 to 8 hours. All doses must be adjusted individually.

Contraindications and precautions
Bethanechol is contraindicated in patients with uncertain strength or integrity of bladder wall; when increased muscular activity of GI or urinary tract is harmful; in mechanical obstructions of GI or urinary tract; in hyperthyroidism, peptic ulcer, latent or active bronchial asthma, cardiac or coronary artery disease, vagotonia, seizure disorder, Parkinson's disease, bradycardia, COPD, and hypotension. Use cautiously in hypertension, vasomotor instability, peritonitis, and other acute inflammatory conditions of GI tract.

Adverse reactions
CNS: headache, malaise.
CV: bradycardia, hypotension, **cardiac arrest**, reflex tachycardia.

‡Available in Australia only
Boldfaced adverse reactions are life-threatening

EENT: lacrimation, miosis.
GI: *abdominal cramps, diarrhea*, salivation, nausea, vomiting, belching, borborygmus, esophageal spasms.
GU: urinary urgency.
SKIN: flushing, sweating.
OTHER: **bronchoconstriction**, increased bronchial secretions.

Interactions
Atropine, cholinergic blockers, procainamide, quinidine: may reverse cholinergic effects. Observe for lack of drug effect.

Nursing considerations
Assessment
- Review the patient's history for a condition that contraindicates the use of bethanechol.
- Obtain a baseline assessment of patient's bladder, colon, or esophageal disorder before initiating bethanechol therapy.
- Be alert for common adverse reactions.
- Evaluate the patient's and family's knowledge about bethanechol.

Planning (Nursing Diagnoses)
Potential nursing diagnoses for the patient receiving bethanechol include:
- Urinary retention related to ineffectiveness of bethanechol to relieve acute postoperative or postpartum nonobstructive urine retention or retention associated with neurogenic atony of urinary bladder.
- Diarrhea related to adverse GI reactions to bethanechol.
- Knowledge deficit related to bethanechol therapy.

Implementation
Preparation and administration
—Never give I.M. or I.V.; could cause circulatory collapse, hypotension, severe abdominal cramping, bloody diarrhea, shock, or cardiac arrest.
—Poor and variable oral absorption requires larger oral doses. Oral and S.C. doses are not interchangeable.
—Check to ensure that all other cholinergics have been discontinued before giving this drug.
—Administer on empty stomach; if taken after meals, may cause nausea and vomiting.

Monitoring
—Monitor the effectiveness of therapy by assessing for symptom relief (for example, patient treated for urine retention is able to void). Drug is usually effective 5 to 15 minutes after injection and 30 to 90 minutes after oral use.
—Monitor vital signs frequently, being especially careful to check respirations.
—Monitor the patient for adverse drug reactions.

—Monitor closely for signs of drug toxicity (sudden change in heart rate, hypotension, respiratory or cardiac arrest), especially with S.C. administration.
—Monitor for diarrhea; if present, assess hydration status frequently.
—Monitor intake and output if used to treat urine retention.
—Monitor the patient for drug interactions.
—Regularly reevaluate the patient's and family's knowledge about bethanechol therapy.

Intervention
—Always have atropine injection readily available and be prepared to give atropine 0.5 mg S.C. or slow I.V. push as ordered, and provide respiratory support if needed.
—If used to treat urine retention, make sure bedpan is readily available.
—Be prepared to insert a rectal tube to help passage of gas if used to prevent abdominal distention and GI distress.
—Obtain an order for an antidiarrheal agent as needed.
—Keep all members of the health care team informed of the patient's response to the drug.

Patient teaching
—Instruct the patient and family about bethanechol, including the dosage, frequency, action, and adverse reactions.
—Tell the patient drug is usually effective 30 to 90 minutes after oral use and 5 to 15 minutes after injection.
—Instruct the patient to take oral dose on an empty stomach.
—Tell the patient to notify the nurse or doctor if adverse reactions develop or questions arise about bethanechol therapy.

Evaluation
In the patient receiving bethanechol, appropriate evaluation statements include:
• Patient's urine retention is relieved.
• Patient reports no evidence of diarrhea.
• Patient and family state an understanding of bethanechol therapy.

SELECTED MAJOR DRUGS: CHOLINERGICS

DRUG, INDICATIONS, AND DOSAGES	SPECIAL PRECAUTIONS

ambenonium (Mytelase)
Symptomatic treatment of myasthenia gravis in patients who cannot take neostigmine bromide or pyridostigmine—
Adults: dosage must be individualized for each patient, but usually ranges from 5 to 25 mg P.O. t.i.d. to q.i.d. Starting dose usually is 5 mg P.O. t.i.d. to q.i.d. Increase gradually and adjust at 1- to 2-day intervals to avoid drug accumulation and overdosage. Usual dosage range is 15 to 100 mg daily, but some patients may require as much as 75 mg b.i.d. to q.i.d.

• Contraindicated in mechanical obstruction of intestine or urinary tract, bradycardia, or hypotension.
• Use with extreme caution in bronchial asthma.
• Use cautiously in seizure disorder, recent coronary occlusion, vagotonia, hyperthyroidism, cardiac arrhythmias, and peptic ulcer.

edrophonium (Enlon, Reversol, Tensilon)
As a curare antagonist (to reverse neuromuscular blocking action)—
Adults: 10 mg I.V. given over 30 to 45 seconds. Dose may be repeated as necessary to 40 mg maximum dosage. Larger dosages may potentiate rather than antagonize effect of curare.
Diagnostic aid in myasthenia gravis (Tensilon test)—
Adults: 1 to 2 mg I.V. within 15 to 30 seconds, then 8 mg if no response (increase in muscular strength).
Children over 34 kg: 2 mg I.V. If no response within 45 seconds, give 1 mg q 45 seconds to maximum of 10 mg.
Children up to 34 kg: 1 mg I.V. If no response within 45 seconds, give 1 mg q 45 seconds to maximum of 5 mg.
Infants: 0.5 mg I.V.
To differentiate myasthenic crisis from cholinergic crisis—
Adults: 1 mg I.V. If no response in 1 minute, repeat dose once. Increased muscular strength confirms myasthenic crisis; no increase or exaggerated weakness confirms cholinergic crisis.
Paroxysmal supraventricular tachycardia—
Adults: 5 to 10 mg I.V. given over 1 minute or less.
Children: 2 mg I.V. Administer slowly.

• Contraindicated in mechanical obstruction of intestine or urinary tract, bradycardia, or hypotension.
• Administer cautiously to patients with hyperthyroidism, cardiac disease, peptic ulcer, and bronchial asthma.
• Always have a cholinergic blocker (such as atropine) available when using as a diagnostic agent.

physostigmine (Antilirium)
To reverse the CNS toxicity associated with tricyclic antidepressant and anticholinergic poisoning—
Adults: 0.5 to 2 mg I.M. or I.V. (1 mg/minute I.V.) repeated as necessary if life-threatening signs recur (coma, seizures, arrhythmias).

• Contraindicated in asthma, gangrene, diabetes, CV disease, or mechanical obstruction of the intestine or urogenital tract or any vagotonic state and in patients receiving choline esters or depolarizing neuromuscular blocking agent (succinylcholine).
• Administer cautiously because of the possibility of hypersensitivity in an occasional patient.

SELECTED MAJOR DRUGS: CHOLINERGICS *continued*

DRUG, INDICATIONS, AND DOSAGES	SPECIAL PRECAUTIONS
pyridostigmine (Mestinon) *Antidote for nondepolarizing neuromuscular blocking agents*— **Adults:** 10 to 20 mg I.V. preceded by atropine 0.6 to 1.2 mg I.V. *Myasthenia gravis*— **Adults:** 60 to 120 mg P.O. q 3 or 4 hours. Usual dosage is 600 mg daily but higher dosage may be needed (up to 1,500 mg daily). Give ⅓ of oral dose I.M. or I.V. Dosage must be adjusted for each patient, depending on response and tolerance of adverse reactions. Alternatively, may give 180 to 540 mg timed-release tablets (1 to 3 tablets) b.i.d., with at least 6 hours between doses.	• Contraindicated in mechanical obstruction of intestine or urinary tract, bradycardia, or hypotension. • Use with extreme caution in bronchial asthma. • Use cautiously in seizure disorder, recent coronary occlusion, vagotonia, hyperthyroidism, cardiac arrhythmias, and peptic ulcer. Avoid large doses in decreased GI motility.

SELF-TEST

1. Mary Graves was admitted to the hospital with a history of muscular weakness and severe generalized fatigue that comes on quickly, most often in the evening. At examination, the doctor noted a ptosis of the eyelids with difficulty in chewing and swallowing and diagnosed myasthenia gravis. The doctor prescribed neostigmine 30 mg P.O. t.i.d. When administering neostigmine, the nurse should:
   a. give the drug with milk or food to decrease GI upset.
   b. avoid awakening the patient at night to administer drug.
   c. observe closely for adverse reactions, which include constipation and dry mouth.
   d. teach the patient to take the medication only if signs of weakness are present.

2. After 2 weeks of treatment with neostigmine, Mrs. Graves begins to experience increased muscle weakness. Her doctor performs a diagnostic test using edrophonium I.V. to determine if her symptoms resulted from toxicity. Which of the following reactions indicate drug toxicity?
   a. Rapid increase in salivation, lacrimation, and sweating
   b. Increase in strength of muscles
   c. Increase in weakness of muscles
   d. Rapid dilation of the pupils

3. Which of the following drugs should the nurse expect to be administered to reverse drug toxicity effects?
   a. Bethanechol
   b. Dopamine
   c. Ergotamine
   d. Atropine

4. On the second day after abdominal surgery, Howard Johns is complaining of severe abdominal distention. Considering that no contraindications apply, which of the following drugs would be most likely to be prescribed for abdominal distention?
   a. Atropine
   b. Morphine
   c. Bethanechol
   d. Edrophonium

Check your answers on page 1066.

CHAPTER 37

CHOLINERGIC BLOCKERS

___

atropine sulfate ◆ glycopyrrolate ◆ scopolamine hydrobromide

___

OVERVIEW

- Cholinergic blockers (also called parasympatholytics) inhibit the action of acetylcholine released by parasympathetic and some sympathetic nerves. Because parasympathetic nerves innervate many organs, parasympatholytic action can be widespread. The effects of parasympatholytics are typically opposite those of parasympathetic stimulation. For example, parasympathetic (vagal) stimulation of the heart decreases heart rate, whereas atropine, a parasympatholytic drug, increases heart rate.
- Parasympatholytic drugs are not organ-specific. The administration of atropine to reverse severe bradycardia, for example, can dry oral and respiratory secretions. (See also Antiarrhythmics, Chapter 20.) Similarly, the use of glycopyrrolate preoperatively to dry oral secretions can produce urine retention, especially in men with prostatic hypertrophy.

MAJOR USES

- Atropine may be used for treatment of poisoning by organic phosphate insecticides and certain mushrooms.
- As preanesthetic medications, atropine, glycopyrrolate, and scopolamine are used to reduce salivary and respiratory secretions.
- Scopolamine may be used to prevent motion sickness.

MECHANISM OF ACTION

- Cholinergic blockers inhibit the effect of acetylcholine—as the neurotransmitter for impulses in the parasympathetic nervous system—at the junction between postganglionic parasympathetic nerve endings and effector organs. These receptor sites are also called muscarinic sites.

ABSORPTION, DISTRIBUTION, METABOLISM, AND EXCRETION

Cholinergic blockers generally are well absorbed from the GI tract. They are widely distributed to body organs innervated by the parasympathetic nervous system and excreted unchanged in the urine.

Atropine and scopolamine are more likely to penetrate the CNS than glycopyrrolate.

GLOSSARY

Neurohormone: hormone that stimulates the neural mechanism.
Neuromuscular junction: joining of a nerve ending and a muscle fiber.
Neuron: nerve cell; the structural unit of the nervous system.
Parasympatholytic: agent that opposes the effects of impulses conveyed by the parasympathetic nervous system; also called anticholinergic or antimuscarinic.

ONSET AND DURATION

All cholinergic blockers take effect within 30 minutes when injected I.M. or S.C. and within 30 to 60 minutes when given orally.

The duration of these agents is from 2 to 6 hours when given I.M. or S.C. and from 4 to 6 hours when given orally. Effects of large doses can last as long as 24 hours.

ADVERSE REACTIONS

Cholinergic blockers produce anticholinergic adverse reactions; such reactions are produced by many other medications as well. Anticholinergic reactions include GI reactions (dry mouth, thirst, constipation, nausea, and vomiting); urinary symptoms (hesitancy and retention); CV reactions (tachycardia, palpitations, and activation of angina); dermatologic reactions (hot, flushed skin); and visual changes (mydriasis, blurred vision, and photophobia). Anticholinergic CNS reactions include headache, restlessness, ataxia, disorientation, hallucinations, delirium, agitation, mental confusion, insomnia, and coma with excessive dosage. (See *Effects of Cholinergic Blockers.*)

EFFECTS OF CHOLINERGIC BLOCKERS

INNERVATED ORGAN	Effect of acetylcholine	Effect of cholinergic blockers
Heart	▼	▲
Bronchioles	▲	▼
GI tract	▲	▼
Bladder	▲	▼
Bladder sphincter	▼	▲
Blood vessels	▼	▲
Sweat and salivary glands	▲	▼

KEY: ▼ = inhibition, relaxation, or dilation; ▲ = constriction or stimulation

ATROPINE SULFATE
(*a' troe peen*)
Classification: cholinergic blocker
Pregnancy risk category C

How supplied
TABLETS: 0.4 mg, 0.6 mg
INJECTION: 0.05 mg/ml, 0.1 mg/ml, 0.3 mg/ml, 0.4 mg/ml, 0.5 mg/ml, 0.6 mg/ml, 0.8 mg/ml, 1 mg/ml, 1.2 mg/ml

Indications and dosage
Symptomatic bradycardia, bradyarrhythmia (junctional or escape rhythm)
ADULTS: usually 0.5 to 1 mg by I.V. push; repeat q 5 minutes to maximum of 2 mg. Lower doses (less than 0.5 mg) can cause bradycardia.
CHILDREN: 0.01 mg/kg I.V. up to maximum of 0.4 mg; or 0.3 mg/m^2 I. V.; may repeat q 4 to 6 hours.

Antidote for anticholinesterase insecticide poisoning
ADULTS: 2 mg I.M. or I.V. repeated hourly until muscarinic symptoms disappear. Severe cases may require up to 6 mg I.M. or I.V. q 1 hour.

Preoperatively for diminishing secretions and blocking cardiac vagal reflexes
ADULTS: 0.4 to 0.6 mg I.M. 45 to 60 minutes before anesthesia.
CHILDREN: 0.01 mg/kg I.M. up to maximum dose of 0.4 mg 45 to 60 minutes before anesthesia.

Treatment of functional GI disorders such as irritable bowel syndrome
ADULTS: 0.4 to 0.6 mg P.O. q 4 to 6 hours.
CHILDREN: 0.01 mg/kg or 0.3 mg/m^2 P.O. (not to exceed 0.4 mg) q 4 to 6 hours.

Contraindications and precautions
Atropine is contraindicated in narrow-angle glaucoma, obstructive uropathy, obstructive disease of GI tract, myasthenia gravis, paralytic ileus, intestinal atony, unstable CV status in acute hemorrhage, and toxic megacolon. Use cautiously in patients with Down's syndrome because such patients are sensitive to this drug.

Adverse reactions
BLOOD: leukocytosis.
CNS: *headache, restlessness*, ataxia, disorientation, hallucinations, delirium, coma, *insomnia, dizziness*; excitement, agitation, and confusion (especially in elderly patients).

Italicized adverse reactions are common

CV: 1 to 2 mg—*tachycardia, palpitations*; greater than 2 mg—**extreme tachycardia**, angina.

EENT: 1 mg—*slight mydriasis*, photophobia; 2 mg—*blurred vision, mydriasis.*

GI: *dry mouth (common even at low doses)*, thirst, *constipation*, nausea, vomiting.

GU: urine retention.

SKIN: hot, flushed skin.

Interactions

Methotrimeprazine: may produce extrapyramidal symptoms. Monitor patient carefully.

Nursing considerations

Assessment
• Review the patient's history for a condition that contraindicates the use of atropine.
• Obtain a baseline assessment of patient's condition for which drug is being prescribed before initiating atropine therapy.
• Be alert for common adverse reactions.
• Evaluate the patient's and family's knowledge about atropine therapy.

Planning (Nursing Diagnoses)
Potential nursing diagnoses for the patient receiving atropine include:
• Potential for injury related to ineffectiveness of atropine to treat indicated condition.
• Pain related to atropine-induced headache.
• Altered oral mucous membrane related to atropine-induced dry mouth.
• Constipation related to adverse GI reactions.
• Knowledge deficit related to atropine therapy.

Implementation

Preparation and administration

— Administer drug exactly as prescribed.

Monitoring

— Monitor the effectiveness of therapy by regularly assessing underlying condition.
— Monitor the patient for adverse drug reactions, which vary considerably with dosage.
— Monitor for toxicity (hyperpyrexia, urine retention, hallucinations, confusion, and other CNS reactions), especially in patients receiving high doses.
— Monitor for initial paradoxical bradycardia with I.V. administration; this effect usually disappears within 2 minutes.
— Monitor for tachycardia in cardiac patients; this effect may precipitate ventricular fibrillation.
— Monitor intake and output. Drug causes urine retention and urinary hesitancy; encourage the patient to void before receiving drug.

— Monitor closely for urine retention in elderly men with benign prostatic hypertrophy.
— Monitor the patient for drug interactions.
— Monitor the patient's compliance with atropine therapy.
— Regularly reevaluate the patient's and family's knowledge about atropine therapy.

Intervention
— Keep physostigmine readily available to treat atropine overdose.
— If atropine-induced headache occurs, obtain an order for a mild analgesic, if appropriate.
— Frequently provide ice chips or sugarless hard candy to relieve dry mouth (except in preoperative patients in whom dry mouth is desired).
— If constipation occurs, obtain an order for a laxative.
— Keep all members of the health care team informed of the patient's response to the drug.

Patient teaching
— Instruct the patient and family about atropine, including dosage, frequency, action, and adverse reactions.
— Teach the patient receiving oral atropine how to handle troublesome reactions, such as constipation and dry mouth.
— Advise the patient to avoid hazardous activities that require mental alertness until CNS reactions are known.
— Encourage the hospitalized patient to ask for assistance when getting out of bed.
— If oral atropine therapy causes headache, advise the patient to take a mild analgesic.
— Tell the patient to notify the nurse or doctor if adverse reactions develop or questions arise about atropine therapy.

Evaluation
In the patient receiving atropine, appropriate evaluation statements include:
• Patient shows relief of signs and symptoms treated by atropine.
• Patient does not experience atropine-induced headache.
• Patient reports relief of dry mouth.
• Patient does not experience constipation.
• Patient and family state an understanding of atropine therapy.

SELECTED MAJOR DRUGS: CHOLINERGIC BLOCKERS

DRUG, INDICATIONS, AND DOSAGES

SPECIAL PRECAUTIONS

glycopyrrolate (Robinul)
To block cholinergic effects of agents used to reverse neuromuscular blockade—
Adults: 0.2 mg I.V. for each 1 mg neostigmine or 5 mg pyridostigmine. May be given I.V. without dilution or may be added to dextrose injection and given by infusion.
Preoperatively to diminish secretions and block cardiac vagal reflexes—
Adults: 0.004 mg/kg of body weight I.M. 30 to 60 minutes before anesthesia.
Adjunctive therapy in peptic ulcers and other GI disorders—
Adults: 1 to 2 mg P.O. t.i.d. or 0.1 mg I.M. t.i.d. or q.i.d. Dosage must be individualized. Maximum P.O. dose is 8 mg daily.

• Contraindicated in narrow-angle glaucoma, obstructive uropathy, obstructive disease of the GI tract, myasthenia gravis, paralytic ileus, intestinal atony, unstable CV status in acute hemorrhage, or toxic megacolon.
• Use cautiously in patients with autonomic neuropathy, hyperthyroidism, coronary artery disease, cardiac arrhythmias, CHF, hypertension, hiatal hernia associated with reflux esophagitis, hepatic or renal disease, and ulcerative colitis and in patients over age 40 because of increased incidence of glaucoma.
• Use cautiously in hot or humid environments. Drug-induced heatstroke is possible.

scopolamine
Postencephalitic parkinsonism and other spastic states—
Adults: 0.5 to 1 mg P.O. t.i.d. to q.i.d.; 0.3 to 0.6 mg S.C., I.M., or I.V. (with suitable dilution) t.i.d. to q.i.d.
Children: 0.006 mg/kg or 0.2 mg/m^2 P.O. or S.C. t.i.d. to q.i.d.
Preoperatively to reduce secretions and block cardiac vagal reflexes—
Adults: 0.4 to 0.6 mg S.C. 30 to 60 minutes before induction of anesthesia.

• Contraindicated in narrow-angle glaucoma, obstructive uropathy, obstructive disease of the GI tract, asthma, chronic pulmonary disease, myasthenia gravis, paralytic ileus, intestinal atony, unstable CV status in acute hemorrhage, or toxic megacolon.
• Use cautiously in patients with autonomic neuropathy, hyperthyroidism, coronary artery disease, cardiac arrhythmias, CHF, hypertension, hiatal hernia associated with reflux esophagitis, hepatic or renal disease, and ulcerative colitis; in patients over age 40 because of the increased incidence of glaucoma; and in children under age 6.
• Use cautiously in hot or humid environments. Drug-induced heatstroke is possible.

SELF-TEST

1. Evelyn Freeman, a 20-year-old college student, was admitted to the emergency department with periumbilical pain. She was diagnosed with acute appendicitis and scheduled for an emergency appendectomy. Preoperative medication orders included atropine 0.4 mg I.M. The nurse understands that atropine is indicated preoperatively to:
   a. improve cardiac contractions.
   b. depress the cerebral cortex.
   c. diminish respiratory secretions.
   d. stimulate vagal responses.

2. When administering atropine and other cholinergic blockers, the nurse must know that these drugs are contraindicated or must be used cautiously in all of the following conditions except:
   a. narrow-angle glaucoma.
   b. myasthenia gravis.
   c. Down's syndrome.
   d. bradycardia.

3. Don Ellis is receiving atropine 0.4 mg P.O. q 4 hours as part of his treatment for irritable bowel syndrome. He complains of dry mouth and constipation. How should his nurse explain these symptoms?
   a. These symptoms are an extension of the drug's pharmacologic action and may be expected.
   b. These symptoms have nothing to do with present drug therapy and should be further investigated.
   c. These symptoms suggest overdose of atropine, and the doctor will probably reduce the dosage.
   d. These symptoms are serious adverse reactions, and the drug should be discontinued immediately.

Check your answers on page 1066.

CHAPTER 38

ADRENERGICS

albuterol ✦ albuterol sulfate ✦ bitolterol mesylate
dobutamine hydrochloride ✦ dopamine hydrochloride ✦ ephedrine sulfate
epinephrine ✦ epinephrine bitartrate ✦ epinephrine hydrochloride
ethylnorepinephrine hydrochloride ✦ isoetharine hydrochloride 1%
isoetharine mesylate ✦ isoproterenol hydrochloride ✦ isoproterenol sulfate
mephentermine sulfate ✦ metaproterenol sulfate ✦ metaraminol bitartrate
norepinephrine bitartrate injection (formerly levarterenol bitartrate)
phenylephrine bitartrate ✦ phenylephrine hydrochloride
phenylpropanolamine hydrochloride ✦ pseudoephedrine hydrochloride
pseudoephedrine sulfate ✦ terbutaline sulfate

OVERVIEW

- Adrenergics (also called sympathomimetics) produce their effect by either mimicking the actions of dopamine, epinephrine, or norepinephrine at receptor sites in the sympathetic nervous system or by displacing natural norepinephrine from neural storage sites. Because these drugs do not stimulate all types of adrenergic receptors equally, their effects and indications for use differ.
- The actions of adrenergics are not organ- or site-specific and may occur at other than the desired sites.
- The sympathetic nervous system innervates numerous organs (for example, the heart, blood vessels, respiratory tract, liver, urinary bladder, and intestines) and significantly affects the regulation of many body functions. When stimulated, sympathetic nerves release norepinephrine (except for sympathetic nerves that innervate sweat glands, which release acetylcholine). Norepinephrine combines with receptor sites on the innervated organ to elicit a response.
- The three major types of receptors within the sympathetic system are alpha, beta, and dopaminergic. Stimulation of alpha receptors causes vasoconstriction and uterine and sphincter contraction. Beta receptors are divided into two subgroups: beta$_1$ and beta$_2$. Beta$_1$ receptors are largely in the heart; when stimulated, they increase the rate and force of MI and the rate of AV node conduction. Beta$_2$ receptors are primarily in the bronchi, blood vessels, and uterus; stimulation produces bronchodila-

GLOSSARY

Adrenergic: activated or transmitted by epinephrine, norepinephrine, or a similar substance.

Alpha-adrenergic receptor: adrenergic receptor of the sympathetic nervous system that responds to norepinephrine and various blocking agents.

Beta-adrenergic receptor: adrenergic receptor of the sympathetic nervous system that responds to epinephrine and various blocking agents.

Catecholamine: class of sympathomimetic neuroregulators that includes dobutamine, dopamine, isoproterenol, norepinephrine, and epinephrine.

Catechol-O-methyl transferase: enzyme diffusely present in all tissues that breaks down catecholamines.

Sympathetic nervous system: adrenergic division of the autonomic nervous system.

Sympathomimetic: agent that produces effects similar to those of impulses conveyed by the adrenergic postganglionic fibers of the sympathetic nervous system.

lation produces bronchodilation, vasodilation, and uterine relaxation, respectively. Dopaminergic receptors are primarily in splanchnic blood vessels; stimulation dilates these vessels.

- The adrenal medulla is a major part of the sympathetic nervous system. During times of danger or acute stress, the sympathetic nervous system can activate the adrenal medulla to release epinephrine into the systemic circulation. Epinephrine activates alpha and beta receptors, ultimately producing physiologic and metabolic effects that prepare the person to cope with the stress (as in the fight-or-flight response).

MAJOR USES

- Dobutamine, dopamine, mephentermine, metaraminol, and norepinephrine raise blood pressure and cardiac output in severely decompensated states, such as cardiogenic shock and heart failure.
- Albuterol, bitolterol, ephedrine, ethylnorepinephrine, isoetharine, isoproterenol, metaproterenol, and terbutaline relieve bronchoconstriction.
- Epinephrine and isoproterenol are used to treat heart block and certain arrhythmias and to restore cardiac rhythm in cardiac arrest.
- Epinephrine and phenylephrine are used to treat anaphylaxis and other allergic reactions.
- Pseudoephedrine and phenylpropanolamine are nasal decongestants; additionally, phenylpropanolamine is used in weight-control aids.

MECHANISM OF ACTION

• Adrenergics stimulate or increase the effect of epinephrine and norepinephrine on alpha- and beta-adrenergic receptors within the sympathetic
nervous system. Effects vary and include bronchodilation, release of
glucose from the liver, increase in heart rate and ventricular contractility,
CNS excitation, dilation (beta effect) of blood vessels in skeletal muscles, and constriction (alpha effect) of blood vessels in cutaneous areas.

ABSORPTION, DISTRIBUTION, METABOLISM, AND EXCRETION

After oral inhalation, albuterol and bitolterol are metabolized in the liver
and excreted primarily by the kidneys.

Dobutamine and dopamine are not absorbed from the GI tract and must
be given parenterally. They're metabolized by the liver to inactive compounds and excreted in urine.

Ephedrine is rapidly absorbed after oral, I.M., or S.C. administration.
Some of the drug is metabolized by the liver; both unchanged compound
and metabolites are excreted in the urine.

Epinephrine and ethylnorepinephrine are not well absorbed from the GI
tract after oral administration. Absorption is efficient, however, after I.M.
or S.C. injection. The drugs are extensively metabolized in the liver and
excreted in the urine.

Isoetharine is rapidly absorbed from the respiratory tract after inhalation. It is partly metabolized by enzymes in the lungs and other tissues.
Both the parent compound and metabolite are excreted in the urine.

Isoproterenol is irregularly absorbed after oral or S.L. administration
but is well absorbed following parenteral administration or oral inhalation.
It is metabolized in the liver and other tissues and excreted in the urine.

Mephentermine is not absorbed from the GI tract and must be given
parenterally. It is metabolized in the liver and excreted in the urine;
excretion is increased in an acidic urine.

Metaproterenol, well absorbed after oral administration, is subject to the
first-pass effect. Conjugates of the parent compound are excreted in the
urine.

Metaraminol is erratically absorbed from the GI tract after being given
orally; therefore, it must be given parenterally. Distribution, metabolism,
and route of excretion are not completely known. Its pharmacologic effects
are stopped by its uptake into body tissues.

Norepinephrine is not absorbed after oral administration and is poorly
absorbed after S.C. injection. The drug is taken up by nerve endings where
it is metabolized; it is also metabolized by the liver and other tissues.
Metabolites are excreted in urine.

Effective when administered orally, pseudoephedrine, phenylephrine,
and phenylpropanolamine are metabolized by the liver. The metabolites
are excreted in the urine. Excretion increases in an acidic urine.

Terbutaline is partially absorbed after oral administration but is well absorbed subcutaneously. It is eliminated in the urine and feces in both metabolized and unchanged forms.

ONSET AND DURATION

Comparing Adrenergic Action summarizes the onset and duration of adrenergics.

ADVERSE REACTIONS

The type and severity of the adverse reactions to adrenergics depend on the medication's specificity for the type of receptor stimulated. Medications that stimulate the alpha receptors predominantly, such as phenylephrine, produce adverse reactions related to alpha stimulation. These reactions include severe peripheral and visceral vasoconstriction, with reduced blood flow to vital organs; decreased renal perfusion; tissue hypoxia; and metabolic acidosis. Bradycardia and decreased cardiac output may also occur. Adverse CNS reactions include restlessness, anxiety, nervousness, weakness, and dizziness. Tremor, respiratory distress, and pallor or blanching of the skin are also adverse reactions related to alpha stimulation.

An adrenergic that produces predominantly beta stimulation, such as isoproterenol, has adverse reactions related to beta stimulation, which are usually cardiovascular in nature. These reactions include tachycardia, cardiac arrhythmias, and precipitation of anginal pain. The beta adrenergics may also produce nervousness, restlessness, insomnia, anxiety, tension, fear, or excitement.

COMPARING ADRENERGIC ACTION

DRUG	ROUTE	ONSET	DURATION
albuterol	inhalation	within 15 minutes; peaks in 1 hour	3 to 4 hours
	P.O.	within 30 minutes	4 to 6 hours
bitolterol	inhalation	3 to 5 minutes; peaks in 30 minutes to 2 hours	4 to 8 hours
dobutamine	I.V.	within 2 minutes	until shortly after end of infusion
dopamine	I.V.	within 5 minutes	less than 10 minutes, or as long as infusion continues

(continued)

COMPARING ADRENERGIC ACTION *continued*

DRUG	ROUTE	ONSET	DURATION
ephedrine	P.O.	less than 1 hour	4 to 12 hours, depending on form of P.O. dosage
epinephrine	I.M. S.C.	3 to 5 minutes	20 to 30 minutes
ethylnorepinephrine	I.M.	3 to 5 minutes	20 to 30 minutes
isoetharine	inhalation	rapid; peaks in 5 to 15 minutes	1 to 4 hours
isoproterenol	I.V	immediate	during infusion
	P.O.	20 minutes	1 hour
mephentermine	I.M.	5 to 15 minutes	1 to 4 hours
	I.V.	immediate	15 to 30 minutes after injection
metaproterenol	inhalation	1 minute; peaks in 1 hour	up to 4 hours
	P.O.	15 minutes; peaks in 1 hour	up to 4 hours
metaraminol	I.M.	within 10 minutes	1 hour
	I.V.	1 to 2 minutes	5 to 15 minutes
	S.C.	5 to 20 minutes	1 hour
norepinephrine	I.V.	immediate	until shortly after end of infusion
phenylephrine	inhalation	2 to 3 minutes	3 hours
	I.M.	10 to 15 minutes	30 minutes to 2 hours
	I.V.	immediate	15 to 20 minutes
	S.C.	10 to 15 minutes	1 hour
phenylpropanolamine	P.O.	15 to 30 minutes	3 hours

DOPAMINE HYDROCHLORIDE
(doe′pa meen)
Intropin, Revimine†‡
Classification: adrenergic
Pregnancy risk category C

How supplied
INJECTION: 40 mg/ml, 80 mg/ml, 160 mg/ml parenteral concentrate for injection for I.V. infusion; 0.8 mg/ml (200 or 400 mg) in dextrose 5%; 1.6 mg/ml (400 or 800 mg) in dextrose 5%; 3.2 mg/ml (800 mg) in dextrose 5% parenteral injection for I.V. infusion.

Indications and dosage
To treat shock and correct hemodynamic imbalances; to improve perfusion to vital organs; to increase cardiac output; to correct hypotension; to treat acute renal failure
ADULTS: 2 to 5 mcg/kg/minute I.V. infusion, up to 50 mcg/kg/minute. Titrate the dosage to the desired hemodynamic and/or renal response.

Contraindications and precautions
Dopamine is contraindicated in uncorrected tachyarrhythmias, pheochromocytoma, or ventricular fibrillation. Use cautiously in patients with occlusive vascular disease, cold injuries, diabetic endarteritis, and arterial embolism; in pregnant patients; and in those taking MAO inhibitors.

Adverse reactions
CNS: headache.
CV: ectopic beats, tachycardia, anginal pain, palpitations, *hypotension.* Less frequently, bradycardia, widening of QRS complex, **conduction disturbances**, vasoconstriction.
GI: nausea, vomiting.
LOCAL: necrosis and tissue sloughing with extravasation.
OTHER: piloerection, dyspnea.

Interactions
Beta blockers: may antagonize dopamine's effects. Notify the doctor.
Ergot alkaloids: extreme elevations in blood pressure. Don't use together.
MAO inhibitors: may cause hypertensive crisis. Avoid if possible.
Phenytoin: may lower blood pressure of dopamine-stabilized patients. Monitor carefully.

Nursing considerations
Assessment
• Review the patient's history for a condition that contraindicates the use of dopamine.

• Obtain a baseline assessment of the patient's underlying condition before initiating dopamine therapy.
• Be alert for common adverse reactions.
• Evaluate the patient's and family's knowledge about dopamine therapy.

Planning (Nursing Diagnoses)
Potential nursing diagnoses for the patient receiving dopamine include:
• Potential for injury related to ineffectiveness of dopamine therapy.
• Altered tissue perfusion (cerebral, cardiopulmonary, and renal) related to dopamine-induced hypotension.
• Impaired tissue integrity related to necrosis and tissue sloughing with extravasation.
• Knowledge deficit related to dopamine therapy.

Implementation
Preparation and administration
—Use large vein, as in the antecubital fossa, to minimize risk of extravasation.
—Don't mix with alkaline solutions. Use dextrose 5% in water (D_5W), 0.9% sodium chloride solution, or combination of D_5W and 0.9% sodium chloride solution. Mix just before use.
—Dopamine solutions deteriorate after 24 hours. Discard at that time or earlier if solution is discolored.
—Do not mix other drugs in I.V. container with dopamine.
—Do not give alkaline drugs (for example, sodium bicarbonate, phenytoin sodium) through I.V. line containing dopamine.
—Use a continuous infusion pump to regulate flow rate.
—Be aware that dopamine is not a substitute for blood or fluid volume deficit. Volume deficit should be corrected before vasopressors such as dopamine are administered.
—Be aware that the patient's response depends on dosage and pharmacologic effect. Dosage of 0.5 to 2 mcg/kg/minute predominantly stimulates dopamine receptors and produces vasodilation. Dosage of 2 to 10 mcg/kg/minute stimulates beta-adrenergic receptors. Higher dosage also stimulates alpha-adrenergic receptors. Most patients are satisfactorily maintained on less than 20 mcg/kg/minute.

Monitoring
—During infusion, monitor the effectiveness of therapy by frequently checking blood pressure, cardiac output, pulse rate, urine output, and color and temperature of extremities.
—Monitor the patient for adverse drug reactions.
—Carefully observe I.V. site for signs of extravasation.
—Monitor ECG for arrhythmias.
—Monitor hydration status if nausea and vomiting occur.
—Monitor the patient for drug interactions.

Intervention
—Titrate infusion rate according to assessment findings, using doctor's guidelines.

—If the patient develops a disproportionate rise in the diastolic pressure (a marked decrease in pulse pressure), decrease infusion rate and observe carefully for further evidence of predominant vasoconstrictor activity, unless such an effect is desired.

—If doses exceed 50 mcg/kg/minute, check urine output often. If urine flow decreases without hypotension, consider reducing dose.

—Be aware that acidosis decreases effectiveness of dopamine.

—If extravasation occurs, stop infusion immediately and call the doctor for instructions; doctor may order infiltration of the area with 5 to 10 mg phentolamine and 10 to 15 ml 0.9% sodium chloride solution to counteract this effect.

—Adverse reactions may require dosage adjustment or discontinuation of the drug.

—Keep all members of the health care team informed of the patient's response to the drug.

Patient teaching

—Instruct the patient (if mentally alert) and family about dopamine, including how it will be administered, the action, and the adverse reactions.

—Emphasize the importance of reporting discomfort at I.V. site immediately.

—Tell the patient to notify the nurse or doctor if adverse reactions develop or questions arise about dopamine therapy.

Evaluation

In the patient receiving dopamine, appropriate evaluation statements include:

• Patient's hemodynamic imbalance is corrected and condition is stabilizing.

• Cerebral, cardiopulmonary, and renal tissue perfusion remains adequate.

• Extravasation does not occur at I.V. site.

• Patient and family state an understanding of dopamine therapy.

SELECTED MAJOR DRUGS: ADRENERGICS

DRUG, INDICATIONS, AND DOSAGES	SPECIAL PRECAUTIONS

albuterol (Proventil, Ventolin)
Prevention and treatment of bronchospasm in patients with reversible obstructive airway disease—
Adults and children over age 13: 1 to 2 inhalations q 4 to 6 hours. More frequent administration or a greater number of inhalations is not recommended. Usual dosage range is 10 to 50 mcg/minute. Or 2 to 4 mg (tablets) P.O. t.i.d. or q.i.d. Maximum dosage is 8 mg q.i.d. Or 4 to 8 mg (sustained-release tablets) P.O. q 12 hours. Maximum dosage is 16 mg b.i.d.
Children ages 6 to 13: 2 mg (1 teaspoonful) P.O. t.i.d. or q.i.d.
Children ages 2 to 5: 0.1 mg/kg P.O. t.i.d., not to exceed 2 mg (1 teaspoonful) t.i.d.
Adults over age 65: 2 mg P.O. t.i.d. or q.i.d.
To prevent exercise-induced asthma—
Adults: 2 inhalations 15 minutes before exercise.
Prevention of premature labor‡—
Adults: initially, 10 mcg/minute by continuous I.V. infusion (use an infusion pump). Dosage should be increased in 10-minute intervals until the desired response is achieved.

• Contraindicated in patients with a history of hypersensitivity to any of the drug's components.
• Use cautiously in CV disorders, including coronary insufficiency and hypertension; in hyperthyroidism or diabetes mellitus; and in patients who are unusually responsive to adrenergics.

dobutamine (Dobutrex)
Refractory heart failure and as adjunct in cardiac surgery—
Adults: 2.5 to 10 mcg/kg/minute as an I.V. infusion. Rarely, infusion rates up to 40 mcg/kg/minute may be needed.

• Contraindicated in idiopathic hypertrophic subaortic stenosis.
• Administer cautiously to patients after acute MI, to pregnant patients, and with drugs likely to cause interactions.

ephedrine (Ephed II)
To correct hypotensive states; to support ventricular rate in Adams-Stokes syndrome—
Adults: 25 to 50 mg I.M. or S.C., or 10 to 25 mg I.V. p.r.n. to maximum of 150 mg daily.
Children: 3 mg/kg S.C. or I.V. daily in four to six divided doses.
Bronchodilator or nasal decongestant—
Adults: 12.5 to 50 mg P.O. b.i.d., t.i.d., or q.i.d. Maximum dosage is 400 mg daily in six to eight divided doses.
Children: 2 to 3 mg/kg P.O. daily in four to six divided doses.

• Contraindicated in porphyria, severe coronary artery disease, cardiac arrhythmias, narrow-angle glaucoma, or psychoneurosis and in patients taking MAO inhibitors.
• Use cautiously in elderly patients and in those with hypertension, hyperthyroidism, nervous or excitable states, CV disease, and prostatic hypertrophy.

epinephrine (Adrenalin, Bronkaid Mist ◇, Primatene Mist ◇, Sus-Phrine)
Bronchospasm, hypersensitivity reactions, anaphylaxis—
Adults: 0.1 to 0.5 ml of 1:1,000 S.C. or I.M. Repeat q 10 to 15 minutes p.r.n. Or 0.1 to 0.25 ml of 1:1,000 I.V.
Children: 0.01 ml (10 mcg) of 1:1,000/kg S.C. Repeat q 20 minutes to 4 hours p.r.n.; 0.005 ml/kg of 1:200 (Sus-Phrine). Repeat q 8 to 12 hours p.r.n.

• Contraindicated in narrow-angle glaucoma, shock (other than anaphylactic shock), organic brain damage, cardiac dilation, or coronary insufficiency. Also contraindicated during general anesthesia with halogenated hydrocarbons or cyclopropane

SELECTED MAJOR DRUGS: ADRENERGICS *(continued)*

DRUG, INDICATIONS, AND DOSAGES

epinephrine *(continued)*
Hemostasis—
Adults: 1:50,000 to 1:1,000, applied topically.
Acute asthmatic attacks (inhalation)—
Adults and children: 1 or 2 inhalations of 1:100 or 2.25% racemic q 1 to 5 minutes until relief is obtained; 0.2 mg/dose usual content.
To prolong local anesthetic effect—
Adults and children: 0.2 to 0.4 ml of 1:1,000 intraspinal; 1:500,000 to 1:50,000 local mixed with local anesthetic.
To restore cardiac rhythm in cardiac arrest—
Adults: 0.5 to 1 mg I.V. or into endotracheal tube. May be given intracardiac if no I.V. or intratracheal route available. Some clinicians advocate higher dose (up to 5 mg), especially in patients who don't respond to usual I.V. dose. After initial I.V. administration, may be infused I.V. at a rate of 1 to 4 mcg/minute.
Children: 10 mcg/kg I.V. or 5 to 10 mcg (0.05 to 0.1 ml of 1:10,000)/kg intracardiac.
  Note: 1 mg = 1 ml of 1:1,000 or 10 ml of 1:10,000.

isoproterenol (Aerolone, Isuprel)
Bronchial asthma and reversible bronchospasm—
Adults: 10 to 20 mg (hydrochloride) S.L. q 6 to 8 hours.
Children: 5 to 10 mg (hydrochloride) S.L. q 6 to 8 hours. Not recommended for children under age 6.
Bronchospasm—
Adults and children: (sulfate) acute dyspneic episodes— 1 inhalation initially. May repeat if needed after 2 to 5 minutes.
  Maintenance dosage is 1 to 2 inhalations q.i.d. to six times daily. May repeat once more 10 minutes after second dose. Not more than three doses should be administered for each attack.
Heart block and ventricular arrhythmias—
Adults: initially, 0.02 to 0.06 mg (hydrochloride) I.V. Subsequent doses 0.01 to 0.2 mg I.V. or 5 mcg/minute I.V.; or 0.2 mg I.M. initially, then 0.02 to 1 mg p.r.n.
Children: (hydrochloride) may give half of initial adult dose.
Shock—
Adults and children: 0.5 to 5 mcg/minute (hydrochloride) by continuous I.V. infusion. Usual concentration is 1 mg (5 ml) in 500 ml dextrose 5% in water. Adjust rate according to heart rate, central venous pressure, blood pressure, and urine flow.

SPECIAL PRECAUTIONS

and in labor (may delay second stage).
• Use with extreme caution in patients with long-standing bronchial asthma and emphysema who have developed degenerative heart disease.
• Use cautiously in elderly patients and in those with hyperthyroidism, angina, hypertension, psychoneurosis, and diabetes.

• Contraindicated in tachycardia caused by digitalis intoxication and in preexisting arrhythmias, especially tachycardia, because chronotropic effect on the heart may aggravate such disorders. Also contraindicated in recent MI.
• Use cautiously in coronary insufficiency, diabetes, or hyperthyroidism.

(continued)

SELECTED MAJOR DRUGS: ADRENERGICS *continued*

DRUG, INDICATIONS, AND DOSAGES	SPECIAL PRECAUTIONS

norepinephrine (Levophed)
To restore blood pressure in acute hypotensive states—
Adults: initially, 8 to 12 mcg/minute I.V. infusion, then adjust to maintain normal blood pressure. Average maintenance dosage is 2 to 4 mcg/minute.

• Contraindicated in mesenteric or peripheral vascular thrombosis, pregnancy, profound hypoxia, hypercapnea, and hypotension from blood volume deficits and during cyclopropane and halothane anesthesia.
• Use cautiously in hypertension, hyperthyroidism, severe cardiac disease, and sulfite sensitivity.
• Use with extreme caution in patients taking MAO inhibitors or tricyclic antidepressants (TCAs).

phenylephrine (Neo-Synephrine)
Hypotensive emergencies during spinal anesthesia—
Adults: initially, 0.2 mg I.V., then subsequent doses of 0.1 to 0.2 mg.
Maintenance of blood pressure during spinal or inhalation anesthesia—
Adults: 2 to 3 mg S.C. or I.M. 3 or 4 minutes before anesthesia.
Children: 0.04 to 0.088 mg/kg S.C. or I.M.
Mild to moderate hypotension—
Adults: 2 to 5 mg S.C. or I.M.; 0.1 to 0.5 mg I.V. Not to be repeated more often than 10 to 15 minutes.
Paroxysmal supraventricular tachycardia—
Adults: initially, 0.5 mg rapid I.V.; subsequent doses should not exceed the preceding dose by more than 0.1 to 0.2 mg and should not exceed 1 mg.
Prolongation of spinal anesthesia—
Adults: 2 to 5 mg added to anesthetic solution.
Severe hypotension and shock (including drug-induced)—
Adults: 10 mg in 500 ml dextrose 5% in water. Start 100 to 180 drops/minute I.V. infusion, then 40 to 60 drops/minute. Adjust to patient response.
Vasoconstrictor for regional anesthesia—
Adults: 1 mg added to 20 ml local anesthetic.

• Contraindicated in narrow-angle glaucoma, hypotension, ventricular tachycardia, severe coronary disease, or CV disease (including MI) and in patients taking MAO inhibitors or TCAs.
• Use with extreme caution in patients with heart disease, hyperthyroidism, diabetes, severe atherosclerosis, bradycardia, partial heart block, myocardial disease, or sulfite sensitivity and in elderly patients.

pseudoephedrine (Sudafed ◇)
Nasal and eustachian tube decongestant—
Adults: 60 mg P.O. q 4 hours. Maximum dosage is 240 mg daily.
Children ages 6 to 12: 30 mg P.O. q 4 hours. Maximum dosage is 120 mg daily.
Children ages 2 to 6: 15 mg P.O. q 4 hours. Maximum dosage is 60 mg daily.

• Contraindicated in severe hypertension or severe coronary artery disease, in patients taking MAO inhibitors, and in breast-feeding women.
• Administer cautiously to patients with hypertension, cardiac disease, diabetes, glaucoma, hy-

◇ Available OTC

SELECTED MAJOR DRUGS: ADRENERGICS *continued*

DRUG, INDICATIONS, AND DOSAGES	SPECIAL PRECAUTIONS
pseudoephedrine *(continued)* **Adults and children over age 12**: 60 to 120 mg (extended-release tablets) P.O. q 12 hours. This form is contraindicated for children under age 12. *Relief of nasal congestion—* **Adults**: 120 mg q 12 hours.	perthyroidism, and prostatic hypertrophy.
terbutaline (Brethine) *Relief of bronchospasm in patients with reversible obstructive airway disease—* **Adults and children over age 11**: 2 inhalations separated by a 60-second interval, repeated q 4 to 6 hours. May also administer 2.5 to 5 mg P.O. q 8 hours or 0.25 mg S.C. *Treatment of premature labor—* **Women**: 0.01 mg/minute by I.V. infusion. Increase by 0.005 mg q 10 minutes up to 0.025 mg/minute or until contractions cease. Or give 0.25 mg S.C. hourly until contractions cease. Maintenance dosage is 5 mg P.O. q 4 hours for 48 hours, then 5 mg q 6 hours.	• Contraindicated in patients with known hypersensitivity to sympathomimetic amines or any component of this drug. • Use cautiously in patients with diabetes, hypertension, hyperthyroidism, severe cardiac disease, and cardiac arrhythmias.

SELF-TEST

1. After a massive MI, Paul Roberts' blood pressure dropped to 80/40 mm Hg, pulse rate increased to 130 beats/minute, and skin became cool and moist. The doctor diagnosed cardiogenic shock and started Mr. Roberts on dopamine 10 mcg/kg/minute. The nurse realizes that dopamine at this rate of dosage will:
   a. stimulate dopamine receptors and produce vasodilation only.
   b. stimulate beta-adrenergic receptors and produce increased rate and force of myocardial contraction.
   c. stimulate alpha-adrenergic receptors and produce vasoconstriction.
   d. block beta-adrenergic responses and produce bronchodilation.

2. When assessing Mr. Roberts, the nurse should make all but which *one* of the following observations?
   a. Vital signs every 5 to 15 minutes
   b. Intake and output
   c. Color and temperature of extremities
   d. Bowel sounds every 4 hours

3. The nurse should be aware that, if Mr. Roberts complains of pain at the site of infusion, she should discontinue the infusion and:
   a. apply cold compresses to the area.
   b. be prepared to infiltrate infusion site with 0.9% sodium chloride solution and phentolamine.
   c. infiltrate infusion site with lactated Ringer's solution and sodium bicarbonate.
   d. apply warm moist compresses to the area.

Check your answers on pages 1066 and 1067.

CHAPTER 39

ADRENERGIC BLOCKERS

Rauwolfia alkaloids
deserpidine ◆ reserpine

Miscellaneous agents
guanethidine monosulfate ◆ guanadrel sulfate

OVERVIEW

- Adrenergic blockers (also called sympatholytics) inhibit the effects of postganglionic sympathetic nerves. Unlike adrenergic receptor blockers (alpha-adrenergic blockers and beta-adrenergic blockers), these drugs do not rely on receptors to achieve their antagonism. Instead, they act directly on the postganglionic nerve endings to reduce the amount of norepinephrine released by each nerve impulse.
- Reserpine, the prototype drug of this class, was first used in the mid-1950s for the treatment of hypertension. An extract of *Rauwolfia serpentina*, a climbing shrub native to India, reserpine is one of the pure alkaloids that can be obtained from the plant. The other purified alkaloid, deserpidine, and the powdered dried root are also commercially available. These agents bind to and gradually destroy the storage vesicles that contain norepinephrine. Therefore, when a sympathetic nerve impulse reaches the nerve ending, less norepinephrine is available to interact with postsynaptic receptors.
- The actions of guanethidine and guanadrel are similar to reserpine; however, these drugs do not enter the CNS. Apparently, the ability to enter the CNS is responsible for some of reserpine's beneficial as well as adverse effects.
- The adrenergic blockers are classified primarily into rauwolfia alkaloids and miscellaneous agents.

MAJOR USES

- Rauwolfia alkaloids, guanethidine, and guanadrel are all used in the treatment of hypertension. Because of the adverse reactions associated with these drugs, they are generally reserved for use only in patients who are unresponsive to other drugs. These agents would not be used as one of the initial steps in the stepped care approach to hypertension.

GLOSSARY

Sympatholytic: agent that opposes the impulses conveyed by the adrenergic postganglionic fibers of the sympathetic nervous system.

MECHANISM OF ACTION

- The rauwolfia alkaloids, deserpidine and reserpine, bind to and gradually destroy the storage vesicles in central and peripheral adrenergic neurons, which contain norepinephrine. The liberated neurotransmitter is metabolized by intraneuronal MAO. Gradually, nerve endings lose their capacity to store and release norepinephrine, serotonin, and dopamine. This process is reversible; however, full recovery of sympathetic function may take days to weeks.
- Guanethidine acts only in peripheral adrenergic neurons. It is taken up by the endings of sympathetic nerves and carried to its site of action by an active transport process. It binds to synaptic storage vesicles and initially may cause a release of norepinephrine (especially after I.V. administration). This initial release may not always occur; it is not usually evident after oral administration. The drug produces sympathetic blockage by preventing the release of norepinephrine after a nerve impulse. Gradually, the neuron loses the ability to store norepinephrine within these vesicles.
- The action of guanadrel is similar to guanethidine, but the two drugs differ in their pharmacokinetics.

ABSORPTION, DISTRIBUTION, METABOLISM, AND EXCRETION

Limited data are available about the pharmacokinetics of deserpidine and reserpine. These drugs and their metabolites are present only in very low concentrations in the serum. Serum levels probably have little impact on their antihypertensive effect because they bind tightly and irreversibly to synaptic storage vesicles. Rauwolfia alkaloids are entirely metabolized.

Absorption of guanethidine is highly variable (3% to 50% of a dose is absorbed). It is rapidly transported to its site of action within sympathetic neurons. About 50% of the drug is eliminated unchanged. Its long elimination half-life (about 5 days) permits once-daily dosing.

Guanadrel is better absorbed (about 85%) and has a short elimination half-life (about 10 hours).

ONSET AND DURATION

The onset and duration of these drugs' effects are not related to either blood or brain levels. Full therapeutic effects do not occur for at least 2 to 3 weeks after daily administration of the drug; the antihypertensive effects persist for days to weeks after the last dose.

Reportedly, after I.M. administration reserpine exerts a hypotensive effect within 2 hours that peaks in 2 to 6 hours. However, parenteral reserpine is no longer commercially available in the United States.

Unlike that produced by the rauwolfia alkaloids, the adrenergic blockade caused by guanethidine is proportional to the plasma concentrations of the drug. The full antihypertensive effect is delayed for 1 to 3 weeks after initiating therapy; after discontinuation of the drug, blood pressure persists at its lowest level for 3 to 4 days and then gradually returns to pretreatment levels over 1 to 3 weeks.

The hypotensive effects of guanadrel have an onset of 30 minutes to 2 hours and peak in 4 to 6 hours. Guanadrel is the shortest acting of these drugs; its effects persist for only 12 to 14 hours.

ADVERSE REACTIONS

All of these drugs can cause CV reactions that are an extension of their pharmacologic effects, commonly, hypotension, orthostatic hypotension, bradycardia, or arrhythmias. Orthostatic hypotension can be worsened by a hot environment. Other adverse reactions include headache, impaired ejaculation, and nasal congestion.

Rauwolfia alkaloids commonly cause drowsiness, fatigue, lethargy, abdominal cramps, nausea, vomiting, and diarrhea. One of the most serious reactions is mental depression, which can lead to hospitalization or suicide. Depression can occur in anyone who takes a rauwolfia alkaloid but seems to occur more often in patients with a history of depression and in those taking relatively high doses (such as 0.25 mg of reserpine daily). Depressive reactions usually develop after 2 to 8 months of therapy.

Guanethidine and guanadrel can cause dizziness, weakness, lassitude, and orthostatic hypotension. Because their effects result in unopposed parasympathetic activity in the GI tract, they may cause frequent bowel movements or explosive diarrhea.

Reportedly, guanethidine has reduced blood glucose levels in patients with diabetes mellitus.

PROTOTYPE: RAUWOLFIA ALKALOIDS

RESERPINE
(re ser′ peen)
Novoreserpine†, Serpalan, Serpasil*
Classification: rauwolfia alkaloid
Pregnancy risk category C

How supplied
TABLETS: 0.1 mg, 0.25 mg, 1 mg

Indications and dosage
Mild to moderate essential hypertension
ADULTS: 0.1 to 0.25 mg P.O. daily.

---

*Liquid form contains alcohol   †Available in Canada only

CHILDREN: 5 to 20 mcg/kg P.O. daily.

Contraindications and precautions

Reserpine is contraindicated in depression. Use cautiously in severe cardiac or cerebrovascular disease, history of seizures, peptic ulcer, ulcerative colitis, gallstones, or mental depressive disorders; in patients undergoing surgery; and in those taking other antihypertensive drugs.

Adverse reactions

CNS: mental confusion, *depression, drowsiness, nervousness, paradoxical anxiety, nightmares*, extrapyramidal symptoms, sedation.
CV: *orthostatic hypotension*, bradycardia, syncope.
EENT: *dry mouth, nasal stuffiness*, glaucoma.
GI: *hyperacidity, nausea, vomiting*, GI bleeding.
SKIN: pruritus, rash.
OTHER: *impotence, weight gain.*

Interactions

MAO inhibitors: may cause excitability and hypertension. Use together cautiously.

Nursing considerations

Assessment

• Review the patient's history for a condition that contraindicates the use of reserpine.
• Obtain a baseline assessment of the patient's blood pressure before initiating reserpine therapy.
• Be alert for common adverse reactions.
• Evaluate the patient's and family's knowledge about reserpine therapy.

Planning (Nursing Diagnoses)

Potential nursing diagnoses for the patient receiving reserpine include:
• Potential for injury related to ineffectiveness of reserpine to lower blood pressure.
• Altered thought processes related to reserpine-induced CNS reactions.
• Knowledge deficit related to reserpine therapy.

Implementation

Preparation and administration
— Administer with meals.

Monitoring
— Monitor the effectiveness of therapy by regularly assessing blood pressure.
— Monitor heart rate regularly for bradycardia.
— Monitor behavior and mental status for evidence of CNS changes, especially depression.
— Monitor the patient for adverse drug reactions.
— Monitor weight and assess for signs of fluid retention (ankle swelling, distended neck veins).
— Monitor the patient for drug interactions.

Italicized adverse reactions are common

— Regularly reevaluate the patient's and family's knowledge about reserpine.

Intervention

— Hold dose and notify the doctor if the patient develops signs of depression, inability to concentrate, anorexia, or detached attitude.
— Hold dose and notify the doctor if the patient develops hypotension or bradycardia.
— Institute safety precautions if adverse CNS reactions occur.
— Assist the patient to a standing position slowly to minimize orthostatic hypotension.
— Provide ice chips or sugarless gum or hard candy to relieve dry mouth.
— Keep all members of the health care team informed of the patient's response to the drug.

Patient teaching

— Instruct the patient and family about reserpine, including the dosage, frequency, action, and adverse reactions.
— Teach the patient about his disease.
— Explain the importance of taking this drug as prescribed even when feeling well.
— Tell the patient not to discontinue this drug suddenly.
— Instruct the patient to check with the doctor or pharmacist before taking any OTC medications.
— Warn the patient that this drug can cause drowsiness. Tell him to avoid hazardous activities that require alertness and coordination until CNS effects of the drug are known.
— Warn the female patient to notify the doctor if she suspects pregnancy.
— Inform the patient that orthostatic hypotension can be minimized by rising slowly and avoiding sudden position changes.
— Instruct the patient that dry mouth can be relieved with sugarless chewing gum or hard candy or ice chips.
— Instruct the patient to contact the doctor if nasal stuffiness is troublesome.
— Instruct the patient to weigh himself daily and notify the doctor if he gains 2 lb in 2 days or observes ankle swelling.
— Advise the patient to have periodic eye examinations because drug can cause glaucoma.
— Warn the male patient that drug may cause impotence.
— Tell the patient to notify the nurse or doctor if adverse reactions develop or questions arise about reserpine therapy.

Evaluation

In the patient receiving reserpine, appropriate evaluation statements include:
• Patient's blood pressure is within normal limits.
• Patient does not display altered thought processes.
• Patient and family state an understanding of reserpine therapy.

GUANETHIDINE MONOSULFATE
(gwahn eth' i deen)
Apo-Guanethidine†, Ismelin
Classification: miscellaneous adrenergic blocker
Pregnancy risk category C

How supplied
TABLETS: 10 mg, 25 mg

Indications and dosage
For moderate to severe hypertension; usually used in combination with other antihypertensives
ADULTS: initially, 10 mg P.O. daily. Increase by 10 mg at weekly to monthly intervals p.r.n. Usual dose is 25 to 50 mg daily. Some patients may require up to 300 mg.
CHILDREN: initially, 200 mcg/kg P.O. daily. Increase gradually q 1 to 3 weeks to maximum of eight times initial dose.

Contraindications and precautions
Guanethidine is contraindicated in pheochromocytoma. Use cautiously in severe cardiac disease, recent MI, cerebrovascular disease, peptic ulcer, impaired renal function, or bronchial asthma or in patients taking other antihypertensives.

Adverse reactions
CNS: *dizziness, weakness, syncope.*
CV: *orthostatic hypotension, bradycardia,* **CHF**, **arrhythmias**.
EENT: *nasal stuffiness.*
GI: *diarrhea.*
OTHER: *edema, weight gain, inhibition of ejaculation.*

Interactions
Levodopa, alcohol: may increase hypotensive effect of guanethidine. Use together cautiously.
MAO inhibitors, ephedrine, norepinephrine, methylphenidate, tricyclic antidepressants, amphetamines, phenothiazines: may inhibit the antihypertensive effect of guanethidine. Adjust dose accordingly.

Nursing considerations
Assessment
• Review the patient's history for a condition that contraindicates the use of guanethidine.
• Obtain a baseline assessment of patient's blood pressure before initiating guanethidine therapy.
• Be alert for common adverse reactions.
• Evaluate the patient's and family's knowledge about guanethidine.

Planning (Nursing Diagnoses)
Potential nursing diagnoses for the patient receiving guanethidine include:
- Potential for injury related to ineffectiveness of guanethidine to lower blood pressure.
- Impaired physical mobility related to guanethidine-induced muscle weakness.
- Diarrhea related to guanethidine's effect on GI tract.
- Knowledge deficit related to guanethidine therapy.

Implementation
Preparation and administration
— Consult with the doctor to discontinue drug 2 to 3 weeks before elective surgery, to reduce the possibility of vascular collapse and cardiac arrest during anesthesia.

Monitoring
— Monitor the effectiveness of therapy by regularly checking blood pressure; be aware that full antihypertensive effect may not appear for 1 to 3 weeks.
— Monitor the patient for adverse drug reactions.
— Monitor heart rate for bradycardia and ECG for arrhythmias.
— Check muscle strength regularly for weakness.
— Monitor for evidence of CHF (crackles, S_3, distended neck veins, ankle swelling, sudden weight gain).
— Monitor for diarrhea.
— Monitor the patient for drug interactions.
— Monitor the patient's compliance with guanethidine therapy.
— Regularly reevaluate the patient's and family's knowledge about guanethidine therapy.

Intervention
— Withhold dose and notify the doctor if hypotension, bradycardia and other arrhythmias, or CHF occurs.
— Institute safety measures if CNS reactions occur.
— Assist the patient with activities if weakness is present.
— Obtain an order for an antidiarrheal agent if diarrhea occurs.
— Assist the patient to standing position slowly to minimize orthostatic hypotension.
— If not contraindicated, restrict the patient's sodium and fluid intake to minimize fluid retention.
— Keep all members of the health care team informed of the patient's response to the drug.

Patient teaching
— Instruct the patient and family about guanethidine, including the dosage, frequency, action, and adverse reactions.
— Teach the patient about his disease. Explain the importance of taking this drug as prescribed, even when he's feeling well. Tell the patient

not to discontinue this drug suddenly but to call the doctor if unpleasant adverse reactions occur.
— Instruct the patient to check with the doctor or pharmacist before taking OTC medications.
— Tell the outpatient to avoid strenuous exercise and warn him that hot showers may cause hypotensive reaction; a hot environment may also potentiate the hypotensive effects of guanethidine.
— Give the patient instructions for a low-sodium diet.
— Inform the patient that orthostatic hypotension can be minimized by rising slowly and avoiding sudden position changes.
— Advise the patient to obtain assistance if muscle weakness occurs and to schedule activities to allow adequate rest.
— Tell the patient to notify the nurse or doctor if adverse reactions develop or questions arise about guanethidine therapy.

Evaluation

In the patient receiving guanethidine, appropriate evaluation statements include:
• Patient's blood pressure is within normal limits.
• Patient does not exhibit muscle weakness.
• Patient does not experience diarrhea.
• Patient and family state an understanding of guanethidine therapy.

SELECTED MAJOR DRUGS: ADRENERGIC BLOCKERS

DRUG, INDICATIONS, AND DOSAGES	SPECIAL PRECAUTIONS
Rauwolfia alkaloid	
deserpidine (Harmonyl) *Mild essential hypertension—* **Adults:** 0.25 mg P.O. daily. No dosing recommendations for children.	• Contraindicated in mental depression. • Use cautiously in severe cardiac or cerebrovascular disease, peptic ulcer, ulcerative colitis, gallstones, or mental depressive disorders; in patients undergoing surgery; and in patients taking other antihypertensives or anticonvulsants.
Miscellaneous agent	
guanadrel (Hylorel) *Treatment of hypertension—* **Adults:** initially, 5 mg P.O. b.i.d. Dosage can be adjusted until blood pressure is controlled. Most patients require doses of 20 to 75 mg daily, usually given b.i.d.; however, tolerance to hypotensive effect may necessitate upward titration of dosage to 100 to 400 mg daily, given in three to four divided doses.	• Contraindicated in known or suspected pheochromocytoma or frank CHF.

COMPARING SELECTED ANTIHYPERTENSIVE COMBINATIONS

TRADE NAME AND CONTENT	SPECIAL CONSIDERATIONS

Adrenergic blocker and diuretic

Chloroserpine-250
reserpine 0.125 mg and
chlorothiazide 250 mg
Diutensin-R
reserpine 0.1 mg and
methyclothiazide 2.5 mg
Enduronyl
deserpidine 0.25 mg and
methyclothiazide 5 mg
Hydropres 25
reserpine 0.125 mg and
hydrochlorothiazide 25 mg
Metatensin #2
reserpine 0.1 mg and
trichlormethiazide 2 mg
Metatensin #4
reserpine 0.1 mg and
trichlormethiazide 4 mg
Oreticyl 25
deserpidine 0.125 mg and
hydrochlorothiazide 25 mg
Rauzide
rauwolfia serpentina 50 mg and
bendroflumethiazide 4 mg
Regroton
reserpine 0.25 mg and
chlorthalidone 50 mg
Renese-R
reserpine 0.25 mg and
polythiazide 2 mg
Salutensin
reserpine 0.125 mg and
hydroflumethiazide 50 mg
Salutensin-Demi
reserpine 0.125 mg and
hydroflumethiazide 25 mg
Serpasil-Esidrix #1
reserpine 0.1 mg and
hydrochlorothiazide 25 mg

• Combine the adrenergic blocking effects of a adrenergic rauwolfia derivative (reserpine, deserpidine, or rauwolfia serpentina) with the diuretic and antihypertensive effects of a thiazide diuretic (chlorothiazide, methyclothiazide, hydrochlorothiazide, polythiazide, trichlormethiazide, bendroflumethiazide) or the thiazide-like diuretic chlorthalidone.
• Used to treat hypertension.
• Fixed combination drugs are not used as initial therapy. Patient's dosage should be titrated to optimal antihypertensive response with the individual drug before the combination is used.

Adrenergic blocker, diuretic, and vasodilator

Ser-Ap-Es,
Serpazide
reserpine 0.1 mg,
hydralazine hydrochloride 25 mg, and
hydrochlorothiazide 15 mg

• Combine the adrenergic neuron blocking effects of reserpine with the vasodilating effect of hydralazine and the antihypertensive and diuretic effects of hydrochlorothiazide.
• Used to treat hypertension.
• Fixed combination is not intended for initial therapy. Patient's dosage should be titrated to

(continued)

COMPARING SELECTED ANTIHYPERTENSIVE COMBINATIONS
continued

TRADE NAME AND CONTENT	SPECIAL CONSIDERATIONS
Adrenergic blocker, diuretic, and vasodilator *(continued)*	
Ser-Ap-Es, *(continued)* **Serpazide**	optimum blood pressure with the individual drugs before the combination is used.
Adrenergic blocker and vasodilator	
Serpasil-Apresoline #1 reserpine 0.1 mg and hydralazine hydrochloride 25 mg **Serpasil-Apresoline #2** reserpine 0.1 mg and hydralazine hydrochloride 5 mg	• Combine the adrenergic blocking effects of reserpine with the vasodilating effect of hydralazine. • Used to treat hypertension. • Fixed combination is not intended for initial therapy. Patient's dosage should be titrated to optimum blood pressure with the individual drugs before the combination is used.

SELF-TEST

1. Ann Zellers, age 42, has mild essential hypertension, for which her doctor prescribed reserpine 0.1 mg P.O. daily. Before instructing her about reserpine, the nurse should check to be sure Mrs. Zellers does not have any conditions that contraindicate the use of this drug. Which of the following conditions contraindicates the use of reserpine?
   a. Depression
   b. Seizure disorder
   c. Peptic ulcer disease
   d. Severe cardiac disease

2. How should the nurse instruct Mrs. Zellers to take reserpine?
   a. With a full glass of water
   b. With a meal
   c. On an empty stomach
   d. At bedtime

3. Mrs. Zellers does not respond well to reserpine. After trials with several other antihypertensive agents and a steady climb in her blood pressure over 6 months, her doctor prescribes clonidine 0.1 mg P.O. b.i.d. with guanethidine 10 mg P.O. daily. Which of the following adverse reactions is associated with guanethidine?
   a. Palpitations
   b. Constipation
   c. Orthostatic hypotension
   d. Anorexia

Check your answers on page 1067.

CHAPTER 40

SKELETAL MUSCLE RELAXANTS

baclofen ✦ carisoprodol ✦ chlorphenesin carbamate ✦ chlorzoxazone
cyclobenzaprine hydrochloride ✦ dantrolene sodium ✦ metaxalone
methocarbamol ✦ orphenadrine citrate

OVERVIEW
- Skeletal muscle relaxants can be divided into two categories: those routinely used to treat painful muscle spasms associated with acute, self-limiting conditions (such as lower back pain) and those used to treat more serious skeletal muscle spasticity associated with disease (such as multiple sclerosis) or spasticity secondary to spinal cord transection. The first category includes all the above drugs except baclofen and dantrolene, the more powerful drugs of the second category. These drugs must not be used for minor clinical problems, but only for their appropriate indications.

MAJOR USES
- Baclofen treats spasticity of multiple sclerosis. It is not recommended for spasticity secondary to stroke or cerebral palsy.
- Carisoprodol, chlorphenesin, chlorzoxazone, cyclobenzaprine, metaxalone, methocarbamol, and orphenadrine are used as adjuncts in the treatment of painful musculoskeletal disorders.
- Oral dantrolene is used to treat spasticity in paraplegia and hemiplegia; both the I.V. and oral forms control malignant hyperthermia.

MECHANISM OF ACTION
- Baclofen's mechanism of action is unclear.
- Carisoprodol, chlorphenesin, chlorzoxazone, cyclobenzaprine, metaxalone, methocarbamol, and orphenadrine reduce transmission of impulses from the spinal cord to skeletal muscle.
- Dantrolene acts directly on skeletal muscle to interfere with intracellular calcium movement.

ABSORPTION, DISTRIBUTION, METABOLISM, AND EXCRETION
All skeletal muscle relaxants are well absorbed after oral administration; all the parenteral forms except dantrolene are well absorbed after I.M. administration. (The parenteral form of dantrolene should be administered only by I.V. infusion.)

GLOSSARY

Relaxation: a reduction of tension, as when a muscle relaxes between contractions.
Spasm: an involuntary muscle contraction of sudden onset.
Spastic: of or pertaining to spasms or other uncontrolled contractions of the skeletal muscles.

These drugs are widely distributed in body tissues, with high concentrations in the brain. Metabolized in the liver, the drugs are excreted by the kidneys as both unchanged parent compound and metabolites.

ONSET AND DURATION
Onset is generally between 30 and 60 minutes, and blood levels peak in 2 to 3 hours. Duration of action is 4 to 6 hours.

ADVERSE REACTIONS
The skeletal muscle relaxants most frequently cause drowsiness, dizziness, and anticholinergic effects, such as dry mouth. CNS reactions include vertigo, ataxia, tremor, headache, nervousness, confusion, depressed mood, and hallucinations. CV reactions include tachycardia and hypotension. Baclofen may exacerbate preexisting psychiatric disturbances or seizures. Dantrolene may cause abnormal liver function tests and, in some cases, fatal or nonfatal hepatitis.

PROTOTYPE: SKELETAL MUSCLE RELAXANTS

CYCLOBENZAPRINE HYDROCHLORIDE
(sye kloe ben' za preen)
Flexeril
Classification: skeletal muscle relaxant
Pregnancy risk category B

How supplied
TABLETS: 10 mg

Indications and dosage
Short-term treatment of muscle spasm
ADULTS: 10 mg P.O. t.i.d. for 7 days. Maximum dosage is 60 mg daily for 2 to 3 weeks.

Contraindications and precautions
Cyclobenzaprine is contraindicated in patients who have received MAO inhibitors within 14 days; during the acute recovery phase of MI; in heart

block, arrhythmias, conduction disturbances, or CHF. Use cautiously in urine retention, narrow-angle glaucoma, increased intraocular pressure, CV disease, impaired hepatic function, and seizures and in elderly or debilitated patients.

Adverse reactions

CNS: *drowsiness*, euphoria, weakness, headache, insomnia, nightmares, paresthesia, dizziness, depression, visual disturbances, seizures.
CV: tachycardia.
EENT: blurred vision, *dry mouth.*
GI: abdominal pain, dyspepsia, peculiar taste, constipation.
GU: urine retention.
SKIN: rash, urticaria, pruritus.
OTHER: in high doses, watch for adverse reactions, such as those of other tricyclic drugs (amitriptyline, imipramine).

Interactions

Cholinergic blockers: enhanced cholinergic effect. Avoid concomitant use.
CNS depressants: excessive CNS depression. Don't use together.

Nursing considerations

Assessment

- Review the patient's history for a condition that contraindicates the use of cyclobenzaprine.
- Obtain a baseline assessment of patient's muscle spasm before therapy.
- Be alert for common adverse reactions.
- Evaluate the patient's and family's knowledge about cyclobenzaprine.

Planning (Nursing Diagnoses)

Potential nursing diagnoses for the patient receiving cyclobenzaprine include:
- Pain related to ineffectiveness of cyclobenzaprine to relieve muscle spasm.
- Injury related to potential for cyclobenzaprine-induced drowsiness.
- Knowledge deficit related to cyclobenzaprine therapy.

Implementation

Preparation and administration
— Do not administer cyclobenzaprine with other CNS depressants.

Monitoring
— Monitor the effectiveness of therapy by regularly assessing the severity and frequency of muscle spasms.
— Monitor the patient for adverse drug reactions.
— Monitor for drowsiness.
— Monitor closely for symptoms of overdose, such as cardiotoxicity (especially in patients receiving high doses).
— Monitor for visual and sleeping disturbances.

Italicized adverse reactions are common

— Monitor for changes in bowel or bladder function, especially constipation or urine retention.

— Monitor for tachycardia.

— Regularly reevaluate the patient's and family's knowledge about cyclobenzaprine.

Intervention

— Notify the doctor immediately if symptoms of overdose occur; have physostigmine readily available as an antidote.

— Be aware that withdrawal symptoms (nausea, headache, and malaise) may follow abrupt discontinuation after long-term use.

— Institute safety precautions until adverse CNS reactions are known.

— Maintain seizure precautions; drug may precipitate seizure activity.

— Keep all members of the health care team informed of the patient's response to the drug.

Patient teaching

— Instruct the patient and family about cyclobenzaprine, including the dosage, frequency, action, and adverse reactions.

— Advise the patient to report urinary hesitancy or urine retention.

— If constipation is troublesome, advise patient to increase fluid intake and use a stool softener.

— Warn the patient to avoid driving and other hazardous activities that require alertness until CNS effects of drug are known. Drowsiness and dizziness usually subside after 2 weeks.

— Tell the patient to avoid alcohol and other CNS depressants during cyclobenzaprine therapy.

— Tell the patient that dry mouth may be relieved with sugarless hard candy or chewing gum or ice chips.

— Tell the patient to notify the nurse or doctor if adverse reactions develop or questions arise about cyclobenzaprine therapy.

Evaluation

In the patient receiving cyclobenzaprine, appropriate evaluation statements include:

• Patient reports muscle spasms have ceased.

• Patient does not experience injury as a result of cyclobenzaprine-induced drowsiness.

• Patient and family state an understanding of cyclobenzaprine therapy.

SELECTED MAJOR DRUGS: SKELETAL MUSCLE RELAXANTS

DRUG, INDICATIONS, AND DOSAGES

SPECIAL PRECAUTIONS

baclofen (Lioresal)
Spasticity in multiple sclerosis, spinal cord injury—
Adults: initially, 5 mg P.O. t.i.d. for 3 days, 10 mg t.i.d. for 3 days, 20 mg t.i.d. for 3 days. Increase according to response up to maximum of 80 mg daily.

- Contraindicated in known hypersensitivity to the drug.
- Use cautiously in impaired renal function, stroke (minimal benefit, poor tolerance), and seizure disorder and when spasticity is used to maintain motor function.

carisoprodol (Rela, Soma)
As an adjunct in acute, painful musculoskeletal conditions—
Adults and children over age 12: 350 mg P.O. t.i.d. and h.s. Not recommended for children under age 12.

- Contraindicated in hypersensitivity to related compounds (for example, meprobamate) or in intermittent porphyria.
- Use cautiously in impaired hepatic or renal function.

chlorzoxazone (Paraflex, Parafon Forte DSC)
As an adjunct in acute, painful musculoskeletal conditions—
Adults: 250 to 750 mg P.O. t.i.d. or q.i.d.
Children: 20 mg/kg P.O. daily in divided doses t.i.d. or q.i.d.

- Contraindicated in impaired hepatic function.
- Use cautiously in history of drug allergies.

dantrolene (Dantrium)
Spasticity and sequelae secondary to severe chronic disorders (multiple sclerosis, cerebral palsy, spinal cord injury, stroke)—
Adults: 25 mg P.O. daily. Increase gradually in increments of 25 mg at 4- to 7-day intervals, up to 100 mg b.i.d. to q.i.d., to maximum of 400 mg daily.
Children: 1 mg/kg daily P.O. in divided doses b.i.d. to q.i.d. Increase gradually as needed by 1 mg/kg daily to maximum of 100 mg q.i.d.
Management of malignant hyperthermia—
Adults and children: initially, 1 mg/kg I.V.; may repeat dose up to cumulative dose of 10 mg/kg.
Prevention or attenuation of malignant hyperthermia in susceptible patients who require surgery—
Adults: 4 to 8 mg/kg P.O. daily in three or four divided doses for 1 to 2 days before procedure. Administer final dose 3 to 4 hours before procedure.
Prevention of recurrence of malignant hyperthermia—
Adults: 4 to 8 mg/kg P.O. daily in four divided doses for up to 3 days after hyperthermic crisis.

The following are considerations for the P.O. form only:
- Contraindicated when spasticity is used to maintain motor function; in spasms; in rheumatic disorders; and in lactation.
- Use with caution in severely impaired cardiac or pulmonary function or preexisting hepatic disease; in women; and in patients over age 35.
- Safety and efficacy in longterm use have not been established; value may be determined by therapeutic trial. Do not give more than 45 days if no benefits are obtained.

metaxalone (Skelaxin)
As an adjunct in acute, painful musculoskeletal conditions—
Adults and children over age 12: 800 mg (2 tablets) t.i.d. to q.i.d.

- Contraindicated in known hypersensitivity to the drug; with known tendency to drug-induced, hemolytic, or other anemias; and with significantly impaired renal or hepatic function.

(continued)

SELECTED MAJOR DRUGS: SKELETAL MUSCLE RELAXANTS
(continued)

DRUG, INDICATIONS, AND DOSAGES	SPECIAL PRECAUTIONS
metaxalone *(continued)*	• Administer cautiously to patients with preexisting liver damage and ensure that serial liver function studies are performed as required; also use cautiously during pregnancy and breast-feeding.
methocarbamol (Robaxin) *As an adjunct in acute, painful musculoskeletal conditions—* **Adults:** 1.5 g P.O. for 2 to 3 days, then 1 g P.O. q.i.d., or not more than 500 mg (5 ml) I.M. into each gluteal region. May repeat q 8 hours. Or 1 to 3 g daily (10 to 30 ml) I.V. directly into vein at 3 ml/minute, or 10 ml may be added to no more than 250 ml of dextrose 5% in water or 0.9% sodium chloride solution. Maximum dosage is 3 g daily. *Supportive therapy in tetanus management—* **Adults:** 1 to 2 g into tubing of running I.V. or 1 to 3 g in infusion bottle q 6 hours. **Children:** 15 mg/kg I.V. q 6 hours.	• Contraindicated in impaired renal function (injectable form), myasthenia gravis, and seizure disorder (injectable form); in children under age 12 (except in tetanus); in patients receiving anticholinesterase agents; and in patients with known hypersensitivity to any of the ingredients. • Administer cautiously to patients with suspected or known seizure disorder and in children under age 12.
orphenadrine (Banflex, Norflex) *As an adjunct in acute, painful musculoskeletal conditions—* **Adults:** 100 mg P.O. b.i.d., or 60 mg I.V. or I.M. q 12 hours p.r.n. For maintenance, switch to oral therapy beginning 12 hours after last parenteral dose.	• Contraindicated in narrow-angle glaucoma; prostatic hypertrophy; pyloric, duodenal, or bladder-neck obstruction; myasthenia gravis; tachycardia; severe hepatic or renal disease; or ulcerative colitis. • Use cautiously in elderly or debilitated patients with cardiac disease; in arrhythmias; in sulfite sensitivity; and in those exposed to high temperatures.

SELF-TEST

1. Samuel Silverberg, a 30-year-old construction worker, strained his back when lifting some building materials. His doctor prescribed bed rest and cyclobenzaprine 10 mg P.O. t.i.d. for 7 days. The nurse understands that this drug is best described as an:
   a. analgesic.
   b. antianxiety agent.
   c. sedative.
   d. skeletal muscle relaxant.

2. In a teaching plan for a patient receiving cyclobenzaprine, the nurse would include all of the following except:
  a. patient should avoid combining alcohol or other depressants with cyclobenzaprine.
  b. patient should be able to return to operating heavy construction machinery within 24 hours after starting medication.
  c. patient should report any problems with voiding to the doctor.
  d. patient should increase fluid intake if constipation is a problem.

3. In teaching Mr. Silverberg about cyclobenzaprine, the nurse informs him that a common adverse reaction is:
  a. drowsiness.
  b. diarrhea.
  c. tinnitus.
  d. bradycardia.

Check your answers on page 1067.

CHAPTER 41

NEUROMUSCULAR BLOCKERS

doxacurium chloride ◆ gallamine triethiodide ◆ metocurine iodide
pancuronium bromide ◆ pipecuronium bromide ◆ succinylcholine chloride
tubocurarine chloride

OVERVIEW

- Potentially dangerous drugs, neuromuscular blockers should be administered either by a doctor or under a doctor's direct supervision. They effectively paralyze skeletal muscle, thereby reducing anesthetic requirements and facilitating manipulation during surgery. However, because they also paralyze muscles essential for respiration (diaphragm and intercostals), mechanical ventilatory support must be available whenever these drugs are administered. Because neuromuscular blockers do not obtund consciousness, they should only be used after the patient is sedated.

MAJOR USES

- Neuromuscular blockers provide muscle relaxation during anesthesia. They facilitate intubation, abdominal surgical procedures, correction of dislocations, and setting of fractures.
- They are also used to control respirations of patients on mechanical ventilators, muscle contraction in electroconvulsive therapy, and muscle spasms in convulsive states (tetanus, status epilepticus, drug intoxication, and black widow spider bites).

MECHANISM OF ACTION

These agents block transmission of nerve impulses at the skeletal neuromuscular junction by one of two mechanisms:

- Succinylcholine (depolarizing agent) prolongs depolarization of the muscle end plate.
- Gallamine, metocurine, pancuronium, tubocurarine, doxacurium, and pipecuronium (nondepolarizing agents) prevent acetylcholine from binding to the receptors on the muscle end plate, thus blocking depolarization.

GLOSSARY

Intubation: passage of a tube through the mouth or nose or into the trachea to ensure a patent airway for the delivery of an anesthetic gas or oxygen.
Neuromuscular blocking agent: a chemical substance that interferes locally with the transmission or reception of impulses from motor nerves to skeletal muscles.
Paralysis: loss of muscle function.

ABSORPTION, DISTRIBUTION, METABOLISM, AND EXCRETION

Neuromuscular blockers are ineffective orally because they're poorly absorbed from the GI tract; they are slowly and unpredictably absorbed from I.M. injection sites. Rapidly distributed from I.V. sites, these drugs (except succinylcholine, which is hydrolyzed by pseudocholinesterase in the blood and liver) are poorly metabolized and remain effective in the body until they are eliminated in urine and—through the bile—in feces as unchanged drug.

ONSET AND DURATION

Gallamine begins to work within 1 to 3 minutes after I.V. administration; its peak effect occurs in about 3 minutes. Duration of action depends on total dosage and number of doses administered.

Metocurine and tubocurarine take effect within 1 to 3 minutes after I.V. administration; duration is 25 to 90 minutes. The drugs accumulate after repeated doses.

Pancuronium's onset occurs within a few minutes after I.V. administration. Its duration of action is 25 to 60 minutes; duration is more prolonged when large doses are given.

Succinylcholine, administered I.V., takes effect in 1 to 3 minutes; its duration of action is only 5 minutes.

Pipecuronium and doxacurium take effect within 5 minutes but exhibit prolonged relaxation (90 minutes or more depending on dose).

ADVERSE REACTIONS

Extensions of the pharmacologic actions are the primary adverse reactions to the neuromuscular blockers. These effects include prolonged apnea and residual muscle weakness. Tubocurarine and—to a lesser extent—metocurine and succinylcholine stimulate histamine release, which causes dermatologic effects of flushing, erythema, pruritus, urticaria, and wheal formation, and pulmonary effects of wheezing and bronchospasm. Hypotension and tachycardia are adverse CV reactions mediated by histamine release. Succinylcholine may cause postoperative pain because it initially produces skeletal muscle fasciculations. Allergic reactions and malignant hyperthermia may also rarely occur.

PANCURONIUM BROMIDE
(pan kyoo roe′ nee um)
Pavulon
Classification: neuromuscular blocker
Pregnancy risk category C

How supplied
INJECTION: 1 mg/ml, 2 mg/ml

Indications and dosage
Adjunct to anesthesia to induce skeletal muscle relaxation; facilitate intubation; lessen muscle contractions in pharmacologically or electrically induced seizures; assist with mechanical ventilation
Dosage depends on anesthetic used, individual needs, and response. Dosages are representative and must be adjusted.
ADULTS: initially, 0.04 to 0.1 mg/kg I.V., then 0.01 mg/kg q 30 to 60 minutes.
CHILDREN OVER AGE 10: initially, 0.04 to 0.1 mg/kg I.V., then ⅕ of initial dose q 30 to 60 minutes.

Contraindications and precautions
Pancuronium is contraindicated in hypersensitivity to bromides and in preexisting tachycardia and in patients for whom even a minor increase in heart rate is undesirable. Use cautiously in elderly or debilitated patients; in those with renal, hepatic, or pulmonary impairment; respiratory depression; myasthenia gravis; myasthenic syndrome of lung cancer or bronchogenic carcinoma; dehydration; thyroid disorders; collagen diseases; porphyria; electrolyte disturbances; hyperthermia; toxemic states; and (in large doses) in those undergoing cesarean section.

Adverse reactions
CV: tachycardia, increased blood pressure.
SKIN: transient rashes.
LOCAL: burning sensation.
OTHER: excessive sweating and salivation, *prolonged dose-related apnea*, wheezing, residual muscle weakness, allergic or idiosyncratic hypersensitivity reactions.

Interactions
Aminoglycoside antibiotics (including amikacin, gentamicin, kanamycin, neomycin, streptomycin); polymyxin antibiotics (polymyxin B sulfate, colistin); clindamycin; quinidine; general anesthetics (such as halothane, enflurane, isoflurane): potentiated neuromuscular blockade, leading to increased skeletal muscle relaxation and possible respiratory paralysis. Use cautiously during surgical and postoperative periods.

Lithium, narcotic analgesics: potentiated neuromuscular blockade, leading to increased skeletal muscle relaxation and possible respiratory paralysis. Use with extreme caution and reduce dose of pancuronium.

Nursing considerations

Assessment

- Review the patient's history for a condition that contraindicates the use of pancuronium.
- Obtain a baseline assessment of skeletal muscle function before therapy.
- Be alert for common adverse reactions.
- Evaluate the patient's and family's knowledge about pancuronium.

Planning (Nursing Diagnoses)

Potential nursing diagnoses for the patient receiving pancuronium include:

- Potential for injury related to adverse drug reactions associated with pancuronium.
- Ineffective breathing pattern related to prolonged dose-related apnea caused by pancuronium.
- Knowledge deficit related to pancuronium therapy.

Implementation

Preparation and administration

- — Pancuronium should be administered only by personnel experienced in airway management.
- — Have emergency respiratory support equipment (endotracheal equipment, ventilator, oxygen, atropine, edrophonium, epinephrine, and neostigmine) on hand before administration.
- — Dose of 1 mg is the approximate therapeutic equivalent of 5 mg tubocurarine.
- — Store in refrigerator. Do not store in plastic containers or syringes, but plastic syringes may be used for administration.
- — Do not mix with barbiturate solutions (precipitate will form); use only fresh solutions.
- — Usually administered together with a cholinergic blocker (such as atropine or glycopyrrolate).
- — If succinylcholine is used, allow effects to subside before giving pancuronium.

Monitoring

- — Monitor the effectiveness of therapy by regularly checking relaxation state of the patient's skeletal muscles; close observation of the patient is mandatory.
- — Closely monitor baseline electrolyte determinations (electrolyte imbalance can potentiate neuromuscular effects) and vital signs (watch respiration and heart rate).
- — Measure intake and output (renal dysfunction may prolong duration of action, since 25% of the drug is unchanged before excretion).

—Monitor respirations and respiratory status closely until patient recovers fully from neuromuscular blockade, as evidenced by tests of muscle strength (hand grip, head lift, and ability to cough).

—Monitor the patient for adverse drug reactions.

—Monitor the patient for drug interactions.

Intervention

—Maintain adequate ventilation through respiratory support equipment throughout drug therapy and provide pulmonary care as indicated.

—Once spontaneous recovery starts, pancuronium-induced neuromuscular blockade may be reversed with an anticholinesterase agent (such as neostigmine or edrophonium).

—Provide emotional support for the intubated patient who is awake.

—Administer pain medication on regular basis (as condition dictates) because the patient will be unable to communicate that pain is present.

—Keep all members of the health care team informed of the patient's response to the drug.

Patient teaching

—Instruct the patient and family about pancuronium, including how the drug will be administered and adverse reactions.

—Reassure the patient that necessary pain management will be provided regularly.

—Inform the patient that drug-induced paralysis will inhibit his ability to communicate but that he will receive continuous monitoring and care.

Evaluation

In the patient receiving pancuronium, appropriate evaluation statements include:

• Patient exhibits no adverse drug reactions.

• Patient maintains adequate ventilation.

• Patient and family state an understanding of pancuronium therapy.

SELECTED MAJOR DRUGS: NEUROMUSCULAR BLOCKERS

DRUG, INDICATIONS, AND DOSAGES	SPECIAL PRECAUTIONS
gallamine (Flaxedil) *Adjunct to anesthesia to induce skeletal muscle relaxation; facilitate intubation, reduction of fractures and dislocations; lessen muscle contractions in pharmacologically or electrically induced seizures; assist with mechanical ventilation—* Dosage depends on anesthetic used, individual needs, and response. Dosages are representative and must be adjusted. **Adults and children over age 1 month:** initially, 1 mg/kg I.V. to maximum of 100 mg, regardless of patient's weight, then 0.5 to 1 mg/kg q 30 to 40 minutes.	• Contraindicated in patients with known hypersensitivity to iodides; in impaired renal function, myasthenia gravis, and shock; and in patients in whom tachycardia may be hazardous. • Use cautiously in elderly or debilitated patients; in hepatic or pulmonary impairment, respiratory depression, myasthenic syndrome of lung cancer or bronchogenic carcinoma, dehy-

SELECTED MAJOR DRUGS: NEUROMUSCULAR BLOCKERS *continued*

DRUG, INDICATIONS, AND DOSAGES	SPECIAL PRECAUTIONS
gallamine *(continued)* **Children under age 1 month but over 5 kg:** initially, 0.25 to 0.75 mg/kg I.V., then may give additional doses of 0.1 to 0.5 mg/kg q 30 to 40 minutes.	dration, thyroid disorders, collagen diseases, porphyria, and electrolyte disturbances; in patients sensitive to sulfites; and in patients undergoing cesarean section.
metocurine (Metubine) *Adjunct to anesthesia to induce skeletal muscle relaxation; facilitate intubation, reduction of fractures and dislocations* — Dosage depends on anesthetic used, individual needs, and response. Dosages are representative and must be adjusted. Administer as sustained injection over 30 to 60 seconds. **Adults:** given cyclopropane — 2 to 4 mg I.V. (2.68 mg average); given ether — 1.5 to 3 mg I.V. (2.1 mg average); given nitrous oxide — 4 to 7 mg I.V. (4.79 mg average). Supplemental injections of 0.5 to 1 mg in 25 to 90 minutes, repeated p.r.n. *Lessen muscle contractions in pharmacologically or electrically induced seizures* — **Adults:** 1.75 to 5.5 mg I.V.	• Contraindicated in patients with known hypersensitivity to iodides and in whom histamine release is a hazard (asthmatic or atopic patients). • Use cautiously in elderly or debilitated patients; in renal, hepatic, or pulmonary impairment, respiratory depression, myasthenia gravis, myasthenic syndrome of lung cancer or bronchogenic carcinoma, dehydration, thyroid disorders, collagen diseases, porphyria, electrolyte disturbances, and hyperthermia; and (in large doses) in patients undergoing cesarean section.
succinylcholine (Anectine) *Adjunct to anesthesia to induce skeletal muscle relaxation; facilitate intubation and assist with mechanical ventilation or orthopedic manipulations (drug of choice); lessen muscle contractions in pharmacologically or electrically induced seizures* — Dosage depends on anesthetic used, individual needs, and response. Dosages are representative and must be adjusted. **Adults:** 25 to 75 mg I.V., then 2.5 mg/minute p.r.n. or 2.5 mg/kg I.M. up to maximum of 150 mg I.M. in deltoid muscle. **Children:** 1 to 2 mg/kg I.M. or I.V. Maximum I.M. dosage is 150 mg. (Children may be less sensitive to succinylcholine than adults.)	• Contraindicated in abnormally low plasma pseudocholinesterase. • Use cautiously in patients with personal or family history of malignant hypertension or hyperthermia; in elderly or debilitated patients; in hepatic, renal, or pulmonary impairment; in respiratory depression, severe burns or trauma, electrolyte imbalances, quinidine or digitalis therapy, hyperkalemia, paraplegia, spinal neuraxis injury, degenerative or dystrophic neuromuscular disease, myasthenia gravis, myasthenic syndrome of lung cancer or bronchogenic carcinoma, dehydration, thyroid disorders, collagen diseases, porphyria, fractures, muscle spasms, glaucoma, eye surgery

(continued)

SELECTED MAJOR DRUGS: NEUROMUSCULAR BLOCKERS *continued*

DRUG, INDICATIONS, AND DOSAGES	SPECIAL PRECAUTIONS
succinylcholine *(continued)*	or penetrating eye wounds, and pheochromocytoma; and (in large doses) in patients undergoing cesarean section.

tubocurarine (Tubarine†)
Adjunct to anesthesia to induce skeletal muscle relaxation; facilitate intubation, orthopedic manipulations—
Dosage depends on anesthetic used, individual needs, and response. Dosages listed are representative and must be adjusted.
Adults: 1 unit/kg or 0.15 mg/kg I.V. slowly over 60 to 90 seconds. Usual initial dose for average-weight patient is 40 to 60 units I.V.; may give 20 to 30 units in 3 to 5 minutes. For longer procedures, give 20 units p.r.n.
Children: 1 unit/kg or 0.15 mg/kg I.V.
Assist with mechanical ventilation—
Adults and children: initially, 0.0165 mg/kg (average 1 mg or 7 units I.V.), then adjust subsequent doses to patient's response.
Lessen muscle contractions in pharmacologically or electrically induced seizures—
Adults and children: 1 unit/kg or 0.15 mg/kg I.V. slowly over 60 to 90 seconds. Initial dose is 20 units (3 mg) less than calculated dose.

• Contraindicated in patients for whom histamine release is a hazard (asthmatics).
• Use cautiously in elderly or debilitated patients; in hepatic or pulmonary impairment, respiratory depression, myasthenia gravis, myasthenic syndrome of lung cancer or bronchogenic carcinoma, dehydration, thyroid disorders, collagen diseases, porphyria, electrolyte disturbances, fractures, and muscle spasms; and (in large doses) in patients undergoing cesarean section.

†Available in Canada only

SELF-TEST

1. During surgery, Marjorie Smith received pancuronium. The nurse understands that Mrs. Smith received this medication:
   a. to improve perfusion to vital organs during surgery.
   b. to prevent postoperative abdominal distention.
   c. to induce skeletal muscle relaxation.
   d. to block cardiac vagal reflexes and diminish secretions.

2. The nurse should be aware that the greatest danger from the use of neuromuscular blocking agents such as pancuronium is:
   a. cardiotoxicity.
   b. apnea and hypoxia.
   c. hepatic damage.
   d. nephrotoxicity.

3. Which one of the following considerations does not apply when a patient is receiving pancuronium?
  a. Do not use plastic syringes for administration.
  b. Monitor respirations closely until patient is fully recovered from neuromuscular blockade.
  c. Do not mix with barbiturate solutions.
  d. Have emergency respiratory support equipment on hand.

Check your answers on page 1067.

CHAPTER 42

ANTIHISTAMINES

astemizole ◆ azatadine maleate ◆ brompheniramine maleate
carbinoxamine maleate ◆ chlorpheniramine maleate
clemastine fumarate ◆ cyproheptadine hydrochloride
dexchlorpheniramine maleate ◆ diphenhydramine citrate
diphenhydramine hydrochloride ◆ diphenylpyraline hydrochloride
doxylamine succinate ◆ methdilazine hydrochloride
promethazine hydrochloride ◆ terfenadine ◆ trimeprazine tartrate
tripelennamine citrate ◆ tripelennamine hydrochloride
triprolidine hydrochloride

OVERVIEW

- Most antihistamines are thought to block the physiologic action of histamine, the humoral compound that causes symptoms associated with allergic reactions. They compete with histamine for receptor sites (by the process of competitive inhibition).
- Many compounds from different chemical classes are called antihistamines. All antihistamines have *qualitatively* similar pharmacologic effects. *Quantitatively,* however, they may differ in potency and range of effect. Drowsiness, an adverse reaction common to most antihistamines, may vary in intensity from drug to drug—and sometimes from patient to patient. Drowsiness results from an effect on histamine or cholinergic receptors in the brain. Astemizole and terfenadine are not associated with drowsiness because their chemical structures prevent them from getting to the CNS.

MAJOR USES

- Antihistamines (except cyproheptadine, methdilazine, and trimeprazine) are used to relieve symptoms of allergy-related rhinitis and conjunctivitis. Antihistamines are also included in combination drug preparations because of the benefits they produce in the treatment of common cold symptoms.
- Cyproheptadine, methdilazine, and trimeprazine are used to treat mild, uncomplicated urticaria or pruritus resulting from allergic dermatoses.
- Diphenhydramine is used as a nighttime sedative. It is also a therapeutic adjunct for anaphylaxis or less severe allergic reactions caused by drugs, blood, or plasma. Additionally, diphenhydramine is used as a local anesthetic in dental procedures.
- Promethazine is used to prevent motion sickness.

GLOSSARY

Allergy: hypersensitivity reaction acquired through exposure to an allergen that results in an increased reaction upon reexposure.
Antihistamine: any substance capable of reducing the physiologic and pharmacologic effects of histamine.
Histamine: powerful tissue substance released during an allergic reaction that dilates capillaries, contracts most smooth muscles, increases heart rate, and stimulates gastric secretions.
Rhinitis: inflammation of nasal mucous membranes.
Rhinorrhea: discharge of thin nasal mucus.
Urticaria: skin reaction characterized by transient wheals that are paler or redder than the surrounding skin and that are commonly accompanied by severe itching; also called hives.

MECHANISM OF ACTION

- Antihistamines compete with histamine for H_1-receptor sites on effector cells. They can prevent but not reverse histamine-mediated responses, particularly histamine's effects on the smooth muscle of the bronchial tubes, GI tract, uterus, and blood vessels.
- Anticholinergic actions of antihistamines dry the nasal mucosa and also relieve vertigo and motion sickness.
- Diphenhydramine, structurally related to local anesthetics, provides anesthesia by preventing initiation and transmission of nerve impulses.

ABSORPTION, DISTRIBUTION, METABOLISM, AND EXCRETION

Antihistamines are well absorbed after oral or parenteral administration. They are distributed to most body tissues, extensively metabolized in the liver, and excreted in the urine as inactive metabolites within 24 hours. The nonsedating antihistamines do not enter the CNS.

ONSET AND DURATION

Antihistamines begin to act within 15 to 30 minutes; blood levels peak in about 1 hour. Duration of action varies, but symptoms are usually relieved for 4 to 6 hours. Action of the sustained-release forms may last 8 to 12 hours.

ADVERSE REACTIONS

Most antihistamines (except astemizole and terfenadine) cause drowsiness, fatigue, and some confusion. They may also cause epigastric distress, postural hypotension, dry mouth, nausea, and vomiting.

The nonsedating antihistamines astemizole and terfenadine cause different reactions. Terfenadine is associated with alopecia, visual disturbances, cough, rash, and itching; astemizole, with headache, increased appetite, weight gain, abdominal pain, and dry mouth.

DIPHENHYDRAMINE HYDROCHLORIDE
(dye fen hye′ dra meen)

Allerdryl†, AllerMax Caplets◊, Beldin◊, Belix◊, Bena-D 10, Bena-D 50◊, Benadryl*◊, Benadryl Complete Allergy◊, Benahist 10, Benahist 50, Ben-Allergin-50, Benaphen◊, Benoject-10, Benoject-50, Benylin Cough*◊, Benylin Pediatric†, Bydramine Cough◊, Compoz◊, Diahist◊, Dihydrex, Diphenacen-50, Diphenadryl◊, Diphen Cough*◊, Diphenhist◊, Dormarex 2◊, Fenylhist◊, Fynex◊, Hydramine*, Hydramyn, Hydril◊, Hyrexin-50, Insomnal†, Nervine Nighttime Sleep-Aid◊, Noradryl, Nordryl, Nytol with DPH◊, SleepEze 3◊, Sominex 2◊, Tusstat*◊, Twilite◊, Wehdryl-10, Wehdryl-50*

Classification: antihistamine
Pregnancy risk category B

How supplied
TABLETS: 25 mg◊, 50 mg◊
CAPSULES: 25 mg◊, 50 mg◊
ELIXIR: 12.5 mg/5 ml (14% alcohol)*◊
SYRUP: 12.5 mg/5 ml◊, 13.3 mg/5 ml (5% alcohol)*◊
INJECTION: 10 mg/ml, 50 mg/ml

Indications and dosage
Rhinitis, allergy symptoms, motion sickness, parkinsonism
ADULTS: 25 to 50 mg P.O. t.i.d. or q.i.d.; or 10 to 50 mg deep I.M. or I.V. Maximum dosage is 400 mg daily.
CHILDREN UNDER AGE 12: 5 mg/kg P.O., deep I.M., or I.V. divided q.i.d. Maximum dosage is 300 mg daily.

Sedation
ADULTS: 25 to 50 mg P.O. or deep I.M. p.r.n.

Nighttime sleep aid
ADULTS: 50 mg P.O. h.s.

Nonproductive cough
ADULTS: 25 mg P.O. q 4 hours (not to exceed 100 mg daily).
CHILDREN AGES 6 TO 12: 12.5 mg P.O. q 4 hours (not to exceed 50 mg daily).
CHILDREN AGES 2 TO 6: 6.25 mg P.O. q 4 hours (not to exceed 25 mg daily).
Note: Children under age 12 should use only as directed by a doctor.

Contraindications and precautions
Diphenhydramine is contraindicated in acute asthmatic attacks. Use cautiously in narrow-angle glaucoma, prostatic hypertrophy, pyloroduodenal and bladder-neck obstruction, and stenosing peptic ulcers; in neonates; and in asthmatic, hypertensive, or cardiac patients.

---

*Liquid form contains alcohol   †Available in Canada only   ◊ Available OTC

Adverse reactions

CNS: *drowsiness,* confusion, insomnia, headache, vertigo (especially in elderly patients).
CV: palpitations.
EENT: diplopia, nasal stuffiness.
GI: *nausea,* vomiting, diarrhea, *dry mouth,* constipation.
GU: dysuria, urine retention.
SKIN: urticaria, photosensitivity.

Interactions

CNS depressants: increased sedation. Use together cautiously.

Nursing considerations

Assessment

- Review the patient's history for a condition that contraindicates the use of diphenhydramine.
- Obtain a baseline assessment of the patient's underlying condition before therapy.
- Be alert for common adverse reactions.
- Evaluate the patient's and family's knowledge about diphenhydramine therapy.

Planning (Nursing Diagnoses)

Potential nursing diagnoses for the patient receiving diphenhydramine include:
- Altered health maintenance related to ineffectiveness of diphenhydramine.
- Potential for injury related to diphenhydramine-induced drowsiness.
- Knowledge deficit related to diphenhydramine therapy.

Implementation

Preparation and administration

— Administer I.M. injection deep into a large muscle.
— Alternate injection sites to prevent irritation.
— If oral forms cause GI distress, administer with food or milk.
— If medication is being used for motion sickness, administer it 30 minutes before travel.

Monitoring

— Monitor the effectiveness of therapy by regularly assessing the patient's condition for relief of symptoms.
— Monitor the degree of drowsiness induced by drug.
— Monitor the patient for other adverse drug reactions. Monitor elderly patients carefully because they are especially vulnerable to reactions such as drowsiness, confusion, insomnia, headaches, and vertigo.
— If bronchial secretions are present, monitor lung sounds and characteristics of the secretions. Ensure adequate fluid intake to decrease the viscosity of the secretions.
— Monitor the patient's intake and output for possible urine retention.
— Monitor the patient for drug interactions.

Italicized adverse reactions are common

—Regularly reevaluate the patient's and family's knowledge about diphenhydramine therapy.

Intervention

—Take safety precautions with all patients, particularly during ambulation. Diphenhydramine is one of the most sedating antihistamines and is often used as a hypnotic.

—Hold medication if the patient is scheduled for allergy skin tests. Diphenhydramine must be discontinued 4 days before testing to preserve the accuracy of the tests.

—Coffee or tea may reduce drowsiness. Sugarless gum or hard candy or ice chips may relieve dry mouth.

—If tolerance develops, another antihistamine may be substituted.

—Keep all members of the health care team informed of the patient's response to the drug.

Patient teaching

—Instruct the patient and family about diphenhydramine, including the dosage, frequency, action, and adverse reactions.

—Explain that drug interactions are likely to occur with simultaneous use of CNS depressants. The patient should seek medical approval before taking any OTC medication.

—Warn the patient against drinking alcoholic beverages during therapy.

—Warn the patient to avoid driving and other hazardous activities that require alertness until the effects of the drug are established. If this becomes a problem, the patient may be able to tolerate terfenadine or astemizole, which are less likely to cause drowsiness.

—Discuss with the patient that allergic rhinitis, conjunctivitis, and urticaria result from particular sources, such as dust and pollen. Such causes of allergy should be identified to prevent future reactions.

—Tell the patient to take the drug with food or milk.

—Tell the patient that coffee or tea may reduce drowsiness and that dry mouth may be relieved with sugarless gum or hard candy or ice chips.

—If the drug is being used for motion sickness, tell the patient to take it 30 minutes before traveling.

—Explain that if an antihistamine becomes ineffective, it is all right to substitute another antihistamine.

—Warn the patient to stop taking the drug 4 days before any allergy skin tests to preserve the accuracy of the tests.

—Tell the patient to avoid sun exposure and to use a sunscreen outdoors to prevent photosensitivity reactions.

—Encourage the patient to notify the doctor of any dysuria or urine retention; tell the patient to notify the doctor if allergy symptoms persist.

—Emphasize the importance of taking the drug exactly as directed.

—Tell the patient to notify the nurse or doctor if adverse reactions develop or questions arise about diphenhydramine therapy.

Evaluation

In the patient receiving diphenhydramine, appropriate evaluation statements include:

• Patient's symptoms are relieved with diphenhydramine.
• Patient does not experience injury as a result of diphenhydramine-induced drowsiness.
• Patient and family state an understanding of diphenhydramine therapy.

SELECTED MAJOR DRUGS: ANTIHISTAMINES

DRUG, INDICATIONS, AND DOSAGES	SPECIAL PRECAUTIONS
astemizole (Hismanal) *Relief of symptoms associated with chronic idiopathic urticaria and seasonal allergic rhinitis—* **Adults and children over age 12:** 10 mg P.O. daily. A loading dose may be given to quickly achieve steady-state plasma levels. Begin therapy at 30 mg on the first day, followed by 20 mg on the second day and 10 mg daily thereafter.	• Contraindicated in patients with known hypersensitivity to astemizole. • Because of its potential for anticholinergic effects, use cautiously in patients with lower respiratory diseases (including asthma) because drying effects can increase the risk of bronchial mucus plug formation. • Use cautiously in patients with hepatic or renal disease. Astemizole is not dialyzable.
azatadine (Optimine, Zadine‡) *Rhinitis, allergy symptoms, chronic urticaria—* **Adults:** 1 to 2 mg P.O. b.i.d. Maximum dosage is 4 mg daily. Not intended for children under age 12.	• Contraindicated in acute asthmatic attacks. • Use cautiously in elderly patients and in patients with increased intraocular pressure, hyperthyroidism, CV or renal disease, hypertension, bronchial asthma, urine retention, prostatic hypertrophy, bladder-neck obstruction, and stenosing peptic ulcers.
brompheniramine (Brombay ◇, Dimetane ◇, Dimetane Extentabs ◇, Histaject Modified) *Rhinitis, allergy symptoms—* **Adults:** 4 to 8 mg P.O. t.i.d. or q.i.d.; or 8 to 12 mg (timed-release) P.O. b.i.d. or t.i.d.; or 5 to 20 mg I.M., I.V., or S.C. q 6 to 12 hours. Maximum dosage is 40 mg daily. **Children over age 6:** 2 to 4 mg P.O. t.i.d. or q.i.d.; or 8 to 12 mg (timed-release) P.O. q 12 hours; or 0.5 mg/kg I.M., I.V., or S.C. in divided doses t.i.d. or q.i.d. **Children under age 6:** 0.5 mg/kg P.O., I.M., I.V., or S.C. in divided doses t.i.d. or q.i.d. *Note:* Children under age 12 should use only as directed by a doctor.	• Contraindicated in acute asthmatic attacks. • Use cautiously in elderly patients; in breast-feeding women; and in patients with increased intraocular pressure, hyperthyroidism, CV or renal disease, hypertension, bronchial asthma, urine retention, prostatic hypertrophy, bladder-neck obstruction, or stenosing peptic ulcers.

(continued)

‡Available in Australia only   ◇ Available OTC

SELECTED MAJOR DRUGS: ANTIHISTAMINES *continued*

DRUG, INDICATIONS, AND DOSAGES	SPECIAL PRECAUTIONS
chlorpheniramine (Aller-Chlor◇, Chlor-Trimeton◇, Chlor-Timeton Repetabs◇, Teldrin◇) *Rhinitis, allergy symptoms —* **Adults:** 4 mg P.O. q 4 hours, not to exceed 24 mg daily; or 8 mg (timed-release) P.O. q 12 hours; or 5 to 40 mg I.M., I.V., or S.C. daily. Give I.V. injection over 1 minute. **Children ages 6 to 12:** 2 mg P.O. q 4 to 6 hours, not to exceed 12 mg daily. Alternatively, may give 8 mg (timed-release) P.O. h.s.. **Children ages 2 to 6:** 1 mg P.O. q 4 to 6 hours. *Note:* Children under age 12 should use only as directed by a doctor.	• Contraindicated in acute asthmatic attacks. • Use cautiously in elderly patients and in patients with increased intraocular pressure, hyperthyroidism, CV or renal disease, hypertension, bronchial asthma, urine retention, prostatic hypertrophy, bladder-neck obstruction, or stenosing peptic ulcers.
dexchlorpheniramine (Dexchlor, Poladex TD, Polaramine, Polaramine Repetabs) *Rhinitis, allergy symptoms, contact dermatitis, pruritus —* **Adults:** 2 mg P.O. q 4 to 6 hours, not to exceed 12 mg daily; or 4 to 6 mg (timed-release) P.O. b.i.d. or t.i.d. **Children ages 6 to 12:** 1 mg P.O. q 4 to 6 hours, not to exceed 6 mg daily; or 4 mg (timed-release tablet) P.O. h.s. **Children ages 2 to 6:** 0.5 mg P.O. q 4 to 6 hours, not to exceed 3 mg daily. *Note:* Children under age 6 should use only as directed by a doctor. Do not use timed-release tablets for children under age 6.	• Contraindicated in acute asthmatic attacks. • Use cautiously in elderly patients and in patients with increased intraocular pressure, hyperthyroidism, CV or renal disease, hypertension, bronchial asthma, urine retention, prostatic hypertrophy, bladder-neck obstruction, or stenosing peptic ulcers.
methdilazine (Dilosyn†, Tacaryl) *Allergic rhinitis; pruritus —* **Adults:** 8 mg P.O. b.i.d. to q.i.d.; or 7.2 mg (chewable tablets) P.O. b.i.d. to q.i.d. **Children over age 3:** 4 mg P.O. b.i.d. to q.i.d.; or 3.6 mg (chewable tablets) P.O. b.i.d. to q.i.d.	• Contraindicated in acute asthmatic attacks. • Use cautiously in elderly or debilitated patients; acutely ill or dehydrated children; and in patients with a history of seizures; pulmonary, hepatic, or CV disease; asthma; hypertension; prostatic hypertrophy; bladder-neck obstruction; CNS depression; or stenosing peptic ulcers.
promethazine (Histantil†, Phenazine, Phenergan, Prothazine‡) *Motion sickness —* **Adults:** 25 mg P.O. b.i.d. **Children:** 1 mg/kg P.O., I.M., or rectally b.i.d. *Nausea —* **Adults:** 12.5 to 25 mg P.O., I.M., or rectally q 4 hours p.r.n. **Children:** 1 mg/kg I.M. or rectally q 4 to 6 hours p.r.n.	• Contraindicated in patients with increased intraocular pressure, intestinal obstruction, prostatic hypertrophy, bladder-neck obstruction, seizure disorder, bone marrow depression, coma, CNS depression, or stenosing peptic ulcers and in neonates and acutely ill or dehydrated children.

†Available in Canada only   ‡Available in Australia only   ◇ Available OTC

SELECTED MAJOR DRUGS: ANTIHISTAMINES *continued*

DRUG, INDICATIONS, AND DOSAGES	SPECIAL PRECAUTIONS
promethazine (Histanil†, Phenazine, Phenergan, Prothazine‡) *(continued)* *Rhinitis, allergy symptoms—* **Adults:** 12.5 mg P.O. q.i.d.; or 25 mg P.O. h.s. *Sedation—* **Adults:** 25 to 50 mg P.O., or I.M. h.s. or p.r.n. **Children:** 12.5 to 25 mg P.O., I.M., or rectally h.s. *Routine preoperative or postoperative sedation or as an adjunct to analgesics—* **Adults:** 25 to 50 mg I.M., I.V., or P.O. **Children:** 12.5 to 25 mg I.M., I.V., or P.O.	• Use cautiously in patients with pulmonary, hepatic, or CV disease; asthma; hypertension; bone marrow depression; in elderly or debilitated patients; or in patients with a history of seizures.
terfenadine (Seldane, Teldane‡) *Rhinitis, allergy symptoms—* **Adults and children over age 12:** 60 mg P.O. b.i.d. **Children ages 6 to 12:** 30 to 60 mg P.O. b.i.d. **Children ages 3 to 5:** 15 mg P.O. b.i.d.	• Contraindicated in patients with known hypersensitivity to terfenadine or any of its ingredients. • Administer cautiously to pregnant or breast-feeding women and children under age 12 because of risk of carcinogenesis, mutagenesis, and impaired fertility.
trimeprazine (Panectyl†, Temaril) *Pruritus—* **Adults:** 2.5 mg P.O. q.i.d.; or 5 mg (timed-release) P.O. b.i.d. **Children ages 3 to 12:** 2.5 mg P.O. h.s. or t.i.d. p.r.n. **Children ages 6 months to 3 years:** 1.25 mg P.O. h.s. or t.i.d. p.r.n. *Note:* Children under age 12 should use only as directed by a doctor.	• Contraindicated in acute asthmatic attacks. • Use cautiously in patients with pulmonary, hepatic, or CV disease; asthma; hypertension; narrow-angle glaucoma; intestinal obstruction; prostatic hypertrophy; bladder-neck obstruction; seizure disorder; bone marrow depression; coma; CNS depression; and stenosing peptic ulcers; in elderly or debilitated patients; or in acutely ill or dehydrated children.
tripelennamine (PBZ, Pelamine) *Rhinitis, allergy symptoms—* **Adults:** 25 to 50 mg P.O. q 4 to 6 hours; or 100 mg (timed-release) P.O. Maximum dosage is 600 mg daily. **Children:** 5 mg/kg P.O. daily in four to six divided doses. Maximum dosage is 300 mg daily.	• Contraindicated in acute asthmatic attacks. • Use cautiously in elderly patients and in patients with increased intraocular pressure, hyperthyroidism, CV or renal disease, hypertension, bronchial asthma, urine retention, prostatic hypertrophy, bladder-neck obstruction, or stenosing peptic ulcers.

†Available in Canada only ‡Available in Australia only

COMPARING ANTIHISTAMINE COMBINATIONS

TRADE NAME AND CONTENT	SPECIAL CONSIDERATIONS
Chlor-Trimeton Decongestant Repetabs ◊ chlorpheniramine maleate 8 mg and pseudoephedrine sulfate 120 mg **Co-Pyronil 2 Pulvules** ◊ **Deconamine** **Dura-Tap/PD** **Fedahist** ◊ **Isoclor** ◊ **Klerist-D** **Napril** ◊ **Pseudo-gest Plus** ◊ **Sudafed Plus** ◊ chlorpheniramine maleate 4 mg and pseudoephedrine sulfate 60 mg	• Combine the antihistamine effect of chlorpheniramine with the sympathomimetic effect of pseudoephedrine. The antihistamine is used to relieve runny nose, itching throat, coughing, sneezing, and watery eyes; the sympathomimetic, to relieve nasal congestion. • Antihistamines may cause a thickening of bronchial secretions and therefore may worsen conditions associated with congestion. They also can cause drowsiness; patients should avoid driving and other hazardous activities that require alertness. • Sympathomimetics should not be used in patients with a history of hypertension.
Actagen ◊ **Actifed** ◊ **Allerfrin** ◊ **Aprodrine** ◊ **Cenafed Plus** ◊ **Genac** ◊ **Trifed** **Triposed** ◊ triprolidine hydrochloride 2.5 mg and pseudoephedrine hydrochloride 60 mg	• Combines the antihistamine effect of triprolidine with the sympathomimetic effect of pseudoephedrine. The antihistamine is used to relieve runny nose, itching throat, coughing, sneezing, and watery eyes; the sympathomimetic, to relieve nasal congestion. • Antihistamines may cause a thickening of bronchial secretions and therefore may worsen conditions that are associated with congestion. They also can cause drowsiness; patients should avoid driving and other hazardous activities that require alertness. • Sympathomimetics should not be used in patients with a history of hypertension.

◊ Available OTC

SELF-TEST

1. Marge Smith, age 52, develops allergic rhinitis. Her doctor prescribes diphenhydramine 25 mg P.O. t.i.d. The nurse should tell Mrs. Smith to watch for which of the following adverse reactions?
   a. Hyperactivity and nervousness
   b. Drowsiness
   c. Orthostatic hypotension
   d. Polyuria

2. If Mrs. Smith were receiving an I.M. antihistamine, such as diphenhydramine, a concern regarding administration would be:
   a. administering the medication before breakfast.
   b. noting the sites used for previous injections.
   c. obtaining a syringe with a 1/2" needle.
   d. checking with the doctor regarding Mrs. Smith's hypotension.

3. Mrs. Smith is scheduled for allergy skin tests. In preparation, her nurse should:
   a. hold the patient's medications for 1 day of testing.
   b. give all medications orally the day of testing.
   c. discontinue the patient's antihistamine 4 days before testing.
   d. administer all medications as usual.

Check your answers on pages 1067 and 1068.

CHAPTER 43

BRONCHODILATORS

Adrenergics
albuterol sulfate ✦ bitolterol mesylate ✦ ephedrine ✦ ephedrine sulfate
ephedrine hydrochloride ✦ epinephrine hydrochloride
ethylnorepinephrine hydrochloride ✦ isoetharine
isoetharine hydrochloride ✦ isoetharine mesylate ✦ isoproterenol
isoproterenol hydrochloride ✦ isoproterenol sulfate
metaproterenol sulfate ✦ pirbuterol acetate ✦ terbutaline sulfate

Anticholinergics
atropine sulfate ✦ ipratropium bromide

Methylxanthines
aminophylline ✦ dyphylline ✦ theophylline
theophylline sodium glycinate

OVERVIEW

- Bronchodilators are used for patients with respiratory diseases, including asthma, bronchitis, and emphysema. Adrenergics (also called sympathomimetics), anticholinergics, and methylxanthines are used in the maintenance therapy of patients with bronchospastic illness; only methylxanthines and adrenergics are used in the emergency treatment of bronchospasm.
- Bronchodilators are classified primarily into adrenergics, anticholinergics, and methylxanthines.

MAJOR USES

- All of these drugs are used to prevent bronchospasm associated with COPD. Because they prevent bronchoconstriction rather than cause bronchodilation, regular use of anticholinergics is effective in the prophylaxis of COPD, but not in the emergency treatment of bronchospasm.

MECHANISM OF ACTION

- Anticholinergics block muscarinic receptors. The bronchodilating agents are administered by inhalation, minimizing absorption into the systemic circulation and thereby decreasing systemic effects. They are useful in preventing vagally mediated bronchoconstriction and are used for prophylaxis of an asthmatic attack rather than treatment of acute bronchoconstriction.
- Adrenergics and methylxanthines cause bronchodilation by acting on the smooth muscle of the bronchial tree. Adrenergic agents act on beta$_2$-ad-

GLOSSARY

Bronchoconstriction: narrowing of the bronchi, resulting in increased airway resistance and decreased airflow in conducting airways.
Bronchodilation: state of relaxed bronchiolar smooth muscle cells, resulting in a widened lumen of the bronchi and bronchioles.
Bronchodilator: substance that relaxes the bronchioles.
Bronchorrhea: excessive secretions from the bronchial mucous membrane.
Methylxanthine: drug group that includes caffeine and theophylline, which act on the CNS.

renergic receptors. When stimulated, these receptors increase the cellular activity of adenylate cyclase, an enzyme that catalyzes the conversion of cellular adenosine triphosphate (ATP) to adenosine 3':5'-cyclic monophosphate (cyclic AMP; cAMP), an intracellular messenger. Cyclic AMP enhances cellular calcium flux, facilitating relaxation of bronchial smooth muscle.

- Aminophylline, also known as theophylline ethylenediamine, is a theophylline salt. This derivative releases free theophylline, which is responsible for the drug's actions, in the plasma. Caffeine and dyphylline are methylxanthine derivatives; they do not release free theophylline. Methylxanthines inhibit phosphodiesterase, the enzyme that breaks down cyclic AMP. They also block adenosine receptors, which may be responsible for some of the drugs' bronchodilating actions. Additionally, they stimulate the respiratory center in the brain, increasing the rate and depth of respiration.

ABSORPTION, DISTRIBUTION, METABOLISM, AND EXCRETION

Anticholinergics are administered by inhalation, limiting their dosage and availability for systemic absorption. Ipratropium is not well absorbed because it is a quaternary ammonium compound. Some of the drug may be swallowed after administration, but it usually is excreted unchanged in the feces.

Methylxanthines are usually well absorbed from the GI tract. Rectal absorption is variable. These drugs are widely distributed, and therapeutic blood levels are well established for theophylline (10 to 20 mcg/ml; higher levels are usually associated with toxicity). Methylxanthines are metabolized in the liver. These metabolites are excreted in the urine.

Most adrenergics are well absorbed from the GI tract and are widely distributed. Some agents, such as albuterol, do not enter the CNS. These drugs are metabolized in the liver and excreted in the urine as metabolites.

ONSET AND DURATION

Little information is available regarding the onset and duration of anticholinergics. Regular daily use of these drugs is required for maximal prophylactic effect.

The onset and duration of methylxanthines depend on serum blood levels. Both theophylline and aminophylline activity depend on serum theophylline levels. In most patients, blood levels of 10 to 20 mcg will produce adequate bronchodilation (some patients may respond at lower levels). Higher levels are associated with toxicity.

After I.V. administration, the onset of theophylline is usually less than 1 hour. For maximum therapeutic effects, a maintenance infusion of theophylline is usually given to patients with moderate to severe bronchospasm. With oral administration, the onset of action and peak drug levels vary according to the formulation of the drug used: immediate-release liquids and tablets provide peak blood levels within 3 to 6 hours; slow-release formulations may not produce peak levels for 8 to 12 hours.

The duration of effect is highly variable, depending on patient responsiveness, physical condition, age, and life-style.

The onset and duration of adrenergics also vary according to route of administration, pharmaceutical formulation, and dosage. (See *Adrenergic Bronchodilators: Pharmacokinetics.*)

ADVERSE REACTIONS

The adrenergic bronchodilators can produce numerous adverse reactions. The alpha agonists (ephedrine and epinephrine) commonly produce cardiovascular reactions, mainly an increase in blood pressure (an important risk in elderly and hypertensive patients), which may result in bradycardia and various degrees of AV block. They may also cause nausea, vomiting, sweating, piloerection, difficult urination, and headache.

The beta agonists (albuterol and bitolterol) frequently cause tachycardia, palpitations, and other arrhythmias. Metabolic reactions include hyperglycemia, increased metabolic rate, and acidosis. Respiratory reactions include increased perfusion of nonfunctioning portions of the lungs (as in COPD) and increased mucus production with development of mucus plugs. Other reactions may include tremor, vertigo, insomnia, sweating, headache, nausea, and vomiting.

The anticholinergics atropine and ipratropium most commonly cause dry mouth and blurred vision. Other reactions may include nausea, GI distress, dizziness, headache, and palpitations.

The methylxanthines aminophylline, dyphylline, and theophylline stimulate the heart and CNS while relaxing smooth muscle, thereby producing adverse reactions that may include hypotension, palpitations, arrhythmias, irritability, nausea and vomiting, urine retention, and headache. Adverse reactions are dose-related and can be controlled by dosage adjustment and monitored via serum theophylline levels.

ADRENERGIC BRONCODILATORS: PHARMACOKINETICS

DRUG	ROUTE	ONSET	PEAK	DURATION
albuterol	inhalation	5 to 15 minutes	30 minutes to 2 hours	3 to 4 hours
	oral	30 minutes	2 to 3 minutes	4 to 6 hours
bitolterol	inhalation	3 to 4 minutes	unknown	5 to 8 hours
ephedrine	oral, nasal	15 to 60 minutes	unknown	2 to 4 hours
	I.V., I.M., S.C.	rapid	rapid	1 hour
epinephrine	S.C.	6 to 15 minutes	variable	1 to 4 hours
	I.M.	variable	variable	1 to 4 hours
	inhalation	3 to 5 minutes	variable	1 to 3 hours
ethylnorepineph-rine	S.C., I.M.	1 to 3 minutes	< 1 hour	1 to 2 hours
isoetharine	inhalation	1 minute	5 to 15 minutes	1 to 4 hours
isoproterenol	S.L.	15 to 30 minutes	variable	1 to 3 hours
	I.V.	immediate	variable	< 1 hour
	inhalation	2 to 5 minutes	variable	0.5 to 2 hours
metaproterenol	oral	15 minutes	1 hour	3 to 4 hours
pirbuterol	inhalation	< 5 minutes	unknown	5 hours
terbutaline	oral	30 minutes	1 to 2 hours	4 to 8 hours
	inhalation	5 to 30 minutes	30 to 60 minutes	3 to 6 hours
	S.C.	5 to 15 minutes	30 to 60 minutes	1.5 to 4 hours

EPINEPHRINE HYDROCHLORIDE
(ep i nef' rin)
Adrenalin Chloride◊, EpiPen, EpiPen Jr., Sus-Phrine
Classification: adrenergic
Pregnancy risk category C

How supplied
AEROSOL INHALER: 160 mcg◊, 200 mcg◊, 250 mcg/metered spray◊
NEBULIZER INHALER: 1% (1:100)†◊, 1.25%†◊, 2.25%†◊
INJECTION: 0.01 mg/ml (1:100,000), 0.1 mg/ml (1:10,000), 0.5 mg/ml (1:2,000), 1 mg/ml (1:1,000) parenteral; 5 mg/ml (1:200) parenteral suspension

Indications and dosage
Bronchospasm, hypersensitivity reactions, anaphylaxis
ADULTS: 0.1 to 0.5 ml of 1:1,000 solution S.C. or I.M., repeated q 10 to 15 minutes p.r.n.; or 0.1 to 0.25 ml of 1:1,000 solution I.V.
CHILDREN: 0.01 ml (10 mcg) of 1:1,000 solution/kg S.C., repeated q 20 minutes to 4 hours p.r.n.; or 0.005 ml/kg of 1:200 (Sus-Phrine), repeated q 8 to 12 hours p.r.n.

Hemostasis
ADULTS: 1:50,000 to 1:1,000, applied topically.

Acute asthmatic attacks (inhalation)
ADULTS AND CHILDREN: 1 or 2 inhalations of 1:100 or 2.25% racemic solution q 1 to 5 minutes until relief is obtained; usual dose contains 0.2 mg.

To prolong local anesthetic effect
ADULTS AND CHILDREN: 0.2 to 0.4 ml of 1:1,000 solution intraspinal; 1:500,000 to 1:50,000 solution mixed with local anesthetic and infiltrated in affected area.

To restore cardiac rhythm in cardiac arrest
ADULTS: 0.5 to 1 mg I.V. or into endotracheal tube. May be given intracardiac if no I.V. route or intratracheal route available. Some clinicians advocate a higher dose (up to 5 mg), especially in patients who don't respond to usual I.V. dose. After initial I.V. administration, may be infused I.V. at a rate of 1 to 4 mcg/minute.
CHILDREN: 10 mcg/kg I.V. or 5 to 10 mcg/kg (0.05 to 0.1 ml of 1:10,000/kg) intracardiac.
Note: 1 mg = 1 ml of 1:1,000 or 10 ml of 1:10,000.

Contraindications and precautions
Epinephrine is contraindicated in narrow-angle glaucoma, shock (other than anaphylactic shock), organic brain damage, cardiac dilation, or coronary insufficiency. It is also contraindicated during general anesthesia

---

with halogenated hydrocarbons or cyclopropane and in labor (may delay second stage). Use with extreme caution in patients with long-standing bronchial asthma and emphysema who have developed degenerative heart disease. Use cautiously in elderly patients and in those with hyperthyroidism, angina, hypertension, psychoneurosis, and diabetes.

Adverse reactions
CNS: *nervousness,* tremor, euphoria, anxiety, coldness of extremities, vertigo, *headache,* sweating, disorientation, agitation; increased rigidity and tremor (in patients with Parkinson's disease).
CV: *palpitations;* widened pulse pressure; hypertension; *tachycardia;* **ventricular fibrillation; CVA;** anginal pain; ECG changes, including a decrease in the T wave amplitude.
METABOLIC: *hyperglycemia,* glycosuria.
OTHER: pulmonary edema, dyspnea, *pallor.*

Interactions
Alpha-adrenergic blockers: hypotension due to unopposed beta-adrenergic effects. Avoid concomitant use.
Beta blockers, such as propranolol: vasoconstriction and reflex bradycardia. Monitor the patient carefully.
Digitalis glycosides, general anesthetics (halogenated hydrocarbons): increased risk of ventricular arrhythmias. Avoid concomitant use.
Doxapram, mazindol, methylphenidate: enhanced CNS stimulation or pressor effects. Avoid concomitant use.
Ergot alkaloids: enhanced vasoconstrictor activity. Avoid concomitant use.
Guanadrel, guanethidine: enhanced pressor effects of epinephrine. Avoid concomitant use.
Levodopa: enhanced risk of cardiac arrhythmias. Monitor closely.
MAO inhibitors: increased risk of hypertensive crisis. Monitor closely.
Tricyclic antidepressants, antihistamines, thyroid hormones: when given with adrenergics, may cause severe adverse cardiac reactions. Avoid giving together.

Nursing considerations
Assessment
• Review the patient's history for a condition that contraindicates the use of epinephrine.
• Obtain a baseline assessment of the patient's cardiopulmonary status by assessing the patient's vital signs, ECG (if ordered), and lung sounds before therapy.
• Be alert for common adverse reactions.
• Evaluate the patient's and family's knowledge about epinephrine therapy.

Planning (Nursing Diagnoses)
Potential nursing diagnoses for the patient receiving epinephrine include:
• Altered health maintenance related to ineffectiveness of epinephrine.
• Altered protection related to epinephrine-induced adverse reactions.
• Knowledge deficit related to epinephrine therapy.

Implementation

Preparation and administration

—Epinephrine should not be mixed with an alkaline solution. Use dextrose 5% in water (D_5W), 0.9% sodium chloride solution, or a combination of D_5W and 0.9% sodium chloride solution.

—Mix the solution just before using it.

—If bronchodilator is administered via inhalant and more than 1 inhalation is ordered, always wait 2 minutes between inhalations.

—If more than one type of inhalant is ordered, always administer the bronchodilator first and wait 5 minutes before administering the other.

—Remember that the patient should not receive more than 12 bronchodilator inhalations in 24 hours.

—Giving the medication on time is extremely important.

—Epinephrine is rapidly destroyed by oxidizing agents, such as iodine, chromates, nitrates, and salts of easily reducible metal (such as iron). Don't mix with other drugs, and don't use discolored solutions.

—Epinephrine solutions deteriorate after 24 hours. Discard the solution after that time, or earlier if the solution is discolored or contains precipitates.

—Store solution in a light-resistant container and do not remove it before use.

—Massage the injection site to counteract possible vasoconstriction.

—Avoid repeated injections at the same site. Repeated local injections can cause local vasoconstriction and necrosis at the site.

—Avoid I.M. administration of oil injection into the buttocks. Gas gangrene may occur because epinephrine reduces oxygen tension of the tissues, encouraging the growth of contaminating organisms.

—Administer the medication around the clock for greatest effectiveness.

Monitoring

—Monitor the effectiveness of therapy by regularly checking the patient's vital signs, ECG pattern (if applicable), and lung sounds. Note changes such as widened pulse pressure, elevated blood pressure, tachycardia, ventricular fibrillation, ECG changes, dyspnea, and crackles in lung fields.

—Monitor for distended neck veins, peripheral edema, and sudden weight gain suggestive of fluid retention.

—Monitor the patient for adverse drug reactions.

—When administered I.V., monitor blood pressure, heart rate, and ECG at start of therapy and frequently thereafter.

—Monitor blood glucose levels regularly because drug may cause hyperglycemia.

—Monitor patients with Parkinson's disease for increased rigidity and tremor.

—Monitor the patient for drug interactions.

—Regularly reevaluate the patient's and family's knowledge about epinephrine therapy.

Intervention

— If blood pressure rises sharply, rapid-acting vasodilators, such as nitrates or alpha-adrenergic blockers, can be given to counteract the marked pressor effects of large doses of epinephrine.

— Hold dose and notify the doctor if CV symptoms, such as palpitations, hypertension, tachycardia, or anginal pain, occur. Also report signs and symptoms of pulmonary edema.

— Notify the doctor if the patient's pulse increases by 20% or more when epinephrine is administered.

— Keep all members of the health care team informed of the patient's response to the drug.

Patient teaching

— Instruct the patient and family about epinephrine, including the dosage, frequency, action, and adverse reactions.

— Tell the patient to always take the medication exactly as prescribed and to take it around the clock.

— Instruct the patient to perform oral inhalation correctly as follows: Clear nasal passages and throat. Breathe out, expelling as much air from the lungs as possible. Place the mouthpiece well into the mouth as the dose from the inhaler is released, and inhale deeply. Hold breath for several seconds, remove the mouthpiece, and exhale slowly.

— If more than one inhalation is ordered, tell the patient to wait at least 2 minutes before repeating the procedure for a second dose.

— Explain why it is necessary to use the bronchodilator first if other inhalants such as a steroid inhaler are prescribed. This allows the bronchodilator to open air passages for maximum effectiveness. Allow 5 minutes between the inhalant treatments.

— Warn the patient to avoid accidentally spraying the inhalant into the eyes, which may cause temporary blurring of vision.

— Tell the patient to reduce the intake of foods containing caffeine, such as coffee, colas, and chocolates, when taking a bronchodilator.

— Instruct the patient to contact the doctor immediately if he experiences a "fluttering" of the heart, rapid beating of the heart, shortness of breath, or chest pain.

— Tell the elderly patient that dizziness may occur at start of the therapy. Therefore, he should take precautions to avoid injury from falls.

— Tell the patient not to self-medicate with any OTC drugs without medical approval while taking this drug.

— Warn the patient against increasing the dosage or frequency of administration. Advise the patient to notify the doctor if the prescribed dosage does not relieve symptoms.

— Show the patient how to check the pulse. Instruct him to check the pulse before and after using a bronchodilator and to call the doctor if his pulse increases more than 20 to 30 beats/minute.

— The patient who has an acute hypersensitivity reaction may require instruction for self-injection of epinephrine at home.

—Tell the patient to notify the nurse or doctor if adverse reactions develop or questions arise about epinephrine therapy.

Evaluation
In the patient receiving epinephrine, appropriate evaluation statements include:
• Patient's cardiopulmonary signs and symptoms are relieved by epinephrine.
• Patient does not experience serious adverse reactions during therapy.
• Patient and family state an understanding of epinephrine therapy.

PROTOTYPE: ANTICHOLINERGICS

IPRATROPIUM BROMIDE
(i pra troe' pee um)
Atrovent
Classification: anticholinergic
Pregnancy risk category B

How supplied
INHALER: each metered dose supplies 18 mcg
SOLUTION FOR NEBULIZER: 0.025% (250 mcg/ml)‡

Indications and dosage
Maintenance treatment of bronchospasm associated with COPD
ADULTS: 2 inhalations (26 mcg) q.i.d. Additional inhalations may be needed. However, total inhalations should not exceed 12 in 24 hours.

Contraindications and precautions
Ipratropium is contraindicated in patients allergic to atropine or its derivatives. Use cautiously in patients with narrow-angle glaucoma, prostatic hypertrophy, or bladder-neck obstruction.

Adverse reactions
CNS: nervousness, dizziness, headache.
CV: palpitations.
EENT: *cough,* blurred vision.
GI: nausea, GI distress, dry mouth.
SKIN: rash.

Interactions
None significant.

Nursing considerations
Assessment
• Review the patient's history for a condition that contraindicates the use of ipratropium.

---

‡Available in Australia only
Italicized adverse reactions are common

- Obtain a baseline assessment of the patient's bronchospasms before initiating therapy.
- Be alert for common adverse reactions.
- Evaluate the patient's and family's knowledge about ipratropium therapy.

Planning (Nursing Diagnoses)
Potential nursing diagnoses for the patient receiving ipratropium include:
- Impaired gas exchange related to ineffectiveness of ipratropium to relieve bronchospasm.
- Sensory/perceptual alterations (visual) related to adverse reaction to ipratropium.
- Knowledge deficit related to ipratropium therapy.

Implementation
Preparation and administration
— The inhalations are usually given q.i.d. Additional inhalations may be needed, but total inhalations should not exceed 12 in 24 hours.
— If the bronchodilator is administered via inhalant and more than one inhalation is ordered, 2 minutes should elapse between inhalations.
— If more than one type of inhalant is ordered, always administer bronchodilator first and wait 5 minutes before administering the other.
— Make sure to give the medication on time to ensure maximal effect.

Monitoring
— Monitor the effectiveness of therapy by regularly assessing the patient's lung fields for bronchospasm.
— Monitor for blurred vision.
— Monitor the patient for adverse drug reactions.
— Regularly reevaluate the patient's and family's knowledge about ipratropium therapy.

Intervention
— Notify the doctor if bronchospasms are not relieved with ipratropium.
— Institute safety precautions if blurred vision or dizziness occurs.
— Remember that ipratropium is not effective for treatment of acute episodes of bronchospasm when rapid response is required.
— Keep all members of the health care team informed of the patient's response to the drug.

Patient teaching
— Instruct the patient and family about ipratropium, including the dosage, frequency, action, and adverse reactions.
— Tell the patient to always take the medication exactly as prescribed and to take it around the clock.
— Instruct the patient to perform oral inhalation correctly as follows: Clear nasal passages and throat. Breathe out, expelling as much air from the lungs as possible. Place the mouthpiece well into the mouth as the dose from the inhaler is released, and inhale deeply. Hold breath for several seconds, remove the mouthpiece, and exhale slowly.

— If more than 1 inhalation is ordered, tell the patient to wait at least 2 minutes before repeating the procedure for a second dose.

— Explain why it is necessary to use the bronchodilator first if other inhalants such as a steroid inhaler are prescribed. This allows the bronchodilator to open air passages for maximum effectiveness. Allow 5 minutes between the inhalant treatments.

— Warn the patient to avoid accidentally spraying the inhalant into the eyes, which may cause temporary blurring of vision.

— Tell the patient to reduce the intake of foods containing caffeine, such as coffee, colas, and chocolates, when taking a bronchodilator.

— Warn the patient to contact the doctor immediately if he experiences a "fluttering" of the heart, rapid beating of the heart, shortness of breath, or chest pain.

— Tell elderly patients that dizziness may occur at the start of therapy. Therefore, they should take precautions to avoid injury from falls.

— Tell the patient not to self-medicate with any OTC drugs without medical approval while taking this drug.

— Warn the patient against increasing the dosage or frequency of administration. Advise the patient to notify the doctor if prescribed dosage does not relieve symptoms.

— Show the patient how to check the pulse. Instruct the patient to check his pulse before and after using a bronchodilator and to call the doctor if his pulse increases more than 20 to 30 beats/minute.

— The patient who has an acute hypersensitivity reaction may require instruction for self-injection of ipratropium at home.

— Warn the patient that this drug is not effective in the treatment of acute episodes of bronchospasm when rapid response is required.

— Tell the patient to notify the nurse or doctor if adverse reactions develop or questions arise about ipratropium therapy.

Evaluation

In the patient receiving ipratropium, appropriate evaluation statements include:

• Patient's bronchospasms are relieved by ipratropium.
• Patient's vision is unaffected by ipratropium therapy.
• Patient and family verbalize an understanding of ipratropium therapy.

THEOPHYLLINE
(thee off´ i lin)
Accurbron*, Aerolate, Aquaphyllin, Asmalix*, Bronkodyl S-R,
Bronkodyl*, Constant-T, Duraphyl, Elixicon, Elixomin*, Elixophyllin
SR, Elixophyllin*, Lanophyllin*, Lixolin, Lodrane, Nuelin-SR‡,
Nuelin‡, Quibron-T/SR, Respbid, Slo-bid Gyrocaps, Slo-Phyllin,
Somophyllin-T, Somophyllin-CRT, Sustaire, Theo-Dur, Theo-Dur
Sprinkle, Theo-Time, Theo-24, Theobid Duracaps, Theobid Jr.,
Theochron, Theolair-SR, Theolair, Theon*, Theophyl-SR, Theospan SR,
Theovent Long-acting, Uniphyl

THEOPHYLLINE SODIUM GLYCINATE
Acet-Am†, Synophylate
Classification: methylxanthine
Pregnancy risk category C

How supplied
theophylline
TABLETS: 100 mg, 125 mg, 200 mg, 225 mg, 250 mg, 300 mg
TABLETS (CHEWABLE): 100 mg
TABLETS (EXTENDED-RELEASE): 100 mg, 200 mg, 250 mg, 300 mg, 400 mg, 500 mg
CAPSULES: 50 mg, 100 mg, 200 mg, 250 mg
CAPSULES (EXTENDED-RELEASE): 50 mg, 60 mg, 65 mg, 75 mg, 100 mg, 125 mg, 130 mg, 200 mg, 250 mg, 260 mg, 300 mg
ELIXIR: 27 mg/5 ml, 50 mg/5 ml
ORAL SOLUTION: 27 mg/5 ml, 53 mg/5 ml
ORAL SUSPENSION: 100 mg/5 ml
SYRUP: 27 mg/5 ml, 50 mg/5 ml
DEXTROSE 5% INJECTION: 200 mg in 50 ml or 100 ml; 400 mg in 100 ml, 250 ml, 500 ml, or 1,000 ml; 800 mg in 500 ml or 1,000 ml
theophylline sodium glycinate
ELIXIR: 110 mg/5 ml (equivalent to 55 mg anhydrous theophylline/5 ml)

Indications and dosage
Prophylaxis and symptomatic relief of bronchial asthma,
bronchospasm of chronic bronchitis, and emphysema
ADULTS: 6 mg/kg P.O. followed by 2 to 3 mg/kg q 4 hours for two doses. Maintenance dosage is 1 to 3 mg/kg q 8 to 12 hours.
CHILDREN AGES 9 TO 16: 6 mg/kg P.O. followed by 3 mg/kg q 4 hours for three doses. Maintenance dosage is 3 mg/kg q 6 hours.

CHILDREN AGES 6 MONTHS TO 9 YEARS: 6 mg/kg P.O. followed by 4 mg/kg q 4 hours for three doses. Maintenance dosage is 4 mg/kg q 6 hours.

Most oral timed-release forms are given q 8 hours. Several products, however, may be given q 24 hours.

Symptomatic relief of bronchial asthma, pulmonary emphysema, and chronic bronchitis

ADULTS: 330 to 660 mg (sodium glycinate) P.O. q 6 to 8 hours after meals.
CHILDREN OVER AGE 12: 220 to 330 mg (sodium glycinate) P.O. q 6 to 8 hours.
CHILDREN AGES 6 TO 12: 330 mg (sodium glycinate) P.O. q 6 hours.
CHILDREN AGES 3 TO 6: 110 to 165 mg (sodium glycinate) P.O. q 6 to 8 hours.

Parenteral theophylline for patient not currently receiving theophylline

ADULTS: loading dose is 4.7 mg/kg I.V. slowly, then maintenance infusion.
ADULTS (NONSMOKERS): 0.55 mg/kg/hour for 12 hours, then 0.35 mg/kg/hour.
OTHERWISE HEALTHY ADULT SMOKERS: 0.79 mg/kg/hour for 12 hours, then 0.63 mg/kg/hour.
OLDER ADULTS WITH COR PULMONALE: 0.47 mg/kg/hour for 12 hours, then 0.24 mg/kg/hour.
ADULTS WITH CHF OR LIVER DISEASE: 0.38 mg/kg/hour for 12 hours, then 0.08 to 0.16 mg/kg/hour.
CHILDREN AGES 9 TO 16: 0.79 mg/kg/hour for 12 hours, then 0.63 mg/kg/hour.
CHILDREN AGES 6 MONTHS TO 9 YEARS: 0.95 mg/kg/hour for 12 hours, then 0.79 mg/kg/hour.

Switch to oral theophylline as soon as the patient shows adequate improvement.

Symptomatic relief of bronchospasm in patients currently receiving theophylline

ADULTS AND CHILDREN: each 0.5 mg/kg I.V. or P.O. (loading dose) will increase plasma levels by 1 mcg/ml. Ideally, dose is based on current theophylline level. In emergency situations, some clinicians recommend a 2.5 mg/kg P.O. dose of rapidly absorbed form if no obvious signs of theophylline toxicity are present.

Contraindications and precautions

Theophylline is contraindicated in patients with known hypersensitivity to xanthine compounds (caffeine, theobromine) and preexisting cardiac arrhythmias, especially tachyarrhythmias. Use cautiously in young children; elderly patients with CHF or other circulatory impairment, cor pulmonale, and renal or hepatic disease; and in peptic ulcer, hyperthyroidism, or diabetes mellitus.

Adverse reactions

CNS: *restlessness, dizziness,* headache, *insomnia,* light-headedness, *seizures,* muscle twitching.
CV: *palpitations,* sinus tachycardia, extrasystoles, flushing, marked hypotension, increase in respiratory rate.

Italicized adverse reactions are common

GI: *nausea, vomiting, anorexia,* bitter aftertaste, dyspepsia, heavy feeling in stomach, diarrhea.
SKIN: urticaria.

Interactions

Barbiturates, phenytoin, rifampin: enhanced metabolism and decreased theophylline blood levels. Monitor for decreased effect.
Beta-adrenergic blockers: antagonism. Propranolol and nadolol, especially, may cause bronchospasms in sensitive patients. Use together cautiously.
Erythromycin, troleandomycin, cimetidine, influenza virus vaccine, oral contraceptives: decreased hepatic clearance of theophylline; increased plasma levels. Monitor for signs of toxicity.

Nursing considerations

Assessment
• Review the patient's history for a condition that contraindicates the use of theophylline.
• Obtain a baseline assessment of the patient's respiratory status before initiating therapy.
• Be alert for common adverse reactions.
• Evaluate the patient's and family's knowledge about theophylline therapy.

Planning (Nursing Diagnoses)
Potential nursing diagnoses for the patient receiving theophylline include:
• Impaired gas exchange related to ineffectiveness of theophylline.
• Fluid volume deficit related to theophylline-induced adverse GI reactions.
• Knowledge deficit related to theophylline therapy.

Implementation
Preparation and administration
— Do not crush extended-release tablets.
— Keep in mind the following dosage guidelines: If theophylline levels are less than 10 mcg/ml, increase dose by about 25% each day. If levels are 20 to 25 mcg/ml, decrease dose by about 10% each day. If levels are 25 to 30 mcg/ml, skip next dose and decrease by 25% each day. If levels are over 30 mcg/ml, skip next two doses and decrease by 50% each day. Repeat serum level determination.
— GI symptoms may be relieved by taking oral drug with full glass of water after meals, although food in stomach delays absorption.
— Habitual cigarette or marijuana smokers may require increased drug dosage because smoking causes the drug to be metabolized faster.
— Be careful not to confuse sustained-release dosage forms with standard-release dosage forms.
— Patients taking Theo-24 brand of theophylline should take it on an empty stomach because food accelerates the drug's absorption.
— Give drug around the clock, using sustained-release product at bedtime as prescribed.

Italicized adverse reactions are common

—Administer I.V. theophylline exactly as prescribed; use infusion pump when administering continuous infusions.

Monitoring

—Monitor the effectiveness of therapy by regularly assessing the patient's respiratory status, especially to evaluate if bronchospasms have been relieved.

—Monitor vital signs; measure and record intake and output. Expected clinical effects include improvement in quality of pulse and respiration.

—Monitor the patient for adverse drug reactions.

—Monitor hydration status if the patient develops GI reactions.

—Monitor serum theophylline measurements, especially in long-term therapy; ideally, levels should be between 10 and 20 mcg/ml. Check levels every 6 months.

—Monitor the patient for drug interactions.

—Regularly reevaluate the patient's and family's knowledge about theophylline therapy.

Intervention

—Notify the doctor if the patient's respiratory status does not improve with theophylline therapy.

—Institute safety precautions if adverse CNS reactions occur.

—Institute seizure precautions until adverse CNS reactions are known.

—Obtain an order for an antiemetic or antidiarrheal if GI reactions occur.

—Help the patient identify nonpharmacologic ways to manage insomnia; if ineffective, obtain an order for a hypnotic.

—Administer a mild analgesic as prescribed for theophylline-induced headache.

—Be prepared to treat theophylline toxicity. Clinical manifestations of overdose include nausea, vomiting, insomnia, irritability, tachycardia, extrasystoles, tachypnea, or tonic-clonic seizures. The onset of toxicity may be sudden and severe, with arrhythmias and seizures as the first signs. Induce emesis except in patients experiencing seizures, then use activated charcoal and cathartics. Treat arrhythmias with lidocaine and seizures with I.V. diazepam; support respiratory tract and CV systems.

—Keep all members of the health care team informed of the patient's response to the drug.

Patient teaching

—Instruct the patient and family about theophylline, including the dosage, frequency, action, and adverse reactions.

—Instruct the patient regarding medication and dosage schedule; if a dose is missed, tell the patient to take it as soon as possible, but not to double up on doses.

—Tell the patient to take the drug at regular intervals as instructed and around the clock.

—Advise the patient of possible signs of toxicity.

—Tell the patient to avoid eating and drinking large quantities of xanthine-containing foods and beverages.

—Warn the elderly patient of dizziness, a common reaction at start of therapy.

—If the patient experiences GI upset with liquid preparations or immediate-release forms, tell him to take the drug with food.

—Warn the patient that OTC remedies may contain ephedrine in combination with theophylline salts; excessive CNS stimulation may result. Tell him to check with the doctor or pharmacist before taking any other medications.

—Warn the patient not to dissolve, crush, or chew slow-release products. To help small children unable to swallow these products to ingest them without chewing, sprinkle the contents of bead-filled capsules over soft food.

—Warn the patient to take the drug regularly, as directed. Patients tend to want to take extra doses.

—Stress the importance of follow-up care and of having theophylline levels checked regularly.

—Tell the patient to notify the nurse or doctor if adverse reactions develop or questions arise about theophylline therapy.

Evaluation

In the patient receiving theophylline, appropriate evaluation statements include:

• Patient's respiratory status is improved with theophylline therapy.

• Patient does not experience adverse GI reactions and maintains adequate hydration.

• Patient and family state an understanding of theophylline therapy.

SELECTED MAJOR DRUGS: BRONCHODILATORS

DRUG, INDICATIONS, AND DOSAGES	SPECIAL PRECAUTIONS
Adrenergics	
albuterol (Proventil, Respolin‡) *Prevention and treatment of bronchospasm in patients with reversible obstructive airway disease—* **Adults and children over age 13:** 1 to 2 inhalations q 4 to 6 hours. More frequent administration or a greater number of inhalations is not recommended. Usual dosage range is 10 to 50 mcg/minute. Or 2 to 4 mg (tablets) P.O. t.i.d. or q.i.d. Maximum dosage is 8 mg q.i.d. (tablets) or 16 mg b.i.d. (extended-release tablets). **Children ages 6 to 13:** 2 mg (1 tsp) P.O. t.i.d. or q.i.d. **Children ages 2 to 5:** 0.1 mg/kg P.O. t.i.d., not to exceed 2 mg (1 tsp) t.i.d. **Adults over age 65:** 2 mg P.O. t.i.d. or q.i.d. *To prevent exercise-induced asthma—* **Adults:** 2 inhalations 15 minutes before exercise.	• No contraindications listed. • Use cautiously in CV disorders, including coronary insufficiency and hypertension; in hyperthyroidism or diabetes mellitus; and in patients who are unusually responsive to adrenergics.

(continued)

SELECTED MAJOR DRUGS: BRONCHODILATORS *continued*

DRUG, INDICATIONS, AND DOSAGES	SPECIAL PRECAUTIONS

Adrenergics *(continued)*

albuterol *(continued)*
Prevention of premature labor‡ —
Adults: initially, 10 mcg/minute by continuous I.V. infusion (use an infusion pump). Dosage should be increased in 10-minute intervals until the desired response is achieved.

ephedrine (Ephed II, Fedrine†)
To correct hypotensive states; to support ventricular rate in Adams-Stokes syndrome—
Adults: 25 to 50 mg I.M. or S.C., or 10 to 25 mg I.V. p.r.n. to maximum of 150 mg daily.
Children: 3 mg/kg S.C. or I.V. daily in four to six divided doses.
Bronchodilator or nasal decongestant—
Adults: 12.5 to 50 mg P.O. b.i.d., t.i.d., or q.i.d. Maximum dosage is 400 mg daily in six to eight divided doses.
Children: 2 to 3 mg/kg P.O. daily in four to six divided doses.

• Contraindicated in porphyria, severe coronary artery disease, cardiac arrhythmias, narrow-angle glaucoma, or psychoneurosis and in patients taking MAO inhibitors.
• Use cautiously in elderly patients and in those with hypertension, hyperthyroidism, nervous or excitable states, CV disease, or prostatic hypertrophy.

isoetharine (Bronkosol)
Bronchial asthma and reversible bronchospasm that may occur with bronchitis and emphysema—
Adults: (hydrochloride) 3 to 7 inhalations by hand nebulizer, or 0.5 ml of 1:3 solution with 0.9% sodium chloride solution by oxygen aerosolization or IPPB.
Adults: (mesylate) 1 to 2 inhalations. Occasionally, more may be required.

• Contraindicated in patients hypersensitive to the drug or any of its ingredients.
• Use cautiously in hyperthyroidism, hypertension, or coronary disease and in sensitivity to sympathomimetics.

isoproterenol (Aerolone, Isuprel)
Bronchial asthma and reversible bronchospasm—
Adults: 10 to 20 mg (hydrochloride) S.L. q 6 to 8 hours.
Children: 5 to 10 mg (hydrochloride) S.L q 6 to 8 hours. Not recommended for children under age 6.
Acute dyspneic episodes of bronchospasm—
Adults and children: 1 inhalation (sulfate) initially. May repeat if needed after 2 to 5 minutes. Maintenance dosage is 1 to 2 inhalations q.i.d. to six times daily. May repeat once more 10 minutes after second dose. Not more than three doses should be administered for each attack.
Heart block and ventricular arrhythmias—
Adults: initially, 0.02 to 0.06 mg (hydrochloride) I.V. Subsequent doses 0.01 to 0.2 mg I.V. or 5 mcg/minute I.V.; or 0.2 mg I.M. initially, then 0.02 to 1 mg p.r.n.
Children: may give half of initial adult dose of isoproterenol hydrochloride.

• Contraindicated in recent MI, in tachycardia caused by digitalis intoxication, and in preexisting arrhythmias, especially tachycardia, because chronotropic effect on the heart may aggravate such disorders.
• Use cautiously in coronary insufficiency, diabetes, or hyperthyroidism.

---

†Available in Canada only   ‡Available in Australia only

SELECTED MAJOR DRUGS: BRONCHODILATORS *continued*

DRUG, INDICATIONS, AND DOSAGES	SPECIAL PRECAUTIONS

Adrenergics *(continued)*

isoproterenol *(continued)*
Shock—
Adults and children: 0.5 to 5 mcg/minute (hydrochloride) by continuous I.V. infusion. Usual concentration is 1 mg (5 ml) in 500 ml dextrose 5% in water. Adjust rate according to heart rate, central venous pressure, blood pressure, and urine flow.

metaproterenol (Alupent, Metaprel)
Acute episodes of bronchial asthma—
Adults and children: 2 to 3 inhalations. Should not repeat inhalations more often than q 3 to 4 hours. Should not exceed 12 inhalations daily.
Bronchial asthma and reversible bronchospasm—
Adults: 20 mg P.O. q 6 to 8 hours.
Children over age 9 or over 27 kg: 20 mg P.O. q 6 to 8 hours (0.4 to 0.9 mg/kg/dose t.i.d.).
Children ages 6 to 9 or less than 27 kg: 10 mg P.O. q 6 to 8 hours (0.4 to 0.9 mg/kg/dose t.i.d.).
Not recommended for children under age 6.

• Contraindicated in tachycardia and arrhythmias associated with tachycardia.
• Use with caution in hypertension, coronary artery disease, hyperthyroidism, and diabetes.

pirbuterol (Maxair)
Prevention and reversal of bronchospasm, asthma—
Adults: 1 or 2 inhalations (0.2 to 0.4 mg) repeated q 4 to 6 hours. Not to exceed 12 inhalations daily.

• Contraindicated in patients with known hypersensitivity to pirbuterol or other adrenergics, and in those with digitalis toxicity or cardiac arrhythmias associated with tachycardia.
• Administer cautiously to patients with CV disorders, including ischemic heart disease, hypertension, or cardiac arrhythmias; hyperthyroidism; diabetes mellitus; or seizure disorders.

terbutaline (Brethine, Bricanyl)
Relief of bronchospasm in patients with reversible obstructive airway disease—
Adults and children over age 11: 2 inhalations separated by a 60-second interval, repeated q 4 to 6 hours. May also administer 2.5 to 5 mg P.O. q 8 hours or 0.25 mg S.C.
Treatment of premature labor—
Women: 0.01 mg/minute by I.V. infusion. Increase by 0.005 mg q 10 minutes up to 0.025 mg/minute or until contractions cease. Or give 0.25 mg S.C. hourly until contractions cease. Maintenance dosage is 5 mg P.O. q 4 hours for 48 hours, then 5 mg q 6 hours.

• Contraindicated in known hypersensitivity to sympathomimetics.
• Use cautiously in patients with diabetes, hypertension, hyperthyroidism, severe cardiac disease, or cardiac arrhythmias.

(continued)

SELECTED MAJOR DRUGS: BRONCHODILATORS *continued*

| DRUG, INDICATIONS, AND DOSAGES | SPECIAL PRECAUTIONS |

Anticholinergics

atropine
Symptomatic bradycardia, bradyarrhythmia (junctional or escape rhythm)—
Adults: usually 0.5 to 1 mg I.V. push; repeat q 5 minutes to maximum of 2 mg. Lower doses (less than 0.5 mg) can cause bradycardia.
Children: 0.01 mg/kg I.V. dose up to maximum of 0.4 mg; or 0.3 mg/m² dose; may repeat q 4 to 6 hours.
Antidote for anticholinesterase insecticide poisoning—
Adults and children: 2 mg I.M. or I.V. repeated hourly until muscarinic symptoms disappear. Severe cases may require up to 6 mg I.M. or I.V. q 1 hour.
Preoperatively to diminish secretions and block cardiac vagal reflexes—
Adults: 0.4 to 0.6 mg I.M. 45 to 60 minutes before anesthesia.
Children: 0.01 mg/kg I.M. up to a maximum dose of 0.4 mg 45 to 60 minutes before anesthesia.
Adjunctive treatment of peptic ulcer disease; treatment of functional GI disorders such as irritable bowel syndrome—
Adults: 0.4 to 0.6 mg P.O. q 4 to 6 hours.
Children: 0.01 mg/kg or 0.3 mg/m² (not to exceed 0.4 mg) q 4 to 6 hours.

• Contraindicated in narrow-angle glaucoma, obstructive uropathy, obstructive disease of GI tract, myasthenia gravis, paralytic ileus, intestinal atony, unstable CV status in acute hemorrhage, and toxic megacolon.
• Use cautiously in patients with Down's syndrome.

Methylxanthines

aminophylline
Symptomatic relief of bronchospasm—
Patients not currently receiving theophylline who require rapid relief of symptoms: loading dose is 6 mg/kg (equivalent to 4.7 mg/kg anhydrous theophylline) I.V. slowly (less than or equal to 25 mg/kg minute), then maintenance infusion.
Adults (nonsmokers): 0.7 mg/kg/hour for 12 hours; then 0.5 mg/kg/hour.
Otherwise healthy adult smokers: 1 mg/kg/hour for 12 hours, then 0.18 mg/kg/hour.
Older patients and adults with cor pulmonale: 0.6 mg/kg/hour for 12 hours, then 0.3 mg/kg/hour.
Adults with CHF or liver disease: 0.5 mg/kg/hour for 12 hours, then 0.1 to 0.2 mg/kg/hour.
Children ages 9 to 16: 1 mg/kg/hour for 12 hours, then 0.8 mg/kg/hour.
Children ages 6 months to 9 years: 1.2 mg/kg/hour for 12 hours, then 1 mg/kg/hour.
Patients currently receiving theophylline: aminophylline infusions of 0.63 mg/kg (0.5 mg/kg anhydrous theophylline) will increase plasma levels of theophylline by 1 mcg/ml. Some clinicians recommend a dose of 3.1 mg/kg (2.5 mg/kg anhydrous theophylline) if no obvious signs of theophylline toxicity are present.

• Contraindicated in patients with known hypersensitivity to xanthine compounds (caffeine, theobromine) and in preexisting cardiac arrhythmias, especially tachyarrhythmias.
• Use cautiously in young children; in elderly patients with CHF or other cardiac or circulatory impairment, cor pulmonale, or hepatic disease; in active peptic ulcer because drug may increase volume and acidity of gastric secretions; and in hyperthyroidism or diabetes mellitus.

SELECTED MAJOR DRUGS: BRONCHODILATORS *continued*

DRUG, INDICATIONS, AND DOSAGES	SPECIAL PRECAUTIONS

Methylxanthines *(continued)*

aminophylline *(continued)*
Chronic bronchial asthma—
Adults: 600 to 1,600 mg P.O. daily divided t.i.d. or q.i.d.
Children: 12 mg/kg P.O. daily divided t.i.d. or q.i.d.

dyphylline
For relief of acute and chronic bronchial asthma and reversible bronchospasm associated with chronic bronchitis and emphysema—
Adults: 15 mg/kg P.O. q 6 hours. I.M. route is rarely used, but patients may receive 250 to 500 mg I.M. injected slowly at 6-hour intervals. Dosage should be decreased in renal insufficiency.

• Contraindicated in hypersensitivity to xanthine compounds (caffeine, theobromine) and in patients with preexisting cardiac arrhythmias, especially tachyarrhythmias.
• Use cautiously in young children; in elderly patients with CHF or other circulatory impairment, cor pulmonale, or renal or hepatic disease; and in peptic ulcer, hyperthyroidism, or diabetes mellitus.

COMPARING BRONCHODILATOR COMBINATIONS

DRUG	SPECIAL CONSIDERATIONS

Duo-Medihaler
isoproterenol hydrochloride 240 mcg and phenylephrine hydrochloride 160 mcg in each metered spray

• Combines the decongestant effect of the sympathomimetic phenylephrine with the bronchodilating effect of isoproterenol.
• Contraindicated in patients with uncontrolled hypertension, recent MI, or severe coronary artery disease. Use with extreme caution in elderly patients and those with thyroid, cardiac, or vascular disease.
• Patients should not administer more than 2 inhalations at any time, more than 6 inhalations in 1 hour, or more than 12 inhalations per 24 hours. The patient who does not get adequate relief from the drug without exceeding these dosage limitations should contact the doctor.

Quibron
theophylline 150 mg and guaifenesin 100 mg

• Combines the bronchodilating effect of the methylxanthine theophylline with the expectorant effect of guaifenesin.
• Contraindicated in patients with known hypersensitivity to any of the components.
• Regular monitoring of serum theophylline levels is advisable to prevent toxicity.
• Use cautiously in patients with CV or thyroid disease, hepatic impairment, or peptic ulcer and in elderly patients.

SELF-TEST

1. David Adams, age 54, has chronic bronchial asthma and came to the emergency department with severe shortness of breath. On physical examination Mr. Adams is found to be in respiratory distress because of bronchospasms inhibiting adequate gas exchange. Among the doctor's orders is a STAT order for epinephrine 0.25 ml of 1:1,000 I.V. Which of the following conditions requires extreme caution when administering epinephrine to a patient such as Mr. Adams?
   a. Narrow-angle glaucoma
   b. Shock
   c. Organic brain damage
   d. Degenerative heart disease

2. After Mr. Adams' recovery from this acute episode, his doctor prescribed ipratropium, 2 inhalations q.i.d., as part of maintenance treatment of bronchospasm associated with COPD. The nurse tells Mr. Adams that he may take additional inhalations as needed but should not exceed how many inhalations in a 24-hour period?
   a. 10
   b. 12
   c. 14
   d. 16

3. Mr. Henry Jones, a 75-year-old retired coal miner, was brought to the emergency room via ambulance, experiencing acute respiratory distress resulting from emphysema and chronic bronchitis. The nurse would expect the drug of choice to be:
   a. epinephrine.
   b. ipratropium.
   c. ephedrine.
   d. theophylline.

Check your answers on page 1068.

CHAPTER 44

MUCOLYTICS, EXPECTORANTS, AND ANTITUSSIVES

Mucolytic
acetylcysteine

Expectorants
guaifenesin ✦ iodinated glycerol ✦ potassium iodide (SSKI) ✦ terpin hydrate

Antitussives
benzonatate ✦ codeine phosphate ✦ codeine sulfate
dextromethorphan hydrobromide ✦ diphenhydramine hydrochloride
hydrocodone bitartrate ✦ hydromorphone hydrochloride

OVERVIEW

- Expectorants may decrease sputum viscosity and ease expectoration. Although they are used to loosen secretions (provide mucolytic action) in chronic pulmonary disorders and the common cold, their therapeutic efficacy is doubtful. Nevertheless, these agents are included in many prescription and OTC cough and cold preparations. These agents should probably be used only in conjunction with a total care plan that includes adequate fluid intake and a cool mist or steam vaporizer.
- Antitussives, or cough suppressants, reduce the frequency of a cough, especially when it is dry and nonproductive. Cough suppression is desirable when a chronic cough produces extreme fatigue (as in lung cancer). Most patients with a common cold don't need antitussives; cough drops will do.
- The mucolytic agent acetylcysteine is used to decrease the viscosity of respiratory tract secretions in chronic pulmonary diseases such as bronchitis, cystic fibrosis, and emphysema.

MAJOR USES

- Expectorants and mucolytics may facilitate expectoration in pneumonia, bronchitis, cystic fibrosis, tuberculosis, emphysema, atelectasis, and bronchial asthma.
- Antitussives suppress nonproductive coughs.
- Acetylcysteine prevents severe liver toxicity following acetaminophen overdose.

GLOSSARY

Antitussive: agent that suppresses or inhibits cough.
Cough (tussis): sudden noisy expulsion of air from the lungs.
Decongestant: agent that reduces swelling of mucous membranes and relieves congestion.
Expectorant: agent that promotes the expulsion of respiratory secretions.
Mucin: mucopolysaccharide or glycoprotein that is the chief constituent of mucus.
Mucociliary clearance mechanism: defense mechanism of the respiratory tract, consisting of ciliated epithelial cells and mucus secretions that trap debris and bacteria and facilitate their removal; also called mucociliary escalator mechanism.
Mucokinesis: movement of mucus in the respiratory tract.
Mucokinetic agent: drug that facilitates mucokinesis.
Mucolytic: having the ability to break down the composition of mucus.
Mucus: coating of the mucous membranes containing glandular secretions, various inorganic salts, desquamated cells, and leukocytes.
Viscid: sticky.

MECHANISM OF ACTION

- Expectorants may increase production of respiratory tract fluids to help liquefy and reduce the viscosity of thick, tenacious secretions.
- Antitussives suppress the cough reflex by direct action on the cough center in the medulla (brain) or by peripheral action on sensory nerve endings. Benzonatate and diphenhydramine also act as local anesthetics.
- Acetylcysteine reduces the viscosity of pulmonary secretions through a chemical interaction involving the drug's sulfhydryl group and mucoproteins in the pulmonary fluid. Acetylcysteine protects the liver following acetaminophen overdose by restoring liver stores of glutathione, a substrate necessary for acetaminophen metabolism.

ABSORPTION, DISTRIBUTION, METABOLISM, AND EXCRETION

All expectorants and antitussives are well absorbed after oral administration, metabolized in the liver, and excreted in the urine. Acetylcysteine acts locally in the respiratory tract. Potassium iodide is also excreted through the respiratory tract.

ONSET AND DURATION

Expectorants and antitussives begin to act within 30 minutes. Their effects generally last 4 to 6 hours; benzonatate, however, may act as long as 8 hours.

ADVERSE REACTIONS

Guaifenesin may cause vomiting, gastric upset, and drowsiness.

The iodine products (iodinated glycerol and potassium iodide) may cause thyroid adenoma, goiter, or myxedema; they have also been associated with GI bleeding, numbness, fatigue, and fever.

The opiate antitussives (codeine and hydrocodone) may cause CNS depression, dizziness, seizures, constipation, nausea, vomiting, palpitations, hypotension, pruritus, and allergic reactions. The nonopiate antitussives are associated with sedation, hypersensitivity reactions, dizziness, and constipation.

Acetylcysteine causes sensitivity reactions, stomatitis, nausea, and rhinorrhea.

PROTOTYPE: MUCOLYTIC

ACETYLCYSTEINE
(a se teel sis' tay een)
Airbron†, Mucomyst, Mucosol, Parvolex†‡
Classification: mucolytic
Pregnancy risk category B

How supplied
SOLUTION: 10%, 20%
INJECTION: 200 mg/ml*†‡

Indications and dosage
Pneumonia, bronchitis, tuberculosis, cystic fibrosis, emphysema, atelectasis (adjunct), complications of thoracic and CV surgery
ADULTS AND CHILDREN: 1 to 2 ml 10% to 20% solution by direct instillation into trachea as often as every hour; or 3 to 5 ml 20% solution; or 6 to 10 ml 10% solution, by mouthpiece t.i.d. or q.i.d.

Acetaminophen toxicity
ADULTS AND CHILDREN: initially, 140 mg/kg P.O., followed by 70 mg/kg q 4 hours for 17 doses (a total of 1,330 mg/kg).

Contraindications and precautions
Acetylcysteine is contraindicated in patients with known hypersensitivity to the drug. Use cautiously in patients with asthma or severe respiratory insufficiency and in elderly or debilitated patients.

Adverse reactions
EENT: *rhinorrhea,* hemoptysis.
GI: stomatitis, *nausea.*
OTHER: *bronchospasm* (especially in asthmatic patients).

Interactions
Activated charcoal: can bind orally administered acetylcysteine, limiting acetylcysteine's effectiveness. Don't use together to treat acetaminophen toxicity.

*Liquid form contains alcohol   †Available in Canada only   ‡Available in Australia only
Italicized adverse reactions are common

Nursing considerations

Assessment
• Review the patient's history for a condition that contraindicates the use of acetylcysteine.
• Obtain a baseline assessment of the patient's respiratory secretions before initiating therapy.
• Be alert for common adverse reactions.
• Evaluate the patient's and family's knowledge about acetylcysteine therapy.

Planning (Nursing Diagnoses)
Potential nursing diagnoses for the patient receiving acetylcysteine include:
• Impaired gas exchange related to ineffectiveness of acetylcysteine.
• Altered oral mucous membranes related to acetylcysteine-induced stomatitis.
• Knowledge deficit related to acetylcysteine therapy.

Implementation

Preparation and administration

— Mucolytics are administered by a nebulizer. Use plastic, glass, stainless steel, or another nonreactive metal when administering the medication by nebulization.
— After opening acetylcysteine, store it in the refrigerator and use it within 96 hours.
— Before aerosol administration, instruct the patient to clear the airway by coughing.
— Be aware that acetylcysteine may have a foul taste or smell that the patient may find distressing.
— Have suction equipment available for the patient, who may have difficulty effectively clearing his air passages.
— Dilute oral doses with cola, fruit juice, or water before administering.
— If the patient vomits within 1 hour of administration of loading or maintenance dose, repeat dose.

Monitoring

— Monitor the effectiveness of therapy by regularly evaluating the patient's sputum production and characteristics.
— Monitor respiratory function closely for bronchospasms.
— Monitor hydration status; record intake and output.
— Monitor the patient for adverse drug reactions.
— Monitor the patient's oral mucous membranes for changes suggestive of stomatitis (swollen gums, ulcers in mouth and throat).
— Monitor the patient for drug interactions.
— Regularly reevaluate the patient's and family's knowledge about acetylcysteine therapy.

Intervention

— Provide the patient with the necessary tissues and waste receptacles for disposing of expectorated respiratory secretions.

— Provide for good oral hygiene for the patient receiving acetylcysteine. If stomatitis develops, alert the doctor and provide supportive care: warm water mouth rinses (antiseptic mouthwashes are contraindicated because they are irritating), application of a topical anesthetic to relieve mouth ulcer pain, and a bland or liquid diet.

— Alert the doctor if respiratory secretions thicken or become purulent or if bronchospasms occur.

— Obtain an order for an antiemetic if nausea is severe.

— Keep all members of the health care team informed of the patient's response to the drug.

Patient teaching

— Instruct the patient and family about acetylcysteine, including the dosage, frequency, action, and adverse reactions.

— Instruct the patient to follow the directions on the medication label exactly. Explain the importance of not taking more of the drug than directed.

— Tell the patient to monitor the type and frequency of his cough and to notify his doctor if the medication has not improved his condition within 10 days. This drug should not be used for prolonged periods unless the patient is under direct medical supervision.

— Tell the patient to increase fluid intake to at least 8 full (8-oz) glasses of fluid per day.

— Encourage the patient to do deep-breathing exercises. The patient should sit properly in a straight chair, take several deep breaths, and then attempt to cough.

— Advise the patient to avoid sources of irritants, such as fumes, smoke, and dust.

— Instruct the patient on the proper use of the nebulizer.

— Warn the patient of unpleasant odor (rotten egg odor of hydrogen sulfide) and explain that increased amounts of liquefied bronchial secretions plus unpleasant odor may cause nausea and vomiting; have the patient rinse mouth with water after nebulizer treatment because it may leave a sticky coating on the oral cavity.

— Tell the patient to notify the nurse or doctor if adverse reactions develop or questions arise about acetylcysteine therapy.

Evaluation

In the patient receiving acetylcysteine, appropriate evaluation statements include:

• Patient's lung sounds are clear with decreased respiratory secretions and decreased frequency and severity of cough.

• Patient's oral mucous membranes remain unchanged with acetylcysteine therapy.

• Patient and family state an understanding of acetylcysteine therapy.

PROTOTYPE: EXPECTORANTS

GUAIFENESIN (GLYCERYL GUAIACOLATE)

(gwye fen' e sin)

Anti-Tuss◊, Balminil Expectorant†◊, Breonesin◊, Colrex
Expectorant*◊, Cremacoat 2◊, Gee-Gee◊, GG-CEN*◊, Glyate*◊,
Glycotuss◊, Glytuss◊, Guiatuss*◊, Halotussin◊, Humibid L.A.◊, Hytuss◊,
Hytuss-2X◊, Malotuss◊, Naldecon Senior EX◊, Nortussin◊, Resyl†,
Robafen◊, Robitussin*◊*

Classification: expectorant
Pregnancy risk category C

How supplied

TABLETS: 100 mg◊, 200 mg◊
CAPSULES: 200 mg◊
SYRUP: 67 mg/5 ml*◊, 100 mg/5 ml*◊

Indications and dosage

Expectorant

ADULTS: 100 to 400 mg P.O. q 4 hours. Maximum is 2,400 mg daily.
CHILDREN AGES 6 TO 12: 100 to 200 mg P.O. q 4 hours. Maximum is 600 mg daily.
CHILDREN AGES 2 TO 5: 50 to 100 mg P.O. q 4 hours. Maximum is 300 mg daily.

Contraindications and precautions

Guaifenesin is contraindicated in patients with known hypersensitivity to the drug.

Adverse reactions

CNS: *drowsiness.*
GI: *vomiting and nausea* (with large doses).

Interactions

Heparin: increased risk of bleeding. Use together cautiously.

Nursing considerations

Assessment

- Review the patient's history for a condition that contraindicates the use of guaifenesin.
- Obtain a baseline assessment of the patient's cough and sputum production before initiating therapy.
- Be alert for common adverse reactions.
- Evaluate the patient's and family's knowledge about guaifenesin.

Planning (Nursing Diagnoses)

Potential nursing diagnoses for the patient receiving guaifenesin include:

---

*Liquid form contains alcohol   **May contain tartrazine   ◊ Available OTC
Italicized adverse reactions are common

• Impaired gas exchange related to ineffectiveness of guaifenesin to loosen and remove secretions.
• Fluid volume deficit related to guaifenesin-induced nausea and vomiting.
• Knowledge deficit related to guaifenesin therapy.

Implementation

Preparation and administration

— Administer drug with a glass of water to help loosen mucus in lungs.

Monitoring

— Monitor the effectiveness of therapy by regularly evaluating the patient's cough and sputum production.
— Monitor hydration status; record intake and output.
— Monitor for drowsiness.
— Monitor the patient for adverse drug reactions.
— Monitor for bleeding if used concurrently with heparin.
— Monitor the patient for drug interactions.
— Regularly reevaluate the patient's and family's knowledge about guaifenesin therapy.

Intervention

— Provide the patient with the necessary tissues and waste receptacles for disposing of expectorated respiratory secretions.
— Provide for good oral hygiene for the patient receiving an expectorant.
— Encourage fluid intake to at least 3,000 ml/day if not contraindicated to help liquefy and reduce the viscosity of thick, tenacious secretions.
— Be aware that guaifenesin may interfere with certain laboratory tests for 5-hydroxyindoleacetic acid and vanillylmandelic acid.
— Encourage deep-breathing exercises.
— Obtain an order for an antiemetic as needed.
— Institute safety precautions if drowsiness occurs.
— Keep all members of the health care team informed of the patient's response to the drug.

Patient teaching

— Instruct the patient and family about guaifenesin, including the dosage, frequency, action, and adverse reactions.
— Instruct the patient to follow the directions on the medication label exactly. Explain the importance of not taking more of the drug than directed.
— Explain that the patient should monitor the type and frequency of his cough and notify his doctor if the medication has not improved his condition within 10 days. This drug should not be used for prolonged periods unless the patient is under direct medical supervision.
— Tell the patient to increase fluid intake to at least 8 full (8-oz) glasses of fluid per 24 hours.
— Encourage the patient to do deep-breathing exercises. The patient should sit properly in a straight chair, take several deep breaths, and then attempt to cough.

—Tell the patient to avoid sources of irritants such as fumes, smoke, and dust.

—Explain that antitussives in some combination products may cause drowsiness or dizziness; therefore, advise caution regarding driving or handling equipment that requires alertness.

—Tell the patient to notify the nurse or doctor if adverse reactions develop or questions arise about guaifenesin therapy.

Evaluation

In the patient receiving guaifenesin, appropriate evaluation statements include:

• Patient's lungs are clear and respiratory secretions and cough are decreased.

• Patient maintains adequate hydration.

• Patient and family state an understanding of guaifenesin therapy.

PROTOTYPE: ANTITUSSIVES

DEXTROMETHORPHAN HYDROBROMIDE
(dex troe meth or' fan)

Balminil D.M.◊, Benylin DM◊, Broncho-Grippol-DM†, Congespirin for Children◊, Delsym◊, DM Cough◊, Hold◊, Koffex†, Mediquell◊, Neo-DM†, Pediacare 1◊, Pertussin 8 Hour Cough Formula◊, Robidex†, Sedatuss†, St. Joseph for Children◊, Sucrets Cough Control Formula◊, Contac Cough & Sore Throat Formula◊, Contac Cough Formula◊, Contac Jr. Children's Cold Medicine◊, Contac Nighttime Cold Medicine◊, Contac Severe Cold Formula Caplets◊, Novahistine DMX Liquid*, Phenergan with Dextromethorphan*, Robitussin-DM*◊, Rondec-DM*◊, Triaminicol Multi-Symptom Cold◊, Trind-DM Liquid*◊, Tussi-Organidin DM Liquid***

Classification: antitussive
Pregnancy risk category C

How supplied

CHEWABLE PIECES: 15 mg◊
LIQUID (SUSTAINED ACTION): 30 mg/5 ml◊
LOZENGES: 5 mg*
SYRUP: 5 mg/5 ml*◊, 7.5 mg/5 ml*◊, 10 mg/5 ml◊, 15 mg/5 ml*◊

Indications and dosage
Nonproductive cough

ADULTS: 10 to 20 mg P.O. q 4 hours, or 30 mg q 6 to 8 hours. Or 60 mg (controlled-release liquid) P.O. b.i.d. Maximum is 120 mg daily.

CHILDREN AGES 6 TO 12: 5 to 10 mg P.O. q 4 hours, or 15 mg q 6 to 8 hours. Or 30 mg (controlled-release liquid) P.O. b.i.d. Maximum is 60 mg daily.

---

*Liquid form contains alcohol   †Available in Canada only   ◊ Available OTC

CHILDREN AGES 2 TO 6: 2.5 to 5 mg P.O. q 4 hours, or 7.5 mg q 6 to 8 hours. Maximum is 30 mg daily.

Contraindications and precautions

Dextromethorphan is contraindicated in patients currently taking—or within 2 weeks of discontinuing—MAO inhibitors.

Adverse reactions

CNS: *drowsiness, dizziness.*
GI: *nausea.*

Interactions

MAO inhibitors: hypotension, coma, hyperpyrexia, and death have occurred. Do not use together.

Nursing considerations

Assessment

• Review the patient's history for a condition that contraindicates the use of dextromethorphan.
• Obtain a baseline assessment of the patient's cough before initiating therapy.
• Be alert for common adverse reactions.
• Evaluate the patient's and family's knowledge about dextromethorphan therapy.

Planning (Nursing Diagnoses)

Potential nursing diagnoses for the patient receiving dextromethorphan include:
• Altered health maintenance related to ineffectiveness of dextromethorphan to relieve cough.
• Potential for injury related to dextromethorphan-induced CNS reactions.
• Knowledge deficit related to dextromethorphan therapy.

Implementation

Preparation and administration

— Do not administer an antitussive such as dextromethorphan to a patient if the effect of the drug may mask an underlying condition.
— Administer dextromethorphan exactly as directed.

Monitoring

— Monitor the effectiveness of therapy by regularly evaluating if the patient's cough is relieved.
— Monitor hydration status; record intake and output.
— Monitor for dizziness and drowsiness.
— Monitor the patient for adverse drug reactions.
— Monitor the patient for drug interactions.
— Regularly reevaluate the patient's and family's knowledge about dextromethorphan therapy.

Intervention

— Notify the doctor if cough is unrelieved with dextromethorphan.

— Encourage the patient to take 2,000 to 3,000 ml of liquids daily.

— Perform percussion and chest vibration during dextromethorphan therapy.

— Institute safety precautions if adverse CNS reactions occur.

— Obtain an order for an antiemetic if nausea persists or becomes severe.

— Keep all members of the health care team informed of the patient's response to the drug.

Patient teaching

— Instruct the patient and family about dextromethorphan, including the dosage, frequency, action, and adverse reactions.

— Instruct the patient to follow the directions on the medication bottle exactly; explain the importance of not taking more of the drug than directed.

— Tell the patient to call the doctor if cough persists more than 7 days.

— Suggest sugarless throat lozenges to decrease throat irritation and resulting cough.

— Advise the patient to use a humidifier to filter out dust, smoke, and air pollutants.

— Tell the patient to notify the nurse or doctor if adverse reactions develop or questions arise about dextromethorphan therapy.

Evaluation

In the patient receiving dextromethorphan, appropriate evaluation statements include:

• Patient's cough is relieved.

• Patient does not experience injury as a result of dextromethorphan-induced CNS reactions.

• Patient and family state an understanding of dextromethorphan therapy.

SELECTED MAJOR DRUGS: EXPECTORANTS AND ANTITUSSIVES

DRUG, INDICATIONS, AND DOSAGES	SPECIAL PRECAUTIONS

Expectorants

iodinated glycerol (Iophen Elixir, Organidin)
Bronchial asthma, bronchitis, emphysema (adjunct) —
Adults: 60 mg (tablets) P.O. q.i.d., or 20 drops (solution) P.O. q.i.d. with fluids, or 5 ml (elixir) P.O. q.i.d.
Children: up to half the adult dose based on child's weight.

• Contraindicated in patients with hypothyroidism or iodine sensitivity and during pregnancy and lactation.
• Administer cautiously to adolescents; acne is possible. Also use cautiously in children with cystic fibrosis.

---

potassium iodide (SSKI)
As expectorant, chronic bronchitis, chronic pulmonary emphysema, bronchial asthma —
Adults: 0.3 to 0.6 ml P.O. q 4 to 6 hours.
Children: 0.25 to 0.5 ml (saturated solution) (1 g/ml) P.O. b.i.d. to q.i.d.
Nuclear radiation protection —
Adults and children: 0.13 ml (SSKI) P.O. immediately before or after initial exposure will block 90% of radioactive iodine. Same dose given 3 to 4 hours after exposure will provide 50% block. Should be administered for up to 10 days under medical supervision.
Infants under age 1: one-half the adult dose.

• Contraindicated in patients with iodine hypersensitivity, tuberculosis, hyperkalemia, acute bronchitis, or hyperthyroidism.
• Administer cautiously to patients sensitive to iodides and to patients receiving potassium-sparing diuretics or potassium supplements.

---

terpin hydrate
Excessive bronchial secretions —
Adults: 5 to 10 ml (elixir) P.O. q 4 to 6 hours.

• Contraindicated in peptic ulcer or severe diabetes mellitus.
• Commonly combined with codeine.
• Use cautiously in patients with conditions that may be worsened by narcotics.

Antitussives

benzonatate (Tessalon)
Nonproductive cough —
Adults and children over age 10: 100 mg P.O. t.i.d., up to 600 mg daily.
Children under age 10: 8 mg/kg P.O. in three to six divided doses.

• Contraindicated in patients with known hypersensitivity to benzonatate or related compounds.
• Administer cautiously to pregnant or breast-feeding women because of risk of carcinogenesis, mutagenesis, or impaired fertility.

---

codeine
Nonproductive cough —
Adults: 10 to 20 mg P.O. q 4 to 6 hours. Maximum dosage is 120 mg daily.
Children ages 6 to 12: 5 to 10 mg P.O. q 4 to 6 hours. Maximum dosage is 60 mg daily.

• Contraindicated in neonates or premature infants and in patients with known hypersensitivity to codeine and any chemically similar drugs.
• Use with extreme caution in

(continued)

SELECTED MAJOR DRUGS: EXPECTORANTS AND ANTITUSSIVES
continued

DRUG, INDICATIONS, AND DOSAGES	SPECIAL PRECAUTIONS

Antitussives *(continued)*

codeine *(continued)*
Children ages 2 to 6: 2.5 to 5 mg P.O. q 4 to 6 hours.
Do not exceed 30 mg daily.

head injury, increased intracranial pressure, increased CSF pressure, hepatic or renal disease, hypothyroidism, Addison's disease, acute alcoholism, seizures, severe CNS depression, bronchial asthma, COPD, respiratory depression, and shock and in elderly or debilitated patients.

---

diphenhydramine (Benadryl ◇, Benylin Cough ◇, Tusstat ◇)
Rhinitis, allergy symptoms, nighttime sedation, motion sickness, antiparkinsonism—
Adults: 25 to 50 mg P.O. t.i.d. or q.i.d.; or 10 to 50 mg deep I.M. or I.V. Maximum dosage is 400 mg daily.
Children under age 12: 5 mg/kg P.O., deep I.M., or I.V. divided q.i.d. Maximum dosage is 300 mg daily.
Sedation—
Adults: 25 to 50 mg P.O. or deep I.M. p.r.n.
As a nighttime sleep aid—
Adults: 50 mg P.O. h.s.
Nonproductive cough—
Adults: 25 mg P.O. q 4 hours (not to exceed 100 mg daily).
Children ages 6 to 12: 12.5 mg P.O. q 4 hours (not to exceed 50 mg daily).
Children ages 2 to 6: 6.25 mg P.O. q 4 hours (not to exceed 25 mg daily).
   Note: Children under age 12 should use only as directed by a doctor.

• Contraindicated in acute asthmatic attacks.
• Administer cautiously to patients with narrow-angle glaucoma, prostatic hypertrophy, pyloroduodenal and bladder-neck obstruction, or stenosing peptic ulcers; to neonates; and to asthmatic, hypertensive, or cardiac patients.

---

hydrocodone
To relieve nonproductive cough—
Adults: 5 to 10 mg P.O. q 4 to 6 hours. Initiate therapy with a 5-mg dose.

• Contraindicated in patients with known hypersensitivity to hydrocodone or phenylpropanolamine; on concurrent MAO inhibitor therapy; with known hypersensitivity to other opioids or sympathomimetics; with heart disease, hypertension, diabetes, or hyperthyroidism; in intracranial lesions; and whenever ventilatory function is depressed.
• Administer cautiously to patients receiving other CNS

SELECTED MAJOR DRUGS: EXPECTORANTS AND ANTITUSSIVES
continued

DRUG, INDICATIONS, AND DOSAGES	SPECIAL PRECAUTIONS
Antitussives *(continued)*	
hydrocodone *(continued)*	depressants or when phenylpro-panolamine is used with other sympathomimetics and MAO inhibitors; to patients at risk of carcinogenesis, mutagenesis, or impaired fertility; during pregnancy or breast-feeding; and in children under age 6.
hydromorphone (Dilaudid) *Moderate to severe pain—* **Adults:** 1 to 6 mg P.O. q 4 to 6 hours, p.r.n. or around the clock; or 2 to 4 mg I.M., S.C., or I.V. q 4 to 6 hours p.r.n., or q 6 to 8 hours around the clock (I.V. dose should be given over 3 to 5 minutes); or 3 mg rectal suppository h.s. p.r.n., or q 6 to 8 hours around the clock. *Cough—* **Adults:** 1 mg P.O. q 3 to 4 hours p.r.n. **Children ages 6 to 12:** 0.5 mg P.O. q 3 to 4 hours p.r.n.	• Contraindicated in increased intracranial pressure and status asthmaticus. • Use with extreme caution in patients with increased CSF pressure, respiratory depression, hepatic or renal disease, hypothyroidism, shock, Addison's disease, acute alcoholism, seizures, head injury, severe CNS depression, brain tumor, bronchial asthma, or COPD; and in elderly or debilitated patients.

COMPARING EXPECTORANT AND ANTITUSSIVE COMBINATIONS

TRADE NAME AND CONTENT	SPECIAL CONSIDERATIONS
Expectorants	
Entex phenylephrine hydrochloride 5 mg, phenylpropanolamine 45 mg, and guaifenesin 200 mg **Entex Liquid** phenylephrine hydrochloride 5 mg/5 ml, phenylpropanolamine 20 mg/5 ml, and guaifenesin 100 mg/5 ml	• Combine the expectorant action of guaifenesin with the decongestant actions of the sympathomimetics phenylpropanolamine and phenylephrine. • Contraindicated in patients with uncontrolled hypertension, those taking MAO inhibitors, and those with known hypersensitivity to the components. • Use cautiously in patients with diabetes, hypertension, CV disease, prostatic hypertrophy, or thyroid disease.

(continued)

COMPARING EXPECTORANT AND ANTITUSSIVE COMBINATIONS
continued

TRADE NAME AND CONTENT	SPECIAL CONSIDERATIONS
Expectorants *(continued)*	
Conex Syrup ◇ **Triaminic Expectorant** ◇ **Theramine Expectorant** ◇ **Triphenyl Expectorant** ◇ guaifenesin 100 mg and phenylpropanolamine 12.5 mg	• Combine the expectorant action of guaifenesin with the decongestant action of the sympathomimetic phenylpropanolamine. • Contraindicated in patients with uncontrolled hypertension, those taking MAO inhibitors, and in those with known hypersensitivity to the drug. • Use cautiously in patients with diabetes, hypertension, CV disease, prostatic hypertrophy, or thyroid disease.
Antitussives	
Vicks Formula 44D ◇ dextromethorphan hydrobromide 10 mg/5 ml and pseudoephedrine hydrochloride 20 mg/5 ml	• Combines the antitussive action of dextromethorphan with the decongestant effect of the sympathomimetic pseudoephedrine. • Contraindicated in patients with uncontrolled hypertension, those taking MAO inhibitors, and those with known hypersensitivity to the drug. • Use cautiously in patients with diabetes, hypertension, CV disease, prostatic hypertrophy, or thyroid disease.
Comtrex ◇ **Kolephrin/DM** ◇ pseudoephedrine hydrochloride 30 mg, chlorpheniramine maleate 2 mg, acetaminophen 325 mg, and dextromethorphan hydrobromide 10 mg	• Combine the antitussive action of dextromethorphan with the decongestant action of the sympathomimetic pseudoephedrine, the drying action of the antihistamine chlorpheniramine, and the analgesic and antipyretic effects of acetaminophen. • Contraindicated in patients with uncontrolled hypertension, those taking MAO inhibitors, and those with known hypersensitivity to any component. • Use cautiously in patients with diabetes, CV or thyroid disease, or prostatic hypertrophy.

◇ Available OTC

SELF-TEST

1. Gwendolyn Pope, age 58, was admitted to the hospital with complaints of fatigue, weakness, dyspnea, malaise, pain in the chest, and a persistent nonproductive cough that she has had for 4 weeks. Shortly after admission, she called for a nurse and insisted that she be given something for her cough. In this situation, the nurse should know that:
   a. an expectorant could be given to this patient to relieve her discomfort from the cough.
   b. a mucolytic could be given to this patient to relieve her discomfort from the cough.
   c. an antitussive could be given to this patient to relieve her discomfort from the cough.
   d. this patient's doctor will probably not prescribe anything for her cough at this time.

2. Mrs. Pope was diagnosed as having a viral upper respiratory tract infection. At this point, the nurse would expect an order for what type of drug for Mrs. Pope's cough?
   a. Antitussive
   b. Antihistamine
   c. Mucolytic
   d. Expectorant

3. If a patient complains of thick, tenacious mucus from the respiratory tract, what type of drug should a nurse expect to see ordered?
   a. Antitussive
   b. Antihistamine
   c. Mucolytic
   d. Expectorant

4. If acetylcysteine is ordered for a patient, the nurse should know that:
   a. the medication should be discarded 24 hours after the vial is opened.
   b. after the medication is opened, it should be stored in the refrigerator.
   c. the medication is available in capsule form and should not be chewed.
   d. this medication should be used with percussion and chest vibration.

5. Which of the following nursing interventions would be considered the most important when the patient is receiving a mucolytic, an expectorant, or an antitussive?
   a. Provide good oral hygiene.
   b. Observe the patient for drowsiness or dizziness.
   c. Obtain a baseline assessment of the patient's respiratory system.
   d. Provide the patient with adequate tissues and waste receptacles.

Check your answers on page 1068.

CHAPTER 45

ANTACIDS

aluminum carbonate ✦ aluminum hydroxide ✦ aluminum phosphate
calcium carbonate ✦ dihydroxyaluminum sodium carbonate
magaldrate (aluminum-magnesium complex)
magnesium hydroxide (milk of magnesia) ✦ magnesium oxide
magnesium trisilicate ✦ sodium bicarbonate

OVERVIEW

- Antacids are used to treat peptic ulcers (localized lesions of the gastric and duodenal mucosa). They may consist of various combinations of aluminum, calcium, and magnesium salts and of magaldrate. But most of them are combinations of aluminum and magnesium salts. Although the antacid properties of the inorganic salts cited have been known for more than 2,000 years, until the modern era their use was mainly empirical and subjective. Today, however, the use and action of the antacids are well-known and medically respected.
- The products vary in their ability to neutralize acid. Adequate doses and proper timing of administration promote healing of duodenal ulcers.
- Many patients on sodium-restricted diets may not realize that the antacids they are taking contain sodium in the form of the salt sodium chloride. Sometimes the sodium content is high enough to aggravate conditions such as CHF and hypertension.

MAJOR USES

- Antacids neutralize gastric acidity and help control ulcer pain. They are also used to treat the retrosternal burning sensation (heartburn) due to reflux esophagitis.

MECHANISM OF ACTION

- Antacids reduce total acid load in the GI tract and elevate gastric pH to reduce pepsin activity. They also strengthen the gastric mucosal barrier and increase esophageal sphincter tone. They do not seem to have a coating effect on ulcers.

ABSORPTION, DISTRIBUTION, METABOLISM, AND EXCRETION

Absorption of antacids varies. Prolonged use of antacids that contain magnesium or calcium may cause systemic absorption of magnesium or calcium ions in toxic quantities. Excessive aluminum antacid therapy can lead to hypophosphatemia. Antacids are distributed throughout the GI tract and are eliminated primarily in feces.

GLOSSARY

Antacid: drug that neutralizes gastric acids.
Pepsin: proteolytic enzyme in gastric juice that acts as a catalyst in protein hydrolysis.
Ulcer: cutaneous or mucosal lesion caused by gradual erosion, disintegration, and necrosis of underlying tissue.

ONSET AND DURATION

Antacids' onset of action is generally immediate. Duration of action is usually only 1 hour when taken on an empty stomach but as long as 3 hours if taken after meals.

ADVERSE REACTIONS

Magnesium-containing antacids, which have a laxative effect, may cause diarrhea. In patients with renal failure, they may cause hypermagnesemia.

Aluminum-containing antacids cause constipation, which may lead to intestinal obstruction. They may also cause aluminum intoxication, osteomalacia, and hypophosphatemia.

Calcium carbonate, magaldrate, sodium bicarbonate, and magnesium oxide may cause rebound hyperacidity and milk-alkali syndrome.

PROTOTYPE: ANTACIDS

ALUMINUM HYDROXIDE
(a loo′ mi num hi drok′ side)
ALternaGEL◊, Alu-Cap◊, Alu-Tab◊, Amphojel◊, Amphotabs‡, Dialume◊, Nephrox◊

Classification: antacid
Pregnancy risk category C

How supplied
TABLETS: 300 mg◊, 600 mg◊
CAPSULES: 475 mg◊, 500 mg◊
ORAL SUSPENSION: 320 mg/5 ml◊, 600 mg/5 ml

Indications and dosage
Antacid
ADULTS: 600 mg P.O. (5 to 10 ml of most products) 1 hour after meals and h.s.; 300- or 600-mg tablet, chewed before swallowing, taken with milk or water five to six times daily after meals and h.s.

Hyperphosphatemia in renal failure
ADULTS: 500 mg to 2 g P.O. b.i.d. to q.i.d.

‡Available in Australia only   ◊ Available OTC

Contraindications and precautions

Aluminum hydroxide is essentially nontoxic but should not be given to any patient taking a prescription antibiotic containing any form of tetracycline. It should be used cautiously in patients who have recently suffered massive upper GI hemorrhage.

Adverse reactions

GI: anorexia, *constipation,* intestinal obstruction.
METABOLIC: hypophosphatemia.

Interactions

Allopurinol, antibiotics (including quinolones and tetracyclines), corticosteroids, diflunisal, digoxin, iron, isoniazid, penicillamine, phenothiazines, ranitidine: decreased pharmacologic effect because absorption may be impaired. Separate administration times.

Nursing considerations

Assessment

- Review the patient's history for a condition that contraindicates the use of aluminum hydroxide.
- Obtain a baseline assessment of the patient's peptic ulcer disease, ulcer pains, or heartburn before therapy.
- Be alert for common adverse reactions.
- Evaluate the patient's and family's knowledge about aluminum hydroxide therapy.

Planning (Nursing Diagnoses)

Potential nursing diagnoses for the patient receiving aluminum hydroxide include:
- Altered health maintenance related to inadequate dosage to reduce or relieve pain.
- Constipation related to drug's binding effect.
- Knowledge deficit related to aluminum hydroxide therapy.

Implementation

Preparation and administration

—Shake suspension well; give with small amount of milk or water to ensure passage to stomach. When administering through nasogastric tube, make sure tube is placed correctly and is patent. After instilling antacid, flush tube with water.
—Administer drug 1 hour after meals and at bedtime. Be sure to schedule other drugs the patient may be receiving as indicated. Do not give other oral medications within 1 to 2 hours of antacid administration.
—May cause enteric-coated drugs to be released prematurely in stomach. Separate doses by 1 hour.
—The tablet form of the medication should be chewed completely before swallowing and followed by a glass of water or milk.
—When administering drug as an antiurolithic, encourage increased fluid intake to enhance drug effectiveness.

Monitoring

— Monitor the effectiveness of therapy by regularly assessing reduction or relief of the patient's ulcer pain or heartburn.
— Monitor the patient for adverse drug reactions.
— Watch long-term, high-dose use in patients on restricted sodium intake.
— Monitor the patient's bowel pattern. Watch for development of constipation, especially in the elderly patient.
— Alternate with magnesium-containing antacids (if the patient does not have renal disease).
— Monitor the patient for drug interactions.
— Periodically monitor serum calcium and phosphate levels; decreased serum phosphate levels may lead to increased serum calcium levels. Observe the patient for signs and symptoms of hypophosphatemia (anorexia, muscle weakness, and malaise).
— Monitor diagnostic test results. Aluminum hydroxide therapy may interfere with imaging techniques using sodium pertechnetate Tc 99m and thus impair evaluation of Meckel's diverticulum. It may also interfere with reticuloendothelial imaging of liver, spleen, and bone marrow using technetium Tc 99m sulfur colloid. Drug may antagonize pentagastrin's effect during gastric acid secretion tests. Aluminum hydroxide may elevate serum gastrin levels and reduce serum phosphate levels.
— Regularly reevaluate the patient's and family's knowledge about aluminum hydroxide therapy.

Intervention

— If the patient develops constipation, notify the doctor and obtain an order for a laxative or stool softener and monitor its effectiveness. Also, if not contraindicated, encourage the patient to eat a high-fiber diet and to drink 8 to 13 8-oz glasses (2 to 3 liters) of water per day to help prevent constipation.
— If the patient is unable to comply with therapy, discuss reasons why and offer suggestions to help the patient improve compliance.
— Keep all members of the health care team informed of the patient's response to the drug.
— Discuss with the patient any emotional factors or dietary habits that may be contributing to the patient's GI problems.

Patient teaching

— Inform the patient and family about aluminum hydroxide, including the dosage, frequency, action, and adverse reactions.
— Explain the disease process and rationale for therapy.
— Caution the patient to take aluminum hydroxide only as directed; to shake suspension well, and to follow with sips of water or juice. Tell the patient receiving the tablet form of the drug to chew the tablets completely before swallowing and, after swallowing, to drink a glass of milk or water.
— As indicated, instruct the patient to restrict sodium intake, drink plenty of fluids, or follow a low-phosphate diet.

— Advise the patient not to switch to another antacid without consulting the doctor.

— Teach the patient how to prevent constipation during therapy.

— Explain the importance of taking these medications as prescribed, and not taking other medications simultaneously.

— Tell the patient to notify the nurse or doctor if adverse reactions develop or questions arise about aluminum hydroxide therapy.

— Warn the patient that these drugs may color his stool white or cause white streaks. Advise the patient to contact the doctor immediately if his stool becomes black.

— Explain to the patient whose sodium intake is restricted that long-term, high-dose usage of aluminum hydroxide is not recommended.

Evaluation
In the patient receiving aluminum hydroxide, appropriate evaluation statements include:

• Patient's ulcer pain or heartburn subsides or is relieved.
• Patient experiences no constipation; maintains normal bowel function during therapy.
• Patient and family state an understanding of aluminum hydroxide therapy.

PROTOTYPE: ANTACIDS

MAGNESIUM HYDROXIDE (MILK OF MAGNESIA)
(mag nee' zhum hi drok' side)

M.O.M.◊

Classification: antacid
Pregnancy risk category B

How supplied
TABLETS: 300 mg◊, 600 mg◊
ORAL SUSPENSION: 7% to 8.5% (approximately 80 mEq magnesium/30 ml)◊

Indications and dosage
Antacid
ADULTS: 5 to 15 ml (milk of magnesia) P.O. t.i.d. or q.i.d.

Constipation, to evacuate bowel before surgery
ADULTS AND CHILDREN OVER AGE 6: 15 to 60 ml P.O.
CHILDREN AGES 2 TO 6: 5 to 15 ml P.O.

Contraindications and precautions
Magnesium hydroxide is contraindicated in patients with abdominal pain, nausea, vomiting, change in bowel habits persisting for over 2 weeks, rectal bleeding, or kidney disease.

◊ Available OTC

Adverse reactions

GI: *abdominal cramping, diarrhea, nausea.*
METABOLIC: fluid and electrolyte disturbances (if used daily).
OTHER: laxative dependence in long-term or excessive use.

Interactions

None significant.

Nursing considerations

Assessment

• Review the patient's history for a condition that contraindicates the use of magnesium hydroxide.
• Obtain a baseline assessment of the patient's peptic ulcer disease, ulcer pain, or heartburn before therapy.
• Be alert for common adverse reactions.
• Evaluate the patient's and family's knowledge about magnesium hydroxide therapy.

Planning (Nursing Diagnoses)

Potential nursing diagnoses for the patient receiving magnesium hydroxide include:
• Potential for injury related to ineffective drug dosage.
• Diarrhea related to the drug's laxative effect.
• Knowledge deficit related to magnesium hydroxide therapy.

Implementation

Preparation and administration

— Before giving for constipation, determine if the patient has adequate fluid intake, exercise, and diet.
— Shake suspension well; give with large amount of water when used as laxative. Give drug at least 1 hour apart from enterically coated medications. When administering through nasogastric tube, make sure tube is placed properly and is patent. After instilling, flush tube with water to ensure passage to stomach and to maintain tube patency.
— For short-term therapy, don't use longer than 1 week.
— Drug produces its laxative effects in 3 to 6 hours. Time drug administration so that it doesn't interfere with scheduled activities or sleep.
— Advise the patient to thoroughly chew any chewable antacid tablets before swallowing and then to drink 6 to 8 oz (180 to 240 ml) of water; with a suspension or regular tablet, to drink 6 to 8 oz of water.

Monitoring

— Monitor the effectiveness of therapy by regularly assessing reduction or relief of the patient's ulcer pain or heartburn.
— Monitor the patient for adverse drug reactions.
— Monitor serum magnesium levels to detect any systemic drug absorption; also monitor for signs and symptoms of hypermagnesemia, especially if the patient has impaired renal function.
— Also monitor serum electrolytes during prolonged use.

— Monitor the patient's intake and output, fluid and electrolyte status, and amount and type of stools. Watch especially for diarrhea resulting from the drug's laxative effects.

— Regularly reevaluate the patient's and family's knowledge about magnesium hydroxide therapy.

Intervention

— If the patient develops diarrhea, notify the doctor and obtain an order for an antidiarrheal. If diarrhea becomes severe, expect to discontinue the antacid as ordered.

— If the patient is unable to comply with therapy, discuss reasons why and offer possible suggestions to help improve compliance.

— Keep all members of the health care team informed of the patient's response to the drug.

Patient teaching

— Instruct the patient and family about magnesium hydroxide, including the dosage, frequency, action, and adverse reactions.

— Explain the disease process and rationale for therapy.

— Caution the patient to avoid overuse to prevent laxative dependence.

— Instruct the patient to shake suspension well.

— Tell the patient to notify the nurse or doctor if adverse reactions develop or questions arise about magnesium hydroxide therapy.

Evaluation

In the patient receiving magnesium hydroxide, appropriate evaluation statements include:

• Patient's ulcer pain or heartburn subsides or is relieved.

• Patient maintains normal bowel function during therapy and does not experience diarrhea.

• Patient and family state an understanding of magnesium hydroxide therapy.

SELECTED MAJOR DRUGS: ANTACIDS

DRUG, INDICATIONS, AND DOSAGES

SPECIAL PRECAUTIONS

aluminum carbonate (Basaljel ◇)
Antacid —
Adults: 5 to 10 ml (suspension) P.O. p.r.n.; 2.5 to 5 ml
(extra-strength suspension) p.r.n.; 1 to 2 tablets p.r.n.;
1 to 2 capsules p.r.n.
*To prevent formation of urinary phosphate stones (with
low-phosphate diet) —*
Adults: 15 to 30 ml (suspension) in water or juice P.O.
1 hour after meals and h.s.; 5 to 15 ml (extra-strength
suspension) in water or juice 1 hour after meals and
h.s.; 2 to 6 tablets or capsules 1 hour after meals and
h.s.

• Use cautiously in elderly patients, especially those with
decreased GI motility (those receiving antidiarrheals, antispas-
modics, or anticholinergics),
dehydration, fluid restriction,
chronic renal disease, and suspected intestinal obstruction.

aluminum phosphate (Phosphaljel ◇)
Antacid —
Adults: 15 to 30 ml (undiluted) P.O. q 2 hours between
meals and h.s.

• Contraindicated in patients
with impaired renal function,
appendicitis, constipation, fecal
impaction, undiagnosed rectal or
GI bleeding, chronic diarrhea,
gastric outlet obstruction, or intestinal obstruction.
• Use cautiously in elderly patients, especially those with
decreased GI motility (those receiving antidiarrheals, antispas-
modics, or anticholinergics),
dehydration, fluid restriction,
chronic renal disease, and suspected intestinal obstruction.

**calcium carbonate (Chooz ◇ , Rolaids Calcium Rich ◇ ,
Titracid ◇ , Tums ◇)**
Antacid —
Adults: 1-g tablet P.O. four to six times daily, chewed
well and taken with water; or 1 g of suspension (5 ml
of most products) 1 hour after meals and h.s.

• Contraindicated in patients
with severe renal disease.
• Use cautiously in elderly patients, especially those with
decreased GI motility (those receiving antidiarrheals, antispas-
modics, or anticholinergics),
dehydration, fluid restriction,
chronic renal disease, and suspected intestinal obstruction.

dihydroxyaluminum sodium carbonate (Rolaids ◇)
Antacid —
Adults: chew 1 to 2 tablets (334 to 668 mg) p.r.n.

• Contraindicated in patients
with renal failure, hypophosphatemia, appendicitis, undiagnosed
rectal or GI bleeding, constipation, fecal impaction, chronic
diarrhea, or intestinal obstruction because drug may exacerbate the symptons associated
with these conditions.
• Use cautiously in elderly patients, especially those with
decreased GI motility (those re-

(continued)

◇ Available OTC

SELECTED MAJOR DRUGS: ANTACIDS *continued*

DRUG, INDICATIONS, AND DOSAGES	SPECIAL PRECAUTIONS
dihydroxyaluminum sodium carbonate *(continued)*	ceiving antidiarrheals, antispasmodics, or anticholinergics), dehydration, fluid restriction, chronic renal disease, and suspected intestinal obstruction.
magaldrate (Lowsium ◇ , Riopan ◇) *Antacid—* **Adults:** 540 to 1,080 mg (5 to 10 ml suspension) P.O. with water between meals and h.s.; 480 to 960 mg (1 to 2 tablets) P.O. with water between meals and h.s.; 480 to 960 mg (1 to 2 chewable tablets) P.O. chewed before swallowing, between meals and h.s.	• Contraindicated in patients with severe renal disease. • Use cautiously in elderly patients, especially those with decreased GI motility (those receiving antidiarrheals, antispasmodics, or anticholinergics), dehydration, fluid restriction, and mild renal impairment.
magnesium oxide (Maox ◇ , Uro-Mag ◇) *Antacid—* **Adults:** 140 mg P.O. with water or milk after meals and h.s. *Laxative—* **Adults:** 4 g P.O. with water or milk, usually h.s. *Oral replacement therapy in mild hypomagnesemia—* **Adults:** 400 to 840 mg P.O. daily. Monitor serum magnesium response.	• Contraindicated in patients with severe renal disease. • Use cautiously in elderly patients and in those with mild renal impairment.
magnesium trisilicate *Relief of acid indigestion—* **Adults:** chew 2 to 4 tablets q.i.d. or as directed by doctor. Tablets should be taken after meals and h.s., or p.r.n.	• Administer cautiously to patients who require sodium restriction.
simethicone (Gas-X ◇ , Mylicon ◇ , Phazyme ◇) *Excess GI tract gas—* **Adults:** 160 to 500 mg P.O. daily in divided doses after each meal and h.s.	• There are no known precautions or contraindications with simethicone use.
sodium bicarbonate (Citrocarbonate ◇ , Soda Mint ◇) *Antacid—* Taken in solution; 3 oz of water/tablet. **Adults:** 1 or 2 tablets q 4 hours p.r.n. **Children:** half the adult dosage.	• Contraindicated in patients on sodium-restricted diets. • Administer cautiously to pregnant or breast-feeding women.

◇ Available OTC

COMPARING ANTACID COMBINATIONS

TRADE NAME AND CONTENT	SPECIAL CONSIDERATIONS
Alka-Seltzer ◇ citric acid 832 mg, sodium bicarbonate 958 mg, and potassium bicarbonate 213 mg per effervescent tablet	• Combines the antacid effects of sodium bicarbonate, potassium bicarbonate, and citric acid. • Contraindicated in patients with known hypersensitivity, asthma, coagulation disorders, CHF, renal failure, edema, or cirrhosis or who require sodium restriction.
Gaviscon Extra Strength Relief Formula ◇ aluminum hydroxide 160 mg and magnesium carbonate 105 mg	• Combines the antacid effects of aluminum hydroxide and magnesium carbonate. • Contraindicated in patients with severe renal disease and in patients who require sodium restriction. • Use cautiously in elderly patients, especially those with decreased GI motility, dehydration, fluid restriction, chronic renal disease, or suspected intestinal obstruction.
Gelusil ◇ aluminum hydroxide 200 mg, magnesium hydroxide 200 mg, and simethicone 20 mg	• Combines the antacid effects of aluminum hydroxide and magnesium hydroxide with the antiflatulent effect of simethicone. • Contraindicated in patients with severe renal disease or who are taking tetracycline. • Use cautiously in elderly patients, especially those with decreased GI motility, dehydration, fluid restriction, chronic renal disease, or suspected intestinal obstruction.
Maalox Plus (Extra Strength) ◇ aluminum hydroxide 500 mg, magnesium hydroxide 340 mg, and simethicone 40 mg	• Combines the antacid effects of aluminum hydroxide and magnesium hydroxide with the antiflatulent effect of simethicone. • Contraindicated in patients with severe renal impairment or who are taking tetracycline. • Use cautiously in elderly patients, especially those with decreased GI motility, dehydration, fluid restriction, chronic renal disease, or suspected intestinal obstruction.
Riopan Plus ◇ magaldrate 540 mg and simethicone 20 mg/5 ml	• Combines the antacid effect of magaldrate and the antiflatulent effect of simethicone. • Contraindicated in patients with severe renal impairment or who are taking tetracycline. • Use cautiously in elderly patients, especially those with decreased GI motility, dehydration, fluid restriction, or mild renal impairment.
Titralac Tablets ◇ calcium carbonate 420 mg and glycine 150 mg	• Combines the antacid effect of calcium carbonate with the smooth pleasant taste of glycine. • Contraindicated in patients with severe renal disease. • Use cautiously in elderly patients, especially those with decreased GI motility, dehydration, fluid restriction, chronic renal disease, or suspected intestinal obstruction.

◇ Available OTC

SELF-TEST

1. Jim Fielding, age 58, has reflux esophagitis for which his doctor prescribed use of an antacid. He asks you how soon after a dose the
antacid will work. You reply:
   a. immediately.
   b. 1 hour.
   c. 2 hours.
   d. 3 hours.

2. Mr. Fielding's prescribed antacid is magnesium hydroxide. You advise him to notify his doctor if he develops:
   a. diarrhea.
   b. constipation.
   c. vomiting.
   d. urine retention.

3. Jane Grant's doctor prescribed aluminum hydroxide. Ms. Grant is also
receiving enterically coated aspirin. When should you administer
the antacid?
   a. at the same time as the aspirin
   b. 1 hour before or after the aspirin
   c. 2 hours before the aspirin
   d. 2 hours after the aspirin

Check your answers on page 1068.

CHAPTER 46

DIGESTANTS

bile salts ◆ dehydrocholic acid ◆ glutamic acid hydrochloride
pancreatin ◆ pancrelipase

OVERVIEW

- Digestants promote digestion in the GI tract. Used in patients lacking such digestive substances as bile salts, gastric acid, or pancreatic enzymes, they can provide replacement therapy in specific deficiencies. The most widely used digestants are bile salts, hydrochloric acid, and the pancreatic enzymes pancreatin and pancrelipase.

MAJOR USES

- Bile salts are used to treat uncomplicated constipation and to help maintain normal cholesterol solubility in the bile. Dehydrocholic acid (synthetic bile salt) increases the solubility of cholesterol, preventing its buildup in recurrent biliary calculi or strictures, recurring noncalculous cholangitis, biliary dyskinesia and chronic partial obstruction of the common bile duct, prolonged drainage from biliary fistulas or drainage of infected bile duct through a T tube, and sclerosing choledochitis. It also prevents bacterial accumulation after biliary tract surgery.
- Glutamic acid hydrochloride counterbalances a deficiency of hydrochloric acid and is used to treat hypochlorhydria and achlorhydria.
- Pancreatin and pancrelipase (enzymes) supplement or replace exocrine pancreatic secretions, which are lacking in such disorders as cystic fibrosis.

MECHANISM OF ACTION

- Bile salts and dehydrocholic acid stimulate bile flow from the liver, promoting normal digestion and absorption of fats, fat-soluble vitamins, and cholesterol.
- Glutamic acid hydrochloride replaces gastric acid and destroys or inhibits growth of putrefactive microorganisms in ingested food.
- Pancreatin and pancrelipase replace endogenous exocrine pancreatic enzymes and aid intestinal digestion of starches, fats, and proteins.

ABSORPTION, DISTRIBUTION, METABOLISM, AND EXCRETION

About 80% to 90% of bile salts are reabsorbed, primarily in the ileum. They return to the liver and reenter the bile acid pool. As natural body

GLOSSARY

Constipation: decreased movement of fecal matter through the large intestine.
Diarrhea: increased frequency or weight and liquidity of stools produced by the rapid movement of fecal matter through the large intestine.
Digestant: drug that promotes digestion in the GI tract.

substances, the rest of the digestants assume the normal physiology of the body.

ONSET AND DURATION
Onset and duration of digestants are variable.

ADVERSE REACTIONS
High dosage of digestants may cause nausea, abdominal cramps, or diarrhea. Extremely high dosage has been associated with hyperuricosuria and hyperuricemia. Excessive dosage of bile salts may cause loose stools and mild cramping.

PROTOTYPE: DIGESTANTS

PANCREATIN
(pan' kree a tin)
Dizymes Tablets◊, Entozyme, Hi-Vegi-Lip Tablets◊, Pancreatin Enseals◊, Pancreatin Tablets◊
Classification: digestant
Pregnancy risk category C

How supplied
Dizymes
TABLETS (ENTERIC-COATED): 250 mg pancreatin, 6,750 units lipase, 41,250 units protease, 43,750 units amylase◊
Hi-Vegi-Lip
TABLETS (ENTERIC-COATED): 2,400 mg pancreatin, 12,000 units lipase, 60,000 units protease, 60,000 units amylase◊
Pancreatin Enseals
TABLETS (ENTERIC-COATED): 1,000 mg pancreatin, 2,000 units lipase, 25,000 units protease, 25,000 units amylase◊
Pancreatin Tablets
TABLETS (ENTERIC-COATED): 325 mg pancreatin, 650 units lipase, 8,125 units protease, 8,125 units amylase◊

◊ Available OTC

Indications and dosage
Exocrine pancreatic secretion insufficiency, digestive aid in cystic fibrosis
ADULTS AND CHILDREN: 1 to 3 tablets P.O. with meals.

Contraindications and precautions
Pancreatin is contraindicated in patients with known hypersensitivity to any of the drug's ingredients or with biliary tract obstruction.

Adverse reactions
GI: *nausea, diarrhea* (with high doses).
OTHER: hyperuricosuria (with high doses).

Interactions
Antacids: may negate pancreatin's beneficial effect. Don't use together.

Nursing considerations
Assessment
- Review the patient's history for a condition that contraindicates the use of pancreatin.
- Obtain a baseline assessment of the patient's digestive distress before therapy.
- Be alert for common adverse reactions.
- Evaluate the patient's and family's knowledge about pancreatin therapy.

Planning (Nursing Diagnoses)
Potential nursing diagnoses for the patient receiving pancreatin include:
- Altered health maintenance related to ineffective drug dosage.
- Noncompliance (medication administration) related to long-term therapy.
- Knowledge deficit related to pancreatin therapy.

Implementation
Preparation and administration
— Use only after confirmed diagnosis of exocrine pancreatic insufficiency. Not effective in GI disorders unrelated to pancreatic enzyme deficiency.
— For maximal effect, administer dose just before or during a meal or snack.
— Tablets may not be crushed or chewed.
— For young children, mix powders (including content of capsule) with applesauce and give with meals.
— Do not mix the drug with foods that contain proteins. Avoid inhalation of powder. Older children may swallow capsules with food.
— Enteric coating on some products may reduce availability of enzyme in upper portion of jejunum.
— Dosage varies according to degree of maldigestion and malabsorption, amount of fat in diet, and enzyme activity of individual preparations.
— Store in airtight containers at room temperature.

Monitoring

—Monitor the effectiveness of therapy by regularly assessing relief of digestive distress when the patient ingests proteins, carbohydrates, and fats.

—Monitor the patient for adverse drug reactions.

—Monitor the patient's bowel habits. Adequate replacement decreases number of bowel movements and improves stool consistency.

—Monitor the patient's diet and eating habits. Diet should balance fat, protein, and carbohydrate intake properly to avoid indigestion.

—Monitor the patient for drug interactions.

—Monitor diagnostic tests. Pancreatin, particularly in large doses, increases serum uric acid concentrations.

—Regularly reevaluate the patient's and family's knowledge about pancreatin therapy.

Intervention

—If the patient is unable to comply with therapy, discuss reasons why and suggest possible methods the patient may use to maintain compliance.

—Keep all members of the health care team informed of the patient's response to the drug.

Patient teaching

—Instruct the patient and family about pancreatin, including the dosage, frequency, action, and adverse reactions.

—Explain disease process and rationale for therapy.

—Explain use of drug and advise storage away from heat and light.

—Be sure the patient or family understands special dietary instructions for the particular disease.

—Tell the patient that adequate replacement of the pancreatic enzyme will decrease the number of bowel movements and improve stool consistency.

—Tell the parents (if the patient is a child) or the patient that the pancreatic enzymes should be taken with all regular meals as well as snacks.

—Warn the patient that digestants interact with antacids, and should not be used together. The patient should not self-medicate with an OTC antacid.

—Warn the patient that eating unbalanced amounts of fat, protein, and starch may cause indigestion.

—If the patient is a child, instruct the parents about the importance of watching the child's appetite and eating habits. The child's appetite will be dramatically decreased and a nutritional problem could develop.

—Tell the parents to clean the enzyme from the child's lips and skin to prevent skin breakdown.

—Tell the parents to notify the doctor if the child experiences diarrhea.

—Symptoms of inadequate pancreatic replacement and excessive intake of fat, such as abdominal cramps and distention; mushy, light-colored stools; foul-smelling gas; rectal seepage of oil; rectal prolapse; or continual weight loss despite a voracious appetite, should be reported to the doctor.

— Inform the patient that he will probably take this drug for the rest of his life.

— Tell the patient to notify the nurse or doctor if adverse reactions develop or questions arise about pancreatin therapy.

Evaluation

In the patient receiving pancreatin, appropriate evaluation statements include:

• Patient maintains normal digestion and shows no signs of digestive distress when ingesting proteins, carbohydrates, and fats.

• Patient complies with prescribed drug regimen.

• Patient and family state an understanding of pancreatin therapy.

SELECTED MAJOR DRUGS: DIGESTANTS

DRUG, INDICATIONS, AND DOSAGES	SPECIAL PRECAUTIONS
dehydrocholic acid (Atrocholin, Decholin) *Insufficient bile production—* **Adults:** 244 to 500 mg P.O. b.i.d. or t.i.d. after meals for 4 to 6 weeks.	• Do not administer to patients who are nauseated or vomiting or who have abdominal pain. • Frequent use may result in dependence on laxatives.
glutamic acid hydrochloride (Acidulin Pulvules) *Hypochlorhydria and achlorhydria—* **Adults:** 1 to 3 capsules P.O. t.i.d. before meals (340 mg to 1 g).	• Do not give to patients with gastric hyperacidity or peptic ulcer disease. • Monitor response to these agents.
pancrelipase (Viokase) *Exocrine pancreatic secretion insufficiency, cystic fibrosis in adults and children, steatorrhea and other disorders of fat metabolism secondary to insufficient pancreatic enzymes—* **Adults and children:** dosage ranges from 1 to 3 capsules or tablets P.O. before or with meals and 1 capsule or tablet with snack; or 1 to 2 powder packets before meals or snacks. Dose must be titrated to patient's response.	• Contraindicated in patients with severe pork hypersensitivity. • Be careful when preparing dosage from powder. Some nurses and caregivers have experienced allergic reactions from the powder's dust.

COMPARING DIGESTANT COMBINATIONS

TRADE NAME AND CONTENT	SPECIAL CONSIDERATIONS
Donnazyme pancreatin 300 mg, pepsin 150 mg, bile salts 150 mg, hyoscyamine sulfate 0.0518 mg, atropine sulfate 0.0097 mg, scopolamine hydrobromide 0.0033 mg, and phenobarbital 8.1 mg	• Combines the anticholinergic and antispasmodic effects of hyoscyamine sulfate, atropine sulfate, and scopolamine hydrobromide and the sedative effect of phenobarbital with natural digestive enzymes (pancreatin and pepsin) plus bile salts. • Contraindicated in patients with glaucoma; obstructive uropathy (for example, bladder neck obstruction due to prostatic hypertrophy); obstructive disease of the GI tract (for example, achalasia, pyloroduodenal stenosis); paralytic ileus; intestinal atony of elderly or debilitated patients; unstable CV status in acute hemorrhage; severe ulcerative colitis, especially if complicated by toxic megacolon; myasthenia gravis; and hiatal hernia associated with reflux esophagitis. • Also contraindicated in patients with known hypersensitivity to any of the drug's ingredients. Phenobarbital is contraindicated in acute intermittent porphyria and in those patients in whom phenobarbital produces restlessness or excitement. • Use cautiously in patients with autonomic neuropathy, hepatic renal disease, hyperthyroidism, coronary heart disease, CHF, cardiac arrhythmias, tachycardia, and hypertension.
Pancrease lipase 4,000 units, protease 25,000 units, and amylase 20,000 units in enteric-coated microspheres	• Combines the effects of the three pancreatic enzymes, lipase, protease, and amylase. • Contraindicated in patients with known hypersensitivity to pork protein. • Use cautiously during pregnancy.

SELF-TEST

1. Michael, a 1-year-old child with cystic fibrosis, has a deficiency of exocrine pancreatic secretion. A digestant is prescribed for him; you know that a digestant:
   a. replaces endogenous bile salts and cholesterol.
   b. replaces endogenous fats, proteins, and carbohydrates.
   c. promotes digestion in the GI tract.
   d. promotes excretion of fats, proteins, and carbohydrates.

2. If pancreatin is prescribed, how should the nurse tell the mother to administer the drug?
   a. Mix powders with applesauce and give with meals.
   b. Mix powders with applesauce and give after meals.
   c. Crush tablet and give with meals.
   d. Crush tablet and give after meals.

3. Which of the following statements made by Michael's mother would indicate successful therapy with pancreatin?
   a. My son was sitting in his crib playing with his truck today when I came to visit.
   b. My son's pain really seems to be eased since treatment with this medication began.
   c. The number of my son's bowel movements has decreased and the consistency has improved.
   d. My son is much more alert.

Check your answers on pages 1068 and 1069.

CHAPTER 47

ANTIDIARRHEALS

bismuth subgallate ♦ bismuth subsalicylate ♦ calcium polycarbophil
difenoxin hydrochloride ♦ diphenoxylate hydrochloride
kaolin and pectin mixtures ♦ loperamide hydrochloride ♦ opium tincture
opium tincture, camphorated

OVERVIEW

- Antidiarrheals reduce the fluidity of the stool and the frequency of defecation.
- Diarrhea is the abnormally frequent passage of watery stools with an average daily weight above 300 g. (Healthy adults have an average daily fecal weight of 100 to 150 g.)
- In the absence of other symptoms, diarrhea usually reflects a minor and transient GI disorder. In more serious conditions, however, it is usually one of several symptoms. Diarrhea may be caused by foods or drugs, laxative abuse, allergies, endocrine dysfunction, malabsorption, neurologic or inflammatory diseases, mechanical obstruction, parasitic infection, gastric resection, or radiation poisoning.

MAJOR USES

- All antidiarrheals are used to treat acute, mild, or chronic stages of nonspecific diarrhea.
- Bismuth subgallate also neutralizes or absorbs fecal odors in patients with a colostomy or ileostomy.
- Loperamide also reduces the volume of ileostomy discharge and decreases daily fecal volume and fluid and electrolyte loss.

MECHANISM OF ACTION

- Bismuth salts have a mild water-binding capacity; they also may absorb toxins and provide protective coating for intestinal mucosa.
- Calcium polycarbophil absorbs free fecal water, thereby producing formed stools.
- Difenoxin, diphenoxylate, loperamide, and opium tinctures increase smooth muscle tone in the GI tract, inhibit motility and propulsion, and diminish digestive secretions. All of these drugs are opiate derivatives; however, loperamide has no analgesic activity and will not produce physical dependence. Commercial preparations containing either difenoxin or diphenoxylate contain subtherapeutic doses of atropine sulfate to discourage drug abuse.

GLOSSARY

Antidiarrheal: drug that decreases the frequency of defecation and water content of the stools.
Diarrhea: increased frequency or weight and liquidity of stools produced by the rapid movement of fecal matter through the large intestine.

• Kaolin and pectin decrease the stool's fluid content by adsorption of bacteria and toxins that may cause diarrhea, although *total* water loss seems to remain the same.

ABSORPTION, DISTRIBUTION, METABOLISM, AND EXCRETION

Adsorbent antidiarrheals (bismuth salts, calcium polycarbophil, and kaolin and pectin) are not systemically absorbed.

Diphenoxylate and difenoxin are well absorbed from the GI tract, metabolized in the liver, and eliminated in both urine and feces. Loperamide is poorly absorbed orally, metabolized in the liver, and eliminated primarily in feces. Opium tinctures are absorbed moderately from the GI tract as morphine, metabolized in the liver, and excreted in urine.

ONSET AND DURATION

Bismuth salts, calcium polycarbophil, and kaolin and pectin begin to act within 30 minutes; their therapeutic effects can last 4 to 6 hours. Diphenoxylate begins to act within 45 to 60 minutes. Its effect lasts as long as 4 hours. Loperamide's peak levels occur in 5 hours after capsule administration and 2.5 hours after liquid administration; elimination half-life is about 10.8 hours (range is 9.1 to 14.4 hours). Opium tinctures begin to act rapidly. Duration of action varies.

ADVERSE REACTIONS

Antidiarrheals that contain atropine (difenoxin and diphenoxylate) may cause anticholinergic effects, such as dryness of the skin and mucous membranes, flushing, hyperthermia, tachycardia, and urine retention. However, because of the small amount of atropine these medications contain, anticholinergic effects are unlikely, except in children.

Many of the associated adverse reactions are difficult to distinguish from the symptoms of the diarrheal syndrome, but include nausea, vomiting, dry mouth, dizziness and light-headedness, drowsiness, headache, tiredness, nervousness, and hypersensitivity reactions.

DIPHENOXYLATE HYDROCHLORIDE
(dye fen ox' i late)
Diphenatol, Lofene, Logen, Lomanate, Lomotil, Lonox, Lo-Trol,
Low-Quel, Nor-Mil*
Classification: antidiarrheal
Controlled substance schedule V
Pregnancy risk category C

How supplied
TABLETS: 2.5 mg (with atropine sulfate 0.025 mg)
LIQUID: 2.5 mg/5 ml (with atropine sulfate 0.025 mg/5 ml)*

Indications and dosage
Acute, nonspecific diarrhea
ADULTS: initially, 1 to 2 tablets or tsp P.O. t.i.d. or q.i.d.; decrease dose to
1 tablet or tsp b.i.d. or t.i.d.
CHILDREN AGES 2 AND OVER: administer according to diphenoxylate com-
ponent. Initially, 0.3 to 0.4 mg/kg P.O. daily in divided doses, or as
follows—
CHILDREN OVER AGE 12: give usual adult dose.
CHILDREN AGES 9 TO 12 (23 TO 55 KG): 1.75 to 2.5 mg P.O. q.i.d.
CHILDREN AGES 6 TO 9 (17 TO 32 KG): 1.25 to 2.5 mg P.O. q.i.d.
CHILDREN AGES 5 TO 6 (16 TO 23 KG): 1.25 to 2.25 mg P.O. q.i.d.
CHILDREN AGES 4 TO 5 (14 TO 20 KG): 1 to 2 mg P.O. q.i.d.
CHILDREN AGES 3 TO 4 (12 TO 16 KG): 1 to 1.5 mg P.O. q.i.d.
CHILDREN AGES 2 TO 3 (11 TO 14 KG): 0.75 to 1.5 mg P.O. q.i.d.

Contraindications and precautions
Diphenoxylate is contraindicated in patients with known hypersensitivity
to diphenoxylate or atropine, obstructive jaundice, and diarrhea associated
with pseudomembranous enterocolitis or enterotoxin-producing bacteria.
Use with special caution in young children and with extreme caution in
patients with advanced hepatorenal disease and abnormal liver function.

Adverse reactions
CNS: *sedation,* dizziness, headache, drowsiness, lethargy, restlessness,
depression, euphoria.
CV: tachycardia.
EENT: mydriasis.
GI: *dry mouth,* nausea, vomiting, abdominal discomfort or distention,
paralytic ileus, anorexia, fluid retention in bowel (may mask depletion of
extracellular fluid and electrolytes, especially in young children treated
for acute gastroenteritis).
GU: urine retention.
SKIN: pruritus, giant urticaria, rash.

---

*Liquid form contains alcohol
Italicized adverse reactions are common

OTHER: possible physical dependence in long-term use, angioedema, respiratory depression.

Interactions

MAO inhibitors: may precipitate hypertensive crisis. Avoid concomitant use.
CNS depressants (such as barbiturates, tranquilizers, and alcohol): increased depressant effect. Use together with caution.

Nursing considerations

Assessment
- Review the patient's history for a condition that contraindicates the use of diphenoxylate.
- Obtain a baseline assessment of the patient's bowel habits, including amount and type of diarrhea, before therapy.
- Be alert for common adverse reactions.
- Evaluate the patient's and family's knowledge about diphenoxylate therapy.

Planning (Nursing Diagnoses)
Potential nursing diagnoses for the patient receiving diphenoxylate include:
- Altered health maintenance related to inadequate dosage to alleviate diarrhea.
- Fluid volume deficit related to decreased intake caused by the adverse GI reactions of an antidiarrheal.
- Knowledge deficit related to diphenoxylate therapy.

Implementation
Preparation and administration
— Administer drug as prescribed.
— Encourage extra fluid intake when administering the drug.
— Drug is a controlled substance schedule V. Follow your institution's policy on the sign out and administration of this drug.
— Withhold drug and notify the doctor if the patient with acute, nonspecific diarrhea shows no improvement in 48 hours.

Monitoring
— Monitor the effectiveness of therapy by regularly assessing the amount, nature, and frequency of the patient's stools.
— Monitor the patient for adverse drug reactions.
— Monitor vital signs, intake and output, and bowel function.
— Monitor fluid and electrolyte status.
— Observe for signs of atropine toxicity.
— Observe for signs of hypoperistalsis, such as anorexia, nausea, abdominal distention, auscultation of high-pitched sounds over the abdomen or absent bowel sounds, percussion of air or fluid over the abdomen, absence of flatus or bowel movements, and vomiting.

—Monitor the patient for drug interactions.

—Monitor diagnostic test results. Diphenoxylate may decrease urine excretion of phenolsulfonphthalein (PSP) during the PSP excretion test; drug may increase serum amylase levels.

—Regularly reevaluate the patient's and family's knowledge about diphenoxylate therapy.

Intervention

—If the patient shows signs of urine retention, such as urinary frequency or a sensation of fullness in the lower abdomen after voiding, notify the doctor. Be prepared to catheterize the patient as prescribed and to reduce the antidiarrheal dosage or administer a different antidiarrheal.

—If signs of hypoperistalsis occur, withhold the next dose and notify the doctor.

—Take safety precautions if drowsiness occurs. For example, place the bed in a low position, keep the side rails up, and supervise ambulation.

—If the patient's vital signs, intake and output, bowel function, or fluid and electrolyte status worsens, notify the doctor.

—Provide the patient with frequent oral hygiene mouth rinses, and suggest the use of sugarless gum or hard candy or ice chips to relieve dry mouth, which he may experience while he is receiving the drug.

—Keep all members of the health care team informed of the patient's response to the drug.

Patient teaching

—Instruct the patient and family about diphenoxylate, including the dosage, frequency, action, and adverse reactions.

—Explain the disease process and rationale for therapy.

—Warn the patient to take drug exactly as ordered and not to exceed recommended dose.

—Advise the patient to maintain adequate fluid intake during course of diarrhea and teach him about diet and fluid replacement.

—Caution the patient to avoid driving while taking this drug because it may cause drowsiness and dizziness; warn the patient to avoid alcohol or any other CNS depressant while taking this drug because additive depressant effects may occur.

—Advise the patient to notify the doctor if drug is not effective within 48 hours.

—Warn the patient that prolonged use may result in tolerance and that taking larger-than-recommended doses may result in drug dependence.

—Instruct the patient to be alert for early warning signs of hypoperistalsis (nausea and anorexia) and toxic megacolon (abdominal distention). If these signs occur, tell the patient to notify the doctor before taking next dose.

—Tell the patient to notify the nurse or doctor if adverse reactions develop or questions arise about diphenoxylate therapy.

—Teach the patient to recognize and report the signs of atropine toxicity, which may require dosage reduction.

—Teach the patient to recognize and report signs or symptoms of urine retention.

Evaluation

In the patient receiving diphenoxylate, appropriate evaluation statements include:

• Patient is free of diarrhea.
• Patient maintains normal fluid balance.
• Patient and family state an understanding of diphenoxylate therapy.

SELECTED MAJOR DRUGS: ANTIDIARRHEALS

DRUG, INDICATIONS, AND DOSAGES	SPECIAL PRECAUTIONS
bismuth subgallate (Devrom ◇), **bismuth subsalicylate (Pepto-Bismol ◇)** *Mild, nonspecific diarrhea—* **Adults:** 1 to 2 tablets (subgallate) P.O. chewed or swallowed whole t.i.d. Or 30 ml or 2 tablets (subsalicylate) P.O. q ½ to 1 hour up to a maximum of eight doses and for no longer than 2 days. **Children ages 9 to 12:** 20 ml or 1 tablet P.O. **Children ages 6 to 9:** 10 ml or ⅔ tablet P.O. **Children ages 3 to 6:** 5 ml or ⅓ tablet P.O. *Prevention and treatment of traveler's diarrhea (turista)—* **Adults:** prophylactically, 60 ml (subsalicylate) P.O. q.i.d. during the first 2 weeks of travel. During acute illness, 30 to 60 ml P.O. q 30 minutes for a total of eight doses. Alternatively, 2 tablets P.O. q.i.d. for up to 3 weeks.	• Contraindicated in patients with a history of hypersensitivity to any of the components. • Administer cautiously and discontinue use if irritation or rectal bleeding occurs or condition persists.
calcium polycarbophil (Equalactin ◇ , FiberCon ◇ , Mitrolan ◇) *Constipation (Equalactin and Mitrolan must be chewed before swallowing)—* **Adults:** 1 g P.O. q.i.d. as required. Maximum is 6 g in 24 hours. **Children ages 6 to 12:** 500 mg P.O. t.i.d. as required. Maximum is 3 g in 24 hours. **Children ages 2 to 6:** 500 mg P.O. b.i.d. as required. Maximum is 1.5 g in 24 hours. *Diarrhea associated with irritable bowel syndrome, as well as acute, nonspecific diarrhea (Mitrolan must be chewed before swallowing)—* **Adults:** 1 g P.O. q.i.d. as required. Maximum is 6 g in 24 hours. **Children ages 6 to 12:** 500 mg P.O. t.i.d. as required. Maximum is 3 g in 24 hours. **Children ages 2 to 6:** 500 mg P.O. b.i.d. as required. Maximum is 1.5 g in 24 hours.	• Contraindicated in patients with signs of GI obstruction. • Drug is used as both a laxative and antidiarrheal; laxative action requires patient to drink plenty of water with each dose. • Administer cautiously. Drug may interact with some forms of tetracycline if taken concomitantly.

(continued)

◇ Available OTC

SELECTED MAJOR DRUGS: ANTIDIARRHEALS *continued*

DRUG, INDICATIONS, AND DOSAGES	SPECIAL PRECAUTIONS
difenoxin with atropine (Lyspafen‡, Motofen) *Adjunct in acute, nonspecific diarrhea and acute exacerbations of chronic functional diarrhea—* **Adults:** initially, 2 mg P.O., then 1 mg P.O. after each loose bowel movement. Total dosage should not exceed 8 mg daily. Not recommended for use longer than 2 days.	• Contraindicated in patients with known hypersensitivity to difenoxin or atropine, in children under age 2, and in patients with diarrhea resulting from pseudomembranous colitis associated with antibiotics. Also contraindicated in patients with jaundice or with diarrhea resulting from organisms that may penetrate the intestinal mucosa (including toxigenic *Escherichia coli, Salmonella,* or *Shigella*).
kaolin and pectin (Kao-Con†, Kaopectate ◇) *Mild, nonspecific diarrhea—* **Adults:** 60 to 120 ml P.O. after each bowel movement. **Children over age 12:** 60 ml P.O. after each bowel movement. **Children ages 6 to 12:** 30 to 60 ml P.O. after each bowel movement. **Children ages 3 to 6:** 15 to 30 ml P.O. after each bowel movement.	• Contraindicated in patients with suspected obstructive bowel lesions.
loperamide (Imodium A-D ◇) *Acute, nonspecific diarrhea—* **Adults:** initially, 4 mg P.O., then 2 mg after each unformed stool. Maximum is 16 mg daily. **Children ages 8 to 12:** 10 ml t.i.d. P.O. on first day. (Subsequent doses of 5 ml/10 kg of body weight may be administered after each unformed stool.) **Children ages 5 to 8:** 10 ml P.O. b.i.d. on first day. **Children ages 2 to 5:** 5 ml P.O. t.i.d. on first day. *Chronic diarrhea—* **Adults:** initially, 4 mg P.O., then 2 mg after each unformed stool until diarrhea subsides. Adjust dosage to individual response.	• Contraindicated in patients with acute diarrhea resulting from poison until toxic material is removed from GI tract, in acute diarrhea caused by organisms that penetrate intestinal mucosa, and when constipation must be avoided. • Use cautiously in severe prostatic hypertrophy, hepatic disease, and history of narcotic dependence.
opium tincture **opium tincture, camphorated (paregoric)** *Acute, nonspecific diarrhea—* **Adults:** 0.6 ml opium tincture (range is 0.3 to 1 ml) P.O. q.i.d. Maximum dosage is 6 ml daily. Or 5 to 10 mg camphorated opium tincture daily b.i.d., t.i.d., or q.i.d. until diarrhea subsides.	• Contraindicated in patients with acute diarrhea resulting from poison until toxic material is removed from GI tract and with diarrhea caused by organisms that penetrate intestinal mucosa. • Use cautiously in asthma, prostatic hypertrophy, hepatic disease, and narcotic dependence.

†Available in Canada only   ‡Available in Australia only   ◇ Available OTC

COMPARING ANTIDIARRHEAL COMBINATIONS

TRADE NAME AND CONTENT	SPECIAL CONSIDERATIONS
Donnagel-PG powdered opium (or equivalent) 24 mg, kaolin 6 g, pectin 142.8 mg, hyoscyamine sulfate 0.1037 mg, atropine sulfate 0.0194 mg, scopolamine hydrobromide 0.0065 mg, sodium benzoate 60 mg (preservative), and alcohol 5%	• Combines the antidiarrheal effects of kaolin, pectin, and opium with the belladonna alkaloids' ability to partly antagonize the occasional cramping effect of opium upon the colon. • Contraindicated in patients with known hypersensitivity to any of the ingredients, glaucoma, or advanced renal or hepatic disease. • Use cautiously in patients with incipient glaucoma, urinary bladder neck obstruction such as prostatic hypertrophy, and in pregnant or breast-feeding women.
Parepectolin opium 15 mg (equivalent to paregoric 3.7 ml), kaolin 5.5 g, pectin 162 mg, and alcohol 0.69%	• Combines the adsorbent effects of kaolin and pectin with the antidiarrheal effect of opium. • Contraindicated in patients with known hypersensitivity to the drug, head injury, or CNS depression. • Use cautiously in patients with renal or hepatic impairment and in elderly patients.

SELF-TEST

1. Jay Bates, age 40, receives diphenoxylate for treatment of acute, nonspecific diarrhea. What is this drug's mechanism of action?
   a. It decreases the stool's fluid content.
   b. It inhibits peristaltic activity.
   c. It suppresses growth of pathogenic microorganisms.
   d. It increases smooth muscle tone in the GI tract, inhibits motility and propulsion, and diminishes digestive secretions.

2. Adverse reactions to antidiarrheals containing atropine may include:
   a. urine retention.
   b. sodium retention.
   c. hyperkalemia.
   d. bradycardia.

3. Mr. Bates' diarrhea has shown no improvement after 48 hours of treatment. What should the nurse do?
   a. Withhold the drug and notify the doctor.
   b. Continue administering the drug as ordered.
   c. Double the ordered dosage.
   d. Cut the ordered dosage in half.

Check your answers on page 1069.

CHAPTER 48

LAXATIVES

bisacodyl ✦ calcium polycarbophil ✦ cascara sagrada
cascara sagrada aromatic fluidextract ✦ cascara sagrada fluidextract
castor oil ✦ docusate calcium ✦ docusate potassium ✦ docusate sodium
glycerin lactulose ✦ magnesium salts ✦ methylcellulose ✦ mineral oil
phenolphthalein ✦ psyllium ✦ senna ✦ sodium phosphates

OVERVIEW

- Laxatives (also historically known as cathartics, drastics, and purgatives) ease the passage of feces from the colon and rectum. The accumulation of feces in the lower bowel results from constipation, which is defined as decreased frequency of fecal elimination, characterized by the passage of hard, dry stools. To alleviate constipation, many people overuse laxatives.
- Laxatives can be classified according to the way they work: hyperosmolar, bulk-forming, saline, lubricant, emollient or stool softener, or stimulant.

MAJOR USES

- Laxatives may relieve or prevent constipation. They are used to evacuate the bowel before rectal or bowel examination, exposure of abdominal X-ray films, barium enema, or various surgical procedures.
- Docusate calcium (formerly dioctyl calcium sulfosuccinate), docusate potassium (formerly dioctyl potassium sulfosuccinate), and docusate sodium (formerly dioctyl sodium sulfosuccinate) are commonly used to soften stools and prevent straining during defecation.
- Lactulose is also used to treat hepatic encephalopathy.

MECHANISM OF ACTION

- Bulk-forming laxatives (psyllium, methylcellulose, calcium polycarbophil) absorb water and expand to increase bulk and moisture content of the stool. The increased bulk encourages peristalsis and bowel movement.
- Emollient laxatives, or stool softeners (docusate calcium, docusate potassium, docusate sodium), reduce surface tension of interfacing liquid contents of the bowel. This mechanism, or detergent activity, promotes incorporation of additional liquid into the stool, forming a softer mass.
- Among the hyperosmolar laxatives, glycerin draws water from the tissues into the feces and thus stimulates evacuation. Lactulose produces an osmotic effect in the colon and is biodegraded by the intestinal flora

GLOSSARY

Cathartic: agent that promotes evacuation of the bowels.
Constipation: decreased movement of fecal matter through the large intestine.
Emollient: drug that softens the stool by increasing the water content of fecal material through a reduction in surface tension of bowel contents.
Laxative: drug that stimulates defecation by forming bulk, stimulating peristalsis, or providing lubrication or chemical irritation.

into lactic, formic, and acetic acids. Distention of the bowel from fluid accumulation promotes peristalsis and bowel movement.

- Saline laxatives (magnesium salts and sodium phosphates) produce an osmotic effect in the small intestine by drawing water into the intestinal lumen. Fluid accumulation produces distention, which then encourages peristalsis and bowel movement. Saline laxatives also promote cholecystokinin secretion, stimulating intestinal motility and inhibiting fluid and electrolyte absorption from the jejunum and ileum.

- The lubricant laxative mineral oil increases water retention in the stool by creating a barrier between the colon wall and feces that prevents colonic reabsorption of fecal water.

- Stimulant laxatives (bisacodyl, cascara sagrada, cascara sagrada aromatic fluidextract, cascara sagrada fluidextract, castor oil, phenolphthalein, and senna) may increase peristalsis by direct effect on the smooth muscle of the intestine. Although the precise mechanism is unknown, stimulant laxatives are thought to either irritate the musculature or stimulate the colonic intramural plexus. These drugs also promote fluid accumulation in the colon and small intestine, increasing the laxative effect.

ABSORPTION, DISTRIBUTION, METABOLISM, AND EXCRETION

Bulk-forming laxatives are not absorbed systemically. Emollient laxatives are systemically absorbed and eliminated in the bile. Among the hyperosmolar laxatives, glycerin suppositories and lactulose are not absorbed systemically. About 20% of the magnesium in magnesium salts is systemically absorbed and excreted in urine. Up to 10% of the sodium content of sodium phosphates in enemas may be absorbed and excreted in urine. Mineral oil, a lubricant laxative, is not significantly absorbed when given in its nonemulsified form; as much as one-half of emulsified mineral oil may be absorbed. Stimulant laxatives are slightly absorbed and are metabolized in the liver. The metabolites are eliminated either in urine or—through the bile—in feces.

ONSET AND DURATION

The action of most laxatives ends after bowel evacuation. Hyperosmolar laxatives, magnesium salts, and sodium phosphates are the most rapid-acting laxatives after oral administration. They usually take effect within 30 minutes to 3 hours. Bulk-forming and emollient laxatives have the slowest onset of action, requiring 12 to 72 hours to produce an effect. The lubricant laxative mineral oil acts within 6 to 8 hours. Stimulant laxatives act within 6 to 12 hours of administration. Their effects usually last less than 24 hours.

ADVERSE REACTIONS

Chronic use of all laxatives can cause "laxative dependence," a condition in which the intestinal musculature is incapable of causing effective peristalsis.

Bulk-forming laxatives may cause flatulence. Esophageal obstruction may occur when these agents are chewed or taken in dry form; therefore, they must be administered in or with a full glass of water or other liquid. They may also cause intestinal obstruction or fecal impaction. Some may contain up to 50% sugar or excessive sodium, which should be considered for patients on restricted diets.

Hyperosmolar and saline laxatives may cause fluid and electrolyte deficits with excessive use. Magnesium salts may cause hypermagnesemia in patients with renal impairment; the sodium phosphates may cause sodium overload.

Emollient laxatives are associated with chronic and abusive use in combination with irritants.

Lubricant laxatives impair the absorption of fat-soluble vitamins (A, D, E, and K). They may cause lipid pneumonia secondary to aspiration, sphincter leakage producing pruritus ani with large doses, and absorption of mineral oil in lymph nodes, intestinal mucosa, liver, and spleen.

Stimulant laxatives can cause gripping, intestinal cramps, increased mucous secretion, and fluid and electrolyte deficiencies (hypokalemia) resulting from excessive catharsis (generally dose-related).

DOCUSATE CALCIUM
(dok′ yoo sate)
Pro-Cal-Sof◊, Surfak◊

DOCUSATE POTASSIUM
Dialose◊, Diocto-K◊, Kasof◊

DOCUSATE SODIUM
*Afko-Lube◊, Colace◊, Coloxyl‡, Coloxyl Enema Concentrate‡, Diocto◊,
Dioeze◊, Diosuccin◊, Dio-Sul◊, Disonate◊, Di-Sosul◊, Doxinate◊, D-S-S◊,
Duosol◊, Genasoft◊, Laxinate 100◊, Modane Soft◊, Pro-Sof◊, Pro-Sof
250◊, Pro-Sof Liquid Concentrate◊, Regulax SS◊, Regutol◊, Stulex◊*
Classification: emollient laxative
Pregnancy risk category C

How supplied
calcium
CAPSULES: 50 mg◊, 240 mg◊
potassium
CAPSULES: 100 mg◊, 240 mg◊
sodium
TABLETS: 50 mg○, 100 mg◊
CAPSULES◊: 50 mg, 60 mg, 100 mg, 240 mg, 250 mg, 300 mg
ORAL LIQUID: 50 mg/ml◊
SYRUP: 50 mg/15 ml◊, 60 mg/15 ml◊
ENEMA CONCENTRATE: 18 g/100 ml (must be diluted)‡

Indications and dosage
Stool softener
ADULTS AND OLDER CHILDREN: 50 to 300 mg (sodium) P.O. daily or 50 to
300 mg (calcium and potassium) P.O. daily until bowel movements are
normal. Alternatively, give enema (where available). Dilute 1:24 with
sterile water before administration, and give 100 to 150 ml (retention
enema), 300 to 500 ml (evacuation enema), or 0.5 to 1.5 liters (flushing
enema).
CHILDREN AGES 6 TO 12: 40 to 120 mg (sodium) P.O. daily.
CHILDREN AGES 3 TO 6: 20 to 60 mg (sodium) P.O. daily.
CHILDREN UNDER AGE 3: 10 to 40 mg (sodium) P.O. daily.
　Higher dosages are for initial therapy. Adjust dosage to individual
response. Usual dosage in children and adults with minimal needs is 50 to
150 mg (sodium) P.O. daily.

Contraindications and precautions
There are no known contraindications to the use of docusate.

Adverse reactions

EENT: throat irritation.

GI: bitter taste, *mild abdominal cramping, diarrhea.*

OTHER: laxative dependence (in long-term or excessive use).

Interactions

Mineral oil: may increase mineral oil absorption and cause lipid pneumonia. Don't administer together.

Nursing considerations

Assessment

• Obtain a baseline assessment of the patient's bowel habits and extent of constipation before therapy.

• Be alert for common adverse reactions.

• Evaluate the patient's and family's knowledge about docusate therapy.

Planning (Nursing Diagnoses)

Potential nursing diagnoses for the patient receiving docusate include:

• Altered health maintenance related to inadequate dosage to prevent constipation.

• Potential for injury related to adverse drug reactions.

• Knowledge deficit related to docusate therapy.

Implementation

Preparation and administration

— Give liquid (but not syrup) in milk, fruit juice, or infant formula to mask bitter taste.

— If giving liquid through nasogastric tube, flush tube afterward to clear it and ensure dispersion into stomach.

— Avoid using docusate sodium in sodium-restricted patients.

— Drug should not be used to treat existing constipation, but rather to prevent it from developing.

— Docusate is the laxative of choice in the patient who should not strain during defecation, such as one recovering from MI or rectal surgery; in disease of rectum and anus that makes passage of firm stool difficult; or in postpartum constipation.

— Drug acts within 24 to 48 hours to produce firm, semisolid stool.

— Discontinue if severe cramping occurs.

— Store at 59° to 86° F (15° to 30° C). Protect liquid from light.

Monitoring

— Monitor the effectiveness of therapy by regularly assessing the patient's bowel habits and number of bowel movements.

— Monitor the patient for adverse drug reactions.

— Monitor for development of diarrhea.

— Monitor the patient for drug interactions.

— Monitor for possible laxative dependence.

— Regularly reevaluate the patient's and family's knowledge about docusate therapy.

Italicized adverse reactions are common

Intervention

—If the patient develops diarrhea, notify the doctor and replace fluids and electrolytes as ordered.
—Keep all members of the health care team informed of the patient's response to the drug.

Patient teaching

—Instruct the patient and family about docusate, including the dosage, frequency, action, and adverse reactions.
—Explain the disease process and rationale for therapy.
—Explain to the patient that drug should not be used to treat existing constipation but rather to prevent constipation.
—Warn the patient to take the medication only as directed.
—Tell the patient to dilute liquid (but not syrup) in juice or other flavored liquid to improve taste.
—Advise the patient that drug should be used only occasionally. The patient should not use drug for more than 1 week without the doctor's knowledge.
—Docusate salts lose their effectiveness over time; advise the patient to report failure of medication.
—Discuss measures the patient can take to prevent constipation. For example, tell the patient that dietary sources of bulk include bran and other cereals, fresh fruit, and vegetables.
—Tell the patient to notify the nurse or doctor if adverse reactions develop or questions arise about docusate therapy.
—Warn the patient that long-term or excessive use can cause laxative dependence.

Evaluation

In the patient receiving docusate, appropriate evaluation statements include:
• Patient maintains normal bowel habits and does not develop constipation.
• Patient experiences no adverse reactions.
• Patient and family state an understanding of docusate therapy.

SELECTED MAJOR DRUGS: LAXATIVES

DRUG, INDICATIONS, AND DOSAGES	SPECIAL PRECAUTIONS
bisacodyl (Biscolax ◇ , Dulcolax ◇) *Chronic constipation; preparation for delivery, surgery, or rectal or bowel examination —* **Adults:** 10 to 15 mg P.O. in evening or before breakfast. Up to 30 mg may be used for thorough evacuation needed for examinations or surgery. **Children age 6 and over:** 5 to 10 mg P.O. **Adults and children over age 2:** 10 mg P.R. **Children under age 2:** 5 mg P.R.	• Contraindicated in patients with abdominal pain, nausea, vomiting, or other symptoms of appendicitis or acute surgical abdomen or in rectal fissures or ulcerated hemorrhoids. • Administer cautiously to pregnant women. • Tablets are enteric-coated. Do not administer with antacids.
cascara sagrada ◇ **cascara sagrada aromatic fluidextract ◇** **cascara sagrada fluidextract ◇** *Acute constipation; preparation for bowel or rectal examination —* **Adults:** 325 mg (cascara sagrada tablets) P.O. h.s.; or 1 ml (fluidextract) daily; or 5 ml (aromatic fluidextract) daily. **Children ages 2 to 12:** half the adult dose. **Children under age 2:** one-fourth the adult dose.	• Contraindicated in patients with abdominal pain, nausea, vomiting, or other symptoms of appendicitis or acute surgical abdomen; acute surgical delirium, fecal impaction, intestinal obstruction, or perforation. • Use cautiously when rectal bleeding is present.
castor oil (Alphamul ◇ , Neoloid ◇) *Preparation for rectal or bowel examination, or surgery; acute constipation (rarely) —* **Adults:** 15 to 60 ml P.O. **Children over age 2:** 5 to 15 ml P.O. **Children under age 2:** 1.25 to 7.5 ml P.O. **Infants:** up to 4 ml P.O. Increased dose produces no greater effect.	• Contraindicated in patients with ulcerative bowel lesions; during menstruation; in abdominal pain, nausea, vomiting, or other symptoms of appendicitis or acute surgical abdomen; in anal or rectal fissures, fecal impaction, or intestinal obstruction or perforation; and in pregnancy. • Use cautiously in rectal bleeding.
glycerin (Fleet Babylax ◇ , Sani-Supp ◇) *Constipation —* **Adults and children over age 6:** 3 g as a rectal suppository; or 5 to 15 ml as an enema. **Children under age 6:** 1 to 1.5 g as a rectal suppository; or 2 to 5 ml as an enema.	• There are no known contraindications or precautions associated with use of glycerin as a laxative.
lactulose (Cephulac, Duphalac) *Constipation —* **Adults:** 15 to 30 ml P.O. daily. *To prevent and treat portal-systemic encephalopathy, including hepatic precoma and coma in patients with severe hepatic disease —* **Adults:** initially, 20 to 30 g (30 to 45 ml) P.O. t.i.d. or q.i.d., until two or three soft stools are produced daily. Usual dosage is 60 to 100 g daily in divided doses. Can also be given by retention enema in at least 100 ml of fluid.	• Contraindicated in low-galactose diet. • Use cautiously in diabetes mellitus.

◇ Available OTC

SELECTED MAJOR DRUGS: LAXATIVES *continued*

DRUG, INDICATIONS, AND DOSAGES	SPECIAL PRECAUTIONS
magnesium salts ◇ *Constipation; to evacuate bowel before surgery—* **Adults and children over age 6:** 15 g (magnesium sulfate) P.O. in glass of water; or 15 to 60 ml (magnesium hydroxide or milk of magnesia) P.O.; or 5 to 10 oz (magnesium citrate) P.O. h.s. **Children ages 2 to 6:** 5 to 15 ml (magnesium hydroxide or milk of magnesia) P.O. *Antacid—* **Adults:** 5 to 15 ml (magnesium hydroxide or milk of magnesia) P.O. t.i.d. or q.i.d.	• Contraindicated in patients with abdominal pain, nausea, vomiting, or other symptoms of appendicitis or acute surgical abdomen; and in myocardial damage, heart block, imminent delivery, fecal impaction, rectal fissures, intestinal obstruction or perforation, or renal disease. • Use cautiously in rectal bleeding.
methylcellulose (Citrucel ◇ **)** *Chronic constipation—* **Adults:** 5 to 20 ml liquid P.O. t.i.d. with a glass of water; or 15 ml syrup P.O. morning and evening. **Children:** 5 to 10 ml P.O. daily or b.i.d.	• Contraindicated in patients with abdominal pain, nausea, vomiting, or other symptoms of appendicitis or acute surgical abdomen and in intestinal obstruction or ulceration, disabling adhesion, or difficulty swallowing.
mineral oil (Agoral Plain ◇ **, Kondremul Plain** ◇ **)** *Constipation; preparation for bowel studies or surgery—* **Adults:** 15 to 30 ml P.O. h.s.; or 120 ml enema. **Children:** 5 to 15 ml P.O. h.s.; or 30 to 60 ml enema.	• Contraindicated in patients with abdominal pain, nausea, vomiting, or other symptoms of appendicitis or acute surgical abdomen and in fecal impaction or intestinal obstruction or perforation. • Use cautiously in young children; in elderly or debilitated patients because of susceptibility to lipoid pneumonitis through aspiration, absorption, and transport from intestinal mucosa; and in rectal bleeding. Enema is contraindicated in children under age 2.
senna (Black-Draught ◇ **, Senokot** ◇ **, X-Prep Liquid** ◇ **)** *Acute constipation, preparation for bowel or rectal examination—* **Adults:** dosage range for Senokot is 1 to 8 tablets P.O.; ½ to 4 tsp granules added to liquid; 1 to 2 suppositories h.s.; 1 to 4 tsp syrup h.s. Dosage range for Black-Draught is 2 tablets or ¼ to ½ level tsp granules mixed with water. **Children over 27 kg:** half the adult dose of tablets, granules, or syrup (Black-Draught tablets and granules not recommended for children). **Children ages 1 month to 1 year:** 1.25 to 2.5 ml Senokot syrup P.O. h.s.	• Contraindicated in patients with ulcerative bowel lesions; in nausea, vomiting, abdominal pain, or other symptoms of appendicitis or acute surgical abdomen; fecal impaction; or intestinal obstruction or perforation.

(continued)

◇ Available OTC

SELECTED MAJOR DRUGS: LAXATIVES *continued*

DRUG, INDICATIONS, AND DOSAGES	SPECIAL PRECAUTIONS
sodium phosphates (Fleet Phospho-Soda ◇) *Relief of constipation—* **Adults:** 4 fl oz P.O.	• Contraindicated in patients with congenital megacolon, imperforate anus, or CHF, as hypernatremic dehydration may occur. • Administer cautiously to patients with impaired renal function, heart disease, or preexisting electrolyte disturbances; in patients on calcium channel blockers, diuretics, or other drugs that may affect electrolyte levels; or in colostomy because hypocalcemia, hyperphosphatemia, hypernatremia, and acidosis may occur.

◇ Available OTC

COMPARING LAXATIVE COMBINATIONS

TRADE NAME AND CONTENT	SPECIAL CONSIDERATIONS
Agoral ◇ **(raspberry or marshmallow)** mineral oil 4.2 g and phenolphthalein 0.2 g	• Combines the lubricating-softening action of mineral oil with the peristaltic action of phenolphthalein. • Contraindicated in patients with known hypersensitivity or in abdominal pain, nausea, or vomiting.
Dialose Plus ◇ docusate potassium 100 mg and casanthranol 30 mg	• Combines the stool softener effect of docusate potassium with the peristaltic activating effect of casanthranol. • Contraindicated in patients with abdominal pain, nausea, or vomiting.
Doxidan ◇ docusate calcium 60 mg and phenolphthalein 65 mg	• Combines the stool softener effect of docusate calcium with the stimulant laxative effect of phenolphthalein. • Contraindicated in patients with abdominal pain, nausea, or vomiting.
Peri-Colace ◇ **(capsules)** docusate sodium 100 mg and casanthranol 30 mg	• Combines the stool softener effect of docusate sodium with the stimulant laxative effect of casanthranol. • Contraindicated in patients with abdominal pain, nausea, or vomiting.

◇ Available OTC

SELF-TEST

1. When administering a laxative to a patient who is recovering from an MI, an emollient laxative is the drug of choice. Why?
   a. Its action prevents straining during defecation.
   b. It works extremely fast.
   c. It stimulates peristaltic movement.
   d. It will be needed for a long time.

2. Stimulant laxatives work by:
   a. increasing water retention in the stool.
   b. increasing peristalsis.
   c. drawing water from the tissues into the feces.
   d. absorbing water.

3. Salvatore Fishman, age 56, complains of a bitter taste when taking docusate. You advise him to:
   a. take the drug with hot tea.
   b. notify his doctor immediately.
   c. stop taking the drug.
   d. take the liquid in milk or fruit juice to mask the bitter taste.

Check your answers on page 1069.

CHAPTER 49

ANTIEMETICS

Antihistamines
buclizine hydrochloride ✦ cyclizine hydrochloride ✦ cyclizine lactate
dimenhydrinate ✦ meclizine hydrochloride
trimethobenzamide hydrochloride

Phenothiazines
prochlorperazine edisylate ✦ prochlorperazine maleate
thiethylperazine maleate

Miscellaneous agents
benzquinamide hydrochloride ✦ diphenidol hydrochloride
metoclopramide hydrochloride ✦ ondansetron hydrochloride ✦ scopolamine

OVERVIEW
- Antiemetics are classified primarily into three groups: antihistamines, phenothiazines, and miscellaneous agents.

MAJOR USES
- Antiemetics are used to prevent and treat nausea, vomiting, and dizziness.

MECHANISM OF ACTION
- Most of these agents act in the CNS on a region known as the chemoreceptor trigger zone (CTZ). The CTZ is a specialized region of sensory neurons located in the area postrema of the medulla oblongata. Although it is located in the CNS, the blood flow to this region is not restricted by the blood-brain barrier. This may enhance the vomiting center's ability to react to toxins in the blood.
- Neurotransmission in the CTZ is mediated by both dopamine- and serotonin-containing neurons. Many antiemetics block these receptors. Other agents act on peripheral neurons to block impulses from reaching the CTZ, thereby blocking the vomiting reflex. For example, anticholinergics such as scopolamine (or drugs with anticholinergic activity, including the antihistamines) act on muscarinic receptors within the labyrinth of the ear to decrease afferent impulses that trigger motion sickness. Ondansetron, a specific serotonin 5-HT3 receptor blocking agent, also acts on 5-HT3 receptors located on vagal afferent nerve terminals within the GI tract. Blocking these receptors may decrease stimulatory impulses from the periphery to the vomiting center.

GLOSSARY

Antiemetic: drug that relieves nausea and vomiting.
Nausea: unpleasant epigastric or abdominal sensation that, in many cases, leads to vomiting.
Vomiting: forcible expulsion of gastric contents through the mouth.

ABSORPTION, DISTRIBUTION, METABOLISM, AND EXCRETION

Benzquinamide is rapidly absorbed after I.M. injection and rapidly distributed in body tissues, with highest concentration in the liver and kidneys. It is metabolized in the liver and eliminated in urine and feces.

Buclizine, cyclizine, dimenhydrinate, and meclizine are well absorbed after either oral or parenteral administration. They are widely distributed in the tissues, metabolized in the liver, and excreted by the kidneys.

Diphenidol is well absorbed after being given orally, is distributed to most body tissues, and is metabolized in the liver. It is eliminated in urine and feces.

Prochlorperazine and thiethylperazine are well absorbed when given orally, parenterally, or rectally. Widely distributed, they are metabolized in the liver and eliminated either in urine or—through the bile—in feces.

Scopolamine is completely and evenly absorbed transdermally. The drug is widely distributed and excreted unchanged in urine.

Trimethobenzamide is well distributed to tissues, metabolized in the liver, and eliminated as both unchanged drug and metabolites in urine and feces.

Ondansetron is administered intravenously. The drug is metabolized in the liver, and metabolites are excreted in the urine.

Metoclopramide is well absorbed after oral administration. Some of the drug is metabolized in the liver. Both metabolites and unchanged drug are found in the urine.

ONSET AND DURATION

Pharmacokinetics of Antiemetics summarizes these drugs' onset and duration.

PHARMACOKINETICS OF ANTIEMETICS

DRUG	ROUTE	ONSET	DURATION
benzquinamide	parenteral	15 to 30 minutes	3 to 4 hours
buclizine	P.O.	30 to 60 minutes	4 to 6 hours
cyclizine	I.M., P.O.	30 to 60 minutes	4 to 6 hours
dimenhydrinate	I.M., P.O., P.R.	30 to 60 minutes	4 to 6 hours
diphenidol	parenteral, P.O.	30 to 40 minutes	4 to 6 hours
meclizine	P.O.	30 to 60 minutes	8 to 24 hours
ondansetron	I.V.	30 minutes	3 to 4 hours
prochlorperazine	parenteral	10 to 20 minutes	3 to 4 hours
	P.O.	30 to 40 minutes	3 to 4 hours (tablet); 10 to 12 hours (extended-release form)
	P.R.	1 hour	3 to 4 hours
scopolamine	transdermal	2 to 8 hours	72 hours
thiethylperazine	P.O.	30 minutes	4 hours
trimethobenzamide	parenteral	15 to 35 minutes	2 to 3 hours
	P.O., P.R.	10 to 40 minutes	3 to 4 hours

ADVERSE REACTIONS

Phenothiazines used in larger dosages as antipsychotics can produce numerous adverse reactions. When used as antiemetics, however, the drugs primarily produce sedation, hypotension, and extrapyramidal effects.

Adverse CNS reactions are among the major problems associated with phenothiazine antiemetics. Mild to moderate sedation occurs in 50% to 80% of the patients who receive these drugs, with chlorpromazine producing the greatest incidence. Tolerance to the sedative effect usually develops over several days of therapy. Confusion may occur, especially in elderly patients. Other adverse CNS reactions associated with phenothiazine antiemetics include anxiety, euphoria, agitation, depression, headache, insomnia, restlessness, and weakness. Because these drugs also can lower the threshold for seizures, they should be used cautiously in patients who are predisposed to seizures.

Adverse anticholinergic reactions typically include dry mouth, blurred vision, constipation, and urine retention.

Hypotension and orthostatic hypotension with tachycardia, syncope, and dizziness frequently occur as adverse reactions to phenothiazine antiemetics. Chlorpromazine produces the highest incidence of hypotensive effects; prochlorperazine and thiethylperazine, the lowest. Tolerance to the hypotensive effects usually develops.

Extrapyramidal reactions to phenothiazine antiemetics may occur. Such reactions usually are dose-related and, therefore, relatively rare with antiemetic doses.

Hypersensitivity reactions can result when phenothiazines are used as antipsychotics, but rarely occur when the drugs are used as antiemetics. Granulocytopenia, although rare, is the most commonly reported adverse hematologic reaction. Phenothiazines also produce many dermatologic effects, especially with long-term therapy. Hypersensitivity reactions manifested as cholestatic jaundice, blood dyscrasia, dermatologic reactions, and photosensitivity have occurred, usually within the first few months of phenothiazine therapy.

Most adverse reactions to antihistamine antiemetics are predictable, mild, and usually easy to control. All antihistamine antiemetics produce some dose-related drowsiness. Reducing the dose may decrease the drowsiness without compromising the antiemetic effect. Paradoxical CNS stimulation has occurred, more often in children than adults. Symptoms of paradoxical CNS stimulation may range from restlessness, insomnia, and euphoria to tremor and even seizures. Other adverse CNS reactions include dizziness, headache, and lassitude.

Antihistamine antiemetics may cause mild nausea or epigastric distress. Administering the drug with food or milk may decrease these symptoms. Anorexia also may occur and last for several weeks from long-term administration of antihistamine antiemetics.

The anticholinergic effect of antihistamine antiemetics may cause constipation. Other anticholinergic effects include dry mouth and throat, dysuria, urine retention, and impotence. The anticholinergic action of antihistamines also may produce visual and auditory disturbances, such as blurred vision or tinnitus.

In addition to these reactions, trimethobenzamide may produce extrapyramidal symptoms, such as acute dystonia and dyskinesia, that require discontinuation of the drug.

Hypersensitivity reactions, as manifested by rashes and photosensitivity, may occur. Blood dyscrasia (including granulocytopenia, hemolytic anemia, leukopenia, thrombocytopenia, and pancytopenia) have occurred rarely.

MECLIZINE HYDROCHLORIDE
(MECLOZINE HYDROCHLORIDE)

(mek′ li zeen)

Ancolan‡, Antivert, Antivert/25◊, Antivert/50, Bonamine†, Bonine◊, Dizmiss◊, Meni-D, Ru-Vert M

Classification: antihistamine
Pregnancy risk category B

How supplied

TABLETS: 12.5 mg, 25 mg◊, 50 mg
TABLETS (CHEWABLE): 25 mg◊
CAPSULES: 15 mg, 25 mg, 30 mg

Indications and dosage

Motion sickness
ADULTS: 25 to 50 mg P.O. 1 hour before travel, repeated daily for duration of journey.

Dizziness
ADULTS: 25 to 100 mg P.O. daily in divided doses. Dosage varies with patient response.

Contraindications and precautions

Meclizine is contraindicated in patients with known hypersensitivity to the drug or other antiemetic antihistamines with a similar chemical structure, such as cyclizine, buclizine, or dimenhydrinate. Use cautiously in patients with narrow-angle glaucoma, asthma, prostatic hypertrophy, or GU or GI obstruction because of anticholinergic effects. Drug may mask signs of intestinal obstruction or brain tumor.

Adverse reactions

CNS: *drowsiness,* fatigue.
EENT: dry mouth, blurred vision.
OTHER: may mask symptoms of ototoxicity, brain tumor, or intestinal obstruction.

Interactions

Aminoglycosides, salicylates, vancomycin, loop diuretics, cisplatin, or other ototoxic drugs: meclizine may mask signs of ototoxicity. Avoid concomitant use.
CNS depressants (alcohol, barbiturates, tranquilizers): increased drowsiness. Avoid concomitant use.

Nursing considerations

Assessment
• Review the patient's history for a condition that contraindicates the use of meclizine.

---

†Available in Canada only   ‡Available in Australia only   ◊ Available OTC
Italicized adverse reactions are common

- Obtain a baseline assessment of the patient's motion sickness or dizziness before therapy.
- Be alert for common adverse reactions.
- Evaluate the patient's and family's knowledge about meclizine therapy.

Planning (Nursing Diagnoses)
Potential nursing diagnoses for the patient receiving meclizine include:
- Potential for injury related to dosage regimen inadequate to relieve or minimize nausea and vomiting.
- Altered thought processes related to CNS depression caused by drug.
- Knowledge deficit related to meclizine therapy.

Implementation
Preparation and administration
— Administer with food or milk to minimize nausea or epigastric distress.
— Tablets may be placed in mouth and allowed to dissolve without water or may be chewed or swallowed whole.
— Abrupt withdrawal of drug after long-term use may cause paradoxical reactions or sudden reversal of improved state.
— For motion sickness, administer 1 hour before travel.
— Safety and efficacy for use in children have not been established. Do not use in children under age 12; infants and children under age 6 may experience paradoxical hyperexcitability.
— This antihistamine has a slower onset and longer duration of action than other antihistamine antiemetics.
— Meclizine should be discontinued 4 days before diagnostic skin tests, to avoid preventing, reducing, or masking test responses.

Monitoring
— Monitor the effectiveness of therapy by regularly assessing for decrease in or relief of the patient's motion sickness or dizziness.
— Monitor the patient for adverse drug reactions. The elderly patient is usually more sensitive to the adverse effects of antihistamines and is especially likely to experience a greater degree of dizziness, sedation, hyperexcitability, dry mouth, and urine retention than the younger patient.
— Monitor for signs and symptoms of drowsiness.
— Monitor the patient for drug interactions.
— Regularly reevaluate the patient's and family's knowledge about meclizine therapy.

Intervention
— If the patient develops dry mouth, offer sugarless chewing gum or hard candy or ice chips.
— If the patient develops drowsiness, take safety precautions, such as placing the bed in the low position and keeping the side rails raised. Notify the doctor and expect to reduce dosage.
— Keep all members of the health care team informed of the patient's response to the drug.

Patient teaching

—Instruct the patient and family about meclizine, including the dosage, frequency, action, and adverse reactions.

—Explain the disease process and rationale for therapy.

—Advise the patient that tablets may be placed in mouth and allowed to dissolve without water or may be chewed or swallowed whole. Tell the patient to take drug with food or milk to minimize nausea or epigastric distress.

—Advise the patient that abrupt withdrawal of drug after long-term use may cause sudden reversal of improved state or paradoxical reactions.

—Warn the patient against driving and other hazardous activities that require alertness until CNS effects of the drug are known.

—Tell the patient not to self-medicate for a condition that persists for more than 24 hours or if currently taking other medications.

—When drug is used for motion sickness, tell the patient to take the medication 1 hour before scheduled travel. Medication may be repeated daily for the duration of the journey.

—Suggest the use of ice chips or sugarless chewing gum or hard candy to relieve dry mouth.

—Tell the patient to notify the nurse or doctor if adverse reactions develop or questions arise about meclizine therapy.

—Instruct the patient to notify the doctor if severe nausea and vomiting persist for more than 24 hours.

—Warn the patient to avoid alcohol or other CNS depressants while taking this drug.

Evaluation

In the patient receiving meclizine, appropriate evaluation statements include:

• Patient's nausea and vomiting has been relieved or minimized.

• Patient maintains normal thought processes; patient experiences no drug-induced drowsiness.

• Patient and family state an understanding of meclizine therapy.

PROCHLORPERAZINE
(proe klor per' a zeen)
Compazine, Stemetil†‡

PROCHLORPERAZINE EDISYLATE
Compazine

PROCHLORPERAZINE MALEATE
Anti-Naus‡, Chlorpazine, Compazine, Stemetil†‡
Classification: phenothiazine
Pregnancy risk category C

How supplied
prochlorperazine
INJECTION: 5 mg/ml
SUPPOSITORIES: 2.5 mg, 5 mg, 25 mg
prochlorperazine edisylate
SYRUP: 1 mg/ml
prochlorperazine maleate
TABLETS: 5 mg, 10 mg, 25 mg
CAPSULES (SUSTAINED-RELEASE): 10 mg, 15 mg, 30 mg

Indications and dosage
Preoperative nausea control
ADULTS: 5 to 10 mg I.M. 1 to 2 hours before induction of anesthetic; repeat once in 30 minutes, if necessary. Or 5 to 10 mg I.V. 15 to 30 minutes before induction of anesthetic (repeat once if necessary); or 20 mg/liter dextrose 5% in water and 0.9% sodium chloride solution by I.V. infusion, added to infusion 15 to 30 minutes before induction. Maximum parenteral dosage is 40 mg daily.

Severe nausea, vomiting
ADULTS: 5 to 10 mg P.O. t.i.d. or q.i.d.; or 15 mg (sustained-release form) P.O. on arising; or 10 mg (sustained-released form) P.O. q 12 hours; or 25 mg P.R. b.i.d.; or 5 to 10 mg I.M. injected deeply into upper outer quadrant of gluteal region. Repeat q 3 to 4 hours p.r.n. Maximum I.M. dosage is 40 mg daily.
CHILDREN 18 TO 39 KG: 2.5 mg P.O. or P.R. t.i.d.; or 5 mg P.O. or P.R. b.i.d. Maximum dosage is 15 mg daily; or 0.132 mg/kg deep I.M. injection. (Control usually obtained with one dose.)
CHILDREN 14 TO 17 KG: 2.5 mg P.O. or P.R. b.i.d. or t.i.d. Maximum dosage is 10 mg daily; or 0.132 mg/kg deep I.M. injection. (Control usually obtained with one dose.)
CHILDREN 9 TO 13 KG: 2.5 mg P.O. or P.R. daily or b.i.d. Maximum dosage is 7.5 mg daily; or 0.132 mg/kg deep I.M. injection. (Control usually obtained with one dose.)

Symptomatic management of psychotic disorders
ADULTS: 5 to 10 mg P.O. t.i.d. or q.i.d.
CHILDREN AGES 2 TO 12: 2.5 mg P.O. or P.R. b.i.d. or t.i.d. Do not exceed 10 mg on day 1. Increase dosage gradually to recommended maximum (if necessary).
CHILDREN AGES 6 TO 12: maximum is 25 mg P.O. daily.
CHILDREN AGES 2 TO 5: maximum is 20 mg P.O. daily.

Symptomatic management of severe psychoses
ADULTS: 10 to 20 mg I.M. May be repeated in 1 to 4 hours. Rarely, patients may receive 10 to 20 mg q 4 to 6 hours. Oral therapy should be instituted after symptoms are controlled.

Management of excessive anxiety
ADULTS: 5 to 10 mg by deep I.M. injection q 3 to 4 hours, not to exceed 40 mg daily; or 5 to 10 mg P.O. t.i.d. or q.i.d. Alternatively, give 15 mg (extended-release capsule) daily or 10 mg (extended-release capsule) q 12 hours.

Contraindications and precautions
Prochlorperazine is contraindicated in patients with known hypersensitivity to phenothiazines, CNS depression, bone marrow suppression, or subcortical damage; during pediatric surgery; in children under age 2; in use of spinal or epidural anesthetic or adrenergic blocking agents; with use of alcohol; and in those in a coma or depression.

Use cautiously in combination with other CNS depressants; in arteriosclerosis or CV disease (may cause sudden drop in blood pressure), exposure to extreme heat or cold (including antipyretic therapy), respiratory disorders, hypocalcemia, seizure disorders or severe reactions to insulin or electroconvulsive therapy, suspected brain tumor, intestinal obstruction, or prostatic hypertrophy; in acutely ill, dehydrated, or vomiting children; in elderly or debilitated patients; and in patients with glaucoma because of increased intraocular pressure, with urine retention, with hepatic or renal dysfunction, with Parkinson's disease, with pheochromocytoma because excessive buildup of neurotransmitters may have adverse CV effects, and with hypocalcemia, which increases the risk of extrapyramidal symptoms.

Adverse reactions
BLOOD: transient leukopenia, **agranulocytosis.**
CNS: extrapyramidal reactions, sedation, pseudoparkinsonism, EEG changes, dizziness.
CV: *orthostatic hypotension,* tachycardia, ECG changes.
EENT: ocular changes, *blurred vision.*
GI: *dry mouth, constipation.*
GU: *urine retention,* dark urine, menstrual irregularities, gynecomastia, inhibited ejaculation.
HEPATIC: cholestatic jaundice.
METABOLIC: hyperprolactinemia.

SKIN: mild photosensitivity, dermal allergic reactions, exfoliative dermatitis.
OTHER: weight gain, increased appetite.

Interactions
Antacids: inhibited absorption of oral phenothiazines. Separate antacid and phenothiazine doses by at least 2 hours.
Antiarrhythmics (quinidine, disopyramide, and procainamide): increased incidence of cardiac arrhythmias and conduction defects. Avoid concomitant use.
Atropine and other anticholinergics (antidepressants, MAO inhibitors, phenothiazines, antihistamines, meperidine, and antiparkinsonian agents): enhanced anticholinergic effects (oversedation, paralytic ileus, visual changes, and severe constipation) and aggravated parkinsonian symptoms. Use together cautiously.
Barbiturates: may decrease phenothiazine effect. Monitor patient for decreased antiemetic effect.
Beta blockers: inhibited prochlorperazine metabolism with increased plasma levels and toxicity. Use together cautiously.
Bromocriptine: reduced effect on prolactin secretion.
Centrally acting antihypertensives (guanethidine, guanabenz, guanadrel, clonidine, methyldopa, and reserpine): inhibited blood pressure response. Use together cautiously.
CNS depressants (alcohol, analgesic barbiturates, narcotics, tranquilizers, anesthetics [general, spinal, or epidural], and parenteral magnesium sulfate): excessive CNS depression (oversedation, respiratory depression, and hypotension). Use together cautiously.
Dopamine, levodopa: decreased effectiveness and increased toxicity of levodopa (by dopamine blockade). Avoid concomitant use.
Lithium: severe neurologic toxicity with an encephalitis-like syndrome and decreased therapeutic response to prochlorperazine. Avoid concomitant use.
Metrizamide: increased risk of seizures. Avoid concomitant use.
Nitrates: hypotension. Use together cautiously.
Phenobarbital, aluminum- and magnesium-containing antacids and antidiarrheals, caffeine, heavy smoking: decreased therapeutic response to prochlorperazine. Monitor effects.
Phenytoin: increased toxicity. Use together cautiously.
Propylthiouracil: increased risk of agranulocytosis. Avoid concomitant use.
Sympathomimetics (including epinephrine, phenylephrine, phenylpropanolamine, ephedrine, and appetite suppressants): decreased stimulatory and pressor effects; may cause epinephrine reversal (hypotensive response to epinephrine). Avoid concomitant use.

Nursing considerations
Assessment
• Review the patient's history for a condition that contraindicates the use of prochlorperazine.

- Obtain a baseline assessment of the patient's nausea and vomiting before therapy.
- Be alert for common adverse reactions.
- Evaluate the patient's and family's knowledge about prochlorperazine therapy.

Planning (Nursing Diagnoses)

Potential nursing diagnoses for the patient receiving prochlorperazine include:
- Potential for injury related to ineffectiveness of drug.
- Impaired physical mobility related to the extrapyramidal effects of the drug.
- Knowledge deficit related to prochlorperazine therapy.

Implementation

Preparation and administration

—The elderly patient should usually receive dosages in the lower range.
—Store in light-resistant container. Slight yellowing does not affect potency; discard very discolored solutions.
—Use only when vomiting can't be controlled by other measures or when only a few doses are required. If more than four doses are needed in a 24-hour period, notify the doctor.
—Drug is not effective in treating motion sickness.
—To prevent contact dermatitis, avoid getting concentrate or injection solution on hands or clothing.
—Dilute syrup with tomato or fruit juice, milk, coffee, carbonated beverage, tea, water, soup, or pudding.
—Do not mix in syringe with another drug.
—Oral formulations may cause stomach upset. Administer with food or fluid.
—Dilute the concentrate in 2 to 4 oz (60 to 120 ml) of water. Store the suppository form in a cool place.
—Give I.V. dose slowly (5 mg/minute). I.M. injection may cause skin necrosis; take care to prevent extravasation. Do not administer subcutaneously.
—Administer I.M. injection deep into the upper outer quadrant of the buttock. Massaging the area after administration may prevent formation of abscesses.
—The sustained-release capsule should be administered upon arising; it should not be crushed or chewed; and it should not be given to children.
—Because this drug may cause hypotension, the patient should remain in bed for 30 to 60 minutes after administration.
—Separate the administration of this drug and of an antacid by at least 2 hours.

Monitoring

—Monitor the effectiveness of therapy by regularly assessing for relief or alleviation of nausea and vomiting.

— Monitor the patient for adverse drug reactions. The elderly patient is at greater risk for adverse reactions, especially tardive dyskinesia, other extrapyramidal effects, and hypotension.

— Watch for orthostatic hypotension, especially when giving I.V. Monitor the patient's blood pressure before and after parenteral administration.

— Monitor for signs and symptoms of extrapyramidal reactions.

— Monitor CBC and liver function studies during prolonged therapy.

— Monitor the patient for drug interactions.

— Monitor diagnostic test results. Prochlorperazine causes false-positive test results for urinary porphyrins, urobilinogen, amylase, and 5-HIAA; it causes false-positive urine pregnancy results in tests using human chorionic gonadotropin as the indicator; it also elevates test results for liver enzymes and protein-bound iodine and causes quinidine-like ECG effects.

— Regularly reevaluate the patient's and family's knowledge about prochlorperazine therapy.

Intervention

— If the patient develops dry mouth, suggest sugarless chewing gum or hard candy or ice chips to help relieve it.

— If the patient develops orthostatic hypotension, advise him to rise slowly when getting up from the bed or chair. If needed, assist the patient to prevent falls.

— If the patient develops signs of extrapyramidal reactions, withhold the drug, notify the doctor immediately, and expect to administer parenteral diphenhydramine 2 mg/kg/minute, a barbiturate, or benztropine.

— If the patient develops dizziness or sedation, take safety precautions; for example, place the bed in the low position, keep side rails up, and assist with ambulation.

— Keep all members of the health care team informed of the patient's response to the drug.

Patient teaching

— Instruct the patient and family about prochlorperazine, including the dosage, frequency, action, and adverse reactions.

— Explain the disease process and rationale for therapy.

— Advise the patient that drug may cause a pink to brown discoloration of urine.

— Explain the risks of dystonic reactions and tardive dyskinesia. Tell the patient to report abnormal body movements promptly.

— Tell the patient to avoid sun exposure and to use a sunscreen when going outdoors, to prevent photosensitivity reactions. (Note that heat lamps and tanning beds also may cause burning of the skin or skin discoloration.)

— Tell the patient to avoid spilling the liquid form. Contact with skin may cause rash and irritation.

— Warn the patient to avoid extremely hot or cold baths and exposure to temperature extremes, sun lamps, or tanning beds; drug may cause thermoregulatory changes.

—Advise the patient to take the drug exactly as prescribed, not to double doses after missing one, and not to share drug with others.

—Tell the patient not to drink alcohol or take other medications that may cause excessive sedation.

—Tell the patient to dilute the concentrate in water; explain the dropper technique of measuring dose; teach correct use of suppository.

—Tell the patient that sugarless chewing gum or hard candy or ice chips can alleviate dry mouth.

—Urge the patient to store this drug safely away from children.

—Tell the patient that interactions are possible with many drugs. Warn him to seek medical approval before taking any OTC medication.

—Warn the patient not to stop taking the drug suddenly and to promptly report difficulty urinating, sore throat, dizziness, or fainting. Reassure the patient that most reactions can be relieved by reducing dose.

—Warn the patient to avoid hazardous activities that require alertness until the drug's effect is established. Reassure the patient that sedative effects subside and become tolerable in several weeks.

—Advise the patient considering breast-feeding to notify her doctor before beginning to breast-feed as drug may enter breast milk.

—Instruct the patient to notify his doctor if severe nausea and vomiting persist for more than 24 hours.

—Tell the patient not to crush or chew sustained-release capsules.

—Explain that orthostatic hypotension may occur and that the patient should change position slowly or remain recumbent for 30 to 60 minutes after taking the drug.

—Tell the patient to notify the nurse or doctor if adverse reactions develop or questions arise about prochlorperazine therapy.

Evaluation

In the patient receiving prochlorperazine, appropriate evaluation statements include:

• Patient experiences reduction or relief of nausea and vomiting and experiences no adverse reactions.

• Patient maintains normal mobility and experiences no extrapyramidal effects.

• Patient and family state an understanding of prochlorperazine therapy.

ONDANSETRON HYDROCHLORIDE
(on dan′ sih tron)
Zofran
Classification: miscellaneous antiemetic
Pregnancy risk category B

How supplied
INJECTION: 2 mg/ml

Indications and dosage
Prevention of nausea and vomiting associated with emetogenic chemotherapy (including high-dose cisplatin)
ADULTS AND CHILDREN OVER AGE 4: administered in three doses of 0.16 mg/kg I.V. Give first dose 30 minutes before administration of chemotherapy; administer subsequent doses 4 and 8 hours after the first dose. Infuse drug over 15 minutes.

Contraindications and precautions
Ondansetron is contraindicated in patients with known hypersensitivity to the drug.

Adverse reactions
CNS: headache.
GI: diarrhea, *constipation.*
METABOLIC: transient elevations in AST (SGOT) and ALT (SGPT) levels.
SKIN: rash.
OTHER: bronchospasm (rare).

Interactions
Drugs that alter hepatic drug metabolizing enzymes, such as phenobarbital or cimetidine: may alter pharmacokinetics of ondansetron. No dosage adjustment appears necessary.

Nursing considerations
Assessment
• Review the patient's history for a condition that contraindicates the use of ondansetron.
• Obtain a baseline assessment of the patient's potential for nausea and vomiting from chemotherapy before therapy.
• Be alert for common adverse reactions.
• Evaluate the patient's and family's knowledge about ondansetron therapy.

Planning (Nursing Diagnoses)

Potential nursing diagnoses for the patient receiving ondansetron include:
• Altered health maintenance related to dosage regimen inadequate to prevent nausea and vomiting.
• Fluid volume deficit related to ineffectiveness of drug.
• Knowledge deficit related to ondansetron therapy.

Implementation

Preparation and administration

—Dilute the drug in 50 ml of dextrose 5% in water injection or 0.9% sodium chloride injection before administration. The drug is also stable for up to 48 hours after dilution in 5% dextrose in 0.9% sodium chloride injection, 5% dextrose in 0.45% sodium chloride injection, and 3% sodium chloride injection.

Monitoring

—Monitor the effectiveness of therapy by regularly assessing for decrease or relief of nausea and/or vomiting.
—Monitor the patient for adverse drug reactions.
—Monitor amount, color, and type of any emesis.
—Monitor the patient's intake and output.
—Monitor serum electrolytes.
—Monitor I.V. site for signs of infiltration and phlebitis.
—Monitor the patient for drug interactions.
—Regularly reevaluate the patient's and family's knowledge about ondansetron therapy.

Intervention

—If the patient develops a fluid volume deficit, notify the doctor and anticipate an order for increasing the patient's fluid intake.
—If the patient develops an electrolyte imbalance, consult with the doctor for appropriate therapy.
—If the patient develops infiltration or phlebitis at I.V. site, discontinue I.V. and restart in another area (preferably the patient's other arm).
—Keep all members of the health care team informed of the patient's response to the drug.

Patient teaching

—Instruct the patient and family about ondansetron, including the dosage, frequency, action, and adverse reactions.
—Explain the disease process and rationale for therapy.
—Instruct the patient to report any nausea and/or vomiting.
—As appropriate, encourage the patient to increase fluid intake.
—Tell the patient to notify the nurse or doctor if adverse reactions develop or questions arise about ondansetron therapy.

Evaluation

In the patient receiving ondansetron, appropriate evaluation statements include:
• Patient experiences no nausea or vomiting.

• Patient maintains normal fluid balance and does not experience nausea or vomiting.
• Patient and family state an understanding of ondansetron therapy.

SELECTED MAJOR DRUGS: ANTIEMETICS

DRUG, INDICATIONS, AND DOSAGES	SPECIAL PRECAUTIONS
Antihistamines	
buclizine (Bucladin-S) *Motion sickness (prevention)* — **Adults:** 50 mg P.O. at least ½ hour before beginning travel. If needed, may repeat another 50 mg after 4 to 6 hours. *Vertigo* — **Adults:** 50 mg P.O., up to 150 mg daily, in severe cases. Maintenance dose is 50 mg b.i.d.	• Contraindicated in pregnant women and in patients with known hypersensitivity to the drug. • Use cautiously in glaucoma, GU or GI obstruction, and elderly males with possible prostatic hypertrophy.
cyclizine hydrochloride (Marezine ◇) **cyclizine lactate, (Marezine, Marzine†)** *Motion sickness (prevention and treatment)* — **Adults:** 50 mg P.O. (hydrochloride) ½ hour before travel, then q 4 to 6 hours p.r.n. to maximum of 200 mg daily; or 50 mg I.M. (lactate) q 4 to 6 hours p.r.n. *Postoperative vomiting* — **Adults:** 50 mg I.M. (lactate) preoperatively or 20 to 30 minutes before expected termination of surgery; then postoperatively 50 mg I.M. (lactate) q 4 to 6 hours, p.r.n. *Motion sickness and postoperative vomiting* — **Children ages 6 to 12:** 3 mg/kg (lactate) I.M. divided t.i.d., or 25 mg (hydrochloride) P.O. q 4 to 6 hours p.r.n. to a maximum of 75 mg daily.	• Use cautiously in glaucoma, GU or GI obstruction, and elderly males with possible prostatic hypertrophy.
dimenhydrinate (Calm X ◇ , Dramamine ◇ , Novodimenate†) *Nausea, vomiting, dizziness of motion sickness (treatment and prevention)* — **Adults:** 50 mg P.O. q 4 hours, or 100 mg q 4 hours if drowsiness is not objectionable; or 50 mg I.M. p.r.n.; or 50 mg I.V. diluted in 10 ml of 0.9% sodium chloride solution, injected over 2 minutes. **Children:** 5 mg/kg P.O. or I.M. divided q.i.d. Maximum dosage is 300 mg daily. Don't use in children under age 2.	• Use cautiously in seizures, narrow-angle glaucoma, and enlargement of prostate gland.
Phenothiazines	
thiethylperazine (Norzine, Torecan) *Nausea and vomiting* — **Adults:** 10 mg P.O., I.M., or P.R. daily, b.i.d., or t.i.d.	• Contraindicated in patients with known hypersensitivity to phenothiazines and in severe CNS depression, hepatic disease, and coma. • Administer cautiously because of onset of seizures and of varied symptom complex.

SELF-TEST

1. Which of the following activities would a patient receiving an antiemetic be advised not to do?
   a. Use the microwave oven
   b. Ride in a car
   c. Walk to the store
   d. Work in the basement doing woodworking

2. Why should the nurse stop a patient's visiting friend from bringing beer into the room of a 3-day postoperative patient who is receiving prochlorperazine?
   a. CNS depressants should not be taken with antiemetics.
   b. It is against hospital policy.
   c. Beer will contribute to the patient's nausea and vomiting.
   d. Beer may cause the patient to become confused when mixed with an antiemetic.

3. When preparing a parenteral dose of prochlorperazine, the nurse became concerned when:
   a. the patient swallowed the drug whole.
   b. the patient's blood pressure rose upon exercising.
   c. she saw an order for an antacid to be administered 2 hours later.
   d. she got some of the medication on her hands while preparing the dose.

Check your answers on page 1069.

CHAPTER 50

ANTICHOLINERGICS

Belladonna alkaloids
atropine sulfate ✦ hyoscyamine sulfate ✦ levorotatory alkaloids of belladonna

Miscellaneous agents
anisotropine methylbromide ✦ clidinium bromide
dicyclomine hydrochloride ✦ glycopyrrolate ✦ hexocyclium methylsulfate
isopropamide iodide ✦ mepenzolate bromide ✦ methantheline bromide
methscopolamine bromide ✦ oxyphencyclimine hydrochloride
propantheline bromide ✦ tridihexethyl chloride

OVERVIEW
- GI anticholinergics may be used to relieve peptic ulcer pain; however, little evidence exists that they heal peptic ulcers. Anticholinergics inhibit GI smooth muscle contraction and delay gastric emptying, thus enhancing the action of antacids. Anticholinergics should not be the sole treatment for ulcers, but rather part of a total therapeutic program.

MAJOR USES
- GI anticholinergics are therapeutic adjuncts for pain associated with peptic ulcers. They are also used to treat irritable colon (mucous colitis, spastic colon, and acute enterocolitis), other functional GI disorders, and neurogenic bowel disturbances, including splenic flexure syndrome and neurogenic colon.

MECHANISM OF ACTION
- GI anticholinergics block the actions of the vagus nerve. By competitively antagonizing the actions of acetylcholine or muscarinic cholinergic receptors, they decrease GI motility and inhibit gastric acid secretion.
- Some agents (including dicyclomine and oxyphencyclimine) exert a nonspecific direct spasmolytic action on smooth muscle. They also possess local anesthetic properties that may be partly responsible for the spasmolysis.

ABSORPTION, DISTRIBUTION, METABOLISM, AND EXCRETION
Most of these agents are rapidly absorbed after oral administration. Because they readily cross the blood-brain barrier, they cause significant adverse CNS reactions. They are metabolized in the liver and eliminated both in urine and—through the bile—in feces.

GLOSSARY

Antacid: drug that neutralizes gastric acids.
Ulcer: cutaneous or mucosal lesion caused by gradual erosion, disintegration, and necrosis of underlying tissue.

Quaternary anticholinergics (including clidinium bromide, glycopyrrolate, isopropamide, mepenzolate bromide, methantheline bromide, propantheline bromide, and tridihexethyl chloride) are poorly and unreliably absorbed after oral administration. Since they *do not* cross the blood-brain barrier, their adverse CNS effects are negligible.

ONSET AND DURATION

Parenteral GI anticholinergics have a quicker onset and shorter duration than oral forms. After oral administration, onset of action is usually 30 to 60 minutes and duration is 4 to 6 hours. Belladonna alkaloids' effects usually last about 4 hours. Effects of the quaternary anticholinergics (except isopropamide) and the tertiary synthetics (except oxyphencyclimine) last 6 hours. Isopropamide and oxyphencyclimine have durations as long as 12 hours.

ADVERSE REACTIONS

GI anticholinergics cause various reactions, especially affecting the GI and GU tracts and ocular function. Adverse GI reactions may include xerostomia, altered taste perception, nausea, vomiting, dysphagia, heartburn, constipation, bloating, and paralytic ileus. GU effects include urine retention, blurred vision, mydriasis, photophobia, cycloplegia, increased intraocular pressure, and dilated pupils. Other reactions include CV, CNS, and dermatologic effects; hypersensitivity; suppression of lactation; nasal congestion; and decreased sweating.

PROTOTYPE: BELLADONNA ALKALOIDS

ATROPINE SULFATE
(a' troe peen)
Classification: belladonna alkaloid
Pregnancy risk category C

How supplied

TABLETS: 0.4 mg, 0.6 mg
INJECTION: 0.05 mg/ml, 0.1 mg/ml, 0.3 mg/ml, 0.4 mg/ml, 0.5 mg/ml, 0.6 mg/ml, 0.8 mg/ml, 1 mg/ml, 1.2 mg/ml

Indications and dosage
Adjunctive treatment of peptic ulcer disease; treatment of functional GI disorders such as irritable bowel syndrome
ADULTS: 0.4 to 0.6 mg P.O. q 4 to 6 hours.
CHILDREN: 0.01 mg/kg or 0.3 mg/m² P.O. (not to exceed 0.4 mg) q 4 to 6 hours.

Contraindications and precautions
Atropine is contraindicated in patients with known hypersensitivity to the drug or other belladonna derivatives. Use cautiously in patients with acute MI because it may promote arrhythmias, including ventricular fibrillation and tachycardia as well as atrial fibrillation; the resulting increase in heart rate may increase myocardial oxygen consumption and worsen myocardial ischemia. Also use cautiously in patients with narrow-angle glaucoma, obstructive uropathy, obstructive GI tract disease, myasthenia gravis, paralytic ileus, intestinal atony, unstable CV status from acute hemorrhage, and toxic megacolon because the drug may worsen these symptoms or disorders.

Interactions
Other anticholinergics or drugs with anticholinergic effects: additive anticholinergic effects. Use with caution.

Adverse reactions
BLOOD: leukocytosis.
CNS: headache, restlessness, ataxia, disorientation, hallucinations, delirium, coma, insomnia, dizziness; excitement, agitation, and confusion (especially in elderly patients).
CV: 1 to 2 mg—tachycardia, palpitations; >2 mg—extreme tachycardia, angina.
EENT: 1 mg—slight mydriasis, photophobia; 2 mg—blurred vision, mydriasis.
GI: *dry mouth* (common even at low doses), *thirst,* constipation, nausea, vomiting.
GU: *urine retention.*
SKIN: hot, flushed skin.

Nursing considerations
Assessment
• Review the patient's history for a condition that contraindicates the use of atropine.
• Obtain a baseline assessment of the patient's GI pain before therapy.
• Be alert for common adverse reactions.
• Evaluate the patient's and family's knowledge about atropine therapy.

Planning (Nursing Diagnoses)
Potential nursing diagnoses for the patient receiving atropine include:
• Altered health maintenance related to ineffectiveness of the drug.
• Potential for injury related to adverse drug reactions.
• Knowledge deficit related to atropine therapy.

Italicized adverse reactions are common

Implementation

Preparation and administration

—When administering drug for adjunctive treatment of peptic ulcer disease or treatment of functional GI disorders such as irritable bowel syndrome, give orally.

—The patient should void before receiving atropine because the drug may cause urine retention.

Monitoring

—Monitor the effectiveness of therapy by regularly assessing for improvement (subsiding or relief) of the patient's peptic ulcer pain or GI discomfort.

—Monitor the patient for adverse drug reactions. Many of the adverse reactions (such as dry mouth and constipation) are an extension of the drug's pharmacologic activity and may be expected. Adverse reactions vary considerably with dosage.

—Watch for tachycardia in cardiac patients. It may precipitate ventricular fibrillation.

—Monitor intake and output. Drug causes urine retention and urinary hesitancy.

—Monitor closely for urine retention in elderly men with benign prostatic hypertrophy.

—Observe for signs of behavioral changes, especially in elderly patients.

—Regularly reevaluate the patient's and family's knowledge about atropine therapy.

Intervention

—If the patient develops dry mouth, provide ice chips or sugarless chewing gum or hard candy. Also provide frequent mouth care if indicated.

—If the patient develops constipation, notify the doctor and obtain an order for a laxative. Also advise the patient about dietary measures to reduce or avoid constipation.

—If the patient develops urine retention, notify the doctor. The patient may need catheterization.

—If the patient is unable to comply with therapy, discuss reasons why and suggest possible methods to help improve compliance.

—Keep all members of the health care team informed of the patient's response to the drug.

Patient teaching

—Instruct the patient and family about atropine, including the dosage, frequency, action, and adverse reactions.

—Explain the disease process and rationale for therapy.

—When used for peptic ulcer pain, instruct the patient about common adverse reactions. Tell the patient which reactions are not harmful, such as dry mouth, constipation, and flushing of the skin.

— Advise the patient to use mouth rinses, sugarless gum or hard candy, ice chips, and frequent oral hygiene for dry mouth.
— Tell the patient to notify the nurse or doctor if adverse reactions develop or questions arise about atropine therapy.

Evaluation
In the patient receiving atropine, appropriate evaluation statements include:
• Patient has complete or partial relief of GI pain.
• Patient experiences no adverse reactions.
• Patient and family state an understanding of atropine therapy.

PROTOTYPE: MISCELLANEOUS GI ANTICHOLINERGICS

PROPANTHELINE BROMIDE
(proe pan' the leen)
Norpanth, Pantheline‡, Pro-Banthine, Propanthel†
Classification: miscellaneous GI anticholinergic
Pregnancy risk category C

How supplied
TABLETS: 7.5 mg, 15 mg

Indications and dosage
Adjunctive treatment of peptic ulcer, irritable bowel syndrome, and other GI disorders; to reduce duodenal motility during diagnostic radiologic procedures
ADULTS: 15 mg P.O. t.i.d. before meals, and 30 mg P.O. h.s. up to 60 mg q.i.d. For elderly patients, 7.5 mg P.O. t.i.d. before meals.

Contraindications and precautions
Propantheline is contraindicated in patients with glaucoma, obstructive disease of the GI tract, obstructive uropathy, intestinal atony of elderly or debilitated patients, severe ulcerative colitis or toxic megacolon complicating ulcerative colitis, unstable CV adjustment in acute hemorrhage, or myasthenia gravis. Drug should not be used by women who are breast-feeding. Use cautiously in elderly patients and in all patients with autonomic neuropathy, hepatic or renal disease, hyperthyroidism, coronary heart disease, CHF, cardiac tachyarrhythmias, hypertension, or hiatal hernia associated with reflux esophagitis.

Adverse reactions
CNS: headache, insomnia, drowsiness, dizziness, *confusion or excitement (in elderly patients),* nervousness, weakness.
CV: *palpitations,* tachycardia.
EENT: *blurred vision,* mydriasis, increased ocular tension, cycloplegia, photophobia.

GI: *dry mouth,* dysphagia, constipation, heartburn, loss of taste, nausea, vomiting, paralytic ileus.
GU: *urinary hesitancy, urine retention,* impotence.
SKIN: urticaria, decreased sweating or possible anhidrosis, other dermal manifestations.
OTHER: fever, allergic reactions.
    Overdosage may cause curare-like symptoms.

Interactions

Antacids: decreased absorption of propantheline. Separate administration times by at least 1 hour.
Anticholinergics and corticosteroids: increased intraocular pressure. Monitor carefully.
Belladonna alkaloids, synthetic or semisynthetic anticholinergics, narcotic analgesics, Type I antiarrhythmics, antihistamines: excessive cholinergic blockade. Use cautiously.
Digoxin: increased serum digoxin levels. Monitor carefully.
Phenothiazines, tricyclic antidepressants (TCAs), or other psychoactive drugs: enhanced sedative effects. Use cautiously.
Potassium supplements (oral): may increase incidence of adverse GI reactions, especially with wax-matrix tablets. Use together cautiously.

Nursing considerations

Assessment
- Review the patient's history for a condition that contraindicates the use of propantheline.
- Obtain a baseline assessment of the patient's GI pain before therapy.
- Be alert for common adverse reactions.
- Evaluate the patient's and family's knowledge about propantheline therapy.

Planning (Nursing Diagnoses)
Potential nursing diagnoses for the patient receiving propantheline include:
- Potential for injury related to inadequate dosage to reduce or alleviate pain.
- Constipation related to adverse GI effects of drug.
- Knowledge deficit related to propantheline therapy.

Implementation
Preparation and administration
— Assess the patient's bowel habits for signs of constipation before administration of the drug.
— Give drug 30 minutes to 1 hour before meals and at bedtime. Bedtime dose can be larger and should be given at least 2 hours after the last meal of the day.
— Drug should not be administered within 1 hour of an antacid or an antidiarrheal.
— Drug may be used with histamine H_2-receptor antagonist to treat Zollinger-Ellison syndrome.

—Propantheline dosage should be titrated until therapeutic effect is obtained or adverse reactions become intolerable.

Monitoring

—Monitor the effectiveness of therapy by regularly assessing for decreased GI pain or relief of GI pain.

—Monitor the patient for adverse drug reactions.

—Monitor vital signs and urine output carefully.

—In elderly patients, monitor level of consciousness.

—Monitor the patient for drug interactions.

—Regularly reevaluate the patient's and family's knowledge about propantheline therapy.

Intervention

—If the patient develops dry mouth, offer sugarless chewing gum or hard candy or ice chips.

—If the patient develops constipation, encourage him to increase exercise, dietary fiber intake, and daily fluid intake (at least 8 full glasses of water per day).

—Keep all members of the health care team informed of the patient's response to the drug.

Patient teaching

—Instruct the patient and family about propantheline, including the dosage, frequency, action, and adverse reactions.

—Explain the disease process and rationale for therapy.

—Instruct the patient to take the medication as it has been prescribed. Even missed doses should be taken unless it is time for the next dose.

—Instruct the patient to swallow tablets whole rather than chewing or crushing them.

—Instruct the patient to avoid driving and other hazardous activities that require alertness if he is drowsy, dizzy, or has blurred vision; to drink plenty of fluids to help prevent constipation; and to report any rash or skin eruption.

—Because the drug may cause hypotension, advise the patient to change positions cautiously.

—Advise the female patient who is breast-feeding to consult with her doctor. Drug may be excreted in breast milk and should not be used in breast-feeding women.

—Advise the patient that sugarless chewing gum or hard candy or ice chips may relieve dry mouth.

—Warn the patient to avoid extreme environmental temperatures. Hot and humid environments should be avoided to prevent a possible heatstroke.

—Tell the patient to notify the nurse or doctor if adverse reactions develop or questions arise about propantheline therapy.

Evaluation

In the patient receiving propantheline, appropriate evaluation statements include:

• Patient's GI pain is reduced or alleviated.
• Patient has no signs or symptoms of constipation.
• Patient and family state an understanding of propantheline therapy.

SELECTED MAJOR DRUGS: ANTICHOLINERGICS

DRUG, INDICATIONS, AND DOSAGES	SPECIAL PRECAUTIONS

Belladonna alkaloid

hyoscyamine (Cystospaz)
GI tract disorders caused by spasm; adjunctive therapy for peptic ulcers—
Adults: 0.125 to 0.25 mg P.O. or S.L. t.i.d. or q.i.d. before meals and h.s.; 0.375 mg (sustained-release form) P.O. q 12 hours; or 0.25 to 0.5 mg (1 to 2 ml) I.V., I.M., or S.C. q 6 hours. (Substitute oral medication when symptoms are controlled.)
Children ages 2 to 10: half the adult dose P.O.

• Contraindicated in patients with known hypersensitivity to anticholinergics, narrow-angle glaucoma, obstructive uropathy, obstructive disease of GI tract, severe ulcerative colitis, myasthenia gravis, paralytic ileus, intestinal atony, unstable CV status in acute hemorrhage, or toxic megacolon.
• Use cautiously in autonomic neuropathy, hyperthyroidism, coronary artery disease, cardiac arrhythmias, CHF, hypertension, hiatal hernia associated with reflux esophagitis, hepatic or renal disease, and ulcerative colitis or in patients over age 40 because of increased incidence of glaucoma.

Miscellaneous GI anticholinergics

anisotropine (Valpin 50)
Adjunctive therapy for peptic ulcers—
Adults: 50 mg P.O. t.i.d. To be effective, should be titrated to individual patient's needs.

• Contraindicated in patients with known hypersensitivity to anticholinergics, narrow-angle glaucoma, obstructive uropathy, obstructive disease of the GI tract, severe ulcerative colitis, myasthenia gravis, paralytic ileus, intestinal atony, unstable CV status in acute hemorrhage, or toxic megacolon.
• Use cautiously in autonomic neuropathy, hyperthyroidism, coronary artery disease, cardiac arrhythmias, CHF, hypertension, hiatal hernia associated with reflux esophagitis, hepatic or renal disease, and ulcerative colitis, or in patients over age 40 because of increased incidence of glaucoma.

clidinium (Quarzan)
Adjunctive therapy for peptic ulcers—
Dosage should be individualized according to severity of symptoms and occurrence of adverse reactions.
Elderly or debilitated patients: 2.5 to 5 mg P.O. t.i.d. or q.i.d. before meals and h.s.

• Contraindicated in patients with known hypersensitivity to anticholinergics, narrow-angle glaucoma, obstructive uropathy, obstructive disease of GI tract, severe ulcerative colitis, myasthenia gravis, paralytic ileus, intestinal atony, unstable CV status in acute hem-

SELECTED MAJOR DRUGS: ANTICHOLINERGICS *continued*

DRUG, INDICATIONS, AND DOSAGES	SPECIAL PRECAUTIONS

Miscellaneous GI anticholinergics *(continued)*

clidinium *(continued)*

orrhage, or toxic megacolon.
• Use cautiously in autonomic neuropathy, hyperthyroidism, coronary artery disease, cardiac arrhythmias, CHF, hypertension, hiatal hernia associated with reflux esophagitis, hepatic or renal disease, and ulcerative colitis, or in patients over age 40 because of increased incidence of glaucoma.

---

glycopyrrolate (Robinul)
To reverse neuromuscular blockade—
Adults: 0.2 mg I.V. for each 1 mg neostigmine or 5 mg pyridostigmine. May be given I.V. without dilution or may be added to dextrose injection and given by infusion.
Preoperatively to diminish secretions and block cardiac vagal reflexes—
Adults: 0.002 mg/lb of body weight I.M. 30 to 60 minutes before anesthesia.
Adjunctive therapy in peptic ulcers and other GI disorders—
Adults: 1 to 2 mg P.O. t.i.d. or 0.1 mg I.M. t.i.d. or q.i.d. Dosage must be individualized. Maximum P.O. dose is 8 mg daily.

• Contraindicated in patients with narrow-angle glaucoma, obstructive uropathy or GI disease, myasthenia gravis, paralytic ileus, intestinal atony, unstable CV status in acute hemorrhage, or toxic megacolon.
• Use cautiously in patients with autonomic neuropathy, hyperthyroidism, coronary artery disease, cardiac arrhythmias, CHF, hypertension, hiatal hernia associated with reflux esophagitis, hepatic or renal disease, or ulcerative colitis and in patients over age 40 because of increased incidence of glaucoma.
• Use cautiously in hot or humid environments. Drug-induced heatstroke is possible.

---

hexocyclium (Tral Filmtabs)
Adjunctive therapy for peptic ulcers and other GI disorders—
Adults: 25 mg P.O. q.i.d. before meals and h.s.

• Contraindicated in patients with known hypersensitivity to anticholinergics, narrow-angle glaucoma, obstructive uropathy, obstructive disease of GI tract, severe ulcerative colitis, myasthenia gravis, paralytic ileus, intestinal atony, unstable CV status in acute hemorrhage, or toxic megacolon.
• Use cautiously in autonomic neuropathy, hyperthyroidism, coronary artery disease, cardiac arrhythmias, CHF, hypertension, hiatal hernia associated with reflux esophagitis, hepatic or renal disease, and ulcerative colitis or in patients over age 40 because of increased incidence of glaucoma.

(continued)

SELECTED MAJOR DRUGS: ANTICHOLINERGICS *continued*

DRUG, INDICATIONS, AND DOSAGES	SPECIAL PRECAUTIONS

Miscellaneous GI anticholinergics *(continued)*

isopropamide (Darbid, Tyrimide‡)
Adjunctive therapy for peptic ulcers, irritable bowel syndrome—
Adults and children over age 12: 5 mg P.O. q 12 hours. Some patients may require 10 mg or more b.i.d. Dosage should be individualized to patient's needs.

• Contraindicated in patients with known hypersensitivity to iodine and to anticholinergics, narrow-angle glaucoma, obstructive uropathy, obstructive disease of GI tract, severe ulcerative colitis, myasthenia gravis, paralytic ileus, intestinal atony, unstable CV status in acute hemorrhage, or toxic megacolon.
• Use cautiously in autonomic neuropathy, hyperthyroidism, coronary artery disease, cardiac arrhythmias, CHF, hypertension, hiatal hernia associated with reflux esophagitis, hepatic or renal disease, and ulcerative colitis or in patients over age 40 because of increased incidence of glaucoma.

mepenzolate (Cantil)
Adjunctive therapy for peptic ulcers, irritable bowel syndrome, and neurologic bowel disturbances—
Adults: 25 to 50 mg P.O. q.i.d. with meals and h.s. Adjust dosage to individual patient's needs.

• Contraindicated in patients with known hypersensitivity to anticholinergics, narrow-angle glaucoma, obstructive uropathy, obstructive disease of GI tract, severe ulcerative colitis, myasthenia gravis, paralytic ileus, intestinal atony, unstable CV status in acute hemorrhage, or toxic megacolon.
• Use cautiously in autonomic neuropathy, hyperthyroidism, coronary artery disease, cardiac arrhythmias, CHF, hypertension, hiatal hernia associated with reflux esophagitis, hepatic or renal disease, and ulcerative colitis or in patients over age 40 because of increased incidence of glaucoma.

methantheline (Banthine)
Adjunctive therapy for peptic ulcers, pylorospasm, spastic colon, biliary dyskinesia, pancreatitis, and certain forms of gastritis—
Adults: 50 to 100 mg P.O. q 6 hours.
Children over age 1: 12.5 to 50 mg P.O. q.i.d.
Children under age 1: 12.5 to 25 mg P.O. q.i.d.
Neonates: 12.5 mg P.O. b.i.d.

• Contraindicated in patients with known hypersensitivity to anticholinergics, narrow-angle glaucoma, obstructive uropathy, obstructive disease of GI tract, severe ulcerative colitis, myasthenia gravis, paralytic ileus, intestinal atony, unstable CV status in acute hemorrhage, or toxic megacolon.
• Use cautiously in autonomic neuropathy, hyperthyroidism, coronary artery disease, cardiac arrhythmias, CHF, hypertension, hiatal hernia associated with reflux esophagitis, hepatic or renal disease, and ulcerative colitis or in patients over age 40 because of increased incidence of glaucoma.

‡Available in Australia only

SELECTED MAJOR DRUGS: ANTICHOLINERGICS *continued*

DRUG, INDICATIONS, AND DOSAGES	SPECIAL PRECAUTIONS

Miscellaneous GI anticholinergics *(continued)*

dicyclomine (Bentyl, Spasmoban†)
Adjunctive therapy for peptic ulcers and other functional GI disorders—
Adults: 10 to 20 mg P.O. t.i.d. or q.i.d.; or 20 mg I.M. q 4 to 6 hours. Always adjust dosage according to patient's needs and response.

• Contraindicated in patients with known hypersensitivity to anticholinergics, obstructive uropathy, obstructive disease of GI tract, severe ulcerative colitis, myasthenia gravis, paralytic ileus, intestinal atony, unstable CV status in acute hemorrhage, or toxic megacolon.
• Use cautiously in autonomic neuropathy, narrow-angle glaucoma, hyperthyroidism, coronary artery disease, cardiac arrhythmias, CHF, hypertension, hiatal hernia associated with reflux esophagitis, hepatic or renal disease, and ulcerative colitis.
• Use cautiously in hot or humid environments. Drug-induced heatstroke is possible.

†Available in Canada only

COMPARING ANTICHOLINERGIC COMBINATIONS

TRADE NAME AND CONTENT	SPECIAL CONSIDERATIONS

Librax Capsules
clidinium bromide 2.5 mg and
chlordiazepoxide hydrochloride 5 mg

• Combines the anticholinergic and spasmolytic effects of clidinium with the anxiolytic effect of chlordiazepoxide.
• Contraindicated in patients with known hypersensitivity to any of the drug's components and with glaucoma, prostatic hypertrophy, and benign bladder neck obstruction.
• Use cautiously in elderly or debilitated patients and in patients with impaired renal or hepatic function or depression.

Donnatal Tablets
atropine sulfate 0.0194 mg,
scopolamine hydrobromide 0.0065 mg,
hyoscyamine hydrobromide or sulfate 0.1037 mg, and
phenobarbital 16.2 mg

• Combines the anticholinergic and antispasmodic effects of atropine, scopolamine, and hyoscyamine hydrobromide or sulfate with the sedatory effect of phenobarbital.
• Contraindicated in patients with glaucoma, obstructive uropathy (for example, bladder neck obstruction due to prostatic hypertrophy); obstructive disease of the GI tract (for example, achalasia, pyloroduodenal stenosis); paralytic ileus, intestinal atony of the elderly or debilitated patient; unstable CV status in acute hemor-

(continued)

COMPARING ANTICHOLINERGIC COMBINATIONS *continued*

TRADE NAME AND CONTENT	SPECIAL CONSIDERATIONS
Donnatal Tablets *(continued)*	rhage; severe ulcerative colitis, especially if complicated by toxic megacolon; myasthenia gravis; and hiatal hernia associated with reflux esophagitis. • Also contraindicated in patients with known hypersensitivity to any of the drug's ingredients. Phenobarbital is contraindicated in acute intermittent porphyria and in those patients in whom phenobarbital produces restlessness and excitement. • Use cautiously with autonomic neuropathy, hepatic or renal disease, hyperthyroidism, coronary heart disease, CHF, cardiac arrhythmias, tachycardia, and hypertension.
Bellergal-S phenobarbital 40 mg, ergotamine tartrate 0.6 mg, and levorotatory alkaloids of belladonna 0.2 mg	• Combines the sympathetic inhibitory effect of ergotamine and the parasympathetic inhibitory effect of levorotatory alkaloids of belladonna with the synergistic effect of phenobarbital. • Contraindicated in patients with peripheral vascular disease, coronary heart disease, hypertension, impaired hepatic or renal function, sepsis, and glaucoma; in pregnant and breast-feeding women; and in those with known hypersensitivity to any of the drug's components. The concomitant administration of ergotamine and dopamine should be avoided because of the increased potential for ischemic vasoconstriction. Phenobarbital is contraindicated in patients with a history of manifest or latent porphyria and in those in whom the drug produces restlessness and excitement. • Use cautiously in bronchial asthma or obstructive uropathy.

SELF-TEST

1. Joe Ryan, age 42, was ordered atropine for adjunctive treatment of his peptic ulcer; after the first dose, he became thirsty, experienced a dry mouth, and was flushed on his face and trunk. His nurse should:
   a. hold the next dose and call the doctor.
   b. administer the next dose and observe the patient.
   c. tell the patient that all of these symptoms are normal and to be expected.
   d. take the patient's vital signs, place him in a prone position, and call the doctor.

2. GI anticholinergics exert their effects by:
   a. healing peptic ulcers.
   b. increasing GI smooth muscle contractions.
   c. inhibiting GI smooth muscle contractions.
   d. increasing gastric emptying.

3. Clarence Duke will take propantheline as part of his treatment for peptic ulcer. You tell him to take this drug:
   a. 30 minutes to 1 hour before meals.
   b. 30 minutes to 1 hour after meals.
   c. with his meals.
   d. with antacids.

Check your answers on pages 1069 and 1070.

CHAPTER 51

ANTIULCER AGENTS

Histamine₂-receptor antagonists

cimetidine ♦ cimetidine hydrochloride ♦ famotidine ♦ nizatidine
ranitidine hydrochloride

Protectants

misoprostol ♦ sucralfate

Acid pump inhibitor

omeprazole

OVERVIEW

- In the past, treatment of peptic ulcer disease involved the use of frequent doses of antacids, anticholinergic therapy, and, in extreme cases, surgery to perform gastric vagotomy.
- Recent advances in understanding of the physiology and pharmacology of gastric acid secretion and mucosal protectant mechanisms has resulted in the introduction of several new drugs, which represent progress in the treatment of peptic ulcer disease. This chapter focuses on these new treatments. (See also Chapter 45, Antacids, and Chapter 50, Anticholinergics, for more information.)
- Antiulcer agents are classified primarily into three groups: histamine₂-receptor (H₂-receptor) antagonists, protectants, and the acid pump inhibitor.

MAJOR USES

- H₂-receptor antagonists (cimetidine, famotidine, nizatidine, ranitidine) are the drugs of choice to treat peptic ulcers; they also promote healing of duodenal and gastric ulcers. These drugs are also used for long-term treatment of pathologic GI hypersecretory conditions, such as Zollinger-Ellison syndrome or hyperhistaminemia. H₂-receptor antagonists are prescribed to reduce gastric acid output and prevent stress ulcers in severely ill patients and in those with reflux esophagitis or upper GI bleeding. The ability of cimetidine to inhibit drug metabolism is currently being evaluated as a potential treatment of acetaminophen overdose. (It may decrease the formation of hepatotoxic metabolites.)
- Protectants include misoprostol and sucralfate. Misoprostol is prescribed to prevent NSAID-induced gastric ulcers in patients at high risk for complications from gastric ulcers. It is under study for other uses as well, including the treatment and prevention of peptic ulcers.

GLOSSARY

Gastrin: hormone secreted by the pyloric mucosa that increases the flow of gastric juices.

Histamine$_2$-receptor antagonist: drug that decreases gastric acid secretion by blocking gastric histamine (H$_2$) receptors.

Ulcer: cutaneous or mucosal lesion caused by gradual erosion, disintegration, and necrosis of underlying tissue.

- Sucralfate is used for short-term treatment (up to 8 weeks) of duodenal ulcers and has also been used successfully for short-term treatment of gastric ulcers. The drug may be prescribed to prevent recurrent, NSAID-induced, and stress ulcers.
- Omeprazole, an acid pump inhibitor, is indicated for short-term treatment of active duodenal ulcers, severe erosive esophagitis diagnosed by endoscopy, or symptomatic esophagitis that responds poorly to usual treatments, such as use of an H$_2$-receptor antagonist. Omeprazole may also be used to treat pathologic hypersecretory conditions, such as Zollinger-Ellison syndrome, multiple endocrine adenomas, and systemic mastocytosis. However, unlike H$_2$-receptor antagonists, omeprazole should not be used for maintenance therapy of peptic ulcer disease because animal studies suggest that long-term exposure to the drug may increase the risk of gastric tumors. More studies are needed to support the long-term safety of the drug in humans.

MECHANISM OF ACTION

- H$_2$-receptor antagonists act by blocking the histamine-receptor sites on the parietal cells of the stomach.
- Misoprostol is a synthetic prostaglandin E$_1$ analog with antisecretory and mucosal protective properties. NSAIDs inhibit prostaglandin synthesis, which may diminish bicarbonate and mucus secretion and promote mucosal damage and ulcer formation in the GI tract. Misoprostol counteracts these effects by replacing the endogenous prostaglandins.
- In an acid environment, sucralfate becomes a pastelike material that is negatively charged, highly viscous, and adhesive. This material binds to the positively charged proteins, such as albumin, fibrinogen, damaged mucosal cells, and dead leukocytes, found at the base of an ulcer. By forming a barrier at the ulcer site, sucralfate protects the ulcer against the ulcerogenic effects of gastric acid, pepsin, and bile. Thus, the ulcer is allowed to heal. The action of sucralfate in actively inhibiting pepsin and in absorbing bile acids also may play a role in its mechanism of action.
- Omeprazole belongs to a unique class of antisecretory compounds known as the substituted benzimidazoles. It suppresses gastric acid formation.

ABSORPTION, DISTRIBUTION, METABOLISM, AND EXCRETION

Cimetidine, nizatidine, and ranitidine are absorbed rapidly and completely from the GI tract; famotidine is absorbed incompletely. Food and antacids may impair the absorption of H_2-receptor antagonists. These drugs are distributed widely throughout the body, although ranitidine is distributed minimally into the CNS. The extent to which famotidine and nizatidine distribute into the CNS is unknown. All H_2-receptor antagonists are only mildly protein-bound.

Cimetidine and ranitidine are metabolized by the liver, but more than 50% of each dose is excreted unchanged in the urine. Famotidine and nizatidine also are metabolized by the liver, with over 70% and 65% of the dose, respectively, being excreted unchanged in the urine. Liver dysfunction increases the bioavailability and slightly prolongs the half-life of cimetidine and ranitidine. Liver dysfunction does not seem to affect nizatidine; its effects on famotidine's half-life are unknown. Nizatidine is metabolized only slightly and is more than 90% bioavailable. A decrease in renal function will prolong the half-lives of H_2-receptor antagonists.

Misoprostol is absorbed extensively and rapidly after oral administration. It is metabolized by de-esterification to misoprostol acid, which is responsible for its clinical activity. Administration with food or antacids may decrease the plasma concentration and total bioavailability, but the decrease does not appear to be clinically significant. Misoprostol acid is 90% protein-bound, has a half-life of 20 to 40 minutes, and does not accumulate with multiple doses. It is excreted primarily in the urine.

The minimal absorption of sucralfate from the GI tract is appropriate because sucralfate exerts its effects locally, rapidly reacting with hydrochloric acid in the GI tract to form a highly condensed, viscous, adhesive pastelike substance that adheres to the gastric mucosa and especially to ulcer sites. The drug is distributed minimally to other areas of the body and is excreted in the feces.

Omeprazole is absorbed rapidly after oral administration. Because omeprazole is affected by stomach acid, the capsules are formulated with delayed-release, enteric-coated granules so that drug absorption begins only after the granules leave the stomach. It undergoes some first-pass metabolism, which reduces the drug's bioavailability to 30% to 40%. About 95% of omeprazole is protein-bound. The drug is metabolized almost completely, and most of its metabolites are excreted in urine.

ONSET AND DURATION

Cimetidine reaches peak concentration levels in about 1 to 1.5 hours; famotidine, nizatidine, and ranitidine, in 1 to 3 hours. The half-life of cimetidine is about 2 hours; famotidine, 2.5 to 4 hours; nizatidine, 0.5 to 3 hours; and ranitidine, 2 to 3 hours. Each of these drugs suppresses gastric acid secretion for 5 to 8 hours after a dose.

After oral administration, misoprostol reaches a peak plasma concentration level in approximately 12 minutes. The drug begins to inhibit gastric acid secretion about 30 minutes after administration. This action persists for at least 3 hours.

The onset of sucralfate is rapid once the drug reaches the GI tract. The duration of action for sucralfate depends on how long the drug remains in contact with its action site. The drug's viscosity, adhesiveness, and affinity for damaged mucosa prolong this contact. Usually, the duration is up to 6 hours after administration.

The plasma concentration of omeprazole peaks 0.5 to 3.5 hours after administration. The onset of action occurs within 1 hour; maximal effects occur within 2 hours. Gastric acid secretion is inhibited by about 50% at 24 hours and lasts for 72 hours. Omeprazole's half-life is short: only 0.5 to 1 hour. Secretion inhibition lasts far longer than would be expected for a drug with such a short half-life, apparently due to its prolonged binding to $H+/K+$ ATPase. When omeprazole is discontinued, acid secretion returns to previous levels gradually over 3 to 5 days.

ADVERSE REACTIONS

H_2-receptor antagonists produce various adverse reactions. Cimetidine and ranitidine may produce headache, dizziness, malaise, myalgia, nausea, diarrhea or constipation, skin rashes, pruritus, loss of libido, and impotence. Cimetidine, however, is more likely to produce these adverse reactions. Cimetidine probably produces sexual dysfunction and gynecomastia through its binding to the androgen receptor. Substituting famotidine, nizatidine, or ranitidine decreases these adverse reactions. Famotidine and nizatidine produce very few adverse reactions, with headache the most frequent reaction (in about 2% of patients), followed by constipation or diarrhea and skin rash.

Reversible confusion, agitation, depression, and hallucinations can result, most commonly in patients receiving cimetidine, especially in severely ill or elderly patients. These reactions, which usually are associated with decreased renal function, also may occur with overdose.

When given by rapid I.V. injection, H_2-receptor antagonists can produce profound bradycardia and other cardiotoxic effects. Pain at the injection site occasionally occurs.

H_2-receptor antagonists rarely cause hypersensitivity reactions. Some patients develop increased hepatic enzyme levels, but this reaction also is rare. Cimetidine has been associated with adverse hematologic reactions, such as thrombocytopenia and granulocytopenia, and with seizures if drug accumulation occurs.

Misoprostol commonly causes adverse GI reactions. Diarrhea occurs in up to 40% of patients. It may be followed by abdominal pain, flatulence, dyspepsia, nausea, and vomiting. Because misoprostol is a prostaglandin, it also may affect the uterus, causing spotting, cramps, hypermenorrhea, and other menstrual disorders. In a pregnant patient, misoprostol therapy may induce miscarriage.

Usually sucralfate is well tolerated. Although typically minor, adverse reactions may become bothersome for the patient. Constipation is the most frequent dose-related adverse reaction, occurring in about 2% of all patients. Nausea and a metallic taste also may accompany the use of sucralfate. Less frequent reactions to this drug may include diarrhea, indigestion, dry mouth, back pain, dizziness, sleepiness, and vertigo. Sucralfate may produce a rash and pruritus, but these reactions are rare.

Omeprazole usually is tolerated well even in the higher dosages used to treat hypersecretory conditions. During clinical trials with omeprazole, the following dose-related adverse reactions were reported in more than 1% of patients: headache, diarrhea, abdominal pain, nausea, vomiting, upper respiratory tract infection, dizziness, rash, constipation, weakness, cough, and back pain. Omeprazole also has been linked to gastric malignancy when used in extremely high dosages in laboratory animals. Therefore, it is recommended only for short-term use.

PROTOTYPE: HISTAMINE$_2$-RECEPTOR ANTAGONISTS

CIMETIDINE
(sye met′ i deen)
Tagamet

CIMETIDINE HYDROCHLORIDE
Tagamet
Classification: histamine$_2$-receptor antagonist
Pregnancy risk category B

How supplied
cimetidine
TABLETS: 200 mg, 300 mg, 400 mg, 800 mg
cimetidine hydrochloride
ORAL LIQUID: 300 mg/5 ml
INJECTION: 150 mg/ml, 200 mg/2 ml‡, 300 mg in 50 ml 0.9% sodium chloride solution

Indications and dosage
Duodenal ulcer (short-term treatment)
ADULTS AND CHILDREN OVER AGE 16: 800 mg P.O. h.s. Alternatively, 400 mg P.O. b.i.d. or 300 mg P.O. q.i.d. (with meals and h.s.). Continue treatment for 4 to 6 weeks unless endoscopy shows healing. Maintenance therapy is 400 mg h.s. Parenteral—300 mg diluted to 20 ml with 0.9% sodium chloride solution or other compatible I.V. solution by I.V. push over 1 to 2 minutes q 6 hours. Or 300 mg diluted in 50 ml 5% dextrose solution or other compatible I.V. solution by I.V. infusion over 15 to 20 minutes q 6 hours. Or 300 mg I.M. q 6 hours (no dilution necessary). To increase dosage, give 300-mg doses more frequently to maximum dosage of 2,400 mg daily.

Duodenal ulcer prophylaxis
ADULTS AND CHILDREN OVER AGE 16: 400 mg P.O. h.s.

Active benign gastric ulcer
ADULTS: 300 mg P.O. q.i.d. with meals and h.s. for up to 8 weeks.

---

‡Available in Australia only

Pathologic hypersecretory conditions (such as Zollinger-Ellison syndrome, systemic mastocytosis, and multiple endocrine adenomas)
ADULTS AND CHILDREN OVER AGE 16: 300 mg P.O. q.i.d. with meals and h.s.; adjust to individual needs. Maximum dosage is 2,400 mg daily. Parenteral—300 mg diluted to 20 ml with 0.9% sodium chloride solution or other compatible I.V. solutions by I.V. push over 1 to 2 minutes q 6 hours. Or 300 mg diluted in 50 ml 5% dextrose solution or other compatible I.V. solution by I.V. infusion over 15 to 20 minutes q 6 hours. To increase dosage, give 300-mg doses more frequently to maximum dosage of 2,400 mg daily.

Contraindications and precautions
Cimetidine is contraindicated in patients with allergy to the drug or cross-sensitivity to other H_2-receptor antagonists. Use cautiously when administering large parenteral doses to patients with asthma because the drug may exacerbate the symptoms of the disease. Also use cautiously when administering to patients with cirrhosis, severely impaired hepatic function, and moderately to severely impaired renal function because drug accumulation may occur.

Adverse reactions
BLOOD: **agranulocytosis**, neutropenia, thrombocytopenia, **aplastic anemia** (rare).
CNS: mental confusion, dizziness, *headaches,* peripheral neuropathy.
CV: bradycardia.
GI: mild and transient diarrhea.
GU: transient elevations in serum creatinine.
HEPATIC: jaundice (rare).
SKIN: acnelike rash, urticaria.
OTHER: hypersensitivity, muscle pain, mild gynecomastia after use longer than 1 month.

Interactions
Antacids: interfere with absorption of cimetidine. Separate cimetidine and antacids by at least 1 hour if possible.
Warfarin, phenytoin, some benzodiazepines, isoniazid, carmustine, tricyclic antidepressants, lidocaine, metronidazole, xanthines (theophylline), propranolol and other beta blockers, and oral contraceptives: inhibited hepatic microsomal enzyme metabolism. Monitor serum levels closely during cimetidine therapy. Dosage reduction may be required.

Nursing considerations
Assessment
• Review the patient's history for a condition that contraindicates the use of cimetidine.
• Obtain a baseline assessment of the patient's GI pain before therapy.
• Be alert for common adverse reactions.
• Evaluate the patient's and family's knowledge about cimetidine therapy.

Planning (Nursing Diagnoses)
Potential nursing diagnoses for the patient receiving cimetidine include:

Italicized adverse reactions are common   Boldfaced adverse reactions are life-threatening

- Potential for injury related to inadequate dosage to relieve GI pain.
- Diarrhea related to adverse drug reactions.
- Knowledge deficit related to cimetidine therapy.

Implementation

Preparation and administration

— I.M. route of administration may be painful.
— I.V. solutions compatible for dilution with cimetidine are 0.9% sodium chloride solution, dextrose 5% and 10% (and combinations of these) in water solutions, lactated Ringer's solution, and 5% sodium bicarbonate injection. Do not dilute with sterile water for injection.
— Hemodialysis reduces blood levels of cimetidine. Schedule cimetidine dose at end of hemodialysis treatment.
— Effectiveness in treatment of gastric ulcers is not as great as in duodenal ulcers.
— Administering tablets with meals will ensure a more consistent therapeutic effect.
— Elderly or debilitated patients may be more susceptible to cimetidine-induced mental confusion.
— I.V. cimetidine is often used in critically ill patients prophylactically to prevent GI bleeding.
— Don't infuse I.V. too rapidly. May cause bradycardia.
— After administration of the liquid via nasogastric tube, tube should be flushed to clear it and ensure drug's passage to stomach.
— Hemodialysis removes cimetidine; schedule dose after dialysis session.
— When administering cimetidine I.V. in 100 ml of diluent solution, do not infuse so rapidly that circulatory overload is produced. Some authorities recommend that the drug be infused over at least 30 minutes to minimize the risk of adverse cardiac reactions. Sometimes drug is administered as continuous I.V. infusion.

Monitoring

— Monitor the effectiveness of therapy by regularly assessing for relief of or decrease in the patient's GI pain.
— Monitor the patient for adverse drug reactions.
— Monitor the patient's stool for type, amount, and color.
— If administering drug I.V., frequently monitor I.V. site for signs of infiltration or phlebitis.
— Monitor for profound bradycardia and other cardiotoxic effects when giving drug rapidly by I.V.
— Evaluate hematologic studies for signs of abnormalities, such as thrombocytopenia and granulocytopenia.
— Monitor blood chemistry results for changes in creatinine and hepatic enzymes, which may reflect changes in the patient's renal or hepatic function.
— Monitor the patient for drug interactions.
— Monitor diagnostic test results. Cimetidine may antagonize pentagastrin's effect during gastric acid secretion tests; it also may

cause false-negative results in skin tests using allergen extracts. Cimetidine therapy increases prolactin, serum alkaline phosphatase, and serum creatinine levels. FD&C blue dye #2 used in Tagamet tablets may impair interpretation of tests for occult blood in gastric content aspirate. Be sure to wait at least 15 minutes after tablet administration before drawing the sample, and follow test manufacturer's instructions closely.

— Regularly reevaluate the patient's and family's knowledge about cimetidine therapy.

Intervention

— If I.V. injection site becomes infiltrated or shows signs of phlebitis, discontinue I.V. and restart in another site. Notify the doctor and, if indicated, apply warm compress to site.

— Take seizure precautions if cimetidine accumulation occurs.

— Take safety precautions if the patient develops dizziness, confusion, or other mental status changes. For example, keep bed in low position, keep side rails up, and supervise the patient's activity.

— If the patient develops diarrhea, notify the doctor and obtain an order for an antidiarrheal. Also encourage the patient to increase his fluid intake.

— If the patient's stool becomes black and tarry, perform a test for occult blood and notify the doctor.

— Keep all members of the health care team informed of the patient's response to the drug.

Patient teaching

— Instruct the patient and family about cimetidine, including the dosage, frequency, action, and adverse reactions.

— Explain the disease process and rationale for therapy.

— Warn the patient to take drug as directed and to continue taking it even after pain subsides, to allow for adequate healing. Remind the patient not to take an antacid within 1 hour of taking drug.

— Remind the patient that, if he's taking cimetidine once daily, he should take it at bedtime for best results.

— Urge the patient to avoid smoking cigarettes, which may increase gastric acid secretion and worsen disease.

— Instruct the patient to avoid sources of GI irritation, such as alcohol, certain foods, and drugs containing aspirin.

— Instruct the patient to report immediately any signs of black, tarry stools; diarrhea; confusion; or rash.

— Advise the female patient considering breast-feeding to consult with her doctor because drug is excreted in breast milk.

— Inform the patient that sexual dysfunction, such as loss of libido and impotence, may occur as an adverse reaction to cimetidine. Advise the patient to notify the doctor if these adverse reactions occur.

— Tell the patient to notify the nurse or doctor if adverse reactions develop or questions arise about cimetidine therapy.

Evaluation
In the patient receiving cimetidine, appropriate evaluation statements include:
• Patient has decrease in or relief of GI pain.
• Patient maintains normal bowel habits and does not experience diarrhea.
• Patient and family state an understanding of cimetidine therapy.

PROTOTYPE: PROTECTANTS

SUCRALFATE
(soo kral′ fate)
Carafate, Sulcrate†
Classification: protectant
Pregnancy risk category B

How supplied
TABLETS: 1 g

Indications and dosage
Short-term (up to 8 weeks) treatment of duodenal ulcer
ADULTS: 1 g P.O. q.i.d. 1 hour before meals and h.s.

Contraindications and precautions
There are no known contraindications to the use of sucralfate.

Adverse reactions
CNS: dizziness, sleepiness.
GI: *constipation,* nausea, gastric discomfort, diarrhea.

Interactions
Antacids: may decrease binding of drug to gastroduodenal mucosa, impairing effectiveness. Don't give within 1 hour of each other.
Orally administered drugs: sucralfate may decrease the bioavailability of other drugs when administered together. Separate administration times by 2 hours.

Nursing considerations
Assessment
• Obtain a baseline assessment of the patient's GI pain before therapy.
• Be alert for common adverse reactions.
• Evaluate the patient's and family's knowledge about sucralfate therapy.

Planning (Nursing Diagnoses)
Potential nursing diagnoses for the patient receiving sucralfate include:
• Potential for injury related to inadequate dosage to reduce or relieve GI pain.
• Constipation related to adverse GI effects of the drug.
• Knowledge deficit related to sucralfate therapy.

Implementation

Preparation and administration

— Sucralfate may inhibit absorption of other drugs. Schedule other medications 2 hours before or after sucralfate.
— Sucralfate is poorly water-soluble. For administration by nasogastric tube, have the pharmacist prepare water-sorbitol suspension of sucralfate. Alternatively, place tablet in 60-ml syringe; add 20 ml water. Let stand with tip up for about 5 minutes, occasionally shaking gently. A suspension will form that may be administered from the syringe. After administration, tube should be flushed several times to ensure that the patient receives the entire dose.
— A patient who has difficulty swallowing a tablet may place it in 15 to 30 ml of water at room temperature, allow it to disintegrate, and then ingest the resulting suspension. This is particularly useful for the patient with esophagitis and painful swallowing.
— Therapy exceeding 8 weeks is not recommended.
— Some experts believe that 2 g b.i.d. is as effective as standard regimen.
— Administer drug on an empty stomach (1 hour before each meal and at bedtime).
— Do not administer this drug within 30 minutes of an antacid. An antacid may interfere with the drug's binding effect.

Monitoring

— Monitor the effectiveness of therapy by regularly assessing relief of or decrease in the patient's GI pain.
— Monitor the patient's bowel habits for signs and symptoms of constipation. Monitor the patient's stool for amount, type, and color.
— Monitor the patient for drug interactions.
— Regularly reevaluate the patient's and family's knowledge about sucralfate therapy.

Intervention

— If the patient develops constipation, notify the doctor and obtain an order for a laxative. Also advise the patient about dietary and other measures he may take to prevent constipation.
— If the patient's stool becomes black and tarry, perform a test for occult blood and notify the doctor of the results.
— Keep all members of the health care team informed of the patient's response to the drug.

Patient teaching

— Instruct the patient and family about sucralfate, including the dosage, frequency, action, and adverse reactions.
— Explain the disease process and rationale for therapy.
— Remind the patient to take the drug on an empty stomach at least 1 hour before meals.
— Advise the patient to continue taking drug as directed, even after pain begins to subside, to ensure adequate healing.

—Tell the patient that he may take an antacid 1 hour before or 1 hour after sucralfate.

—Warn the patient not to take drug longer than 8 weeks.

—Urge the patient to avoid smoking because it may increase gastric acid secretion and worsen disease.

—Instruct the patient to avoid sources of GI irritation, such as alcohol, certain foods, and drugs containing aspirin.

—Instruct the patient to immediately report any signs of black, tarry stools; diarrhea; confusion; or rash.

—Tell the patient to notify the nurse or doctor if adverse reactions develop or questions arise about sucralfate therapy.

Evaluation

In the patient receiving sucralfate, appropriate evaluation statements include:

• Patient experiences complete or partial relief of GI pain.

• Patient does not experience constipation.

• Patient and family state an understanding of sucralfate therapy.

PROTOTYPE: ACID PUMP INHIBITOR

OMEPRAZOLE

(oh me′ pray zol)

Prilosec

Classification: acid pump inhibitor
Pregnancy risk category C

How supplied

CAPSULES (DELAYED-RELEASE): 20 mg

Indications and dosage

Severe erosive esophagitis; symptomatic, poorly responsive gastroesophageal reflux disease (GERD)

ADULTS: 20 mg P.O. daily for 4 to 8 weeks. Patients with GERD should have failed initial therapy with an H_2-receptor antagonist.

Pathologic hypersecretory conditions (such as Zollinger-Ellison syndrome)

ADULTS: initially, 60 mg P.O. daily, with dosage titrated according to patient response. Dosage exceeding 80 mg daily should be administered in divided doses. Dosages up to 120 mg t.i.d. have been administered. Therapy should continue as long as clinically indicated.

Contraindications and precautions

Omeprazole is contraindicated in patients with known hypersensitivity to the drug or any component of the enteric formulation. Prolonged (2-year) studies in rats revealed a dose-related increase in gastric carcinoid tumors; studies in humans have not detected a risk from short-term exposure to the drug. Further study is needed to assess the impact of sustained hypergastrinemia and hypochlorhydria. According to the manufacturer, duration of omeprazole therapy should not exceed the recommended period.

Adverse reactions

CNS: headache, dizziness.
GI: diarrhea, abdominal pain, nausea, vomiting, constipation, flatulence.
RESPIRATORY: cough.
SKIN: rash.
OTHER: back pain.

Interactions

Diazepam, warfarin, and phenytoin: decreased hepatic clearance, possibly leading to increased serum levels. Monitor closely.
Ketoconazole, iron derivatives, and ampicillin esters: may exhibit poor bioavailability in patients taking omeprazole because optimal absorption of these drugs requires a low gastric pH. Avoid concomitant use.

Nursing considerations

Assessment

• Review the patient's history for a condition that contraindicates the use of omeprazole.
• Obtain a baseline assessment of the patient's disease before therapy.
• Be alert for common adverse reactions.
• Evaluate the patient's and family's knowledge about omeprazole therapy.

Planning (Nursing Diagnoses)

Potential nursing diagnoses for the patient receiving omeprazole include:
• Altered health maintenance related to ineffectiveness of drug.
• Noncompliance (medication administration) related to long-term therapy.
• Knowledge deficit related to omeprazole therapy.

Implementation

Preparation and administration

—Capsules should be swallowed whole and not opened or crushed.
—Omeprazole increases its own bioavailability with repeated administration. The drug is labile in gastric acid, and less drug is lost to hydrolysis as the drug increases gastric pH.
—Dosage adjustments are not required for renal or hepatic impairment.

Monitoring

—Monitor the effectiveness of therapy by regularly assessing for decreased GI reflux (heartburn).
—Monitor the patient's stool for amount, type, and color.
—Monitor the patient for drug interactions.
—Monitor diagnostic test results. Serum gastrin levels rise in most patients during the first 2 weeks of therapy.

— Regularly reevaluate the patient's and family's knowledge about omeprazole therapy.

Intervention

— If the patient's stool becomes black and tarry, perform a test for occult blood and notify the doctor of results.
— If the patient develops an adverse reaction, consult with doctor for appropriate treatment and provide supportive care as indicated.
— If the patient is unable to comply with therapy, discuss reasons why and suggest possible methods to help improve compliance.
— Keep all members of the health care team informed of the patient's response to the drug.

Patient teaching

— Instruct the patient and family about omeprazole, including the dosage, frequency, action, and adverse reactions.
— Explain the disease process and rationale for therapy.
— Explain the importance of taking the drug exactly as prescribed.
— Tell patient to take drug before meals and not to crush the capsule.
— Tell the patient to notify the nurse or doctor if adverse reactions develop or questions arise about omeprazole therapy.

Evaluation

In the patient receiving omeprazole, appropriate evaluation statements include:
• Patient obtains relief of or decrease in GI reflux (heartburn).
• Patient is compliant with therapy and completes entire prescribed regimen.
• Patient and family state an understanding of omeprazole therapy.

SELECTED MAJOR DRUGS: ANTIULCER AGENTS

DRUG, INDICATIONS, AND DOSAGES	SPECIAL PRECAUTIONS
Histamine$_2$-receptor (H$_2$-receptor) antagonists	
famotidine (Pepcid) *Duodenal ulcer—* **Adults:** for acute therapy, 40 mg P.O. daily h.s. For maintenance therapy, 20 mg P.O. daily h.s. *Pathologic hypersecretory conditions (such as Zollinger-Ellison syndrome)—* **Adults:** 20 mg P.O. q 6 hours. As much as 160 mg q 6 hours may be administered. *Hospitalized patients with intractable ulcers or hypersecretory conditions, or patients who cannot take oral medication—* **Adults:** 20 mg I.V. q 12 hours.	• Contraindicated in patients with allergy to the drug. • Use cautiously in severely impaired hepatic function because inadequate hepatic metabolism may cause accumulation of the drug and toxic effects.

SELECTED MAJOR DRUGS: ANTIULCER AGENTS *continued*

DRUG, INDICATIONS, AND DOSAGES	SPECIAL PRECAUTIONS
Histamine₂-receptor (H₂-receptor) antagonists *(continued)*	

nizatidine (Axid)
Active duodenal ulcer—
Adults: 300 mg P.O. daily h.s. Alternatively, may give 150 mg b.i.d. If creatinine clearance is 20 to 50 ml/min/1.73 m², give 150 mg daily; if creatinine clearance is < 20 ml/min/1.73 m², give 150 mg every other day.
Maintenance therapy for duodenal ulcer patients—
Adults: 150 mg P.O. daily h.s. If creatinine clearance is 20 to 50 ml/min/1.73 m², give 150 mg every other day; if creatinine clearance is < 20 ml/min/1.73 m², give 150 mg q 3 days.

• Contraindicated in patients with known hypersensitivity to the drug.
• Use cautiously in patients with known hypersensitivity to other H₂-receptor antagonists.

---

ranitidine hydrochloride (Zantac)
Duodenal and gastric ulcer (short-term treatment); pathologic hypersecretory conditions, such as Zollinger-Ellison syndrome—
Adults: 150 mg P.O. b.i.d. or 300 mg h.s. Doses up to 6.3 g daily may be prescribed in patients with Zollinger-Ellison syndrome. Drug also may be administered parenterally—50 mg I.V. or I.M. q 6 to 8 hours.
Maintenance therapy in duodenal ulcer—
Adults: 150 mg P.O. h.s.
Gastroesophageal reflux disease—
Adults: 150 mg P.O. b.i.d.

• Contraindicated in patients with allergy to the drug.
• Use cautiously in impaired hepatic function; dosage adjustment may be necessary in impaired renal function.

Protectant	

misoprostol (Cytotec)
Prevention of gastric ulcer induced by NSAIDs—
Adults: 200 mcg P.O. q.i.d. with meals and h.s. Dosage may be reduced to 100 mg P.O. q.i.d. in patients who cannot tolerate this dosage.
Duodenal ulcer—
Adults: 200 mg P.O. q.i.d. with meals and h.s.

• Contraindicated in pregnant women because of its abortifacient property. Patients must be warned about this potential and be advised not to give the drug to anyone else. Should not be used in women of childbearing age unless they require NSAID therapy and are at high risk for developing gastric ulcers.
• Also contraindicated in patients with allergy to prostaglandin derivatives.

SELF-TEST

1. Lucy Kenmore, age 35, takes large doses of an NSAID for rheumatoid arthritis. To prevent NSAID-induced ulcers, her doctor prescribes sucralfate 1 g P.O. q.i.d. How does sucralfate produce its therapeutic effects?
   a. It neutralizes the acid content of the stomach.
   b. It binds to the ulcer, forming a protective barrier.
   c. It decreases gastric acid secretion.
   d. It allows fluids to cleanse the ulcer site.

2. During acute flare-ups, Mr. Davis takes 150 mg of ranitidine P.O. b.i.d. How does this H_2-receptor antagonist exert its therapeutic effects?
   a. By increasing the absorption of stomach acid by the intestinal contents
   b. By decreasing the effectiveness of stomach alkalies in buffering acids
   c. By inhibiting the gastrocolic reflex, which is necessary for gastrin secretion
   d. By blocking the stimulant action of histamine on acid-secreting cells in the stomach

3. Because Mr. Davis also takes an antacid, how should the nurse administer these other medications?
   a. By an alternate route
   b. Shortly before the antacid
   c. 30 minutes after the antacid
   d. 1 to 2 hours before or after the antacid

Check your answers on page 1070.

CHAPTER 52

CORTICOSTEROIDS

___

Glucocorticoids
beclomethasone dipropionate ✦ betamethasone
betamethasone acetate and betamethasone sodium phosphate
betamethasone sodium phosphate ✦ cortisone acetate ✦ dexamethasone
dexamethasone acetate ✦ dexamethasone sodium phosphate
hydrocortisone ✦ hydrocortisone acetate ✦ hydrocortisone cypionate
hydrocortisone retention enema ✦ hydrocortisone sodium phosphate
hydrocortisone sodium succinate ✦ methylprednisolone
methylprednisolone acetate ✦ methylprednisolone sodium succinate
paramethasone acetate ✦ prednisolone ✦ prednisolone acetate
prednisolone sodium phosphate ✦ prednisolone tebutate ✦ prednisone
triamcinolone ✦ triamcinolone acetonide ✦ triamcinolone diacetate
triamcinolone hexacetonide

Mineralocorticoid
fludrocortisone acetate

___

OVERVIEW

- Corticosteroids mimic hormones produced naturally by the adrenal cortex. The corticosteroids described in this chapter are organic or synthetic compounds used to treat adrenocortical disorders, produce immunosuppression, and reduce inflammation. Corticosteroids are divided into three groups according to their primary physiologic actions: the glucocorticoids, which produce effects regulating carbohydrate, fat, and protein metabolism and have anti-inflammatory activity; the mineralocorticoids, which produce effects regulating electrolyte and water metabolism; and the adrenal androgens and estrogens, which produce hormonal effects. (For a complete discussion of these, see Chapter 53, Androgens and Anabolic Steroids, and Chapter 54, Estrogens and Progestins.)
- This chapter discusses the two major categories of corticosteroids: the glucocorticoids and the mineralocorticoids.

MAJOR USES

- Glucocorticoids have multiple clinical uses, including:
- —treatment of adrenal insufficiency (Addison's disease)
- —treatment of hypercalcemia resulting from breast cancer, multiple myeloma, sarcoidosis, or vitamin D intoxication (but not hyperparathyroidism)

GLOSSARY

Anabolism: constructive metabolism characterized by the conversion of simple substances into the more complex compounds of living matter.

Catabolism: complex metabolic process in which the oxidation of carbohydrates, fats, and proteins liberates energy for use in work, storage, or heat production.

Corticosteroid: any one of the natural or synthetic hormones associated with the adrenal cortex that influences or controls key physiologic processes, such as carbohydrate and protein metabolism, electrolyte and water balance, and the functions of the cardiovascular system, skeletal muscle, kidneys, and other organs.

Glucocorticoid: adrenocorticoid hormone that increases gluconeogenesis, exerts an anti-inflammatory effect, and influences many body functions.

Metabolism: aggregate of all chemical processes in living organisms that result in growth, generation of energy, elimination of wastes, and other bodily functions, as they relate to the distribution of nutrients in the blood after digestion.

Mineralocorticoid: adrenocorticoid secreted by the adrenal cortex that maintains normal blood volume, promotes sodium and water retention, and increases urinary excretion of potassium and hydrogen ions.

— topical treatment of dermatologic and ocular inflammations, such as exfoliative dermatitis, uncontrollable eczema, cutaneous sarcoidosis, and Stevens-Johnson syndrome (see Chapter 86, Topical Corticosteroids)

— systemic or inhalation therapy for respiratory diseases, including status asthmaticus, refractory bronchial asthma, berylliosis, Löffler's syndrome , and lipid pneumonitis

— relief of inflammation in rheumatic fever, rheumatoid arthritis, collagen diseases (systemic lupus erythematosus, dermatomyositis, and periarteritis nodosa), and nephrotic syndrome

— suppression of inflammatory reaction in allergic dermatoses, food and drug allergies, asthma, ulcerative colitis, and vasculitis

— diagnosis of endocrine disorders such as Cushing's syndrome and certain adrenocortical tumors

— emergency treatment of shock and anaphylactic reactions

— immunosuppression and relief of inflammation in organ and tissue transplants to prevent rejection

— adjunctive treatment of leukemias, lymphomas, and myelomas

— relief of cerebral edema resulting from neurosurgical procedures, head trauma, or brain tumors.

— adjunctive treatment of spinal cord injury.

- Mineralocorticoids are used to treat salt-losing forms of adrenogenital syndrome (congenital adrenal hyperplasia) after electrolyte balance is restored. In combination with glucocorticoids, they are used to treat adrenal insufficiency (Addison's disease).

MECHANISM OF ACTION

- Glucocorticoids (beclomethasone, betamethasone, cortisone, dexamethasone, hydrocortisone, methylprednisolone, paramethasone, prednisolone, prednisone, and triamcinolone) influence protein metabolism by increasing protein catabolism, decreasing use of amino acids for protein synthesis, and converting amino acids to glucose. Conversion of amino acids to glucose results in accelerated protein breakdown, and in muscle weakness and wasting. Interference with wound healing, immunosuppression, temporary growth arrest, and osteoporosis may also be related to protein catabolism.
- Glucocorticoids influence fat metabolism by inducing lipogenesis, which decreases adipose tissue formation. In high doses they cause fat redistribution—fat loss from the extremities and fat accumulation in the neck, back, and cheeks.
- The glucocorticoids influence carbohydrate metabolism by stimulating conversion of amino acids to glucose and decreasing peripheral utilization of glucose. This raises blood glucose levels, which triggers pancreatic release of insulin. Prolonged treatment in patients with controlled diabetes may cause resistance to exogenous insulin and necessitate adjustment of insulin levels.
- Glucocorticoids also block fibroblast formation, collagen deposition, capillary proliferation, increased capillary permeability in response to tissue trauma, microvascular dilation, plasma exudation, migration of polymorphonuclear leukocytes into inflamed areas, and phagocytosis. Glucocorticoids stabilize cell membranes and inhibit release of proteolytic enzymes, preventing normal inflammatory response. They also have an antilymphocytic action in the treatment of some neoplasms.
- Glucocorticoids may also potentiate the vasoconstriction produced by norepinephrine in treatment of shock; however, their use is somewhat controversial. They inhibit release of pituitary corticotropin, leading to adrenocortical suppression; and they lower blood calcium levels by antagonizing vitamin D effects on calcium absorption from the bowel and by decreasing calcium reabsorption from bone in multiple myeloma.
- Mineralocorticoids (fludrocortisone) increase sodium reabsorption and potassium and hydrogen secretion at the nephron's distal convoluted tubule. They also increase water retention, resulting in increased plasma volume and elevated blood pressure.

ABSORPTION, DISTRIBUTION, METABOLISM, AND EXCRETION

Most corticosteroids are efficiently absorbed from the GI tract. Water-soluble esters (for example, hydrocortisone sodium succinate and dexamethasone sodium phosphate) achieve rapid and high blood levels when given parenterally. Aqueous suspensions (such as hydrocortisone acetate or methylprednisolone acetate) are slowly absorbed after I.M. injection.

Corticosteroids are rapidly distributed to all body tissues, metabolized in the liver, and excreted in urine.

ONSET AND DURATION

Oral corticosteroids usually begin to act within 6 hours. Aqueous suspensions and solutions in oil have slow onset after I.M. administration; they produce low, prolonged blood levels (days to weeks). Aqueous solutions given I.V. have a rapid onset.

Some glucocorticoids (for example, betamethasone and dexamethasone) have a prolonged duration of action (more than 48 hours). Consequently, they should not be used in alternate-day therapy.

ADVERSE REACTIONS

Because corticosteroids strongly influence most systems of the body, they produce varied adverse reactions.

Fluid and electrolyte disturbances—ranging from mild edema and sodium retention to CHF—can occur, depending on the dose, duration of therapy, and the patient's underlying physical status. Such fluid and electrolyte disturbances may result from the mineralocorticoid activity of most glucocorticoids. Metabolic alkalosis, hypocalcemia, or hypokalemia can lead to other problems, including ECG changes, arrhythmias, hypotension, or hypertension.

Muscle weakness or myopathy, weakening of the skeletal system leading to pathologic fractures of the long bones or vertebral compression fractures, can also occur. GI disturbances are common, especially after oral administration. Nausea, vomiting, increased appetite, weight gain, and peptic ulcers may also result. Peptic ulcers are most likely to develop in patients with a history of peptic ulcer disease or in those who are taking other drugs irritating to the GI tract.

Endocrine disturbances, including menstrual irregularities, growth suppression in children, cushingoid signs (moon face, buffalo hump, central obesity), or decreased carbohydrate tolerance may occur, depending on the dose and duration of therapy.

Other effects include dermatologic disturbances (fragile skin, acne, hirsutism, impaired wound healing, or rash), ophthalmic changes (elevated intraocular pressure, exophthalmos, or posterior subcapsular cataracts), anaphylactoid or hypersensitivity reactions, malaise, aggravated infections, or leukocytosis.

PROTOTYPE: GLUCOCORTICOIDS

HYDROCORTISONE
(hye droe kor' ti sone)
Cortef, Cortenema, Hycort†, Hydrocortone

HYDROCORTISONE ACETATE
Biosone, Cortamed, Cortifoam, Hydrocortone Acetate

HYDROCORTISONE CYPIONATE
Cortef

HYDROCORTISONE SODIUM PHOSPHATE
Hydrocortone Phosphate

HYDROCORTISONE SODIUM SUCCINATE
A-HydroCort, Solu-Cortef
Classification: glucocorticoid
Pregnancy risk category C

How supplied
hydrocortisone
TABLETS: 5 mg, 10 mg, 20 mg
INJECTION: 25 mg/ml, 50 mg/ml suspension
ENEMA: 100 mg/60 ml
hydrocortisone acetate
INJECTION: 25 mg/ml, 50 mg/ml suspension
ENEMA: 10% aerosol foam (provides 90 mg/application)
hydrocortisone cypionate
ORAL SUSPENSION: 10 mg/5 ml
hydrocortisone sodium phosphate
INJECTION: 50 mg/ml
hydrocortisone sodium succinate
INJECTION: 100-mg, 250-mg, 500-mg, 1,000-mg vial

Indications and dosage
Severe inflammation, adrenal insufficiency
ADULTS: 5 to 30 mg P.O. b.i.d., t.i.d., or q.i.d. (as much as 80 mg P.O. q.i.d. may be given in acute situations); or initially, 100 to 250 mg (succinate) I.M. or I.V., then 50 to 100 mg I.M., as indicated; or 15 to 240 mg (phosphate) I.M. or I.V. q 12 hours; or 5 to 75 mg (acetate) into joints and soft tissue as a single dose. Dosage varies with size of joint. Often local anesthetics are injected with dose.
Shock
ADULTS: 500 mg to 2 g (succinate) I.M. or I.V. q 2 to 6 hours.
CHILDREN: 0.16 to 1 mg/kg (phosphate or succinate) I.M. or I.V., daily to t.i.d.

Adjunctive treatment of ulcerative colitis and proctitis
ADULTS: 1 enema (100 mg) nightly for 21 days.

Contraindications and precautions
Hydrocortisone is contraindicated in patients with systemic fungal infections. Use cautiously in patients with GI ulceration or renal disease, hypertension, osteoporosis, varicella, vaccinia, exanthema, diabetes mellitus, Cushing's syndrome, thromboembolic disorders, seizures, myasthenia gravis, metastatic cancer, CHF, tuberculosis, ocular herpes simplex, hypoalbuminemia, emotional instability or psychotic tendencies, and in children.

Adverse reactions
Most adverse reactions to corticosteroids are dose- or duration-dependent.
CNS: *euphoria, insomnia*, psychotic behavior, pseudotumor cerebri.
CV: **CHF**, hypertension, edema.
EENT: cataracts, glaucoma.
GI: peptic ulcer, GI irritation, increased appetite.
METABOLIC: possible hypokalemia, hyperglycemia and carbohydrate intolerance, growth suppression in children.
SKIN: delayed wound healing, acne, various skin eruptions.
OTHER: muscle weakness, pancreatitis, hirsutism, susceptibility to infections. Acute adrenal insufficiency may occur with increased stress (infection, surgery, or trauma) or abrupt withdrawal after long-term therapy.
Withdrawal symptoms: rebound inflammation, fatigue, weakness, arthralgia, fever, dizziness, lethargy, depression, fainting, orthostatic hypotension, dyspnea, anorexia, hypoglycemia. Sudden withdrawal may be fatal.

Interactions
Barbiturates, phenytoin, rifampin: decreased corticosteroid effect. Corticosteroid dose may need to be increased.
Immunizations: immunosuppressive effect may depress response to immunizations. Postpone elective immunizations if possible.
Indomethacin, aspirin: increased risk of GI distress and bleeding. Give together cautiously.
Insulin: glucocorticoid effect may alter insulin requirements. Monitor glucose levels closely.

Nursing considerations
Assessment
- Review the patient's history for a condition that contraindicates the use of hydrocortisone.
- Obtain a baseline assessment of the patient's underlying condition before initiating hydrocortisone therapy.
- Be alert for common adverse reactions.
- Evaluate the patient's and family's knowledge about hydrocortisone.

Planning (Nursing Diagnoses)
Potential nursing diagnoses for the patient receiving hydrocortisone include:

- Impaired tissue integrity related to ineffective dosing regimen of hydrocortisone.
- Altered protection related to adverse reactions associated with hydrocortisone.
- Knowledge deficit related to hydrocortisone therapy.

Implementation

Preparation and administration
— Do not use the acetate form for I.V. use.
— Do not confuse hydrocortisone sodium succinate (Solu-Cortef) with methylprednisolone sodium succinate (Solu-Medrol).
— Do not use injectable forms for alternate-day therapy.
— Gradually reduce drug dosage after long-term therapy.
— Always titrate to lowest effective dose as prescribed.
— Give a daily dose in the morning for better results and less toxicity.
— Give I.M. injection deep into gluteal muscle. Rotate injection sites to prevent muscle atrophy. Avoid S.C. injection, because atrophy and sterile abscesses may occur.
— Give oral dose with food when possible to avoid GI upset.
— Enema may produce same systemic effects as other forms of hydrocortisone. If enema therapy must exceed 21 days, discontinue gradually by reducing administration to every other night for 2 or 3 weeks.

Monitoring
— Monitor the effectiveness of therapy by regularly assessing the patient for signs and symptoms of the underlying condition.
— Monitor the patient for adverse drug reactions.
— Monitor the patient's weight, blood pressure, blood glucose level, and serum electrolyte levels regularly.
— Monitor the patient for infection. Drug may mask or exacerbate infections.
— Monitor the patient's stress level. Stress (fever, trauma, surgery, or emotional problems) may increase adrenal insufficiency. Dose may have to be increased.
— Monitor the patient's mental status for depression or psychotic episodes, especially in high-dose therapy.
— Monitor the patient's skin for petechiae.
— Monitor growth in infants and children on long-term therapy.
— Monitor patients receiving immunizations for decreased antibody response.
— Monitor the patient for early signs of adrenal insufficiency or cushingoid signs.
— Monitor the patient for drug interactions.
— Regularly reevaluate the patient's and family's knowledge about hydrocortisone.

Intervention
— Notify the doctor immediately if serious adverse drug reactions occur.

—Unless contraindicated, give the patient a low-sodium diet high in potassium and protein. Potassium supplement may be needed. Watch for additional potassium depletion from diuretics and amphotericin B.

—Never withdraw drug abruptly after long-term therapy; sudden withdrawal may be fatal.

—Expect to increase dosage during times of physiologic stress (trauma, surgery, or infection).

—Keep all members of the health care team informed of the patient's response to the drug.

Patient teaching

—Inform the patient and family about hydrocortisone, including the dosage, frequency, action, and adverse reactions.

—Be sure that the patient understands the need to take hydrocortisone as prescribed. Give the patient instructions on what to do if a dose is inadvertently missed.

—Warn the patient not to discontinue the drug abruptly or without the doctor's approval.

—Inform the patient of the possible therapeutic and adverse effects of the drug so that he may report complications to the doctor as soon as possible.

—Tell the patient to carry medical alert identification indicating the need for supplemental adrenocorticoids during stress.

—Teach the patient to recognize signs of early adrenal insufficiency (fatigue, muscular weakness, joint pain, fever, anorexia, nausea, dyspnea, dizziness, and fainting) and to notify the doctor promptly if they occur.

—Warn patients on long-term therapy about cushingoid signs, which may develop regardless of route of administration.

—Tell the patient to notify the nurse or doctor if adverse reactions develop or questions arise about hydrocortisone therapy.

Evaluation

In the patient receiving hydrocortisone, appropriate evaluation statements include:

• Patient does not demonstrate impaired tissue integrity while receiving hydrocortisone therapy.

• Patient does not experience serious adverse reactions associated with hydrocortisone.

• Patient and family state an understanding of hydrocortisone therapy.

FLUDROCORTISONE ACETATE
(floo droe kor′ ti sone)
Florinef
Classification: mineralocorticoid
Pregnancy risk category C

How supplied
TABLETS: 0.1 mg

Indications and dosage
Adrenal insufficiency (partial replacement), adrenogenital syndrome
ADULTS: 0.1 to 0.2 mg P.O. daily.

Contraindications and precautions
Fludrocortisone is contraindicated in patients with hypertension, CHF, or cardiac disease. Use cautiously in patients with Addison's disease.

Adverse reactions
CV: *sodium and water retention*, hypertension, cardiac hypertrophy, edema.
METABOLIC: hypokalemia.

Interactions
None significant.

Nursing considerations
Assessment
- Review the patient's history for a condition that contraindicates the use of fludrocortisone.
- Obtain a baseline assessment of the patient's adrenal insufficiency or adrenogenital syndrome before initiating fludrocortisone therapy.
- Be alert for common adverse reactions.
- Evaluate the patient's and family's knowledge about fludrocortisone therapy.

Planning (Nursing Diagnoses)
Potential nursing diagnoses for the patient receiving fludrocortisone include:
- Altered protection related to ineffectiveness of fludrocortisone.
- Fluid volume excess related to potential sodium and water retention.
- Knowledge deficit related to fludrocortisone therapy.

Implementation
Preparation and administration
—Give oral dose as prescribed.
—Expect to use fludrocortisone with cortisone or hydrocortisone in patients with adrenal insufficiency.

Monitoring

— Monitor the effectiveness of therapy by regularly assessing the patient for signs and symptoms of adrenal insufficiency.
— Monitor the patient for adverse drug reactions.
— Monitor the patient's blood pressure and serum electrolyte levels regularly. Weigh the patient daily.
— Regularly reevaluate the patient's and family's knowledge about fludrocortisone.

Intervention

— Report any significant patient weight gain, edema, hypertension, or severe headaches to the doctor.
— Unless contraindicated, give the patient a low-sodium diet high in potassium and protein. Potassium supplement may be needed.
— Keep all members of the health care team informed of the patient's response to the drug.

Patient teaching

— Inform the patient and family about fludrocortisone, including the dosage, frequency, action, and adverse reactions.
— Teach the patient to recognize signs of electrolyte imbalance: muscle weakness, paresthesia, numbness, fatigue, anorexia, nausea, altered mental status, increased urination, altered heart rhythm, severe or continuing headaches, unusual weight gain, or swelling of the feet.
— Tell the patient to take missed doses as soon as possible, unless it is almost time for the next dose, and not to double doses.
— Tell the patient to notify the nurse or doctor if adverse reactions develop or questions arise about fludrocortisone therapy.

Evaluation

In the patient receiving fludrocortisone, appropriate evaluation statements include:
• Patient's dosage regimen relieves signs and symptoms of mineralocorticoid insufficiency.
• Patient does not develop sodium and water retention.
• Patient and family state an understanding of fludrocortisone therapy.

SELECTED MAJOR DRUGS: CORTICOSTEROIDS

DRUG, INDICATIONS, AND DOSAGES	SPECIAL PRECAUTIONS

Glucocorticoids

beclomethasone dipropionate (Beclovent)
Steroid-dependent asthma —
Adults: 2 to 4 inhalations t.i.d. or q.i.d. Maximum dosage is 20 inhalations daily.
Children age 6 to 12: 1 to 2 inhalations t.i.d. or q.i.d. Maximum dosage is 10 inhalations daily.

• Contraindicated in status asthmaticus, in asthma controlled by bronchodilators or other noncorticosteroids alone, or for nonasthmatic bronchial diseases.

betamethasone (Celestone)
betamethasone acetate and betamethasone sodium phosphate (Celestone Soluspan)
betamethasone sodium phosphate (Celestone Phosphate)
Severe inflammation or immunosuppression —
Adults: 0.6 to 7.2 mg P.O. daily; or 0.5 to 9 mg (sodium phosphate) I.M., I.V., or into joint or soft tissue daily; or 1.5 to 12 mg (sodium phosphate-acetate suspension) into joint or soft tissue q 1 to 2 weeks, p.r.n.
Prevention of neonatal respiratory distress syndrome —
Pregnant women: 12 mg I.M. Celestone Soluspan 36 to 48 hours before premature delivery. Repeat in 24 hours.

• Contraindicated in systemic fungal infections.
• Use cautiously in patients with GI ulceration or renal disease, hypertension, osteoporosis, varicella, vaccinia, exanthema, diabetes mellitus, Cushing's syndrome, thromboembolic disorders, seizure disorders, myasthenia gravis, CHF, tuberculosis, ocular herpes simplex, hypoalbuminemia, and emotional instability or psychotic tendencies.

cortisone acetate (Cortone Acetate)
Adrenal insufficiency, allergy, inflammation —
Adults: 25 to 300 mg P.O. or I.M. daily or on alternate days. Dosages highly individualized, depending on severity of disease.

• Contraindicated in systemic fungal infections.
• Use cautiously in patients with GI ulceration or renal disease, hypertension, osteoporosis, varicella, vaccinia, exanthema, diabetes mellitus, Cushing's syndrome, thromboembolic disorders, seizure disorders, myasthenia gravis, CHF, tuberculosis, ocular herpes simplex, hypoalbuminemia and emotional instability or psychotic tendencies.

dexamethasone (Decadron, Hexadrol)
dexamethasone acetate (Dalalone D.P., Decadron-LA)
dexamethasone sodium phosphate (Decadron Phosphate, Hexadrol Phosphate)
Cerebral edema —
Adults: initially, 10 mg (phosphate) I.V., then 4 to 6 mg I.M. q 6 hours for 2 to 4 days, then tapered over 5 to 7 days.
Children: initially, 0.5 to 1.5 mg/kg I.V. daily; then 0.2 to 0.5 mg/kg I.V. daily in divided doses q 6 hours.
Inflammatory conditions, allergic reactions, neoplasms —
Adults: 0.25 to 4 mg P.O. b.i.d., t.i.d., or q.i.d.; or 4 to 16 mg (acetate) I.M. into joint or soft tissue q 1 to 3

• Contraindicated in systemic fungal infections and for alternate-day therapy.
• Use cautiously in patients with GI ulceration or renal disease, hypertension, osteoporosis, varicella, vaccinia, exanthema, diabetes mellitus, Cushing's syndrome, thromboembolic disorders, seizure disorders, myasthenia gravis, metastatic cancer, CHF, tuberculosis, ocular herpes simplex,

(continued)

SELECTED MAJOR DRUGS: CORTICOSTEROIDS *continued*

DRUG, INDICATIONS, AND DOSAGES	SPECIAL PRECAUTIONS

Glucocorticoids *(continued)*

dexamethasone *(continued)*
weeks; or 0.8 to 1.6 mg (acetate) intralesionally q 1 to 3 weeks.
Shock—
Adults: 1 to 6 mg/kg (phosphate) I.V. single dosage; or 40 mg I.V. q 2 to 6 hours, p.r.n.
Dexamethasone suppression test—
Adults: 0.5 mg P.O. q 6 hours for 48 hours.

hypoalbuminemia, emotional instability or psychotic tendencies, and in children.

---

methylprednisolone (Medrol)
methylprednisolone acetate (Depo-Medrol)
methylprednisolone sodium succinate (Solu-Medrol)
Severe inflammation or immunosuppression—
Adults: 2 to 60 mg P.O. in four divided doses; or 40 to 80 mg (acetate) I.M. daily; 10 to 250 mg (succinate) I.M. or I.V. q 4 hours; or 4 to 30 mg (acetate) into joints and soft tissues, p.r.n.
Children: 117 mcg to 1.66 mg/kg (succinate) I.V. in three or four divided doses.
Shock—
Adults: 100 to 250 mg (succinate) I.V. at 2- to 6-hour intervals.
To decrease residual damage following spinal cord trauma—
Adults: 30 mg/kg I.V. as a bolus injection within 8 hours of the injury, followed by a continuous infusion of 5.4 mg/hour over the next 23 hours.

• Contraindicated in systemic fungal infections.
• Use cautiously in patients with GI ulceration or renal disease, hypertension, osteoporosis, varicella, vaccinia, exanthema, diabetes mellitus, Cushing's syndrome, thromboembolic disorders, seizure disorders, myasthenia gravis, metastatic cancer, CHF, tuberculosis, ocular herpes simplex, hypoalbuminemia, and emotional instability or psychotic tendencies.

---

paramethasone acetate (Haldrone)
Inflammatory conditions—
Adults: 0.5 to 6 mg P.O. t.i.d. or q.i.d.
Children: 58 to 800 mcg/kg P.O. daily divided t.i.d. or q.i.d.

• Contraindicated in systemic fungal infections and alternate-day therapy.
• Use cautiously in patients with GI ulceration or renal disease, hypertension, osteoporosis, varicella, vaccinia, exanthema, diabetes mellitus, Cushing's syndrome, thromboembolic disorders, seizure disorders, myasthenia gravis, metastatic cancer, CHF, tuberculosis, ocular herpes simplex, hypoalbuminemia, and emotional instability or psychotic tendencies.

SELECTED MAJOR DRUGS: CORTICOSTEROIDS *continued*

DRUG, INDICATIONS, AND DOSAGES	SPECIAL PRECAUTIONS

Glucocorticoids *(continued)*

prednisolone (Cortalone, Delta-Cortef)
prednisolone acetate (Predalone 50, Predate 50)
prednisolone sodium phosphate (Hydeltrasol, Predate-S)
prednisolone tebutate (Hydeltra T.B.A., Predate T.B.A.)
Severe inflammation or immunosuppression—
Adults: 2.5 to 15 mg P.O. b.i.d., t.i.d., or q.i.d.; 2 to 30 mg I.M. (acetate, phosphate) or I.V. (phosphate) q 12 hours; or 2 to 30 mg (phosphate) into joints, lesions, and soft tissue as a single dose; or 4 to 40 mg (tebutate) into joints and lesions; or 0.25 to 1 ml (acetate-phosphate suspension) into joints weekly, p.r.n.

• Contraindicated in systemic fungal infections.
• Use cautiously in patients with GI ulceration or renal disease, hypertension, osteoporosis, varicella, vaccinia, exanthema, diabetes mellitus, Cushing's syndrome, thromboembolic disorders, seizure disorders, myasthenia gravis, metastatic cancer, CHF, tuberculosis, ocular herpes simplex, hypoalbuminemia, and emotional instability or psychotic tendencies.

prednisone (Deltasone, Orasone)
Severe inflammation or immunosuppression—
Adults: 2.5 to 15 mg P.O. b.i.d., t.i.d., or q.i.d. Maintenance dosage given once daily or every other day. Dosage must be individualized.
Children: 0.14 to 2 mg/kg P.O. daily divided q.i.d.
Acute exacerbations of multiple sclerosis—
Adults: 200 mg P.O. daily for 1 week, then 80 mg every other day for 1 month.

• Contraindicated in systemic fungal infections.
• Use cautiously in patients with GI ulceration or renal disease, hypertension, osteoporosis, varicella, vaccinia, exanthema, diabetes mellitus, Cushing's syndrome, thromboembolic disorders, seizure disorders, myasthenia gravis, metastatic cancer, CHF, tuberculosis, ocular herpes simplex, hypoalbuminemia, and emotional instability or psychotic tendencies.

triamcinolone (Aristocort, Kenacort)
triamcinolone acetonide (Kenaject-40, Kenalog)
triamcinolone diacetate (Aristocort Forte, Kenacort)
triamcinolone hexacetonide (Aristospan Intra-articular, Aristospan Intralesional)
Severe inflammation or immunosuppression—
Adults: 4 to 48 mg P.O. daily divided b.i.d., t.i.d., or q.i.d., or 40 mg I.M. (diacetate or acetonide) weekly; or 5 to 48 mg (diacetate or acetonide) into lesions; or 2 to 40 mg (diacetate or acetonide) into joints and soft tissue; or up to 0.5 mg (hexacetonide) per square inch of affected skin intralesionaly; or 2 to 20 mg (hexacetonide) intra-articular or intrasynovially. Often, a local anesthetic is injected into the joint with triamcinolone.
Steroid-dependent asthma—
Adults: 2 inhalations t.i.d. to q.i.d. Maximum dosage is 16 inhalations daily.
Children age 6 to 12: 1 to 2 inhalations t.i.d. to q.i.d. Maximum dosage is 12 inhalations daily.

• Contraindicated in systemic fungal infections.
• Use cautiously in patients with GI ulceration or renal disease, hypertension, osteoporosis, varicella, vaccinia, exanthema, diabetes mellitus, Cushing's syndrome, thromboembolic disorders, seizure disorders, myasthenia gravis, metastatic cancer, CHF, tuberculosis, ocular herpes simplex, hypoalbuminemia, and emotional instability or psychotic tendencies.

SELF-TEST

1. Jason Chir, age 64, has been admitted to your unit for major surgery tomorrow. His history records that he has been taking oral corticosteroids for 12 years for adrenal insufficiency. He is to have nothing by mouth after midnight. As his nurse you should:
   a. withhold all medication for 24 hours.
   b. administer the oral medication before surgery.
   c. contact the doctor for a decreased amount of corticosteroid to be given via a parenteral route.
   d. contact the doctor for an increased amount of corticosteroid to be given via a parenteral route.

2. Because of the corticosteroid therapy, after surgery Mr. Chir will require careful nursing assessment and intervention to:
   a. detect an infection.
   b. prevent hypoglycemia.
   c. prevent hypercalcemia.
   d. prevent an allergic reaction to the dressing tape.

3. After surgery, Mr. Chir's laboratory results indicate a mineralocorticoid deficiency. His doctor prescribes fludrocortisone acetate 0.1 mg P.O. daily. Which of the following adverse reactions commonly occurs with this drug?
   a. hypotension
   b. sodium and water retention
   c. drowsiness
   d. skin rash

Check your answers on page 1070.

CHAPTER 53

ANDROGENS AND ANABOLIC STEROIDS

Androgens

danazol ✦ fluoxymesterone ✦ methyltestosterone ✦ testosterone
testosterone cypionate ✦ testosterone enanthate ✦ testosterone propionate

Anabolic steroids

nandrolone decanoate ✦ nandrolone phenpropionate ✦ oxandrolone
oxymetholone ✦ stanozolol

OVERVIEW

- Androgens (danazol, fluoxymesterone, methyltestosterone, and testosterone and its salts) include both the organic and the synthetic steroids that stimulate growth of the male accessory sex organs, promoting development of secondary sex characteristics such as facial and body hair, deep voice, and skeletal muscle. Testosterone, the primary natural androgen in humans, is produced by the interstitial cells of the testes under the stimulation of luteinizing hormone from the pituitary. A smaller amount of testosterone is secreted by the adrenal cortex in both sexes and by the ovaries in females.

- Anabolic steroids (nandrolone decanoate, nandrolone phenpropionate, oxandrolone, oxymetholone, and stanozolol) are synthetic compounds structurally related to testosterone. They promote tissue-building and reverse tissue-depleting processes. They have an advantage over testosterone, its esters, and synthetic androgens when anabolic rather than androgenic activity is desired. Despite their preponderant anabolic properties, their residual androgenic activity may produce some virilization in female patients if large doses are administered for long periods.

- This chapter discusses androgens and anabolic steroids.

MAJOR USES

- Androgens in androgen-deficient males combat hypogonadism of either primary origin (for example, Klinefelter's syndrome or myotonic dystrophy) or secondary origin (for example, pituitary tumors or pituitary insufficiency, and selective gonadotropin deficiencies, such as eunuchoidism). They're also used to treat oligospermia and impotence.

- Androgens in women may palliate androgen-responsive, advanced inoperable breast cancer in patients who have been in menopause for more than 1 year but less than 5 years, or who have an estrogen-dependent tumor.

GLOSSARY

Anabolic: promoting general body growth.
Androgenic: producing masculine characteristics.
Eunuchoidism: deficiency of the function of male hormone or its formation by the testes.
Gonadotropin: hormonal substance that stimulates the ovaries or testes.
Gynecomastia: excessive development of male mammary glands.

- Androgens are also used to treat certain gynecologic conditions (for example, uterine hemorrhage, dysmenorrhea, and menopausal syndrome).
- Danazol, a synthetic androgen, is therapeutic for fibrocystic breast disease. It is also used to treat refractory endometriosis.
- Anabolic steroids promote weight gain in patients who are underweight due to predisposing catabolic states. An adequate dietary regimen should be established to maximize tissue-building.
- Anabolic steroids also correct corticosteroid catabolism and reverse the profound negative nitrogen balance that occurs as a result of corticosteroid therapy.
- As adjunctive therapy, anabolic steroids may be effective in senile and postmenopausal osteoporosis as well as refractory anemias associated with chronic disease.
- Androgens and anabolic steroids improve athletic performance (ergogenic effect), but the medical risks associated with their use far outweigh any benefits. Most athletic organizations have outlawed their use, and random testing for the presence of these drugs is commonly performed at major competitive events. The Drug Enforcement Agency has classified these drugs as controlled substance schedule III.

MECHANISM OF ACTION

- Androgens are simply exogenous replacements that stimulate target tissues to develop normally in androgen-deficient males.
- Anabolic steroids stimulate cellular protein synthesis in debilitated patients. The resulting positive nitrogen balance promotes anabolism. Anabolic steroids also promote a sense of well-being in debilitated patients, which may encourage the patient to eat more and gain weight.
- Anabolic steroids improve calcium balance and decrease bone resorption. They also enhance erythropoiesis by stimulating secretion of renal or extrarenal erythropoietin and by directly stimulating heme synthesis, an action potentiated by erythropoietin.

ABSORPTION, DISTRIBUTION, METABOLISM, AND EXCRETION

Testosterone and anabolic steroids are well absorbed from the GI tract. However, because most of these drugs undergo rapid degradation in the liver (because of first-pass effect), they are not effective when given orally. Administering testosterone buccally or sublingually circumvents the drug's hepatic degradation. Methyltestosterone and fluoxymesterone resist hepatic metabolism because they are alkylated in the 17-alpha position; they are therefore the only orally active androgens. Testosterone cypionate and testosterone enanthate are dissolved in oil and injected intramuscularly.

All androgens and anabolic steroids are metabolized in the liver and excreted primarily by the kidneys.

ONSET AND DURATION

Onset of action of the androgens and anabolic steroids is difficult to determine because subjective response varies. Hematologic and other objective responses are not apparent for at least 3 months.

Nandrolone decanoate and nandrolone phenpropionate given I.M. have durations of 3 to 4 weeks and 1 to 2 weeks, respectively. Testosterone cypionate and testosterone enanthate have effects that last as long as 4 weeks. Testosterone propionate dissolved in oil has a shorter action than the other two ester analogs; however, its 2- to 3-day duration supplies the effect of daily injections of testosterone alone. Subcutaneous implantation of testosterone pellets prolongs action up to 6 months.

ADVERSE REACTIONS

Both androgens and anabolic steroids can cause the following adverse reactions:

In females, androgens and anabolic steroids cause menstrual irregularities, inhibition of gonadotropin secretion, and virilization, including deepening of voice and clitoral enlargement (usually not reversible). If administered during pregnancy, androgens cause virilization of external genitalia of the female fetus.

In males, these drugs cause gynecomastia, excessive frequency and duration of penile erections, inhibition of testicular function, testicular atrophy, impotence, chronic priapism, decreased ejaculatory volume, epididymitis, bladder irritability, and prepubertal phallic enlargement. Oligospermia may occur at high doses.

Other adverse reactions to both androgens and anabolic steroids include rashes, skeletal malformations, fluid and electrolyte disturbances, nausea, vomiting, hallucinations, and anaphylactoid reactions. An increased risk of hepatocellular carcinoma is associated with prolonged use of both androgens and anabolic steroids.

TESTOSTERONE
(tess toss'ter one)

Andro 100, Andronaq-50, Histerone 50, Histerone 100, Malogen,
Testaqua, Testoject 50, Testoject LA

Classification: androgen
Controlled substance schedule III
Pregnancy risk category X

How supplied
INJECTION (AQUEOUS SUSPENSION): 25 mg/ml, 50 mg/ml, 100 mg/ml
PELLETS (STERILE) FOR SUBCUTANEOUS IMPLANTATION: 75 mg

Indications and dosage
Eunuchoidism, eunuchism, male climacteric symptoms
ADULTS: 10 to 25 mg I.M. two to five times weekly. Once dosage is
established, patient may be switched to subcutaneous pellets (150 to 450
mg) implanted every 3 to 6 months.

Breast cancer in women 1 to 5 years postmenopausal
WOMEN: 100 mg I.M. three times weekly as long as improvement is
maintained.

Contraindications and precautions
Testosterone is contraindicated in women of childbearing potential because of the risk of possible virilization of female infant; in elderly,
asthenic men who may react adversely to androgen overstimulation; in
men with prostatic or breast cancer; in patients with hypercalcemia;
cardiac, hepatic, or renal decompensation; benign prostatic hypertrophy
with obstruction; conditions aggravated by fluid retention; or hypertension; and in premature infants. Use cautiously in patients with MI or
coronary artery disease, and in prepubertal boys.

Adverse reactions
ANDROGENIC: in women—*acne, edema, oily skin, weight gain, hirsutism,*
hoarseness, clitoral enlargement, decreased or increased libido; in prepubertal boys—premature epiphyseal closure, acne, priapism, growth of
body and facial hair, phallic enlargement; in postpubertal men—testicular
atrophy, oligospermia, decreased ejaculatory volume, impotence,
gynecomastia, epididymitis.
CV: edema.
GI: gastroenteritis, nausea, vomiting, constipation, diarrhea, change in
appetite.
GU: bladder irritability.
HEPATIC: reversible jaundice.
HYPOESTROGENIC: in women—flushing; sweating; vaginitis with itching,
drying, burning, or bleeding; menstrual irregularities.

Italicized adverse reactions are common

LOCAL: pain at injection site, induration, irritation and sloughing with pellet implantation, edema.
OTHER: hypercalcemia.

Interactions

Insulin: glucocorticoid effect may alter insulin requirements. Monitor blood glucose levels.
Oral anticoagulants: increased risk of bleeding. Monitor for adverse effects and adjust dosage as ordered.

Nursing considerations

Assessment

- Review the patient's history for a condition that contraindicates the use of testosterone.
- Obtain a baseline assessment of the patient's underlying condition before initiating testosterone therapy.
- Be alert for common adverse reactions.
- Evaluate the patient's and family's knowledge about testosterone therapy.

Planning (Nursing Diagnoses)

Potential nursing diagnoses for the patient receiving testosterone include:
- Sexual dysfunction related to ineffectiveness of testosterone used to treat male sexual disorders.
- Body image disturbance related to adverse reactions associated with testosterone.
- Fluid volume excess related to potential for edema caused by testosterone.
- Knowledge deficit related to testosterone therapy.

Implementation

Preparation and administration

— Store I.M. preparations at room temperature. If crystals appear, warming and shaking the bottle will usually disperse them.
— Inject deep into upper outer quadrant of gluteal muscle. Rotate injection sites to prevent muscle atrophy.

Monitoring

— Monitor the effectiveness of therapy by regularly assessing the patient's underlying condition for improvement.
— Monitor the patient for adverse drug reactions.
— Monitor the patient with metastatic breast cancer for hypercalcemia, which usually indicates progression of bone metastases.
— Monitor liver function studies regularly.
— Monitor prepubertal boys by X-ray for rate of bone maturation.
— Monitor for ecchymotic areas, petechiae, or abnormal bleeding in patients receiving concomitant anticoagulant therapy. Monitor prothrombin time. Monitor the patient's weight routinely for fluid retention.

— Monitor the patient for nutritional deficiencies if adverse GI reactions occur.
— Monitor the injection site for local reactions such as induration, irritation and sloughing (with pellet implantation), or edema.
— Monitor female patients for signs of excessive virilization.
— Regularly reevaluate the patient's and family's knowledge about testosterone.

Intervention

— Report signs of virilization in females so the doctor can reevaluate treatment.
— Therapeutic response in breast cancer is usually apparent within 3 months. Monitor for signs of therapeutic response or disease progression.
— Give the patient a diet high in calories and protein unless contraindicated. Give small, frequent feedings. Also implement salt restriction if edema occurs and expect to administer a diuretic concurrently, if needed.
— Carefully evaluate results of laboratory studies, because many laboratory results may be altered during therapy and for 2 to 3 weeks after therapy ends.
— Obtain an order for an antiemetic, antidiarrheal, or laxative, as indicated.
— Keep all members of the health care team informed of the patient's response to the drug.

Patient teaching

— Inform the patient and family about testosterone, including the dosage, frequency, action, and adverse reactions.
— Explain to female patients that virilization may occur. Tell these patients to report androgenic effects immediately. Stopping the drug will prevent further androgenic changes, but will probably not reverse those already present.
— Tell female patients to report menstrual irregularities; discontinue therapy pending determination of the cause.
— Advise male patients to report too frequent or persistent penile erections to the doctor.
— Advise the patient to report persistent GI distress, diarrhea, or the onset of jaundice.
— Tell the patient to notify the nurse or doctor if adverse reactions develop or questions arise about testosterone therapy.

Evaluation

In the patient receiving testosterone, appropriate evaluation statements include:
• Patient reports satisfactory sexual function.
• Patient states acceptance of altered body image as a result of testosterone therapy.
• Patient does not develop fluid retention.

• Patient and family state an understanding of testosterone therapy.

PROTOTYPE: ANABOLIC STEROIDS

OXANDROLONE
(ox an'droe lone)
Anavar, Lonavar‡
Classification: anabolic steroid
Controlled substance schedule III
Pregnancy risk category X

How supplied
TABLETS: 2.5 mg

Indications and dosage
To combat catabolic effects of corticosteroid therapy, osteoporosis, prolonged immobilization, and debilitated states
ADULTS: 2.5 mg P.O. b.i.d., t.i.d., or q.i.d., up to 20 mg daily for 2 to 4 weeks.
CHILDREN: 0.25 mg/kg P.O. daily in divided doses for 2 to 4 weeks.
   Continuous therapy should not exceed 3 months.

Contraindications and precautions
Oxandrolone is contraindicated in patients with prostatic hyperplasia with obstruction; prostatic and male breast cancer; cardiac, hepatic, or renal decompensation; hypercalcemia; nephrosis; and in premature infants. Use oxandrolone cautiously in prepubertal boys, patients with diabetes or coronary disease, and patients taking corticotropin, corticosteroids, or anticoagulants.

Adverse reactions
ANDROGENIC: in women—*acne, edema, oily skin, weight gain, hirsutism, hoarseness,* clitoral enlargement, decreased or increased libido; in prepubertal boys—premature epiphyseal closure, acne, priapism, growth of body and facial hair, phallic enlargement; in postpubertal men—testicular atrophy, oligospermia, decreased ejaculatory volume, impotence, gynecomastia, epididymitis.
CV: edema.
GI: gastroenteritis, nausea, vomiting, constipation or diarrhea, change in appetite.
GU: bladder irritability.
HEPATIC: reversible jaundice, hepatotoxicity.
HYPOESTROGENIC: in women—flushing; sweating; vaginitis with itching, drying, burning, or bleeding; menstrual irregularities.
OTHER: hypercalcemia.

Interactions
Anticoagulants: increased risk of bleeding. Use together cautiously.

---

‡Available in Australia only
Italicized adverse reactions are common

Corticotropin, corticosteroids: increased risk of excessive sodium retention and edema. Use together cautiously.

Hypoglycemic agents: androgens may alter blood glucose levels. Dosage adjustments may be necessary.

Nursing considerations

Assessment

- Review the patient's history for a condition that contraindicates the use of oxandrolone.
- Obtain a baseline assessment of the catabolic effects of the patient's underlying condition before initiating oxandrolone therapy.
- Be alert for common adverse reactions.
- Evaluate the patient's and family's knowledge about oxandrolone.

Planning (Nursing Diagnoses)

Potential nursing diagnoses for the patient receiving oxandrolone include:

- Altered protection related to continued catabolic effects caused by ineffectiveness of oxandrolone.
- Body image disturbance related to adverse reactions associated with oxandrolone.
- Fluid volume excess related to potential for edema caused by oxandrolone therapy.
- Knowledge deficit related to oxandrolone therapy.

Implementation

Preparation and administration

— Check that in children, therapy is preceded by X-ray of wrist bones to establish level of bone maturation. During treatment, bone maturation may proceed more rapidly than linear growth; dosage should be intermittent and X-rays taken periodically.
— Administer with food or meals if GI upset occurs.

Monitoring

— Monitor the effectiveness of therapy by regularly assessing the patient's condition.
— Monitor the patient for hypercalcemia and obtain calcium levels regularly.
— Monitor the patient for adverse drug reactions.
— Monitor female patients for signs of virilization.
— Monitor the patient for symptoms of jaundice, which may be reversed by dosage adjustment. Periodic liver function tests should be performed.
— Monitor the patient on concomitant anticoagulant therapy for ecchymotic areas, petechiae, or abnormal bleeding. Monitor prothrombin time.
— Monitor boys under age 7 for precocious sexual development.
— Monitor the patient's weight routinely for fluid retention.
— Monitor the patient for nutritional deficiencies if adverse GI reactions occur.

— Regularly reevaluate the patient's and family's knowledge about oxandrolone.

Intervention

— Report signs of virilization in females to the doctor.

— Be aware that therapeutic response in breast cancer is usually apparent within 3 months. Monitor for signs of therapeutic response or disease progression.

— Give the patient a diet high in calories and protein unless contraindicated. Give small, frequent feedings. Also implement salt restriction if edema occurs; expect to administer a diuretic concurrently, if needed.

— Carefully evaluate results of laboratory studies. Many laboratory results may be altered during therapy and for 2 to 3 weeks after therapy ends.

— Obtain an order for an antiemetic, antidiarrheal, or laxative, as indicated.

— Keep all members of the health care team informed of the patient's response to the drug.

Patient teaching

— Inform the patient and family about oxandrolone, including the dosage, frequency, action, and adverse reactions.

— Tell the patient to take drug with food or meals if GI upset occurs.

— Tell female patients to report menstrual irregularities; therapy should be discontinued pending etiologic determination.

— Explain to female patients that virilization may occur. Tell these patients to report such effects immediately.

— Stress importance of not abusing drug to enhance athletic performance.

— Tell the patient to notify the nurse or doctor if adverse reactions develop or questions arise about oxandrolone therapy.

Evaluation

In the patient receiving oxandrolone, appropriate evaluation statements include:

• Patient exhibits less catabolic activity.

• Patient states acceptance of body image changes caused by oxandrolone therapy.

• Patient does not develop fluid retention.

• Patient and family state an understanding of oxandrolone therapy.

SELECTED MAJOR DRUGS: ANDROGENS AND ANABOLIC STEROIDS

DRUG, INDICATIONS, AND DOSAGES	SPECIAL PRECAUTIONS

Androgens

danazol (Cyclomen, Danocrine)
Mild endometriosis—
Women: initially, 100 to 200 mg P.O. b.i.d. Subsequent dosage based on patient response.
Moderate to severe endometriosis—
Women: 400 mg P.O. b.i.d. uninterrupted for 3 to 6 months; may continue for 9 months.
Fibrocystic breast disease—
Women: 100 to 400 mg P.O. daily in two divided doses uninterrupted for 2 to 6 months.
Prevention of hereditary angioedema—
Adults: 200 mg P.O. b.i.d. to t.i.d., continued until favorable response is achieved. Then dosage should be decreased by half at 1- to 3-month intervals.

• Contraindicated in undiagnosed abnormal vaginal bleeding, or in impaired renal, cardiac, or hepatic function.
• Use cautiously in patients with seizure disorders or migraine headache.

fluoxymesterone (Android-F, Halotestin)
Hypogonadism and impotence caused by testicular deficiency—
Adults: 2 to 10 mg P.O. daily.
Palliation of breast cancer in women—
Women: 15 to 30 mg P.O. daily in divided doses. All dosages should be individualized and reduced to minimum when effect is noted.
Postpartum breast engorgement—
Women: 2.5 mg P.O. followed by 5 to 10 mg daily for 5 days.

• Contraindicated in prostatic hyperplasia with obstruction; male breast or prostatic cancer; cardiac, hepatic, or renal decompensation; nephrosis; hypercalcemia; and in premature infants.
• Use cautiously in prepubertal boys; patients with diabetes or coronary disease; and patients taking corticotropin, corticosteroids, or anticoagulants.

methyltestosterone (Android, Metandren)
Postpartum breast engorgement—
Women: 80 mg P.O. daily, or 40 mg buccal daily for 3 to 5 days.
Breast cancer in women 1 to 5 years postmenopausal—
Women: 200 mg P.O. daily, or 100 mg buccal daily.
Eunuchoidism and eunuchism, male climacteric symptoms—
Men: 10 to 40 mg P.O. daily, or 5 to 20 mg buccal daily.
Postpubertal cryptorchidism—
Adolescent boys: 30 mg P.O. daily, or 15 mg buccal daily.

• Contraindicated in women of childbearing potential (possible virilization of female fetus); in elderly, asthenic men, who may react adversely to androgen overstimulation; and in hypercalcemia; cardiac, hepatic, or renal decompensation; prostatic or breast cancer in men; benign prostatic hyperplasia with obstruction; conditions aggravated by fluid retention; hypertension; and in premature infants.
• Use cautiously in patients with MI or coronary artery disease.

oxymetholone (Anadrol)
Aplastic anemia—
Adults and children: 1 to 5 mg/kg P.O. daily. Dosage highly individualized; response not immediate. Trial of 3 to 6 months required.
Osteoporosis, catabolic conditions—
Adults: 5 to 15 mg P.O. daily, or up to 30 mg P.O. daily.

• Contraindicated in prostatic hyperplasia with obstruction; prostatic and male breast cancer; cardiac, hepatic, or renal decompensation; nephrosis; and in premature infants.
• Use cautiously in prepubertal

SELECTED MAJOR DRUGS: ANDROGENS AND ANABOLIC
STEROIDS *continued*

DRUG, INDICATIONS, AND DOSAGES	SPECIAL PRECAUTIONS

Androgens *(continued)*

oxymetholone *(continued)*
Children over age 6: up to 10 mg P.O. daily.
Children under age 6: 1.25 mg P.O. daily up to q.i.d.
Continuous therapy should not exceed 30 days in children; 90 days in any patient.

boys; patients with diabetes or coronary diseases; and patients taking corticotropin, corticosteroids, or anticoagulants.

stanozolol (Winstrol)
Prevention of hereditary angioedema—
Adults: 2 mg P.O. t.i.d. to 4 mg P.O. q.i.d. for 5 days initially. Dosage is gradually reduced at intervals of 1 to 3 months to a dosage of 2 mg daily.
Children age 6 to 12: administer up to 2 mg P.O. daily.
Children under age 6: 1 mg P.O. daily.
  Note: Stanozolol should be used in children only during an acute attack.

• Contraindicated in prostatic hyperplasia with obstruction; prostatic and male breast cancer; cardiac, hepatic, or renal decompensation; nephrosis; and in premature infants.
• Use cautiously in prepubertal boys; patients with diabetes or coronary disease; and patients taking corticotropin, corticosteroids, or anticoagulants.

testosterone cypionate (Andro-Cyp, Depotest)
testosterone enanthate (Android-T, Testone L.A.)
testosterone propionate (Testex)
Eunuchism, eunuchoidism, deficiency after castration and male climacteric—
Men: 200 to 400 mg (cypionate or enanthate) I.M. q 4 weeks; or 10 to 25 mg (propionate) I.M. two to four times weekly.
Oligospermia—
Men: 100 to 200 mg (cypionate or enanthate) I.M. q 4 to 6 weeks.
Metastatic breast cancer—
Women: 50 to 100 mg (propionate) I.M. three times weekly; or 200 to 400 mg (cypionate or enanthate) I.M. q 2 to 4 weeks.
Postmenopausal or primary osteoporosis—
Adults: 200 to 400 mg (enanthate) I.M. q 4 weeks.

• Contraindicated in women of childbearing potential (possible virilization of female fetus); in patients with hypercalcemia; cardiac, hepatic, or renal decompensation; prostatic or breast cancer in men; benign prostatic hyperplasia with obstruction; conditions aggravated by fluid retention; or hypertension; in elderly, asthenic men, who may react adversely to androgen overstimulation; and in premature infants.
• Use cautiously in patients with MI or coronary artery disease and in prepubertal boys.

Anabolic steroids

nandrolone decanoate (Anabolin LA-100, Deca-Durabolin)
nandrolone phenpropionate (Anabolin-IM, Durabolin)
Severe debility or disease states, refractory anemias—
Adults: 100 to 200 mg (decanoate) I.M. weekly. Therapy should be intermittent.
Tissue-building—
Adults: 50 to 100 mg (decanoate) I.M. q 3 to 4 weeks.
Children age 2 to 13: 25 to 50 mg (decanoate) I.M. q 3 to 4 weeks.
Control of metastatic breast cancer—
Adults: 25 to 50 mg (phenpropionate) I.M. weekly.
Children age 2 to 13: 12.5 to 25 mg (phenpropionate) I.M. every 2 to 4 weeks.

• Contraindicated in prostatic hyperplasia with obstruction; male breast and prostatic cancer; cardiac, hepatic, or renal decompensation; nephrosis; and in premature infants.
• Use cautiously in prepubertal boys; patients with diabetes or coronary disease; and patients taking corticotropin, corticosteroids, or anticoagulants.

SELF-TEST

1. Caroline Jamison, age 52 and 2 years postmenopausal, has an estrogen-dependent tumor. Her medication includes testosterone, an androgen. As her nurse, you teach her the adverse reactions to this medication. Adverse reactions to testosterone therapy in a female include:
   a. weight loss.
   b. hypertension.
   c. hirsutism.
   d. gynecomastia.

2. Thomas Johy, age 62, is severely underweight and generally debilitated. His doctor has just prescribed oxandrolone, an anabolic steroid. As his nurse, you teach him the adverse reactions to this medication. Common adverse reactions to oxandrolone in a male include:
   a. testicular hypertrophic changes.
   b. increased ejaculatory volume.
   c. impotence.
   d. weight gain.

3. At discharge, Mr. Johy requests "some extra anabolic steroid pills to share with my grandson who wants to play pro football." Which of the following is the best response the nurse can make?
   a. "I will ask the doctor to prescribe a larger number."
   b. "That is a very common thing to say. The doctor has written a prescription for more than you will need, so you should be able to share a few with your grandson."
   c. "Your grandson will need to find another source."
   d. "Anabolic steroids are a prescription drug and have serious adverse reactions that require careful monitoring. You should not share this or any other prescription drug."

Check your answers on page 1070.

CHAPTER 54

ESTROGENS AND PROGESTINS

Estrogens
chlorotrianisene ✦ dienestrol ✦ diethylstilbestrol
diethylstilbestrol diphosphate ✦ esterified estrogens ✦ estradiol
estradiol cypionate ✦ estradiol valerate
estrogenic substances, conjugated ✦ estrone ✦ ethinyl estradiol
quinestrol

Progestins
hydroxyprogesterone caproate ✦ levonorgestrel
medroxyprogesterone acetate ✦ norethindrone ✦ norethindrone acetate
norgestrel ✦ progesterone

Oral contraceptives
ethinyl estradiol and ethynodiol diacetate
ethinyl estradiol and levonorgestrel ✦ ethinyl estradiol and norethindrone
ethinyl estradiol and norethindrone acetate ✦ ethinyl estradiol and norgestrel
mestranolol and norethindrone

OVERVIEW

- Estrogens are organic compounds that occur naturally in humans and animals; they are also produced synthetically. They can be chemically classified as either steroidal or nonsteroidal estrogens.
- Steroidal estrogens include all natural estrogens (estradiol and estrone), esters of natural estrogens (estradiol cypionate, estradiol valerate, and esterified estrogens), a conjugate of natural estrogens (conjugated estrogenic substances), and a semisynthetic estrogen (ethinyl estradiol).
- Nonsteroidal estrogens comprise the synthetic estrogens (chlorotrianisene, dienestrol, diethylstilbestrol, diethylstilbestrol diphosphate, and quinestrol).
- Estrogens traditionally have been described as agents that produce estrus, whether or not they are derived from the ovaries. Secreted mainly by the ovarian follicles, they are also secreted in large amounts by the placenta, in smaller quantities by the testes, and—in both sexes—by the adrenal cortex.

GLOSSARY

Contraception: technique for the prevention of pregnancy by means of a medication, device, or method that blocks or alters one or more of the processes of reproduction so that sexual union can occur without impregnation.

Estrogen: one of a group of hormonal steroid compounds that promote the development of female secondary sex characteristics. During the menstrual cycle, estrogen renders the female genital tract suitable for fertilization, implantation, and nutrition of the early embryo.

Progesterone: hormone produced by the corpus luteum and adrenal cortex during the luteal phase of the menstrual cycle that prepares the uterus for reception of the fertilized ovum.

- The reproductive physiochemistry of estrogens in women parallels that of androgens in men. Estrogens are responsible for the development of secondary sex characteristics in women. They promote growth and development of the vagina, uterus, and fallopian tubes; enlargement of the breasts; molding of the body contours; and closure of the epiphyses of the long bones. They also promote growth of axillary and pubic hair, and pigmentation of the skin of the nipples and genital region. They stimulate estrus and produce changes in the genital tract and mammary glands during pregnancy.

- Metabolic activities of estrogens occur in three areas: estrogens reduce blood cholesterol by altering lipid metabolism, they exert a protein anabolic action, and they promote sodium and water retention.

- The natural hormone progesterone and its synthetic derivatives are called progestogens or progestins; they produce the characteristic endometrial changes that favor pregnancy (gestation). Progesterone is secreted mainly by the corpus luteum after ovulation (during the last half of the menstrual cycle). Large amounts are also secreted by the placenta. Smaller quantities are produced by both the mature follicle before ovulation (during the first half of the menstrual cycle) and the adrenal cortex.

- Progestins trigger glandular and vascular development, which results in the endometrial swelling essential for implantation of the fertilized ovum. If implantation doesn't occur, the sharp drop in the progesterone level at the end of the menstrual cycle helps start menstruation.

- Progestins also relax uterine smooth muscle. During pregnancy, increased progesterone secretion prevents premature uterine contractions and allows the pregnancy to continue to term. Along with estrogen, progestins aid growth and development of the alveolar duct system in the mammary glands.

- Progestins promote protein catabolism and sodium and water retention.

- Oral contraceptives are popular, effective, and convenient to use. They may produce serious reactions in women with certain risk factors.

Currently, two recognized classes of oral contraceptives are being marketed: an estrogen-progestin combination and a progestin-only "minipill." The combination tablets contain a synthetic estrogen compound (ethinyl estradiol or mestranol) and a synthetic progestin (ethynodiol diacetate, norethindrone, norethindrone acetate, norethynodrel, or norgestrel). They are taken for 21 days of the menstrual cycle (usually days 5 through 24). Natural steroids aren't used because large doses would be required to achieve the same pharmacologic effect as the synthetics. The progestin-only pill contains either norethindrone or norgestrel and is taken once daily every day of the menstrual cycle. The minipill is not widely used because it frequently causes menstrual irregularities. Although slightly less effective than the combination product, it may suffice for the patient who has to avoid the use of estrogen or for whom pregnancy is not life-threatening.

- An implantable progestin-only contraceptive system is also available. Levonorgestrel is encapsulated in an inert, flexible implantable device which is inserted intradermally in the posterior aspect of the upper arm. This system has several advantages: Patient compliance is not a factor in providing reliable contraception; the implantable system is effective for up to 5 years; and the effect of the drug is rapidly reversed when the capsules are removed.
- This chapter discusses the three major categories of estrogens and progestins: estrogens, progestins, and oral contraceptives.

MAJOR USES

- Estrogens are used as replacement therapy in menopause, pituitary failure (to stimulate development of secondary sex characteristics), and after radical hysterectomy. They are used to treat atrophic changes in the lower genital tract (as in atrophic vaginitis or kraurosis vulvae) that are caused by chronic estrogen deficiency. Estrogens can initiate menstrual periods and relieve secondary amenorrhea (as in female hypogonadism, female castration, and primary ovarian failure). They are used in the palliation and inhibition of androgen-dependent primary tumors with soft-tissue metastases (for example, inoperable cancer of the prostate and breast in males and inoperable postmenopausal breast carcinoma). Progestins relieve dysfunctional uterine bleeding, amenorrhea, and dysmenorrhea. Norethindrone and norethindrone acetate are used to treat endometriosis.
- As oral contraceptives, norethindrone, norethindrone acetate, and norgestrel are used alone or in combination with estrogens. Oral contraceptives are used to prevent pregnancy or to treat such menstrual cycle disorders as endometriosis and hypermenorrhea.

MECHANISM OF ACTION

- Estrogens replace endogenous hormones to maintain normal hormonal balance. They suppress lactation by inhibiting prolactin secretion from the anterior pituitary and antagonize the action of androgens that stimulate growth of tumor tissue.

- Progestins mimic the body's production of progesterone to reestablish a normal menstrual cycle in patients with amenorrhea. They promote glandular and vascular development of the endometrium by restoring progesterone levels. Progestins suppress ovulation possibly by inhibiting pituitary gonadotropin secretion. They also form a thick cervical mucus that is relatively impermeable to sperm.

- Oral contraceptives (estrogen-progestin combinations) inhibit ovulation through a negative feedback mechanism directed at the hypothalamus. They may also prevent transport of the ovum through the fallopian tubes. In oral contraceptives, the estrogen component suppresses secretion of follicle-stimulating hormone, blocking follicular development and ovulation. The progestin component suppresses luteinizing hormone secretion so ovulation can't occur even if the follicle develops. Progestin thickens cervical mucus, which interferes with sperm migration, and also causes endometrial changes that prevent implantation of the fertilized ovum.

ABSORPTION, DISTRIBUTION, METABOLISM, AND EXCRETION

Estrogens are readily absorbed from the GI tract, distributed to all body tissues, metabolized in the liver, and excreted primarily in urine. Small amounts are also eliminated—through the bile—in feces. Ethinyl estradiol is well absorbed when given orally. Most of it is metabolized in the liver. Because metabolism is slow, the drug retains its high intrinsic potency.

Estradiol is rapidly metabolized (oxidized) in the liver to estrone, which is subsequently converted to estriol.

Progestins are rapidly absorbed, distributed to all tissues, metabolized in the liver, and excreted in urine.

Oral contraceptives are rapidly and completely absorbed from the GI tract and distributed to all body tissues. They are metabolized in the liver and excreted in urine.

ONSET AND DURATION

Estrogens begin to act immediately. Oral estrogens (except chlorotrianisene) have a short duration of action; daily doses are usually needed. Chlorotrianisene is a long-acting drug because it's stored in adipose tissue and released only gradually. Parenteral estrogens have a longer duration of action than the oral preparations; their effect may last several days.

Onset and duration of progestins vary with the disorder, the progestin given, and whether the progestin is administered with, after, or without an estrogen. Generally, however, onset is fastest when estrogens are given first; duration is longest when the slow-release ("depot") forms (injection in oil, for example) are used.

Oral contraceptives containing estrogens with progestins begun on day 5 of the menstrual cycle theoretically provide complete protection if taken on schedule. But alternative protection is recommended for at least the first 7 days of therapy since ovulation and conception are still possible during this time. Progestin-only products must be started on day 1 of the cycle and are taken daily.

Duration of contraceptive effect is about 1 day; therefore, strict compliance is necessary to ensure effectiveness. For complex endocrine, metabolic, and acne disorders, several months of treatment may be needed to obtain a satisfactory response.

Blood levels of levonorgestrel peak within 24 hours after insertion of the implant system and decline gradually over the next 3 months. Contraceptive efficacy averages fewer than 1 pregnancy per 100 women through 5 years.

ADVERSE REACTIONS

Adverse reactions to estrogens are similar to those produced by oral contraceptives. They commonly include breakthrough bleeding, spotting, change in menstrual flow, dysmenorrhea, premenstrual-like syndrome, amenorrhea during and after treatment, increase in size of uterine fibromas, vaginal candidiasis, change in cervical erosion and degree of cervical secretion, cystitis-like syndrome, hemolytic uremic syndrome, and endometrial cystic hyperplasia. GI, dermatologic, ophthalmic, and CNS reactions may also occur (mood changes, insomnia).

Adverse reactions to progestins include breakthrough bleeding, spotting, change in menstrual flow, amenorrhea, changes in cervical erosion and cervical secretions, breast changes (including tenderness), virilization of the female fetus, edema, weight change, allergic rash with or without pruritus, and acne. A small percentage of patients develop local reactions at the injection site.

Serious adverse reactions to estrogen-progestin combinations include thrombophlebitis and thrombosis, pulmonary embolism, MI, Raynaud's disease, arterial thromboembolism, cerebral hemorrhage, hypertension, gallbladder disease, congenital anomalies, liver tumors and other hepatic lesions with or without intra-abdominal bleeding, and hepatocellular carcinoma.

GI reactions include nausea and vomiting, abdominal cramps, bloating, and cholestatic jaundice. Breast changes, skin rash, mental depression, edema, and weight gain or weight loss may also occur.

PROTOTYPE: ESTROGENS

CONJUGATED ESTROGENS
(ess'troe jenz)
C.E.S.†, C.S.D.†, Premarin, Progens Tabs
Classification: estrogen
Pregnancy risk category X

How supplied
TABLETS: 0.3 mg, 0.625 mg, 0.9 mg, 1.25 mg, 2.5 mg
INJECTION: 25 mg/5 ml
VAGINAL CREAM: 0.625 mg/g

Indications and dosage

Abnormal uterine bleeding (hormonal imbalance)
WOMEN: 25 mg I.V. or I.M. Repeat in 6 to 12 hours.

Breast cancer (at least 5 years after menopause)
WOMEN: 10 mg P.O. t.i.d. for 3 months or more.

Castration, primary ovarian failure, and osteoporosis
WOMEN: 1.25 mg P.O. daily in cycles of 3 weeks on, 1 week off.

Hypogonadism
WOMEN: 2.5 mg P.O. b.i.d. or t.i.d. for 20 consecutive days each month.

Menopausal symptoms
WOMEN: 0.3 to 1.25 mg P.O. daily in cycles of 3 weeks on, 1 week off.

Postpartum breast engorgement
WOMEN: 3.75 mg P.O. q 4 hours for five doses or 1.25 mg P.O. q 4 hours for 5 days.

Atrophic vaginitis, kraurosis vulvae associated with menopause
WOMEN: 2 to 4 g intravaginally or topically once daily in cycles of 3 weeks on, 1 week off.

Inoperable prostatic cancer
MEN: 1.25 to 2.5 mg P.O. t.i.d.

Contraindications and precautions

Conjugated estrogens are contraindicated in patients with thrombophlebitis or thromboembolic disorders, or with undiagnosed abnormal vaginal bleeding, and in pregnant women. Use cautiously in patients with hypertension, gallbladder disease, bone diseases, blood dyscrasia, or migraine.

Adverse reactions

CNS: headache, dizziness, chorea, depression, libido changes, lethargy.
CV: thrombophlebitis; **thromboembolism; hypertension;** edema; **increased risk of stroke, pulmonary embolism**, and **MI**.
EENT: worsening of myopia or astigmatism, intolerance to contact lenses.
GI: *nausea*, vomiting, abdominal cramps, bloating, diarrhea, constipation, anorexia, increased appetite, weight changes, pancreatitis.
GU: in women—breakthrough bleeding, altered menstrual flow, dysmenorrhea, amenorrhea, cervical erosion, altered cervical secretions, enlargement of uterine fibromas, vaginal candidiasis; in men—gynecomastia, testicular atrophy, impotence.
HEPATIC: cholestatic jaundice.
METABOLIC: hyperglycemia, hypercalcemia, folic acid deficiency.
SKIN: melasma, urticaria, acne, seborrhea, oily skin, flushing (when given rapidly I.V.), hirsutism or hair loss.
OTHER: breast changes (tenderness, enlargement, secretion), leg cramps.

Interactions

None significant.

Nursing considerations
Assessment
- Review the patient's history for a condition that contraindicates the use of conjugated estrogens and related compounds.
- Obtain a baseline assessment of the patient's underlying condition before initiating therapy with conjugated estrogens.
- Be alert for common adverse reactions.
- Evaluate the patient's and family's knowledge about estrogen therapy.

Planning (Nursing Diagnoses)
Potential nursing diagnoses for the patient receiving conjugated estrogens include:
- Altered health maintenance related to ineffectiveness of conjugated estrogens.
- Altered cerebral, peripheral, pulmonary, or myocardial tissue perfusion related to potential for conjugated estrogens to cause thromboembolism.
- Knowledge deficit related to therapy with conjugated estrogens.

Implementation
Preparation and administration
—Refrigerate parenteral solution before reconstituting. Agitate gently after adding diluent.
—Be aware that I.M. or I.V. use is preferred for rapid treatment of dysfunctional uterine bleeding or reduction of surgical bleeding.
—Administer oral preparations at mealtimes or bedtime (if only one daily dose is required) to minimize nausea.

Monitoring
—Monitor the effectiveness of therapy by regularly assessing the patient's signs and symptoms.
—Monitor patient for thromboemboli formation by noting any changes in cerebral or cardiopulmonary function or peripheral circulation.
—Monitor the patient's blood glucose, calcium, and folic acid levels for alterations.
—Monitor the patient for adverse drug reactions.
—Monitor the patient's mental status for depression.
—Monitor the patient's hydration status if GI reactions occur.
—Monitor for abnormal GU function.
—Monitor for evidence of cholestatic jaundice.
—Regularly reevaluate the patient's and family's knowledge about conjugated estrogens.

Intervention
—Withhold drug and notify the doctor if a thromboembolic event is suspected; be prepared to provide supportive care as indicated.
—Alert the pathologist if a specimen is obtained during estrogen therapy.
—Be prepared to adjust a diabetic patient's therapeutic regimen if blood glucose levels rise during therapy with conjugated estrogens.
—Institute safety measures if adverse CNS reactions occur.

— Obtain an order for an antiemetic, antidiarrheal, or laxative agent, as
needed.
— Prepare the patient for body changes that may occur, such as hair loss.
— Keep all members of the health care team informed of the patient's
response to the drug.

— Inform the patient and family about conjugated estrogens, including
the dosage, frequency, action, and adverse reactions.
— Warn the patient to report immediately abdominal pain; pain, numbness, or stiffness in legs or buttocks; pressure or pain in chest; shortness
of breath; severe headaches; visual disturbances such as blind spots,
flashing lights, or blurriness; vaginal bleeding or discharge; breast
lumps; swelling of hands or feet; yellow skin and sclera; dark urine;
and light-colored stools.
— Tell male patients on long-term therapy about possible gynecomastia
and impotence, which will disappear when therapy is terminated.
— Explain to patients on cyclic therapy for postmenopausal symptoms
that, although withdrawal bleeding may occur in week off drug, fertility
has not been restored; ovulation does not occur.
— Teach female patients how to perform routine breast self-examination.
— Teach the patient that medical supervision is essential during prolonged
therapy with conjugated estrogens.
— Inform the patient that nausea, when present, usually disappears with
continued therapy. Nausea can be relieved by taking medication at
mealtimes or bedtime (if only one daily dose is required).
— Tell diabetic patients to report symptoms of hyperglycemia or glycosuria.
— Teach the patient how to apply estrogen ointments locally. Explain
what symptoms may occur in a systemic reaction to estrogen ointment.
— Tell patients who are planning to breast-feed not to take conjugated
estrogens.
— Tell patients who become pregnant during therapy with conjugated
estrogens to stop taking the drug immediately because it may adversely
affect the fetus.
— Give the patient the package insert describing adverse reactions to
conjugated estrogens, and also provide verbal explanation.
— Tell the patient to notify the nurse or doctor if adverse reactions develop
or questions arise about therapy with conjugated estrogens.

In patients receiving conjugated estrogens, appropriate evaluation state-
ments may include:
• Patient exhibits improved health as a result of estrogens therapy.
• Patient does not experience a thromboembolic event during estrogens
therapy.
• Patient and family state an understanding of estrogen therapy.

PROGESTERONE

(proe jess'ter one)

Gesterol 50, Progestaject-50, Progestasert, Progestilin†

Classification: progestin

Pregnancy risk category X

How supplied

INJECTION (IN OIL): 50 mg/ml

INTRAUTERINE DEVICE: 38 mg within a T-shaped device

Indications and dosage

Amenorrhea

WOMEN: 5 to 10 mg I.M. daily for 6 to 8 days.

Dysfunctional uterine bleeding

WOMEN: 5 to 10 mg I.M. daily for 6 days.

Contraception (as part of intrauterine device [IUD])

WOMEN: 1 IUD containing 38 mg progesterone inserted into the uterine cavity. Contraceptive effect lasts 1 year.

Contraindications and precautions

Progesterone is contraindicated in patients with thromboembolic disorders, breast cancer, undiagnosed abnormal vaginal bleeding, severe hepatic disease, or incomplete abortion. Use cautiously in patients with diabetes mellitus, seizure disorder, migraine, cardiac or renal disease, asthma, or mental illness.

Adverse reactions

CNS: dizziness, migraine headache, lethargy, depression.

CV: hypertension, thrombophlebitis, **pulmonary embolism, edema.**

GI: nausea, vomiting, abdominal cramps.

GU: breakthrough bleeding, dysmenorrhea, amenorrhea, cervical erosion or abnormal secretions, uterine fibromas, vaginal candidiasis.

HEPATIC: cholestatic jaundice.

METABOLIC: hyperglycemia.

SKIN: melasma, rash.

LOCAL: pain at injection site.

OTHER: breast tenderness, enlargement, or secretion; decreased libido.

Interactions

Rifampin: decreased progesterone effects. Monitor for diminished therapeutic response.

Nursing considerations
Assessment
• Review the patient's history for a condition that contraindicates the use of progesterone.
• Obtain a baseline assessment of the patient's uterine bleeding problem or premenstrual syndrome before initiating progesterone therapy.
• Be alert for common adverse reactions.
• Evaluate the patient's and family's knowledge about progesterone.

Planning (Nursing Diagnoses)
Potential nursing diagnoses for the patient receiving progesterone include:
• Altered health maintenance related to ineffectiveness of progesterone.
• Impaired gas exchange related to potential for progesterone-induced pulmonary embolism.
• Fluid volume excess related to progesterone-induced edema.
• Knowledge deficit related to progesterone therapy.

Implementation
Preparation and administration
— Give oil solutions (peanut oil or sesame oil) deep I.M.
— Rotate injection sites.
— Expect to administer preliminary estrogen treatment in patients with menstrual disorders.
— Food and Drug Administration regulations require that before receiving their first dose, patients read the package insert describing possible adverse reactions to progesterone. Provide verbal explanations as well.
— Prepare the patient for Progestasert insertion as directed by doctor.

Monitoring
— Monitor the effectiveness of therapy by regularly assessing the degree of uterine bleeding or symptoms of premenstrual syndrome (PMS).
— Monitor the patient for breathing difficulty and sudden changes in respiratory status.
— Monitor the patient for adverse drug reactions.
— Monitor injection sites frequently for evidence of irritation.
— Monitor the patient's blood pressure for elevation.
— Monitor frequently for breakthrough bleeding or abnormal vaginal secretions.
— Regularly monitor the patient's blood glucose level.
— Monitor the patient for drug interactions, especially with rifampin.
— Monitor hydration status if GI reactions occur.
— Monitor the patient's weight for sudden increases suggestive of fluid retention.
— Monitor the patient's compliance with progesterone therapy.
— Regularly reevaluate the patient's and family's knowledge about progesterone.

Intervention

— Progesterone should be discontinued if hypersensitivity, thromboembolic or thrombotic disorders, visual disturbances, migraine headache, or severe depression occurs. Notify doctor immediately. Be prepared to provide supportive treatment as indicated.

— Expect to adjust the diabetic patient's treatment regimen if hyperglycemia occurs.

— Keep all members of the health care team informed of the patient's response to the drug.

Patient teaching

— Inform the patient and family about progesterone, including the dosage, frequency, action, and adverse reactions.

— Advise the patient to discontinue therapy and call the doctor immediately if migraine or visual disturbances occur, or if sudden severe headache or vomiting develops.

— Teach the patient how perform breast self-examination.

— Tell the patient receiving progesterone she should have a full physical examination, including a gynecologic exam and a Papanicolaou test, every 6 to 12 months.

— Tell the patient to check with her doctor promptly if period is missed or unusual bleeding occurs, and to discontinue drug immediately and check with her doctor if she suspects she is pregnant.

— Advise the patient who misses a dose to take the missed dose as soon as possible or omit it, and not to double-dose.

— Tell the patient that GI distress may subside after a few cycles.

— Inform the patient that progesterone may cause possible dental problems (tenderness, swelling, or bleeding of gums). Advise the patient to brush and floss teeth, massage gums, and have the dentist clean teeth regularly. The patient should check with the dentist if there are questions about care of teeth or gums or if tenderness, swelling or bleeding of gums occurs.

For the patient using Progestasert:

— Inform the patient that bleeding and cramping may occur for a few weeks after insertion.

— Advise the patient to contact the doctor if abnormal or excessive bleeding, severe cramping, abnormal vaginal discharge, fever, or flu-like syndrome occurs.

— Teach the patient how to check for proper placement of IUD.

— Tell the patient that the progesterone supply in the IUD is depleted in 1 year and the device must be changed at that time. Pregnancy risk increases if the patient relies on progesterone-depleted device for contraception.

— Inform the patient of the adverse reactions to IUD use: uterine perforation, increased risk of infection, pelvic inflammatory disease, ectopic pregnancy, abdominal cramping, increased menstrual flow, and expulsion of the device.

— Tell the patient to notify the nurse or doctor if adverse reactions develop or questions arise about progesterone therapy.

Evaluation

In the patient receiving progesterone, appropriate evaluation statements include:
• Patient's health status is improved with progesterone therapy.
• Patient does not experience a pulmonary embolism.
• Patient does not exhibit fluid retention.
• Patient and family state an understanding of progesterone therapy.

PROTOTYPE: ESTROGENS AND PROGESTINS

ETHINYL ESTRADIOL AND NORETHINDRONE
(eth' in il ess tra dye'ole and nor eth in'drone)

Monophasic: Brevicon 21-day, Brevicon 28-day, Genora 0.5/35, Genora 1/35, ModiCon, N.E.E. 1/35, Nelova 0.5/35E, Nelova 1/35E, Norcept-E 1/35, Norethin 1/35 E, Norinyl 1+35, Ortho-Novum 1/35, Ovcon-35, Ovcon-50
Biphasic: Nelova 10/11, Ortho-Novum 10/11
Triphasic: Ortho-Novum 7/7/7, Tri-Norinyl

Classification: estrogen and progestin
Pregnancy risk category X

How supplied

TABLETS: ethinyl estradiol 35 mcg and norethindrone 0.4 mg (Ovcon-35); ethinyl estradiol 35 mcg and norethindrone 0.5 mg (Brevicon, Genora 0.5/35, Modicon, Nelova 0.5/35E); ethinyl estradiol 35 mcg and norethindrone 1 mg (Genora 1/35, N.E.E. 1/35, Nelova 1/35E, Norcept-E 1/35, Norethin 1/35E, Norinyl 1+35, Ortho-Novum 1/35); ethinyl estradiol 50 mcg and norethindrone 1 mg (Ovcon-50)

Indications and dosage

Contraception

WOMEN: 1 tablet P.O. daily, beginning on day 5 of menstrual cycle (first day of menstrual flow is day 1). With 20- and 21-tablet packages, new dosing cycle begins 7 days after last tablet taken. With 28-tablet packages, dosage is 1 tablet daily without interruption; extra tablets are placebos or contain iron. If only one or two doses are missed, dosage may continue on schedule. If three or more doses are missed, remaining tablets in monthly package must be discarded and another contraceptive method substituted. If next menstrual period doesn't begin on schedule, rule out pregnancy before starting new dosing cycle. If menstrual period begins, start new dosing cycle 7 days after last tablet was taken. If all doses have been taken on schedule and one menstrual period is missed, continue dosing cycle. If two consecutive menstrual periods are missed, pregnancy test is required before new dosing cycle is started.

Biphasic oral contraceptives
WOMEN: 1 color tablet P.O. daily for 10 days, followed by next color tablet for 11 days.

Triphasic oral contraceptives
WOMEN: 1 tablet P.O. daily in the sequence specified by the brand.

Contraindications and precautions
The combination product ethinyl estradiol and norethindrone is contraindicated in patients with thromboembolic disorders, cerebrovascular or coronary artery disease, myocardial infarction, known or suspected cancer of breasts or reproductive organs, benign or malignant liver tumors, undiagnosed abnormal vaginal bleeding, known or suspected pregnancy, or lactation; and in adolescents with incomplete epiphyseal closure. They are also contraindicated in women age 35 or older who smoke more than 15 cigarettes a day, and in all women over age 40.

Use cautiously in patients with systemic lupus erythematosus, hypertension, mental depression, migraine, seizure disorders, asthma, diabetes mellitus, amenorrhea, scanty or irregular menstrual periods, fibrocystic breast disease, family history (mother, grandmother, sister) of breast or genital tract cancer, or renal or gallbladder disease. Report development or worsening of these conditions to the doctor. Prolonged therapy is inadvisable in women who plan to become pregnant.

Adverse reactions
CNS: *headache, dizziness,* depression, libido changes, lethargy, migraine.
CV: **thromboembolism,** hypertension, edema.
EENT: worsening of myopia or astigmatism, intolerance to contact lenses.
GI: *nausea,* vomiting, abdominal cramps, bloating, diarrhea, constipation, anorexia, changes in appetite, weight gain, bowel ischemia, pancreatitis.
GU: *breakthrough bleeding,* granulomatous colitis, dysmenorrhea, amenorrhea, cervical erosion or abnormal secretions, enlargement of uterine fibromas, vaginal candidiasis.
HEPATIC: gallbladder disease, cholestatic jaundice, liver tumors.
METABOLIC: hyperglycemia, hypercalcemia, folic acid deficiency.
SKIN: rash, acne, seborrhea, oily skin, erythema multiforme, hyperpigmentation.
OTHER: *breast tenderness,* enlargement, and secretion.

Interactions
Barbiturates, anticonvulsants, rifampin: may diminish contraceptive effectiveness. Use supplemental form of contraception.

Nursing considerations
Assessment
• Review the patient's history for a condition that contraindicates the use of ethinyl estradiol and norethindrone.
• Obtain a baseline assessment of the patient's pregnancy status before initiating oral contraceptive therapy.
• Be alert for common adverse reactions.

• Evaluate the patient's and family's knowledge about ethinyl estradiol and norethindrone therapy.

Planning (Nursing Diagnoses)

Potential nursing diagnoses for the patient receiving ethinyl estradiol and norethindrone include:

• Altered protection related to ineffectiveness of ethinyl estradiol and norethindrone.
• Altered cerebral, pulmonary, or peripheral tissue perfusion related to drug-induced thromboembolism.
• Knowledge deficit related to ethinyl estradiol and norethindrone therapy.

Implementation

Preparation and administration

— Ensure that the patient has been properly instructed about the drug before first dose is administered.

Monitoring

— Monitor the effectiveness of therapy by regularly assessing that pregnancy has not occurred; have pregnancy test performed if menstruation does not occur when expected.
— Monitor the patient's blood glucose, calcium, and folic acid levels regularly.
— Monitor the patient's mental status for CNS changes such as depression.
— Monitor the patient for adverse drug reactions.
— Regularly monitor blood pressure and weight.
— Monitor hydration status if GI reactions occur.
— Regularly monitor the patient for breakthrough bleeding or abnormal vaginal secretions.
— Monitor the patient for drug interactions.
— Regularly reevaluate the patient's and family's knowledge about ethinyl estradiol and norethindrone.

Intervention

— Alert the doctor immediately if a thromboembolic event is suspected and be prepared to provide supportive care as indicated.
— Evaluate laboratory study findings carefully. Anticipate increases in serum bilirubin, alkaline phosphatase, AST (SGOT), ALT (SGPT), and protein-bound iodine levels and decreases in glucose tolerance and urinary excretion of 17-hydroxycorticosteroids.
— Keep all members of the health care team informed of the patient's response to the drug.

Patient teaching

— Inform the patient about ethinyl estradiol and norethindrone, including the dosage, frequency, action, and adverse reactions.
— Warn the patient that headache, nausea, dizziness, breast tenderness, spotting, and breakthrough bleeding are common at first. These should

diminish after three to six dosing cycles (months). However, breakthrough bleeding in patients taking high-dose estrogen-progestin combinations for menstrual disorders may necessitate dosage adjustment.

— Advise the patient to use an additional method of birth control for the first week of administration in the initial cycle.

— Tell the patient to take tablets at the same time each day for efficacy of medication; nighttime dosing may reduce incidence of nausea and headaches.

— If one menstrual period is missed and tablets have been taken on schedule, tell the patient to continue taking them. If two consecutive menstrual periods are missed, tell the patient to stop drug and have a pregnancy test performed. Progestins may cause birth defects if taken early in pregnancy.

— Teach the patient to keep tablets in original container and to take them in correct (color-coded) sequence.

— Suggest that the patient take the drug with or immediately after food to reduce nausea.

— Stress importance of annual Papanicolaou smears and gynecologic examinations while taking ethinyl estradiol and norethindrone.

— Warn the patient of possible delay in achieving pregnancy when drug is discontinued.

— Advise the patient of increased risks associated with simultaneous use of cigarettes and oral contraceptives.

— Instruct the patient to weigh herself at least twice weekly and to report any sudden weight gain or edema to the doctor.

— Warn the patient to avoid exposure to ultraviolet light or prolonged exposure to sunlight; chloasma seems to be aggravated by sunlight. With anticipated exposure (as in summer), taking pill at bedtime will reduce daytime levels of circulating hormone.

— Many doctors recommend that women not become pregnant within 2 months after stopping oral contraceptive therapy. Advise the patient to check with her doctor about how soon pregnancy may be safely attempted after ethinyl estradiol and norethindrone therapy is stopped.

— Inform the patient that oral contraceptives decrease viscosity of the cervical mucus and increase susceptibility to vaginal infections. Good hygienic practices are essential.

— Instruct the patient to ask her doctor for another form of contraception if she is receiving ampicillin, anticonvulsants, phenylbutazone, rifampin, or tetracycline, because intermittent bleeding and unwanted pregnancy might result from effect of drug interactions.

— Instruct the patient about missed doses. For monophasic and biphasic cycles—20-, 21-, or 24-day dosing schedule, if one regular dose is missed, take tablet as soon as possible; if remembered on the next day, take 2 tablets, then continue regular dosing schedule. If two consecutive doses are missed, take 2 tablets daily for next 2 days, then resume regular dosing schedule. If 3 consecutive days are missed, discontinue drug and substitute other contraceptive method until period begins or pregnancy is ruled out. Then start new cycle of tablets. For 28-day

dosing schedule, follow instructions for 21-day dosing schedule; if one of the last 7 tablets is missed, be sure to take first tablet of next month's cycle on regularly scheduled day. For triphasic cycle—21-day dosing schedule, if one dose is missed, take dose as soon as possible; if remembered on the next day, take 2 tablets, then continue regular dosing schedule while using additional method of contraception for remainder of cycle. If two consecutive doses are missed, take 2 tablets daily for next 2 days, then continue regular schedule while using additional contraceptive method for remainder of cycle. If three consecutive doses are missed, discontinue drug and use other contraceptive method until period begins or pregnancy is ruled out. Then start new cycle of tablets. For 28-day dosing schedule, follow instructions for 21-day dosing schedule; if one of the last 7 tablets was missed, be sure to take first tablet of next month's cycle on regularly scheduled day.
— Tell the patient to notify the nurse or doctor if adverse reactions develop or questions arise about ethinyl estradiol and norethindrone therapy.

Evaluation
In the patient receiving ethinyl estradiol and norethindrone, appropriate evaluation statements include:
• Patient does not become pregnant.
• Patient does not experience a thromboembolic event during ethinyl estradiol and norethindrone therapy.
• Patient and family state an understanding of ethinyl estradiol and norethindrone therapy.

SELECTED MAJOR DRUGS: ESTROGENS AND PROGESTINS

DRUG, INDICATIONS, AND DOSAGES	SPECIAL PRECAUTIONS
Estrogens	
chlorotrianisene (TACE) *Prostatic cancer—* **Men:** 12 to 25 mg P.O. daily. *Atrophic vaginitis—* **Women:** 12 to 25 mg P.O. daily for 30 to 60 days. *Female hypogonadism—* **Women:** 12 to 25 mg P.O. for 21 days, followed by one dose of progesterone 100 mg I.M. or 5 days of oral progestin given concurrently with last 5 days of chlorotrianisene (for example, medroxyprogesterone 5 to 10 mg). *Menopausal symptoms—* **Women:** 12 to 25 mg P.O. daily for 30 days or cyclic (3 weeks on, 1 week off).	• Contraindicated in thrombophlebitis or thromboembolic disorders, cancer of breast, reproductive organs or genitals; undiagnosed abnormal vaginal bleeding; and pregnancy. • Use cautiously in patients with hypertension, asthma, mental depression, bone diseases, blood dyscrasia, gallbladder disease, migraine, seizure disorders, diabetes mellitus, amenorrhea, heart failure, hepatic or renal dysfunction, and family history (mother, grandmother, sister) of breast or genital tract cancer.

SELECTED MAJOR DRUGS: ESTROGENS AND PROGESTINS *continued*

DRUG, INDICATIONS, AND DOSAGES	SPECIAL PRECAUTIONS

Estrogens *(continued)*

dienestrol (DV)
Atrophic vaginitis and kraurosis vulvae—
Postmenopausal women: 1 to 2 intravaginal applications of vaginal cream daily for 1 to 2 weeks (as directed), then half that dose for the same period. A maintenance dosage of 1 applicatorful one to three times weekly may be ordered.

• Contraindicated in thrombophlebitis or thromboembolic disorders; cancer of breast, reproductive organs, or genitals; undiagnosed abnormal vaginal bleeding; and pregnancy.
• Use cautiously in patients with menstrual irregularities or endometriosis.

diethylstilbestrol (DES)
Hypogonadism, castration, primary ovarian failure—
Women: 0.2 to 0.5 mg P.O. daily.
Menopausal symptoms—
Women: 0.1 to 2 mg P.O. daily in cycles of 3 weeks on, 1 week off.
Postcoital contraception ("morning-after pill")—
Women: 25 mg P.O. b.i.d. for 5 days, starting within 72 hours after coitus.
Postpartum breast engorgement—
Women: 5 mg P.O. daily or t.i.d. up to total dose of 30 mg.
Prostatic cancer—
Men: initially, 1 to 3 mg P.O. daily; may be reduced to 1 mg P.O. daily, or 5 mg I.M. twice weekly initially, followed by up to 4 mg I.M. twice weekly. Or 50 to 200 mg (diphosphate) P.O. t.i.d.; or 0.25 to 1 g I.V. daily for 5 days, then once or twice weekly.
Breast cancer—
Men and postmenopausal women: 15 mg P.O. daily.

• Contraindicated in thrombophlebitis or thromboembolic disorders, undiagnosed abnormal vaginal bleeding, and pregnancy.
• Use cautiously in patients with hypertension, asthma, mental depression, bone disease, migraine, seizure disorders, blood dyscrasia, diabetes mellitus, gallbladder disease; amenorrhea, heart failure, hepatic or renal dysfunction, and in patients with family history (mother, grandmother, sister) of breast or genital tract cancer.

esterified estrogens (Menest)
Inoperable prostatic cancer—
Men: 1.25 to 2.5 mg P.O. t.i.d.
Breast cancer—
Men and postmenopausal women: 10 mg P.O. t.i.d. for 3 or more months.
Hypogonadism, castration, primary ovarian failure—
Women: 2.5 mg P.O. daily to t.i.d. in cycles of 3 weeks on, 1 week off.
Menopausal symptoms—
Women: average 0.3 to 3.75 mg P.O. daily in cycles of 3 weeks on, 1 week off.

• Contraindicated in thrombophlebitis or thromboembolic disorders, undiagnosed abnormal vaginal bleeding, and pregnancy.
• Use cautiously in patients with history of hypertension, mental depression, gallbladder disease, migraine, seizure disorders, diabetes mellitus, amenorrhea, or family history (mother, grandmother, sister) of breast or genital tract cancer.

(continued)

SELECTED MAJOR DRUGS: ESTROGENS AND PROGESTINS *continued*

DRUG, INDICATIONS, AND DOSAGES	SPECIAL PRECAUTIONS

Estrogens *(continued)*

estradiol (Estrace, Estraderm)
estradiol cypionate (Estro-Cyp, Estrofem)
estradiol valerate (Delestrogen, Estraval)
Menopausal symptoms, hypogonadism, castration, primary ovarian failure—
Women: 1 to 2 mg P.O. daily, in cycles of 21 days on, 7 days off; or one transdermal system (0.05 mg) applied twice weekly.
Kraurosis vulvae—
Women: 1 to 1.5 mg I.M. once or more per week.
Atrophic vaginitis—
Women: 2 to 4 g intravaginal applications of cream daily for 1 to 2 weeks. When vaginal mucosa is restored, begin maintenance dosage of 1 g one to three times weekly.
Menopausal symptoms—
Women: 1 to 5 mg (cypionate) I.M. q 3 to 4 weeks, or 5 to 20 mg (valerate) I.M., repeated once after 2 to 3 weeks.
Postpartum breast engorgement—
Women: 10 to 25 mg (valerate) I.M. at end of first stage of labor.
Inoperable breast cancer—
Women: 10 mg P.O. t.i.d. for 3 months.
Treatment of moderate to severe symptoms of menopause, female hypogonadism, female castration, primary ovarian failure, and atrophic conditions caused by deficient endogenous estrogen production—
Women: place one Estraderm transdermal patch on trunk of the body twice weekly. Administer on a cyclic schedule (3 weeks on, 1 week off).
Inoperable prostatic cancer—
Men: 30 mg (valerate) I.M. q 1 to 2 weeks, or 1 to 2 mg P.O. t.i.d.

• Contraindicated in thrombophlebitis or thromboembolic disorders, cancer of breast or reproductive organs, undiagnosed abnormal vaginal bleeding, and pregnancy.
• Use cautiously in patients with hypertension, mental depression, bone diseases, blood dyscrasia, migraine, seizure disorders, diabetes mellitus, amenorrhea, heart failure, hepatic or renal dysfunction, or family history (mother, grandmother, sister) of breast or genital tract cancer.

estrone (Estronol, Theelin Aqueous)
Atrophic vaginitis and menopausal symptoms—
Women: 0.1 to 0.5 mg I.M. two or three times weekly.
Female hypogonadism and primary ovarian failure—
Women: 0.1 to 1 mg I.M. weekly in single or divided doses.
Inoperable prostatic cancer—
Men: 2 to 4 mg I.M. two to three times weekly.

• Contraindicated in thrombophlebitis or thromboembolic disorders, cancer of breast or reproductive organs, undiagnosed abnormal vaginal bleeding, and pregnancy.
• Use cautiously in patients with hypertension, mental depression, migraine, seizure disorders, diabetes mellitus, amenorrhea, hepatic or renal dysfunction, or family history (mother, grandmother, sister) of breast or genital tract cancer.

SELECTED MAJOR DRUGS: ESTROGENS AND PROGESTINS *continued*

DRUG, INDICATIONS, AND DOSAGES	SPECIAL PRECAUTIONS

Estrogens *(continued)*

ethinyl estradiol (Estinyl, Feminone)
Breast cancer (at least 5 years postmenopausal)—
Women: 1 mg P.O. t.i.d.
Hypogonadism—
Women: 0.05 mg P.O. daily to t.i.d. for 2 weeks a month, followed by 2 weeks progesterone therapy; continue for 3 to 6 monthly dosing cycles, followed by 2 months rest.
Menopausal symptoms—
Women: 0.02 to 0.05 mg P.O. daily for cycles of 3 weeks on, 1 week off.
Postpartum breast engorgement—
Women: 0.5 to 1 mg P.O. daily for 3 days, then taper over 7 days to 0.1 mg and discontinue.
Inoperable prostatic cancer—
Men: 0.15 to 2 mg P.O. daily.

• Contraindicated in thrombophlebitis or thromboembolic disorders, undiagnosed abnormal vaginal bleeding, and pregnancy.
• Use cautiously in patients with hypertension, mental depression, bone diseases, migraine, seizure disorders, blood dyscrasia, diabetes mellitus, amenorrhea, heart failure, hepatic or renal dysfunction, or family history (mother, grandmother, sister) of breast or genital tract cancer.

quinestrol (Estrovis)
Moderate to severe vasomotor symptoms associated with menopause, and for atrophic vaginitis, kraurosis vulvae, female hypogonadism, female castration, and primary ovarian failure—
Women: 100 mcg P.O. daily for 7 days, followed by 100 mcg weekly as maintenance dosage beginning 2 weeks after treatment starts. Dosage may be increased to 200 mcg weekly.

• Contraindicated in thrombophlebitis or thromboembolic disorders, cancer of breast or reproductive organs, undiagnosed abnormal vaginal bleeding, and pregnancy.
• Use cautiously in patients with hypertension, mental depression, migraine, seizure disorders, diabetes mellitus, amenorrhea, hepatic or renal dysfunction, or family history (mother, grandmother, sister) of breast or genital tract cancer.

Progestins

hydroxyprogesterone caproate (Duralutin, Hyroxon)
Menstrual disorders—
Women: 125 to 375 mg I.M. q 4 weeks. Stop after four cycles.
Uterine cancer—
Women: 1 to 5 g I.M. weekly.

• Contraindicated in thromboembolic disorders, breast cancer, undiagnosed abnormal vaginal bleeding, severe hepatic disease, missed abortion, or in pregnant women.
• Use cautiously in patients with diabetes mellitus, seizure disorders, migraine, cardiac or renal disease, asthma, or mental illness.

(continued)

SELECTED MAJOR DRUGS: ESTROGENS AND PROGESTINS *continued*

DRUG, INDICATIONS, AND DOSAGES	SPECIAL PRECAUTIONS

Progestins *(continued)*

medroxyprogesterone acetate (Depo-Provera, Provera)
Abnormal uterine bleeding due to hormonal imbalance—
Women: 5 to 10 mg P.O. daily for 5 to 10 days beginning on day 16 of menstrual cycle. If patient has received estrogen, give 10 mg P.O. daily for 10 days beginning on day 16 of cycle.
Secondary amenorrhea—
Women: 5 to 10 mg P.O. daily for 5 to 10 days.
Endometrial or renal carcinoma—
Adults: 400 mg to 1 g I.M. weekly.

• Contraindicated in thromboembolic disorders, breast cancer, undiagnosed abnormal vaginal bleeding, missed abortion, hepatic dysfunction, or in pregnant women.
• Use cautiously in patients with diabetes mellitus, seizure disorders, migraine, cardiac or renal disease, asthma, or mental illness.

norethindrone acetate (Aygestin, Norlutate)
Amenorrhea, abnormal uterine bleeding—
Women: 5 to 20 mg P.O. daily on days 5 to 25 of menstrual cycle; or 2.5 to 10 mg (acetate) P.O. daily on days 5 to 25 of menstrual cycle.
Endometriosis—
Women: 10 mg P.O. daily for 14 days, then increase by 5 mg P.O. daily q 2 weeks up to 30 mg daily; or 5 mg (acetate) P.O. daily for 14 days, then increase by 2.5 mg daily q 2 weeks up to 15 mg daily.
Contraception—
Women: initiate therapy with 0.35 mg P.O. on the first day of menstruation. Then, 0.35 mg P.O. daily.

• Contraindicated in thromboembolic disorders, breast cancer, undiagnosed abnormal vaginal bleeding, severe hepatic disease, missed abortion, or in pregnant women.
• Use cautiously in patients with diabetes mellitus, seizure disorders, migraine, cardiac or renal failure, asthma, or mental illness.

norgestrel (Ovrette)
Contraception—
Women: 0.075 mg P.O. daily.

• Contraindicated in thromboembolic disorders, breast cancer, undiagnosed abnormal vaginal bleeding, severe hepatic disease, missed abortion, or in pregnant women.
• Use cautiously in patients with diabetes mellitus, seizure disorders, migraine, cardiac or renal failure, asthma, or mental illness.

COMPARING ESTROGEN AND PROGESTIN COMBINATIONS

TRADE NAME	ESTROGEN COMPONENT	PROGESTIN COMPONENT
Monophasic products		
Demulen 1/35	ethinyl estradiol 35 mcg	ethynodiol diacetate 1 mg
Demulen 1/50	ethinyl estradiol 50 mcg	ethynodiol diacetate 1 mg
Levlen Nordette	ethinyl estradiol 30 mcg	levonorgestrel 0.15 mg
Ovcon-35	ethinyl estradiol 35 mcg	norethindrone 0.4 mg
Brevicon Genora 0.5/35 ModiCon Nelova 0.5/35E	ethinyl estradiol 35 mcg	norethindrone 0.5 mg
Genora 1/35 N.E.E. 1/35 Nelova 1/35E Norcept-E 1/35 Norethin 1/35E Norinyl 1 + 35 Ortho-Novum 1/35	ethinyl estradiol 35 mcg	norethindrone 1 mg
Ovcon-50	ethinyl estradiol 50 mcg	norethindrone 1 mg
Loestrin 21 1/20	ethinyl estradiol 20 mcg	norethindrone acetate 1 mg
Loestrin 21 1.5/30	ethinyl estradiol 30 mcg	norethindrone acetate 1.5 mg
Norlestrin 21 1/50	ethinyl estradiol 50 mcg	norethindrone acetate 1 mg
Norlestrin 21 2.5/50	ethinyl estradiol 50 mcg	norethindrone acetate 2.5 mg
Lo/Ovral	ethinyl estradiol 30 mcg	norgestrel 0.3 mg
Ovral	ethinyl estradiol 50 mcg	norgestrel 0.5 mg

(continued)

COMPARING ESTROGEN AND PROGESTIN COMBINATIONS *continued*

TRADE NAME	ESTROGEN COMPONENT	PROGESTIN COMPONENT
Monophasic products *(continued)*		
Genora 1/50 Nelova 1/50M Norethin 1/50M Norinyl 1 + 50 Ortho-Novum 1/50	mestranol 50 mcg	norethindrone 1 mg
Biphasic products		
Nelova 10/11 Ortho-Novum 10/11	*Phase I (10 days)* ethinyl estradiol 35 mcg *Phase II (11 days)* ethinyl estradiol 35 mcg	*Phase I (10 days)* norethindrone 0.5 mg *Phase II (11 days)* norethindrone 1 mg
Triphasic products		
Tri-Levlen Triphasil	*Phase I (6 days)* ethinyl estradiol 35 mcg *Phase II (5 days)* ethinyl estradiol 35 mcg *Phase III (10 days)* ethinyl estradiol 35 mcg	*Phase I (6 days)* levonorgestrel 0.05 mg *Phase II (5 days)* levonorgestrel 0.075 mg *Phase III (10 days)* levonorgestrel 0.125 mg
Tri-Norinyl	*Phase I (7 days)* ethinyl estradiol 35 mcg *Phase II (9 days)* ethinyl estradiol 35 mcg *Phase III (5 days)* ethinyl estradiol 35 mcg	*Phase I (7 days)* norethindrone 0.5 mg *Phase II (9 days)* norethindrone 1 mg *Phase III (5 days)* norethindrone 0.5 mg
Ortho-Novum 7/7/7	*Phase I (7 days)* ethinyl estradiol 35 mcg *Phase II (7 days)* ethinyl estradiol 35 mcg *Phase III (7 days)* ethinyl estradiol 35 mcg	*Phase I (7 days)* norethindrone 0.5 mg *Phase II (7 days)* norethindrone 0.75 mg *Phase III (7 days)* norethindrone 0.5 mg

SELF-TEST

1. Because Phyllis Carey, age 51, has been experiencing distressing menopausal symptoms, her doctor has prescribed estrogen replacement. Your patient teaching about the new medication will include:
a. how and when to perform breast self-examination.
b. informing her that increased libido may occur.
c. stating that fertility and ovulation are restored.
d. telling her to report hearing changes to her doctor.

2. Ms. Carey should be monitored for which of the following adverse reactions?
a. pulmonary embolism
b. seizures
c. orthostatic hypotension
d. hypoglycemia

3. Helen Vaughn, age 35, will receive progesterone for severe PMS symptoms. Her nurse should instruct her that potential adverse reactions to progesterone include which of the following?
a. edema
b. orthostatic hypotension
c. constipation
d. manic behavior

4. Louise Jeffiner, age 21, gave birth to her first child 6 weeks ago and has now requested oral contraceptives to facilitate family planning. Her nurse should instruct her on the correct dosage cycle. Which of the following statements is correct?
a. If 2 or more consecutive days' doses are missed, effective contraception will resume as soon as the missed doses are taken.
b. Missed mid-cycle doses greatly increase the likelihood of pregnancy.
c. Cigarette smoking reduces the incidence of adverse reactions regardless of the total effective dosage.
d. An every-morning dosage schedule typically produces the fewest adverse reactions.

Check your answers on page 1070.

CHAPTER 55

GONADOTROPINS

chorionic gonadotropin, human (HCG) ♦ gonadorelin acetate
gonadorelin hydrochloride ♦ menotropins ♦ nafarelin acetate

OVERVIEW

- Gonadotropins are hormones that stimulate both male and female go-
  nads. Human chorionic gonadotropin (HCG) originates in the placenta.
  Human menopausal gonadotropin (HMG or menotropins) is an extract
  of both luteinizing hormone (LH) and follicle-stimulating hormone
  (FSH), two gonadotropins that originate in the pituitary gland.
- HCG and menotropins are purified preparations obtained from the urine
  of pregnant and postmenopausal women, respectively.
- Gonadorelin acetate and gonadorelin hydrochloride are synthetic preparations that mimic the action of luteinizing hormone-releasing hormone
  (LHRH). Nafarelin acetate also mimics the action of LHRH, but it acts
  on the pituitary to decrease FSH and LH release.

MAJOR USES

- HCG, menotropins, and gonadorelin acetate induce ovulation in infertile
  women when anovulation is not due primarily to ovarian failure.
- HCG is used to treat cryptorchidism not due to anatomic obstruction.
  Stimulation of androgen secretion by HCG leads to the development of
  secondary sex characteristics and may promote testicular descent. HCG
  is also therapeutic for hypogonadism secondary to pituitary deficiency
  in males.
- Gonadorelin hydrochloride is a diagnostic agent used to test the
  gonadotropins' functional capacity and response.
- Nafarelin acetate is used to treat endometriosis.

MECHANISM OF ACTION

- HCG, when given on the day after the last dose of menotropins, serves
  as a substitute for LH to stimulate ovulation of an HMG-prepared follicle.
  HCG also promotes secretion of androgens by stimulating production of
  testosterone by the interstitial cells of the testes (Leydig's cells).
- Menotropins, when administered to women who have not had primary
  ovarian failure, mimic FSH in inducing follicular growth and LH in
  aiding follicular maturation.
- Gonadorelin is a synthetic LH-releasing hormone.

GLOSSARY

Anovulation: failure of the ovaries to produce, mature, or release eggs because of ovarian immaturity or postmaturity, altered ovarian function, or a disturbance of the interaction of the hypothalamus, pituitary gland, and ovary caused by stress or disease.
Cryptorchidism: failure of one or both of the testes to descend into the scrotum.
Gonadotropin: hormonal substance that stimulates gonadal function.

• Nafarelin, an LH-releasing hormone analog, acts on the pituitary to decrease the release of FSH and LH. The decreased ovarian stimulation and circulating estrogens relieve the symptoms associated with endometriosis.

ABSORPTION, DISTRIBUTION, METABOLISM, AND EXCRETION

Gonadotropins are administered parenterally or nasally because oral doses are destroyed by digestive enzymes. They're distributed throughout the body, with highest concentrations in the ovaries and testes.

Gonadorelin acetate is administered I.V. with an ambulatory infusion pump over 21 days. It is rapidly cleared from the plasma and excreted from the urine as peptide fragments. HCG is partly degraded in the body but is largely excreted in urine.

Menotropins are not excreted and may undergo total degradation in the body.

Nafarelin acetate is administered as a nasal spray and is rapidly absorbed from the nasal mucosa. It is bound to plasma proteins and probably metabolized by peptidases. Approximately 3% of the dose is excreted unchanged in urine.

ONSET AND DURATION

Gonadotropin blood levels peak 6 hours after injection. Duration of action varies widely because the half-lives of these agents range from 4 to 70 hours.

ADVERSE REACTIONS

HCG, gonadorelin acetate, gonadorelin hydrochloride, and menotropins may cause ovarian hyperstimulation, ovarian enlargement, hypersensitivity reactions, and occasional gynecomastia in men. The gonadotropins may also cause CNS effects (depression, insomnia, restlessness). Multiple pregnancy may also occur in women using these drugs to induce ovulation.

Nafarelin acetate has been associated with decreased bone density. It is recommended for use for only 6 months in women over age 18; retreatment is not recommended. Nafarelin is also associated with breast engorgement, nasal irritation, and slight elevations of plasma cholesterol.

MENOTROPINS
(men oh troe'pins)
Pergonal
Classification: gonadotropin
Pregnancy risk category C

How supplied
INJECTION: 75 IU of LH and 75 IU of FSH activity per ampule; 150 IU of LH and 150 IU of FSH activity per ampule.

Indications and dosage
Anovulation
WOMEN: 75 IU each of FSH and LH I.M. daily for 9 to 12 days, followed by HCG 10,000 units I.M. 1 day after last dose of menotropins. Repeat for one to three menstrual cycles until ovulation occurs.

Infertility with ovulation
WOMEN: 75 IU each of FSH and LH I.M. daily for 9 to 12 days, followed by HCG 10,000 units I.M. 1 day after last dose of menotropins. Repeat for two menstrual cycles and then increase to 150 IU each FSH and LH I.M. daily for 9 to 12 days, followed by HCG 10,000 units I.M. 1 day after last dose of menotropins. Repeat for two menstrual cycles.

Infertility
MEN: 75 IU each of FSH and LH I.M. three times weekly (given concomitantly with HCG 2,000 units I.M. twice weekly) for at least 4 months.

Contraindications and precautions
Menotropins are contraindicated in patients with ovarian failure, high urinary gonadotropin levels, thyroid or adrenal dysfunction, pituitary tumor, abnormal uterine bleeding, or ovarian cysts or enlargement, and in pregnant women. Use with caution and with close monitoring in order to prevent ovarian hyperstimulation.

Adverse reactions
BLOOD: hemoconcentration with fluid loss into abdomen.
GI: nausea, vomiting, diarrhea.
GU: in women—**ovarian enlargement with pain and abdominal distention,** multiple births, ovarian hyperstimulation syndrome (sudden ovarian enlargement, ascites with or without pain, pleural effusion); in men—*gynecomastia.*
OTHER: fever.

Interactions
None significant.

Nursing considerations
Assessment
• Review the patient's history for a condition that contraindicates the use of menotropins and related compounds.
• Obtain a baseline assessment of the patient's infertility problems before initiating therapy with menotropins.
• Be alert for common adverse reactions.
• Evaluate the patient's and family's knowledge about menotropins.

Planning (Nursing Diagnoses)
Potential nursing diagnoses for the patient receiving menotropins include:
• Altered role performance related to ineffectiveness of menotropins to treat infertility.
• Pain related to ovarian enlargement induced by menotropins.
• Knowledge deficit related to therapy with menotropins.

Implementation
Preparation and administration
—Reconstitute with 1 to 2 ml sterile 0.9% sodium chloride for injection. Use immediately.
—Rotate injection sites to prevent muscle atrophy.

Monitoring
—Regularly monitor the effectiveness of therapy by determining if conception has occurred.
—Closely monitor the patient's response to therapy: this is critical to ensure adequate ovarian stimulation without hyperstimulation (sudden ovarian enlargement, ascites or pleural effusion).
—Monitor the patient for adverse drug reactions.
—Monitor for abdominal pain and discomfort, which may indicate ovarian enlargement.
—Monitor the patient's hydration status if GI reactions occur.
—Monitor the patient for temperature elevation.
—Regularly reevaluate the patient's and family's knowledge about menotropins.

Intervention
—Menotropins should be discontinued if ovarian hyperstimulation syndrome or abdominal pain occurs or if ovaries become abnormally enlarged.
—Obtain an order for an antiemetic or antidiarrheal agent as needed.
—Keep all members of the health care team informed of the patient's response to the drug.

Patient teaching
—Inform the patient and family about menotropins, including the dosage, frequency, action, and adverse reactions.
—Teach the patient signs and tests that indicate time of ovulation, such as increase in basal body temperature and change in the appearance and volume of cervical mucus.

—Warn the patient to report immediately symptoms of ovarian hyper-stimulation syndrome: abdominal distention and pain, dyspnea, and vaginal bleeding.

—Tell the patient that multiple births are possible.

—In patients being treated for infertility, encourage daily intercourse from day before HCG is given until ovulation occurs.

—Advise the patient that she should be examined at least every other day for signs of excessive ovarian stimulation during therapy and for 2 weeks after treatment ends.

—Tell the patient to notify the nurse or doctor if adverse reactions develop or questions arise about therapy with menotropins.

Evaluation

In the patient receiving menotropins, appropriate evaluation statements include:

• Patient becomes pregnant.

• Patient does not experience abdominal pain.

• Patient and family state an understanding of menotropins therapy.

SELECTED MAJOR DRUGS: GONADOTROPINS

DRUG, INDICATIONS, AND DOSAGES	SPECIAL PRECAUTIONS
chorionic gonadotropin, human (Chorex, Pregnyl) *Anovulation and infertility—* **Women:** 10,000 units I.M. 1 day after last dose of men-otropins. *Hypogonadism—* **Men:** 500 to 1,000 units I.M. three times weekly for 3 weeks, then twice weekly for 3 weeks; or 4,000 units I.M. three times weekly for 6 to 9 months, then 2,000 units three times weekly for 3 more months. *Nonobstructive cryptorchidism—* **Boys age 4 to 9:** 5,000 units I.M. every other day for four doses.	• Contraindicated in pituitary hypertrophy or tumor, prostatic cancer, and early puberty (usual onset is between ages 10 and 13). • Use cautiously in patients with seizure disorders, migraine, asthma, or cardiac or renal disease.
gonadorelin acetate (Lutrepulse) *To induce ovulation in women with primary hypotha-lamic amenorrhea—* **Women:** 5 mcg I.V. q 90 minutes for 21 days using am-bulatory infusion pump. If no response after three treatment intervals, dosage may be increased.	• Contraindicated in patients hy-persensitive to the drug, with conditions that could be compli-cated by pregnancy (such as a pituitary prolactinoma), in pa-tients anovulatory from any cause other than a hypotha-lamic disorder, or with ovarian cysts.
gonadorelin hydrochloride (Factrel) *Evaluation of the functional capacity and response of gonadotropic hormones—* **Women:** 100 mcg S.C. or I.V. In women for whom the phase of the menstrual cycle can be established, per-form the test between day 1 and day 7.	• Although no hypersensitivity reactions have been reported to date, use cautiously in patients who are allergic to other drugs. Keep epinephrine readily avail-able.

SELECTED MAJOR DRUGS: GONADOTROPINS *continued*

DRUG, INDICATIONS, AND DOSAGES

nafarelin acetate (Synarel)
Management of endometriosis; pain relief and reduction of endometriotic lesions—
Women: usual daily dose is 400 mcg administered as one 200-mcg spray into one nostril in a.m. and one 200-mcg spray into the other nostril in p.m. If menstruation persists after 2 months, may increase dose to 800 mcg daily as 1 spray in each nostril in a.m. and 1 spray in each nostril in p.m.
Note: Recommended duration of therapy is 6 months. Retreatment is not recommended; safety data for retreatment is not available. Clinical experience is limited to women age 18 and older.

SPECIAL PRECAUTIONS

• Contraindicated in patients with known hypersensitivity to LHRH and LHRH agonist analogs, with undiagnosed abnormal vaginal bleeding, and in patients who are or may become pregnant or who are breast-feeding.

SELF-TEST

1. After a history and medical work-up, Ellen Gila, age 32, begins therapy with menotropins for anovulation. How will menotropins alter the hormonal balance to enhance her fertility?
   a. Menotropins mimic thyroid-stimulating hormone.
   b. Menotropins decrease HCG levels.
   c. Menotropins mimic FSH.
   d. Menotropins decrease LH levels.

2. In explaining the potential adverse reactions to menotropins to Ms. Gila, the nurse should include:
   a. constipation.
   b. ovarian enlargement with pain and abdominal distention.
   c. dizziness and lethargy.
   d. virilization.

3. Ms. Gila should be warned about which of the following as a possible consequence of therapy with menotropins?
   a. multiple births
   b. early menopause
   c. dysmenorrhea
   d. infertility

Check your answers on page 1071.

ANTIDIABETIC AGENTS AND GLUCAGON

━━━━━━━━━

Insulins
insulin injection (regular, crystalline zinc)
prompt insulin zinc suspension (semilente)
isophane insulin suspension (NPH) ✦ insulin zinc suspension (lente)
isophane (NPH) 70%, regular insulin 30%
protamine zinc insulin suspension
extended insulin zinc suspension (ultralente)

Sulfonylureas
acetohexamide ✦ chlorpropamide ✦ glipizide ✦ glyburide
tolazamide ✦ tolbutamide

Hyperglycemic agent
glucagon

━━━━━━━━━

OVERVIEW

- Antidiabetic drugs supply exogenous insulin or stimulate production of endogenous insulin in patients with diabetes mellitus. Endogenous insulin, produced by beta cells of the pancreatic islets of Langerhans, and commercial insulin, obtained from beef and pork pancreases or synthesized using recombinant DNA technology, lower glucose levels.
- The sulfonylureas (acetohexamide, chlorpropamide, glipizide, glyburide, tolazamide, and tolbutamide) are synthetic antidiabetic drugs given orally to stimulate insulin secretion in patients with diabetes who have some beta cell function. They have no value in patients with no functional beta cell tissue.
- Glucagon, a hormone normally produced by alpha cells of the pancreatic islets, raises blood glucose levels by stimulating glycogenolysis and glyconeogenesis. It thus reverses insulin-induced hypoglycemia in patients with adequate hepatic glycogen stores.
- This chapter discusses the two types of antidiabetic agents, insulins and sulfonylureas, as well as the hyperglycemic agent, glucagon.

GLOSSARY

Diabetes mellitus: metabolic disorder in which the ability to metabolize carbohydrates is lost because of decreased insulin secretion; characterized by hyperglycemia, glycosuria, polyuria, polydipsia, polyphagia, emaciation, and weakness.
Gluconeogenesis: carbohydrate formation from protein molecules.
Glycogenolysis: breakdown of the polysaccharide glycogen in body tissues.
Hyperglycemia: abnormally high blood glucose level.
Hypoglycemia: abnormally low blood glucose level.
Lipoatrophy: wasting of the body's fatty tissues.
Lipodystrophy: disturbance of fat metabolism involving regional loss of subcutaneous fat.
Lipohypertrophy: excessive enlargement of fatty tissues.
Lipolysis: fat breakdown.

MAJOR USES

- Insulin supplements or replaces endogenous insulin in the treatment of diabetes mellitus, especially insulin-dependent (Type I) diabetes. It's used in non–insulin-dependent (Type II) diabetes mellitus if sulfonylureas are ineffective.
- Sulfonylureas are used to treat Type II diabetes mellitus that is inadequately controlled by diet alone. Chlorpropamide is also used to treat diabetes insipidus.
- Glucagon is used in emergencies to reverse insulin-induced hypoglycemia in patients with diabetes mellitus.

MECHANISM OF ACTION

- Insulin increases glucose transport across muscle and fat cell membranes to reduce blood glucose levels. It promotes conversion of glucose to its storage form, glycogen; triggers amino acid uptake and conversion to protein in muscle cells and inhibits protein degradation; stimulates triglyceride formation and inhibits release of free fatty acids from adipose tissue; and stimulates lipoprotein lipase activity, which converts circulating lipoproteins to fatty acids.
- Sulfonylureas stimulate insulin release from the pancreatic beta cells, promote peripheral tissue glucose utilization, and reduce glucose output by the liver. Chlorpropamide also exerts an antidiuretic effect in patients with pituitary-deficient diabetes insipidus.
- Glucagon raises blood glucose levels by promoting catalytic depolymerization of hepatic glycogen to glucose.

ABSORPTION, DISTRIBUTION, METABOLISM, AND EXCRETION

Insulin, because it is destroyed in the GI tract, is generally administered by S.C. injection. It is absorbed directly from the injection site into the bloodstream. Absorption rate depends on insulin type, concentration, dose, volume, vascularity at the injection site, and the patient's physical activity pattern. Vigorous exercise, for example, accelerates absorption and metabolism from an injection in the thigh, but not from an injection in the arm. Insulin is distributed throughout extracellular fluid and metabolized in the liver (primary site) and in the kidneys and muscles (secondary sites). Only small quantities of insulin are excreted in urine.

Of the sulfonylureas, acetohexamide and tolazamide are metabolized to active metabolites and excreted in urine. Chlorpropamide is excreted in urine, primarily unchanged. Glipizide, glyburide, and tolbutamide are metabolized to inactive metabolites and excreted in urine.

Glucagon is rapidly absorbed after parenteral administration, metabolized mainly in the liver, and excreted in urine.

ONSET AND DURATION

See *Comparing Actions of Antidiabetic Drugs and Glucagon* for the onset, peak, and duration of these drugs.

ADVERSE REACTIONS

The most common adverse reactions to insulin are related to the drug's metabolic effects. Hypoglycemia can occur if changes in diet or activity levels are not considered when administering the typical daily dose.

Other reactions usually occur at the administration site and can include lipodystrophy, itching, swelling, redness, stinging, or warmth. Allergic reactions to pork or beef insulin can also occur. The availability of human insulin has reduced the risk of such allergy.

Sulfonylureas can cause metabolic disturbances, including hypoglycemia, and allergic reactions, such as rash, fever, pruritus, erythema multiforme, exfoliative dermatitis, joint pain, leukopenia, and bronchospasm. Hematologic disturbances may include granulocytopenia, thrombocytopenia, agranulocytosis, and hemolytic anemia in patients with G6PD deficiency. GI disturbances, including nausea and vomiting, are common.

Long-term (5- to 8-year) studies have compared the results of oral sulfonylurea therapy with those of diet alone or diet plus insulin. Patients taking certain oral sulfonylureas exhibited increased cardiovascular mortality as compared to the other groups; however, there is some controversy regarding the interpretation of these studies.

Glucagon has been associated with nausea, vomiting, and light-headedness.

COMPARING ACTIONS OF ANTIDIABETIC DRUGS AND GLUCAGON

PREPARATION	ONSET	PEAK	DURATION
Rapid-acting insulins			
Insulin injection (regular, crystalline zinc)			
Regular Iletin I	½ to 1 hr	2 to 4 hr	6 to 8 hr
Regular Insulin	½ hr	2½ to 5 hr	8 hr
Pork Regular Iletin II	½ to 1 hr	2 to 4 hr	6 to 8 hr
Beef Regular Iletin II	½ to 1 hr	2 to 4 hr	6 to 8 hr
Regular (concentrated) Iletin II	½ hr	Variable	Up to 24 hr
Velosulin	½ hr	1 to 3 hr	8 hr
Purified Pork Insulin	½ hr	2½ to 5 hr	8 hr
Humulin R	½ to 1 hr	2 to 4 hr	6 to 8 hr
Novolin R	½ hr	2½ to 5 hr	8 hr
Prompt insulin zinc suspension (semilente)			
Semilente Iletin I	1 to 3 hr	3 to 8 hr	10 to 16 hr
Semilente Insulin	1½ hr	5 to 10 hr	16 hr
Semilente Purified Pork Prompt Insulin	1½ hr	5 to 10 hr	16 hr
Intermediate-acting insulins			
Isophane insulin suspension (NPH)			
NPH Iletin I	2 hr	6 to 12 hr	18 to 26 hr
NPH Insulin	1½ hr	4 to 12 hr	24 hr
Beef NPH Iletin II	2 hr	6 to 12 hr	18 to 26 hr
Pork NPH Iletin II	2 hr	6 to 12 hr	18 to 26 hr
NPH Purified Pork Isophane Insulin	1½ hr	4 to 12 hr	24 hr
Insulatard NPH	1½ hr	4 to 12 hr	24 hr
Humulin N	1 to 2 hr	6 to 12 hr	18 to 24 hr
Novolin N	1½ hr	4 to 12 hr	24 hr

(continued)

COMPARING ACTIONS OF ANTIDIABETIC DRUGS AND GLUCAGON
continued

PREPARATION	ONSET	PEAK	DURATION
Intermediate-acting insulins *(continued)*			
Insulin zinc suspension (lente)			
Lente Iletin I	2 to 4 hr	6 to 12 hr	18 to 26 hr
Lente Insulin	2½ hr	7 to 15 hr	24 hr
Beef Lente Iletin II	2 to 4 hr	6 to 12 hr	18 to 26 hr
Pork Lente Iletin II	2 to 4 hr	6 to 12 hr	18 to 26 hr
Lente Purified Pork Insulin	2½ hr	7 to 15 hr	22 hr
Humulin L	1 to 3 hr	6 to 12 hr	18 to 21 hr
Novolin L	2½ hr	7 to 15 hr	22 hr
Isophane (NPH) 70%, regular insulin 30%			
Humulin 70/30	½ hr	4 to 8 hr	24 hr
Mixtard Human 70/30	½ hr	4 to 8 hr	24 hr
Novolin 70/30	½ hr	4 to 8 hr	24 hr
Mixtard	½ hr	4 to 8 hr	24 hr
Long-acting insulins			
Protamine zinc insulin suspension			
Protamine Zinc & Iletin I	4 to 8 hr	14 to 24 hr	28 to 36 hr
Beef Protamine Zinc & Iletin II	4 to 8 hr	14 to 24 hr	28 to 36 hr
Pork Protamine Zinc & Iletin II	4 to 8 hr	14 to 24 hr	28 to 36 hr
Extended insulin zinc suspension (ultralente)			
Ultralente Iletin I	4 to 8 hr	14 to 24 hr	28 to 36 hr
Ultralente Insulin	4 hr	10 to 30 hr	36 hr
Ultralente Purified Beef Insulin	4 hr	10 to 30 hr	36 hr

COMPARING ACTIONS OF ANTIDIABETIC DRUGS AND GLUCAGON
continued

PREPARATION	ONSET	PEAK	DURATION
Long-acting insulins *(continued)*			
Sulfonylureas			
Acetohexamide	1 hr	4 to 5 hr	12 to 24 hr
Chlorpropamide	1 hr	3 to 6 hr	40 to 60 hr
Glipizide	½ to 1½ hr	1 to 3 hr	10 to 24 hr
Glyburide	2 to 4 hr	2 to 4 hr	24 hr
Tolazamide	4 to 6 hr	4 to 6 hr	10 to 14 hr
Tolbutamide	1 hr	4 to 6 hr	6 to 12 hr
Hyperglycemic agent			
Glucagon	10 to 15 min	30 min	1 to 1½ hr

PROTOTYPE: INSULINS

INSULIN INJECTION (REGULAR INSULIN, CRYSTALLINE ZINC INSULIN)
(in'su lin)

Actrapid HM‡, Actrapid HM Penfill‡, Actrapid MC‡, Actrapid MC Penfill‡, Beef Regular Iletin II◊, Humulin R◊, Hypurin Neutral‡, Insulin 2‡, Novolin R◊, Novolin R Penfill◊, Pork Regular Iletin II◊, Regular (concentrated) Iletin II, Regular Iletin I◊, Regular Purified Pork Insulin◊, Velosulin◊, Velosulin Human‡, Velosulin Insuject◊

Classification: exogenous insulin
Pregnancy risk category B

How supplied
INJECTION (FROM BEEF AND PORK): 40 units/ml◊, 100 units/ml◊ (Regular Iletin I◊)
INJECTION (HUMAN): 100 units/ml (Actrapid HM‡, Humulin R◊, Novolin R◊, Velosulin◊, Velosulin Human‡; 100 units/ml in 1.5-ml cartridge system (Actrapid HM Penfill‡, Novolin R Penfill◊)
INJECTION (FROM PORK): 100 units/ml◊
INJECTION (PURIFIED BEEF): 100 units/ml (Beef Regular Iletin II◊, Hypurin Neutral‡, Insulin 2‡)

---

‡Available in Australia only   ◊ Available OTC

INJECTION (PURIFIED PORK): 100 units/ml (Actrapid MC‡, Pork Regular Iletin II◊, Regular Purified Pork Insulin◊, Velosulin◊); 100 units/ml in 1.5-ml cartridge system‡ (Actrapid MC Penfill‡); 100 units/ml in 2-ml cartridge system‡ (Velosulin Insuject‡); 500 units/ml (Regular [Concentrated] Iletin II)

Indications and dosage
Diabetic ketoacidosis (use regular insulin only)
ADULTS: 25 to 150 units I.V. immediately; then additional doses may be given q 1 hour based on blood glucose level until patient is out of acidosis; then give S.C. q 6 hours. Alternative dosage schedule: 50 to 100 units I.V. and 50 to 100 units S.C. immediately; additional doses may be given q 2 to 6 hours based on blood glucose levels; or 0.33 units/kg I.V. bolus, followed by 7 to 10 units/hour I.V. by continuous infusion. Continue infusion until blood glucose level drops to 250 mg/dl, then start S.C. insulin q 6 hours.
CHILDREN: 0.5 to 1 unit/kg in two divided doses, one given I.V. and the other S.C., followed by 0.5 to 1 unit/kg I.V. q 1 to 2 hours; or 0.1 unit/kg I.V. bolus, then 0.1 unit/kg I.V. hourly by continuous infusion until blood glucose level drops to 250 mg/dl; then start S.C. insulin.

Insulin-dependent (Type I) diabetes mellitus, ketosis-prone diabetics, diabetes mellitus inadequately controlled by diet and oral antidiabetic agents
ADULTS AND CHILDREN: therapeutic regimen prescribed by doctor and adjusted according to patient's blood and urine glucose concentrations.

Contraindications and precautions
I.V. administration of concentrated regular insulin (500 units/ml) is contraindicated.

Adverse reactions
METABOLIC: *hypoglycemia,* hyperglycemia (rebound, or Somogyi, effect).
SKIN: urticaria.
LOCAL: *lipoatrophy, lipohypertrophy,* itching, swelling, redness, stinging, warmth at injection site.
OTHER: **anaphylaxis.**

Interactions
Alcohol, beta blockers, clofibrate, fenfluramine, MAO inhibitors, salicylates, tetracycline: prolonged hypoglycemic effect. Monitor blood glucose level carefully.
Corticosteroids, thiazide diuretics: diminished insulin response. Monitor for hyperglycemia.

Nursing considerations
Assessment
• Review the patient's history for a condition that contraindicates the use of beef or pork insulin, such as hypersensitivity.
• Obtain a baseline assessment of the patient's blood glucose level before initiating insulin therapy.

• Be alert for common adverse reactions.
• Evaluate the patient's and family's knowledge about insulin therapy as well as other aspects of diabetes treatment that may affect insulin therapy.

Planning (Nursing Diagnoses)
Potential nursing diagnoses for the patient receiving insulin include:
• Altered health maintenance related to inadequate dosage or frequency of insulin administration.
• Potential for injury related to insulin-induced hypoglycemia.
• Impaired tissue integrity related to insulin injections.
• Knowledge deficit related to insulin therapy.

Implementation

Preparation and administration

— Accuracy of measurement is very important, especially with regular insulin concentrated. Use aids, such as a magnifying sleeve or dose magnifier to improve accuracy.
— Be aware that the dosage is always expressed in USP units.
— Do not interchange beef, pork, or human insulins; a dosage adjustment may be required.
— Regular insulin may be mixed with NPH or lente insulins in any proportion. However, in vitro binding will occur over time until an equilibrium is reached. Administer these mixtures immediately after preparation or after stability occurs (15 minutes for NPH regular, 24 hours for lente regular) to minimize variability in patient response. Note that switching from separate injections to a prepared mixture also may alter the patient's response.
— Store insulin in a cool area. Refrigeration is desirable but not essential, except with regular insulin concentrated.
— Do not use insulin that has changed color or becomes clumped or granular in appearance.
— Check expiration date on vial before using contents.
— Some patients may develop insulin resistance and require large insulin doses to control symptoms of diabetes. U-500 insulin is available as Regular (concentrated) Iletin I for such patients. Never store U-500 insulin in same area with other insulin preparations because of the danger of severe overdose if given accidentally to other patients. U-500 insulin must be administered with a U-100 syringe because no syringes are made specifically for this drug.
— Human insulin may be advantageous in patients who are allergic to pork or beef forms. Otherwise, these insulins offer no advantage. Humulin is synthesized by a genetically altered strain of *Escherichia coli*. Novolin brands are derived by enzymatic alteration of pork insulin.
— Administer drug by S.C. route because it allows slower absorption and causes less pain than I.M. injections. Patients with juvenile-onset diabetes mellitus as well as ketosis-prone, severely ill, and newly diagnosed diabetics with very high blood glucose levels may require hospitalization and I.V. treatment with regular fast-acting insulin.

—When injecting insulin S.C., insert needle at a 90-degree angle unless 1 inch of subcutaneous tissue cannot be bunched together; then insert at a 45-degree angle. You do not need to aspirate before injection.

—Press but do not rub site after injection. Rotate injection sites. Record sites to avoid overuse of one area. However, some diabetics may achieve better control if the injection site is rotated within the same anatomic region.

Monitoring

—Monitor the effectiveness of therapy by regularly checking the patient's blood glucose levels. Monitor blood glucose levels more frequently if the patient is under stress, unstable, pregnant, or is a recently diagnosed or unstable diabetic.

—Monitor the patient for signs and symptoms of both hyperglycemia and hypoglycemia; note time and circumstances associated with each.

—Monitor the patient for adverse drug reactions.

—Monitor the patient's urine ketone levels when blood glucose levels are elevated.

—Monitor injection sites for local reactions such as lipoatrophy or lipohypertrophy.

—Monitor for drug interactions.

—Regularly reevaluate the patient's and family's knowledge about insulin injection.

Intervention

—Notify the doctor if sudden changes in blood glucose levels occur, if they are dangerously high or low, or if ketosis is present.

—Be prepared to provide supportive measures if diabetic ketoacidosis or hyperglycemic, hyperosmolar, nonketotic coma occurs.

—Treat a hypoglycemic reaction with an oral form of rapid-acting glucose if the patient is awake or with glucagon or I.V. glucose if the patient cannot be aroused. Follow up treatment with a complex carbohydrate snack when patient is awake, and determine cause of the reaction.

—Be sure that other treatment measures, such as diet and exercise programs, are being used appropriately. Expect to adjust insulin dosage when other aspects of treatment regimen are altered.

—Discuss with the doctor how to approach issues of noncompliance.

—Treat lipoatrophy or lipohypertrophy according to prescribed protocol.

—Keep all members of the health care team informed of the patient's response to the drug.

Patient teaching

—Inform the patient and family about insulin injection, including the dosage, type, concentration, frequency, peak action time, and adverse reactions.

—Teach the patient how to draw up insulin and self-administer S.C. dose.

—Teach the patient the preferred injection sites, the importance of site rotation, and how to rotate sites.

—Teach the patient how to store insulin and injection equipment.

—Advise the patient not to change the order of mixing insulins nor the model or brand of syringe or needle used.

—Be sure the patient knows that insulin therapy relieves symptoms but does not cure the disease.

—Tell the patient about the nature of the disease and the importance of the therapeutic regimen (adhering to a specific diet, losing weight, following exercise programs, maintaining personal hygiene, avoiding infection, and properly timing injection and meals).

—Emphasize the importance of regular mealtimes and that meals must not be omitted.

—Teach the patient that blood glucose testing is an essential guide to correct dosage and to therapeutic success. Instruct patient how to self-test blood glucose.

—Emphasize the importance of recognizing hypoglycemic symptoms (including nervousness, shakiness, and confusion) because insulin-induced hypoglycemia is hazardous and may cause brain damage if prolonged.

—Advise the patient to always wear medical alert identification, to carry ample insulin supply and syringes on trips, to have carbohydrates (sugar or candy) on hand for emergency, and to note any time-zone changes for dosage schedule when traveling.

—Tell the patient that use of marijuana may increase insulin requirements.

—Cigarette smoking decreases the absorption of insulin administered subcutaneously. Advise the patient not to smoke within 30 minutes after insulin injection.

—Tell the patient to notify the nurse or doctor if adverse reactions develop or questions arise about insulin injection therapy.

Evaluation

In the patient receiving insulin injection, appropriate evaluation statements include:

• Patient's blood glucose level is normal.
• Patient recognizes hypoglycemia early and treats hypoglycemic episodes effectively before injury occurs.
• Patient's injection sites do not exhibit altered tissue integrity.
• Patient and family state an understanding of insulin therapy and demonstrate correct insulin administration.

PROTOTYPE: SULFONYLUREAS

GLYBURIDE
(glye'byoor ide)
DiaBeta, Euglucon†, Micronase
Classification: *sulfonylurea*
Pregnancy risk category B

How supplied
TABLETS: 1.25 mg, 2.5 mg, 5 mg

Indications and dosage
Adjunct to diet to lower blood glucose level in patients with non–insulin-dependent diabetes mellitus (Type II)
ADULTS: initially, 2.5 to 5 mg P.O. daily administered with breakfast. Patients who are more sensitive to sulfonylureas should be started at 1.25 mg daily. Usual maintenance dosage is 1.25 to 20 mg daily, given either as a single dose or in divided doses.

To replace insulin therapy
ADULTS: if insulin dosage is more than 40 units daily, patient may be started on 5 mg glyburide daily in addition to 50% of the insulin dosage.

Contraindications and precautions
Glyburide is contraindicated in patients with diabetic ketoacidosis, with or without coma. Use cautiously in patients with sulfonamide hypersensitivity and severe renal impairment.

Adverse reactions
GI: nausea, epigastric fullness, heartburn.
HEPATIC: *cholestatic jaundice.*
METABOLIC: *hypoglycemia.*
SKIN: rash, pruritus, *facial flushing.*

Interactions
Anabolic steroids, chloramphenicol, clofibrate, guanethidine, MAO inhibitors, oral anticoagulants, phenylbutazone, salicylates, sulfonamides: increased hypoglycemic activity. Monitor blood glucose level.
Beta blockers, clonidine: prolonged hypoglycemic effect and masked symptoms of hypoglycemia. Use together cautiously.
Corticosteroids, glucagon, rifampin, thiazide diuretics: decreased hypoglycemic response. Monitor blood glucose level.

Nursing considerations
Assessment
• Review the patient's history for a condition that contraindicates the use of glyburide and related compounds.
• Obtain a baseline assessment of the patient's blood glucose level before initiating glyburide therapy.

---

† Available in Canada only
Italicized adverse reactions are common

• Be alert for common adverse reactions.
• Evaluate the patient's and family's knowledge about glyburide therapy.

Planning (Nursing Diagnoses)

Potential nursing diagnoses for the patient receiving glyburide include:
• Altered health maintenance related to ineffectiveness of glyburide to control blood glucose.
• Potential for injury related to glyburide-induced hypoglycemia.
• Knowledge deficit related to glyburide therapy.

Implementation

Preparation and administration

— Administer once-daily doses with breakfast.
— Be aware that to improve control in patients receiving 10 mg/day or more, divided doses are usually given before the morning and evening meals.
— Consider that some patients taking glyburide may be controlled effectively on a once-daily regimen, whereas others show better response with divided dosing.
— Remember that in elderly, debilitated, or malnourished patients or those with renal or liver dysfunction, glyburide therapy should start with 1.25 mg once a day.

Monitoring

— Monitor the effectiveness of therapy by regularly checking patient's blood glucose levels. Monitor blood glucose levels more frequently if the patient is under stress, has difficulty controlling blood glucose levels, or is newly diagnosed.
— Monitor the patient for signs and symptoms of both hyperglycemia and hypoglycemia; note time and circumstances of each reaction.
— Monitor the patient for adverse drug reactions. Glyburide is a second-generation sulfonylurea that appears to cause fewer adverse reactions than first-generation drugs.
— Monitor the patient for drug interactions.
— When substituting glyburide for chlorpropamide, monitor the patient closely during the first week because of the prolonged retention of chlorpropamide in the body.
— Monitor the patient for cardiovascular dysfunction, because sulfonylureas have been associated with an increased risk of cardiovascular mortality as compared to diet or diet and insulin therapy.
— Regularly reevaluate the patient's and family's knowledge about glyburide.

Intervention

— Notify the doctor if blood glucose levels remain elevated or frequent episodes of hypoglycemia occur.
— Treat a hypoglycemic reaction with an oral form of rapid-acting glucose if the patient is awake or with glucagon or I.V. glucose if the patient cannot be aroused. Follow up treatment with a complex carbohydrate snack when patient is awake, and determine cause of reaction.

— Be sure other treatment measures, such as diet and exercise programs, are being used appropriately.

— Discuss with the doctor how to approach noncompliance issues.

— Keep all members of the health care team informed of the patient's response to the drug.

Patient teaching

— Inform the patient and family about glyburide, including the dosage, frequency, action, and adverse reactions.

— Emphasize to the patient the importance of following the prescribed diet, exercise, and medical regimens.

— Tell the patient to take the medication at the same time each day. If a dose is missed, it should be taken immediately, unless it's almost time to take the next dose. Instruct the patient not to take double doses.

— Advise the patient to avoid alcohol while taking glyburide. Remind him that many foods and nonprescription medications contain alcohol.

— Encourage the patient to wear medical alert identifiction.

— Tell the patient to take drug with food; once-daily dosage should be taken with breakfast.

— Teach the patient how to monitor blood glucose and urine glucose levels as prescribed.

— Teach the patient how to recognize the signs and symptoms of hyper-glycemia and hypoglycemia and what to do if they occur.

— Stress the importance of compliance and close follow-up with glyburide therapy.

— Tell the patient to notify the nurse or doctor if adverse reactions develop or questions arise about glyburide therapy.

Evaluation

In the patient receiving glyburide, appropriate evaluation statements include:

• Patient's blood glucose level is normal.

• Patient recognizes hypoglycemia early and treats hypoglycemic episodes effectively before injury occurs.

• Patient and family state an understanding of glyburide therapy.

PROTOTYPE: HYPERGLYCEMIC AGENT

GLUCAGON
(gloo'ka gon)
Classification: hyperglycemic agent
Pregnancy risk category B

How supplied
POWDER FOR INJECTION: 1 mg (1 unit)/vial, 10 mg(10 units)/vial

Indications and dosage
Coma of insulin-shock therapy
ADULTS: 0.5 to 1 mg S.C., I.M., or I.V. 1 hour after coma develops; may repeat within 25 minutes, if necessary. In very deep coma, also give glucose 10% to 50% I.V. for faster response. When patient responds, give additional carbohydrate immediately.

Severe insulin-induced hypoglycemia during diabetic therapy
ADULTS AND CHILDREN: 0.5 to 1 mg S.C., I.M., or I.V.; may repeat q 20 minutes for two doses, if necessary. If coma persists, give dextrose 10% to 50% I.V.

Diagnostic aid for radiologic examination
ADULTS: 0.25 to 2 mg I.V. or I.M. before initiation of radiologic procedure.

Contraindications and precautions
Glucagon is contraindicated in patients with known hypersensitivity to it or in patients with pheochromocytoma. Administer cautiously to patients with a history suggestive of insulinoma or pheochromocytoma.

Adverse reactions
GI: nausea, vomiting.
OTHER: hypersensitivity.

Interactions
Phenytoin: inhibited glucagon-induced insulin release. Use together cautiously.

Nursing considerations
Assessment
• Review the patient's history for a condition that contraindicates the use of glucagon.
• Obtain a baseline assessment of the patient's blood glucose level before initiating glucagon therapy.
• Evaluate the patient's and family's knowledge about glucagon therapy.

Planning (Nursing Diagnoses)
Potential nursing diagnoses for the patient receiving glucagon include:
• Altered health maintenance related to ineffectiveness of glucagon to raise blood glucose level sufficiently to alleviate hypoglycemia.
• Knowledge deficit related to glucagon therapy.

Implementation
Preparation and administration
— Administer by parenteral route as recommended in hospital protocol or doctor's order.
— Repeat dose within 25 minutes, as needed.
— Use dextrose solution for I.V. drip infusion, as glucagon is compatible with it; drug forms a precipitate in chloride solutions.

Monitoring
— Monitor the effectiveness of therapy by checking patient's blood glucose level after administration and noting patient's response.
— Monitor the patient for adverse drug reactions.
— Monitor for drug interactions, especially with phenytoin.
— Regularly reevaluate the patient's and family's knowledge about glucagon therapy.

Intervention
— Notify the doctor that patient's hypoglycemic episode required glucagon use. Be prepared to provide emergency intervention if patient does not respond to glucagon administration.
— Be aware that unstable hypoglycemic diabetics may not respond to glucagon. Give dextrose I.V. instead.
— It is vital to arouse the patient from coma as quickly as possible and to give additional carbohydrates orally to prevent secondary hypoglycemic reactions.
— Identify the cause of the hypoglycemic episode and determine if the patient is able to recognize early warning signs (may be blunted in patients with chronic diabetes or masked by other drug therapies).
— If the patient experiences nausea and vomiting from glucagon administration and cannot retain some form of sugar for 1 hour, notify the doctor.
— Keep all members of the health care team informed of the patient's response to the drug.

Patient teaching
— Inform the patient and family about glucagon, including when to use, dosage, frequency, action, and adverse reactions.
— Teach the patient how to mix and inject the medication properly, using an appropriate-sized syringe and injecting at a 90-degree angle.
— Recommend that the patient use medication within 3 months after mixing and store the mixed solution in refrigerator. Patient should store unmixed medication at room temperature and not in the bathroom, which often becomes hot and humid.
— Instruct family members how to administer glucagon and how to recognize hypoglycemia. Urge them to call a doctor immediately in emergencies.
— Tell the patient to expect a response usually within 20 minutes after injection and that injection may be repeated if no response occurs. Tell the patient to seek medical assistance if second injection is needed.
— Tell the patient to notify the nurse or doctor if adverse reactions develop or questions arise about glucagon therapy.

Evaluation
In the patient receiving glucagon, appropriate evaluation statements include:
• Patient's blood glucose level returns to normal.

• Patient and family state an understanding of glucagon therapy and demonstrate appropriate administration techniques.

SELECTED MAJOR DRUGS: ORAL ANTIDIABETIC AGENTS

DRUG, INDICATIONS, AND DOSAGES	SPECIAL PRECAUTIONS
acetohexamide (Dymelor) *Adjunct to diet to lower blood glucose in patients with non–insulin-dependent diabetes mellitus (Type II)—* **Adults:** initially, 250 mg P.O. daily before breakfast; may increase dosage q 5 to 7 days (by 250 to 500 mg) as needed to maximum of 1.5 g daily, divided b.i.d. to t.i.d. before meals. *To replace insulin therapy—* **Adults:** if insulin dosage is less than 20 units daily, insulin may be stopped and oral therapy started with 250 mg P.O. daily before breakfast, increased as above if needed. If insulin dosage is 20 to 40 units daily, start oral therapy with 250 mg P.O. daily before breakfast, while reducing insulin dosage 25% to 30% daily or every other day, depending on response to oral therapy.	• Contraindicated in patients with Type I (insulin-dependent) diabetes mellitus; in diabetes adequately controlled by diet; and in Type II diabetes complicated by ketosis, acidosis, diabetic coma, Raynaud's disease, gangrene, renal or hepatic impairment, or thyroid or other endocrine dysfunction. • Use cautiously in patients with sulfonamide hypersensitivity.
chlorpropamide (Diabinese) *Adjunct to diet to lower blood glucose in patients with non–insulin-dependent diabetes mellitus (Type II)—* **Adults:** 250 mg P.O. daily with breakfast or in divided doses if GI disturbances occur. First dosage increase may be made after 5 to 7 days because of extended duration of action; then dosage may be increased q 3 to 5 days by 50 to 125 mg, if needed, to maximum of 750 mg daily. **Adults over age 65:** initial dose should be between 100 and 125 mg P.O. daily. *To change from insulin to oral therapy—* **Adults:** if insulin dosage is less than 40 units daily, insulin may be stopped and oral therapy started as above. If insulin dosage is 40 units or more daily, start oral therapy as above with insulin reduced 50%. Further insulin reductions should be made according to patient response.	• Contraindicated in patients with Type I (insulin-dependent) diabetes mellitus; in diabetes adequately controlled by diet; and in Type II diabetes complicated by fever, ketosis, acidosis, diabetic coma, major surgery, severe trauma, Raynaud's disease, gangrene, renal or hepatic impairment, or thyroid or other endocrine dysfunction. • Use cautiously in patients with sulfonamide hypersensitivity.
glipizide (Glucotrol) *Adjunct to diet to lower blood glucose in patients with non–insulin-dependent diabetes mellitus (Type II)—* **Adults:** initially, 5 mg P.O. daily given before breakfast. Elderly patients or those with liver disease may be started on 2.5 mg. Usual maintenance dosage is 10 to 15 mg. Maximum recommended daily dosage is 40 mg. *To replace insulin therapy—* **Adults:** if insulin dosage is more than 20 units daily, patient may be started at usual dosage in addition to 50% of the insulin. If insulin dosage is less than 20 units, insulin may be discontinued.	• Contraindicated in patients with diabetic ketoacidosis, with or without coma. • Use cautiously in patients with renal or hepatic disease or sulfonamide hypersensitivity.

(continued)

SELECTED MAJOR DRUGS: ORAL ANTIDIABETIC AGENTS *continued*

DRUG, INDICATIONS, AND DOSAGES	SPECIAL PRECAUTIONS
tolazamide (Tolinase) *Adjunct to diet to lower blood glucose in patients with non–insulin-dependent diabetes mellitus (Type II)* — **Adults:** initially, 100 mg P.O. daily with breakfast if fasting blood sugar (FBS) under 200 mg/dl; or 250 mg if FBS is over 200 mg/dl. May adjust dosage at weekly intervals by 100 to 250 mg. Maximum dosage is 500 mg b.i.d. before meals. **Adults over age 65:** 100 mg P.O. daily *To change from insulin to oral therapy* — **Adults:** if insulin dosage is under 20 units daily, insulin may be stopped and oral therapy started at 100 mg P.O. daily with breakfast. If insulin dosage is 20 to 40 units daily, insulin may be stopped and oral therapy started at 250 mg P.O. daily with breakfast. If insulin dosage is over 40 units daily, decrease insulin 50% and start oral therapy at 250 mg P.O. daily with breakfast. Increase dosages as above.	• Contraindicated in patients with Type I (insulin-dependent) diabetes mellitus; in diabetes adequately controlled by diet; and in Type II diabetes complicated by fever, ketosis, acidosis, or coma, major surgery, severe trauma, Raynaud's disease, renal or hepatic impairment, or thyroid or other endocrine dysfunction. • Administer cautiously in sulfonamide hypersensitivity and in elderly, debilitated, or malnourished patients.
tolbutamide (Orinase) *Stable, maturity-onset (Type II), nonketotic diabetes mellitus uncontrolled by diet alone and previously untreated* — **Adults:** initially, 1 to 2 g P.O. daily as single dose or divided b.i.d. to t.i.d. May adjust dosage to maximum of 3 g daily. *To change from insulin to oral therapy* — **Adults:** if insulin dosage is under 20 units daily, insulin may be stopped and oral therapy started at 1 to 2 g P.O. daily. If insulin dosage is 20 to 40 units daily, insulin is reduced 30% to 50% and oral therapy started as above. If insulin dosage is over 40 units daily, insulin is decreased 20% and oral therapy started as above. Further reductions in insulin are based on patient's response to oral therapy.	• Contraindicated in patients with Type I (insulin-dependent) diabetes mellitus; in diabetes adequately controlled by diet; and in Type II diabetes complicated by fever, ketosis, acidosis, or coma, major surgery, severe trauma, Raynaud's disease, renal or hepatic impairment, thyroid or other endocrine dysfunction, or pregnancy. • Administer cautiously in patients with sulfonamide hypersensitivity.

SELF-TEST

1. Barry Morton, age 53, has just started treatment with glyburide 2.5 mg P.O. daily. He had been diagnosed with diabetes mellitus 6 years ago and tells his nurse that "I am glad to be starting on pills. I hated watching my diet." Which of the following is the best response to Mr. Morton?

a. The oral antidiabetic agents work with diet and exercise to help keep your glucose within normal limits; they do not replace correct diet.

b. I can understand your relief about fewer diet restrictions.

c. It is important that you continue to gain weight.

d. If you gain enough weight, you may be able to stop the oral antidiabetic agent.

2. The nurse should tell Mr. Morton to take glyburide:
   a. with water.
   b. with breakfast.
   c. at bedtime.
   d. with an antacid.

3. Jerry Levine, age 31, is newly diagnosed with insulin-dependent diabetes mellitus. You include the signs and symptoms of hyperglycemia and hypoglycemia in your patient teaching. Which of the following signs and symptoms occur with hypoglycemia?
   a. urine ketone spillage
   b. nervousness, shakiness, and mental changes
   c. polyuria and polydipsia
   d. fruity breath odor

4. Joan Dougherty, age 22, has difficulty maintaining normal blood glucose levels and has been encouraged by her doctor to have glucagon available for emergencies. Which one of the following statements regarding glucagon is true?
   a. Glucagon is normally produced in the liver.
   b. Glucagon increases the serum glucose level.
   c. Glucagon works with insulin to improve glucose control.
   d. The severe adverse reactions to glucagon limit its usefulness.

Check your answers on page 1071.

CHAPTER 57

THYROID HORMONES

levothyroxine sodium (T$_4$ or L-thyroxine sodium)
liothyronine sodium (T$_3$) ♦ liotrix ♦ thyroglobulin
thyroid USP (desiccated)
thyrotropin (thyroid-stimulating hormone, or TSH)

OVERVIEW

- Thyroid hormones are produced and stored in the follicles of the thyroid gland. Their synthesis and release are regulated by thyrotropin, also known as thyroid-stimulating hormone (TSH), which is secreted by the anterior pituitary gland. Increased blood levels of thyroid hormones inhibit release of pituitary TSH. Through this negative feedback mechanism, they homeostatically control further increases in thyroid hormone.
- Thyroid extract was once the treatment of choice for hypothyroidism. This substance, the desiccated thyroid gland of animals, contains liothyronine (T$_3$) and tetraiodothyronine or levothyroxine (T$_4$) as well as other organic materials. It is no longer used.
- Thyroglobulin is a purified extract of a hog's thyroid gland that is standardized on the basis of iodine content and metabolic activity. Thyroid USP (desiccated) is a cleaned, dried, and powdered thyroid gland obtained from animal (usually hog) sources.
- Liothyronine and levothyroxine are the purified forms of the naturally occurring hormone; levothyroxine is usually used for replacement therapy in thyroid-deficient patients.

MAJOR USES

- Thyroid hormones are used as replacement therapy in patients with diminished or absent thyroid function. They prevent goiter and hypothyroidism in patients receiving antithyroid drugs for thyrotoxicosis. They are also used to treat confirmed hypothyroidism and to supply replacement therapy in primary and secondary myxedema, myxedema coma, cretinism, and simple nontoxic goiter. Levothyroxine is the preferred agent for thyroid hormone replacement therapy.
- Thyroglobulin and thyroid USP are used to treat certain thyrotropin-dependent carcinomas of the thyroid.
- Thyrotropin is used in combination with radioactive iodine to treat thyroid tumors and is also used in differential diagnosis of subclinical hypothyroidism and low thyroid reserve.

GLOSSARY

Cretinism: condition of deficient growth and mental development resulting from severe congenital hypothyroidism.
Euthyroidism: condition of normal thyroid function.
Hypothyroidism: state of low serum thyroid hormone level, resulting from hypothalamic, pituitary, or thyroid insufficiency.
Myxedema: condition resulting from hypothyroidism and characterized by dry, waxy, nonpitting edema; abnormal mucin deposits in the skin; swollen lips; and a thickened nose.
Thyroglobulin: iodine-containing protein in the colloid of thyroid gland follicles, which stores thyroid hormones.
Thyrotropin: anterior pituitary hormone that stimulates the thyroid gland.

MECHANISM OF ACTION

- Thyroid hormones stimulate the metabolism of all body tissues by accelerating the rate of cellular oxidation. They enhance carbohydrate and protein biosynthesis by glyconeogenesis, which increases the mobilization and utilization of glycogen stores. They also affect lipid metabolism levels in the liver and blood.
- Thyrotropin stimulates the uptake of radioactive iodine in patients with thyroid carcinoma. It also promotes thyroid hormone production by the anterior pituitary.

ABSORPTION, DISTRIBUTION, METABOLISM, AND EXCRETION

Levothyroxine, liothyronine, thyroglobulin, and thyroid USP are efficiently absorbed from the GI tract. Liothyronine is better absorbed, however, than levothyroxine. Levothyroxine, well distributed to all body tissues, is partially metabolized in the liver. Both the metabolite and the unchanged hormone are passed into the bile. The metabolite is eliminated in feces; the small amount of free levothyroxine is recycled to the liver.

Liothyronine's metabolism is unclear. Liothyronine releases iodine into the body tissues. The thyroid then uses this iodine for synthesis of additional levothyroxine and liothyronine. Some of the iodine released by liothyronine is either excreted in urine or eliminated through the bile in feces.

ONSET AND DURATION

Full onset of action of levothyroxine, liotrix, thyroglobulin, and thyroid USP takes 1 to 3 weeks, although a response may be noted after several days. Levothyroxine generally has the slowest onset (several days) and a half-life of 6½ days. It has a long duration: its action may persist for weeks after therapy is terminated.

Liothyronine has a relatively rapid onset of action (a few hours), and its half-life is less than 3 days. Its action persists for several days.

ADVERSE REACTIONS

The most common adverse reaction is hyperthyroidism, which is most likely due to therapeutic overdosage. Common symptoms include nervousness, insomnia, tremor, tachycardia, nausea, and headache. Other reactions may include weight loss, menstrual irregularities, sweating, heat intolerance, and fever.

PROTOTYPE: THYROID HORMONES

LEVOTHYROXINE SODIUM (T₄ or L-THYROXINE SODIUM)

(lee voe thye rox′een)
Eltroxin†, Levothroid, Levoxine, Synthroid**, Synthrox
Classification: thyroid hormone
Pregnancy risk category A

How supplied

TABLETS: 25 mcg, 50 mcg, 75 mcg, 100 mcg, 125 mcg, 150 mcg, 175 mcg, 200 mcg, 300 mcg
INJECTION: 200 mcg/vial, 500 mcg/vial

Indications and dosage

Cretinism
CHILDREN UNDER AGE 1: initially 0.025 to 0.05 mg P.O. daily, increased by 0.05 mg P.O. q 2 to 3 weeks to total daily dosage of 0.1 to 0.4 mg P.O.

Myxedema coma
ADULTS: 0.2 to 0.5 mg I.V. If no response in 24 hours, additional 0.1 to 0.3 mg I.V. After condition stabilizes, oral maintenance dosage is 0.1 to 0.4 mg daily.

Thyroid hormone replacement
ADULTS: initially, 0.025 to 0.1 mg P.O. daily, increased by 0.05 to 0.1 mg P.O. q 1 to 4 weeks until desired response. Maintenance dosage is 0.1 to 0.4 mg daily. May be administered I.V. or I.M. when oral ingestion is precluded for long periods.
ADULTS OVER AGE 65: 0.025 mg P.O. daily. May be increased by 0.025 mg at 3- to 4-week intervals, depending on response.
CHILDREN: initially, maximum 0.05 mg P.O. daily, gradually increased by 0.025 to 0.05 mg P.O. q 1 to 4 weeks until desired response.

Contraindications and precautions

Levothyroxine is contraindicated in patients with acute MI, thyrotoxicosis (except with antithyroid drugs), or uncorrected adrenal insufficiency (thyroid hormones increase tissue demand for adrenocortical hormone and may cause acute adrenal crisis). Use with extreme caution in patients with angina pectoris, hypertension, or other cardiovascular disorders; renal insufficiency; or ischemic states.

---

†Available in Canada only   **May contain tartrazine

Adverse reactions

Adverse reactions to thyroid hormones are extensions of their pharmacologic properties and reflect patient sensitivity to them. Signs of overdosage may include the following reactions.

CNS: *nervousness, insomnia, tremor.*

CV: *tachycardia,* palpitations, **arrhythmias,** angina pectoris, hypertension.

GI: change in appetite, nausea, diarrhea.

OTHER: headache, leg cramps, weight loss, sweating, heat intolerance, fever, menstrual irregularities.

Interactions

Anticoagulants: increased risk of bleeding. Monitor closely. Dosage adjustments may be necessary.

Cholestyramine and colestipol: levothyroxine absorption impaired. Separate doses by 4 to 5 hours.

I.V. phenytoin: free-thyroid release. Monitor for tachycardia.

Nursing considerations

Assessment

- Review the patient's history for a condition that contraindicates the use of levothyroxine.
- Obtain a baseline assessment of the patient's thyroid status before initiating levothyroxine therapy.
- Be alert for common adverse reactions.
- Evaluate the patient's and family's knowledge about levothyroxine therapy.

Planning (Nursing Diagnoses)

Potential nursing diagnoses for the patient receiving levothyroxine include:

- Potential activity intolerance related to ineffective dosage of levothyroxine.
- Decreased cardiac output related to potential adverse cardiovascular reactions caused by levothyroxine overdose.
- Knowledge deficit related to levothyroxine therapy.

Implementation

Preparation and administration

— Be aware that when changing from levothyroxine to liothyronine, the doctor will stop levothyroxine and begin liothyronine. The dose of liothyronine will be increased slowly after residual effects of levothyroxine have disappeared. When changing from liothyronine to levothyroxine, the doctor will start levothyroxine several days before withdrawing liothyronine to avoid relapse.

— Prepare I.V. dose immediately before injection. Do not mix with other I.V. solutions.

— Protect drug from moisture and light.

— Administer as a single dose before breakfast.

Monitoring

—Monitor the effectiveness of therapy by regularly checking thyroid function studies and assessing the patient for signs and symptoms of thyroid dysfunction.

—Monitor the patient for signs of overdosage.

—Monitor the patient's temperature, pulse rate, and blood pressure regularly for alterations such as fever, tachycardia, or hypertension.

—Monitor the patient for adverse drug reactions.

—Monitor the patient's hydration status if adverse GI reactions occur.

—Monitor the patient for weight loss.

—Monitor prothrombin time; patients taking these hormones usually require less anticoagulant.

—Monitor for aggravation of concurrent diseases, such as Addison's disease or diabetes mellitus.

—Monitor the patient with a history of lactose intolerance, who may be sensitive to Levothroid, which contains lactose.

—Monitor the patient for hypersensitivity. Synthroid tablets may contain tartrazine, a dye that causes allergic reactions in susceptible individuals.

—Monitor the patient for drug interactions.

—Regularly reevaluate the patient's and family's knowledge about levothyroxine.

Intervention

—Withhold drug and notify the doctor if the patient develops signs of overdosage. Be prepared to treat overdosage with antithyroid drugs.

—Assist the patient with activities as needed until a euthyroid state is achieved.

—Obtain an order for an antiemetic or antidiarrheal agent, as needed.

—Administer a mild analgesic as prescribed if drug-induced headache occurs.

—Keep the patient dry if profuse sweating occurs.

—Keep all members of the health care team informed of the patient's response to the drug.

Patient teaching

—Inform the patient and family about levothyroxine, including the dosage, frequency, action, and adverse reactions.

—Instruct the patient to take the medication at the same time each day; encourage morning dosing to avoid insomnia.

—Tell the patient to notify doctor if he experiences headache, diarrhea, nervousness, excessive sweating, heat intolerance, chest pain, increased pulse rate, or palpitations.

—Advise the patient not to store the drug in warm, humid areas, such as the bathroom, to prevent deterioration of the drug.

—Tell the patient who has achieved a stable response not to change product brands, because they are not all bioequivalent.

—Warn female patients that levothyroxine may cause menstrual irregularities.

— Stress the importance of taking the drug exactly as prescribed and of receiving follow-up care.

— Tell the patient to notify the nurse or doctor if adverse reactions develop or questions arise about levothyroxine therapy.

Evaluation

In the patient receiving levothyroxine, appropriate evaluation statements include:

• Patient is able to perform activities without assistance.

• Patient does not exhibit signs and symptoms of levothyroxine overdosage.

• Patient and family state an understanding of levothyroxine therapy.

SELECTED MAJOR DRUGS: THYROID HORMONES

DRUG, INDICATIONS, AND DOSAGES	SPECIAL PRECAUTIONS
liothyronine sodium (Cytomel) *Cretinism—* **Children age 3 and older:** 50 to 100 mcg P.O. daily. **Children under age 3:** 5 mcg P.O. daily, increased by 5 mcg q 3 to 4 days until desired response occurs. *Myxedema—* **Adults:** initially, 5 mcg P.O. daily, increased by 5 to 10 mcg q 1 to 2 weeks. Maintenance dosage is 50 to 100 mcg daily. *Nontoxic goiter—* **Adults:** initially, 5 mcg P.O. daily; may be increased by 12.5 to 25 mcg daily q 1 to 2 weeks. Usual maintenance dosage is 75 mcg daily. **Adults over age 65:** initially, 5 mcg P.O. daily, increased by 5-mcg increments at weekly intervals until desired response occurs. **Children:** initially, 5 mcg P.O. daily, increased by 5-mcg increments at weekly intervals until desired response occurs. *Thyroid hormone replacement—* **Adults:** initially, 25 mcg P.O. daily, increased by 12.5 to 25 mcg q 1 to 2 weeks until satisfactory response occurs. Usual maintenance dosage is 25 to 75 mcg daily. *T_3 suppression test to differentiate hyperthyroidism from euthyroidism—* **Adults:** 75 to 100 mcg P.O. daily for 7 days.	• Contraindicated in patients with MI, thyrotoxicosis (except when administered with antithyroid drugs), or uncorrected adrenal insufficiency (thyroid hormones increase tissue demand for corticotropin and may cause acute adrenal crisis). • Use with extreme caution in patients with angina pectoris, hypertension, or other cardiovascular disorders; renal insufficiency; or ischemic states.
thyroglobulin (Proloid) *Cretinism and juvenile hypothyroidism—* **Children age 1 and older:** dosage may approach adult dosage (60 to 180 mg P.O. daily), depending on response. **Children age 4 to 12 months:** 60 to 80 mg P.O. daily. **Children age 1 to 4 months:** initially, 15 to 30 mg P.O. daily, increased at 2-week intervals. Usual maintenance dosage is 30 to 45 mg P.O. daily.	• Contraindicated in patients with MI, thyrotoxicosis (except when administered with antithyroid drugs), or uncorrected adrenal insufficiency (thyroid hormones increase tissue demand for corticotropin and may cause acute adrenal crisis). • Use with extreme caution in

(continued)

SELECTED MAJOR DRUGS: THYROID HORMONES *continued*

DRUG, INDICATIONS, AND DOSAGES	SPECIAL PRECAUTIONS
thyroglobulin *(continued)* *Hypothyroidism or myxedema—* **Adults:** initially, 15 to 30 mg P.O. daily, increased by 15 to 30 mg at 2-week intervals until desired response occurs. Usual maintenance dosage is 60 to 180 mg P.O. daily, as a single dose. **Adults over age 65:** initially, 7.5 to 15 mg P.O. daily; dosage is doubled at 6- to 8-week intervals until desired response is obtained.	patients with angina pectoris, hypertension, or other cardiovascular disorders; renal insufficiency; or ischemic states.
thyroid USP (desiccated) (Armour Thyroid, S-P-T, Thyrar) *Adult hypothyroidism—* **Adults:** initially, 60 mg P.O. daily, increased by 60 mg q 30 days until desired response occurs. Usual maintenance dosage is 60 to 180 mg P.O. daily, as a single dose. **Adults over age 65:** 7.5 to 15 mg P.O. daily; dosage is doubled at 6- to 8-week intervals. *Adult myxedema—* **Adults:** 16 mg P.O. daily. May double dosage q 2 weeks to maximum 120 mg. *Cretinism and juvenile hypothyroidism—* **Children age 1 and older:** dosage may approach adult dosage (60 to 180 mg P.O. daily), depending on response. **Children age 4 to 12 months:** 30 to 60 mg P.O. daily. **Children age 1 to 4 months:** initially, 15 to 30 mg P.O. daily, increased at 2-week intervals. Usual maintenance dosage is 30 to 45 mg P.O. daily.	• Contraindicated in patients with MI, thyrotoxicosis (except when administered with antithyroid drugs), or uncorrected adrenal insufficiency (thyroid hormones increase tissue demand for corticotropin and may cause acute adrenal crisis). • Use with extreme caution in patients with angina pectoris, hypertension, or other cardiovascular disorders; renal insufficiency; or ischemic states.
thyrotropin (Thytropar) *Diagnosis of thyroid cancer remnant with I[131] after surgery—* **Adults:** 10 IU I.M. or S.C. for 3 to 7 days. *Differential diagnosis of primary and secondary hypothyroidism—* **Adults:** 10 IU I.M. or S.C. for 1 to 3 days. *In PBI or I[131] uptake determinations for differential diagnosis of subclinical hypothyroidism or low thyroid reserve—* **Adults:** 10 IU I.M. or S.C. *Therapy for thyroid carcinoma (local or metastatic) with I[131]—* **Adults:** 10 IU I.M. or S.C. for 3 to 8 days. *To determine thyroid status of patient receiving thyroid—* **Adults:** 10 IU I.M. or S.C. for 1 to 3 days.	• Contraindicated in patients with coronary thrombosis and untreated Addison's disease. • Use cautiously in patients with angina pectoris, CHF, hypopituitarism, or adrenocortical suppression.

COMPARING THYROID HORMONE COMBINATIONS

THYROID EQUIVALENT	TRADE NAME	LIOTRIX COMPONENTS T₃	T₄
15 mg (¼ grain)	Thyrolar-¼	3.1 mcg	12.5 mcg
30 mg (½ grain)	Thyrolar-½ Euthroid-½	6.25 mcg 7.5 mcg	25 mcg 30 mcg
60 mg (1 grain)	Thyrolar-1 Euthroid-1	12.5 mcg 15 mcg	50 mcg 60 mcg
120 mg (2 grains)	Thyrolar-2 Euthroid-2	25 mcg 30 mcg	100 mcg 120 mcg
180 mg (3 grains)	Thyrolar-3 Euthroid-3	37.5 mcg 60 mcg	150 mg 180 mcg

SELF-TEST

1. Martha Stymo, age 48, has just begun treatment of hypothyroidism with levothyroxine 0.025 mg P.O. daily. As you assess Ms. Stymo, which of the following would indicate a therapeutic response to the drug?
   a. weight gain
   b. lethargy
   c. complaints of depression
   d. an increase in activity

2. As you assess Ms. Stymo, which of the following would indicate an overdosage of the drug?
   a. constipation
   b. bradycardia
   c. drowsiness
   d. nervousness or tremor

3. Ms. Stymo also has a history of a seizure disorder. If Ms. Stymo were to receive I.V. phenytoin while taking levothyroxine, which of the following drug interactions could occur?
   a. free-thyroid release
   b. reduced effectiveness of levothyroxine
   c. increased potency of phenytoin
   d. delayed excretion of levothyroxine

Check your answers on page 1071.

CHAPTER 58

THYROID HORMONE ANTAGONISTS

iodine ♦ radioactive iodine (sodium iodide) [131]I
methimazole ♦ propylthiouracil (PTU)

OVERVIEW
- Thyroid hormone antagonists, or antithyroid agents, are used to treat hyperthyroidism. Some antagonists, such as iodine and the thioamides (methimazole and propylthiouracil), have reversible effects and may be used in a young patient or one in whom hyperthyroidism is not necessarily permanent. They do not permanently affect the thyroid, but control hormone production until spontaneous remission of hyperthyroidism.
- Radiation therapy (with radioactive iodine) and thyroidectomy (partial or total) are definitive treatments for hyperthyroidism. Both procedures are reserved for adults who may not respond to milder agents; unfortunately, both carry a long-term risk of hypothyroidism.

MAJOR USES
- Iodine, methimazole, and propylthiouracil are used to treat hyperthyroidism (Graves' disease, multinodular goiter, and thyroiditis) in children, pregnant women, and patients in whom the condition is permanent or in whom thyroidectomy is contraindicated. These agents also help prepare patients for thyroidectomy and are effective for thyrotoxic crisis.
- Iodine combats lethal thyrotoxic crisis in adults and neonates. It is used preoperatively to decrease vascularity of the thyroid gland. It may also be used to produce thyroid-blocking effects during a radiation emergency. Radioactive iodine is usually therapeutic for hyperthyroidism in adults when surgical treatment is contraindicated. However, it is not used in pregnant women. Radioactive iodine is also used as a diagnostic tracer in thyroid function disorders and as a therapeutic adjunct after thyroidectomy for thyroid cancer. It causes ablation of any residual thyroid tissue. It can also be used to treat thyroid-cancer metastases.

MECHANISM OF ACTION
- Iodine inhibits thyroid hormone formation by blocking iodotyrosine and iodothyronine synthesis. It also limits iodide transport into the thyroid gland and blocks thyroid hormone release.
- Radioactive iodine limits thyroid hormone secretion by destroying thyroid tissue. The affinity of thyroid tissue for radioactive iodine facilitates uptake of the drug by metastatic thyroid tissue.

GLOSSARY

Hyperthyroidism: state of accelerated thyroid function with unknown cause.
Iodism: toxicity from excessive ingestion of iodine, characterized by glandular atrophy, coryza, frontal headache, emaciation, weakness, and skin eruptions.
Thyroiditis: thyroid gland inflammation.
Thyrotoxicosis: disorder caused by thyroid gland overactivity; hyperthyroidism.

• The thioamides inhibit oxidation of iodine in the thyroid gland, blocking iodine's ability to combine with tyrosine to form levothyronine. They may also prevent the coupling of monoiodotyrosine and diiodotyrosine to form levothyroxine and triiodothyronine.

ABSORPTION, DISTRIBUTION, METABOLISM, AND EXCRETION

Methimazole and propylthiouracil are readily absorbed from the GI tract and metabolized in the liver. Their metabolites are excreted in urine; however, 35% of propylthiouracil is excreted unchanged.

Iodine and radioactive iodine is rapidly absorbed. It is trapped in the thyroid gland within 30 minutes of oral administration and incorporated into the thyroid follicles; it is excreted in urine.

ONSET AND DURATION

Action of the thioamides may not be apparent for days or weeks—until the stored supply of thyroid hormones is depleted. The half-life of propylthiouracil is 2 hours; that of methimazole, 6 to 9 hours. After correction of the abnormally high metabolic rate (as in hyperthyroidism), the half-lives of these drugs may increase, allowing lower doses. Patients with severe hyperthyroidism respond most rapidly, usually in 1 or 2 days.

Radioactive iodine's action may not begin for weeks, so watch for potentially serious thyrotoxic reactions that may occur during the first few days of treatment. Radioactive iodine has a half-life of 8 days.

Iodine's effects are evident within 24 hours after administration. Peak effects occur after 10 to 15 days of daily dosing.

ADVERSE REACTIONS

Therapeutic doses of thyroid hormone antagonists can cause fever, chills, sore throat, weakness, backache, swelling of ankles or feet, or joint pain. Toxic doses can cause constipation; cold intolerance; dry, puffy skin; headache; sleepiness; muscle aches; and unusual weight gain.

Methimazole and propylthiouracil may cause agranulocytosis. Therefore, close monitoring of WBC count is recommended, at least for the first 3 months of therapy. Other severe reactions may include aplastic anemia, hepatitis, or exfoliative dermatitis.

METHIMAZOLE
(meth im′a zole)
Tapazole
Classification: thyroid hormone antagonist
Pregnancy risk category D

How supplied
TABLETS: 5 mg, 10 mg

Indications and dosage
Hyperthyroidism
ADULTS: 5 mg P.O. t.i.d. if mild; 10 to 15 mg P.O. t.i.d. if moderately severe; and 20 mg P.O. t.i.d. if severe. Continue until patient is euthyroid, then start maintenance dosage of 5 mg daily to t.i.d. Maximum dosage 150 mg daily.
CHILDREN: 0.4 mg/kg P.O. daily in divided doses q 8 hours. Continue until patient is euthyroid, then start maintenance dosage of 0.2 mg/kg daily in divided doses q 8 hours.

Preparation for thyroidectomy
ADULTS AND CHILDREN: same doses as for hyperthyroidism until patient is euthyroid; then iodine may be added for 10 days before surgery.

Thyrotoxic crisis
ADULTS AND CHILDREN: same doses as for hyperthyroidism, with concomitant iodine therapy and propranolol.

Contraindications and precautions
Methimazole is contraindicated in patients with known hypersensitivity to the drug and during lactation. Use cautiously in pregnancy.

Adverse reactions
BLOOD: **agranulocytosis,** leukopenia, thrombocytopenia (appear to be dose-related).
CNS: headache, drowsiness, vertigo.
GI: diarrhea, nausea, vomiting (may be dose-related).
HEPATIC: jaundice.
SKIN: rash, urticaria, skin discoloration.
OTHER: arthralgia, myalgia, salivary gland enlargement, loss of taste, drug fever, lymphadenopathy.

Interactions
None significant.

Nursing considerations
Assessment
• Review the patient's history for a condition that contraindicates the use of methimazole.

Boldfaced adverse reactions are life-threatening

- Obtain a baseline assessment of the patient's thyroid function before initiating methimazole therapy.
- Be alert for common adverse reactions.
- Evaluate the patient's and family's knowledge about methimazole.

Planning (Nursing Diagnoses)

Potential nursing diagnoses for the patient receiving methimazole include:
- Altered health maintenance related to ineffectiveness of methimazole to control hyperthyroid signs and symptoms.
- Diarrhea related to methimazole-induced GI reaction.
- Knowledge deficit related to methimazole therapy.

Implementation

Preparation and administration

— Store in light-resistant container.
— Give with meals to reduce adverse GI reactions.

Monitoring

— Monitor the effectiveness of therapy by regularly assessing patient's thyroid function studies and signs and symptoms for hyperthyroidism. Be aware that euthyroidism may take several months to develop.
— Monitor the patient for adverse drug reactions.
— Monitor for signs of hypothyroidism (mental depression; cold intolerance; hard, nonpitting edema). Dosage adjustment may be required.
— Monitor CBC periodically to detect impending leukopenia, thrombocytopenia, and agranulocytosis. Dosage that exceeds 30 mg/day increases the risk of agranulocytosis.
— Monitor the patient's hydration status if GI reactions occur.
— Monitor skin color for changes.
— Monitor the patient's temperature for drug-induced fever.
— Regularly reevaluate the patient's and family's knowledge about methimazole.

Intervention

— Withhold methimazole therapy if severe rash or enlarged cervical lymph nodes develop.
— Notify the doctor if the patient shows signs and symptoms of hypothyroidism; if so, dosage reduction will be required.
— Institute safety precautions if adverse CNS reactions occur.
— Obtain an order for an antiemetic or antidiarrheal agent, as needed.
— Keep all members of the health care team informed of the patient's response to the drug.

Patient teaching

— Inform the patient and family about methimazole, including the dosage, frequency, action, and adverse reactions.
— Tell the patient to take drug at regular intervals around the clock and to take it at the same time each day in relation to meals.
— If GI upset occurs, tell the patient to take drug with meals.

—Tell the patient to ask doctor whether he should use iodized salt or eat shellfish during treatment.

—Warn the patient not to use self-prescribed cough medicines; many contain iodine.

—Tell the patient to notify doctor promptly if fever, sore throat, malaise, unusual bleeding, yellowing of eyes, nausea, or vomiting occurs.

—Advise the patient not to store drug in bathroom; heat and humidity cause it to deteriorate.

—Have the patient check with the doctor before undergoing surgery (including dental surgery).

—Teach the patient how to recognize the signs of hyperthyroidism and hypothyroidism and what to do if they occur.

—Tell the patient to notify the nurse or doctor if adverse reactions develop or questions arise about methimazole therapy.

Evaluation

In the patient receiving methimazole, appropriate evaluation statements include:

• Patient is euthyroid with methimazole therapy.

• Patient does not experience diarrhea.

• Patient and family state an understanding of methimazole therapy.

SELECTED MAJOR DRUGS: THYROID HORMONE ANTAGONISTS

DRUG, INDICATIONS, AND DOSAGES	SPECIAL PRECAUTIONS
strong iodine solution (Lugol's Solution) *Preparation for thyroidectomy—* **Adults and children:** Strong Iodine Solution, USP, 0.1 to 0.3 ml P.O. t.i.d., or Potassium Iodide Solution, USP, 5 drops in water P.O. t.i.d. after meals for 2 to 3 weeks before surgery. *Thyrotoxic crisis—* **Adults and children:** Strong Iodine Solution, USP, 1 ml in water P.O. t.i.d. after meals. *Radiation protectant for thyroid gland—* **Adults:** 100 to 150 mg P.O. 24 hours before and for 3 to 10 days after radiation exposure *Expectorant—* **Adults:** 0.3 to 0.6 ml SSKI diluted in water t.i.d. or q.i.d.	• Contraindicated in patients with tuberculosis, iodide hypersensitivity, or hyperkalemia; after meals that contain excessive starch; and in patients with laryngeal edema or swelling of salivary glands.
propylthiouracil (PTU) *Hyperthyroidism—* **Adults:** 100 mg P.O. t.i.d.; up to 300 mg q 8 hours have been used. Continue until patient is euthyroid, then start maintenance dosage of 100 mg daily to t.i.d. **Children over age 10:** 100 mg P.O. t.i.d. Continue until patient is euthyroid, then start maintenance dosage of 25 mg t.i.d. to 100 mg b.i.d. **Children ages 6 to 10:** 50 to 150 mg P.O. divided q 8 hours.	• Use cautiously in pregnant women because they may require less drug as pregnancy progresses. Monitor thyroid function studies closely. Thyroid hormone replacement may be added to regimen. Drug may be discontinued during last few weeks of pregnancy.

SELECTED MAJOR DRUGS: THYROID HORMONE ANTAGONISTS
continued

DRUG, INDICATIONS, AND DOSAGES	SPECIAL PRECAUTIONS
propylthiouracil *(continued)* *Preparation for thyroidectomy—* **Adults and children:** same doses as for hyperthyroidism; then iodine may be added 10 days before surgery. *Thyrotoxic crisis—* **Adults and children:** same doses as for hyperthyroidism, with concomitant iodine therapy and propranolol.	
radioactive iodine (sodium iodide) (Iodotope Therapeutic) *Hyperthyroidism—* **Adults:** usual dosage is 4 to 10 mCi P.O., based on weight of thyroid gland and thyroid uptake. Treatment may be repeated after 6 weeks, depending on thyroxine level. *Thyroid cancer—* **Adults:** 50 to 150 mCi P.O. Dosage based on estimated malignant thyroid tissue and metastatic tissue as determined by total body scan. Treatment may be repeated.	• Contraindicated in pregnant and breast-feeding women unless used to treat thyroid cancer.

SELF-TEST

1. Brendan Bonae, age 58, is taking methimazole for treatment of hyperthyroidism. You will explain that the potential adverse reactions to this new medication include:
   a. hyperglycemia.
   b. an enhanced sense of taste.
   c. nausea, vomiting, and diarrhea.
   d. arrhythmias.

2. Patient teaching about methimazole should include:
   a. types of drug interactions.
   b. need to increase use of iodized salt in diet.
   c. importance of taking drug at bedtime.
   d. symptoms of hypothyroidism and hyperthyroidism that the patient should monitor for.

3. At his doctor's request, you instruct Mr. Bonae to avoid iodized salt. Why would this be necessary?
   a. Iodized salt would counteract the effects of the drug.
   b. Iodized salt would decrease the maintenance dosage.
   c. Iodized salt would increase the incidence of adverse reactions.
   d. Iodized salt would alter the medication's excretion.

Check your answers on page 1071.

CHAPTER 59

PITUITARY HORMONES

corticotropin (ACTH) ◆ cosyntropin ◆ desmopressin acetate
lypressin ◆ somatrem ◆ somatropin ◆ vasopressin (antidiuretic hormone)

OVERVIEW

- The pituitary hormones fall into three groups according to use: Corticotropin and cosyntropin are used to diagnose primary adrenal insufficiency; somatrem and somatropin are recombinant human growth hormones. They spur growth in patients with pituitary growth deficiency. Vasopressin and its synthetic derivatives, desmopressin acetate and lypressin regulate water balance in patients with diabetes insipidus. All these hormones are either natural pituitary extracts or synthetic derivatives.
- The pituitary gland is the most complex endocrine structure in the body. Its two major divisions are the anterior lobe (adenohypophysis) and the posterior lobe (neurohypophysis). Except for melanocyte-stimulating hormone—which is not commercially available—and somatotropin (human growth hormone), the anterior lobe secretes tropic (primary) hormones that activate other organs (target glands) to secrete their characteristic hormones, called genic (secondary) hormones.
- Extract from the posterior lobe may be divided into two active components: vasopressin (primarily associated with pressor and antidiuretic activities) and oxytocin (primarily associated with pronounced uterine-contracting and milk-releasing action). For more information on oxytocin, see Chapter 88, Oxytocics and Tocolytics.

MAJOR USES

- Corticotropin and cosyntropin act as screening agents for primary adrenal insufficiency.
- Desmopressin, lypressin, and vasopressin combat symptoms of central diabetes insipidus.
- Somatrem and somatropin are used to treat growth impairment due to growth hormone deficiency.

MECHANISM OF ACTION

- Corticotropin and cosyntropin, by replacing the body's own tropic hormone, stimulate the adrenal cortex to secrete its entire spectrum of hormones.

GLOSSARY

Diabetes insipidus: metabolic disorder characterized by extreme polyuria and polydipsia from deficient secretion of antidiuretic hormone
(ADH) or the inability of kidney tubules to respond to ADH.

- Desmopressin, lypressin, and vasopressin increase the permeability of
the renal tubular epithelium to adenosine monophosphate and water; the
epithelium promotes reabsorption of water and produces a concentrated
urine (antidiuretic hormone effect).
- Lypressin and vasopressin cause contraction of smooth muscle in the
vascular bed (vasopressor effect). Vasopressin also causes contraction
of smooth muscle in the GI tract.
- Somatrem and somatropin stimulate linear growth in patients with
pituitary growth deficiency by various mechanisms. These include facilitating intracellular transport of amino acids; increasing intestinal absorption and urinary excretion of calcium; increasing renal tubular
reabsorption of phosphorus and decreasing that of calcium; promoting
synthesis of collagen and chondroitin, which form cartilage; and inhibiting intracellular glucose metabolism.

ABSORPTION, DISTRIBUTION, METABOLISM, AND EXCRETION

Corticotropin is destroyed in the GI tract after oral administration but is
well absorbed parenterally. The parenteral form is well distributed and
inactivated in body tissues and excreted in urine.

Cosyntropin is destroyed by the proteolytic enzymes of the GI tract and
so must be given either I.M. or I.V. It is inactivated in the tissues and
excreted in urine.

Desmopressin and lypressin, because they are inactivated in the GI tract
by the enzyme trypsin, are given intranasally. Absorption through the nasal
mucosa is usually adequate but is decreased in patients with nasal congestion, rhinitis, or upper respiratory tract infection.

Desmopressin and lypressin are distributed throughout the extracellular
fluid, metabolized in the liver and kidneys, and excreted in urine.

Somatrem and somatropin are destroyed in the GI tract after oral
administration but are well distributed to the body tissues after S.C. or I.M.
administration. They are metabolized in the liver and excreted in urine.

Vasopressin is distributed throughout the extracellular fluid, metabolized in the liver and kidneys, and excreted in urine.

ONSET AND DURATION

Corticotropin begins to work within 5 minutes and lasts 3 to 25 hours,
depending on dose and route of administration.

Cosyntropin, as reflected by plasma cortisol levels, has an onset within
5 minutes, peaks within 1 hour, and lasts 4 hours.

Desmopressin and lypressin take effect within 1 hour. Desmopressin peaks in 1 to 5 hours and lasts 8 to 20 hours. Lypressin lasts 3 to 8 hours.

Somatrem and somatropin take effect immediately; their action lasts several days.

Vasopressin (aqueous solution) takes effect within 1 hour and lasts 2 to 8 hours when given subcutaneously, and 6 to 12 hours when given I.V.

ADVERSE REACTIONS

The most common adverse reactions to the pituitary hormones reflect an extension of their pharmacologic effects.

Adverse reactions to corticotropin and cosyntropin are related to prolonged use, which may result in hypothalamic-pituitary-adrenal axis suppression, increased risk of hypersensitivity reactions, posterior subscapular cataracts, and glaucoma. These agents are also potent immunosuppressants; prolonged high-dose therapy is associated with an increased risk of infection. These agents may also cause metabolic disturbances, including fluid and electrolyte imbalances. They are usually well tolerated when used as diagnostic agents.

Vasopressin and its derivatives (desmopressin and lypressin) can cause water intoxication secondary to excessive fluid retention. These drugs can precipitate anginal pain; in higher doses, they can cause MI. They cause vasoconstriction, which can raise blood pressure or cause alterations in local tissue integrity. Desmopressin, given intranasally, can cause local burning or pain. Vasopressin derivatives administered I.V. can cause severe vasoconstriction and local tissue necrosis if the infusion extravasates.

PROTOTYPE: PITUITARY HORMONES

DESMOPRESSIN ACETATE
(des moe press'in)
DDAVP, Minirin‡, Stimate
Classification: pituitary hormone
Pregnancy risk category B

How supplied
NASAL SOLUTION: 0.1 mg/ml
INJECTION: 4 mcg/ml

Indications and dosage
Nonnephrogenic diabetes insipidus, temporary polyuria and polydipsia associated with pituitary trauma
ADULTS: 0.1 to 0.4 ml intranasally daily in one to three doses. Adjust morning and evening doses separately for adequate diurnal rhythm of water turnover. Alternatively, may administer injectable form in dosage

of 0.5 to 1 ml I.V. or S.C. daily, usually in two divided doses.
CHILDREN AGE 3 MONTHS TO 12 YEARS: 0.05 to 0.3 ml intranasally daily in one or two doses.

Treatment of hemophilia A and von Willebrand's disease
ADULTS AND CHILDREN: 0.3 mcg/kg diluted in normal saline and infused I.V. slowly over 15 to 30 minutes. May repeat dose if necessary as indicated by laboratory response and the patient's clinical condition.

Primary nocturnal enuresis
CHILDREN AGE 5 AND OLDER: initially, 20 mcg intranasally h.s. Adjust dose according to response. Maximum recommended dose is 40 mcg daily.

Contraindications and precautions
Desmopressin is contraindicated in patients with known hypersensitivity to the drug. Use with caution in patients with coronary artery insufficiency or hypertensive cardiovascular disease.

Adverse reactions
CNS: headache.
CV: slight rise in blood pressure at high doses.
EENT: nasal congestion, rhinitis.
GI: nausea.
GU: vulval pain.
OTHER: flushing.

Interactions
None significant.

Nursing considerations
Assessment
- Review the patient's history for a condition that contraindicates the use of desmopressin.
- Obtain a baseline assessment of the patient's underlying condition before initiating desmopressin therapy.
- Be alert for common adverse reactions.
- Evaluate the patient's and family's knowledge about desmopressin.

Planning (Nursing Diagnoses)
Potential nursing diagnoses for the patient receiving desmopressin include:
- Fluid volume deficit related to ineffectiveness or improper administration of desmopressin for treatment of diabetes insipidus.
- Knowledge deficit related to desmopressin therapy.

Implementation
Preparation and administration
— Check expiration date before administering.
— When intranasal route is prescribed, administer desmopressin through a flexible catheter called a rhinyle. Draw up the correct dosage into the catheter, and insert one end into the patient's nose. The patient blows on the other end to deposit the drug into the nasal cavity.

— When desmopressin is used to treat diabetes insipidus, dosage or frequency of administration may be adjusted according to the patient's fluid output; adjust morning and evening doses separately for adequate diurnal rhythm of water turnover.

— For treating nocturnal enuresis, the recommended method of administration is one-half of the calculated dose in each nostril.

— Do not administer a desmopressin injection to treat hemophilia A with Factor VIII levels of 0% to 5%, or in severe cases of von Willebrand's disease.

Monitoring

— Monitor the effectiveness of therapy by regularly monitoring the patient's intake and output, serum and urine osmolality, and urine specific gravity for treatment of diabetes insipidus or alleviation of symptoms of other disorders.

— Monitor the patient for adverse drug reactions.

— Monitor for early signs of water intoxication—drowsiness, listlessness, headache, confusion, anuria, and weight gain—to prevent seizures, coma, and death.

— Monitor the patient's weight daily and observe for edema.

— Monitor carefully for hypertension during high-dose treatment.

— Regularly reevaluate the patient's and family's knowledge about desmopressin.

Intervention

— Adjust the patient's fluid intake to reduce risk of water intoxication and of sodium depletion, especially in young or elderly patients.

— Overdose may cause oxytocic or vasopressor activity. Withhold drug as prescribed until effects subside. Furosemide may be administered if fluid retention is excessive.

— Be aware that intranasal use can cause changes in the nasal mucosa resulting in erratic, unreliable absorption. Report any patient's worsening condition to doctor, who may prescribe injectable DDAVP.

— Administer a mild analgesic for drug-induced headache, if not contraindicated.

— Offer patient ice chips or frequent sips of water if nausea occurs. If nausea persists or becomes severe, obtain an order for an antiemetic.

— Keep all members of the health care team informed of the patient's response to the drug.

Patient teaching

— Inform the patient and family about desmopressin, including the dosage, frequency, action, and adverse reactions.

— Some patients may have difficulty measuring and inhaling drug into nostrils. Teach them correct administration technique, then evaluate their proficiency at drug administration and accurate measurement on return visits.

— Emphasize that the patient should not increase or decrease dosage unless instructed by doctor.

— Review methods for measuring fluid output with patient.

— Tell the patient to contact doctor if signs of water intoxication (drowsiness, listlessness, headache, or shortness of breath) develop.

— Advise the patient to wear medical alert identification.

— Instruct the patient to clear nasal passages before administering drug. This clears area for absorption of the drug.

— Teach patients using S.C. desmopressin to rotate injection sites to prevent tissue damage.

— Nasal congestion, allergic rhinitis, or upper respiratory infections may impair drug absorption. Advise the patient to report such conditions to the doctor because they may require dosage adjustment.

— Tell the patient to notify the nurse or doctor if adverse reactions develop or questions arise about desmopressin therapy.

— Tell patient to store drug away from heat and direct light. Do not store in bathroom, where heat and moisture can cause drug to deteriorate.

Evaluation

In the patient receiving desmopressin, appropriate evaluation statements include:

• Patient achieves normal fluid and electrolyte balance.

• Patient and family state an understanding of desmopressin therapy.

SELECTED MAJOR DRUGS: PITUITARY HORMONES

DRUG, INDICATIONS, AND DOSAGES	SPECIAL PRECAUTIONS
corticotropin (ACTH, Acthar, Cortrophin Gel) *Diagnostic test of adrenocortical function—* **Adults:** up to 80 units I.M. or S.C. in divided doses; or a single dose of repository form; or 10 to 25 units (aqueous form) in 500 ml dextrose 5% in water I.V. over 8 hours, between blood samplings. Individual dosages generally vary with adrenal glands' sensitivity to stimulation as well as with specific disease. Infants and younger children require larger doses per kilogram than do older children and adults. *For therapeutic use—* **Adults:** 40 units S.C. or I.M. in four individual doses (aqueous); 40 units q 12 to 24 hours (gel or repository form).	• Contraindicated in patients with scleroderma, osteoporosis, systemic fungal infections, ocular herpes simplex, recent surgery, peptic ulcer, CHF, hypertension, sensitivity to pork and pork products, adrenocortical hyperfunction or primary insufficiency, or Cushing's syndrome. • Use cautiously in pregnant or breast-feeding women; in patients being immunized; and in those with latent tuberculosis or tuberculin reactivity, hypothyroidism, cirrhosis, infection, acute gouty arthritis, emotional instability or psychotic tendencies, diabetes, renal insufficiency, or myasthenia gravis.
lypressin (Diapid) *Nonnephrogenic diabetes insipidus—* **Adults and children:** 1 or 2 sprays (approximately 2 USP posterior pituitary pressor units/spray) in either or both nostrils q.i.d. and an additional dose h.s., if needed, to prevent nocturia. If usual dosage is inadequate, in-	• Contraindicated in patients with known hypersensitivity to lypressin. • Use cautiously in patients with coronary artery disease.

(continued)

SELECTED MAJOR DRUGS: PITUITARY HORMONES *continued*

DRUG, INDICATIONS, AND DOSAGES	SPECIAL PRECAUTIONS

lypressin *(continued)*
crease frequency of administration, not the number of sprays.

---

vasopressin (antidiuretic hormone) (Pitressin)
Nonnephrogenic, nonpsychogenic diabetes insipidus—
Adults: 5 to 10 units I.M. or S.C. b.i.d. to q.i.d., p.r.n.; or intranasally (aqueous solution used as spray or applied to cotton balls) in individualized doses, based on response.
Children: 2.5 to 10 units I.M. or S.C. b.i.d. to q.i.d., p.r.n.; or intranasally (aqueous solution used as spray or applied to cotton balls) in individualized doses.
Postoperative abdominal distention—
Adults: initially, 5 units I.M., then q 3 to 4 hours, increasing dose to 10 units, if needed. Reduce dose proportionately for children.
To expel gas before abdominal X-ray—
Adults: inject 10 units S.C. 2 hours before, then again 30 minutes before X-ray. Enema before first dose may also help to eliminate gas.
Upper GI tract hemorrhage—
Adults: 0.2 to 0.4 units/minute by intra-arterial injection.

• Contraindicated in patients with chronic nephritis with nitrogen retention.
• Use cautiously in children or elderly patients, pregnant women, and those with seizure disorders, migraine, asthma, CV disease, or fluid overload.

SELF-TEST

1. Amelia Primig, age 42, is diagnosed with diabetes insipidus, for which her doctor prescribes intranasal desmopressin. Which of the following conditions require cautious use of this agent?
   a. diabetes mellitus
   b. hypertensive cardiovascular disease
   c. asthma
   d. renal failure

2. Your patient teaching about potential adverse reactions to desmopressin should include which of the following?
   a. nasal congestion
   b. seizures
   c. hypotension
   d. hypercalcemia

3. What should the nurse tell Ms. Primig to do when administering intranasal desmopressin?
   a. She should clear the nasal passages.
   b. She should lie down to administer drug.
   c. She should drink a glass of water.
   d. She should blow nose immediately afterward.

Check your answers on pages 1071 and 1072.

CHAPTER 60

CALCITONIN AND HYPOCALCEMIC AGENTS

calcitonin (human) ◆ calcitonin (salmon) ◆ etidronate disodium
gallium nitrate

OVERVIEW

- The body has an exceptional capacity to ensure normal serum calcium levels. Normally, calcium homeostasis is regulated by the kidneys and GI tract. When these regulatory mechanisms fail (for example, because of cancer), drug therapy may be necessary to restore normal calcium levels.
- Calcitonin is a hormone secreted by the parafollicular cells of the thyroid gland. It immediately lowers higher-than-normal serum calcium levels.
- Etidronate, a synthetic compound, acts primarily on the bones to lower serum calcium levels.
- Gallium nitrate reduces blood calcium levels by an unknown mechanism. It apparently decreases osteolysis, thereby reducing calcium resorption from bone.

MAJOR USES

- Calcitonin reduces serum calcium levels in acute hypercalcemia.
- Calcitonin and etidronate combat Paget's disease (osteitis deformans).
- Gallium nitrate is used to treat symptomatic cancer-related hypercalcemia unresponsive to other treatments.

MECHANISM OF ACTION

- Calcitonin and etidronate decrease osteoclastic activity by inhibiting osteolysis. They also decrease mineral release and matrix or collagen breakdown in bone.
- Gallium nitrate decreases osteolysis. By preventing calcium release as bone is resorbed, it decreases serum calcium levels.

ABSORPTION, DISTRIBUTION, METABOLISM, AND EXCRETION

Calcitonin is well absorbed after S.C. or I.M. administration. Because it's destroyed in the GI tract, it must be given parenterally. Calcitonin is metabolized by the kidneys and excreted in urine.

Etidronate is absorbed from the GI tract. It is excreted in the urine as unchanged drug. A small amount is excreted in the feces.

Gallium nitrate is administered I.V. It is not metabolized and is primarily excreted in the urine.

ONSET AND DURATION

Calcitonin's onset after I.V. administration is 15 minutes; its duration is 30 minutes to 12 hours. After I.M. or S.C. injection, onset is 4 hours and duration is 8 to 24 hours.

Etidronate begins to work after 1 to 3 months. Maximal therapeutic activity occurs in about 6 months.

Gallium nitrate effect is usually evident within 5 days of daily therapy.

ADVERSE REACTIONS

Calcitonin and related agents can cause hypocalcemia as an extension of their pharmacologic effects. Because such hypocalcemia can be severe and life-threatening, close supervision of therapy, with frequent monitoring of serum calcium levels, is recommended. Alterations of other serum electrolytes (such as bicarbonate or phosphate) may also occur. Many patients with Paget's disease experience increased bone pain after treatment with these agents.

About 50% of patients treated with calcitonin (salmon) develop circulating antibodies to the drug within 2 to 18 months of initiating therapy. Commonly, this has little impact on therapy; however, some patients develop resistance to the hypocalcemic effects of the drug because of this immune response. This immune effect is rare with etidronate disodium.

Gallium nitrate can cause severe renal insufficiency, especially in patients treated with nephrotoxic antineoplastic medications, and requires close monitoring of renal function.

PROTOTYPE: CALCITONIN

CALCITONIN (HUMAN)
(kal si toe′nin)
Cibacalcin

CALCITONIN (SALMON)
Calcimar, Miacalcin
Classification: calcitonin
Pregnancy risk category B

How supplied
INJECTION: 0.5 mg/vial (human); 100 IU/ml, 200 IU/ml (salmon)

Indications and dosage
Paget's disease of bone (osteitis deformans)
ADULTS: initially, 100 IU of calcitonin (salmon) S.C. or I.M. daily. Maintenance dosage is 50 to 100 IU daily or every other day. Alternatively, give calcitonin (human) 0.5 mg S.C. daily. If patient improvement is sufficient, dosage may be reduced to 0.25 mg daily two or three times per week. Some patients may need as much as 1 mg daily.

Hypercalcemia
ADULTS: 4 IU/kg of calcitonin (salmon) I.M. q 12 hours.

Postmenopausal osteoporosis
ADULTS: 100 IU of calcitonin (salmon) I.M. or S.C. daily

Contraindications and precautions
Calcitonin is contraindicated in patients allergic to calcitonin (salmon) or its gelatin diluent. It is not recommended for breast-feeding women, or women who are or may become pregnant. Safe use in children has not been established.

Adverse reactions
CNS: *headaches.*
GI: transient nausea with or without vomiting, diarrhea, anorexia.
GU: transient diuresis.
METABOLIC: hyperglycemia, hypocalcemia.
LOCAL: inflammation at injection site, rashes.
OTHER: *facial flushing;* swelling, tingling, and tenderness of hands; unusual taste sensation; **anaphylaxis.**

Interactions
None significant.

Nursing considerations
Assessment
- Review the patient's history for a condition that contraindicates the use of calcitonin (human).
- Obtain a baseline assessment of the patient's serum calcium level before initiating calcitonin therapy.
- Be alert for common adverse reactions.
- Evaluate the patient's and family's knowledge about calcitonin therapy.

Planning (Nursing Diagnoses)
Potential nursing diagnoses for the patient receiving calcitonin include:
- Injury related to potential ineffective calcitonin dosage.
- Altered protection related to potential for calcitonin-induced anaphylaxis.
- Knowledge deficit related to calcitonin therapy.

Implementation
Preparation and administration
— Administer a skin test, as ordered, before beginning therapy.

— If possible, administer drug at bedtime to minimize nausea and vomiting.
— Use the freshly reconstituted solution within 2 hours.
— Be aware that the S.C. route is the preferred method of administration.

Monitoring

— Monitor the effectiveness of therapy by regularly checking the patient's serum calcium levels.
— Monitor the patient for signs of hypocalcemic tetany during therapy (muscle twitching, tetanic spasms, and seizures if hypocalcemia is severe), or watch for signs of hypercalcemic relapse: bone pain, renal calculi, polyuria, anorexia, nausea, vomiting, thirst, constipation, lethargy, bradycardia, muscle hypotonicity, pathologic fracture, psychosis, and coma.
— Be aware that periodic examinations of urine sediment are advisable.
— Be aware that periodic serum alkaline phosphatase and 24-hour urine hydroxyproline levels should be determined to evaluate drug effect.
— Monitor the patient for adverse reactions.
— Monitor the patient's compliance with calcitonin therapy.
— Regularly reevaluate the patient's and family's knowledge about calcitonin.

Intervention

— Systemic allergic reactions are possible since calcitonin is a protein. Keep epinephrine handy when administering.
— Remember that patients with good initial clinical response to calcitonin who suffer relapse should be evaluated for antibody formation response to the hormone protein.
— Keep parenteral calcium available during the first doses in case hypocalcemic tetany occurs.
— Keep all members of the health care team informed of the patient's response to the drug.

Patient teaching

— Inform the patient and family about calcitonin, including the dosage, frequency, action, and adverse reactions.
— Teach the patient how to self-administer calcitonin, and assist patient until proper technique is achieved.
— Tell the patient to handle missed doses as follows: With daily dosing—take as soon as possible; do not double up on doses. With every other day dosing—take missed dose as soon as possible, then resume alternate-day therapy.
— Stress the importance of regular visits to the doctor to assess progress.
— If calcitonin is being taken to treat postmenopausal osteoporosis, remind patient to take adequate calcium and vitamin D supplements.
— Tell patients in whom calcitonin loses its hypocalcemic activity that further medication or increased dosages will be of no value.

— Facial flushing and warmth occur in 20% to 30% of all patients within minutes of injection and usually last about 1 hour. Reassure the patient that this is a transient effect.

— Tell the patient to notify the nurse or doctor if adverse reactions develop or questions arise about calcitonin therapy.

Evaluation

In the patient receiving calcitonin, appropriate evaluation statements include:

• Patient's serum calcium levels are normal.

• Patient does not experience anaphylaxis.

• Patient and family state an understanding of calcitonin therapy.

SELECTED MAJOR DRUGS: HYPOCALCEMIC AGENTS

DRUG, INDICATIONS, AND DOSAGES	SPECIAL PRECAUTIONS
etidronate disodium (Didronel) *Symptomatic Paget's disease—* **Adults:** 5 mg/kg P.O. daily as a single dose 2 hours before a meal with water or juice. Patient should not eat for 2 hours after dose. May give up to 10 mg/kg daily in severe cases. Maximum dosage is 20 mg/kg daily. *Heterotopic ossification in spinal cord injuries—* **Adults:** 20 mg/kg P.O. daily for 2 weeks, then 10 mg/kg P.O. daily for 10 weeks. Total treatment period is 12 weeks. *Heterotopic ossification after total hip replacement—* **Adults:** 20 mg/kg P.O. daily for 1 month before total hip replacement and for 3 months afterward.	• Use cautiously in enterocolitis or impaired renal function.
gallium nitrate (Ganite) *Symptomatic, unresponsive hypercalcemia caused by cancer—* **Adults:** 200 mg/m² I.V. daily for 5 consecutive days or until serum calcium level is normal. Administer as a constant infusion over 24 hours. Lower doses (100 mg/m²) may be given to patients with mild hypercalcemia.	• Contraindicated in patients with severe renal impairment. Keep in mind the association of hypercalcemia with decreased renal function in cancer patients. • The drug should *not* be used in patients with asymptomatic hypercalcemia (generally, serum calcium levels of < 12 mg/dl).

SELF-TEST

1. Jackie Sellers, age 62, has Paget's disease and takes calcitonin (human) 0.5 mg S.C. daily. Which of the following conditions would contraindicate the use of calcitonin?
   a. diabetes mellitus
   b. allergy to gelatin
   c. asthma
   d. osteoporosis

2. Mrs. Sellers complains that this drug causes nausea and vomiting. The nurse should advise Mrs. Sellers to:
   a. take the drug at bedtime.
   b. request that the doctor change route of administration.
   c. request that the dosage be lowered.
   d. use the reconstituted solution within 4 hours after mixing.

3. Which drug should be kept readily available in case of a systemic allergic reaction to calcitonin (human)?
   a. parenteral calcium
   b. calcitonin (salmon)
   c. epinephrine
   d. etidronate disodium

Check your answers on page 1072.

CHAPTER 61

DIURETICS

Thiazide and thiazide-like diuretics
bendroflumethiazide ✦ benzthiazide ✦ chlorothiazide ✦ chlorthalidone
cyclothiazide ✦ hydrochlorothiazide ✦ hydroflumethiazide ✦ indapamide
methylclothiazide ✦ metolazone ✦ polythiazide ✦ quinethazone
trichlormethiazide

Potassium-sparing diuretics
amiloride hydrochloride ✦ spironolactone ✦ triamterene

Loop diuretics
bumetanide ✦ ethacrynate sodium ✦ ethacrynic acid ✦ furosemide

Miscellaneous diuretics
acetazolamide ✦ acetazolamide sodium ✦ dichlorphenamide ✦ mannitol
methazolamide ✦ urea (carbamide)

OVERVIEW
• Diuretics reduce the body's total volume of water and salt by increasing their excretion in urine. This occurs mainly because diuretics impair sodium chloride reabsorption in the renal tubules. Diuretics can be classified according to chemical structure (thiazide and thiazide-like drugs), the site of sodium- and water-depleting effects on the nephrons (loop diuretics), and pharmacologic activity (potassium-sparing and miscellaneous diuretics).
• Diuretics can be classified primarily into four groups: thiazide and thiazide-like, potassium-sparing, loop, and miscellaneous.

MAJOR USES
• Most diuretics (except the miscellaneous diuretics, including mannitol, urea, and carbonic anhydrase inhibitors) are used to treat essential hypertension. Thiazide and thiazide-like diuretics are often used in the initial therapy of essential hypertension because they are both effective and well-tolerated by most patients. Similarly, most diuretics (except mannitol, urea, and carbonic anhydrase inhibitors) are used to treat edema associated with CHF or hepatic or renal disease.
• Because of their rapid onset of action and potent diuretic actions, loop diuretics (also known as high-ceiling diuretics) are also used for conditions such as acute pulmonary edema that require a rapid, substantial diuretic effect.

GLOSSARY

Diuresis: increased formation and excretion of urine.
Diuretic: drug or other substance tending to promote the formation and excretion of urine.
Edema: abnormal accumulation of fluid in the interstitial spaces of tissues, pericardial sac, intrapleural space, peritoneal cavity, or joint capsules.
Electrolyte: element or compound that when melted or dissolved in water or other solvent, dissociates into ions and is able to conduct an electrical current. Common electrolytes measured in clinical settings include bicarbonate, calcium, chloride, magnesium, phosphates, potassium, and sodium.

- Carbonic anhydrase inhibitors (acetazolamide, dichlorphenamide, and methazolamide) are mild diuretics that are used for other conditions. Because they inhibit the enzymes necessary to produce the aqueous humor of the eye, they are useful in the treatment of glaucoma. They are also used as adjuncts in the treatment of certain seizure disorders, although tolerance to their anticonvulsant action develops very rapidly. Acetazolamide is used to prevent acute high-altitude sickness in mountain climbers attempting rapid ascent.
- Mannitol and urea are used to reduce intracranial pressure in patients with hydrocephalus or head injury. They are also used to rapidly decrease intraocular pressure in patients with glaucoma.

MECHANISM OF ACTION

- The thiazide and thiazide-like diuretics increase urine excretion of sodium and water by inhibiting sodium reabsorption in the cortical diluting site of the ascending loop of Henle. They also increase urine excretion of chloride, potassium, and—to a lesser extent—bicarbonate ions.
- Loop diuretics inhibit reabsorption of sodium and chloride at the proximal portion of the ascending loop of Henle, enhancing water excretion. These potent diuretics can be effective in patients with markedly reduced glomerular filtration rates (in whom other diuretics usually fail).
- Potassium-sparing diuretics reduce the loss of potassium ions in the urine. Spironolactone antagonizes the hormone aldosterone in the distal tubule, increasing excretion of sodium and water but sparing potassium. Triamterene and amiloride depress sodium reabsorption and potassium secretion by direct action on the distal segment of the nephron. This reduces potassium excretion.
- Among miscellaneous diuretics, mannitol increases the osmotic pressure of glomerular filtrate, inhibiting tubular reabsorption of water and electrolytes. Similarly, urea rapidly increases blood tonicity, which results in passage of fluid from the tissue (including the brain) to the blood.
- Carbonic anhydrase inhibitors, by enzymatic blocking, promote renal excretion of sodium, potassium, bicarbonate, and water. Bicarbonate ion

excretion makes the urine alkaline; blood bicarbonate levels are accordingly reduced, leading to metabolic acidosis. In this condition, the carbonic anhydrase inhibitors become less effective as diuretics. (Carbonic anhydrase inhibitors also decrease secretion of aqueous humor in the eye, thereby lowering intraocular pressure, but this mechanism is unrelated to their diuretic action.)

- Like the thiazides, indapamide produces diuresis by inhibiting sodium reabsorption in the cortical diluting site of the ascending loop of Henle. Indapamide also has a direct vasodilating effect that may be a result of calcium channel-blocking action.

ABSORPTION, DISTRIBUTION, METABOLISM, AND EXCRETION

Thiazides and thiazide-like diuretics are all well absorbed from the GI tract, well distributed to the body tissues, and excreted primarily unchanged in urine. Indapamide is rapidly absorbed from the GI tract, distributed to body tissues, and extensively metabolized. The drug and its metabolites are excreted in the urine and feces.

Potassium-sparing diuretics are administered orally. Spironolactone is absorbed from the GI tract, distributed to body tissues, metabolized in the liver, and eliminated in both urine and feces. Amiloride and triamterene are absorbed from the GI tract, partially bound to plasma proteins, distributed to body tissues, and rapidly excreted unchanged in urine.

Among loop diuretics, ethacrynic acid is rapidly absorbed after oral administration, metabolized in the liver, and excreted by the kidneys. Ethacrynate sodium is administered parenterally. Its metabolism and excretion are the same as those of ethacrynic acid. Bumetanide is well absorbed from the GI tract; both metabolites and unchanged drug are excreted in urine. Furosemide is partially (about 60%) absorbed from the GI tract; a small amount is metabolized. Both metabolites and unchanged drug are excreted in urine.

Among miscellaneous diuretics, mannitol is poorly absorbed after oral administration and must be given I.V. It remains in the extracellular fluid, is filtered by the glomeruli, and is excreted unchanged in urine. Urea is well absorbed after oral administration, but it is seldom given orally because of its unpleasant taste. After I.V. administration, it is distributed to intracellular and extracellular fluids, including CSF. Urea is hydrolyzed in the GI tract by bacterial ureases and excreted by the kidneys.

Carbonic anhydrase inhibitors are absorbed from the GI tract after oral administration and are distributed throughout body tissue.

Acetazolamide is excreted unchanged in urine, but other carbonic anhydrase inhibitors are partially metabolized and eliminated in both urine and feces.

ONSET AND DURATION

Thiazides and thiazide-like diuretics begin to act 1 to 2 hours after oral administration. Most of them have a duration of action of 12 to 24 hours, but several act as long as 36 to 72 hours. I.V. chlorothiazide takes effect within 15 minutes after administration and has a duration of 2 hours.

Indapamide begins to act 1 to 2 hours after administration. Its duration of action is 24 hours.

Among the potassium-sparing diuretics, spironolactone's onset occurs gradually over 2 to 3 days, but a loading dose may be used for faster effect. The drug continues to act for 2 to 3 days. Triamterene begins to act in 2 to 4 hours and has a duration of up to 24 hours. Maximal therapeutic effect may not occur during the first few days of therapy. Amiloride begins to act within 2 hours, reaches a peak effect between 6 to 10 hours, and has a duration of 24 hours.

Among loop diuretics, ethacrynic acid begins to act 30 minutes after oral administration and has a duration of up to 12 hours. Ethacrynate sodium, after I.V. administration, begins to act within 5 minutes. Its duration is 2 hours. After oral administration, bumetanide and furosemide begin to act in 30 to 60 minutes and have a duration of 6 to 8 hours. After I.V. administration, onset occurs within 5 minutes, and the drugs have a duration of 2 hours. After I.M. injection, they begin to act within 30 minutes and have a duration of 6 to 8 hours.

Among the miscellaneous diuretics, mannitol begins to act 15 to 30 minutes after I.V. administration; diuresis occurs in 1 to 3 hours. Duration is 4 to 6 hours, but it may reduce CSF pressure for up to 8 hours. Urea begins to act 1 to 2 hours after I.V. administration and has a duration of 3 to 10 hours.

Carbonic anhydrase inhibitors begin to act 1 to 3 hours after oral administration and have a duration of 8 to 12 hours. The timed-release form of acetazolamide, however, acts as long as 24 hours; methazolamide acts for up to 18 hours. After I.V. administration, acetazolamide has an onset within 2 minutes and a duration of 4 to 5 hours.

ADVERSE REACTIONS

The most common adverse reaction to thiazide and loop diuretics is potassium depletion; in most patients, it is usually mild and rarely causes symptoms. However, potassium depletion is an important consideration in patients receiving digitalis glycosides because a low potassium level increases the cardiotoxicity of these agents. Hypokalemia may be associated with hypochloremic alkalosis, especially in patients with other losses of potassium and chloride such as vomiting and diarrhea. Dilutional hyponatremia may occur. Hyperuricemia may occur but is usually asymptomatic, except in patients predisposed to gout or chronic renal failure.

Thiazides and thiazide-like diuretics can produce hyperglycemia, glycosuria, and elevated triglyceride and cholesterol levels. GI reactions include anorexia, nausea, and pancreatitis. CV reactions can include orthostatic hypotension and volume depletion; electrolyte disturbances can include dehydration, hypocalcemia, and hypomagnesemia. Rare reactions to the thiazides and loop diuretics include agranulocytosis, leukopenia, and thrombocytopenia. When rapidly given I.V. or in high I.V. dosage, the loop diuretics have been associated with ototoxicity which may lead to deafness, especially when aminoglycoside antibiotics are used concomitantly.

Amiloride, spironolactone, and triamterene are all potassium-sparing diuretics and, as a result, may cause hyperkalemia. Other reactions are mild and occur infrequently. They may include nausea, vomiting, anorexia, headache, and dizziness. Some reactions are specific to individual agents: amiloride has been known to cause impotence; spironolactone has caused gynecomastia in men and breast soreness and mental disturbances in women; and triamterene has caused anaphylaxis, photosensitivity, and megaloblastic anemia.

Carbonic anhydrase inhibitors produce metabolic disturbances similar to those associated with loop and thiazide diuretics. Such reactions are uncommon except for hyperchloremic acidosis, which is an extension of these agents' pharmacologic action.

Nonmetabolic reactions may include aplastic anemia, agranulocytosis, thrombocytopenia or leukopenia, nausea, vomiting, drowsiness, paresthesia, transient myopia, crystalluria, and renal calculi.

The most severe adverse reaction to mannitol and urea is fluid and electrolyte imbalance. Accumulation of mannitol and urea can result in an expansion of extracellular fluid, which may result in circulatory overload, worsening CHF, pulmonary edema, water intoxication, and tachycardia. Mild reactions include headache, nausea, vomiting, and necrotic sloughing with extravasation.

PROTOTYPE: THIAZIDE DIURETICS

HYDROCHLOROTHIAZIDE
(hye droe klor oh thye' a zide)
Apo-Hydro†, Dichlotride‡, Diuchlor H†, Esidrix, HydroDIURIL, Mictrin, Novohydrazide†, Oretic, Urozide†
Classification: thiazide diuretic
Pregnancy risk category D

How supplied
TABLETS: 25 mg, 50 mg, 100 mg
ORAL SOLUTION: 10 mg/ml, 100 mg/ml

Indications and dosage
Edema
ADULTS: initially, 25 to 100 mg P.O. daily or intermittently for maintenance dosage.
CHILDREN OVER AGE 6 MONTHS: 2.2 mg/kg P.O. daily in divided doses b.i.d.
CHILDREN UNDER AGE 6 MONTHS: up to 3.3 mg/kg P.O. daily in divided doses b.i.d.

Hypertension
ADULTS: 25 to 100 mg P.O. daily as a single dose or in divided doses. Daily dosage is increased or decreased according to blood pressure response.

---

†Available in Canada only   ‡Available in Australia only

Contraindications and precautions
Hydrochlorothiazide is contraindicated in patients with anuria or known hypersensitivity to other thiazides or to sulfonamides because thiazides are sulfonamide derivatives. Use cautiously in patients with severe renal disease, impaired hepatic function, and progressive hepatic disease; and also in elderly patients because they are especially susceptible to excessive diuresis.

Adverse reactions
BLOOD: **aplastic anemia, agranulocytosis**, leukopenia, thrombocytopenia.
CNS: dizziness, vertigo, paresthesia, headache, restlessness, hepatic encephalopathy.
CV: *volume depletion and dehydration,* orthostatic hypotension.
GI: anorexia, nausea, pancreatitis, vomiting, cramping, diarrhea.
METABOLIC: fluid and electrolyte imbalances, including *hypokalemia,* dilutional hyponatremia and hypochloremia, metabolic alkalosis, hypercalcemia; *asymptomatic hyperuricemia* and gout; hyperglycemia and impairment of glucose tolerance.
SKIN: dermatitis, photosensitivity, rash.
OTHER: hypersensitivity reactions, such as pneumonitis and vasculitis, elevated serum cholesterol.

Interactions
Cholestyramine, colestipol: decreased intestinal absorption of thiazides. Keep doses as separate as possible.
Diazoxide: increased antihypertensive, hyperglycemic, and hyperuricemic effects. Use together cautiously.
NSAIDs: decreased diuretic effectiveness. Avoid concomitant use.

Nursing considerations
Assessment
• Review the patient's history for a condition that contraindicates the use of hydrochlorothiazide.
• Obtain a baseline assessment of blood pressure, serum electrolytes, urine output, weight, and peripheral edema before initiating hydrochlorothiazide therapy.
• Be alert for common adverse reactions.
• Evaluate the patient's and family's knowledge about hydrochlorothiazide therapy.

Planning (Nursing Diagnoses)
Potential nursing diagnoses for the patient receiving hydrochlorothiazide include:
• Fluid volume excess related to ineffectiveness of hydrochlorothiazide to relieve edema.
• Altered urinary elimination related to hydrochlorothiazide therapy.
• Knowledge deficit related to hydrochlorothiazide therapy.

Implementation

Preparation and administration
— Read order and drug label carefully before administration.
— If possible, give drug early in the day to prevent nocturia.
— Chart drug administration and related observations.

Monitoring
— Monitor the effectiveness of therapy by regularly checking blood pressure, urine output, and weight.
— Monitor serum electrolytes, BUN, creatinine, glucose, and uric acid levels.
— Monitor CBC, differential, and platelet count.
— Monitor the patient for adverse drug reactions.
— For the patient receiving concomitant digitalis therapy, monitor for increased risk of digitalis toxicity.
— Monitor for signs of hypokalemia (for example, muscle weakness and cramps).
— Monitor the diabetic patient's insulin requirements because hydrochlorothiazide has hyperglycemic effects.
— Monitor skin turgor and mucous membranes for signs of fluid volume deficit.
— Monitor the patient for drug interactions.
— Regularly reevaluate the patient's and family's knowledge about hydrochlorothiazide therapy.

Intervention
— Hold drug and notify the doctor if hypersensitivity reactions occur.
— Keep accurate records of intake and output, blood pressure, and weight.
— Provide frequent skin and mouth care to relieve dryness from diuretic therapy.
— Answer the patient's call bells promptly; make sure bathroom or bed pan is easily accessible.
— Use safety precautions to minimize risk of falling due to hypotension.
— In the patient undergoing tests of parathyroid function, hold thiazide and thiazide-like drugs before these tests are performed.
— Be aware that optimal antihypertensive effect may not occur for 3 to 4 weeks after beginning of therapy with hydrochlorothiazide.
— Keep all members of the health care team informed of the patient's response to the drug.
— Elevate the patient's legs to aid reduction of peripheral edema.
— Administer potassium supplements as indicated.

Patient teaching
— Instruct the patient and family about hydrochlorothiazide, including the dosage, frequency, action, and adverse reactions.
— Teach the patient and family to identify and report signs of hypersensitivity reaction and hypokalemia.

—Teach the patient and family to monitor the patient's fluid volume by recording daily weight and intake and output.

—Inform the patient that optimal therapeutic response may not occur until several weeks after beginning hydrochlorothiazide therapy.

—Teach the patient to avoid foods high in sodium and to choose foods high in potassium.

—Advise the patient to change positions slowly, especially when rising to standing position, to avoid dizziness and fainting due to orthostatic hypotension.

—Advise the patient to minimize risks of photosensitivity reaction by using a sunscreen when outdoors.

—Advise the diabetic patient that insulin dosage may require adjustment.

—Tell the patient to notify the nurse or doctor if adverse reactions develop or questions arise about hydrochlorothiazide therapy.

—Advise the patient who is taking digitalis that the drug's potassium-depleting effect may increase the risk of digitalis toxicity.

—Advise the patient to take hydrochlorothiazide early in the day to avoid interruptions of sleep due to nocturia.

Evaluation

In the patient receiving hydrochlorothiazide, appropriate evaluation statements include:

• Patient is free of edema.

• Patient demonstrates adjustment of life-style to deal with altered patterns of urinary elimination.

• Patient and family state an understanding of hydrochlorothiazide therapy.

PROTOTYPE: POTASSIUM-SPARING DIURETICS

SPIRONOLACTONE
(speer on oh lak' tone)
Aldactone, Novospiroton†, Spirotone‡
Classification: potassium-sparing diuretic
Pregnancy risk category D

How supplied
TABLETS: 25 mg, 50 mg, 100 mg

Indications and dosage

Edema
ADULTS: 25 to 200 mg P.O. daily in divided doses.
CHILDREN: initially, 3.3 mg/kg P.O. daily in divided doses. Dosage is adjusted according to response.

Hypertension
ADULTS: 50 to 100 mg P.O. daily in divided doses.

Treatment of diuretic-induced hypokalemia

ADULTS: 25 to 100 mg P.O. daily when oral potassium supplements are considered inappropriate.

Detection of primary hyperaldosteronism

ADULTS: 400 mg P.O. daily for 4 days (short test) or 3 to 4 weeks (long test). If hypokalemia and hypertension are corrected, a presumptive diagnosis of primary hyperaldosteronism is made.

Contraindications and precautions

Spironolactone is contraindicated in anuria, acute or progressive renal insufficiency, or hyperkalemia. Use cautiously in fluid or electrolyte imbalances, impaired renal function, and hepatic disease. Mild acidosis may occur, which may be dangerous in patients with hepatic cirrhosis. Also use cautiously in elderly patients, who are more susceptible to excessive diuresis. Breast cancer has been reported in some patients taking spironolactone, but a cause-and-effect relationship is not confirmed. Warn against taking drug indiscriminately.

Adverse reactions

CNS: headache.
CV: arrhythmias.
GI: anorexia, nausea, diarrhea.
METABOLIC: *hyperkalemia,* dehydration, hyponatremia, transient elevation in BUN levels, acidosis.
SKIN: urticaria.
OTHER: gynecomastia in men; breast soreness and menstrual disturbances in women.

Interactions

Angiotensin converting enzyme (ACE) inhibitors, potassium supplements: concomitant use may result in hyperkalemia. Don't use together.
Aspirin: possible blocked spironolactone effect. Watch for diminished spironolactone response.
Digoxin: may alter digoxin clearance and increase risk of toxicity. Monitor digoxin levels.
Diuretics, antihypertensives: spironolactone may enhance the effects of these drugs. Dosage should be reduced at least 50% when spironolactone is added to the drug regimen.

Nursing considerations

Assessment

• Review the patient's history for a condition that contraindicates the use of spironolactone.
• Obtain a baseline assessment of blood pressure, urine output, weight, serum electrolytes, and peripheral edema before initiating spironolactone therapy.
• Be alert for common adverse reactions.
• Evaluate the patient's and family's knowledge about spironolactone therapy.

Planning (Nursing Diagnoses)
Potential nursing diagnoses for the patient receiving spironolactone include:
- Fluid volume excess related to ineffectiveness of spironolactone to relieve edema.
- Altered urinary elimination related to spironolactone therapy.
- Injury related to potential hyperkalemia caused by spironolactone therapy.
- Knowledge deficit related to spironolactone therapy.

Implementation
Preparation and administration
— Read orders and drug label carefully before administration.
— Give spironolactone with meals to enhance absorption.
— Chart drug administration and related observations.

Monitoring
— Monitor the effectiveness of therapy by regularly checking urine output, blood pressure, weight, and evidence of edema.
— Monitor the patient for adverse drug reactions.
— Monitor BUN and serum electrolyte levels, especially potassium level.
— Monitor for signs of hyperkalemia: muscle weakness and cramps, paresthesia, diarrhea, and cardiac arrhythmias.
— Monitor skin turgor and mucous membranes for signs of fluid volume depletion.
— Monitor the patient for drug interactions.
— Monitor the patient's compliance with spironolactone therapy.
— Regularly reevaluate the patient's and family's knowledge about spironolactone therapy.

Intervention
— Hold drug and notify the doctor if hyperkalemia or dehydration occurs.
— Keep accurate record of intake and output, and blood pressure.
— Weigh the patient daily.
— Provide frequent skin and mouth care to relieve dryness caused by diuretic therapy.
— Answer the patient's call bells promptly; make sure bathroom or bed pan is easily accessible.
— Use safety precautions to prevent the risk of injury from falls.
— Elevate the patient's legs to reduce peripheral edema.
— Keep all members of the health care team informed of the patient's response to the drug.

Patient teaching
— Instruct the patient and family about spironolactone, including the dosage, frequency, action, and adverse reactions.
— Teach the patient and family to identify and report signs of hyperkalemia.

— Teach the patient and family to monitor the patient's fluid volume by recording daily weight and intake and output.

— Advise the patient to avoid excessive intake of foods high in potassium and of potassium-containing sodium substitutes.

— Instruct the patient to avoid concomitant use of potassium supplements.

— Advise the patient to change positions slowly, especially when rising to a standing position, to avoid dizziness and fainting due to orthostatic hypotension.

— Tell the patient to take spironolactone with meals and, if possible, early in the day to avoid interruption of sleep due to nocturia.

— Tell the patient to notify the nurse or doctor if adverse reactions develop or questions arise about spironolactone therapy.

Evaluation

In the patient receiving spironolactone, appropriate evaluation statements include:

• Patient is free of edema.

• Patient demonstrates adjustment of life-style to deal with altered patterns of urinary elimination.

• Patient's serum potassium remains within normal range.

• Patient and family state an understanding of spironolactone therapy.

PROTOTYPE: LOOP DIURETICS

FUROSEMIDE
(fur oh' se mide)

Apo-Furosemide†, Furomide M.D., Furoside†, Lasix*, Lasix Special†, Myrosemide*, Novosemide†, Urex, Urex-M‡, Uritol†

Classification: loop diuretic
Pregnancy risk category C

How supplied
TABLETS: 20 mg, 40 mg, 80 mg, 500 mg†
ORAL SOLUTION: 8 mg/ml, 10 mg/ml, 50 mg/ml
INJECTION: 10 mg/ml

Indications and dosage
Acute pulmonary edema
ADULTS: 40 mg I.V. injected slowly; then 40 mg I.V. in 1 to 1½ hours if needed.

Edema
ADULTS: 20 to 80 mg P.O. daily in the morning, with second dose given in 6 to 8 hours; carefully titrated up to 600 mg daily if needed. Or 20 to 40 mg I.M. or I.V., increased by 20 mg q 2 hours until desired response is achieved. I.V. dose should be given slowly over 1 to 2 minutes.

---

*Liquid form contains alcohol   †Available in Canada only   ‡Available in Australia only

Hypertension

ADULTS: 40 mg P.O. b.i.d. Adjust dose according to response.
INFANTS AND CHILDREN: 2 mg/kg P.O. daily, increased by 1 to 2 mg/kg in 6 to 8 hours if needed; carefully titrated up to 6 mg/kg daily if needed.

Hypertensive crisis, acute renal failure

ADULTS: 100 to 200 mg I.V. over 1 to 2 minutes.

Chronic renal failure

ADULTS: initially, 80 mg P.O. daily. Increase by 80 to 120 mg daily until desired response is achieved.

Contraindications and precautions

Furosemide is contraindicated in patients with known hypersensitivity to furosemide. Use cautiously in cardiogenic shock complicated by pulmonary edema; anuria, renal insufficiency, hepatic coma, or electrolyte imbalances; and in patients receiving digitalis. Drug is not routinely administered to women of childbearing age because its safety in pregnancy hasn't been established.

Adverse reactions

BLOOD: **agranulocytosis**, leukopenia, thrombocytopenia.
CV: *volume depletion and dehydration, orthostatic hypotension.*
EENT: tinnitus or transient deafness with too-rapid I.V. injection.
GI: abdominal discomfort and pain, diarrhea (with oral solution).
METABOLIC: *fluid and electrolyte imbalances, including hypokalemia, hypochloremic alkalosis, dilutional hyponatremia, hypocalcemia, and hypomagnesemia; asymptomatic hyperuricemia; hyperglycemia and impairment of glucose tolerance.*
SKIN: dermatitis.

Interactions

Aminoglycoside antibiotics: potentiated ototoxicity. Use together cautiously.
Antihypertensives: furosemide may potentiate antihypertensive effects. Use cautiously.
Chloral hydrate: sweating, flushing, and variable blood pressure with I.V. furosemide. Administer furosemide slowly, and monitor closely for adverse effects.
Clofibrate: enhanced furosemide effects. Use cautiously.
Digitalis: may cause digitalis toxicity. Use cautiously.
Indomethacin: inhibited diuretic response. Use cautiously.

Nursing considerations

Assessment

• Review the patient's history for a condition that contraindicates the use of furosemide.
• Obtain a baseline assessment of urine output, vital signs, serum electrolytes, breath sounds, peripheral edema, and weight before initiating furosemide therapy.
• Be alert for common adverse reactions.

• Evaluate the patient's and family's knowledge about furosemide therapy.

Planning (Nursing Diagnoses)

Potential nursing diagnoses for the patient receiving furosemide include:
• Fluid volume excess related to ineffectiveness of furosemide to relieve edema.
• Altered urinary elimination related to diuretic therapy (frequency, urgency).
• Injury related to potential furosemide-induced fluid and electrolyte imbalance.
• Knowledge deficit related to furosemide therapy.

Implementation

Preparation and administration

— Read orders and drug label carefully before administration.
— Check injectable preparation for discoloration (yellow); discard if present.
— Check patency of I.V. line and site before administration of I.V. furosemide.
— Give I.V. dose over 1 to 2 minutes to avoid transient hearing impairment.
— Avoid parenteral route of administration in infants and children if possible.
— Give P.O. or I.M. preparations early in the morning to avoid nocturia. Give second doses in early afternoon.
— Store tablets in light-resistant container to avoid discoloration.
— Store oral furosemide solution in refrigerator to ensure drug stability.
— Chart administration of drug and related observations.

Monitoring

— Monitor the effectiveness of therapy by regularly checking urine output, weight, peripheral edema, and breath sounds.
— Monitor the patient for adverse drug reactions.
— Monitor ECG for arrhythmias.
— Monitor serum electrolytes and BUN levels.
— Monitor vital signs: hypotension, dyspnea, tachycardia, and fever may indicate dehydration.
— In the diabetic patient, monitor serum glucose.
— In the patient with gout, monitor serum uric acid.
— In the patient receiving digitalis, monitor for signs of digitalis toxicity.
— Monitor for signs of hypokalemia (muscle weakness and cramping).
— Monitor the patient for drug interactions.
— Monitor skin turgor and mucous membranes for signs of fluid volume depletion.
— Regularly reevaluate the patient's and family's knowledge about furosemide therapy.

Intervention

— Hold drug and notify the doctor if hypersensitivity or adverse reactions occur.
— Keep accurate record of intake and output.
— Weigh the patient daily.
— Elevate the patient's legs to aid decrease of peripheral edema.
— Encourage diet low in sodium and high in potassium.
— Provide frequent skin and mouth care to relieve dryness caused by diuretic therapy.
— Answer the patient's call bells promptly; make sure bathroom or bed pan are easily accessible.
— Use safety precautions to avoid risk of falls from hypotension.
— Use written communication for the patient who experiences drug-related deafness.
— Keep all members of the health care team informed of the patient's response to the drug.

Patient teaching

— Instruct the patient and family about furosemide therapy, including the dosage, frequency, action, and adverse reactions.
— Teach the patient and family to identify and report signs of hypersensitivity or furosemide toxicity (ringing ears, severe abdominal pain, sore throat, or fever).
— Teach the diabetic patient receiving furosemide to monitor blood glucose.
— Teach the patient receiving furosemide and digitalis to be aware of signs of digitalis toxicity and to store these drugs separately to avoid risk of dosage error.
— Teach the patient to monitor fluid volume by daily weight and intake and output.
— Encourage the patient to avoid foods high in sodium and to choose foods high in potassium.
— Advise the patient to change positions slowly, especially when rising to a standing position, to avoid dizziness due to orthostatic hypotension.
— Advise the patient to limit alcohol intake and strenuous exercise in warm weather.
— Advise the patient to take furosemide early in the day to avoid sleep interruption from nocturia.
— Tell the patient to notify the nurse or doctor if adverse reactions develop or questions arise about furosemide therapy.

Evaluation

In the patient receiving furosemide, appropriate evaluation statements include:
• Patient is free of edema.
• Patient demonstrates adjustment of life-style to deal with altered patterns of urinary elimination.
• Patient's serum electrolytes remain within normal limits.

• Patient and family state an understanding of furosemide therapy.

MANNITOL
(man' i tole)
Osmitrol†
Classification: *osmotic diuretic*
Pregnancy risk category C

How supplied
INJECTION: 5%, 10%, 15%, 20%, 25%

Indications and dosage
Test dose for marked oliguria or suspected inadequate renal function
ADULTS AND CHILDREN OVER AGE 12: 200 mg/kg or 12.5 g as a 15% or 20% solution I.V. over 3 to 5 minutes. Response is adequate if 30 to 50 ml urine/hour is excreted over 2 to 3 hours.

Treatment of oliguria
ADULTS AND CHILDREN OVER AGE 12: 50 to 100 g I.V. as a 15% to 20% solution over 90 minutes to several hours; dosage is adjusted to maintain output of 30 to 50 ml urine/hour.

Prevention of oliguria or acute renal failure following toxic drugs (such as chemotherapeutic agents) or poisoning
ADULTS AND CHILDREN OVER AGE 12: 50 to 100 g I.V. of a concentrated (5% to 25%) solution, at a rate to maintain output of 100 to 500 ml urine/hour.

To reduce intraocular pressure or intracranial pressure
ADULTS AND CHILDREN OVER AGE 12: 0.25 to 2 g/kg I.V. as a 15% to 25% solution over 30 to 60 minutes.

Contraindications and precautions
Mannitol is contraindicated in anuria, severe pulmonary congestion, frank pulmonary edema, severe CHF, severe dehydration, metabolic edema, progressive renal disease or dysfunction, progressive heart failure during administration, or active intracranial bleeding except during craniotomy.

Adverse reactions
CNS: **rebound increase in intracranial pressure 8 to 12 hours after diuresis**, *headache,* confusion.
CV: transient expansion of plasma volume during infusion, causing circulatory overload and **pulmonary edema**; tachycardia; angina-like chest pain.
EENT: blurred vision, rhinitis.
GI: *thirst,* nausea, vomiting.
GU: urine retention.

METABOLIC: *fluid and electrolyte imbalance,* water intoxication, cellular dehydration.

Interactions

None significant.

Nursing considerations

Assessment

- Review the patient's history for a condition that contraindicates the use of mannitol.
- Obtain a baseline assessment of hourly urine output; vital signs, including central venous pressure (CVP); breath sounds; serum electrolytes; and peripheral edema before initiating mannitol therapy.
- Be alert for common adverse reactions.
- Evaluate the patient's and family's knowledge about mannitol therapy.

Planning (Nursing Diagnoses)

Potential nursing diagnoses for the patient receiving mannitol include:
- Fluid volume excess related to ineffectiveness of or adverse reaction to mannitol therapy.
- Altered urinary elimination related to diuretic therapy.
- Knowledge deficit related to mannitol therapy.

Implementation

Preparation and administration

— Read orders and drug label carefully before administration.
— Always give mannitol infusions via an in-line filter and with an infusion pump.
— Check patency of the I.V. line and infusion site before and during administration of mannitol.
— Test for marked oliguria or suspected inadequate renal function (see "Indications and dosage").
— For maximum intraocular pressure reduction before surgery, give 1 to 1½ hours preoperatively.
— Solution often crystallizes, especially at low temperatures. To redissolve, warm bottle in hot water bath and shake vigorously. Cool to body temperature before giving. Concentrations greater than 15% have greater tendency to crystallize. Do not use solution with undissolved crystals.
— Do not administer with whole blood; agglutination will occur.
— Chart drug administration and related observations.

Monitoring

— Monitor the effectiveness of therapy by regularly checking hourly urine output, vital signs, breath sounds, and CVP readings.
— Monitor the patient for adverse drug reactions.
— Regularly monitor serum and urine levels of sodium and potassium.
— Weigh the patient daily, if possible.
— Monitor renal function studies.

— Monitor for signs of rebound increased intracranial pressure (headache and confusion) as indicated.
— Monitor I.V. line patency and infusion site to prevent infiltration of mannitol and possible local edema and tissue necrosis.
— Monitor skin turgor and mucous membranes for signs of fluid volume deficit.
— Monitor the patient's extremities for peripheral edema.

Intervention

— Hold dose and notify the doctor immediately if adverse reactions occur.
— Keep accurate record of intake and output, vital signs, and CVP measurement.
— Provide frequent skin and mouth care to relieve dryness caused by mannitol therapy.
— Frequently check I.V. site for infiltration. If extravasation of mannitol occurs, elevate the extremity, apply warm moist compress, and notify the doctor.
— Use safety precautions to avoid risk of injury from falls.
— A urethral catheter is inserted in the comatose or incontinent patient because therapy is based on strict evaluation of intake and output. In the patient with a urethral catheter, use an hourly urometer collection bag to facilitate accurate evaluation of output.
— Reorient the confused patient to person, time, and place.
— If peripheral edema is present, elevate the patient's extremities.
— Keep all members of the health care team informed of the patient's response to the drug.

Patient teaching

— Instruct the patient and family about mannitol, including the dosage, frequency, action, and adverse reactions.
— Teach the patient to avoid foods high in sodium.
— Tell the patient he may feel thirsty or experience mouth dryness, and emphasize importance of drinking only the amount of fluids provided, as ordered by the doctor.
— With initial doses, warn the patient to change positions slowly, especially when rising from a lying or sitting position, to prevent dizziness from orthostatic hypotension.
— Instruct the patient to tell the doctor immediately if he experiences pain in the chest, back, or legs; shortness of breath; or apnea.
— Tell the patient to notify the nurse or doctor if adverse reactions develop or questions arise about mannitol therapy.

Evaluation

In the patient receiving mannitol, appropriate evaluation statements include:
• Patient is free of edema.
• Patient demonstrates coping behaviors and comfort in dealing with altered patterns of urinary elimination.
• Patient and family state an understanding of mannitol therapy.

SELECTED MAJOR DRUGS: DIURETICS

DRUG, INDICATIONS, AND DOSAGES	SPECIAL PRECAUTIONS

Thiazide and thiazide-like diuretics

benzthiazide (Aquatag, Exna, Marazide)
Edema —
Adults: 50 to 200 mg P.O. daily or in divided doses.
Children: 1 to 4 mg/kg P.O. daily in three divided doses.
Hypertension —
Adults: 50 mg P.O. daily b.i.d., t.i.d., or q.i.d., adjusted to patient response.

• Contraindicated in patients with anuria or known hypersensitivity to benzthiazide or other sulfonamide derivatives.
• Administer cautiously to patients with severe renal disease, impaired hepatic function, or progressive liver disease and to pregnant or breast-feeding women.

chlorothiazide (Diachlor, Diuril)
Edema, hypertension —
Adults: 500 mg to 2 g P.O. or I.V. daily or in two divided doses.
Diuresis —
Children over age 6 months: 20 mg/kg P.O. or I.V. daily in divided doses.
Children under age 6 months: may require 30 mg/kg P.O. or I.V. daily in two divided doses.

• Contraindicated in patients with anuria or known hypersensitivity to chlorothiazide or other sulfonamide derivatives and in breast-feeding women.
• Administer cautiously to patients with severe renal disease, impaired hepatic function, or progressive liver disease and during pregnancy.

chlorthalidone (Hygroten, Novothalidone†)
Edema, hypertension —
Adults: 25 to 100 mg P.O. daily, or 100 mg three times weekly or on alternate days.
Children: 2 mg/kg P.O. three times weekly.

• Contraindicated in patients with anuria or known hypersensitivity to thiazides or other sulfonamide derivatives.
• Administer cautiously to patients with severe renal disease, progressive hepatic disease, and impaired hepatic function.

cyclothiazide (Anhydron)
Edema —
Adults: 1 to 2 mg P.O. daily. May be used on alternate days as maintenance dosage.
Children: 0.02 to 0.04 mg/kg P.O. daily.
Hypertension —
Adults: 2 mg P.O. daily, up to 2 mg b.i.d. or t.i.d.

• Contraindicated in patients with anuria or known hypersensitivity to other thiazides or other sulfonamide derivatives.
• Administer cautiously to patients with severe renal disease, impaired hepatic function, and progressive hepatic disease.

indapamide (Lozol)
Edema, hypertension —
Adults: 2.5 mg P.O. as a single daily dose taken in the morning. Dosage may be increased to 5 mg daily.

• Contraindicated in patients with anuria or known hypersensitivity to other sulfonamide derivatives.
• Use cautiously in patients with severe renal disease, impaired hepatic function, and progressive hepatic disease.

†Available in Canada only

SELECTED MAJOR DRUGS: DIURETICS *continued*

DRUG, INDICATIONS, AND DOSAGES	SPECIAL PRECAUTIONS

Thiazide and thiazide-like diuretics *(continued)*

metolazone (Diulo, Zaroxolyn)
Edema (heart failure) —
Adults: 5 to 10 mg P.O. daily.
Edema (renal disease) —
Adults: 5 to 20 mg P.O. daily.
Hypertension —
Adults: 2.5 to 5 mg P.O. daily. Maintenance dosage determined by patient's blood pressure.

• Contraindicated in patients with anuria; hepatic coma or precoma; or known hypersensitivity to thiazides or other sulfonamide derivatives.
• Use cautiously in hyperuricemia or gout and severely impaired renal function.

trichlormethiazide (Metahydrin, Naqua)
Edema —
Adults: 1 to 4 mg P.O. daily or in two divided doses.
Hypertension —
Adults: 2 to 4 mg P.O. daily.

• Contraindicated in patients with anuria or known hypersensitivity to other thiazides or other sulfonamide derivatives.
• Use cautiously in severe renal disease and impaired hepatic function.

Potassium-sparing diuretics

amiloride (Midamor)
Hypertension; edema associated with CHF, usually in patients who are also taking thiazide or other potassium-wasting diuretics —
Adults: usual dosage is 5 mg P.O. daily. Dosage may be increased to 10 mg daily, if necessary. As much as 20 mg daily can be given.

• Contraindicated in patients with elevated serum potassium levels (greater than 5.5 mEq/liter). Don't administer to patients receiving other potassium-sparing diuretics, such as spironolactone and triamterene. Also contraindicated in anuria.
• Use cautiously in patients with renal impairment because potassium retention is increased.

triamterene (Dyrenium)
Diuresis —
Adults: initially, 100 mg P.O. b.i.d. after meals. Total dosage should not exceed 300 mg daily.

• Contraindicated in patients with anuria, severe or progressive renal disease or dysfunction, severe hepatic disease, or hyperkalemia.
• Use cautiously in patients with impaired hepatic function, diabetes mellitus, during pregnancy, or in breast-feeding women.

(continued)

SELECTED MAJOR DRUGS: DIURETICS *continued*

DRUG, INDICATIONS, AND DOSAGES	SPECIAL PRECAUTIONS

Loop diuretics

bumetanide (Bumex)
Edema (CHF, hepatic and renal disease) —
Adults: 0.5 to 2 mg P.O. daily. If diuretic response is not adequate, a second or third dose may be given at 4- to 5-hour intervals. Maximum dosage is 10 mg daily. May be administered parenterally when P.O. not feasible. Usual initial dose is 0.5 to 1 mg I.V. or I.M. If response is not adequate, a second or third dose may be given at 2- to 3-hour intervals. Maximum dosage is 10 mg daily.

• Contraindicated in patients with anuria hepatic coma or severe electrolyte depletion.
• Use cautiously in patients with hepatic cirrhosis and ascites. Supplemental potassium or potassium-sparing diuretics may be used to prevent hypokalemia and metabolic alkalosis in these patients.
• Use cautiously in patients with depressed renal function.

ethacrynate sodium
ethacrynic acid (Edecrin)
Acute pulmonary edema —
Adults: 50 to 100 mg (ethacrynate sodium) I.V. slowly over several minutes.
Edema —
Adults: 50 to 200 mg P.O. daily. Refractory cases may require up to 200 mg b.i.d.
Children: initial dose is 25 mg P.O., cautiously, increased in 25-mg increments daily until desired effect is achieved.

• Contraindicated in patients with anuria and in infants.
• Use cautiously in patients with electrolyte abnormalities. If electrolyte imbalance, azotemia, or oliguria develops, may require discontinuation of drug.

Miscellaneous diuretics

acetazolamide (Diamox)
Narrow-angle glaucoma —
Adults: 250 mg P.O. q 4 hours; or 250 mg P.O., I.M., or I.V. b.i.d. for short-term therapy.
Open-angle glaucoma —
Adults: 250 mg daily to 1 g P.O., I.M., or I.V. daily in divided doses q.i.d.
Prevention or amelioration of acute mountain sickness —
Adults: 250 mg P.O. q 8 to 12 hours.
Myoclonic, refractory generalized tonic-clonic or absence, or mixed seizures —
Adults: 375 mg P.O., I.M., or I.V. daily up to 250 mg q.i.d. Alternatively, use sustained-release form 250 to 500 mg P.O. daily or b.i.d. Initial dosage when used with other anticonvulsants usually is 250 mg daily.
Children: 8 to 30 mg/kg P.O. daily in divided doses t.i.d. or q.i.d. Maximum dosage is 1.5 g daily, or 300 to 900 mg/m² daily.

• Contraindicated for long-term use in chronic noncongestive narrow-angle glaucoma; also in patients with hyponatremia or hypokalemia, renal or hepatic disease or dysfunction, adrenal gland failure, or hyperchloremic acidosis.
• Use cautiously in patients with respiratory acidosis, emphysema, chronic pulmonary disease, and in those receiving other diuretics.

SELECTED MAJOR DRUGS: DIURETICS *continued*

DRUG, INDICATIONS, AND DOSAGES	SPECIAL PRECAUTIONS

Miscellaneous diuretics *(continued)*

dichlorphenamide (Daranide)
Adjunct in glaucoma —
Adults: initially, 100 to 200 mg P.O., followed by 100 mg q 12 hours until desired response obtained. Maintenance dosage is 25 to 50 mg P.O. b.i.d. or t.i.d. Give miotics concomitantly.

• Contraindicated in patients with hepatic insufficiency, renal failure, adrenocortical insufficiency, hyperchloremic acidosis, depressed sodium or potassium levels, severe pulmonary obstruction with inability to increase alveolar ventilation, or Addison's disease.
• Long-term use is contraindicated in patients with severe, absolute, or chronic noncongestive narrow-angle glaucoma.
• Use cautiously in patients with respiratory acidosis; monitor blood pH and blood gases.

methazolamide (Neptazane)
Open-angle glaucoma or preoperatively in obstructive or narrow-angle glaucoma —
Adults: 50 to 100 mg P.O. b.i.d. or t.i.d.

• Contraindicated for long-term use in chronic noncongestive narrow-angle glaucoma; in severe or absolute glaucoma; and in those patients with depressed serum sodium or potassium levels, renal or hepatic disease or dysfunction, adrenal gland dysfunction, or hyperchloremic acidosis.
• Use cautiously in patients with respiratory acidosis, emphysema, and chronic pulmonary disease.

urea (carbamide) (Ureaphil)
Intracranial or intraocular pressure —
Adults: 1 to 1.5 g/kg as a 30% solution by slow I.V. infusion over 1 to 2½ hours.
Maximum adult daily dosage is 120 g. To prepare 135 ml of 30% solution, mix contents of 40-g vial of urea with 105 mg dextrose 5% or 10% in water or 10% invert sugar in water. Each ml of 30% solution provides 300 mg urea.
Children over age 2: 0.5 to 1.5 g/kg by slow I.V. infusion.
Children under age 2: as little as 0.1 g/kg by slow I.V. infusion. Maximum rate is 4 ml/minute.

• Contraindicated in patients with severely impaired renal function, marked dehydration, frank hepatic failure, or active intracranial bleeding.
• Use cautiously in pregnant or breast-feeding women, and in those with cardiac disease, hepatic impairment, and sickle cell disease with CNS involvement.

COMPARING DIURETIC COMBINATIONS

TRADE NAME AND CONTENT	SPECIAL CONSIDERATIONS
Moduretic amiloride 5 mg and hydrochlorothiazide 50 mg **Aldactazide 25/25** **Spirozide** spironolactone 25 mg and hydrochlorothiazide 25 mg **Aldactazide 50/50** spironolactone 50 mg and hydrochlorothiazide 50 mg **Dyazide** triamterene 50 mg and hydrochlorothiazide 25 mg **Maxzide-25** triamterene 37.5 mg and hydrochlorothiazide 25 mg **Maxzide** triamterene 75 mg and hydrochlorothiazide 50 mg	• Combine the diuretic and antihypertensive actions of hydrochlorothiazide, a thiazide diuretic, and amiloride, spironolactone, or triamterene, potassium-sparing diuretics. They lower blood pressure and cause diuresis without significant loss of potassium. • Fixed combination products are not indicated for initial use. Patient's dosage should be titrated to the desired antihypertensive effect with individual drugs before a combination product is used.

SELF-TEST

1. Michael Murray was admitted to the hospital with sepsis and acute renal failure. His doctor prescribed an I.V. aminoglycoside antibiotic (gentamicin) for the infection and an I.V. loop diuretic (furosemide) to help maintain Mr. Murray's urine output. With this combination of medications, which of the following assessments is especially important?
   a. Measure the patient's blood pressure frequently.
   b. Assess the I.V. injection site before administering each dose of drug.
   c. Monitor CBC results daily.
   d. Evaluate the patient for ringing in the ears or decreased hearing acuity.

2. Avery Sharp was recently diagnosed as having hypertension. Her doctor prescribed hydrochlorothiazide 2 weeks ago to lower her blood pressure. Mrs. Sharp has been monitoring her blood pressure at home and is discouraged because her blood pressure readings have not decreased as much as she hoped they would. What should the nurse tell her?
   a. The full antihypertensive effect of hydrochlorothiazide may not occur for 3 to 4 weeks after initiation of therapy.
   b. She is probably taking the drug incorrectly.
   c. She should stop taking the medication because it is unlikely it will help her.
   d. She should contact her doctor and ask him to prescribe an additional antihypertensive.

3. While in the hospital for an acute MI, Angela Perry is started on hydrochlorothiazide and spironolactone for treatment of hypertension. The nurse's discharge instructions should advise Mrs. Perry to:
   a. contact her doctor if blood pressure control is not achieved in 2 to 3 days.
   b. take spironolactone between meals to increase absorption.
   c. watch for signs of hypokalemia and include potassium-rich foods in her diet.
   d. watch for signs of hyperkalemia and avoid high-potassium foods.

4. Gerald Harris develops profound hypotension after repair of a ruptured abdominal aortic aneurysm. His doctor prescribes mannitol 100 g I.V. to be given over 2 hours. When administering mannitol to an oliguric patient, the nurse should closely monitor the patient for signs of:
   a. hyperkalemia.
   b. hyperglycemia.
   c. circulatory overload.
   d. cellular dehydration.

Check your answers on page 1072.

CHAPTER 62

ACIDIFIER AND ALKALINIZERS

Acidifier
ammonium chloride

Alkalinizers
sodium bicarbonate ✦ sodium lactate ✦ tromethamine

OVERVIEW
- Acidifiers and alkalinizers may correct acid-base imbalances in metabolic disorders. In severe metabolic alkalosis, acidifiers may be given to lower blood pH. In metabolic acidosis, alkalinizers raise blood pH.

MAJOR USES
- Acidifiers are used to treat metabolic alkalosis.
- Alkalinizers are used to treat metabolic acidosis. Sodium bicarbonate and sodium lactate may also alkalinize the urine. This blocks tubular reabsorption of acidic drugs and increases their excretion. Alkalinizing the urine can be part of the treatment of aspirin or phenobarbital overdose.

MECHANISM OF ACTION
- Acidifiers increase free hydrogen ion concentration.
- Alkalinizers decrease free hydrogen ion concentration. Sodium bicarbonate restores the buffering capacity of the body. Sodium lactate is metabolized to sodium bicarbonate before it can produce a buffering effect. Tromethamine combines with hydrogen ions and associated acid anions; the resulting salts are excreted by the kidneys.

ABSORPTION, DISTRIBUTION, METABOLISM, AND EXCRETION
Ammonium chloride and sodium bicarbonate are rapidly and well absorbed orally. Sodium lactate and tromethamine are administered I.V. Ammonium chloride and sodium bicarbonate can be administered either orally or I.V.

Ammonium chloride and sodium lactate are metabolized in the liver. Ammonium chloride is excreted in urine. Tromethamine is not metabolized and is excreted in urine.

GLOSSARY

Metabolic acidosis: decreased serum pH caused by an excess of hydrogen ions in the extracellular fluid.
Metabolic alkalosis: increased serum pH caused by excess bicarbonate in the extracellular fluid.
Systemic acidifier: agent that decreases serum pH level.
Systemic alkalinizer: agent that increases serum pH level.
Urinary acidifier: agent that decreases urine pH level.
Urinary alkalinizer: agent that increases urine pH level.

ONSET AND DURATION
Onset is rapid after oral administration and immediate after I.V. administration. Duration of action varies, depending on use and the underlying disease.

ADVERSE REACTIONS
Adverse reactions to ammonium chloride result from too-rapid I.V. infusion or ammonia toxicity. Severe reactions include hypocalcemic tetany, EEG abnormalities, and alternating episodes of depression and excitation. Metabolic reactions can include acidosis, hyperchloremia, hypokalemia, and hyperglycemia.

The alkalinizers can produce metabolic reactions, such as alkalosis, hyperkalemia, and—with the sodium salts—hypernatremia. Tromethamine may also cause respiratory depression and hypoglycemia.

Adverse reactions with both acidifiers and alkalinizers can be minimized by careful monitoring of serum electrolytes and clinical parameters.

PROTOTYPE: ACIDIFIER

AMMONIUM CHLORIDE
(a moe' nee um klor' ide)
Classification: acidifier
Pregnancy risk category B

How supplied
TABLETS: 500 mg ◊
TABLETS (ENTERIC-COATED): 500 mg ◊, 1,000 mg
INJECTION: 2.14% (0.4 mEq/ml), 26.75% (5 mEq/ml)

Indications and dosage
Metabolic alkalosis
ADULTS AND CHILDREN: I.V. dose (in mEq) is equal to the serum chloride deficit (in mEq/ml) multiplied by the extracellular fluid volume (estimated

as 20% of the body weight in kg). One-half the calculated volume should be given; then the patient should be reassessed.

As an acidifying agent
ADULTS: 4 to 12 g P.O. daily in divided doses.
CHILDREN: 75 mg/kg P.O. daily in four divided doses.

Contraindications and precautions
Ammonium chloride is contraindicated in severe hepatic or renal dysfunction. Use cautiously in pulmonary insufficiency or cardiac edema or in infants.

Adverse reactions
CNS: headache, confusion, progressive drowsiness, periods of excitement alternating with depression, coma, hyperventilation, calcium-deficient tetany, twitching, hyperreflexia, EEG abnormalities.
CV: bradycardia.
GI: (with oral dose) *gastric irritation, nausea, vomiting,* thirst, anorexia, retching.
GU: glycosuria.
METABOLIC: *electrolyte imbalances, acidosis,* hyperchloremia, hypokalemia, hyperglycemia.
SKIN: rash, pallor.
LOCAL: pain at injection site.
OTHER: irregular respirations with periods of apnea.

Interactions
Spironolactone: systemic acidosis. Use together cautiously. Incompatible with milk and other alkaline solutions.

Nursing considerations
Assessment
• Review the patient's history for a condition that contraindicates the use of ammonium chloride.
• Obtain a baseline assessment of rate and depth of respirations, urine pH and output, serum electrolytes, and carbon dioxide–combining power before initiating ammonium chloride therapy.
• Be alert for common adverse reactions.
• Evaluate the patient's and family's knowledge about ammonium chloride therapy.

Planning (Nursing Diagnoses)
Potential nursing diagnoses for the patient receiving ammonium chloride include:
• Altered health maintenance related to inadequate dosage regimen of ammonium chloride.
• Fluid volume deficit related to drug-induced adverse GI reactions.
• Altered protection related to potential drug-induced acidosis and electrolyte imbalance.
• Knowledge deficit related to ammonium chloride therapy.

Italicized adverse reactions are common

Implementation

Preparation and administration

— Read order and drug label carefully before administering ammonium chloride.

— For I.V. administration, check patency of I.V. line and infusion site; check infusion pump functioning.

— Dilute a concentrated solution of ammonium chloride (26.75%) before administration. Add 100 to 200 mg (20 to 40 ml) of the solution to 500 or 1,000 ml of 0.9% sodium chloride injection.

— In adults, administer ammonium chloride solution via infusion pump, not exceeding 5 ml/minute.

— Decrease rate of infusion if pain at infusion site occurs.

— Give oral ammonium chloride after meals to decrease adverse GI reactions.

— Enteric-coated tablets may minimize GI symptoms but are absorbed erratically.

— Chart administration of drug and related observations.

Monitoring

— Monitor the effectiveness of therapy by regularly checking respiratory rate and depth, urine output and pH, serum electrolytes, partial pressure of carbon dioxide in arterial blood (PCO_2), and sodium bicarbonate (HCO_3^-).

— Monitor the patient for adverse drug reactions.

— Monitor for signs of metabolic acidosis: CNS depression, Kussmaul's respirations, headache, and confusion.

— Monitor renal and hepatic function.

— Monitor mental and neurologic status.

— Monitor the patient for drug interactions.

— Monitor vital signs. Hypotension, tachycardia, dyspnea, and fever may indicate fluid volume deficit.

— Regularly reevaluate the patient's and family's knowledge about ammonium chloride therapy.

Intervention

— Hold drug and notify the doctor if acidosis occurs.

— Institute safety and seizure precautions.

— Avoid sedative-hypnotics if the patient develops decreased respiratory rate or CNS depression.

— Maintain accurate record of intake and output.

— Weigh the patient daily.

— Provide frequent skin and mouth care.

— Reorient the patient to person, place, and time as indicated.

— Obtain an order for an antiemetic if adverse GI reactions occur.

— Keep all members of the health care team informed of the patient's response to the drug.

Patient teaching
—Instruct the patient and family about ammonium chloride, including the dosage, frequency, action, and adverse reactions.
—Instruct the patient to take oral ammonium chloride with meals to avoid GI symptoms.
—Advise the patient to avoid taking drug with milk or other alkaline solutions.
—Teach the patient to avoid excessive use of sodium bicarbonate and other prescribed or OTC alkaline substances.
—Teach the patient and family to identify and report the signs of metabolic acidosis: headache, confusion, CNS depression, and Kussmaul's respirations.
—Tell the patient to notify the nurse or doctor if adverse reactions develop or questions arise about ammonium chloride therapy.

Evaluation
In the patient receiving ammonium chloride, appropriate evaluation statements include:
• Patient's metabolic alkalosis is resolved.
• Patient does not experience adverse GI reactions.
• Patient's acid-base balance and electrolyte levels become normal.
• Patient and family state an understanding of ammonium chloride therapy.

PROTOTYPE: ALKALINIZERS

SODIUM BICARBONATE
(so' dee um bi kar' boe nate)
Classification: alkalinizer
Pregnancy risk category C

How supplied
TABLETS: 300 mg◊, 325 mg◊, 600 mg◊, 650 mg◊
INJECTION: 4% (2.4 mEq/5 ml), 4.2% (5 mEq/10 ml), 5% (297.5 mEq/500 ml), 7.5% (8.92 mEq/10 ml and 44.6 mEq/50 ml), 8.4% (10 mEq/10 ml and 50 mEq/50 ml)

Indications and dosage
Cardiac arrest
ADULTS AND CHILDREN: 7.5% or 8.4% solution, 1 mEq/kg I.V. bolus followed by 0.5 mEq/kg q 10 minutes depending on arterial blood gas (ABG) values. Further dosages based on ABG values. If ABG values are unavailable, use 0.5 mEq/kg q 10 minutes until spontaneous circulation returns.
INFANTS UP TO AGE 2: 4.2% solution by I.V. infusion. Rate not to exceed 8 mEq/kg daily.

Metabolic acidosis
ADULTS AND CHILDREN: dosage depends on blood carbon dioxide (CO_2) content, pH, and the patient's clinical condition. Generally, 2 to 5 mEq/kg I.V. infused over a 4- to 8-hour period.

Systemic or urinary alkalinization
ADULTS: 325 mg to 2 g P.O. q.i.d.
CHILDREN: 12 to 120 mg/kg P.O. daily.

Antacid
ADULTS: 300 mg to 2 g P.O. chewed and taken with glass of water.

Contraindications and precautions
Sodium bicarbonate is contraindicated in patients with hypertension or tendency toward edema; in patients who are losing chlorides by vomiting or from continuous GI suction; in patients who are receiving diuretics known to produce hypochloremic alkalosis; in patients on sodium-restricted diets; and in those with renal disease.

Sodium bicarbonate is not routinely recommended for use in cardiac arrest because it may produce a paradoxical acidosis from CO_2 production. It should not be routinely administered during the early stages of CPR unless preexisting acidosis is clearly present. May be used at health care team leader's discretion after such interventions as defibrillation, cardiac compression, and administration of first-line drugs. Use cautiously with enteric-coated drugs (may cause premature release in stomach).

Adverse reactions
GI: *gastric distention, belching,* flatulence.
GU: renal calculi or crystals.
METABOLIC: (with overdose) alkalosis, hypernatremia, hyperkalemia, hyperosmolarity.
LOCAL: extravasation, which can cause tissue necrosis and sloughing.
OTHER: **intracellular acidosis** (with high dosage).

Interactions
Catecholamines, such as norepinephrine and dopamine: inactivation when I.V. solutions are mixed. Don't mix in the same I.V. container.

Nursing considerations
Assessment
- Review the patient's history for a condition that contraindicates the use of sodium bicarbonate.
- Obtain a baseline assessment of ABG values, serum electrolytes, and urine pH and output before initiating sodium bicarbonate therapy.
- Be alert for common adverse reactions.
- Evaluate the patient's and family's knowledge about sodium bicarbonate therapy.

Planning (Nursing Diagnoses)
Potential nursing diagnoses for the patient receiving sodium bicarbonate include:

Italicized adverse reactions are common   Boldfaced adverse reactions are life-threatening

- Altered health maintenance related to ineffective dosage regimen of sodium bicarbonate.
- Altered protection related to sodium bicarbonate overdose.
- Knowledge deficit related to sodium bicarbonate therapy.

Implementation

Preparation and administration

— Read order and drug label carefully before administration.
— Sodium bicarbonate may be mixed with other I.V. solutions except those containing dopamine or norepinephrine.
— Check patency of I.V. line and infusion site before administration.
— Dose is usually administered in I.V. bolus form q 10 minutes as needed.
— Give oral preparation with a full glass of water.
— Do not administer oral sodium bicarbonate with milk or other alkaline solutions.
— Chart drug administration and related observations.

Monitoring

— Monitor the effectiveness of therapy by regularly checking ABGs, serum electrolytes, and urine pH and output.
— Monitor the patient for adverse drug reactions.
— Monitor vital signs: tachycardia, hypotension, dyspnea, and fever may indicate fluid volume deficit.
— Monitor skin turgor and mucous membranes to indicate fluid volume deficit.
— Monitor for signs of metabolic alkalosis (indicates overdose).
— Monitor mental and neurologic status.
— Monitor the patient for drug interactions.
— Regularly reevaluate the patient's and family's knowledge about sodium bicarbonate therapy.

Intervention

— Hold dose and notify the doctor if drug overdose occurs.
— Frequently check I.V. site and patency; if infiltration results in extravasation of sodium bicarbonate to surrounding tissues, elevate the extremity, apply heat, and consult the doctor for additional orders.
— Maintain accurate record of intake and output.
— Weigh the patient daily.
— Provide frequent skin and mouth care to relieve skin and mucous membrane dryness.
— Encourage oral intake of fluids if the patient is alert.
— Institute safety precautions due to potential weakness and altered thought processes.
— Reorient the patient to person, place, and time as needed.
— Keep all members of the health care team informed of the patient's response to the drug.

Patient teaching
— Instruct the patient and family about sodium bicarbonate, including the dosage, frequency, action, and adverse reactions.
— Teach the patient and family to identify and report signs of metabolic alkalosis (overdose).
— Teach the patient and family to monitor the patient's fluid volume by weighing the patient daily and recording his fluid intake and urine output.
— Advise the patient not to take oral sodium bicarbonate with milk or other alkaline solutions.
— Discourage use of sodium bicarbonate as an antacid or with the use of other antacid preparations containing sodium.
— Teach the patient to avoid foods high in sodium.
— Tell the patient to notify the nurse or doctor if adverse reactions develop or questions arise about sodium bicarbonate therapy.

Evaluation
In the patient receiving sodium bicarbonate, appropriate evaluation statements include:
• Patient's metabolic alkalosis is resolved.
• Patient does not experience signs and symptoms of sodium bicarbonate overdose.
• Patient and family state an understanding of sodium bicarbonate therapy.

SELECTED MAJOR DRUGS: ALKALINIZERS

DRUG, INDICATIONS, AND DOSAGES	SPECIAL PRECAUTIONS
sodium lactate *Alkalinize urine —* **Adults:** 30 ml of ⅙ M solution/kg of body weight I.V. given in divided doses over 24 hours. *Metabolic acidosis —* **Adults:** usually given as ⅙ M injection (167 mEq lactate/liter) I.V. Dosage depends on degree of bicarbonate deficit.	• Contraindicated in patients with severe hepatic and renal disease, respiratory alkalosis, or acidosis associated with congenital heart disease with persistent cyanosis.
tromethamine (Tham) *Metabolic acidosis (associated with cardiac bypass surgery or cardiac arrest) —* **Adults:** dosage depends on degree of bicarbonate deficit. Calculate as follows: ml of 0.3 M tromethamine solution required = weight in kg × bicarbonate deficit (mEq/liter). Additional therapy based on serial determinations of existing bicarbonate deficit. **Children:** calculate dosage as above. Give slowly over 3 to 6 hours. Additional therapy based on degree of acidosis. Total 24-hour dosage should not exceed 33 to 40 ml/kg.	• Contraindicated in patients with anuria, uremia, chronic respiratory acidosis, or during pregnancy (except in acute, life-threatening situations). • Use cautiously in patients with renal disease and poor urine output. Monitor ECG and serum potassium in these patients.

SELF-TEST

1. Bruce Barrett is admitted to the hospital with hepatic cirrhosis complicated by a severe metabolic alkalosis. His medical history reveals Type II diabetes, angina pectoris, and COPD. Although ammonium chloride can be used to treat Mr. Barrett's acid-base imbalance, it is contraindicated because of his:
   a. hepatic cirrhosis.
   b. diabetes mellitus.
   c. angina pectoris.
   d. chronic obstructive pulmonary disease.

2. Christina Carter has just been resuscitated after a cardiac arrest. She received sodium bicarbonate by I.V. push during resuscitation to correct severe acidosis. The nurse who administered the sodium bicarbonate observed infiltration of Ms. Carter's peripheral I.V. site. The remainder of the dosage was given through an alternative site. Now that Ms. Carter is more stable, what should her nurse do to treat the site of sodium bicarbonate infiltration?
   a. The nurse should discontinue the I.V. No further treatment is necessary.
   b. She should discontinue the I.V., elevate the arm, apply heat, and contact Ms. Carter's doctor for further orders.
   c. She should discontinue the I.V., elevate the arm, and apply ice packs for 2 hours.
   d. She should discontinue the I.V. and inject phentolamine (Regitine) subcutaneously around the area of infiltration.

3. For which of the following adverse reactions should the nurse monitor Ms. Carter?
   a. Arrhythmias
   b. Drowsiness
   c. Metabolic alkalosis
   d. Hyponatremia

Check your answers on page 1072.

CHAPTER 63

HEMATINICS

ferrous fumarate ✦ ferrous gluconate ✦ ferrous sulfate ✦ iron dextran

OVERVIEW

- Hematinics are iron-containing compounds that increase both the hemo-globin level and the number of RBCs. Iron is necessary for formation of hemoglobin, which transports oxygen within the RBCs from the lungs to the tissues. Iron deficiency, which can lead to decreased hemoglobin synthesis and decreased RBC production, may result from blood loss or inadequate iron intake during accelerated growth or pregnancy. Al-though many expensive forms of iron therapy are available, ferrous sulfate is the cheapest and most effective.

MAJOR USES

- Iron preparations supplement depleted iron stores. As a daily dietary supplement, 10 to 18 mg of elemental iron for adults and 4 to 8 mg for children are sufficient. Patients with iron deficiency may require 90 to 200 mg of elemental iron daily.

MECHANISM OF ACTION

- After absorption into the blood, iron is immediately bound to transferrin, a plasma protein that transports iron. Transferrin carries iron to bone marrow, where it's used during hemoglobin synthesis. Some iron is also used during synthesis of myoglobin or other nonhemoglobin heme units.

ABSORPTION, DISTRIBUTION, METABOLISM, AND EXCRETION

The absorption of iron is complex and influenced by many factors, including the iron salt given, iron stores in the body, degree of erythropoi-esis, drug dose, and diet.

Absorption occurs mainly in the duodenum after oral administration, although a small amount is typically absorbed as well in the proximal jejunum. Healthy persons absorb about 10% of the iron present in their diets, whereas patients with iron deficiency may absorb as much as 30% of dietary iron in an attempt to replace body stores of this element.

When given therapeutically, the ferrous form of iron is better absorbed orally than the ferric form. Patients with iron deficiency absorb as much as 60% of an iron dose. When total body stores of iron are large, absorption is diminished. After I.M. injection, 60% of the iron is absorbed after 3 days and up to 90% is absorbed after 1 to 3 weeks. When administered I.V., all of the iron is absorbed immediately.

GLOSSARY

Anemia: disorder characterized by a decrease in hemoglobin in the blood to levels below the normal range.
Erythropoiesis: production of RBCs.
Erythropoietin: glycoprotein produced by the kidneys that stimulates RBC production.
Ferritin: one of the complexes in which iron is stored in the body.
Hematinic: agent capable of improving blood quality by increasing hemoglobin level and number of RBCs.
Hemoglobin: oxygen-carrying pigment of the RBCs.
Transferrin: trace protein present in the blood that is essential in iron transport.

Iron is stored in the bone marrow (2,400 mg) and liver (800 mg in males, 300 mg in females). The remainder is bound to plasma proteins and contained in muscles (myoglobin) and certain enzymes.

Iron metabolism is a closed system: the body conserves and reuses most of the iron that's liberated by hemoglobin destruction. Elimination of iron is minimal: 500 mcg to 2 mg are lost daily, primarily as cells exfoliated from the skin, GI mucosa, nails, and hair. Only trace amounts of iron are secreted in bile or excreted in sweat. Women normally lose 12 to 30 mg of iron during each menstrual period.

ONSET AND DURATION

With therapeutic doses of iron salts, symptoms of iron deficiency usually improve within 2 to 3 days. Peak reticulocytosis (formation of new RBCs) occurs in 5 to 10 days, and the hemoglobin level rises after 2 to 4 weeks. Normal hemoglobin values are usually attained in 2 months, unless blood loss continues.

ADVERSE REACTIONS

The usual dosage of oral iron commonly produces constipation, dark stools, diarrhea, nausea, or epigastric pain. These reactions can be minimized by taking the drug between or after meals or by administering lower doses at shorter intervals.

Fatal anaphylaxis has been reported with the parenteral administration (I.M. or I.V.) of iron dextran, commonly within the first few minutes of administration; this reaction is most often associated with sudden respiratory difficulty, sometimes with CV collapse.

Other reactions to iron dextran may include local reactions at injection sites; nausea, vomiting, and disturbances in taste; headache, weakness, dizziness; arthralgia and myalgia; and flushing and hypotension with rapid I.V. administration.

FERROUS SULFATE
(fer' us sul' fate)

Feosol*◊, Fer-In-Sol*◊, Feritard‡, Fero-Grad†, Fero-Gradumet◊, Ferospace◊, Ferralyn Lanacaps◊, Fespan‡, Irospan◊, Mol-Iron*◊, Novoferrosulfat†, Slow-Fe

Classification: hematinic
Pregnancy risk category A

How supplied
Ferrous sulfate is 20% elemental iron; dried and powdered (exsiccated), it is about 32% elemental iron.
TABLETS: 195 mg◊, 300 mg◊, 325 mg◊; 200 mg (exsiccated)◊
TABLETS (EXTENDED-RELEASE): 160 mg (exsiccated)◊
CAPSULES: 150 mg◊, 225 mg◊, 250 mg◊, 390 mg; 190 mg (exsiccated)◊
CAPSULES (EXTENDED-RELEASE): 525 mg◊; 150 mg◊, 167 mg (exsiccated)◊
ELIXIR: 220 mg/5 ml◊
LIQUID: 75 mg/0.6 ml◊
SYRUP: 90 mg/5 ml

Indications and dosage
Iron deficiency
ADULTS: 325 mg P.O. t.i.d. or q.i.d. Alternatively, give 1 extended-release capsule (160 or 525 mg) P.O. b.i.d.
CHILDREN: 5 mg/kg P.O. t.i.d., increased to 10 mg/kg P.O. t.i.d. p.r.n. and as tolerated.

Prophylaxis for iron deficiency
PREGNANT WOMEN: 150 to 300 mg P.O. daily in divided doses.
PREMATURE OR UNDERNOURISHED INFANTS: 1 to 2 mg/kg P.O. daily (as elemental iron) in divided doses.

Contraindications and precautions
Ferrous sulfate is contraindicated in patients with hemosiderosis and hemochromatosis. Use cautiously in peptic ulcer, ulcerative colitis, and regional enteritis. Also use cautiously on long-term basis.

Adverse reactions
GI: *nausea,* vomiting, *constipation, black stools.*
OTHER: elixir may stain teeth.

Interactions
Antacids, cholestyramine resin, pancreatic extracts, vitamin E: decreased iron absorption. Separate doses if possible.
Chloramphenicol: watch for delayed response to iron therapy.
Tetracyclines, ciprofloxacin and other quinolone antibiotics: decreased absorption of these antibiotics. Separate administration times by at least 2 hours.

---

*Liquid form contains alcohol   †Available in Canada only   ‡Available in Australia only   ◊ Available OTC
Italicized adverse reactions are common

Vitamin C: may increase iron absorption. Beneficial drug interaction.

Nursing considerations

Assessment

• Review the patient's history for a condition that contraindicates the use of ferrous sulfate.
• Obtain a baseline assessment of the patient's hemoglobin and reticulocyte counts before therapy.
• Be alert for common adverse reactions.
• Evaluate the patient's and family's knowledge about ferrous sulfate therapy.

Planning (Nursing Diagnoses)

Potential nursing diagnoses for the patient receiving ferrous sulfate include:

• Altered health maintenance related to ineffective dosing regimen of ferrous sulfate to correct iron deficiency.
• Constipation related to adverse effects of ferrous sulfate on the GI tract.
• Knowledge deficit related to ferrous sulfate therapy.

Implementation

Preparation and administration

— Administer between meals if possible.
— If GI upset occurs, give with food.
— Dilute liquid preparations in juice or water but not in milk or antacids. Diluting liquid preparations in or giving tablets with orange juice promotes iron absorption.
— Administer iron elixirs through straw to avoid staining of teeth.

Monitoring

— Monitor the effectiveness of therapy by regularly evaluating the patient's hemoglobin and reticulocyte counts.
— Monitor the patient for constipation; record color and amount of stool.
— Monitor the patient for adverse drug reactions.
— Monitor the patient for drug interactions.
— Regularly reevaluate the patient's and family's knowledge about ferrous sulfate therapy.

Intervention

— Notify the doctor if hemoglobin and reticulocyte count do not improve with ferrous sulfate therapy.
— If not contraindicated, encourage the patient to increase intake of fiber and fluid and to exercise regularly to prevent constipation. If constipation occurs despite these measures, obtain a laxative order.
— Keep all members of the health care team informed of the patient's response to the drug.

Patient teaching

— Instruct the patient and family about ferrous sulfate, including the dosage, frequency, action, and adverse reactions.

— Tell the patient to take drug between meals; if GI upset occurs, to take with food. If GI upset persists, tell the patient to ask the doctor about enteric-coated products.

— Tell the patient to dilute liquid preparations in or take tablets with orange juice to promote iron absorption.

— Instruct the patient taking iron elixir to use a straw to avoid staining of teeth.

— Tell the patient to continue regular dosing schedule if he misses a dose and not to double the dose.

— Warn parents of the potential for iron poisoning in children and to store drug out of children's reach.

— Teach the patient measures to prevent constipation.

— Alert the patient that drug may turn stools black but that this effect is harmless.

— Stress importance of follow-up care.

— Instruct the patient to eat foods that are rich in iron.

— Tell the patient to notify the nurse or doctor if adverse reactions develop or questions arise about ferrous sulfate therapy.

Evaluation

In the patient receiving ferrous sulfate, appropriate evaluation statements include:

• Patient's hemoglobin and reticulocyte counts are normal.

• Patient's bowel pattern remains unchanged.

• Patient and family state an understanding of ferrous sulfate therapy.

SELECTED MAJOR DRUGS: HEMATINICS

DRUG, INDICATIONS, AND DOSAGES	SPECIAL PRECAUTIONS
ferrous fumarate (Femiron ◇, Feostat ◇) *Iron deficiency —* **Adults:** 200 mg P.O. t.i.d. or q.i.d. **Children:** 3 mg/kg P.O. t.i.d., increased to 6 mg/kg P.O. t.i.d. p.r.n. and as tolerated.	• Contraindicated in patients with hemosiderosis or hemo-chromatosis. • Use cautiously in patients with peptic ulcer, regional enteritis, and ulcerative colitis. Also use cautiously when given on long-term basis.
ferrous gluconate (Fergon ◇, Ferralet ◇) *Iron deficiency —* **Adults:** 300 to 325 mg P.O. q.i.d., increased to 650 mg q.i.d. p.r.n. and as tolerated. **Children ages 2 and over:** 8 mg/kg P.O. t.i.d., increased to 16 mg P.O. t.i.d. p.r.n. and as tolerated.	• Contraindicated in patients with peptic ulcer, regional enteritis, ulcerative colitis, hemosid-erosis, or hemochromatosis. • Use cautiously when given on long-term basis.

(continued)

◇ Available OTC

SELECTED MAJOR DRUGS: HEMATINICS *continued*

DRUG, INDICATIONS, AND DOSAGES	SPECIAL PRECAUTIONS
iron dextran (Imferon) *Iron deficiency—* **Adults:** test dose (0.5 ml) is required before administration. I.M. (by Z-track)—inject 0.5-ml test dose. If no reactions, next daily dose should ordinarily not exceed 0.5 ml (25 mg) for infants under 5 kg; 1 ml (50 mg), for children under 9 kg; 2 ml (100 mg), for patients under 50 kg; 5 ml (250 mg), for patients over 50 kg. I.V. push—inject 0.5-mg test dose. If no reaction, within 2 to 3 days the dosage may be raised to 2 ml I.V. daily, 1 ml/minute undiluted and infused slowly until total dose is achieved. No single dose should exceed 100 mg. I.V. infusion—dosages are expressed in terms of elemental iron. Dilute in 250 to 1,000 ml of 0.9% sodium chloride solution; dextrose increases local vein irritation. Infuse test dose of 25 mg slowly over 5 minutes. If no reaction occurs in 5 minutes, infusion may be started. Infuse total dose slowly over approximately 6 to 12 hours.	• Contraindicated in all anemias other than iron-deficiency anemia. • Use with extreme caution in patients with impaired hepatic function or rheumatoid arthritis. • I.M. or I.V. injections of iron are advisable only for patients for whom oral administration is impossible or ineffective.

COMPARING HEMATINIC COMBINATIONS

TRADE NAME AND CONTENT	SPECIAL CONSIDERATIONS
Fermalox ◇ ferrous sulfate 200 mg, magnesium hydroxide 100 mg, and dried aluminum hydroxide 100 mg	• Combines the effect of the iron preparation ferrous sulfate with the antacid effects of magnesium hydroxide and dried aluminum hydroxide. • Contraindicated in patients with hemochromatosis, hemosiderosis, hemolytic anemia, or known hypersensitivity to any component of the drug. • Use cautiously in patients with peptic ulcer, ulcerative colitis, or regional enteritis and in long-term use.
Ferocyl ◇ **Ferro-Sequels** ◇ ferrous fumarate 150 mg and docusate sodium 100 mg	• Combine the effect of the iron preparation ferrous fumarate with the stool softening effect of docusate sodium. • Contraindicated in patients with hemochromatosis, hemosiderosis, hemolytic anemia, or known hypersensitivity to any component of the drug and with concomitant mineral oil. • Use cautiously in patients with peptic ulcer, ulcerative colitis, or regional enteritis and in long-term use.

◇ Available OTC

SELF-TEST

1. Elvira Engels, age 33, has iron-deficiency anemia. Her doctor prescribed ferrous sulfate 325 mg P.O. q.i.d. Mrs. Engels can expect her symptoms of iron deficiency to improve after:
   a. 24 hours.
   b. 2 to 3 days.
   c. 1 week.
   d. 1 month.

2. Which of the following adverse reactions commonly occurs with ferrous sulfate administration?
   a. Diarrhea
   b. Constipation
   c. Gastric ulceration
   d. Regional enteritis

3. The nurse should teach Mrs. Engels to:
   a. take the drug with orange juice.
   b. avoid concomitant ingestion of complex B vitamins.
   c. immediately follow ingestion of drug with 30 ml of an antacid.
   d. eat a diet high in vitamin K.

Check your answers on pages 1072 and 1073.

CHAPTER 64

ANTICOAGULANTS

dicumarol ◆ heparin calcium ◆ heparin sodium ◆ warfarin sodium

OVERVIEW
- Anticoagulants impede clotting by preventing fibrin formation.
- Anticoagulants are given to patients at risk for developing clots (thromboses). These drugs are also used to prevent clot enlargement or fragmentation (thromboembolism).
- Oral anticoagulants include the coumarin derivatives warfarin sodium and dicumarol. Heparin is not active after oral administration.

MAJOR USES
- All anticoagulants are used to treat pulmonary emboli and deep-vein thrombosis (DVT) and to reduce thrombus formation after cardiac valve replacement surgery.
- Heparin is administered subcutaneously in low doses (minidoses) to prevent DVT and pulmonary embolism.
- Oral anticoagulants are also used in rheumatic heart disease with valvular damage and in atrial arrhythmias that impair hemodynamics.

MECHANISM OF ACTION
- Heparin accelerates formation of an antithrombin III-thrombin complex. It inactivates thrombin and prevents conversion of fibrinogen to fibrin.
- The oral anticoagulants inhibit vitamin K–dependent activation of clotting factors II, VII, IX, and X, which are formed in the liver.

ABSORPTION, DISTRIBUTION, METABOLISM, AND EXCRETION
Heparin is not absorbed from the GI tract and must be administered parenterally. Although absorption after S.C. injection varies greatly among patients, heparin is generally well absorbed and is usually administered by this route. Warfarin is well absorbed from the GI tract; dicumarol is incompletely absorbed.

Heparin is distributed widely in the blood. Oral anticoagulants are 98% bound to plasma proteins, primarily albumin, and are widely distributed in body tissues.

Although the metabolism of heparin is not completely clear, most of the drug seems to be removed from circulation by the reticuloendothelial cells. However, some heparin is probably metabolized by the liver. Up to 50% of the drug is excreted unchanged in urine. Oral anticoagulants are largely

GLOSSARY

Activated partial thromboplastin time (APTT): screening test to evaluate the intrinsic coagulation pathway (except Factor VII and Factor XIII) and common pathway and to monitor heparin therapy.

Anticoagulant: substance that suppresses, delays, or negates blood coagulation.

Antiplatelet: substance that interferes with activity of blood platelets.

Coagulation: conversion of blood from a liquid, free-flowing state to a semisolid gel. Although coagulation, or clotting, can occur within an intact vessel, the process usually starts with tissue damage and exposure of the blood to air.

Embolus: clot or other plug (composed of fat, bone, or another substance foreign to blood) that is totally or partially dislodged from its site of origin and moved by blood flow to a more distant narrow site in the circulatory system, where it may obstruct flow.

Partial thromboplastin time (PTT): screening test to evaluate the intrinsic coagulation pathway (except Factors VII and XIII) and the common pathway and to monitor heparin therapy; less sensitive than APTT.

Prothrombin: glycoprotein converted to thrombin by extrinsic thromboplastin during the second stage of blood coagulation; also called coagulation Factor II.

Prothrombin time (PT): screening test to evaluate the extrinsic coagulation pathway and common pathway and to monitor oral anticoagulant therapy.

Thrombin: enzyme derived from prothrombin that converts fibrinogen to fibrin.

Thrombin time: qualitative test to measure the functional fibrinogen level.

metabolized in the liver and excreted in the urine and feces as inactive metabolites.

ONSET AND DURATION

Heparin begins to act immediately, with peak effects occurring within minutes. Clotting time returns to normal within 2 to 6 hours.

Oral anticoagulants are detectable in the blood within 1 hour after administration, and blood levels usually peak within 12 hours. However, oral anticoagulants require 1 to 3 days to produce therapeutic anticoagulation, even though they alter prothrombin time (PT) the first day of therapy. The average course of therapy is 3 to 6 months, but the anticoagulants should be used for the shortest period necessary. Durations vary from 1 to 14 days.

To reverse the effects of oral anticoagulants, vitamin K_1 (phytonadione) may be used to overcome the pharmacologic effects of these drugs. However, there is a substantial delay until the liver can synthesize new blood factors. If necessary, transfusions may be given.

ADVERSE REACTIONS

The most common adverse reaction to heparin therapy is hemorrhage. The effect is an extension of the drug's pharmacologic action. Major bleeding is more commonly associated with high dose and intermittent I.V. injection than with low dose or continuous infusion therapy. Bleeding may occur at any site but can be minimized by careful patient management. If an overdose occurs, protamine sulfate may be used to reverse the effects of heparin.

Thrombocytopenia may occur in patients on heparin and is usually mild, but requires discontinuation of heparin if significant.

Allergic reactions to heparin are rare and may be manifested by fever, chills, urticaria, pruritus, bronchospasm, and anaphylactoid reactions, including shock.

Hemorrhage is also the most common adverse reaction to oral anticoagulants and may range from minor local petechiae to major hemorrhages. This adverse reaction is an extension of their pharmacologic actions. Massive bleeding most often involves the GI or GU tract but can occur elsewhere, such as in the liver, lungs, or CNS. The risk of bleeding may be minimized by careful monitoring and frequent determinations of PT.

Necrosis or gangrene of tissues has also been reported with oral anticoagulants and principally occurs in women within 2 to 10 days after beginning therapy. If necrosis is suspected, the drug should be discontinued.

Other reported adverse reactions include nausea, vomiting, anorexia, dermatitis, urticaria, alopecia, and fever. Rarely, agranulocytosis, nephropathy, and increases in liver function tests occur. Frequent monitoring of hematologic, renal, and hepatic function should be performed.

Concurrent administration of other drugs may result in drug interactions. Before starting any concurrent drug therapy, consult personnel knowledgeable in this field.

PROTOTYPE: ANTICOAGULANTS

HEPARIN CALCIUM
(hep' a rin)
Calcilean, Calciparine, Caprin‡, Uniparin-Ca‡

HEPARIN SODIUM
Hepalean†, Hep-Lock, Liquaemin Sodium, Uniparin‡
Classification: anticoagulant
Pregnancy risk category C

How supplied

Products are derived from beef lung or porcine intestinal mucosa.
calcium
AMPULE: 12,500 units/0.5 ml; 20,000 units/0.8 ml
SYRINGE: 5,000 units/0.2 ml

---

sodium
CARPUJECT: 5,000 units/ml
DISPOSABLE SYRINGES: 1,000 units/ml, 2,500 units/ml, 5,000 units/ml, 7,500 units/ml, 10,000 units/ml, 20,000 units/ml, 40,000 units/ml
PREMIXED I.V. SOLUTIONS: 1,000 units in 500 ml 0.9% sodium chloride solution; 2,000 units in 1,000 ml 0.9% sodium chloride solution; 12,500 units in 250 ml 0.45% sodium chloride solution; 25,000 units in 250 ml 0.45% sodium chloride; 25,000 units in 500 ml 0.45% sodium chloride solution; 10,000 units in 100 ml dextrose 5% in water (D_5W); 12,500 units in 250 ml D_5W; 25,000 units in 250 ml D_5W; 25,000 units in 500 ml D_5W
UNIT-DOSE AMPULES: 1,000 units/ml, 5,000 units/ml, 10,000 units/ml
VIALS: 1,000 units/ml, 2,500 units/ml, 5,000 units/ml, 7,500 units/ml, 10,000 units/ml, 15,000 units/ml, 20,000 units/ml, 40,000 units/ml
heparin sodium flush
DISPOSABLE SYRINGES: 10 units/ml, 100 units/ml
VIALS: 10 units/ml, 100 units/ml

Indications and dosage
Deep-vein thrombosis DVT, MI
ADULTS: initially, 5,000 to 7,500 units I.V. push; then adjust dose according to partial thromboplastin time (PTT) results and give dose I.V. q 4 hours (usually 4,000 to 5,000 units); or 5,000 to 7,500 units I.V. bolus, then 1,000 units/hour by I.V. infusion pump. Wait 8 hours after bolus dose and adjust hourly rate according to PTT.

Pulmonary embolism
ADULTS: initially, 7,500 to 10,000 units I.V. push; then adjust dose according to PTT results and give dose I.V. q 4 hours (usually, 4,000 to 5,000 units); or 7,500 to 10,000 units I.V. bolus, then 1,000 units/hour by I.V. infusion pump. Wait 8 hours after bolus dose and adjust hourly rate according to PTT.

Prophylaxis of embolism
ADULTS: 5,000 units S.C. q 12 hours.

Open-heart surgery
ADULTS: (total body perfusion) 150 to 300 units/kg by continuous I.V. infusion.

Treatment of pulmonary emboli; prevention and treatment of DVT
CHILDREN: initially, 50 units/kg I.V. drip. Maintenance dose is 100 units/kg I.V. drip q 4 hours. Constant infusion—20,000 units/m^2 daily. Dosages adjusted according to PTT.
    Note: Heparin dosing is highly individualized, depending on disease state, age, and renal and hepatic status.

As an I.V. flush to maintain patency of indwelling I.V. catheters
10 to 100 units as an I.V. flush. Not intended for therapeutic use.

Contraindications and precautions
Heparin is conditionally contraindicated in active bleeding; blood dyscrasia; bleeding tendencies, such as hemophilia, thrombocytopenia, or he-

patic disease with hypoprothrombinemia; suspected intracranial hemorrhage; suppurative thrombophlebitis; inaccessible ulcerative lesions (especially of GI tract); open ulcerative wounds; extensive denudation of skin; and ascorbic acid deficiency and other conditions causing increased capillary permeability; during or after brain, eye, or spinal cord surgery; during continuous tube drainage of stomach or small intestine; in subacute bacterial endocarditis; shock; advanced renal disease; threatened abortion; and severe hypertension. Although the use of heparin is clearly hazardous in these conditions, a decision to use it depends on the comparative risk of failure to treat the coexisting thromboembolic disorder.

Use cautiously during menses; in patients with mild hepatic or renal disease or alcoholism; in patients whose occupations carry a risk of physical injury; immediately postpartum; and in patients with a history of allergies, asthma, or GI ulcers.

Adverse reactions
BLOOD: *hemorrhage with excessive dosage, overly prolonged clotting time,* thrombocytopenia.
LOCAL: irritation, mild pain.
OTHER: **"white clot" syndrome**; hypersensitivity reactions, including chills, fever, pruritus, rhinitis, burning of feet, conjunctivitis, lacrimation, arthralgia, urticaria.

Interactions
Anticoagulants, oral: additive anticoagulation. Monitor PT and PTT.
Salicylates: increased anticoagulant effect. Don't use together.

Nursing considerations
Assessment
• Review the patient's history for a condition that contraindicates the use of heparin.
• Obtain a baseline assessment of the patient's clotting ability and underlying thromboembolic condition before therapy.
• Be alert for common adverse reactions.
• Evaluate the patient's and family's knowledge about heparin therapy.

Planning (Nursing Diagnoses)
Potential nursing diagnoses for the patient receiving heparin include:
• Altered health maintenance related to ineffective dosage of heparin to prevent thromboembolic events.
• Altered protection related to increased risk of bleeding with heparin therapy.
• Knowledge deficit related to heparin therapy.

Implementation
Preparation and administration
—Heparin is available in various concentrations. Check order and vial carefully.
—Low-dose injections are given sequentially deep into S.C. fat between iliac crests in lower abdomen. Inject drug slowly subcutaneously into

fat pad. Leave needle in place for 10 seconds after injection; then withdraw needle. Alternate site every 12 hours—right for morning, left for evening.

—Don't massage after S.C. injection.

—I.M. administration is not recommended.

—I.V. administration is preferred because of long-term effect and irregular absorption when given subcutaneously. Whenever possible, administer I.V. heparin with an infusion pump for maximum safety.

—Concentrated heparin solutions (greater than 100 units/ml) can irritate blood vessels.

—In the elderly patient, heparin therapy should begin at lower dosage.

—Check constant I.V. infusions regularly, even when pumps are in good working order, to prevent overdosage or underdosage.

—Give on time; try not to skip a dose or "catch up" with an I.V. containing heparin. If I.V. is out, restart it as soon as possible and reschedule bolus dose immediately.

—Never piggyback other drugs into an infusion line while heparin infusion is running. Many antibiotics and other drugs inactivate heparin. Never mix any drug with heparin in syringe when bolus therapy is used.

—Abrupt withdrawal may cause increased coagulability. Usually, heparin therapy is followed by oral anticoagulants for prophylaxis.

Monitoring

—Monitor the effectiveness of therapy by regularly measuring PTT carefully. Anticoagulation is present when PTT values are 1.5 to 2 times control values.

—When intermittent I.V. therapy is used, always draw blood ½ hour before next scheduled dose to avoid falsely elevated PTT.

—Blood for PTT can be drawn any time after 8 hours of initiation of continuous I.V. heparin therapy. Never draw blood for PTT from I.V. tubing of heparin infusion or from vein of infusion; falsely elevated PTT will result. Always draw blood from opposite arm.

—Monitor platelet counts regularly. Thrombocytopenia caused by heparin may be associated with a type of arterial thrombosis known as "white clot" syndrome.

—Regularly monitor the patient for bleeding gums, bruises on arms or legs, petechiae, nosebleeds, melena, tarry stools, hematuria, and hematemesis. Also monitor for signs of bleeding at injection site.

—Monitor the patient for adverse drug reactions.

—Monitor for hypersensitivity reaction, such as chills, fever, pruritus, rhinitis, burning of feet, conjunctivitis, lacrimation, arthralgia, or urticaria, especially at the start of therapy.

—Monitor the patient for drug interactions.

—Regularly reevaluate the patient's and family's knowledge about heparin therapy.

Intervention

—Institute bleeding precautions. For example, place notice above the patient's bed to inform I.V. team or laboratory personnel to apply pressure dressings after taking blood; to avoid excessive I.M. injections of other drugs to prevent or minimize hematomas; and, if possible, to avoid all I.M. injections.

—Withhold drug and notify the doctor immediately if hypersensitivity reaction occurs.

—If a new thromboembolic event occurs, also notify the doctor to discuss change in dosage; provide emergency supportive care as indicated.

—Keep protamine sulfate readily available to neutralize heparin effects in case of overdose resulting in bleeding.

—Keep all members of the health care team informed of the patient's response to the drug.

Patient teaching

—Instruct the patient and family about heparin, including the dosage, frequency, action, and adverse reactions.

—Teach proper injection technique if the patient or family will be administering the drug.

—Tell the patient to watch for evidence of bleeding, such as nosebleeds, hematuria, and easy bruising, and for signs of peripheral vascular ischemia, such as muscle pain, numbness, and coldness of extremities; stress importance of notifying the doctor at once if any such signs occur.

—Tell the patient to avoid OTC medications containing aspirin, other salicylates, or drugs that may interact with heparin.

—Instruct the patient to take bleeding precautions while receiving heparin therapy, such as using a soft toothbrush, shaving with an electric razor, and avoiding injury.

—Tell the patient to notify the nurse or doctor if adverse reactions develop or questions arise about heparin therapy.

Evaluation

In the patient receiving heparin, appropriate evaluation statements include:
• Patient does not develop additional thromboembolisms.
• Patient does not develop abnormal bleeding.
• Patient and family state an understanding of heparin therapy.

PROTOTYPE: COUMARIN DERIVATIVES

WARFARIN SODIUM
(war′ far in)
Coumadin, Panwarfin**, Warfilone Sodium†
Classification: coumarin derivative
Pregnancy risk category D

How supplied
TABLETS: 2 mg, 2.5 mg, 5 mg, 7.5 mg, 10 mg
INJECTION: 50 mg/vial

Indications and dosage
Treatment of pulmonary emboli; prevention and treatment of DVT, MI, rheumatic heart disease with heart valve damage, atrial arrhythmias
ADULTS: 10 to 15 mg P.O. for 3 days, then dosage based on daily PT readings. Usual maintenance dosage is 2 to 10 mg P.O. daily. Alternate regimen—initially, 40 to 60 mg P.O. daily; then 2 to 10 mg daily based on PT determinations.

Warfarin is also available for I.V. use (50 mg/vial). Reconstitute with sterile water for injection. I.V. form is rarely used and may be in periodic short supply.

Contraindications and precautions
Warfarin is contraindicated in bleeding or hemorrhagic tendencies resulting from open wounds, visceral cancer, GI ulcers, severe hepatic or renal disease, severe uncontrolled hypertension, subacute bacterial endocarditis, or vitamin K deficiency and after recent surgery involving the eye, brain, or spinal cord. Use cautiously in patients with diverticulitis, colitis, mild or moderate hypertension, or mild or moderate hepatic or renal disease; in women who are breast-feeding; in patients with drainage tubes in any orifice or with regional or lumbar block anesthesia; or in any condition increasing risk of hemorrhage.

Adverse reactions
BLOOD: *hemorrhage with excessive dosage,* leukopenia.
GI: paralytic ileus, intestinal obstruction (both resulting from hemorrhage), diarrhea, vomiting, cramps, nausea.
GU: excessive uterine bleeding.
SKIN: dermatitis, urticaria, rash, necrosis, alopecia.
OTHER: fever.

Interactions
Acetaminophen: increased bleeding possible with chronic (greater than 2 weeks) therapy with acetaminophen. Monitor very carefully.
Amiodarone, chloramphenicol, clofibrate, diflunisal, thyroid drugs, heparin, anabolic steroids, cimetidine, disulfiram, glucagon, inhalation anesthetics, metronidazole, quinidine, influenza vaccine, sulindac, sulfinpyrazone, sulfonamides: increased PT. Monitor carefully for bleeding.

---

†Available in Canada only   **May contain tartrazine
Italicized adverse reactions are common

Consider anticoagulant dosage reduction.

Barbiturates: inhibition of hypoprothrombinemic effect of anticoagulants. If barbiturates are withdrawn, reduce anticoagulant dose; inhibition may last weeks after barbiturate is withdrawn, but fatal hemorrhage can occur when inhibiting effect disappears.

Cholestyramine: decreased response when administered too close together. Administer 6 hours after oral anticoagulants.

Ethacrynic acid, indomethacin, mefenamic acid, oxyphenbutazone, phenylbutazone, salicylates: increased PT; ulcerogenic effects. Don't use together.

Glutethimide, chloral hydrate: increased or decreased PT. Avoid use if possible, or monitor carefully.

Griseofulvin, haloperidol, ethchlorvynol, carbamazepine, paraldehyde, rifampin: decreased PT with reduced anticoagulant effect. Monitor carefully.

Nursing considerations

Assessment
• Review the patient's history for a condition that contraindicates the use of warfarin.
• Obtain a baseline assessment of the patient's clotting ability and underlying thromboembolism, if present, before therapy.
• Be alert for common adverse reactions.
• Evaluate the patient's and family's knowledge about warfarin therapy.

Planning (Nursing Diagnoses)
Potential nursing diagnoses for the patient receiving warfarin include:
• Altered health maintenance related to ineffective dosage of warfarin to prevent thromboembolic events.
• Altered protection related to increased risk of bleeding with warfarin therapy.
• Knowledge deficit related to warfarin therapy.

Implementation

Preparation and administration
— Administer drug at same time daily.
— Double-check dosage to prevent medication error.

Monitoring
— Monitor the effectiveness of therapy by regularly doing PT determinations essential for proper control. High incidence of bleeding is seen when PT exceeds 2.5 times control values. Doctors usually try to maintain PT at 1.5 to 2 times normal.
— Because warfarin has a slow onset of action, heparin is usually given during first few days of treatment. When heparin is being given simultaneously, don't draw blood for PT within 5 hours of intermittent I.V. heparin administration. However, blood for PT may be drawn at any time during continuous heparin infusion.

—Regularly monitor the patient for bleeding gums, bruises on arms or legs, petechiae, nosebleeds, melena, tarry stools, hematuria, and hematemesis.

—Monitor the patient for adverse drug reactions.

—Monitor breast-feeding infants of mothers taking warfarin for unexpected bleeding.

—Monitor WBC count for leukopenia.

—Monitor bowel sounds and patterns for evidence of serious GI upset, such as paralytic ileus or intestinal obstruction.

—Monitor the female patient for excessive uterine bleeding.

—Monitor for temperature elevation.

—Monitor for skin changes, such as dermatitis, urticaria, rash, necrosis, or alopecia.

—Monitor the patient for drug interactions.

—Regularly reevaluate the patient's and family's knowledge about warfarin therapy.

Intervention

—Fever and skin rash signal severe adverse reactions. Withhold drug and call the doctor immediately.

—Keep parenteral vitamin K handy to neutralize warfarin effect in case of bleeding.

—Food and enteric feedings that contain vitamin K may cause inadequate anticoagulation. Provide diet low in vitamin K; read enteric feeding labels carefully.

—Institute bleeding precautions.

—Keep all members of the health care team informed of the patient's response to the drug.

Patient teaching

—Instruct the patient and family about warfarin, including the dosage, frequency, action, and adverse reactions.

—Explain the disease process and rationale for therapy; stress importance of complying with recommended amount and timing of dosage and of keeping follow-up appointments.

—Stress importance of taking a missed dose as soon as possible. If the missed dose is not remembered until the next day, the patient should not take it; doubling the dose can cause bleeding. Tell the patient to notify the doctor of any missed doses.

—Tell the patient to carry a card that identifies him as a potential bleeder, and to inform any doctors or dentists who may be treating him.

—Tell the patient and family to watch for bruising and other signs of increased bleeding and to notify the doctor immediately of these or other severe complications; heavier-than-usual menses may also necessitate dosage adjustment.

—Warn the patient to avoid OTC products containing aspirin, other salicylates, or drugs that may interact with the anticoagulant, causing an increase in action of drug, and to check with the doctor or pharmacist before stopping or starting any medication.

—Explain that PT is increased by fever, long periods of hot weather, malnutrition, diarrhea, and exposure to X-rays.

—Advise the patient not to substantially alter daily intake of leafy green vegetables (asparagus, broccoli, cabbage, lettuce, turnip greens, spinach, watercress) or of fish, pork or beef liver, green tea, or tomatoes; these foods contain vitamin K and widely varying daily intake may alter the drug's anticoagulant effect.

—Explain that smoking may also increase dosage requirement because of changes in metabolism; light to moderate alcohol intake does not significantly alter PT.

—Advise the patient to take special precautions against cutting or bruising his skin, for example, by using an electric razor when shaving and a soft toothbrush to prevent gum irritation.

—Tell the patient to notify the nurse or doctor if adverse reactions develop or questions arise about warfarin therapy.

Evaluation
In the patient receiving warfarin, appropriate evaluation statements include:
• Patient's PT determination falls within therapeutic limits.
• Patient does not exhibit bleeding.
• Patient and family state an understanding of warfarin therapy.

SELECTED MAJOR DRUG: ANTICOAGULANT

DRUG, INDICATIONS, AND DOSAGES	SPECIAL PRECAUTIONS
Coumarin derivative	
dicumarol	• Contraindicated in patients with hemo-
Treatment of pulmonary emboli; prevention and treatment of deep-vein thrombosis, MI, rheumatic heart disease with heart valve damage, atrial arrhythmias —	philia, thrombocytopenic purpura, leukemia with pronounced bleeding tendency, open wounds or ulcers, impaired hepatic or renal function, severe hypertension, acute nephri-
Adults: 200 to 300 mg P.O. on first day, 25 to 200 mg P.O. daily thereafter, based on prothrombin times.	tis, or subacute bacterial endocarditis.
	• Use with extreme caution (if at all) in psychiatric, debilitated, or cachectic pa- tients.
	• Use cautiously during menses, during use of any drainage tube, and in any patient in whom slight bleeding is dangerous.
	• Use cautiously when adding or stopping any drug for patient receiving anticoagu- lants. May change the clotting status and result in hemorrhage.

SELF-TEST

1. Sam Raymond, age 47, is admitted to a medical/surgical unit for treatment of acute thrombophlebitis in his left calf. His doctor ordered strict bed rest and I.V. heparin 5,000-unit bolus, followed by 1,000 units/hour. Heparin is the anticoagulant of choice for Mr. Raymond because:
   a. it reduces clot formation caused by platelet aggregation in the arterial system.
   b. it has an immediate anticoagulant effect.
   c. it suppresses the synthesis of vitamin K–dependent clotting factors.
   d. it breaks down the clots in the veins by stimulating fibrinolysis.

2. To determine the anticoagulant effect of heparin, which blood test will be measured regularly during therapy?
   a. Prothrombin time
   b. Clotting times
   c. Partial thromboplastin time
   d. Platelet count

3. In preparation for discharge, Mr. Raymond begins to take oral warfarin while the heparin infusion continues. Why doesn't the doctor discontinue the heparin immediately?
   a. Warfarin's onset of action is delayed, taking several days to achieve therapeutic concentration levels.
   b. Warfarin is not as effective as heparin in dissolving already formed thrombi.
   c. The risk of drug interactions with warfarin is reduced when warfarin is given with heparin.
   d. The doctor wants to assess whether Mr. Raymond will have gastric discomfort commonly associated with warfarin.

Check your answers on page 1073.

CHAPTER 65

BLOOD DERIVATIVES

albumin 5% ✦ albumin 25% ✦ antihemophilic factor
anti-inhibitor coagulant complex ✦ factor IX complex ✦ plasma protein fraction

OVERVIEW

- Most blood products (except whole blood) are prepared from pooled, donated blood or plasma. Certain standards must be followed regarding the size of the donor pool. Each unit is screened for both hepatitis B surface antigen and human immunodeficiency virus (HIV). Certain blood derivatives, such as I.V. immune globulin products, are further processed to inactivate HIV.
- Albumin (also called normal serum albumin) and plasma protein fraction are made from pooled normal human blood, plasma, or serum; albumin is also obtained from human placentas. Both preparations furnish means for stabilizing the body's hemodynamic mechanisms in hypovolemic shock or hypoproteinemia, or both.
- Since the late 1970s, all 25% solutions of albumin have had to contain 130 to 160 mEq of sodium/liter. Despite the discontinuation of high-sodium forms of albumin many years ago, the term "salt poor" has persisted.
- Current techniques allow separation of freshly donated whole blood into its component fractions: human RBCs, plasma, platelets, granulocytes, human $RH_o(D)$ immune globulin, albumin, and plasma protein. Because each component can correct a particular hematologic deficiency, use of whole blood is seldom needed. Whole blood is indicated only when a patient has lost considerable quantities of blood within a short time.
- Component transfusion—the technique of administering specific components rather than whole blood to a patient—has several advantages. Besides providing deficiency-specific therapy, the technique expands the potential usefulness of a single blood donation and helps ease the chronic shortage of blood.

MAJOR USES

- Blood derivatives act as plasma expanders in hypovolemic shock caused by burns, trauma, sepsis, or surgical procedures. They are also used to treat hypoproteinemia associated with malnutrition, toxemia of pregnancy, or prematurity.
- Albumin is used to treat hypoproteinemia associated with hepatic cirrhosis and nephrotic syndrome.
- Some blood derivatives (antihemophilic factor, factor IX complex) are used to replace missing clotting factors in patients with hereditary coagulopathies.

MECHANISM OF ACTION

- Albumin 25% provides intravascular oncotic pressure in a 5:1 ratio, which causes a shift of fluid from interstitial spaces to the circulation and slightly increases plasma protein concentration.
- Albumin 5% and plasma protein fraction supply colloid to the blood and expand plasma volume.
- Antihemophilic factor and factor IX complex are components of normal human plasma that are necessary for blood clot formation.
- Anti-inhibitor coagulant complex contains clotting factors. About 10% of patients with factor VIII deficiency (hemophilia A) produce inhibitors to factor VIII.

ABSORPTION, DISTRIBUTION, METABOLISM, AND EXCRETION

Since these blood derivatives are given only by the I.V. route, absorption is complete; they are rapidly distributed in the blood.

ONSET AND DURATION

Adequate patient response to albumin usually occurs within 15 to 30 minutes. Duration of therapy with albumin and plasma protein fraction varies not only with the patient, but also with the abnormality or condition that is being treated.

ADVERSE REACTIONS

Adverse reactions to albumin, blood derivatives, and plasma protein fraction products are uncommon but may result from allergy or protein overload. Such reactions may include fever, chills, nausea, vomiting, urticaria, and effects on heart rate, blood pressure, and respiratory rate. Albumin is more purified than plasma protein fraction and is less likely to cause hypotension. Vascular overload may also result from too-rapid administration of large doses of these agents.

PROTOTYPE: BLOOD DERIVATIVES

ALBUMIN 5%
(al byu′ min)
Albuminar-5, Albutein 5%, Buminate 5%, Plasbumin-5

ALBUMIN 25%
Albuminar-25, Albutein 25%, Buminate 25%, Plasbumin-25
Classification: blood derivative
Pregnancy risk category C

How supplied
INJECTION: 5%, in 50-ml, 250-ml, 500-ml, and 1,000-ml bottles; 25%, in 10-ml, 20-ml, and 50-ml bottles

Indications and dosage

Shock
ADULTS: initially, 500 ml (5% solution) by I.V. infusion; repeat q 30 minutes p.r.n. Dosage varies with patient's condition and response.
CHILDREN: 25% to 50% adult dose in nonemergency.

Hypoproteinemia
ADULTS: 1,000 to 1,500 ml (5% solution) by I.V. infusion daily; maximum rate is 5 to 10 ml/minute. Or 25 to 100 g (25% solution) by I.V. infusion daily; maximum rate is 3 ml/minute. Dosage varies with patient's condition and response.

Burns
ADULTS AND CHILDREN: dosage varies according to extent of burn and patient's condition. Usually maintain plasma albumin at 2 to 3 g/100 ml.

Hyperbilirubinemia
INFANTS: 1 g albumin (4 ml 25%)/kg before transfusion.

Contraindications and precautions
Albumin is contraindicated in severe anemia or heart failure. Use cautiously in low cardiac reserve, absence of albumin deficiency, and restricted sodium intake.

Adverse reactions
CV: *vascular overload after rapid infusion,* hypotension, altered pulse rate.
GI: increased salivation, nausea, vomiting.
SKIN: urticaria.
OTHER: chills, fever, altered respiration.

Interactions
None significant.

Nursing considerations

Assessment
• Review the patient's history for a condition that contraindicates the use of albumin.
• Obtain a baseline assessment of the patient's underlying condition before therapy.
• Be alert for common adverse reactions.
• Evaluate the patient's and family's knowledge about albumin therapy.

Planning (Nursing Diagnoses)
Potential nursing diagnoses for the patient receiving albumin include:
• Altered health maintenance related to ineffective dosage regimen of albumin to correct underlying condition being treated.
• Fluid volume overload related to rapid infusion of albumin.
• Knowledge deficit related to albumin therapy.

Implementation

Preparation and administration

— Do not give more than 250 g in 48 hours.
— The patient should be properly hydrated before infusion of solution.
— Avoid rapid I.V. infusion. Specific rate is individualized according to the patient's age, condition, and diagnosis.
— Dilute with sterile water for injection. 0.9% sodium chloride solution, or dextrose 5% in water injection. Use solution promptly; contains no preservatives. Discard unused solution.
— Don't use cloudy solutions or those containing sediment. Solution should be clear amber color.
— Freezing may cause bottle to break. Follow storage instructions on bottle.

Monitoring

— Monitor the effectiveness of therapy by regularly monitoring vital signs, intake and output, hemoglobin, hematocrit, and serum protein and electrolyte levels during therapy.
— Monitor for signs of vascular overload (heart failure or pulmonary edema).
— Monitor the patient for adverse drug reactions.
— Monitor for hypersensitivity reactions, such as urticaria, chills, and fever.
— Monitor hydration status if increased salivation, nausea, and vomiting occur.
— Regularly reevaluate the patient's and family's knowledge about albumin therapy.

Intervention

— Be prepared to treat vascular overload and provide supportive care if it occurs.
— If not contraindicated, obtain an order for an antiemetic if nausea and vomiting occur.
— Keep all members of the health care team informed of the patient's response to the drug.

Patient teaching

— Instruct the patient and family about albumin, including the dosage, frequency, action, and adverse reactions.
— Emphasize the importance of alerting the nurse promptly if any adverse reactions occur.

Evaluation

In the patient receiving albumin, appropriate evaluation statements include:
• Patient's underlying clinical condition is improved.
• Vascular overload does not occur.
• Patient and family state an understanding of albumin therapy.

BLOOD DERIVATIVES AND OTHER AGENTS TO CONTROL BLEEDING

Blood derivatives and miscellaneous drugs listed below are used to control bleeding of various causes.

DRUG, INDICATIONS, AND DOSAGES	SPECIAL PRECAUTIONS

Blood derivatives

antihemophilic factor (AHF, Factor VIII [Hemofilm, Koa'te-HS, Koa'te-HT, Monoclate])
Bleeding from Factor VIII deficiency—
Adults and children: 10 to 20 IU/kg I.V. push or infusion q 8 to 24 hours, calculated by this formula:
AHF dosage = body weight (in kg) x desired Factor VIII (% of normal) x 0.5.

- Ensure that the patient's blood is typed and crossmatched as prescribed for possible transfusion.
- Monitor the patient's vital signs frequently. If tachycardia develops, reduce the flow rate or stop administration and notify the doctor.
- Monitor the patient for hypersensitivity reactions.
- Use only a plastic syringe to administer I.V. Drug may interact with a glass syringe.
- Monitor coagulation study results before and during therapy.
- Refrigerate concentrate until use but not after reconstitution. Before reconstituting, bring concentrate and diluent bottles to room temperature. Use the reconstituted solution within 3 hours.
- Do not mix with other I.V. solutions.

Factor IX complex (Konyne, Profilnine, Proplex)
Bleeding caused by Factor IX deficiency (hemophilia B or Christmas disease) or anticoagulant overdose—
Adults and children: 10 to 20 units/kg daily; for anticoagulant overdose, 15 units/kg calculated by this formula:
Factor IX dosage = 1 unit/kg x body weight (in kg) x desired increase (% of normal).

- Ensure that the patient's blood is typed and crossmatched as prescribed to treat possible hemorrhage.
- Observe the patient for hypersensitivity reactions. Slow the infusion and notify the doctor if a hypersensitivity reaction occurs.
- Monitor the patient's vital signs frequently.
- Avoid rapid infusion, which may cause tingling sensations, fever, chills, or headache.
- Reconstitute with 20 ml sterile water. Keep refrigerated until ready to use but warm to room temperature before reconstituting.
- Do not administer with other I.V. solutions.

BLOOD DERIVATIVES AND OTHER AGENTS TO CONTROL BLEEDING
continued

DRUG, INDICATIONS, AND DOSAGES	SPECIAL PRECAUTIONS

Blood derivatives *(continued)*

anti-inhibitor coagulant complex (Auto-plex T, Feiba VH Immuno)
Bleeding or surgery in a patient with Factor VIII inhibitors —
Adults: 25 to 100 Factor VIII correctional units/kg I.V., repeated after 6 hours if the patient shows no improvement.

• Contraindicated in patients with signs of fibrinolysis and in those with DIC or normal coagulation.
• Assess fibrinogen levels before the infusion begins, and then monitor them periodically.
• Administer the drug at the prescribed infusion rate, which may be as fast as 10 ml/minute. If headache, flushing, and rapid pulse occur, however, decrease the rate to 2 ml/minute.
• Keep epinephrine 1:1,000 available to manage an acute hypersensitivity reaction.

Miscellaneous agents

aminocaproic acid (Amicar)
Excessive bleeding resulting from hyperfibrinolysis —
Adults: initially 5 g P.O. or slow I.V. infusion followed by 1 to 1.25 g/hour; maximum dosage, 30 g daily.

• Contraindicated in patients with active intravascular clotting.
• Dilute with sterile water, 0.9% sodium chloride solution, dextrose 5% in water, or Ringer's solution.
• Monitor coagulation study results.

tranexamic acid (Cyklokapron)
Reduction or prevention of hemorrhage in hemophilia patients; reduction of need for replacement therapy for tooth extraction —
Adults: 10 mg/kg I.V. immediately before tooth extraction or 25 mg/kg P.O. t.i.d. to q.i.d. for 1 day before tooth extraction; then 25 mg/kg P.O. t.i.d. to q.i.d. for 2 to 8 days afterward.

• Contraindicated in patients with subarachnoid hemorrhage or defective color vision that prevents detection of toxicity.
• I.V. tranexamic acid is compatible with most I.V. solutions.
• Do not mix with blood or penicillin.

topical thrombin (Thrombinar, Thrombostat)
Adjunct to hemostasis in surgery —
Adults: apply dry powder or solution, as needed.

• Contraindicated in patients with known allergy to bovine products.
• Do not inject this drug.

(continued)

BLOOD DERIVATIVES AND OTHER AGENTS TO CONTROL BLEEDING
continued

DRUG, INDICATIONS, AND DOSAGES	SPECIAL PRECAUTIONS
Miscellaneous agents *(continued)*	
topical thrombin *(continued)*	• Prepare the solution with sterile distilled water or 0.9% sodium chloride solution for irrigation. Solutions with a concentration of 100 units/ml commonly are used, but concentrations of 1,000 to 2,000 units/ml may be required to stop bleeding from liver or spleen lacerations.

SELF-TEST

1. John Evans, age 18, was admitted to the emergency department after an automobile accident. He has extensive trauma to his abdomen and both legs. His blood pressure is 70/40 mm Hg and his heart rate is 150 beats/minute. His doctor initially prescribed albumin 5%, 500 ml by I.V. infusion. How soon can another dose be given?
   a. In 15 minutes
   b. In 30 minutes
   c. In 1 hour
   d. In 4 hours

2. Which serious adverse reaction should the nurse monitor for when administering albumin?
   a. Vascular overload
   b. Seizures
   c. Hypertensive crisis
   d. Hemorrhage

3. Which of the following parameters should be monitored during albumin therapy?
   a. Serum protein and electrolytes, hemoglobin, and hematocrit
   b. Serum creatinine, BUN, and alkaline phosphatase levels
   c. Cardiac enzymes
   d. Liver enzymes

Check your answers on page 1073.

CHAPTER 66

THROMBOLYTIC AGENTS

alteplase ◆ anistreplase ◆ streptokinase ◆ urokinase

OVERVIEW
- Thrombolytic agents are effective in treating acute and extensive epi-sodes of thrombotic disorders. Before administering these agents, how-ever, be aware of the increased risk of hemorrhage that attends their use. Although major bleeding is a possible complication of treatment, bruis-ing and oozing of blood at the incision site and surgical trauma are more likely. Because of the inherent risk of hemorrhage, thrombolytic therapy should be accompanied by close laboratory monitoring.

MAJOR USES
- All of these agents can be used to treat an MI. When administered soon after the onset of symptoms, thrombolytic agents lyse thrombi that block coronary arteries and cause the MI.
- Alteplase, streptokinase, and urokinase are used to treat acute, massive pulmonary emboli. Streptokinase is also used to dissolve acute, extensive deep-vein thrombi and acute arterial thromboemboli.

MECHANISM OF ACTION
- Thrombolytic agents activate plasminogen and convert it to plasmin, which degrades fibrin clots, fibrinogen, and other plasma proteins.
- Alteplase, sometimes called recombinant tissue plasminogen activator (rT-PA), is a synthetically derived form of the naturally occurring enzyme that initiates thrombolysis. Unlike the nonspecific proteolytic enzyme streptokinase, which activates both tissue-bound and circulating plasminogen, alteplase mimics the fibrin-bound tissue plasminogen and causes local thrombolysis.
- Streptokinase activates plasminogen in a two-step process. Plasminogen and streptokinase form a complex that exposes the plasminogen-activat-ing site. Plasminogen is converted to plasmin by cleavage of the peptide bond.
- Anistreplase, sometimes called anisoylated plasminogen-streptokinase activator complex (APSAC), is derived from human Lys-plasminogen and streptokinase. It is slightly different from the naturally occurring complex that forms in the blood after administration of streptokinase.

GLOSSARY

Fibrin: major element of a blood clot; insoluble protein formed from fibrinogen by thrombin action.
Fibrin degradation products (FDPs): substances that result from plasmin action on fibrin; also called fibrin split products (FSPs).
Fibrinogen: high-molecular-weight plasma protein that is converted to fibrin through thrombin action; also called coagulation Factor I.
Fibrinolysis: breakdown of fibrin by the proteolytic enzyme, plasmin.
Plasmin: highly specific proteolytic enzyme that dissolves fibrin clots.
Plasminogen: inactive precursor of plasmin.
Thrombolysis: breakdown of preformed thrombin by local plasmin action.

Additionally, the active portion of the enzyme is temporarily blocked with a chemical entity known as an anisoyl group; after administration, the drug spontaneously activates within the bloodstream or the thrombus. It causes the endogenous fibrinolytic system to produce plasmin, which degrades fibrin clots, fibrinogen, and other plasma proteins.
• Urokinase activates plasminogen by directly cleaving peptide bonds at two different sites.

ABSORPTION, DISTRIBUTION, METABOLISM, AND EXCRETION

Thrombolytic agents are administered only by I.V. infusion and are distributed throughout the body. Their metabolism and excretion have not been fully explained. Alteplase, which is administered by I.V. infusion, is rapidly cleared from the plasma within 10 minutes of discontinuing an infusion. Metabolism is primarily hepatic; over 85% of the drug is excreted in the urine as metabolites.

ONSET AND DURATION

All thrombolytic agents begin to act immediately. Alteplase, streptokinase, and urokinase must be infused at a constant dosage level to maintain therapeutic effectiveness. Anistreplase is given I.V. push. The drug is slowly cleared from the plasma, and the half-life of the drug's fibrinolytic activity is about 90 minutes.

When used to lyse coronary artery thrombi, the time to peak effect for most thrombolytic agents is about 45 minutes after injection. Thrombolysis may continued for 6 to 12 hours after injection, but the hyperfibrinolytic state induced by these drugs may persist for 2 days or more.

ADVERSE REACTIONS

Thrombolytic agents may cause severe and spontaneous external or internal bleeding or oozing from puncture sites. They may also cause mild allergic reactions; serious anaphylactoid reactions are more common with streptokinase. Febrile reactions have been reported; they should not be treated with aspirin or antiplatelet drugs. Rapid lysis of coronary artery thrombi may be associated with a reperfusion-related cardiac arrhythmia. Such arrhythmia is usually transient but occasionally may require treatment.

Thrombolytic agents may cause hypotension unrelated to bleeding or anaphylaxis. It is usually transient but may require reduction of drug dosage.

PROTOTYPE: THROMBOLYTIC AGENTS

STREPTOKINASE
(strep toe kye' nase)
Kabikinase, Streptase
Classification: *thrombolytic agent*
Pregnancy risk category C

How supplied
INJECTION: 100,000 IU, 250,000 IU, 600,000 IU, 750,000 IU, 1,500,000 IU in vials for reconstitution

Indications and dosage
Arteriovenous cannula occlusion
250,000 IU in 2 ml I.V. solution by I.V. pump infusion into each occluded limb of the cannula over 25 to 35 minutes. Clamp off cannula for 2 hours. Then aspirate contents of cannula; flush with 0.9% sodium chloride solution and reconnect.

Venous thrombosis, pulmonary embolism, and arterial thrombosis and embolism
ADULTS: loading dose is 250,000 IU I.V. infusion over 30 minutes. Sustaining dose is 100,000 IU/hour I.V. infusion for 72 hours for deep-vein thrombosis and 100,000 IU/hour over 24 to 72 hours by I.V. infusion pump for pulmonary embolism.

Lysis of coronary artery thrombi after acute MI
ADULTS: 1,500,000 units I.V. infused over 60 minutes. Alternatively, may be administered by coronary artery catheter. Loading dose is 20,000 IU via coronary catheter, followed by a maintenance infusion of 2,000 IU/minute for 60 minutes.

Contraindications and precautions
Streptokinase is contraindicated in patients with ulcerative wounds, active internal bleeding, or recent CVA; recent trauma with possible internal injuries; visceral or intracranial malignancy; ulcerative colitis; diverticulitis; severe hypertension; acute or chronic hepatic or renal insufficiency; uncontrolled hypocoagulation; chronic pulmonary disease with cavitation; subacute bacterial endocarditis or rheumatic valvular disease; or recent cerebral embolism, thrombosis, or hemorrhage. Also contraindicated

within 10 days after intra-arterial diagnostic procedure or any surgery, including liver or kidney biopsy, lumbar puncture, thoracentesis, paracentesis, or extensive or multiple cutdowns.

Use cautiously when treating arterial emboli that originate from left side of heart because of danger of cerebral infarction.

Adverse reactions

BLOOD: *bleeding,* low hematocrit.

CV: transient lowering or elevation of blood pressure.

EENT: periorbital edema.

SKIN: urticaria.

LOCAL: phlebitis at injection site.

OTHER: hypersensitivity to drug, *anaphylaxis, fever,* musculoskeletal pain, minor breathing difficulty, bronchospasms, angioneurotic edema.

Interactions

Anticoagulants: concurrent use with streptokinase not recommended. Reversing the effects of oral anticoagulants must be considered before beginning therapy; heparin must be stopped and its effect allowed to diminish.

Aspirin, dipyridamole, indomethacin, phenylbutazone, drugs affecting platelet activity: increased risk of bleeding. Combined therapy with low-dose aspirin (162.5 mg) or dipyridamole has improved acute and long-term results.

Nursing considerations

Assessment

• Review the patient's history for a condition that contraindicates the use of streptokinase.

• Obtain a baseline assessment of the patient's partial thromboplastin time (PTT) and prothrombin time (PT) before initiating streptokinase therapy.

• Be alert for serious adverse reactions.

• Evaluate the patient's and family's knowledge about streptokinase therapy.

Planning (Nursing Diagnoses)

Potential nursing diagnoses for the patient receiving streptokinase include:

• Altered tissue perfusion (venous or arterial) related to ineffectiveness of streptokinase.

• Altered protection related to adverse reactions associated with streptokinase therapy.

• Knowledge deficit related to streptokinase therapy.

Implementation

Preparation and administration

—Before initiating therapy, draw blood to determine PTT and PT. Rate of I.V. infusion depends on thrombin time and streptokinase resistance.

—If the patient has had either a recent streptococcal infection or recent treatment with streptokinase, a higher loading dose may be necessary.

— To prepare I.V. solution: reconstitute each vial with 5 ml 0.9% sodium chloride solution for injection. Further dilute to 45 ml. Don't shake; roll gently to mix. Use within 24 hours. Store at room temperature in powder form; refrigerate after reconstitution.

— Should be used only by doctors with wide experience in thrombotic disease management and only where clinical and laboratory monitoring can be performed.

— Thrombolytic therapy in the patient with acute MI is associated with decreased infarct size, improved ventricular function, and decreased incidence of CHF. Streptokinase must be administered within 6 hours of the onset of symptoms for optimal effect.

— I.M. injections are contraindicated during streptokinase therapy.

Monitoring

— Monitor the effectiveness of therapy by frequently checking the patient's response; for example, if an extremity is involved, monitor pulses, color, and sensation in extremities every hour.

— Monitor the patient for excessive bleeding every 15 minutes for the first hour, every 30 minutes for the second through eighth hours, then once every shift.

— Monitor the patient for adverse drug reactions.

— Monitor PTT, PT, hemoglobin, and hematocrit.

— Monitor vital signs frequently. Watch for significant changes in blood pressure.

— Monitor for signs of hypersensitivity.

— Monitor respiratory status for breathing difficulty and bronchospasms.

— Monitor the patient for drug interactions.

Intervention

— If serious bleeding is evident, stop therapy and notify the doctor immediately. Pretreatment with heparin or drugs affecting platelet activity causes high risk of bleeding, but may improve long-term results. Monitor closely.

— Have typed and crossmatched packed RBCs and whole blood ready to treat possible hemorrhage.

— Keep aminocaproic acid available to treat bleeding. Corticosteroids are used to treat allergic reactions.

— Therapy need not be discontinued for minor allergic reactions that can be treated with antihistamines or corticosteroids; about one third of patients experience a slight temperature elevation, and some have chills. Symptomatic treatment with acetaminophen (but not aspirin or other salicylates) is indicated if temperature reaches 104° F (40° C). Some doctors pretreat patients with corticosteroids, repeating doses during therapy, to minimize pyrogenic or allergic reactions.

— If minor bleeding can be controlled by local pressure, do not decrease dose because that makes more plasminogen available for conversion to plasmin.

— Effectiveness of I.V. or intracoronary instillation to prevent extension of myocardial infarct decreases rapidly after 5 to 6 hours.

— Antibodies to streptokinase can persist for 3 to 6 months or longer after the initial dose; if further thrombolytic therapy is needed, consider urokinase.

— Heparin by continuous infusion is usually started within 1 hour after stopping streptokinase. Use an infusion pump to administer heparin.

— Bruising is more likely during therapy; avoid unnecessary handling of the patient. Side rails should be padded.

— Maintain the involved extremity in straight alignment to prevent bleeding from the infusion site.

— Keep venipuncture sites to a minimum; use pressure dressing on puncture sites for at least 15 minutes.

— Keep a laboratory flow sheet on the patient's chart.

— Before using streptokinase to clear an occluded arteriovenous cannula, try flushing with heparinized 0.9% sodium chloride solution.

— Keep all members of the health care team informed of the patient's response to the drug.

Patient teaching

— Instruct the patient and family about streptokinase, including the dosage, frequency, action, and adverse reactions.

— Tell the patient to keep the involved extremity in straight alignment to prevent bleeding.

— To prevent bruising, warn the patient to avoid bumping side rails.

— Tell the patient to notify the nurse or doctor if adverse reactions develop or questions arise about streptokinase therapy.

Evaluation

In the patient receiving streptokinase, appropriate evaluation statements include:

• Patient exhibits normal tissue perfusion.

• Patient does not develop serious adverse reactions, such as bleeding or hypersensitivity.

• Patient and family state an understanding of streptokinase therapy.

SELECTED MAJOR DRUGS: THROMBOLYTIC AGENTS

DRUG, INDICATIONS, AND DOSAGES	SPECIAL PRECAUTIONS
alteplase (Actilyse‡, Activase) *Lysis of thrombi obstructing coronary arteries in acute MI—* **Adults:** 100 mg by I.V. infusion over 3 hours as follows: 60 mg in the first hour, of which 6 to 10 mg is given as a bolus over the first 1 to 2 minutes. Then 20 mg/hour infusion for 2 hours. Smaller adults (< 65 kg) should receive a dose of 1.25 mg/kg in a similar fashion (60% in the first hour, with 10% as a bolus; then 20% of the total dose/hour for 2 hours).	• Contraindicated in patients with active internal bleeding, intracranial neoplasm, arteriovenous malformation, aneurysm, or severe uncontrolled hypertension. Also contraindicated in patients with a history of CVA, recent (within 2 months) intraspinal or intracranial trauma or surgery, or known hemorrhagic diathesis.

‡Available in Australia only

SELECTED MAJOR DRUGS: THROMBOLYTIC AGENTS *continued*

DRUG, INDICATIONS, AND DOSAGES	SPECIAL PRECAUTIONS
anistreplase (Eminase) *Lysis of cornary artery thrombi after acute MI* — **Adults:** 30 units I.V. over 2 to 5 minutes. Administer by direct injection.	• Contraindicated in patients with active internal bleeding, a history of CVA, recent (within the past 2 months) intraspinal or intracranial trauma or surgery, aneurysm, arteriovenous malformation, intracranial neoplasm, or known hemorrhagic diathesis. • Consider risk-benefit ratio in patients with recent (within 10 days) major surgery, trauma (including cardiopulmonary resuscitation), or GI or GU bleeding; cerebrovascular disease or hypertension (systolic ≥ 180 mm Hg or diastolic ≥ 110 mm Hg, or both); mitral stenosis, atrial fibrillation, or other condition that may lead to left heart thrombus; acute pericarditis or subacute bacterial endocarditis; septic thrombophlebitis; or diabetic hemorrhagic retinopathy; in those ages 75 and over; and in those receiving anticoagulants.
urokinase (Abbokinase, Ukidan‡, Win-Kinase) *Lysis of acute, massive pulmonary emboli and lysis of pulmonary emboli accompanied by unstable hemodynamics* — **Adults:** for I.V. infusion only by constant infusion pump that will deliver a total volume of 195 ml. Priming dose — 4,400 IU/kg of urokinase-0.9% sodium chloride solution admixture given over 10 minutes. Follow with 4,400 IU/kg hourly for 12 to 24 hours. Total volume should not exceed 200 ml. Follow therapy with continuous I.V. infusion of heparin, then oral anticoagulants. *Coronary artery thrombosis* — **Adults:** after a bolus dose of heparin ranging from 2,500 to 10,000 units, infuse 6,000 IU/minute of urokinase into the occluded artery for up to 2 hours. Average total dosage is 500,000 IU. *Venous catheter occlusion* — Instill 5,000 IU into occluded line, wait 5 minutes, then aspirate. Repeat aspiration attempts q 5 minutes for 30 minutes. If not patent after 30 minutes, cap line and let urokinase work for 30 to 60 minutes before aspirating. May require second instillation.	• Contraindicated in patients with ulcerative wounds, active internal bleeding, or CVA; recent trauma with possible internal injuries; during visceral or intracranial malignancy; during pregnancy and first 10 days postpartum; in ulcerative colitis; diverticulitis; severe hypertension; acute or chronic hepatic or renal insufficiency; uncontrolled hypocoagulation; chronic pulmonary disease with cavitation; subacute bacterial endocarditis or rheumatic valvular disease; or recent cerebral embolism, thrombosis, or hemorrhage. Also contraindicated within 10 days after intra-arterial diagnostic procedures or any surgery, including liver or kidney biopsy, lumbar puncture, thoracentesis, paracentesis, or extensive or multiple cutdowns.

‡Available in Australia only

SELF-TEST

1. Rodney Peters, age 56, has been admitted to the emergency department with a diagnosis of an acute MI. Symptoms began 3 hours ago. His doctor plans to administer I.V. streptokinase immediately. Streptokinase works by:
   a. preventing further thrombus formation at the infarction site.
   b. lysing the clot by activating plasminogen.
   c. decreasing the size of the clot by decreasing platelet aggregation.
   d. blocking synthesis of vitamin K–dependent clotting factors.

2. During the infusion of streptokinase, it is essential that the nurse assess Mr. Peters frequently for:
   a. pulmonary edema.
   b. bleeding from puncture sites.
   c. decreased electrolyte levels, particularly potassium.
   d. hyperglycemia.

3. A major contraindication to thrombolytic therapy is:
   a. mild hypertension.
   b. active internal bleeding.
   c. abdominal surgery 6 months ago.
   d. diagnosis of acute MI 4 to 6 hours after onset of chest pain.

Check your answers on page 1073.

CHAPTER 67

ALKYLATING AGENTS

busulfan ◆ carboplatin ◆ carmustine (BCNU)
chlorambucil ◆ cisplatin (cis-platinum) ◆ cyclophosphamide
dacarbazine (DTIC) ◆ ifosfamide ◆ lomustine (CCNU)
mechlorethamine hydrochloride (nitrogen mustard) ◆ melphalan
pipobroman ◆ streptozocin ◆ thiotepa ◆ uracil mustard

OVERVIEW

• Alkylating agents are anticancer or antitumor drugs developed from nitrogen mustard or its derivatives as a result of military research. Because these compounds produce bone marrow depression and atrophy of lymphoid tissue, they were first used to treat malignant lymphomas and leukemias. But ever since the introduction of mechlorethamine, the first nitrogen mustard, an intensive search for more potent and less toxic agents has been underway. Alkylating agents act during any phase of cellular activity, giving them an advantage over more specific antineoplastics, which are effective only during a single phase. This makes their toxicity nonspecific.

MAJOR USES

• Alkylating agents are used to treat carcinomas, sarcomas, lymphomas, and leukemias. They are also used to treat polycythemia vera.

MECHANISM OF ACTION

• Alkylating agents cross-link strands of cellular DNA, causing an imbalance of growth that leads to cell death.

ABSORPTION, DISTRIBUTION, METABOLISM, AND EXCRETION

Busulfan, chlorambucil, cyclophosphamide, lomustine, melphalan, pipobroman, and uracil mustard are absorbed from the GI tract after oral administration. All other alkylating agents must be administered intravenously.

All alkylating agents are distributed widely to body tissues. Carmustine, lomustine, and thiotepa diffuse into the CSF and cross the blood-brain barrier.

All alkylating agents except thiotepa are metabolized in the liver and excreted in the urine as either active or inactive metabolites. Thiotepa is excreted unchanged by the kidneys.

GLOSSARY

Alkylation: linkage between a substance and DNA that causes irreversible inhibition of the DNA molecule by enzyme modification.

Alopecia: loss of hair.

Carcinogenesis: cancer production.

Carcinoma: malignant neoplasm composed of epithelial cells, which tends to infiltrate surrounding tissues and leads to metastases.

Cell cycle: division pattern of cells characterized by five phases: nonproliferation, G_0; presynthesis, G1; DNA synthesis, S; RNA production, G2; and mitosis, M1 (cell division).

Cell-cycle-nonspecific: capable of acting during several or all cell-cycle stages.

Leukemia: malignant disorder of the blood-forming organs marked by increased leukocytes and leukocyte precursors in the blood and bone marrow.

Leukopenia: deficiency of leukocytes in the blood, usually below $5,000/mm^3$.

Lymphoma: neoplastic disorder of lymphoid tissue.

Polycythemia vera: myeloproliferative disease characterized by increased RBCs and total blood volume, usually associated with splenomegaly, leukocytosis, thrombocytosis, and bone marrow hyperactivity.

Sarcoma: malignant neoplasm composed of a substance similar to embryonic connective tissue.

Thrombocytopenia: decreased number of platelets.

ONSET AND DURATION

Therapeutic activity varies with the alkylating agent, disease, and patient response.

ADVERSE REACTIONS

Adverse drug reactions common to all the alkylating agents involve suppression of varying degrees of the various blood cell lines. Leukopenia and thrombocytopenia occur most frequently; anemia is less common. Other common adverse reactions are alopecia, nausea, vomiting, diarrhea, stomatitis of varying degrees, and hepatotoxicity.

Some agents have specific adverse reactions. Busulfan can cause an Addison-like wasting syndrome, gynecomastia, and an irreversible pulmonary fibrosis. Melphalan, like busulfan, may cause pneumonitis and pulmonary fibrosis.

Carboplatin may exhibit CNS toxicity, such as peripheral neuropathy, ototoxicity, dizziness, and confusion.

Cisplatin can cause severe nausea and vomiting; both cisplatin and streptozocin can cause renal toxicity evidenced by azotemia and proteinuria; this renal toxicity is more prolonged and severe with repeated courses of therapy.

Cyclophosphamide and ifosfamide can both cause severe hemorrhagic cystitis. This may be minimized by adequate hydration and the concomitant use of mesna when using ifosfamide. Cyclophosphamide may exhibit cardiotoxicity when used in combination with doxorubicin.

A flulike syndrome may begin 7 days after the administration of dacarbazine and may last 7 to 21 days after therapy is stopped.

Some adverse reactions may seem trivial, such as the metallic taste seen with nitrogen mustard or cisplatin, but these may impair the patient's ability to maintain an adequate caloric intake by mouth.

PROTOTYPE: ALKYLATING AGENTS

CYCLOPHOSPHAMIDE
(sye kloe foss' fa mide)
Cycoblastin, Cytoxan, Cytoxan Lyophilized, Endoxan-Asta‡, Neosar, Procytox†
Classification: alkylating agent
Pregnancy risk category D

How supplied
TABLETS: 25 mg, 50 mg
INJECTION: 100 mg, 200 mg, 500 mg, 1 g, 2 g in single-dose vials

Indications and dosage
Breast, head, neck, lung, and ovarian cancer; Hodgkin's disease; chronic lymphocytic leukemia; chronic myelocytic leukemia; acute lymphoblastic leukemia; neuroblastoma; retinoblastoma; non-Hodgkin's lymphomas; multiple myeloma; mycosis fungoides; sarcomas
ADULTS: initially, 40 to 50 mg/kg I.V. in divided doses over 2 to 5 days; then adjust for maintenance. Or 1 to 5 mg/kg P.O. daily, depending on patient tolerance. Maintenance dosage is 1 to 5 mg/kg P.O. daily, or 10 to 15 mg/kg I.V. q 7 to 10 days, or 3 to 5 mg/kg I.V. twice weekly.
CHILDREN: 2 to 8 mg/kg or 60 to 250 mg/m^2 P.O. or I.V. daily for 6 days (dosage depends on susceptibility of neoplasm). Maintenance dosage is 2 to 5 mg/kg or 60 to 150 mg/m^2 P.O. twice weekly.

Contraindications and precautions
Cyclophosphamide is contraindicated in patients with serious bacterial, viral, or fungal infections, especially varicella-zoster infections. Use cyclophosphamide with extreme caution in patients with leukopenia, thrombocytopenia, impaired hepatic or renal function, tumor cell infiltration of the bone marrow, or previous treatment with radiation or other cytotoxic agents.

Adverse reactions
BLOOD: *leukopenia* (nadir between days 8 to 15, recovery in 17 to 28 days), thrombocytopenia, anemia.

---

†Available in Canada only   ‡Available in Australia only
Italicized adverse reactions are common

CV: **cardiotoxicity** (with very high doses and in combination with doxorubicin).
GI: *anorexia, nausea and vomiting* (beginning within 6 hours, lasting 4 hours), stomatitis, mucositis.
GU: *gonadal suppression* (may be irreversible), *hemorrhagic cystitis,* bladder fibrosis, nephrotoxicity.
METABOLIC: *hyperuricemia;* SIADH (with high doses).
OTHER: reversible *alopecia* in 50% of patients, especially with high doses; skin and nail hyperpigmentation; secondary malignancies; **pulmonary fibrosis** (high doses).

Interactions
Barbiturates: increased pharmacologic effect and enhanced cyclophosphamide toxicity due to induction of hepatic enzymes. Avoid concomitant use.
Cardiotoxic drugs: additive adverse cardiac effects. Monitor closely.
Corticosteroids, chloramphenicol: reduced activity of cyclophosphamide. Use together cautiously.
Succinylcholine: may cause apnea. Don't use together.

Nursing considerations
Assessment
• Review the patient's history for a condition that contraindicates the use of cyclophosphamide.
• Obtain a baseline assessment of the patient's CBC and differential, intake and output, ECG, and vital signs as well as the patient's underlying cancerous state before initiating therapy.
• Be alert for common adverse reactions.
• Evaluate the patient's and family's knowledge about cyclophosphamide therapy.

Planning (Nursing Diagnoses)
Potential nursing diagnoses for the patient receiving cyclophosphamide include:
• Altered health maintenance related to ineffectiveness of cyclophosphamide to halt cancer progression.
• Infection related to potential cyclophosphamide-induced leukopenia.
• Altered oral mucous membranes related to stomatitis and esophagitis.
• Fluid volume deficit related to potential nausea and vomiting.
• Body image disturbance related to potential alopecia and hyperpigmentation of the skin and nails.
• Knowledge deficit related to cyclophosphamide therapy.

Implementation
Preparation and administration
— Read order and drug label carefully before administration.
— Dosage modification may be required in severe leukopenia, thrombocytopenia, malignant cell infiltration of bone marrow, recent radiation therapy or chemotherapy, or hepatic or renal disease.

— Follow institutional policy for handling hazardous materials to minimize carcinogenic, mutagenic, and teratogenic risks.

— Lyophilized preparation is much easier to reconstitute. Request this form from the pharmacy when preparing I.V. Drug is usually mixed in pharmacy.

— Reconstituted solution is stable for 6 days if refrigerated or 24 hours at room temperature.

— Check reconstituted solution for small particles. Filter solution if necessary.

— Label all syringes containing cyclophosphamide "FOR I.V. USE ONLY."

— Check I.V. line patency and infusion site before administration.

— Check patient's I.D. band and ask patient's name before administration.

— Can be given by direct I.V. push into a running I.V. line or by infusion in 0.9% sodium chloride solution or dextrose 5% in water.

— Chart drug administration and related observations.

Monitoring

— Monitor the effectiveness of cyclophosphamide therapy by regularly monitoring changes in signs and symptoms as well as appropriate diagnostic studies for the type of cancer being treated.

— Regularly monitor CBC and differential, uric acid levels, and renal and hepatic studies.

— Monitor the patient for adverse drug reactions.

— Monitor urine output and note amount and color for evidence of hemorrhagic cystitis and other adverse GU reactions.

— Monitor for signs of bleeding (melena, ecchymosis, petechiae), especially when thrombocytopenia is present.

— Monitor hydration status, especially if adverse GI reactions occur.

— Monitor respiratory status and pulmonary function studies for evidence of pulmonary fibrosis.

— Monitor ECG for arrhythmia, ST segment changes, and other signs of cardiotoxicity, especially with high doses or in combination with doxorubicin.

— Monitor the patient for drug interactions.

— Periodically reevaluate the patient's and family's knowledge about cyclophosphamide.

Intervention

— Premedicate the patient with an antiemetic to decrease nausea and vomiting before cyclophosphamide administration.

— Provide a private room and use reverse isolation precautions for patients with compromised immune systems.

— Keep accurate records of intake and output and daily weight.

— Encourage fluid intake (3 liters daily) to prevent hemorrhagic cystitis. Don't give drug at bedtime, when voiding is too infrequent to avoid cystitis.

— Encourage patients to void every 1 to 2 hours while awake to minimize risk of hemorrhagic cystitis.
— If hemorrhagic cystitis occurs, discontinue drug. Remember that cystitis can occur months after therapy has been stopped.
— To prevent hyperuricemia with resulting uric acid nephropathy, administer allopurinol with adequate hydration.
— Avoid all I.M. injections when platelet count is below 100,000/mm³.
— Institute safety precautions to minimize risk of bleeding due to injury.
— Provide frequent mouth care with a soft toothbrush and mild mouthwash to minimize trauma to oral mucosa.
— Use a topical oral anesthetic to soothe lesions if stomatitis occurs.
— Discontinue cyclophosphamide if diarrhea occurs.
— Encourage the patient to maintain adequate caloric intake; offer frequent small meals.
— Offer emotional support and opportunities to express feelings about changes in body image.
— Keep all members of the health care team informed of the patient's response to the drug.

Patient teaching

— Inform the patient and family about cyclophosphamide, including the dosage, frequency, action, and adverse reactions.
— Teach the patient and family to identify and report signs of infection and bleeding.
— Teach the patient and family protective measures to conserve the patient's energy and prevent infection: maintaining a balanced diet; eating frequent, small meals; maintaining fluid intake of at least 3 liters/day; allowing adequate rest; avoiding fatigue; and avoiding exposure to people with colds or other infections.
— Advise the patient that alopecia and hyperpigmentation of nails and skin may occur, but are reversible.
— Advise both male and female patients to practice contraception while taking this drug and for 4 months after; drug is potentially teratogenic.
— Teach the patient and family good mouth care strategies, using a soft toothbrush, mild mouthwash, and oral anesthetic solution.
— Tell the patient to notify the nurse or doctor if adverse reactions develop or questions arise about cyclophosphamide therapy.

Evaluation

In the patient receiving cyclophosphamide, appropriate evaluation statements include:
• Patient's diagnostic studies reveal a positive response to cyclophosphamide administration.
• Patient is free of infection.
• Patient demonstrates healing or absence of alterations in oral mucosa.
• Patient's input equals output, and patient demonstrates no signs of fluid volume deficit.
• Patient verbalizes feelings about changes in body image and demonstrates coping behaviors.

• Patient and family state an understanding of cyclophosphamide treatment regimen.

SELECTED MAJOR DRUGS: ALKYLATING AGENTS

DRUG, INDICATIONS, AND DOSAGES	SPECIAL PRECAUTIONS
busulfan (Myleran) *Chronic myelocytic (granulocytic) leukemia—* **Adults:** 4 to 8 mg P.O. daily, up to 12 mg P.O. daily until WBC count falls to 15,000/mm³; stop drug until WBC count rises to 50,000/mm³, then resume treatment as before; or 4 to 8 mg P.O. daily until WBC count falls to 10,000 to 20,000/mm³, then reduce daily dosage as needed to maintain WBC count at this level (usually 2 mg daily). **Children:** 0.06 to 0.12 mg/kg or 2.3 to 4.6 mg/m² P.O. daily; adjust dosage to maintain WBC count at 20,000/mm³, but never less than 10,000/mm³.	• Contraindicated in patients whose chronic myelogenous leukemia has demonstrated prior resistance to this drug. • Use cautiously in patients recently given other myelosuppressive drugs or radiation treatment, and in those with depressed neutrophil or platelet count.
carmustine (BiCNU) *Brain, colon, and stomach cancer; Hodgkin's disease; non-Hodgkin's lymphomas; melanomas; multiple myeloma; and hepatoma—* **Adults:** 75 to 100 mg/m² I.V. by slow infusion daily for 2 days; repeat q 6 weeks if platelet count is above 100,000/mm³ and WBC count is above 4,000/mm³. Dosage is reduced 50% when WBC count is less than 2,000/mm³ and platelet count is less than 25,000/mm³. Alternatively, give 200 mg/m² I.V. by slow infusion as a single dose, repeated q 6 to 8 weeks, or 40 mg/m² I.V. by slow infusion for 5 consecutive days, repeated q 6 weeks.	• Contraindicated in patients with known hypersensitivity to the drug. • Use cautiously because of the risk of carcinogenesis, mutagenesis, or impaired fertility. Avoid use in pregnant or breast-feeding women.
chlorambucil (Leukeran) *Chronic lymphocytic leukemia, diffuse lymphocytic lymphoma, nodular lymphocytic lymphoma, Hodgkin's disease, ovarian carcinoma, mycosis fungoides—* **Adults:** 0.1 to 0.2 mg/kg P.O. daily for 3 to 6 weeks, then adjust for maintenance (usually 2 mg daily). **Children:** 0.1 to 0.2 mg/kg or 4.5 mg/m² P.O. daily as a single dose or in divided doses.	• Contraindicated in patients whose disease has resisted prior treatment with this agent, and in those with known hypersensitivity to the drug. • Administer cautiously.
cisplatin (Platamine‡, Platinol) *Adjunctive therapy in metastatic testicular cancer—* **Men:** 20 mg/m² I.V. daily for 5 days. Repeat q 3 weeks for three cycles or longer. *Adjunctive therapy in metastatic ovarian cancer—* **Women:** 100 mg/m² I.V., repeated q 4 weeks; or 50 mg/m² I.V. q 3 weeks with concurrent doxorubicin therapy. Give as I.V. infusion in 2 liters 0.9% sodium chloride solution with 37.5 g mannitol over 6 to 8 hours. *Treatment of advanced bladder cancer—* **Adults:** 50 to 70 mg/m² I.V. q 3 to 4 weeks. Patients who have received other antineoplastics or radiation therapy should receive 50 mg/m² q 4 weeks. *Note:* Prehydration and mannitol diuresis may reduce renal toxicity and ototoxicity significantly.	• Contraindicated in patients with preexisting renal impairment, myelosuppression, hearing impairment, or known hypersensitivity to cisplatin or other platinum-containing compounds. • Use cautiously: peripheral blood counts should be monitored weekly, and liver function tests and neurologic examinations should be performed regularly.

(continued)

‡Available in Australia only

SELECTED MAJOR DRUGS: ALKYLATING AGENTS *continued*

| DRUG, INDICATIONS, AND DOSAGES | SPECIAL PRECAUTIONS |

dacarbazine (DTIC-Dome)
Metastatic malignant melanoma —
Adults: 2 to 4.5 mg/kg or 70 to 160 mg/m² I.V. daily for 10 days, then repeat q 4 weeks as tolerated; or 250 mg/m² I.V. daily for 5 days, repeated at 3-week intervals.
Hodgkin's disease —
Adults: 150 mg/m² I.V. daily (in combination with other agents) for 5 days, repeated q 4 weeks; or 375 mg/m² on the first day of a combination regimen, repeated q 15 days.

• Contraindicated in patients with known hypersensitivity to the drug.
• Use cautiously in pregnant or breast-feeding women.

mechlorethamine (Mustargen)
Breast, lung, and ovarian cancer; Hodgkin's disease; non-Hodgkin's lymphomas; diffuse lymphocytic lymphoma —
Adults: 0.4 mg/kg or 10 mg/m² I.V. as a single dose or in divided doses q 3 to 6 weeks. Give through running I.V. infusion. Dosage is reduced to 0.2 to 0.4 mg/kg in patients who have undergone previous radiation or chemotherapy. Dosage is based on ideal or actual body weight, whichever is less.
Neoplastic effusions —
Adults: 0.4 mg/kg intracavitarily.
Mycosis fungoides —
Adults: topical solution or ointment applied to lesion. Topical preparations must be compounded by pharmacist; drug concentration, frequency of application, and duration of therapy will vary according to patient tolerance and response. Mechlorethamine ointments of 0.01% to 0.02% and topical solutions containing 10 mg in each 50 to 60 ml have been used.

• Contraindicated in pregnant or breast-feeding women or those with a known infectious disease or previous anaphylactic reaction to the drug.
• Use with extreme caution in patients with chronic lymphatic leukemia.
• Use with caution in patients undergoing radiation therapy or receiving other cytotoxic agents in alternating courses; use cautiously in patients with leukopenia, thrombocytopenia, or anemia caused by tumor invasion of the bone marrow.
• Be careful to prevent extravasation. Mechlorethamine may cause a moderate to severe painful local injury that is difficult to treat. If extravasation occurs, local infiltration with sodium thiosulfate (⅙ molar solution) and ice packs may be used.

streptozocin (Zanosar)
Treatment of metastatic islet cell carcinoma of the pancreas; colon cancer; exocrine pancreatic tumors; and carcinoid tumors —
Adults and children: 500 mg/m² I.V. for 5 consecutive days q 6 weeks until maximum benefit or toxicity is observed. Alternatively, 1,000 mg/m² at weekly intervals for the first 2 weeks. Don't exceed a single dose of 1,500 mg/m².

• Contraindicated in preexisting renal disease.
• Use cautiously because of the risk of mutagenesis, carcinogenesis, or impaired fertility. Avoid use in pregnant or breast-feeding women.

SELECTED MAJOR DRUGS: ALKYLATING AGENTS *continued*

DRUG, INDICATIONS, AND DOSAGES	SPECIAL PRECAUTIONS
thiotepa (Thiotepa Parenteral) *Breast and ovarian cancer; lymphomas and bronchogenic carcinomas —* **Adults and children over age 12:** 0.2 mg/kg I.V. daily for 4 to 5 days at intervals of 2 to 4 weeks. *Bladder tumor —* **Adults and children over age 12:** 60 mg in 60 ml water instilled into bladder for 2 hours once weekly for 4 weeks. *Neoplastic effusions —* **Adults and children over age 12:** 0.6 to 0.8 mg/kg intracavitarily, p.r.n. Stop drug or decrease dosage if WBC count is below 4,000/mm³ or if platelet count is below 150,000/mm³. *Malignant meningeal neoplasms —* **Adults:** 1 to 10 mg/m² intrathecally once or twice weekly.	• Contraindicated in preexisting hepatic, renal, or bone marrow damage. • Use cautiously in bone marrow suppression and renal or hepatic dysfunction.

SELF-TEST

1. Molly Malone, age 36, is receiving cyclophosphamide 2 mg/kg P.O. daily as maintenance therapy for ovarian cancer. Which of the following laboratory tests should be monitored closely?
   a. Serum calcium levels
   b. Serum glucose levels
   c. White blood cell count
   d. Estrogen levels

2. Which of the following disorders requires discontinuation of cyclophosphamide therapy?
   a. Hypertension
   b. Serious bacterial infection
   c. Diabetes mellitus
   d. Seizures

3. Which of the following nursing interventions should be used during cyclophosphamide therapy?
   a. Give drug at bedtime.
   b. Maintain seizure precautions.
   c. Encourage fluid intake of at least 3 liters/day.
   d. Limit sodium intake.

Check your answers on pages 1073 and 1074.

CHAPTER 68

ANTIMETABOLITES

cytarabine (ara-C) ◆ floxuridine ◆ fluorouracil (5-fluorouracil, 5-FU)
hydroxyurea ◆ mercaptopurine ◆ methotrexate ◆ methotrexate sodium
thioguanine (6-thioguanine, 6-TG)

OVERVIEW

- Antimetabolites, the first group of antineoplastics designed specifically as antitumor agents, function in one of two ways: as replacements for cellular components or as enzyme inhibitors. When they replace a necessary component in a cellular compound, the resulting cell product fails to function, blocking cell division. When antimetabolites inhibit a key enzyme reaction, they interfere with cellular metabolism.
- Antimetabolites can be further classified as folic acid antagonists (methotrexate and methotrexate sodium), purine antagonists (mercaptopurine and thioguanine), and pyrimidine antagonists (cytarabine, floxuridine, and fluorouracil). Hydroxyurea also functions as an antimetabolite but cannot be assigned to any group.

MAJOR USES

- Antimetabolites are used to treat carcinomas (mostly of the breast and GI tract), trophoblastic tumors such as choriocarcinomas and hydatidiform moles, medulloblastomas, and osteogenic sarcomas.

MECHANISM OF ACTION

- All the antimetabolites interfere with DNA synthesis; they do so using different mechanisms, as follows.
- Mercaptopurine and thioguanine inhibit purine synthesis.
- Cytarabine, floxuridine, and fluorouracil inhibit pyrimidine synthesis.
- Hydroxyurea inhibits ribonucleotide reductase.
- Methotrexate prevents reduction of folic acid to tetrahydrofolate by binding to dihydrofolate reductase.

ABSORPTION, DISTRIBUTION, METABOLISM, AND EXCRETION

Hydroxyurea, mercaptopurine, methotrexate, and thioguanine are well absorbed when given orally. Cytarabine, floxuridine, and fluorouracil are not absorbed after oral administration and must be given parenterally. However, fluorouracil can be administered orally in local treatment of some GI carcinomas.

GLOSSARY

Anemia: blood disorder characterized by a deficiency of erythrocytes, hemoglobin, or volume of packed RBCs.

Antimetabolite: substance having a molecular structure similar to an essential metabolite but inhibiting or opposing its action.

Immunosuppressant: ability of a substance to suppress the immune response.

Medulloblastoma: malignant brain tumor with a tendency to spread in the meninges; most common in the cerebellum of children.

Osteogenic: pertaining to the deep layer of periosteum from which bone is formed.

Rheumatoid arthritis: chronic systemic disease of unknown etiology characterized by joint inflammation and connective tissue changes in related structures, leading to crippling deformities.

Stomatitis: mouth inflammation that may affect the buccal mucosa, palate, tongue, floor of the mouth, and gingivae.

Trophoblastic tumors: tumors affecting the outer, ectodermal epithelium of the mammalian blastocyst or chorion and chorionic villi.

All antimetabolites are distributed widely in body tissues and fluids, metabolized in the liver, and excreted in urine, largely as inactive metabolites.

ONSET AND DURATION

Therapeutic activity varies with the antimetabolite, disease, and patient response.

ADVERSE REACTIONS

Antimetabolites commonly cause thrombocytopenia, neutropenia, and, to a lesser extent, anemia. Other reactions that occur with varying frequency and severity include nausea, vomiting, diarrhea, dysphagia, and stomatitis. Most of these agents will mildly elevate results of liver function studies and cause jaundice.

Cytarabine can cause a flulike syndrome at all dosages, and can cause neurotoxicity at high dosages. Floxuridine can also cause various CNS symptoms, including ataxia, vertigo, and seizures. Fluorouracil, a metabolite of floxuridine, has been known to cause acute cerebellar syndrome.

Mercaptopurine can cause hepatic necrosis. Methotrexate can cause acute (elevated liver function test results) and chronic (hepatic fibrosis) hepatotoxicity, and may also cause pulmonary interstitial infiltrates.

FLUOROURACIL
(5-fluorouracil, 5-FU)
(flure oh yoor′ a sill)
Adrucil, Efudex, Fluoroplex
Classification: antimetabolite
Pregnancy risk category D

How supplied
INJECTION: 50 mg/ml in 10-ml ampules
CREAM: 1% in 30-g tubes, 5% in 25-g tubes
TOPICAL SOLUTION: 1% in 30-ml bottles; 2%, 5% in 10-ml droppers

Indications and dosage
Colon, rectal, breast, ovarian, cervical, bladder, liver, and pancreatic cancer
ADULTS: 12.5 mg/kg I.V. daily for 3 to 5 days q 4 weeks; or 15 mg/kg I.V. weekly for 6 weeks. (Dosages recommended based on lean body weight.) Maximum single recommended dose is 800 mg, although higher single doses (up to 1.5 g) have been used. The injectable form has been given orally but is not recommended.

Multiple actinic (solar) keratoses; superficial basal cell carcinoma
ADULTS: apply cream or topical solution b.i.d.

Contraindications and precautions
Fluorouracil is contraindicated in patients with poor nutritional state, depressed bone marrow function, or potentially serious infections. Use with caution in patients with a history of high-dose pelvic irradiation, previous use of alkylating agents, widespread tumor involvement of bone marrow, or impaired hepatic or renal function.

Adverse reactions
BLOOD: *leukopenia* (WBC nadir 9 to 14 days after first dose), thrombocytopenia (platelet nadir in 7 to 14 days), anemia.
CNS: acute cerebellar syndrome.
GI: stomatitis, GI ulcer (may precede leukopenia), *nausea, vomiting, and diarrhea* in 30% to 50% of patients.
SKIN: (I.V. use) dermatitis, hyperpigmentation (especially in blacks), nail changes, pigmented palmar creases.
LOCAL: erythema, pain, burning, scaling, pruritus; (topical use) contact dermatitis, hyperpigmentation, soreness, suppuration, swelling.
OTHER: *reversible alopecia* in 5% to 20% of patients, weakness, malaise.

Interactions
Leucovorin: may result in increased effectiveness and toxicity. Monitor patient carefully.

Italicized adverse reactions are common

Nursing considerations

Assessment
- Review the patient's history for a condition that contraindicates the use of fluorouracil.
- Obtain a baseline assessment of WBC count and differential, platelets, nutritional status, and weight, and the patient's underlying cancerous state before initiating therapy.
- Be alert for common adverse reactions.
- Evaluate the patient's and family's knowledge about fluorouracil therapy.

Planning (Nursing Diagnoses)
Potential nursing diagnoses for the patient receiving fluorouracil include:
- Altered health maintenance related to ineffectiveness of fluorouracil to halt cancer.
- Infection related to potential fluorouracil-induced leukopenia.
- Altered oral mucous membranes related to stomatitis and esophagitis caused by fluorouracil therapy.
- Fluid volume deficit related to potential nausea, vomiting, or diarrhea caused by fluorouracil therapy.
- Knowledge deficit related to fluorouracil therapy.

Implementation
Preparation and administration
— Read order and drug label carefully before administering fluorouracil.
— Fluorouracil is sometimes ordered as 5-fluorouracil or 5-FU. The numeral 5 is part of the drug name; don't confuse it with dosage units.
— Follow institutional policy for handling hazardous materials to minimize carcinogenic, mutagenic, and teratogenic risks.
— Don't refrigerate fluorouracil.
— Don't use cloudy solution. If crystals form, redissolve by warming.
— Solution is more stable in plastic I.V. bags than in glass bottles. Use plastic I.V. containers for administering continuous infusions.
— Fluorouracil is sometimes administered via hepatic arterial infusion in treatment of hepatic metastases.
— Check I.V. line patency and site before administering fluorouracil.
— Check the patient's I.D. band and ask the patient's name before administration.
For topical application:
— Avoid occlusive dressings, because they increase the risk of inflammatory reactions in adjacent normal skin.
— Apply with caution near eyes, nose, and mouth.
— Expect to use 1% concentration on the face. Higher concentrations are used for thicker-skinned areas or resistant lesions.
— Expect to use 5% strength for superficial basal cell carcinoma confirmed by biopsy.
— Chart drug administration and related observations.

Monitoring

— Monitor the effectiveness of fluorouracil therapy by checking patient's response, exhibited by reduction in tumor size.

— Monitor WBC and platelet counts daily. Drug should be discontinued when WBC count is below 3,500/mm³ and platelet count is below 100,000/mm³.

— Monitor the patient for adverse drug reactions.

— Regularly monitor renal and hepatic function.

— Monitor the patient for signs of bleeding (ecchymosis, petechiae, melena, hematuria) if platelet count is abnormal.

— Monitor the patient's skin for local changes.

— Monitor the patient for signs of infection (fever, chills, fatigue) if WBC count is below normal.

— Monitor hydration status if adverse GI reactions occur.

— Monitor the patient for drug interactions.

— Periodically reevaluate the patient's and family's knowledge about fluorouracil.

Intervention

— Notify the doctor and discontinue fluorouracil if the patient develops intractable vomiting, diarrhea, stomatitis or esophagitis, GI ulceration or bleeding, or hemorrhage.

— Premedicate the patient with an antiemetic to decrease nausea and vomiting.

— Provide a private room and use reverse isolation precautions for patients with compromised immune systems.

— Keep accurate records of intake and output and daily weight.

— Provide frequent mouth care with a soft toothbrush and mild mouthwash to avoid trauma to oral mucosa.

— Use a topical oral anesthetic to soothe lesions if stomatitis occurs.

— Encourage the patient to maintain adequate caloric and fluid intake; offer frequent, small meals.

— Avoid I.M. injections to decrease risk of bleeding.

— Offer the patient emotional support and opportunities for expressing feelings about changes in body image.

— Keep all members of the health care team informed of the patient's response to the drug.

Patient teaching

— Inform the patient and family about fluorouracil, including the dosage, frequency, action, and adverse reactions.

— Teach the patient and family how to identify and report signs of infection.

— Teach the patient and family protective measures to conserve the patient's energy and prevent infection: maintaining a balanced diet; eating frequent, small meals; allowing adequate rest; avoiding exposure to people with colds or other infections; and maintaining adequate oral fluid intake.

—Tell the patient that alopecia and skin changes are usually reversible.

—Warn patients receiving topical fluorouracil that treated area may be unsightly during therapy and for several weeks after therapy. Complete healing may take 1 or 2 months.

—Instruct the patient and family members to wear gloves when applying the topical preparation and to avoid occlusive dressings.

—Tell the patient to use with caution on areas near eyes, nose, and mouth.

—Instruct the patient and family to wash hands thoroughly after handling fluorouracil cream or solution.

—Warn the patient that ingestion and systemic absorption may cause leukopenia, thrombocytopenia, stomatitis, diarrhea, GI ulceration or bleeding, or hemorrhage.

—Tell the patient to store drug away from children.

—Tell the patient to notify the nurse or doctor if adverse reactions develop or questions arise about fluorouracil therapy.

Evaluation

In the patient receiving fluorouracil, appropriate evaluation statements include:

• Patient's tumor is decreased as a result of fluorouracil therapy.
• Patient is free of infection.
• Patient demonstrates healing or absence of alterations in oral mucosa.
• Patient's intake equals output, and patient has no signs of fluid volume deficit.
• Patient and family state an understanding of fluorouracil therapy.

SELECTED MAJOR DRUGS: ANTIMETABOLITES

DRUG, INDICATIONS, AND DOSAGES	SPECIAL PRECAUTIONS
cytarabine (Alexan‡, Cytosar-U) *Acute myelocytic and other acute leukemias—* **Adults and children:** 200 mg/m² by continuous I.V. infusion daily for 5 days. *Meningeal leukemias and meningeal neoplasms—* **Adults and children:** 10 to 30 mg/m² intrathecally q 4 days.	• Use cautiously in patients receiving other drugs that depress bone marrow function. • Drug may increase risk of infection. Patient should report fever, sore throat, or other symptoms of infection.
floxuridine (FUDR) *Brain, breast, head, neck, liver, gallbladder, and bile duct cancer—* **Adults:** 0.1 to 0.6 mg/kg by intra-arterial infusion daily (use pump for continuous, uniform rate); or 0.4 to 0.6 mg/kg into hepatic artery daily.	• Contraindicated in patients in a poor nutritional state, and in those with depressed bone marrow function or potentially serious infections.

(continued)

‡Available in Australia only

SELECTED MAJOR DRUGS: ANTIMETABOLITES *continued*

DRUG, INDICATIONS, AND DOSAGES	SPECIAL PRECAUTIONS

hydroxyurea (Hydrea)
Melanoma; resistant chronic myelocytic leukemia; recurrent, metastatic, or inoperable ovarian cancer—
Adults: 80 mg/kg P.O. as single dose q 3 days; or 20 to 30 mg/kg P.O. daily.

- Contraindicated in patients with marked bone marrow depression, as evidenced by leukopenia (WBC count $< 2,500/$ mm^3), thrombocytopenia (platelet count $< 100,000/$mm^3), or severe anemia.
- Use with caution in patients with renal dysfunction. Discontinue if WBC count is less than 3,500/mm^3 or if platelet count is less than 100,000/mm^3.

mercaptopurine (Purinethol)
Acute lymphoblastic leukemia (in children), acute myeloblastic leukemia, chronic myelocytic leukemia—
Adults: 80 to 100 mg/m^2 P.O. daily as a single dose up to 5 mg/kg daily. Maintenance dosage is usually 1.5 to 2.5 mg/kg P.O. daily.
Children: 70 mg/m^2 P.O. daily. Maintenance dosage is usually 1.5 to 2.5 mg/kg P.O. daily.

- Contraindicated unless a diagnosis of acute lymphatic leukemia has been established and the patient's doctor is knowledgeable in assessing response to chemotherapy.
- Use cautiously in pregnant or breast-feeding women.

methotrexate
methotrexate sodium (Folex, Mexate, Rheumatrex)
Trophoblastic tumors (choriocarcinoma, hydatidiform mole)—
Adults: 15 to 30 mg P.O. or I.M. daily for 5 days. Repeat after 1 or more weeks, according to response or toxicity.
Acute lymphoblastic and lymphatic leukemia—
Adults and children: 3.3 mg/m^2 P.O., I.M., or I.V. daily for 4 to 6 weeks or until remission occurs; then 20 to 30 mg/m^2 P.O. or I.M. twice weekly.
Meningeal leukemia—
Adults and children: 10 to 15 mg/m^2 intrathecally q 2 to 5 days until CSF is normal. Use only 20-, 50-, or 100-mg vials of powder with no preservatives; dilute using 0.9% sodium chloride injection *without* preservatives or Elliot's B solution. Use only new vials of drug and diluent. Use immediately.
Burkitt's lymphoma (Stage I or Stage II)—
Adults: 10 to 25 mg P.O. daily for 4 to 8 days with 1-week rest intervals.
Lymphosarcoma (Stage III)—
Adults: 0.625 to 2.5 mg/kg P.O., I.M., or I.V. daily.
Mycosis fungoides—
Adults: 2.5 to 10 mg P.O. daily or 50 mg I.M. weekly; or 25 mg I.M. twice weekly.
Psoriasis—
Adults: 10 to 25 mg P.O., I.M., or I.V. as single weekly dose.

- Contraindicated in pregnant women with psoriasis, rheumatoid arthritis, or neoplastic disease unless the potential benefit outweighs the risk to the fetus; in breast-feeding women; in patients with psoriasis or rheumatoid arthritis along with alcoholism, alcoholic liver disease, or other chronic liver disease; in those with overt or laboratory evidence of immunodeficiency syndromes; with preexisting blood dyscrasia,·such as bone marrow hypoplasia, leukopenia, thrombocytopenia, or significant anemia; and in patients with known hypersensitivity to methotrexate.
- Dosage modification may be required in patients with impaired hepatic or renal function, bone marrow suppression, aplasia, leukopenia, thrombocytopenia, or anemia.
- Use cautiously in patients with infection, peptic ulcer, or ulcerative colitis, and in very young, elderly, or debilitated patients.

SELECTED MAJOR DRUGS: ANTIMETABOLITES *continued*

DRUG, INDICATIONS, AND DOSAGES	SPECIAL PRECAUTIONS
methotrexate *(continued)* *Rheumatoid arthritis—* **Adults:** initially, 7.5 mg P.O. weekly, either in a single dose or divided as 2.5 mg P.O. q 12 hours for three doses once a week. Dosage may be gradually increased to a maximum of 20 mg weekly.	
thioguanine (Lanvis†) *Acute leukemia, chronic granulocytic leukemia—* **Adults and children:** initially, 2 mg/kg P.O. daily (usually calculated to nearest 20 mg); then increased gradually to 3 mg/kg daily if no toxic effects occur.	• Contraindicated in patients whose disease has resisted previous treatment with this drug. • Administer cautiously because of the risk of drug interactions, carcinogenesis, mutagenesis, and impaired fertility; use cautiously in pregnant or breast-feeding women.

†Available in Canada only

SELF-TEST

1. Celia Cirano has breast cancer and takes fluorouracil 12.5 mg/kg I.V. daily for 3 to 5 days every 4 weeks. She asks the nurse how the drug works. The nurse tells Mrs. Cirano that fluorouracil is a member of the antimetabolite group of antineoplastic agents, which act primarily by:
   a. interfering with DNA synthesis.
   b. destroying essential amino acids.
   c. changing cell hormonal balance.
   d. blocking enzyme production.

2. Laurence Kaye, age 68, is receiving fluorouracil for the treatment of liver cancer. Which of the following reactions should the nurse anticipate and monitor for?
   a. Seizures
   b. Depressed reflexes
   c. Nausea, vomiting, and diarrhea
   d. Joint pain

3. Which of the following conditions requires cautious use of fluorouracil?
   a. Cardiomyopathy
   b. Asthma
   c. Colitis
   d. Impaired renal function

Check your answers on page 1074.

CHAPTER 69

ANTIBIOTIC ANTINEOPLASTIC AGENTS

bleomycin sulfate ✦ dactinomycin (actinomycin D)
daunorubicin hydrochloride ✦ doxorubicin hydrochloride ✦ mitomycin
plicamycin (mithramycin) ✦ procarbazine hydrochloride

OVERVIEW
- Antibiotic antineoplastic agents are isolated from naturally occurring microorganisms that inhibit bacterial growth. But unlike the anti-infective drugs they are related to, antibiotic antineoplastic agents can disrupt the functioning of both the host's cells and bacterial cells. Although procarbazine is not an antibiotic, it's included in this group because its action is similar.

MAJOR USES
- Bleomycin, dactinomycin, doxorubicin, mitomycin, and procarbazine are used mainly to treat carcinomas, sarcomas, and lymphomas.
- Daunorubicin is used to treat acute leukemias.
- Plicamycin is used specifically to treat testicular carcinoma and hypercalcemia from various causes.

MECHANISM OF ACTION
- Bleomycin inhibits DNA synthesis and causes splitting of single- and double-stranded DNA.
- Dactinomycin, daunorubicin, doxorubicin, and plicamycin interfere with DNA-dependent RNA synthesis by intercalation.
- Plicamycin also inhibits osteocytic activity, blocking calcium and phosphorus resorption from bone.
- Mitomycin acts like an alkylating agent, cross-linking strands of DNA. This causes an imbalance of cell growth, leading to cell death.
- Procarbazine inhibits DNA, RNA, and protein synthesis.

ABSORPTION, DISTRIBUTION, METABOLISM, AND EXCRETION
Procarbazine is well absorbed after oral administration. All the other drugs must be given parenterally.

All are distributed to most body tissues and organs, especially the liver, spleen, kidneys, lungs, and heart. Plicamycin is the only antibiotic antineoplastic agent that crosses the blood-brain barrier in significant amounts.

The antibiotic antineoplastic agents are generally metabolized in the liver. Their inactive metabolites are eliminated in urine or through the bile in feces.

ONSET AND DURATION
Therapeutic activity varies with the drug, disease, and patient response.

ADVERSE REACTIONS
The hematologic reactions to the antibiotic antineoplastic agents range from minimal effects with bleomycin, and thrombocytopenia and bleeding with plicamycin, to severe bone marrow depression with the other agents of this class. Other reactions to these agents commonly include nausea, vomiting, alopecia, diarrhea, and stomatitis. They vary in severity with each agent.

Dermatologic and pulmonary reactions are among the most common effects of bleomycin; changes in skin texture and coloration of palmar and plantar skin occur in 8% of patients. Pulmonary fibrosis occurs in 10% of patients. Anaphylaxis may also occur in 1% to 6% of patients.

Dactinomycin produces skin changes, including erythema, desquamation, and acnelike lesions.

Daunorubicin and doxorubicin are associated with unique cardiotoxicity: irreversible cardiomyopathy with ECG changes, arrhythmias, pericarditis, and myocarditis. Severe cellulitis and tissue sloughing follow extravasation of doxorubicin, daunorubicin, mitomycin, or dactinomycin.

PROTOTYPE: ANTIBIOTIC ANTINEOPLASTIC AGENTS

DOXORUBICIN HYDROCHLORIDE
(dox oh roo′ bi sin)
Adriamycin, Adriamycin PFS, Adriamycin RDF
Classification: antibiotic antineoplastic agent
Pregnancy risk category D

How supplied
INJECTION (PRESERVATIVE-FREE): 2 mg/ml
POWDER FOR INJECTION: 10-mg, 20-mg, 50-mg vials

Indications and dosage
Dosage and indications may vary. Check patient's protocol with doctor.

Bladder, breast, cervical, head, neck, liver, lung, ovarian, prostatic, stomach, testicular, and thyroid cancer; Hodgkin's disease; acute lymphoblastic and myeloblastic leukemia; Wilms' tumor; neuroblastomas; lymphomas; sarcomas

ADULTS: 60 to 75 mg/m^2 I.V. as single dose q 3 weeks; or 30 mg/m^2 I.V. in single daily dose, days 1 to 3 of 4-week cycle. Alternatively, 20 mg/m^2 I.V. once weekly or 30 mg^2 I.V. on 3 successive days, repeated q 4 weeks. Maximum cumulative dose is 550 mg/m^2.

Contraindications and precautions

Doxorubicin is contraindicated in patients with marked myelosuppression induced by previous treatments with anti-tumor agents or radiation, in those with preexisting heart disease, and in those who have received treatment with the total cumulative doses of doxorubicin or daunorubicin. Use with caution in patients with hepatic dysfunction, in those receiving other cytotoxic drugs, or those receiving doxorubicin for the first time.

Adverse reactions

BLOOD: *leukopenia,* especially **agranulocytosis,** during days 10 to 15, with recovery by day 21; **thrombocytopenia**.

CV: **cardiac depression**, seen in such ECG changes as sinus tachycardia, T wave flattening, ST segment depression, voltage reduction; *arrhythmias* in 11% of patients; irreversible **cardiomyopathy** (sometimes with pulmonary edema), with mortality of 30% to 75%.

GI: *nausea, vomiting, diarrhea,* ulceration and necrosis of the colon, stomatitis, esophagitis.

GU: enhancement of cyclophosphamide-induced bladder injury, *transient red urine.*

SKIN: hyperpigmentation of skin, especially in previously irradiated areas.

LOCAL: severe cellulitis or tissue sloughing if drug extravasates, phlebosclerosis.

OTHER: hyperpigmentation of nails and dermal creases, complete alopecia within 3 to 4 weeks (hair may regrow 2 to 5 months after drug is stopped), hypersensitivity—fever, chills, urticaria, anaphylaxis, cross-sensitivity to lincomycin.

Interactions

Heparin: may form a precipitate. Don't mix together.
Myelosuppressive agents, cyclophosphamide, radiation therapy: additive toxicity. Monitor patient closely.
Streptozocin: increased and prolonged blood levels. Dosage may have to be adjusted.

Nursing considerations

Assessment

• Review the patient's history for a condition that contraindicates the use of doxorubicin.
• Obtain a baseline assessment of the patient's CBC and differential; platelet count; ALT, AST, alkaline phosphatase, and bilirubin levels;

---

cardiac status, including ECG; and the patient's underlying cancerous state before initiating therapy.
• Be alert for common adverse reactions.
• Evaluate the patient's and family's knowledge about doxorubicin therapy.

Planning (Nursing Diagnoses)

Potential nursing diagnoses for the patient receiving doxorubicin include:
• Altered health maintenance related to ineffectiveness of doxorubicin to arrest cancer growth.
• Infection related to potential immunosuppressive effects of doxorubicin.
• Decreased cardiac output related to cardiac depression.
• Body image disturbance related to alopecia and changes in skin pigmentation.
• Fluid volume deficit related to potential nausea and vomiting.
• Knowledge deficit related to doxorubicin therapy.

Implementation

Preparation and administration

— Read order and drug label carefully before administering. Use extreme caution to avoid confusing doxorubicin with daunorubicin (which is a similar reddish color).
— Follow institutional policy for handling hazardous materials to minimize carcinogenic, mutagenic, and teratogenic risks for personnel.
— Label all syringes containing doxorubicin "FOR I.V. USE ONLY." Never give intramuscularly or subcutaneously.
— Refrigerated, reconstituted solution is stable for 48 hours; at room temperature, it's stable for 24 hours.
— Dosage modification may be required in patients with myelosuppression or impaired cardiac or hepatic function.
— Expect to use the alternative dosage schedule (once-weekly dosing), which has been found to lower the incidence of cardiomyopathy.
— Dosage must be decreased if serum bilirubin level is increased.
— Check the patient's I.D. band and ask patient's name before administering.
— Check I.V. line patency and site before administering.
— Avoid extravasation; inject slowly by I.V. push into tubing of freely flowing infusion. Don't place I.V. line over joints or in extremities with poor venous or lymphatic drainage.
— Chart administration of drug and related observations.

Monitoring

— Monitor the effectiveness of therapy by regularly checking patient's tumor response through diagnostic studies.
— Monitor CBC and differential, and platelet counts for evidence of immunosuppression.
— Monitor the patient for adverse drug reactions.
— Monitor the patient's oral cavity for evidence of stomatitis or esophagitis.

—Monitor AST, ALT, alkaline phosphatase, uric acid, and bilirubin levels for changes reflecting hepatic dysfunction.

—Monitor ECG for arrhythmia, tachycardia, or ST wave changes.

—Monitor cardiac function studies for evidence of cardiomyopathy.

—Monitor the patient for signs of infection (fever, sore throat, or fatigue).

—Monitor the patient for signs of bleeding (epistaxis, petechiae, melena, or hematuria).

—Monitor the patient for signs of CHF, including dyspnea, cyanosis, jugular vein distention, decreased peripheral pulses, edema, and changes in mental status.

—Monitor the patient's hydration status if adverse GI reactions occur.

—Monitor the patient for drug interactions.

—Periodically reevaluate the patient's and family's knowledge about doxorubicin.

Intervention

—Premedicate the patient with an antiemetic to decrease nausea and vomiting.

—Stop drug or slow rate of infusion if tachycardia develops.

—Stop drug immediately if signs of CHF appear. Prevent CHF by limiting cumulative dose to 550 mg/m^2, or 450 mg/m^2 if the patient is also receiving cyclophosphamide or irradiation to cardiac area.

—If extravasation occurs, discontinue I.V. immediately and apply ice to area for 24 to 48 hours. Some clinicians will infiltrate the area with a parenteral corticosteroid. The area should be monitored closely. Because the extravasation reaction may be progressive, early consultation with a plastic surgeon may be advisable.

—If vein streaking occurs, slow administration rate. However, if welts occur, stop administration and report to doctor.

—Provide private room and use reverse isolation precautions for patients with compromised immune systems.

—Keep accurate records of intake and output and weight.

—Provide frequent mouth care, using a soft toothbrush and mild mouthwash to avoid trauma to oral mucosa.

—Encourage the patient to maintain adequate caloric and fluid intake; offer frequent, small meals.

—Offer emotional support and opportunities to express feelings about changes in body image.

—Keep all members of the health care team informed of the patient's response to the drug.

Patient teaching

—Inform the patient and family about doxorubicin, including the dosage, frequency, action, and adverse reactions.

—Teach the patient and family how to identify and report signs of hypersensitivity, infection, and CHF.

SELECTED MAJOR DRUGS **865**

— Teach the patient and family protective measures to conserve energy and prevent infection: consume a balanced diet; get adequate rest; avoid fatigue; and avoid people with colds or other infectious conditions.
— Advise the patient that hyperpigmentation of skin and nails may occur, especially in previously irradiated areas.
— Warn the patient that alopecia will occur, but tell him that it is usually reversible.
— Warn the patient that urine will be orange to red for 1 to 2 days. Explain that this is not blood; it is caused by the appearance of the drug in the urine.
— Tell the patient to notify the nurse or doctor if adverse reactions develop or questions arise about doxorubicin therapy.

Evaluation
In the patient receiving doxorubicin, appropriate evaluation statements include:
• Patient's tumor size decreases with doxorubicin therapy.
• Patient is infection-free.
• Patient demonstrates no signs of decreased cardiac output.
• Patient expresses feelings about changes in body image and demonstrates coping behaviors.
• Patient's intake equals output, and patient demonstrates no signs of fluid volume deficit.
• Patient and family state an understanding of doxorubicin therapy.

SELECTED MAJOR DRUGS: ANTIBIOTIC ANTINEOPLASTIC AGENTS

DRUG, INDICATIONS, AND DOSAGES

bleomycin (Blenoxane)
Dosage and indications may vary. Check patient's protocol with doctor.
Cervical, esophageal, head, neck, and testicular cancer—
Adults: 10 to 20 units/m² I.V., I.M., or S.C. one or two times weekly to total of 300 to 400 units.
Hodgkin's disease—
Adults: 10 to 20 units/m² I.V., I.M., or S.C. one or two times weekly. After 50% response, maintenance dose is 1 unit I.M. or I.V. daily or 5 units I.M. or I.V. weekly.
Lymphomas—
Adults: first two doses should be 2 units or less I.V., I.M., or S.C., and patient should be monitored for any allergic reaction. If no reaction occurs, then follow above dosing schedule.

SPECIAL PRECAUTIONS

• Contraindicated in patients who have demonstrated a hypersensitive or idiosyncratic reaction to the drug.
• Use cautiously in patients with renal or pulmonary impairment.

(continued)

SELECTED MAJOR DRUGS: ANTIBIOTIC ANTINEOPLASTIC AGENTS
continued

DRUG, INDICATIONS, AND DOSAGES	SPECIAL PRECAUTIONS
dactinomycin (Cosmegen) Dosage and indications may vary. Check patient's protocol with doctor. *Melanomas, sarcomas, trophoblastic tumors in women, testicular cancer—* **Adults:** 500 mcg I.V. daily for 5 days, not to exceed 15 mg/kg or 400 to 600 mg/m² daily; wait 2 to 4 weeks and repeat. Or 2 mg I.V. single weekly dose for 3 weeks; wait for bone marrow recovery, then repeat in 3 to 4 weeks. *Wilms' tumor, rhabdomyosarcoma, Ewing's sarcoma—* **Children:** 15 mcg/kg I.V. daily for 5 days. Maximum dosage is 500 mcg daily. Wait for bone marrow recovery.	• Contraindicated in renal, hepatic, or bone marrow impairment. • Use cautiously within 2 months of irradiation for the treatment of right-sided Wilms' tumor, because hepatomegaly and elevated AST levels have been noted. Administer cautiously because of the risk of carcinogenesis, mutagenesis, and impaired fertility; use with caution in children and in pregnant or breast-feeding women.
daunorubicin (Cerubidin‡, Cerubidine) Dosage and indications may vary. Check patient's protocol with doctor. *Remission induction in acute nonlymphocytic leukemia (myelogenous, monocytic, erythroid)—* **Adults:** as a single agent, 60 mg/m² I.V. daily on days 1, 2, and 3 q 3 to 4 weeks; in combination, 45 mg/m² I.V. daily on days 1, 2, and 3 of the first course and on days 1 and 2 of subsequent courses with cytosine arabinoside infusions. *Note:* Dose should be reduced if hepatic or renal function is impaired.	• Use cautiously in patients with myelosuppression and impaired cardiac, renal, or hepatic function.
mitomycin (Mutamycin) Dosage and indications may vary. Check patient's protocol with doctor. *Breast, colon, head, neck, lung, pancreatic, and stomach cancer; malignant melanoma—* **Adults:** 2 mg/m² I.V. daily for 5 days. Stop drug for 2 days, then repeat dosage for 5 more days; or 20 mg/m² as a single dose. Repeat cycle in 6 to 8 weeks. Stop drug if WBC count is less than 4,000/mm³ or platelet count is less than 75,000/mm³.	• Contraindicated in patients who have demonstrated a hypersensitive or idiosyncratic reaction to the drug and in patients with thrombocytopenia, coagulation disorders, or increased bleeding from other causes. • Administer cautiously because of the risk of bone marrow suppression, (thrombocytopenia and leukopenia) and the risk of renal and other toxicity. Use cautiously in pregnant women.
plicamycin (Mithracin) Dosage and indications may vary. Check patient's protocol with doctor. *Hypercalcemia associated with advanced malignancy—* **Adults:** 25 mcg/kg I.V. daily for 1 to 4 days. *Testicular cancer—* **Men:** 25 to 30 mcg/kg I.V. daily for up to 10 days (based on ideal body weight or actual weight, whichever is less).	• Contraindicated in thrombocytopenia and in coagulation and bleeding disorders. • Use cautiously in patients with hepatic and renal dysfunction and in those who have received abdominal or mediastinal radiation because such patients may be more susceptible to the drug's toxic effects.

‡Available in Australia only

SELECTED MAJOR DRUGS: ANTIBIOTIC ANTINEOPLASTIC AGENTS
continued

DRUG, INDICATIONS, AND DOSAGES	SPECIAL PRECAUTIONS
procarbazine (Matulane, Natulan†‡) Dosage and indications may vary. Check patient's protocol with doctor. *Hodgkin's disease, lymphomas, brain and lung cancer—* **Adults:** 2 to 4 mg/kg P.O. daily in a single dose or divided doses for the first week. Then, 4 to 6 mg/kg daily until WBC count falls below 4,000/mm³ or platelet count falls below 100,000/mm³. After bone marrow recovers, resume maintenance dosage of 1 to 2 mg/kg/day. **Children:** 50 mg/m² P.O. daily for first week, then 100 mg/m² until response or toxicity occurs. Maintenance: 50 mg/m² P.O. daily after bone marrow recovery.	• Contraindicated in patients with known hypersensitivity to the drug or inadequate marrow reserve as demonstrated by bone marrow aspiration. • Use cautiously in patients with leukopenia, thrombocytopenia, anemia, or impaired hepatic or renal function.

†Available in Canada only   ‡Available in Australia only

SELF-TEST

1. Donald Smith is receiving doxorubicin (Adriamycin) as part of a combination regimen to treat cancer of the bladder. When assessing Mr. Smith, the nurse should pay particular attention to which of the following body systems?
   a. Hepatobiliary
   b. Pulmonary
   c. Endocrine
   d. Cardiac

2. When giving I.V. doxorubicin to Mr. Smith, the nurse needs to monitor for:
   a. confusion.
   b. extravasation.
   c. thrombophlebitis.
   d. hypercalcemia.

3. Which of the following effects should the nurse warn Mr. Smith to expect after doxorubicin therapy?
   a. Orange to red urine for 1 to 2 days due to presence of drug in urine
   b. Weight gain
   c. Numbness and tingling in extremities
   d. Double vision

Check your answers on page 1074.

CHAPTER 70

ANTINEOPLASTICS ALTERING HORMONE BALANCE

aminoglutethimide ✦ estramustine phosphate sodium ✦ flutamide
goserelin acetate ✦ leuprolide acetate ✦ megestrol acetate ✦ mitotane
tamoxifen citrate ✦ testolactone ✦ trilostane

OVERVIEW

- Synthetic sex hormones, such as megestrol and testolactone, counterbalance the tumor-stimulating effects of endogenous sex hormones.
- Tamoxifen is not a synthetic hormone, but an estrogen antagonist. Mitotane, also not a hormone, is useful in managing cancer of the adrenal cortex.
- Aminoglutethimide is an antisteroid drug that's used for the treatment of Cushing's syndrome.
- Trilostane inhibits adrenocorticoid synthesis.
- Estramustine is a combination of nitrogen mustard and estradiol and is used in treatment of patients with advanced prostatic cancer.
- Flutamide inhibits androgen uptake or binding of the nucleus of cells.
- Goserelin and leuprolide are luteinizing hormone-releasing hormone (LHRH) analogs and decrease the release of follicle-stimulating hormone and luteinizing hormone, which in turn decrease testosterone levels.
- These drugs are especially useful in treating cancer because they inhibit neoplastic growth in specific tissues without directly causing cytotoxicity.

MAJOR USES

- Tamoxifen and testolactone are used as palliatives in postmenopausal metastatic breast cancer. Tamoxifen is also used to treat advanced breast cancer in premenopausal women and breast cancer in men, and has been used to stimulate ovulation in women with oligomenorrhea or amenorrhea who previously used oral contraceptives.
- Estramustine is indicated for the palliative treatment of patients with advanced prostate carcinoma.
- Flutamide, goserelin, and leuprolide are used to treat advanced carcinoma of the prostate.
- Megestrol is a palliative in both breast and endometrial cancer.
- Mitotane is a palliative in inoperable adrenocortical carcinoma.

GLOSSARY

Amenorrhea: absence of menstruation.
Cushing's syndrome: endocrine disorder caused by adrenocortical hormone excess from adrenocortical tumor or hyperplasia, basophilic adenoma of the pituitary, certain tumors of nonendocrine origin, or administration of adrenocortical hormones.
Cytotoxicity: ability of a substance to destroy or poison cells.
Oligomenorrhea: abnormally infrequent menstruation.
Osseous: composed of or resembling bone.
Palliative: providing relief but not cure.
Pancytopenia: deficiency of all cellular elements in the blood.

- Trilostane and aminoglutethimide suppress adrenal function in some patients with Cushing's syndrome or adrenal cancer.

MECHANISM OF ACTION

- Aminoglutethimide blocks conversion of cholesterol to delta-5-pregnenolone in the adrenal cortex, inhibiting the synthesis of glucocorticoids, mineralocorticoids, and other steroids.
- Megestrol and testolactone change the tumor's hormonal environment and alter the neoplastic process.
- Estramustine acts by its ability to bind selectively to a protein present in the human prostate. The exact mechanism is unknown.
- Mitotane selectively destroys adrenocortical tissue and hinders extra-adrenal metabolism of cortisol.
- Trilostane blocks steroid synthesis within the adrenal cortex.
- Tamoxifen acts as an estrogen antagonist.
- Flutamide is an antiandrogen. It blocks androgen uptake into target cells or inhibits the binding of androgens within the nucleus of target cells.
- Goserelin and leuprolide are analogs of naturally occurring LHRH. They occupy and eventually desensitize pituitary LHRH receptors, which results in decreased gonadotropin secretion and reduced gonadal steroidogenesis.

ABSORPTION, DISTRIBUTION, METABOLISM, AND EXCRETION

Most of the antineoplastics that alter hormone balance are well absorbed after oral administration and distributed widely in body tissues. Leuprolide is slowly absorbed after I.M. or S.C. injection. Goserelin is administered as a subcutaneous implant in the upper abdominal wall; the drug is slowly absorbed from the implanted pellet, and serum levels peak in 12 to 15 days. Mitotane is partially absorbed when given orally (about 40%).

All of these antineoplastics are metabolized in the liver and excreted in urine. Aminoglutethimide is excreted mainly unchanged in the urine or feces.

ONSET AND DURATION
Therapeutic activity varies with the drug, disease, and patient response.

ADVERSE REACTIONS
Trilostane and aminoglutethimide produce different adverse reactions even though they both inhibit adrenal steroid production. Trilostane's major adverse reaction, diarrhea, occurs in about 16% of patients. Less frequently trilostane causes burning of oral or nasal mucosa, flushing, and headache. Aminoglutethimide produces adverse reactions in 50% to 67% of patients. Severe reactions include transient leukopenia or severe pancytopenia, hypotension, and tachycardia. Skin rash may occur in as many as 17% of patients but is often reversible with continued therapy.

Testolactone, an androgen, produces few adverse reactions. Among those reported are anorexia, nausea and vomiting, glossitis, paresthesia, maculopapular rash, erythema, edema, hypertension, and alopecia.

Flutamide, an antiandrogen, produces significant reactions, especially in combination with the LHRH agonists leuprolide and goserelin. In patients treated with such combination therapy, 61% reported hot flashes; 36%, loss of libido; 33%, impotence; 12%, diarrhea; 11%, nausea and vomiting; and 9%, gynecomastia. Other reactions include rash, photosensitivity, and elevations in hepatic enzymes.

Megestrol may cause carpal tunnel syndrome, alopecia, breast tenderness, nausea, vomiting, and backache. Dysfunctional uterine bleeding may follow cessation of therapy because of the drug's progestin-like activity.

Estramustine, a unique combination of estradiol and nornitrogen mustard, produces significant adverse reactions. Cardiovascular, pulmonary, and hematologic reactions are the most severe and can cause MI, CVA, pulmonary emboli, edema, CHF, leukopenia, and thrombocytopenia. Nausea, vomiting, gynecomastia, and breast tenderness can also be significant.

Adverse reactions to tamoxifen are infrequent and can usually be controlled by dosage adjustment without compromising disease control. Most frequently, such reactions include hot flashes and nausea and vomiting; less frequently, vaginal discharge or bleeding; infrequently, hypercalcemia and temporary bone or tumor pain.

Goserelin and leuprolide are LHRH analogs that produce adverse reactions related to their pharmacologic effects. Both drugs are usually well tolerated and infrequently require cessation of therapy. Most disturbing to the patient are sexual dysfunction, decreased libido, and hot flashes. These drugs also cause worsening of CHF, hypertension, edema, gout, and hyperglycemia, and occasionally nausea, vomiting, dizziness, headache, insomnia, and some skin reactions.

Mitotane produces anorexia, nausea and vomiting, and diarrhea in up to 80% of patients; depression manifested by dizziness, vertigo, lethargy, and somnolence in 40%; and transient skin rash that subsides with continuation of therapy in 15%.

TAMOXIFEN CITRATE
(ta moxé i fen)
Nolvadex, Nolvadex D†‡, Tamofen†, Tamone†
Classification: estrogen antagonist
Pregnancy risk category D

How supplied
TABLETS: 10 mg, 15.2 mg†‡, 20 mg†
TABLETS (FILM-COATED): 30.4 mg

Indications and dosage
Advanced premenopausal and postmenopausal breast cancer
WOMEN: 10 mg P.O. b.i.d.
Also used to treat breast cancer in men and advanced ovarian cancer in women.

Contraindications and precautions
Tamoxifen is contraindicated during pregnancy, and in patients hypersensitive to the drug. Use cautiously in patients with preexisting leukopenia or thrombocytopenia.

Adverse reactions
BLOOD: transient fall in WBC or platelet counts.
EYE: retinopathy, corneal changes, decreased visual acuity.
GI: *nausea (in 10% of patients), vomiting,* anorexia.
GU: vaginal discharge and bleeding.
METABOLIC: hypercalcemia.
SKIN: rash.
OTHER: temporary bone or tumor pain, *hot flashes,* exacerbation of pain from osseous metastases, weight gain.

Interactions
Antacids or H₂ antagonists: may raise gastric pH and cause premature dissolution of the drug in the stomach and gastric irritation. Avoid concomitant use.
Oral contraceptives: may interfere with the drug's therapeutic effect. Monitor patient carefully.

Nursing considerations
Assessment
• Obtain a baseline assessment of CBC and differential, platelet count, visual acuity, and patient's underlying cancerous state before initiating therapy.
• Be alert for common adverse reactions.
• Evaluate the patient's and family's knowledge about tamoxifen therapy.

Planning (Nursing Diagnoses)

Potential nursing diagnoses for the patient receiving tamoxifen include:

- Altered health maintenance related to ineffectiveness of tamoxifen to halt cancer.
- Altered protection related to immunosuppressive effects of tamoxifen.
- Pain related to tamoxifen-induced bone or tumor pain.
- Altered nutrition: less than body requirements, related to nausea, vomiting, and anorexia.
- Sensory or perceptual alterations (visual) related to potential retinopathy and corneal changes.
- Knowledge deficit related to tamoxifen therapy.

Implementation

Preparation and administration

— Read order and drug label carefully before administration.

— Administer medication on time despite nausea; if vomiting becomes a problem, premedicate patient with an antiemetic.

— Chart drug administration and related observations.

Monitoring

— Monitor the effectiveness of therapy by regularly checking tumor size and rate of growth through appropriate studies.

— Monitor the patient for adverse drug reactions.

— Monitor the patient's weight, hydration, and nutritional status if adverse GI reactions occur.

— Monitor serum calcium level. Tamoxifen may compound hypercalcemia related to bone metastases.

— Monitor for changes in visual acuity.

— Monitor CBC and differential and platelet counts for evidence of immunosuppression.

— In men receiving tamoxifen for breast cancer, monitor for gynecomastia.

— Monitor the patient for drug interactions.

— Monitor the patient for infection if leukopenia occurs; observe for fever, chills, or purulent drainage or sputum.

— Monitor for bleeding (bruising, epistaxis, or hematuria) if the patient's platelet count drops.

— Monitor for bone or tumor pain.

— Monitor for hot flashes, especially at start of therapy.

— Periodically reevaluate the patient's and family's knowledge about tamoxifen.

Intervention

— Use analgesics to control bone or tumor pain as indicated and prescribed.

— Use safety precautions to minimize risk of injury due to changes in visual acuity.

— Provide comfort measures to relieve hot flashes: environmental temperature control, skin care, and adequate intake of oral fluids.

—Encourage the patient to maintain adequate caloric intake. Offer frequent, small meals and supplemental forms of nourishment as needed.
—Institute infection and bleeding precautions if immunosuppression occurs.
—Keep all members of the health care team informed of the patient's response to the drug.

Patient teaching

—Inform the patient and family about tamoxifen, including the dosage, frequency, action, and adverse reactions.
—Advise the patient that short-term therapy with tamoxifen induces ovulation. Recommend mechanical contraception.
—Reassure the patient that bone pain during therapy usually indicates that the drug will produce a good response; tell the patient to request an analgesic from doctor.
—Instruct patient and family in comfort measures to relieve hot flashes: controlling environmental temperature, avoiding alcohol and tobacco, maintaining oral fluid intake, and dressing in layers of clothing to accommodate changes in perceived body temperature.
—Stress the importance of regular eye examinations to detect visual changes.
—Teach the patient and family protective measures to conserve the patient's energy and prevent infection or bleeding: allowing adequate rest, avoiding fatigue, and avoiding exposure to people with colds or other infections.
—Instruct the patient to eat a high caloric diet and how to manage nausea, anorexia, and vomiting; stress importance of continuing medication despite adverse GI reactions. Tell the patient to notify doctor if vomiting occurs shortly after a dose is taken.
—Tell the patient to notify the nurse or doctor if adverse reactions develop or questions arise about tamoxifen therapy.

Evaluation

In the patient receiving tamoxifen, appropriate evaluation statements include:
• Patient's tumor size is decreasing with tamoxifen therapy.
• Patient's WBC and platelet counts are normal.
• Patient is free of pain.
• Patient consumes adequate calories and demonstrates no weight loss.
• Patient demonstrates no visual alterations.
• Patient and family state an understanding of tamoxifen therapy.

SELECTED MAJOR DRUGS: ANTINEOPLASTICS ALTERING HORMONE BALANCE

DRUG, INDICATIONS, AND DOSAGES	SPECIAL PRECAUTIONS
flutamide (Eulexin) *Treatment of metastatic prostatic carcinoma (stage D_2) in combination with LHRH analogs such as leuprolide acetate—* **Men:** 250 mg P.O. q 8 hours.	• Contraindicated in patients with known hypersensitivity to flutamide. • Administer cautiously because of the risk of drug interactions, carcinogenesis, mutagenesis, and impaired fertility.
goserelin (Zoladex) *Palliative treatment of advanced prostate cancer—* **Men:** 1 implant S.C. q 28 days into the upper abdominal wall.	• Use cautiously in patients with ureteral obstruction or spinal cord compression and in children; administer cautiously because of the risk of carcinogenesis, mutagenesis, and impaired fertility.
leuprolide (Lucrin‡, Lupron, Lupron Depot) *Management of advanced prostate cancer—* **Men:** 1 mg S.C. daily. Alternatively, give 7.5 mg I.M. (depot injection) monthly.	• Use cautiously in patients with metastatic vertebral lesions or urinary tract obstruction; administer cautiously because of the risk of carcinogenesis, mutagenesis, and impaired fertility.
megestrol (Megace, Megostat‡) *Breast cancer—* **Women:** 40 mg P.O. q.i.d. *Endometrial cancer—* **Women:** 40 to 320 mg P.O. daily in divided doses.	• Contraindicated as a diagnostic test for pregnancy. • Use cautiously in patients with history of thrombophlebitis.
testolactone (Teslac) *Advanced postmenopausal breast cancer—* **Women:** 250 mg P.O. q.i.d.	• Contraindicated in male breast cancer and in premenopausal women. • Use cautiously in children and in pregnant or breast-feeding women; administer cautiously because of the risk of carcinogenesis, mutagenesis, impaired fertility, and drug or laboratory test interactions.

‡Available in Australia only

SELF-TEST

1. Barbara Breyer, age 58, has breast cancer and is about to begin treatment with tamoxifen. During initial assessment, the nurse should especially note a baseline assessment of:
   a. blood pressure.
   b. muscle strength.
   c. visual acuity.
   d. breath sounds.

2. When reviewing Mrs. Breyer's blood work, the nurse should be aware of CBC, differential, platelet count, and:
   a. sodium level.
   b. bilirubin level.
   c. calcium level.
   d. magnesium level.

3. In explaining the mechanism of action of tamoxifen to Mrs. Breyer, the nurse states that tamoxifen is a hormone-altering antineoplastic agent that is specifically antagonistic to:
   a. progesterone.
   b. estrogen.
   c. thyroid stimulating hormone.
   d. testosterone.

Check your answers on page 1074.

CHAPTER 71

MISCELLANEOUS ANTINEOPLASTIC AGENTS

asparaginase (L-asparaginase) ◆ etoposide (VP-16)
mitoxantrone hydrochloride ◆ vinblastine sulfate ◆ vincristine sulfate

OVERVIEW

- Vinblastine and vincristine are used as palliative treatment of various malignant neoplastic conditions. Closely related derivatives of the periwinkle plant, they are referred to as vinca alkaloids.
- Etoposide, a podophyllin derivative, is prescribed primarily as a treatment for testicular cancer.
- Asparaginase, derived from *Escherichia coli* and a number of other sources, is usually given in combination with other antineoplastic drugs as initial therapy of acute nonlymphocytic leukemia.

MAJOR USES

- Vinblastine, vincristine, and asparaginase furnish supplemental or adjunctive therapy for acute lymphocytic leukemia (ALL).
- Mitoxantrone primarily is used in the treatment of acute nonlymphocytic leukemia (ANLL).
- Etoposide and the vinca alkaloids are used as palliative therapy for lymphomas, leukemias, sarcomas, and some carcinomas.

MECHANISM OF ACTION

- Asparaginase destroys the amino acid asparagine, which is needed for protein synthesis in ALL. This leads to death of the leukemic cell.
- Vinca alkaloids and etoposide arrest mitosis in metaphase, blocking cell division.
- Mitoxantrone is a non–cell-cycle-specific agent that reacts with DNA to produce a cytotoxic effect.

ABSORPTION, DISTRIBUTION, METABOLISM, AND EXCRETION

Although all the miscellaneous antineoplastics are rapidly cleared from the blood and distributed in body tissues, they penetrate the blood-brain barrier poorly.

Asparaginase is well absorbed after I.M. injection; it can also be administered I.V. Its metabolism and route of excretion are unknown. Only trace amounts are excreted in urine.

Mitoxantrone and vinca alkaloids are given I.V. only. They are extensively metabolized in the liver and eliminated both in urine and—through the bile—in feces.

ONSET AND DURATION
Therapeutic activity varies with the drug, disease, and patient response.

ADVERSE REACTIONS
All of these antineoplastic agents suppress factors and cell lines commonly found in blood; most cause leukopenia, thrombocytopenia, and mild anemia. Asparaginase can also cause hypofibrinogenemia and may depress other clotting factors.

All of the agents can cause vomiting, nausea, and other GI reactions. Asparaginase can cause azotemia, hyperglycemia, hemorrhagic pancreatitis, and anaphylaxis (relatively common).

Etoposide may cause hypotension with rapid infusion; mitoxantrone produces arrhythmias, tachycardia, and CHF.

The vinca alkaloids (vincristine and vinblastine) commonly cause neurotoxicity, including peripheral neuropathy, loss of deep tendon reflexes, paresthesia, muscle pain, and weakness. Their GI reactions may include ileus that can mimic a surgical abdomen. Bronchospasm may occur.

PROTOTYPE: VINCA ALKALOIDS

VINCRISTINE SULFATE
(vin kris' teen)
Oncovin, Vincasar PFS
Classification: vinca alkaloid
Pregnancy risk category D

How supplied
INJECTION: 1 mg/ml in 1-ml, 2-ml, and 5-ml multiple-dose vials; 1 mg/ml in 1-ml and 2-ml preservative-free vials; 1 mg/ml in 1-ml and 2-ml syringes

Indications and dosage
Acute lymphoblastic and other leukemias, Hodgkin's disease, lymphosarcoma, reticulum cell sarcoma, neuroblastoma, rhabdomyosarcoma, Wilms' tumor, osteogenic and other sarcomas, lung and breast cancer
ADULTS: 1 to 2 mg/m^2 I.V. weekly.
CHILDREN: 1.5 to 2 mg/m^2 I.V. weekly. Maximum single dosage (adults and children) is 2 mg.

Contraindications and precautions

Vincristine is contraindicated in patients with hypertrophic interstitial neuropathy (Dejerine-Sottas disease), the demyelinating form of Charcot-Marie-Tooth syndrome. Use cautiously in patients with jaundice, hepatic dysfunction, neuromuscular disease, or infection, and in those treated with other neurotoxic and oncolytic agents. Use with caution in children, who are more resistant to neurotoxicity.

Adverse reactions

BLOOD: rapidly reversible mild anemia and leukopenia.

CNS: peripheral neuropathy, sensory loss, loss of deep tendon reflexes, paresthesia, wristdrop and footdrop, ataxia, cranial nerve palsies (headache, jaw pain, hoarseness, vocal cord paralysis, visual disturbances), muscle weakness and cramps, depression, agitation, insomnia; some neurotoxicities may be permanent.

EENT: diplopia, optic and extraocular neuropathy, ptosis.

GI: constipation, cramps, ileus that mimics surgical abdomen, *nausea, vomiting,* anorexia, stomatitis, weight loss, dysphagia.

GU: urine retention, SIADH.

LOCAL: severe local reaction when extravasated, phlebitis, cellulitis.

OTHER: **acute bronchospasm,** *reversible alopecia* (up to 71% of patients).

Interactions

Asparaginase: decreased hepatic clearance of vincristine. Monitor carefully for signs of toxicity.

Calcium channel blockers: enhanced vincristine accumulation in cells. Monitor for signs of toxicity.

Digoxin: decreased digoxin effects. Monitor serum digoxin level.

Mitomycin: possibly increased frequency of bronchospasm and acute pulmonary reactions. Monitor patient carefully.

Nursing considerations

Assessment

- Review the patient's history for a condition that contraindicates the use of vincristine.
- Obtain a baseline assessment of CBC and differential, muscle tone and reflexes, bowel and bladder elimination patterns, nutritional status, vital signs, and patient's underlying cancerous state before initiating therapy.
- Be alert for common adverse reactions.
- Evaluate the patient's and family's knowledge about vincristine therapy.

Planning (Nursing Diagnoses)

Potential nursing diagnoses for the patient receiving vincristine include:

- Altered health maintenance related to ineffectiveness of vincristine to halt cancer growth.
- Body image disturbance related to alopecia and weight loss.
- Impaired physical mobility related to toxic effects of vincristine on neuromuscular system.
- Altered nutrition: less than body requirements, related to inability to ingest foods due to vincristine-induced nausea, vomiting, and stomatitis.

- Constipation related to adverse GI reactions to vincristine.
- Altered oral mucous membranes related to vincristine-induced stomatitis.
- Knowledge deficit related to vincristine therapy.

Implementation

Preparation and administration

— Read order and drug label carefully before administration of drug. Use extreme caution to avoid confusing vincristine with vinblastine.

— Follow institutional policy for handling hazardous materials to minimize risk to personnel.

— All vials contain 1 mg/ml solution and should be refrigerated. The 5-ml vials are for multiple-dose use only. Don't administer entire vial to a patient as a single dose.

— Check opened vials for discoloration and particles.

— Label all syringes containing vincristine "FOR I.V. USE ONLY." Never give vincristine I.M. or S.C.

— Check patient's I.D. band and ask patient's name before administration.

— Check I.V. site and patency of line before administration.

— Vincristine may be injected directly into a vein or into a running I.V. infusion slowly over 1 minute.

— Vincristine may also be added to 50 ml of dextrose 5% in water or 0.9% sodium chloride solution and infused over 15 minutes.

— Chart administration of drug and related observations.

Monitoring

— Monitor the effectiveness of therapy by regularly checking CBC and differential, and tumor size and rate of growth with appropriate studies.

— Monitor for presence of petechiae, epistaxis, melena, or hematuria if platelet count drops.

— Monitor respiratory status; be alert for life-threatening bronchospasm.

— Monitor the patient for adverse drug reactions.

— Monitor bowel sounds regularly; monitor bowel function.

— Monitor urine output, noting decreased or absent urine flow suggestive of urine retention.

— Monitor for depression of Achilles tendon reflex, numbness, tingling, footdrop or wristdrop, difficulty in walking alone, slapping gait, or difficulty walking on heels.

— Monitor for visual changes.

— Monitor weight, nutritional status, and hydration status if adverse GI reactions occur.

— Monitor electrolyte levels and urine output for evidence of SIADH.

— Monitor the I.V. site for extravasation.

— Monitor the patient for drug interactions.

— Monitor the patient's compliance with vincristine therapy.

— Periodically reevaluate the patient's and family's knowledge about vincristine.

Intervention

— Discontinue drug and notify doctor if serious adverse reactions occur.
— If infiltration of I.V. results in extravasation of vincristine, stop infusion, apply ice packs to the site every 2 hours for 24 hours, and notify doctor.
— Provide a private room and reverse isolation for patients with compromised immune systems.
— Institute safety precautions to minimize risk of injury due to impaired mobility and sensory alterations.
— Help patient to turn every 2 hours and provide skin care, especially over areas with bony prominences, as needed.
— Provide frequent mouth care. Use a soft toothbrush and mild mouthwash to avoid injury to oral mucous membranes.
— Give stool softeners or laxatives and encourage fluid intake to treat constipation.
— Provide range-of-motion (ROM) exercises to joints (unless medically contraindicated), progressing from passive to active as needed.
— Provide support while patient is walking.
— Encourage the patient to maintain adequate caloric intake; offer small, frequent meals and supplemental feedings.
— Administer an antiemetic as needed.
— Provide the patient emotional support and opportunities to express feelings about body image.
— Keep all members of the health care team informed of the patient's response to the drug.

Patient teaching

— Inform the patient and family about vincristine, including the dosage, frequency, action, and adverse reactions.
— Advise the patient that burning or stinging at I.V. site during administration is common.
— Advise the patient that alopecia may occur, but is usually reversible.
— Teach the patient and family protective measures to consume energy and prevent infections: getting adequate rest, avoiding fatigue, maintaining a balanced diet and adequate fluid intake, avoiding exposure to people with colds or other infections, and using support while walking to avoid risk of injury due to falls.
— Encourage adequate fluid intake to increase urine output and facilitate excretion of uric acid.
— Tell the patient to notify the nurse or doctor if adverse reactions develop or questions arise about vincristine therapy.

Evaluation

In the patient receiving vincristine, appropriate evaluation statements include:
• Patient demonstrates decrease in tumor size.
• Patient verbalizes feelings about changes in body image and demonstrates coping behaviors.

- Patient maintains muscle strength, ROM, and reflexes within normal range.
- Patient consumes adequate number of calories daily and demonstrates no weight loss.
- Patient maintains regular bowel patterns.
- Patient's oral mucous membranes remain normal throughout vincristine therapy.
- Patient and family state an understanding of vincristine therapy.

SELECTED MAJOR DRUGS: MISCELLANEOUS ANTINEOPLASTIC AGENTS

DRUG, INDICATIONS, AND DOSAGES	SPECIAL PRECAUTIONS
asparaginase (Elspar, Kidrolase†) *Acute lymphocytic leukemia (when used along with other drugs)* — **Adults and children:** 1,000 IU/kg I.V. daily for 10 days, injected over 30 minutes or by slow I.V. push; or 6,000 IU/m² I.M. at intervals specified in protocol. *Sole induction agent for acute lymphocytic leukemia* — **Adults and children:** 200 IU/kg I.V. daily for 28 days.	• Contraindicated in pancreatitis and known hypersensitivity to the drug unless desensitized. • Use cautiously in patients with preexisting hepatic dysfunction.
etoposide (VePesid) *Small-cell carcinoma of the lung, acute nonlymphocytic leukemia, lymphosarcoma, Hodgkin's disease, testicular carcinoma* — **Adults:** 45 to 75 mg/m² I.V. or P.O. daily for 3 to 5 days repeated q 3 to 5 weeks; or 200 to 250 mg/m² I.V. or P.O. weekly; or 125 to 140 mg/m² I.V. or P.O. daily three times a week q 5 weeks.	• Contraindicated in patients with known hypersensitivity to the drug. • Use cautiously in children and in pregnant or breast-feeding women because of the risk of carcinogenesis, mutagenesis, and impaired fertility.
mitoxantrone (Novantrone) *Combination initial therapy for acute nonlymphocytic leukemia (ANLL)* — **Adults:** 12 mg/m² I.V. daily on days 1 through 3, in combination with cytosine arabinoside 100 mg/m² daily on days 1 through 7. If a repeat course is necessary, mitoxantrone should be given on days 1 and 2 with cytosine arabinoside administered on days 1 through 5.	• Contraindicated in patients with known hypersensitivity to the drug. • Use cautiously in patients with prior exposure to anthracyclines or other cardiotoxic drugs.
vinblastine (Velban, Velbe‡) *Breast or testicular cancer, Hodgkin's and non-Hodgkin's lymphomas, choriocarcinoma, lymphosarcoma, neuroblastoma, mycosis fungoides, histiocytosis* — **Adults and children:** 0.1 mg/kg or 3.7 mg/m² I.V. weekly or q 2 weeks. May be increased to maximum dosage (adults) of 0.5 mg/kg or 18.5 mg/m² I.V. weekly according to response. Dosage should not be repeated if WBC count is less than 4,000/mm³.	• Contraindicated in severe leukopenia or bacterial infection. • Use cautiously in patients with jaundice or hepatic dysfunction.

SELF-TEST

1. Laureen Keller, age 62, is receiving vincristine for the treatment of Hodgkin's disease. An important part of the nurse's assessment of Mrs. Keller is:
   a. auscultating heart sounds.
   b. checking deep tendon reflexes.
   c. monitoring blood pressure.
   d. assessing skin turgor.

2. The correct route of administration of vincristine is:
   a. intrathecally.
   b. orally.
   c. intramuscularly.
   d. intravenously.

3. During treatment with vincristine, the nurse should monitor Mrs. Keller for:
   a. seizures.
   b. acute bronchospasm.
   c. hypotensive episodes.
   d. cardiac arrhythmias.

Check your answers on page 1074.

CHAPTER 72

IMMUNOSUPPRESSANTS

azathioprine ✦ cyclosporine ✦ levamisole hydrochloride
lymphocyte immune globulin (antithymocyte globulin [equine])
muromonab-CD3

OVERVIEW
• The immunosuppressants, a chemically distinct group, have common uses because of their ability to suppress the immune system. The idea of using drugs to suppress the body's immune response was considered nearly 100 years ago, but the actual development and use of such drugs is recent, coinciding with the development of organ transplantation. In combination with corticosteroids, the immunosuppressants have been used to prevent and treat organ transplant rejection. Immunosuppressants have also been used experimentally to treat many diseases that have an autoimmune origin.

MAJOR USES
• The immunosuppressants are mainly used with corticosteroids to prevent organ transplant rejection after kidney, liver, heart, lung, pancreas, or bone marrow transplantation.
• Azathioprine provides immunosuppression in kidney transplants and is used to treat severe, refractory rheumatoid arthritis.
• Cyclosporine provides prophylaxis of organ rejection in kidney, liver, bone marrow, and heart transplants.
• Levamisole is used for adjuvant treatment of Duke's stage C colon cancer (with fluorouracil) after surgical resection.
• Lymphocyte immune globulin and muromonab-CD3 are used to prevent acute renal allograft rejection.

MECHANISM OF ACTION
• Immunosuppressants block the normal immune response, suppress cell-mediated hypersensitivity, and alter the production of antibodies.
• Azathioprine inhibits purine synthesis.
• Cyclosporine inhibits the action of T cells.
• Muromonab-CD3 is an IgG antibody that reacts in the T-cell membrane with a molecule (CD3) needed for antigen recognition. This drug depletes the blood of CD3-positive T cells, which leads to restoration of allograft function and reverses transplant rejection.
• Levamisole appears to restore depressed immune function and may potentiate the actions of monocytes and macrophages and enhance T-cell responses.

GLOSSARY

Autoimmunity: abnormal reactivity of the body to its own tissue.
Immunosuppression: inhibition of the body's immune response to foreign substances.
T helper cell: cell released by T cells in response to an antigen that activates other T cells, B cells, and macrophages.
T suppressor cell: cell released by T cells in response to an antigen that prevents other T cells from producing an excessive immune response that might damage the body severely.

• Lymphocyte immune globulin inhibits cell-mediated immune responses by either altering T-cell function or eliminating antigen-reactive T cells.

ABSORPTION, DISTRIBUTION, METABOLISM, AND EXCRETION

Azathioprine is well absorbed from the GI tract; oral absorption of cyclosporine is variable and incomplete. Approximately 30% of a cyclosporine dose is absorbed, and increases with increased dosage and duration of treatment. Whenever possible, azathioprine and cyclosporine should be administered orally, but both agents may also be administered I.V. Lymphocyte immune globulin and muromonab-CD3 are only administered I.V.

The distribution of azathioprine is not fully understood, but the drug is 30% protein-bound. Cyclosporine and muromonab-CD3 are widely distributed throughout the body; cyclosporine is highly bound to lipoproteins. The distribution of lymphocyte immune globulin has not been completely determined.

Both cyclosporine and azathioprine are metabolized in the liver. Azathioprine is metabolized to the active metabolite mercaptopurine, which is excreted in the urine. Cyclosporine is excreted in the bile.

Muromonab-CD3 is consumed by the circulating T cells. Little is known of the metabolic fate of lymphocyte immune globulin except that it is excreted in the urine.

Levamisole is well absorbed from the GI tract. It is metabolized in the liver and excreted in the urine. The elimination half-life of the drug is about 16 hours.

ONSET AND DURATION

The onset of action of the immunosuppressants occurs soon after administration, but the full effect is not evident for several days. Azathioprine's full effect may take as long as 4 to 8 weeks. Because these drugs have long half-lives, once-daily administration is possible. The clinical effects of the immunosuppressants persist for a long time after the drugs are eliminated until the immune system can regenerate itself.

ADVERSE REACTIONS

The immunosuppressants have multisystem toxic effects and should be administered only under the close supervision of a clinical expert familiar with their effects. These drugs suppress the body's ability to mount an immune response.

Azathioprine produces adverse GI reactions—nausea, vomiting, diarrhea, and mouth ulcerations—as well as leukopenia or thrombocytopenia from bone marrow depression.

Cyclosporine causes significant nephrotoxicity, evidenced by increased BUN and serum creatinine levels; this complicates differentiation between organ rejection and toxicity reactions. Common adverse reactions to cyclosporine include hyperkalemia, hypertension, tremor, gingival hyperplasia, hirsutism, and GI complaints (nausea, vomiting, diarrhea, and abdominal distention). Occasionally, cyclosporine causes sinusitis, gynecomastia, hearing loss, tinnitus, hyperglycemia, muscle pain, and edema. Hepatotoxicity has been reported during the first month of high-dose treatment.

Lymphocyte immune globulin most consistently causes fever and chills. Approximately 20% of patients receiving lymphocyte immune globulin experience myelosuppression in the form of leukopenia or thrombocytopenia. Lymphocyte immune globulin can also cause nausea, vomiting, erythema, and pruritus; rarely, it can produce hypotension, hypertension, tachycardia, edema, pulmonary edema, and renal artery stenosis.

Muromonab-CD3 most commonly causes fever and chills, usually during the first 2 days of therapy. Other reactions include dyspnea, chest pain, nausea, vomiting, diarrhea, and, rarely, a potentially fatal pulmonary edema.

The most serious adverse reaction to levamisole therapy is agranulocytosis, which can be fatal. A flulike syndrome usually precedes the onset of agranulocytosis, but some patients are asymptomatic. Other reactions include nausea, vomiting, stomatitis, diarrhea, and anorexia.

PROTOTYPE: IMMUNOSUPPRESSANTS

CYCLOSPORINE
(CYCLOSPORIN)
(*sye′kloe spor een*)
Sandimmun‡, Sandimmune
Classification: immunosuppressant
Pregnancy risk category C

How supplied
ORAL SOLUTION: 100 mg/ml in 50-ml bottles
INJECTION: 50 mg/ml in 5-ml ampules

---

‡Available in Australia only

Indications and dosage
Prophylaxis of organ rejection in kidney, liver, bone marrow, and heart transplants
ADULTS AND CHILDREN: 15 mg/kg P.O. 4 to 12 hours before transplantation. Continue this daily dosage postoperatively for 1 to 2 weeks. Then, gradually reduce dosage by 5% a week to maintenance level of 5 to 10 mg/kg/day. Alternatively, administer 4 to 5 mg/kg I.V. 4 to 12 hours before transplantation. Postoperatively, repeat this dosage daily until the patient can tolerate oral solution.

Contraindications and precautions
Cyclosporine I.V. is contraindicated in patients with known hypersensitivity to cyclosporine or other components of the solution. Because of the possibility of hyperkalemia, cyclosporine should not be used concomitantly with potassium-sparing diuretics.

Adverse reactions
CNS: tremor, headache.
CV: hypertension.
GI: gum hyperplasia, nausea, vomiting, diarrhea, oral thrush.
GU: nephrotoxicity.
HEPATIC: hepatotoxicity.
SKIN: hirsutism, acne.
OTHER: sinusitis, flushing.

Interactions
Aminoglycosides, amphotericin B, co-trimoxazole, NSAIDs: increased risk of nephrotoxicity. Monitor renal function.
Azathioprine, corticosteroids, cyclophosphamide, verapamil: increased immunosuppression. Monitor for toxicity and infection.
Carbamazepine, isoniazid, phenobarbital, phenytoin, rifampin: possible decreased immunosuppressant effect. May need to increase cyclosporine dosage.
Ketoconazole, amphotericin B, cimetidine, diltiazem, erythromycin, imipenem-cilastatin, metoclopramide, prednisolone: may increase blood levels of cyclosporine. Monitor for increased toxicity.

Nursing considerations
Assessment
• Review the patient's history for a condition that contraindicates the use of cyclosporine.
• Obtain a baseline assessment of the status of the patient's immune response before initiating therapy.
• Be alert for common adverse reactions.
• Evaluate the patient's and family's knowledge about cyclosporine therapy.

Planning (Nursing Diagnoses)
Potential nursing diagnoses for the patient receiving cyclosporine include:
• Injury related to potential adverse drug reactions.

- Altered protection related to immunosuppression caused by long-term therapy.
- Knowledge deficit related to cyclosporine therapy.

Implementation

Preparation and administration

— Expect to administer cyclosporine concomitantly with adrenal corticosteroids.
— Measure oral doses carefully in an oral syringe or supplied pipette. To increase palatability, mix with whole milk, chocolate milk, or orange juice. Use a glass container to minimize adherence to container walls. Stir well and have the patient drink it immediately. Do not allow drug to stand before administering it to the patient.
— Dose should be given once daily in the morning. Administer the drug at the same time each day.
— Administer drug with meals if it causes nausea.
— If administering cyclosporine I.V., dilute the I.V. concentrate immediately before use. Dilute each milliliter of cyclosporine for I.V. infusion in 20 to 100 ml of 0.9% sodium chloride solution or dextrose 5% in water immediately before administration. Infuse over 2 to 6 hours. Ensure that the solution is free of particulate matter and discoloration. If it is not, discard it and start over.

Monitoring

— Monitor the effectiveness of cyclosporine therapy by regularly assessing for successful transplantation and no evidence of organ rejection.
— Monitor the patient for signs of infection.
— Monitor the patient for adverse drug reactions.
— Cyclosporine may cause nephrotoxicity. Monitor BUN and serum creatinine levels. Nephrotoxicity may develop 2 to 3 months after transplant surgery.
— Monitor liver function tests for hepatotoxicity, which usually occurs during the first month after an organ transplant.
— Absorption of oral cyclosporine can be erratic. Monitor cyclosporine blood levels at regular intervals.
— Monitor the patient for drug interactions.
— Monitor diagnostic test results. Cyclosporine therapy may alter the patient's CBC and differential and may increase serum lipid levels; elevated BUN and serum creatinine levels and elevated liver function test results may signal nephrotoxicity or hepatotoxicity.
— Periodically reevaluate the patient's and family's knowledge about cyclosporine.

Intervention

— Take infection control measures, such as maintaining reverse isolation.
— If the patient develops signs of infection, notify the doctor for appropriate therapy. Provide supportive care as appropriate.
— If the patient develops signs of organ or graft rejection, notify the doctor immediately.

— If the patient shows signs of nephrotoxicity (elevated BUN and serum creatinine levels), notify the doctor and expect to administer a reduced dosage of cyclosporine.

— If the patient shows signs of hepatotoxicity, notify the doctor.

— If the patient becomes noncompliant with therapy, discuss reasons why and suggest methods to help maintain compliance.

— Keep all members of the health care team informed of the patient's response to the drug.

Patient teaching

— Inform the patient and family about cyclosporine, including the dosage, frequency, action, and adverse reactions.

— Explain the disease process and rationale for therapy.

— Encourage compliance with therapy and follow-up visits.

— Stress to patient that therapy should not be stopped without doctor's approval.

— Tell the patient to swish and swallow nystatin four times daily to prevent thrush.

— If hirsutism occurs, tell the patient she may use a depilatory.

— Advise the patient that the oral solution can be made more palatable by diluting with room-temperature milk, chocolate milk, or orange juice.

— Advise the patient of the need for repeated laboratory tests while taking cyclosporine.

— Inform the patient that he will be more susceptible to infection and may develop lymphoma from immunosuppression. Advise the patient of precautions he must take to prevent infection—for example, avoiding crowds and exposure to people who have infections.

— Advise the patient to postpone any immunizations until after therapy is ended.

— Advise women to avoid breast-feeding while taking cyclosporine because it is excreted in human milk.

— Advise female patients to avoid conception during therapy and for up to 4 months afterward.

— Tell the patient to notify the nurse or doctor if adverse reactions develop or questions arise about cyclosporine therapy.

Evaluation

In the patient receiving cyclosporine, appropriate evaluation statements include:

• Patient develops no adverse reactions, and accepts organ or graft transplant.

• Patient does not develop infection.

• Patient and family state an understanding of cyclosporine therapy.

SELECTED MAJOR DRUGS: IMMUNOSUPPRESSANTS

DRUG, INDICATIONS, AND DOSAGES	SPECIAL PRECAUTIONS
azathioprine (Imuran, Thioprine‡) *Immunosuppression in renal transplants —* **Adults and children:** initially, 3 to 5 mg/kg P.O. or I.V. daily, usually beginning on the day of transplantation. Maintain at 1 to 3 mg/kg daily (dosage varies considerably according to patient response). *Treatment of severe, refractory rheumatoid arthritis —* **Adults:** initially, 1 mg/kg P.O. taken as a single dose or as two doses. If patient response is not satisfactory after 6 to 8 weeks, dosage may be increased by 0.5 mg/kg daily (up to a maximum of 2.5 mg/kg daily) at 4-week intervals.	• Contraindicated in patients with known hypersensitivity to the drug and in pregnant patients. • Use cautiously in patients with hepatic or renal dysfunction; in patients receiving cadaveric kidneys, who may have decreased elimination; and in rheumatoid arthritis patients previously treated with alkylating agents — cyclophosphamide, chlorambucil, or melphalan — who are at increased risk of neoplasia.
levamisole (Ergamisol) *Adjuvant treatment of Dukes' stage C colon cancer (with fluorouracil) after surgical resection —* **Adults:** 50 mg P.O. q 8 hours for 3 days. Therapy should begin no sooner than 7 days and no later than 30 days after surgery, providing that the patient is out of the hospital, ambulating, and maintaining normal oral nutrition; has well-healed wounds; and has recovered from any postoperative complications. Fluorouracil (450 mg/m² I.V. daily) is given for 5 days starting 21 to 34 days after surgery. Maintenance dosage is 50 mg P.O. q 8 hours for 3 days q 2 weeks for 1 year. Given in conjunction with fluorouracil maintenance therapy (450 mg/m² by rapid I.V. push once a week beginning 28 days after the initial 5-day course for 1 year).	• Contraindicated in patients with known hypersensitivity to the drug. • Use cautiously; closely monitor hematologic status because the drug is associated with sometimes-fatal agranulocytosis.
lymphocyte immune globulin (antithymocyte globulin [equine], ATG) (Atgam) *Prevention of acute renal allograft rejection —* **Adults and children:** 15 mg/kg I.V. daily for 14 days followed by alternate-day dosing for 14 days; the first dose should be given within 24 hours of transplantation. *Treatment of acute renal allograft rejection —* **Adults and children:** 10 to 15 mg/kg I.V. daily for 14 days followed by alternate-day dosing for 14 days. Therapy should be initiated when rejection is diagnosed.	• Contraindicated in patients who have had a severe systemic reaction during therapy with this drug or with another equine immunoglobulin G preparation. • Use cautiously in patients receiving additional immunosuppressive therapy (e.g., corticosteroids, azathioprine) because of the increased potential for infection.
muromonab-CD3 (Orthoclone OKT-3) *Treatment of acute allograft rejection in renal transplant patients —* **Adults:** 5 mg I.V. bolus once daily for 10 to 14 days. **Children:** 2.5 mg I.V. bolus once daily for 10 to 14 days.	• Contraindicated in patients with fluid overload, as evidenced by chest X-ray or weight gain greater than 3% within the week before treatment.

‡Available in Australia only

SELF-TEST

1. Lou Cherry, age 45, has just received a kidney transplant. To prevent transplant rejection, his doctor prescribed treatment with a corticosteroid and cyclosporine 15 mg/kg P.O. daily. Which of the following reactions should the nurse assess for?
   a. Hypotension
   b. Nephrotoxicity
   c. Cardiac arrhythmias
   d. Urticaria

2. The primary use of an immunosuppressant is to:
   a. treat infection.
   b. prevent infection.
   c. treat anaphylaxis.
   d. prevent organ transplant rejection.

3. When administering oral cyclosporine to Mr. Cherry, the nurse should:
   a. mix the drug with milk, chocolate milk, or orange juice, then give after drug stands for 15 minutes.
   b. mix the drug with milk, chocolate milk, or orange juice, then give immediately.
   c. administer the drug at bedtime.
   d. administer the drug at variable times during the day.

Check your answers on pages 1074 and 1075.

VACCINES AND TOXOIDS

Vaccines
bacille Calmette-Guérin (BCG) vaccine ✦ cholera vaccine
Haemophilus b (HIB) conjugate vaccines
hepatitis B vaccine, recombinant
influenza virus vaccines, trivalent types A & B
measles, mumps, and rubella virus (MMR) vaccine, live
measles (rubeola) and rubella virus vaccine, live attenuated
measles (rubeola) virus vaccine, live attenuated ✦ meningitis vaccine
mumps virus vaccine, live ✦ plague vaccine
pneumococcal vaccine, polyvalent ✦ poliovirus vaccine, inactivated (IPV)
poliovirus vaccine, live, oral, trivalent (TOPV)
rabies vaccine, human diploid cell (HDCV)
rubella and mumps virus vaccine, live
rubella virus vaccine, live attenuated ✦ typhoid vaccine
yellow fever vaccine

Toxoids
diphtheria and tetanus toxoids, adsorbed
diphtheria and tetanus toxoids and pertussis vaccine (DTP)
tetanus toxoid, adsorbed ✦ tetanus toxoid, fluid

OVERVIEW

- Vaccines and toxoids provide an acquired immunity (the power to overcome an infection) caused by the formation of antibodies in response to an antigen exposure.
- Vaccines are suspensions of killed or weakened (attenuated) microorganisms used to provide immunity against an infectious disease. Toxoids contain bacterial exotoxin that has lost its toxicity but can still stimulate the formation of antibodies to provide immunity.
- Immunization with vaccines and toxoids can prevent and sometimes eradicate commonly occurring communicable diseases.

MAJOR USES

- Vaccines and toxoids provide active immunity to bacteria or viruses and thus are used to prevent certain childhood viral diseases (such as measles, mumps, and rubella) and certain other infectious diseases (such as pneumococcal pneumonia and hepatitis B). They are also used to prevent diseases transmitted through injuries or animal bites (such as tetanus and rabies).

GLOSSARY

Acquired immunity: any form of immunity that is not innate and is obtained during life.

Active immunity: form of acquired immunity that results from the production of antibodies in the cells.

Poliomyelitis: infectious disease caused by one of the three polioviruses.

Tetanus: acute, potentially fatal infection of the CNS caused by the exotoxin tetanospasmin, which is elaborated by an anaerobic bacillus, *Clostridium tetani.*

Toxoid: toxin that has been treated with chemicals or with heat to weaken its toxic effect but that retains its antigenic power. It's given to produce immunity by stimulating the creation of antibodies.

Vaccine: suspension of attenuated or killed microorganisms administered to induce active immunity to infectious disease.

MECHANISM OF ACTION

• Both vaccines and toxoids initiate the formation of specific antibodies to the administered antigen by stimulating the body's antigen-antibody mechanism.

ABSORPTION, DISTRIBUTION, METABOLISM, AND EXCRETION

Most vaccines are administered parenterally because digestion after oral administration may destroy the antigenic component. Poliovirus vaccine is administered orally because the virus must multiply in the GI tract to provide immunity. The distribution, metabolism, and excretion of most vaccines have not been well characterized.

ONSET AND DURATION

The onset of active immunity is not immediate, and therefore these agents should not be used when acute immunity is needed. Instead they are used to prevent certain communicable diseases. Antibody production reaches immunity-producing levels in a few days and lasts for years.

ADVERSE REACTIONS

The adverse reactions associated with vaccines and toxoids are usually mild and range from local reactions at the site of injection to mild systemic reactions. Local reactions include erythema, induration, tenderness, and itching at the injection site. DPT immunization may sometimes also produce a sterile abscess.

Mild systemic reactions include fever in 50% of children after DPT immunization and a transient rash, lymphadenopathy, and fever after MMR immunization; reactions to HDCV immunization include headache, nausea, dizziness, and muscle and abdominal pain; influenza vaccines commonly produce fever, malaise, and myalgia within the first 24 hours, lasting up to 1 to 2 days after immunization. Because many vaccines are grown in egg culture, they can cause anaphylactic reactions in anyone allergic to eggs.

TOPV, a live virus vaccine, usually produces no predictable reactions; however, when given to immunocompromised patients, its administration has resulted in poliomyelitis.

Rarely, MMR has produced subacute sclerosing panencephalitis and blindness associated with optic neuritis.

Rubella vaccine has transmitted rubella, which presents a risk for birth defects when given to pregnant patients.

HIB immunization has been associated with unpredictable seizures, rashes, and sleep disturbances.

PROTOTYPE: VACCINES

POLIOVIRUS VACCINE, LIVE, ORAL, TRIVALENT
(poe lee oh vye′ russ)
Orimune
Classification: vaccine
Pregnancy risk category C

How supplied
ORAL VACCINE: mixture of three viruses (types 1, 2, and 3), grown in monkey kidney tissue culture, in 0.5-ml single-dose Dispettes

Indications and dosage
Poliovirus immunization
ADULTS: TOPV should not be given to persons ages 18 and over who have not received at least one prior dose of TOPV. Inactivated poliovirus vaccine (IPV) should be used if polio vaccination is indicated.
INFANTS: 0.5 ml at ages 2 months, 4 months, and 18 months. Optional dose may be given at 6 months.

Poliovirus immunization (primary series)
ADULTS, ADOLESCENTS, AND OLDER CHILDREN: two doses (0.5 ml each) administered 8 weeks apart; third dose 6 to 12 months after second dose.
INFANTS: 0.5 ml at ages 2 months, 4 months, and 18 months. Optional dose may be given at 6 months when substantial risk of exposure exists.
SUPPLEMENTARY: All children entering elementary school (ages 4 to 6) who have completed the primary series should receive a single follow-up dose of TOPV. Booster vaccination beyond elementary school is not routinely recommended.

Persons traveling to countries with endemic or epidemic poliomyelitis who previously completed a primary series should receive a single follow-up dose of TOPV. This vaccine should not be administered to infants under age 6 weeks.

Contraindications and precautions
Parenteral administration of live poliovirus vaccines is strongly contraindicated. Vaccine must not be administered to patients with immune deficiency or altered immune states, or to members of families with immunodeficient members. Vaccination should usually be avoided in pregnant women unless immediate protection against poliomyelitis is needed. Administration of the vaccine should be postponed or avoided during any acute illness, advanced debilitation, or persistent vomiting or diarrhea.

Adverse reactions
SYSTEMIC: paralytic poliomyelitis (extremely rare).

Interactions
Immune serum globulin, whole blood, plasma: antibodies in serum may interfere with immune response. If possible, don't use vaccine within 3 months of transfusion.

Nursing considerations
Assessment
- Review the patient's history for a condition that contraindicates the use of TOPV.
- Obtain a baseline assessment of the patient's polio immunization status before vaccination with TOPV.
- Be alert for the development of paralytic poliomyelitis, an extremely rare adverse reaction.
- Evaluate the patient's and family's knowledge about oral poliovirus vaccine therapy.

Planning (Nursing Diagnoses)
Potential nursing diagnoses for the patient receiving oral poliovirus vaccine include:
- Impaired physical mobility related to rare occurrence of paralytic poliomyelitis with poliovirus vaccine use.
- Noncompliance (immunization schedule) related to length of time between doses of poliovirus vaccine.
- Knowledge deficit related to oral poliovirus vaccine therapy.

Implementation
Preparation and administration
— Obtain a thorough history of allergies, especially to antibiotics, and of reactions to immunizations.
— Check the parents' immunization history when they bring in a child for the vaccine; this is an excellent time for parents to receive booster immunizations.
— Adults and immunocompromised persons who have not been vaccinated should receive subcutaneous IPV (IPOL, Poliovax) in three doses, given 1 month apart, before other household contacts are immunized with TOPV.

— Keep vaccine in freezer until used. The sorbitol content of the vaccine may permit the drug to remain fluid in temperatures as low as 7° F (−14° C). It may be refrigerated up to 30 days once thawed, if unopened. Opened vials may be refrigerated up to 7 days.

— Color change from pink to yellow has no effect on the efficacy of the vaccine as long as the vaccine remains clear. Yellow color results from storage at low temperatures.

— This vaccine is not for parenteral use. Dose may be administered directly or mixed with distilled water, chlorine-free tap water, simple syrup U.S.P., or milk. It also may be placed on bread, cake, or a sugar cube.

— Avoid administration of vaccine shortly after immune globulin unless such a procedure is unavoidable.

— Comply with the requirements of The National Childhood Vaccine Injury Act of 1986 (as amended in 1987): report the manufacturer and lot number of the administered vaccine in the vaccine recipient's permanent record, along with the date of administration and the name, address, and title of the person giving the vaccine. Also, report the occurrence of any of the events listed in the Vaccine Injury Table to a health department or to the FDA; these include paralytic poliomyelitis in a nonimmunodeficient recipient within 35 days of vaccination, or within 6 months in an immunodeficient patient; any vaccine-associated community case of paralytic poliomyelitis; or any acute complication or sequelae (including death) of these events.

Monitoring

— Monitor the effectiveness of TOPV therapy by determining that the patient does not develop polio.

— Monitor the patient for the rare development of paralytic poliomyelitis.

— Monitor the patient for drug interactions.

— Periodically reevaluate the patient's and family's knowledge about oral poliovirus vaccine.

Intervention

— If the patient develops signs and symptoms of paralytic poliomyelitis, notify the doctor immediately.

— If the patient does not comply with the immunization schedule, discuss reasons why and methods the patient or appropriate family member may use to maintain compliance.

— Keep all members of the health care team informed of the patient's response to the drug.

Patient teaching

— Inform the patient and family about TOPV, including the dosage, frequency, action, and adverse reactions.

— Explain the disease process and rationale for therapy.

— Advise the patient that the risk of vaccine-associated paralysis is extremely small for those receiving the vaccine, susceptible family members, and other close contacts (about 1 case per 2.6 million doses given).

— Advise the immunized patient to avoid close contact with all persons with altered immune status for at least 6 to 8 weeks.
— Tell the patient to notify the nurse or doctor if adverse reactions develop or questions arise about poliovirus vaccine.

Evaluation
In the patient receiving oral poliovirus vaccine, appropriate evaluation statements include:
• Patient maintains normal physical mobility.
• Patient remains compliant with immunization schedule.
• Patient and family state an understanding of oral poliovirus vaccine therapy.

PROTOTYPE: TOXOIDS

TETANUS TOXOID, ADSORBED
(tet' ah nus tok' soid)

TETANUS TOXOID, FLUID
Classification: toxoid
Pregnancy risk category C

How supplied
adsorbed
INJECTION: 5 to 10 Lf units of inactivated tetanus/0.5-ml dose, in 0.5-ml syringes and 5-ml vials
fluid
INJECTION: 4 to 5 Lf units of inactivated tetanus/0.5-ml dose, in 0.5-ml syringes and 7.5-ml vials

Indications and dosage
Primary immunization
ADULTS AND CHILDREN: 0.5 ml adsorbed formulation I.M. 4 to 6 weeks apart for two doses, then a third dose 1 year after the second dose. Booster dosage is 0.5 ml I.M. q 10 years. Alternatively, give 0.5 ml fluid formulation I.M. or S.C. 4 to 8 weeks apart for three doses, then a fourth dose 6 to 12 months after the third dose. Booster dosage is 0.5 ml I.M. or S.C. q 10 years.

Tetanus prophylaxis in wound management
ADULTS AND CHILDREN: in patients with history of primary immunization, booster less than 10 years ago, and a clean wound—none required; in patients with history of primary immunization, booster more than 10 years ago, and a clean wound—0.5 ml adsorbed formulation I.M.; in patients with history of primary immunization or booster more than 5 years ago, and a dirty (tetanus-prone) wound—booster dose (0.5 ml) adsorbed formulation I.M.; in patients with incomplete or unknown immunization history—0.5 ml adsorbed formulation I.M., followed by complete primary

immunization; in patients with no history of primary immunization—initiate primary immunization.

Concurrent use of tetanus immune globulin depends on primary immunization history, the type of wound, and care received for the wound.

Contraindications and precautions

Tetanus toxoid is contraindicated in patients with known hypersensitivity to any component of the vaccine, including thimerosal, in those who experienced any adverse CNS reactions to the product, and during any acute febrile illness or infection. Routine immunization should be deferred during an outbreak of poliomyelitis, except in patients with an injury that increases the risk of tetanus.

Tetanus toxoid should not be given more frequently than every 10 years to a person who experienced Arthus-type hypersensitivity or fever over 39.4° C (103° F) after a previous dose of tetanus toxoid; it should not be administered by I.M. injection to patients with thrombocytopenia or any coagulation disorder, unless the potential benefit clearly outweighs the risk.

Patients with impaired immune responsiveness due to immunosuppressants, HIV infection, or other causes may show reduced antibody response to immunization. Administration of the toxoid may be deferred in patients receiving immunosuppressive therapy.

Adverse reactions

CNS: **seizures; encephalopathy;** neuropathies, including Guillain-Barré syndrome.
CV: tachycardia, hypotension.
SYSTEMIC: slight fever, chills, malaise, aches and pains, flushing, urticaria, pruritus, **anaphylaxis.**
LOCAL: *erythema, tenderness,* induration, nodule or sterile abscess formation, subcutaneous atrophy.
OTHER: erythema multiforme or other rash, arthralgias.

Interactions

Chloramphenicol, corticosteroids, immunosuppressants: concomitant use may impair the immune response to tetanus toxoid. Avoid elective immunization under these circumstances.

Nursing considerations

Assessment

- Review the patient's history for a condition that contraindicates the use of tetanus toxoid.
- Obtain a baseline assessment of the patient's tetanus immunization status and wound history before initiating tetanus toxoid therapy.
- Be alert for common adverse reactions.
- Evaluate the patient's and family's knowledge about tetanus toxoid therapy.

Planning (Nursing Diagnoses)

Potential nursing diagnoses for the patient receiving tetanus toxoid include:

- Potential for injury related to inadequate dosage regimen.
- Pain related to I.M. injection.
- Knowledge deficit related to tetanus toxoid therapy.

Implementation

Preparation and administration

— Before administering this toxoid, inform the parent, guardian, or adult patient of the benefits and risks of immunization against tetanus.

— Obtain a thorough history of allergies and reactions to immunizations. Determine tetanus immunization status and date of last tetanus immunization.

— Keep epinephrine solution 1:1,000 available to treat allergic reactions.

— Do not confuse this drug with tetanus immune globulin. These toxoids are used to prevent, not treat, tetanus infections.

— Store at 2° to 8° C (36° to 46° F). Do not freeze.

— Preferably, tetanus immunization should be completed and maintained using multiple-antigen preparations appropriate for the patient's age, such as DTP, DT, or Td.

— Shake vial vigorously to ensure a uniform suspension before withdrawing the dose. Inspect for particulate matter and discoloration before administering.

— The preferred I.M. injection site is the deltoid or midlateral thigh in adults and children and the midlateral thigh in infants.

— Comply with the requirements of The National Childhood Vaccine Injury Act of 1986 (as amended in 1987): report the manufacturer and lot number of the administered toxoid in the toxoid recipient's permanent record, along with the date of administration and the name, address, and title of the person giving the toxoid. Also, report the occurrence of any of the events listed in the Vaccine Injury Table to a health department or to the FDA; these include anaphylaxis or anaphylactic shock within 24 hours, encephalopathy or encephalitis within 7 days, residual seizure disorder, any acute complication or sequelae (including death) of those events, or any other event that would contraindicate giving further doses of the toxoid.

Monitoring

— Monitor the effectiveness of tetanus toxoid therapy by assessing for prevention of tetanus.

— Monitor the patient for adverse drug reactions.

— Monitor for pain or tenderness at the injection site.

— Monitor the patient for drug interactions.

Intervention

— If the patient develops pain or tenderness at the injection site, notify the doctor and obtain an order for acetaminophen.

— If the patient does not comply with the immunization schedule, discuss reasons why and suggest methods patient may use to maintain compliance—for example, marking on a calendar the date of the next scheduled immunization.

—If the patient develops an adverse reaction, notify the doctor for appropriate treatment and provide supportive care as appropriate.

—Keep all members of the health care team informed of the patient's response to the drug.

Patient teaching

—Inform the patient and family about tetanus toxoid, including the dosage, frequency, action, and adverse reactions.

—Explain the disease process and rationale for therapy.

—Tell the patient to expect discomfort at the injection site and a nodule that may develop there and persist for several weeks after immunization. Patient also may develop fever, general malaise, or body aches and pains. Recommend acetaminophen to alleviate these effects.

—Advise the patient not to use hot or cold compresses at the injection site because this may increase the severity of the local reaction.

—Tell the patient that immunization requires a series of injections. Stress the importance of keeping scheduled appointments for subsequent doses.

—Tell the patient to notify the nurse or doctor if adverse reactions develop or questions arise about tetanus toxoid therapy.

Evaluation

In the patient receiving tetanus toxoid, appropriate evaluation statements include:

• Patient does not develop tetanus.

• Patient has no pain at injection site, or pain has been alleviated.

• Patient and family state an understanding of tetanus toxoid therapy.

SELECTED MAJOR DRUGS: VACCINES AND TOXOIDS

DRUG, INDICATIONS, AND DOSAGES	SPECIAL PRECAUTIONS
Vaccines	
BCG vaccine *Tuberculosis exposure, cancer immunotherapy—* **Adults and children age 3 months and over:** 0.1 ml (intradermal) or 0.2 to 0.3 ml (percutaneous) applied to cleansed area of skin followed by application of multiple-puncture disk. **Children under age 3 months:** 0.05 ml (intradermal).	• Contraindicated in hypogammaglobulinemia, burns, after positive tuberculin reaction (when meant for use as immunoprophylactic after exposure to tuberculosis), in immunosuppressed patients, after fresh smallpox vaccination, and in patients receiving corticosteroid therapy. • Use cautiously in patients with chronic skin disease. Inject in area of healthy skin only.

(continued)

SELECTED MAJOR DRUGS: VACCINES AND TOXOIDS *continued*

DRUG, INDICATIONS, AND DOSAGES	SPECIAL PRECAUTIONS

Vaccines *(continued)*

cholera vaccine
Primary immunization—
Adults and children over age 10: two doses (0.5 ml each) I.M. or 1 ml S.C., 1 week to 1 month apart, before traveling in cholera area. Booster is 0.5 ml q 6 months as long as protection is needed.
Children ages 5 to 10: 0.3 ml I.M. or S.C.
Children ages 6 months to 4 years: 0.2 ml I.M. or S.C. Boosters of same dose should be given q 6 months as long as protection is needed.

• Contraindicated in patients receiving corticosteroid therapy and in immunosuppressed patients.
• Defer immunization in acute illness.

hepatitis B vaccine (Engerix-B, Recombivax HB)
Immunization against infection from all known subtypes of hepatitis B, primary preexposure prophylaxis against hepatitis B, or postexposure prophylaxis (when given with hepatitis B immune globulin)—
Engerix-B
Adults and children over age 10: initially, 20 mcg I.M. repeated in 30 days, with a third dose 6 months after the initial dose.
Neonates and children up to age 10: initially, 10 mcg pediatric formulation I.M., repeated in 30 days, with a third dose 6 months after the initial dose.
Adults undergoing dialysis or receiving immunosuppressant therapy: initially, 40 mcg I.M. (divided into two doses and administered at different sites). Repeat in 30 days, with a final dose 6 months after the initial dose.
Note: Certain populations (neonates born to infected mothers, persons recently exposed to the virus, and travelers to high-risk areas) may receive the vaccine on an abbreviated schedule, with the initial dose followed by a second dose in 1 month, and the third dose after 2 months. For prolonged maintenance of protective antibody titers, a booster dose is recommended 12 months after the initial dose.
Recombivax HB
Adults: initially, 10 mcg I.M., repeated in 30 days, with a third dose 6 months after the initial dose.
Children ages 11 to 19: initially, 5 mcg pediatric formulation I.M., repeated in 30 days, with a third dose 6 months after the initial dose.
Neonates (born to HB_sAg-negative mothers) and children under age 11: initially, 2.5 mcg pediatric formulation I.M., repeated in 30 days, with a third dose 6 months after the initial dose.
Neonates born to HB_sAg-positive mothers: initially, 5 mcg pediatric formulation I.M., repeated in 30 days, with a third dose 6 months after the initial dose.
Adults undergoing dialysis or receiving immunosuppressant therapy: initially, 40 mcg dialysis formulation I.M., repeated in 30 days, with a final dose 6 months after the initial dose.

• Contraindicated in patients with known hypersensitivity to yeast or to any other component of the vaccine.
• Use cautiously in any patient with serious, active infection; in those with compromised cardiac or pulmonary status; and in those for whom a febrile or systemic reaction could pose a serious risk.

SELECTED MAJOR DRUGS: VACCINES AND TOXOIDS *continued*

DRUG, INDICATIONS, AND DOSAGES	SPECIAL PRECAUTIONS

Vaccines *(continued)*

Haemophilus b conjugate vaccine (ProHIBIT, Pedvax HIB, HibTITER) *Immunization against HIB infection—* Dosage varies with product used and age of child. Optimal schedules are as follows: *ProHIBIT* **Children ages 15 months to 5 years:** 0.5 ml I.M. *Pedvax HIB* **Children age 2 months:** 0.5 ml I.M. Repeat at ages 4 months and 12 months. *HibTITER* **Children age 2 months:** 0.5 ml I.M. Repeat at ages 4 months, 6 months, and 15 months.	• Contraindicated in immunosuppressed patients. Defer immunization in acute illness. • Use cautiously during pregnancy because of the risk of carcinogenesis, mutagenesis, and impairment of fertility. • Ensure that the injection does not enter a blood vessel.
influenza virus; vaccine, trivalent types A and B (whole and split virus; Flu-Imune, Fluogon, Fluzone) *Influenza prophylaxis—* **Adults and children over age 12:** 0.5 ml whole or split virus I.M. Only one dose is required. **Children ages 3 to 12:** 0.5 ml split virus I.M. Repeat dose in 4 weeks unless child has been previously vaccinated. **Children ages 6 to 35 months:** 0.25 ml split virus I.M. Repeat dose in 4 weeks unless child has been previously vaccinated.	• Contraindicated in patients with known hypersensitivity to eggs. Defer immunization in acute respiratory or other active infection. • Use cautiously in patients with a history of sulfite allergy.
measles, mumps, and rubella virus vaccine, live (MMR II) *Routine immunization—* **Children:** 1 vial S.C. A two-dose schedule is recommended, with the first dose given at age 15 months (age 12 months in high-risk areas) and the second dose given when the child enters school (kindergarten or first grade). *Measles outbreak control—* **Children:** if cases are occurring in children under age 1, immunize children as young as age 6 months. All students and their siblings should be revaccinated if they are without documentation of measles immunity. **Adults:** school personnel born in or after 1957 should be revaccinated if they are without proof of measles immunity. If the outbreak is in a medical facility, all workers born in or after 1957 should be revaccinated if they are without proof of immunity. Revaccination should be considered for persons born before 1957 as well.	• Contraindicated in immunosuppressed patients; in those with cancer, blood dyscrasias, gamma globulin disorders, fever, or active, untreated tuberculosis; and in those undergoing corticosteroid or radiation therapy. • Use cautiously in patients with known hypersensitivity to neomycin, chickens, ducks, eggs, or feathers. • Defer immunization in acute illness.
measles (rubeola) virus vaccine, live attenuated (Attenuvax) *Immunization—* **Children ages 15 months to puberty:** 1 vial (1,000 units) S.C.	• Contraindicated in immunosuppressed patients; in those with cancer, blood dyscrasias, gamma globulin disorders, fever, or active, untreated tuberculo-

(continued)

SELECTED MAJOR DRUGS: VACCINES AND TOXOIDS *continued*

DRUG, INDICATIONS, AND DOSAGES	SPECIAL PRECAUTIONS

Vaccines *(continued)*

measles virus vaccine *(continued)*

sis; and during corticosteroid or radiation therapy.
• Use cautiously in patients with known hypersensitivity to neomycin, chickens, ducks, eggs, or feathers; a history of febrile seizures; or cerebral injury.
• Defer immunization in acute illness.

meningitis vaccine (Menomune-A/C)
Meningococcal meningitis prophylaxis—
Adults and children over age 2: 0.5 ml S.C.

• Contraindicated in immunosuppressed patients.
• Defer immunization in acute illness.

mumps virus vaccine, live
Immunization—
Adults and children over age 1: 1 vial (5,000 units) S.C.

• Contraindicated in immunosuppressed patients; in those with cancer, blood dyscrasias, gamma globulin disorders, or active, untreated tuberculosis; and during corticosteroid or radiation therapy; and in pregnant women.
• Use cautiously in patients with known hypersensitivity to neomycin, chickens, ducks, eggs, or feathers.
• Defer immunization in acute or febrile illness and for 3 months after transfusions or treatment with immune serum globulin.

plague vaccine
Primary immunization and booster—
Adults and children over age 10: 1 ml I.M. followed by 0.2 ml in 4 weeks, then 0.2 ml 6 months after the first dose. Booster dosage is 0.1 to 0.2 ml q 6 months while in plague area.
Children ages 5 to 10: ⅗ adult primary or booster dose.
Children ages 1 to 4: ⅖ adult primary or booster dose.
Children under age 1: ⅕ adult primary or booster dose.

• Contraindicated in immunosuppressed patients.
• Defer immunization in respiratory infection.
• Use cautiously in children, during pregnancy, and in patients at risk of drug interactions.

pneumococcal vaccine, polyvalent (Pneumovax 23)
Pneumococcal immunization—
Adults and children over age 2: 0.5 mg I.M. or S.C. Not recommended for children under age 2.

• Contraindicated in patients with known hypersensitivity to any component of the vaccine and in revaccination of adults. In patients with Hodgkin's dis-

SELECTED MAJOR DRUGS: VACCINES AND TOXOIDS *continued*

DRUG, INDICATIONS, AND DOSAGES	SPECIAL PRECAUTIONS
Vaccines *(continued)*	
pneumococcal vaccine, polyvalent *(continued)*	ease immunized less than 7 to 10 days before immunosuppressive therapy, postimmunization antibody levels have been found to be below preimmunization levels; therefore, such use is contraindicated. • Also contraindicated in patients with Hodgkin's disease who have received extensive chemotherapy or nodal irradiation because they have impaired antibody response to a 12-valent pneumococcal vaccine. • Use cautiously in patients with severely compromised cardiac or pulmonary function, in whom a systemic reaction would pose a significant risk.
rabies vaccine, human diploid cell (HDCV; Imovax) *Postexposure antirabies immunization—* **Adults and children:** five doses (1 ml each) I.M. Give first dose as soon as possible after exposure; give an additional dose on days 3, 7, 14, and 28 after first dose. *Preexposure antirabies prophylaxis for persons in high-risk groups—* **Adults and children:** three doses (1 ml each) I.M. Give first dose on the first day of therapy, second dose on day 7, and third dose on either day 21 or 28. Alternatively, give 0.1 ml intradermally on the same dosage schedule.	• Postpone immunization for preexposure prophylaxis in patients with febrile illness. • Use cautiously in patients with known hypersensitivity to neomycin or other components of the vaccine.
rubella and mumps virus vaccine, live (Biavax II) *Measles and mumps immunization—* **Adults and children over age 1:** 1 vial (1,000 units) S.C.	• Contraindicated in immunosuppressed patients; in those with cancer, blood dyscrasias, gamma globulin disorders, fever, or active, untreated tuberculosis; in those undergoing corticosteroid or radiation therapy; and in pregnant women. • Use with caution in patients with known hypersensitivity to neomycin, chickens, ducks, eggs, or feathers. • Defer immunization in acute illness and after administration of immune serum globulin, blood, or plasma.

(continued)

SELECTED MAJOR DRUGS: VACCINES AND TOXOIDS *continued*

DRUG, INDICATIONS, AND DOSAGES	SPECIAL PRECAUTIONS
Vaccines *(continued)*	
rubella virus vaccine, live attenuated (Meruvax II) *Measles immunization—* **Adults and children over age 1:** 1 vial (1,000 units) S.C.	• Contraindicated in immunosuppressed patients; in those with cancer, blood dyscrasias, gamma globulin disorders, fever, or active, untreated tuberculosis; or those undergoing corticosteroid or radiation therapy. • Use cautiously in patients with known hypersensitivity to neomycin, chickens, ducks, eggs, or feathers. • Defer immunization in acute illness and after administration of human immune serum globulin, blood, or plasma.
typhoid vaccine *Primary immunization—* **Adults and children over age 10:** 0.5 ml S.C., repeated in 4 weeks. Booster dosage is 0.5 ml S.C. q 3 years. **Children ages 6 months to 10 years:** 0.25 ml S.C., repeated in 4 weeks. Booster dosage is 0.25 ml S.C. q 3 years.	• Contraindicated in patients receiving corticosteroid therapy. • Defer immunization in acute illness.
yellow fever vaccine (YF Vax) *Primary immunization—* **Adults and children over age 6 months:** 0.5 mg deep S.C.; booster dosage is 0.5 mg S.C. q 10 years.	• Contraindicated in patients with known hypersensitivity to chickens or eggs, in those with gamma globulin deficiency or cancer, in immunosuppressed patients, in those undergoing corticosteroid or radiation therapy, and in pregnant women. Also contraindicated in infants under age 9 months except in high-risk areas.
Toxoids	
diphtheria and tetanus toxoids, adsorbed (DT) *Primary immunization—* **Adults and children over age 7:** use adult strength; 0.5 ml I.M. 4 to 6 weeks apart for two doses, with a third dose 1 year later. Booster dosage is 0.5 ml I.M. q 10 years. **Children ages 1 to 6:** use pediatric strength; 0.5 ml I.M. at least 4 weeks apart for two doses. Give booster dosage 6 to 12 months after the second injection. If the final immunizing dose is given after the 7th birthday, use the adult strength. **Infants ages 6 weeks to 1 year:** use pediatric strength; 0.5 ml I.M. at least 4 weeks apart for three doses. Give booster dose 6 to 12 months after third injection.	• Contraindicated in immunosuppressed patients and in those undergoing radiation or corticosteroid therapy. • Defer immunization in respiratory illness or polio outbreaks, or in acute illness except in emergency. • Use single antigen during polio outbreaks. In children under age 6, use only when DPT is contraindicated because of pertussis component.

SELECTED MAJOR DRUGS: VACCINES AND TOXOIDS *continued*

DRUG, INDICATIONS, AND DOSAGES	SPECIAL PRECAUTIONS
Toxoids *(continued)*	
diphtheria, tetanus toxoids and pertussis vaccine (DPT) *Primary immunization—* **Children ages 6 weeks to 6 years:** 0.5 ml I.M. 2 months apart for three doses, with a fourth dose 1 year later. Booster dosage is 0.5 ml I.M. when starting school. Not advised for adults or children over age 6.	• Contraindicated in patients receiving corticosteroids, in immunosuppressed patients, and in those with a history of seizures. • Defer immunization in acute febrile illness. • Children with preexisting neurologic disorders should not receive pertussis component. Children with previous adverse CNS reactions to any DPT injection shouldn't receive pertussis component in any succeeding injection. Diphtheria and tetanus toxoids should be given instead.
diphtheria toxoid, adsorbed, pediatric (DT) *Diphtheria immunization—* **Children under age 6:** 0.5 ml I.M. 6 to 8 weeks apart for two doses, with a third dose 1 year later. Booster dosage is 0.5 ml I.M. at 5- to 10-year intervals. Not advised for adults or for children over age 6; instead, use adult strength of diphtheria toxoid (usually available as diphtheria and tetanus toxoids, adsorbed).	• Contraindicated in patients with known hypersensitivity to any component of the product, including thimerosal; and in patients with adverse CNS reactions to it. • Defer immunization during any febrile illness or acute infection, and in pregnant women.

SELF-TEST

1. Beverly Batts brought her infant to the well-baby clinic. Her pediatrician explained that the infant should receive the poliovirus vaccine. Vaccines and toxoids provide:
   a. acquired immunity.
   b. passive immunity.
   c. negative immunity.
   d. positive immunity.

2. By which of the following routes should poliovirus vaccine be administered?
   a. Oral only
   b. Oral or subcutaneous injection
   c. Oral or intramuscular injection
   d. Subcutaneous injection or intramuscular injection

3. Herbert Walker, after stepping on a rusty nail, came to the emergency department for a tetanus toxoid injection. The preferred site of tetanus toxoid administration for an adult is:
   a. deltoid only.
   b. midlateral thigh only.
   c. deltoid or midlateral thigh.
   d. gluteus medius only.

Check your answers on page 1075.

CHAPTER 74

ANTITOXINS AND ANTIVENINS

Antitoxins
botulism antitoxin, bivalent equine ✦ diphtheria antitoxin, equine
tetanus antitoxin (TAT), equine

Antivenins
black widow spider antivenin ✦ crotaline (rattlesnake) antivenin, polyvalent
Micrurus fulvius (coral snake) antivenin

OVERVIEW
• Antitoxins and antivenins combine with and neutralize toxins produced
by plants or microorganisms and venoms produced by animals. These
preparations are made from immunoglobulins isolated from the blood of
horses inoculated with the specific toxins or venoms.

MAJOR USES
• Antitoxins are used to prevent and treat bacterial infections: botulism
(botulism antitoxin), diphtheria (diphtheria antitoxin), and tetanus (tetanus antitoxin).
• Antivenins are used to treat the symptoms of bites by the black widow
spider (black widow spider antivenin), rattlesnake (crotaline antivenin),
and coral snake (*M. fulvius* antivenin).

MECHANISM OF ACTION
• Antitoxins and antivenins provide passive immunity (immunity conferred by the administration of preformed antibodies).
• These agents bind to and neutralize the specific toxins and venoms for
which they are administered.

ABSORPTION, DISTRIBUTION, METABOLISM, AND EXCRETION
Not applicable.

ONSET AND DURATION
The onset of action of antitoxins and antivenins is immediate. The duration
of the resulting immunity is unknown.

GLOSSARY

Antitoxin: subgroup of antisera usually prepared from the serum of horses immunized against a particular toxin-producing organism.
Antivenin: suspension of venom-neutralizing antibodies prepared from the serum of immunized horses.
Toxin: poison, usually one produced by or occurring in a plant or microorganism.
Venom: toxic fluid substance secreted by some snakes, arthropods, and other animals and transmitted by their stings or bites.

ADVERSE REACTIONS

Because all antitoxins and antivenins are derived from nonhuman proteins, anaphylactic reactions are a possibility and must be watched for. These products can also cause serum sickness reactions evidenced by urticaria, pruritus, malaise, and arthralgia, which can occur as long as 5 to 13 days after administration.

PROTOTYPE: ANTITOXINS

TETANUS ANTITOXIN (TAT), EQUINE

(tet' ah nus an ti tok' sin)
Classification: antitoxin
Pregnancy risk category D

How supplied
INJECTION: not less than 400 units/ml in 1,500-unit and 20,000-unit vials

Indications and dosage
Tetanus prophylaxis
PATIENTS OVER 30 KG: 3,000 to 5,000 units I.M. or S.C.
PATIENTS UNDER 30 KG: 1,500 to 3,000 units I.M. or S.C.

Tetanus treatment
ADULTS AND CHILDREN: 10,000 to 20,000 units injected into wound. Give additional 40,000 to 100,000 units I.V. Start tetanus toxoid at same time but at different site and with a different syringe.

Contraindications and precautions
Use with caution in patients with known hypersensitivity to equine preparations. Sensitivity testing should be performed in all persons, regardless of their history of exposure to the antitoxin.

Adverse reactions

SYSTEMIC: joint pain, *hypersensitivity*, **anaphylaxis**, *serum sickness*, skin rash.

LOCAL: *pain,* numbness.

Interactions

None significant.

Nursing considerations

Assessment

- Review the patient's history for a condition that contraindicates the use of tetanus antitoxin.
- Obtain a baseline assessment of the patient's wound and tetanus prophylaxis history before administering tetanus antitoxin.
- Be alert for serious adverse reactions.
- Evaluate the patient's and family's knowledge about tetanus antitoxin therapy.

Planning (Nursing Diagnoses)

Potential nursing diagnoses for the patient receiving tetanus antitoxin include:

- Injury related to potential inadequate tetanus antitoxin dosage.
- Altered health status related to adverse reactions to tetanus antitoxin.
- Knowledge deficit related to tetanus antitoxin.

Implementation

Preparation and administration

—Test for sensitivity before giving. Give 0.1 ml as a 1:1,000 dilution in 0.9% sodium chloride solution intradermally.

—Use only when tetanus immune globulin (human) is not available.

—Obtain an accurate patient history of allergies, especially to horses, and of reaction to immunization.

—Give preventive dose to those who have had two or fewer injections of tetanus toxoid and who have tetanus-prone injuries more than 24 hours old.

Monitoring

—Monitor the effectiveness of tetanus antitoxin therapy by assessing the patient for signs of tetanus. If given to treat tetanus, monitor for signs of improvement.

—Monitor the patient for adverse drug reactions.

—Monitor for pain at the injection or infusion site.

—Periodically reevaluate the patient's and family's knowledge about tetanus antitoxin.

Intervention

—If the patient develops signs and symptoms of anaphylaxis, notify the doctor immediately for appropriate treatment. Be prepared to administer epinephrine and provide supportive care, as appropriate.

—If the patient develops other adverse reactions, notify the doctor for appropriate treatment. Provide supportive care, as appropriate.

—Keep all members of the health care team informed of the patient's response to the drug.

Patient teaching

—Inform the patient and family about tetanus antitoxin, including the dosage, frequency, action, and adverse reactions.

—Explain the disease process and rationale for therapy.

—Advise the patient that he may experience pain at injection site.

—Advise mothers of infants to discontinue breast-feeding temporarily until the effects of the toxin subside; patients should also discontinue breast-feeding if symptoms of serum sickness develop.

—Tell the patient to notify the nurse or doctor if adverse reactions develop or questions arise about tetanus antitoxin therapy.

Evaluation

In the patient receiving tetanus antitoxin, appropriate evaluation statements include:

• Patient does not develop tetanus.

• Patient experiences no adverse reactions.

• Patient and family state an understanding of tetanus antitoxin therapy.

PROTOTYPE: ANTIVENINS

BLACK WIDOW SPIDER ANTIVENIN

(blak' wid'oh spied' er ant ee ven' in)

Antivenin (Latrodectus mactans)

Classification: antivenin

Pregnancy risk category C

How supplied

INJECTION: combination package—1 vial of antivenin (6,000 units/vial), one 2.5-ml vial of diluent (sterile water for injection), and one 1-ml vial of normal horse serum (1:10 dilution) for sensitivity testing

Indications and dosage

Black widow spider bite

ADULTS AND CHILDREN: 2.5 ml (1 vial) I.M. in anterolateral thigh or deltoid muscle. If symptoms do not subside in 1 to 3 hours, dose may be repeated. Antivenin also may be given I.V. in 10 to 50 ml of 0.9% sodium chloride solution over 15 minutes (the preferred route for severe cases, such as patients in shock or those under age 12).

Contraindications and precautions

Before treatment with any product prepared from horse serum, carefully review the patient's history, emphasizing prior exposure to horse serum and any allergies. Serious illness and even death could follow the use of horse serum in a sensitive patient.

Adverse reactions

SYSTEMIC: hypersensitivity, **anaphylaxis**, serum sickness.
LOCAL: *pain*, erythema, urticaria.

Interactions

None significant.

Nursing considerations

Assessment

• Review the patient's history for a condition that contraindicates the use of black widow spider antivenin.
• Obtain a baseline assessment of the patient's black widow spider bite before administering black widow spider antivenin.
• Be alert for serious adverse reactions.
• Evaluate the patient's and family's knowledge about black widow spider antivenin therapy.

Planning (Nursing Diagnoses)

Potential nursing diagnoses for the patient receiving black widow spider antivenin include:
• Injury related to potential ineffectiveness of black widow spider antivenin.
• Altered health maintenance related to adverse reactions.
• Knowledge deficit related to black widow spider antivenin therapy.

Implementation

Preparation and administration

— Immobilize the patient; splint the bitten limb to prevent spread of venom.
— Obtain an accurate patient history of allergies, especially to horses, and of reactions to immunization.
— Earliest possible use of antivenin is recommended for best results.
— Test the patient for sensitivity (against a control of 0.9% sodium chloride solution in opposing extremity) before giving antivenin. Give 0.02 ml of the 1:10 dilution of horse serum into (not under) the skin. Read results after 10 minutes. *Positive reaction:* Wheal with or without pseudopodia and surrounding erythema. If skin sensitivity test is positive, consider a conjunctival test and desensitization schedule.
— For the conjunctival test in adults, instill 1 drop of a 1:10 dilution of horse serum into the conjunctival sac; for children, 1 drop of 1:100 dilution. Itching of the eye and reddening of the conjunctiva within 10 minutes indicate a positive reaction.

Monitoring

— Monitor the effectiveness of antivenin therapy by assessing for relief of, or decrease in, the symptoms related to a black widow spider bite.
— Monitor the patient for adverse drug reactions.

—Check vital signs every 30 minutes for 1 to 3 hours.

—Observe for signs of serum sickness for 8 to 12 days after administering antivenin.

—Monitor spider bite site. A black widow spider bite induces painful muscle spasms. Local muscle cramps begin from 15 minutes to several hours after the bite. The exact sequence of symptoms depends somewhat on the location of the bite. The neurotoxic venom acts on the myoneural junctions or on the nerve endings, causing an ascending motor paralysis or destruction of the peripheral nerve endings. The groups of muscles most frequently affected at first are those of the thigh, shoulder, and back. The pain eventually becomes more severe, spreading to the abdomen, and weakness and tremor usually develop. The abdominal muscles assume a boardlike rigidity, but tenderness is slight.

—Monitor patient for associated symptoms and abnormalities: thoracic respiration; restlessness and anxiety; feeble pulse; cold, clammy skin; labored breathing and speech; light stupor; and delirium may occur. Seizures also may occur, particularly in small children. The patient's temperature may be normal or slightly elevated. Urine retention, shock, cyanosis, nausea and vomiting, insomnia, and cold sweats also have been reported.

—The symptoms of black widow spider bite increase in severity for several hours, perhaps for a day, and then very slowly become less severe, gradually passing in 2 or 3 days except in fatal cases. Residual symptoms such as general weakness, tingling, nervousness, and transient muscle spasm may persist for weeks or months after recovery from the acute stage.

—Periodically reevaluate the patient's and family's knowledge about black widow spider antivenin.

Intervention

—If the patient develops anaphylaxis, apply tourniquet above site of I.M. injection.

—Keep epinephrine solution 1:1,000 available to treat allergic reactions.

—Continually assess the patient's respiratory status; if signs of respiratory paralysis occur, notify the doctor immediately. If the patient develops respiratory arrest, begin CPR and call a code.

—Provide seizure precautions. If the patient develops seizures, stay with the patient, provide protective care, and notify the doctor immediately.

—If the patient develops pain or muscle spasms at the bite site, obtain an order for an analgesic. If ordered, administer 10 ml of 10% calcium gluconate I.V. to control muscle pain p.r.n. Warm baths may also be helpful.

—Find out when the patient received last tetanus immunization, because many clinicians order a tetanus booster after black widow spider bites.

—Keep all members of the health care team informed of the patient's response to the drug.

Patient teaching

—Inform the patient and family about black widow spider antivenin, including the dosage, frequency, action, and adverse reactions.

—Inform the patient that allergic reactions to the antivenin may cause a rash, joint swelling or pain, fever, or difficulty breathing.

—Encourage the patient to report any unusual reactions.

—Explain that residual effects of the spider bite (general weakness, tingling of the extremities, nervousness, and muscle spasm) may persist for weeks or months.

—Advise women who are breast-feeding to discontinue breast-feeding temporarily until effects of the venom subside; patient should also discontinue breast-feeding if symptoms of serum sickness develop.

—Tell the patient to notify the nurse or doctor if adverse reactions develop or questions arise about black widow spider antivenin.

Evaluation

In the patient receiving black widow spider antivenin, appropriate evaluation statements include:

• Patient's symptoms resulting from black widow spider bite are relieved.

• Patient experiences no adverse reactions.

• Patient and family state an understanding of black widow spider antivenin therapy.

SELECTED MAJOR DRUGS: ANTITOXINS AND ANTIVENINS

DRUG, INDICATIONS, AND DOSAGES	SPECIAL PRECAUTIONS
Antitoxins	
botulism antitoxin, bivalent equine *Botulism—* **Adults and children:** 1 vial I.V. stat and q 4 hours, p.r.n., until patient's condition improves. Dilute antitoxin 1:10 in dextrose 5% or 10% in water or 0.9% sodium chloride solution. Give first 10 ml of dilution over 5 minutes; after 15 minutes, rate may be increased.	• Use cautiously in patients with known hypersensitivity to equine products. The risk of using the drug must be weighed against benefit.
diphtheria antitoxin, equine *Diphtheria prevention—* **Adults and children:** 1,000 to 5,000 units I.M. *Diphtheria treatment—* **Adults and children:** 20,000 to 80,000 units or more slow I.V. Additional doses may be given in 24 hours. I.M. route may be used in mild cases.	• Because this product is derived from horses immunized with diphtheria toxin, an intradermal or scratch skin test and a conjunctival test for sensitivity to equine serum (against a control of 0.9% sodium chloride solution) should be performed before administering diphtheria antitoxin. If the sensitivity test is positive, check desensitization schedule.

(continued)

SELECTED MAJOR DRUGS: ANTITOXINS AND ANTIVENINS *continued*

DRUG, INDICATIONS, AND DOSAGES	SPECIAL PRECAUTIONS
Antivenins	

crotaline (rattlesnake) antivenin, polyvalent
Crotalid (rattlesnake) bite—
Adults and children: initially, 10 to 50 ml or more I.M. or S.C., depending on severity of bite and patient response. If large amount of venom, 70 to 100 ml I.V. directly into superficial vein. Subsequent doses based on patient's response; may give 10 ml q 30 minutes to 2 hours, p.r.n. If bite is in extremity, inject part of initial dose at various sites around limb above swelling; don't inject in finger or toe. The smaller the patient, the larger the initial dose.

• Contraindicated in patients with a history of allergy or a positive sensitivity test to horse serum. However, the risk of administering antivenin must be weighed against the risk of withholding it, because severe envenomation can be fatal.

Micrurus fulvius (coral snake) antivenin
Eastern and Texas coral snake bite—
Adults and children: 3 to 5 vials slow I.V. through running infusion of 0.9% sodium chloride solution. Give first 1 to 2 ml over 3 to 5 minutes, and watch for signs of allergic reaction. If no signs develop, continue injection. Up to 10 vials may be needed.

• Use cautiously in patients with a history of hypersensitivity to equine products. Risk of administering drug must be weighed against benefit.
• Not effective for Sonoran or Arizona coral snake bites.

SELF-TEST

1. Julia Jefferson, age 30, was bitten by a black widow spider and came to the emergency department for treatment. Besides monitoring for signs of anaphylaxis and serum sickness, the nurse should monitor for which of the following conditions after administering black widow spider antivenin?
   a. Acute renal failure
   b. Cardiac arrhythmias
   c. Acute liver failure
   d. Respiratory paralysis and seizures

2. Richard Ellis requires tetanus prophylactic therapy. Tetanus antitoxin, equine, should be administered:
   a. concomitantly with tetanus immune globulin.
   b. only when tetanus immune globulin is not available.
   c. only to those who have received tetanus toxoid.
   d. after the administration of tetanus toxoid.

3. Antitoxins and antivenins provide:
  a. active immunity.
  b. passive immunity.
  c. a negative immune response.
  d. a positive immune response.

Check your answers on page 1075.

CHAPTER 75

IMMUNE SERUMS

antirabies serum, equine ♦ hepatitis B immune globulin, human
immune globulin intramuscular ♦ immune globulin intravenous
rabies immune globulin, human ♦ Rh$_O$(D) immune globulin, human
tetanus immune globulin, human ♦ varicella-zoster immune globulin (VZIG)

OVERVIEW

- Immune serums provide passive immunity (by administration of pre-formed antibodies) to treat various infectious diseases or to suppress antibody formation, as in Rh incompatibility.
- Immune serums are obtained from hyperimmunized human or animal donors or pooled plasma. They are used only for prophylaxis against the infectious disease or Rh incompatibility for which they are administered.

MAJOR USES

- Immune serums are used to prevent infectious diseases (rabies, hepatitis, and varicella).
- Rh$_O$(D) immune globulin prevents the formation of antibodies in Rh-negative mothers of Rh-positive infants or in transfusion accidents.

MECHANISM OF ACTION

- Immune serums contain preformed antibodies against specific organisms or toxins of disease. These antibodies confer a passive immunity against specific toxins or viruses. Rh$_O$(D) immune globulin suppresses the active antibody response and prevents the formation of antibodies after exposure to Rh-positive blood.

ABSORPTION, DISTRIBUTION, METABOLISM, AND EXCRETION

Not applicable.

ONSET AND DURATION

The onset of passive immunity is immediate but its duration is temporary, generally lasting for 3 to 4 weeks.

ADVERSE REACTIONS

Adverse reactions associated with immune serums vary from local pain and discomfort at the injection site to anaphylaxis. Other adverse reactions may include rash, fever, urticaria, headache, malaise, muscle stiffness, and erythema.

GLOSSARY

Anaphylaxis: life-threatening allergic reaction of a person to a foreign protein or other substance.

Passive immunity: form of acquired immunity resulting from antibodies that are transmitted naturally through the placenta to a fetus or through the colostrum to an infant, or artificially by injection of antiserum for treatment or prophylaxis.

Rabies: acute, usually fatal, viral disease of the CNS transmitted from animals to people by infected blood, tissue, or most commonly saliva.

Serum sickness: type of immune complex hypersensitivity occurring 6 to 12 days after injection with foreign serum; characterized by edema, fever, inflammation of the blood vessels and joints, and urticaria.

PROTOTYPE: IMMUNE SERUMS

ANTIRABIES SERUM, EQUINE
(ant ee ray' bees sere' um eek' wine)
Classification: immune serum
Pregnancy risk category C

How supplied
INJECTION: 125 IU/ml in 1,000-unit vial

Indications and dosage
Rabies exposure
ADULTS AND CHILDREN: 40 to 55 IU/kg at time of first dose of rabies vaccine. Use half of dose to infiltrate wound area. Give remainder I.M. Don't give rabies vaccine and antirabies serum in same syringe or at same site. For wounds that involve mucous membranes, the entire dose should be administered I.M.

Contraindications and precautions
Antirabies serum is contraindicated in patients with a history of allergic symptoms or known hypersensitivity to horse serum.

Adverse reactions
SYSTEMIC: immediate—pruritus, sneezing, coughing, wheezing, generalized urticaria, *marked hypotension*; delayed—serum sickness within 6 to 12 days in at least 40% of adult patients (reaction rates for children are lower); symptoms include skin eruptions, arthralgia, pruritus, lymphadenopathy, fever, headache, malaise, abdominal pain, and **anaphylaxis**.
LOCAL: pain, erythema, urticaria.

Italicized adverse reactions are common   Boldfaced adverse reactions are life-threatening

Interactions

Corticosteroids and immunosuppressive agents: interfere with response to antirabies serum. Avoid during postexposure immunization period.

Nursing considerations

Assessment

• Review the patient's history for a condition that contraindicates the use of antirabies serum.
• Obtain a baseline assessment of the patient's exposure to rabies before administering antirabies serum.
• Be alert for anaphylaxis and other adverse reactions.
• Evaluate the patient's and family's knowledge about antirabies serum therapy.

Planning (Nursing Diagnoses)

Potential nursing diagnoses for the patient receiving antirabies serum, equine, include:
• Altered health maintenance related to ineffectiveness of antirabies serum.
• Injury related to potential anaphylaxis.
• Knowledge deficit related to antirabies serum therapy.

Implementation

Preparation and administration

— Perform a sensitivity test before giving I.M. dose. Dilute antirabies serum to 1:100 or 1:1,000 with 0.9% sodium chloride solution for injection. Inject 0.1 ml of 1:100 dilution (or 0.05 ml of 1:1,000 dilution in patient with a history of allergy) intradermally on inner forearm. Give 0.1 ml of 0.9% sodium chloride solution intradermally in other arm as a control. Read within 30 minutes. *Positive reaction:* Wheal of 10 mm or more and erythematous flare of 20 × 20 mm. If the patient tests positive for hypersensitivity to horse serum, desensitize the patient before giving antirabies serum. Consult doctor or pharmacist for method.
— Equine antirabies serum is used primarily when rabies immune globulin, human, is not available.
— Up to 50% of a dose should be infiltrated around the wound, if possible.
— Obtain history of the animal bite, allergies (especially to equine serum and to eggs), and previous reactions to immunization.
— Do not confuse this drug with rabies vaccine, a suspension of attenuated or killed microorganisms used to confer long-term active immunity. This immune serum provides immediate short-term passive immunity. These two drugs are often administered together prophylactically after exposure to known or suspected rabid animals.
— Ask the patient when he received last tetanus immunization, because many doctors order a tetanus booster after exposure to rabies.
— Because untreated rabies can be fatal, use of antirabies serum during pregnancy appears justified. No fetal risk from antirabies serum use has been reported to date.

— Store between 2° and 8° C (36° to 46° F). Do not freeze.

Monitoring

— Monitor the effectiveness of antirabies serum therapy by regularly assessing for signs of rabies.
— Monitor the patient for adverse drug reactions.
— Monitor the patient for drug interactions.
— Periodically reevaluate the patient's and family's knowledge about antirabies serum, equine.

Intervention

— Notify the doctor immediately if the patient begins to develop signs of rabies.
— If the patient develops anaphylaxis, notify the doctor immediately and be prepared to administer epinephrine. Keep 1:1,000 solution readily available.
— If the patient develops signs of serum sickness, notify the doctor immediately for appropriate therapy. Provide supportive care as indicated.
— Keep all members of the health care team informed of the patient's response to the serum.

Patient teaching

— Inform the patient and family about antirabies serum, including the dosage, frequency, action, and adverse reactions.
— Explain the disease process and rationale for therapy.
— Explain to the patient that the body takes approximately 1 week to develop immunity to rabies after the vaccine is given. He is receiving antirabies serum to provide antibodies in his blood for immediate protection against rabies.
— Inform the patient that reactions to antirabies serum may develop up to 12 days after administration and are related to the product's source, namely horses. Have him immediately report skin changes, difficulty breathing, headache, swollen lymph nodes, and joint pain.
— Tell the patient to take acetaminophen to relieve headache, joint pain, or other minor discomfort after antirabies serum injection.
— Tell the patient to notify the nurse or doctor if adverse reactions develop or questions arise about antirabies serum therapy.

Evaluation

In the patient receiving antirabies serum, equine, appropriate evaluation statements include:
• Patient does not develop rabies.
• Patient does not experience anaphylaxis.
• Patient and family state an understanding of antirabies serum therapy.

SELECTED MAJOR DRUGS: IMMUNE SERUMS

DRUG, INDICATIONS, AND DOSAGES	SPECIAL PRECAUTIONS
hepatitis B immune globulin, human (H-BIG, HyperHep) *Hepatitis B exposure—* **Adults and children:** 0.06 ml/kg I.M. within 7 days after exposure. Repeat 28 days after exposure. **Neonates born to HB,Ag-positive women:** 0.5 ml within 12 hours of birth. Repeat dose at ages 3 months and 6 months.	• Contraindicated in patients with known hypersensitivity to any component of the product. • Use cautiously in patients with a history of systemic allergic reactions to human immune globulin preparations, and in pregnant or breast-feeding women.
immune globulin intramuscular (IGIM; Gamastan, Gammar) **immune globulin intravenous (IGIV; Gamimune N, Gammagard, Sandoglobulin, Venoglobulin-1)** *Agammaglobulinemia or hypogammaglobulinemia—* **Adults:** 30 to 50 ml I.M. monthly. Alternatively, administer 100 mg/kg Gamimune N I.V. once a month. Infuse at 0.01 to 0.02 ml/kg/min for 30 minutes. Or administer 200 mg/kg Sandoglobulin I.V. once a month. Infuse initially at 0.5 to 1 ml/min; after 15 to 30 minutes, increase infusion rate to 1.5 to 2.5 ml/min for remainder of infusion. **Children:** 20 to 40 ml I.M. monthly. *Hepatitis A exposure—* **Adults and children:** 0.02 ml/kg I.M. as soon as possible after exposure. Up to 0.06 ml/kg may be given for prolonged exposure. *Post-transfusion hepatitis B—* **Adults and children:** 10 ml I.M. within 1 week after transfusion and 10 ml I.M. 1 month later. *Measles exposure—* **Adults and children:** 0.02 ml/kg I.M. within 6 days after exposure. *Modification of measles—* **Adults and children:** 0.04 ml/kg I.M. within 6 days after exposure. *Measles vaccine complications—* **Adults and children:** 0.02 to 0.04 ml/kg I.M. *Poliomyelitis exposure—* **Adults and children:** 0.3 to 0.4 ml/kg I.M. within 7 days after exposure. *Chicken pox exposure—* **Adults and children:** 0.2 to 1.3 ml/kg I.M. as soon as exposed. *Rubella exposure in first trimester of pregnancy—* **Women:** 0.2 to 0.4 ml/kg I.M. as soon as exposed. *Prophylaxis in primary immunodeficiencies—* **Adults and children:** 100 mg/kg Gamimune by I.V. infusion monthly. Infuse at 0.01 to 0.02 ml/kg/min for 30 minutes, increasing to 0.04 ml/min for remainder of infusion.	• Contraindicated in isolated immunoglobulin A (IgA) deficiency, severe thrombocytopenia, or any coagulation disorder that could contraindicate I.M. injections; and in patients with known hypersensitivity to thimerosal. • Use cautiously in patients with a history of systemic allergic reactions to human immune globulin preparations, and in pregnant women.

SELECTED MAJOR DRUGS: IMMUNE SERUMS *continued*

DRUG, INDICATIONS, AND DOSAGES	SPECIAL PRECAUTIONS
immune globulin *(continued)* *Idiopathic thrombocytopenic purpura —* **Adults:** 0.4 g/kg Gamimune N or Sandoglobulin I.V. for 5 consecutive days, or 1 g/kg Gammagard I.V. Additional doses may be given based on response. Give up to three doses (every other day) if necessary. Or give 1.5 g/kg Venoglobulin I.V. daily for 2 to 7 days.	
rabies immune globulin, human (Hyperab, Imogan) *Rabies exposure —* **Adults and children:** 20 IU/kg I.M. at time of first dose of rabies vaccine. Use half of dose to infiltrate wound area. Give remainder I.M. Don't give rabies vaccine and rabies immune globulin in same syringe or at same site.	• Repeated doses contraindicated after rabies vaccine is started. • Use with caution in patients with history of systemic allergic reactions to human immune globulin preparations, in patients with known hypersensitivity to thimerosal, in those with thrombocytopenia or other bleeding disorders, and in pregnant women.
Rh$_o$(D) immune globulin, human (RhoGAM) *Rh exposure —* **Women (postabortion, postmiscarriage, ectopic pregnancy, or postpartum):** transfusion unit or blood bank determines fetal packed RBC volume entering woman's blood, then gives 1 vial I.M. if fetal packed RBC volume is less than 15 ml. More than 1 vial may be required if there is large fetomaternal hemorrhage. Must be given within 72 hours after delivery or miscarriage. *Transfusion accidents —* **Adults and children:** consult blood bank or transfusion unit at once. Must be given within 72 hours. *Postabortion or postmiscarriage to prevent Rh antibody formation —* **Women:** consult transfusion unit or blood bank. 1 microdose vial will suppress immune reaction to 2.5 ml Rh$_o$(D)-positive RBCs. Ideally should be given within 3 hours, but may be given up to 72 hours after abortion or miscarriage.	• Contraindicated in Rh$_o$(D)-positive or D^u-positive patients and those previously immunized to Rh$_o$(D) blood factor. • Use cautiously in patients with history of systemic allergic reactions to human immune globulin preparations; in patients with known hypersensitivity to thimerosal; in those with isolated immunoglobulin A (IgA) deficiency, or thrombocytopenia or other bleeding disorders; and in pregnant women.
tetanus immune globulin, human (Homo-Tet, Hyper-Tet) *Tetanus exposure —* **Adults and children:** 250 to 500 units I.M. *Tetanus treatment —* **Adults and children:** single doses of 3,000 to 6,000 units I.M. have been used. Optimal dosage schedules have not been established. Don't give at same site as toxoid.	• There are no contraindications to the use of tetanus immune globulin. • Use with caution in patients with a history of systemic allergic reactions to human immune globulin preparations; in patients with known hypersensitivity to thimerosal; in those with severe thrombocytopenia or any coagulation disorder; and in pregnant women.

(continued)

SELECTED MAJOR DRUGS: IMMUNE SERUMS *continued*

DRUG, INDICATIONS, AND DOSAGES	SPECIAL PRECAUTIONS
varicella-zoster immune globulin (VZIG) *Passive immunization of susceptible immunodeficient patients after exposure to varicella (chicken pox or herpes zoster)*— **Children to 10 kg:** 125 units I.M. **Children 10.1 to 20 kg:** 250 units I.M. **Children 20.1 to 30 kg:** 375 units I.M. **Children 30.1 to 40 kg:** 500 units I.M. **Adults and children over 40 kg:** 625 units I.M.	• Contraindicated in patients with a history of severe reaction to human immune serum globulin or severe thrombocytopenia.

SELF-TEST

1. An immune serum acts by providing:
   a. active immunity.
   b. passive immunity.
   c. enhancement of antibody formation.
   d. suppression of antigen formation.

2. Kathy Star, age 12, received antirabies serum, equine, after she was bitten by a raccoon. How long should her mother watch for signs and symptoms of serum sickness?
   a. 1 to 2 days after receiving the drug
   b. 2 to 6 days
   c. 6 to 12 days
   d. 14 to 28 days

3. After administering antirabies serum, equine, the nurse should monitor for:
   a. anaphylaxis.
   b. hypotension.
   c. seizures.
   d. polyuria.

Check your answers on page 1075.

CHAPTER 76

BIOLOGICAL RESPONSE MODIFIERS

epoetin alfa (erythropoietin) ◆ filgrastim (G-CSF)
interferon alfa-2a, recombinant ◆ interferon alfa-2b, recombinant
interferon alfa-n3 ◆ sargramostim (GM-CSF)

OVERVIEW
• Biological response modifiers are a new class of drugs that are products of recombinant DNA technology. These agents are synthetic versions of naturally occurring growth factors or immunomodulators.

MAJOR USES
• Epoetin alfa is used to treat anemia caused by reduced production of endogenous erythropoietin, especially in end-stage renal disease, and is an adjunct to treatment of HIV-infected patients with anemia secondary to zidovudine therapy. Epoetin alfa has also been used to correct the hemostatic defect associated with uremia. Additional clinical trials are investigating the agent for treatment of the anemia seen in cancer patients undergoing chemotherapy and patients with rheumatoid arthritis. It is also being investigated for facilitating autologous blood transfusion by helping to produce more units of blood before surgery.
• Filgrastim (granulocyte colony stimulating factor, or G-CSF) is used to decrease the incidence of infection in patients with nonmyeloid malignancies who are receiving myelosuppressive antineoplastic agents.
• Interferon alfa-2a, recombinant, is used to treat hairy-cell leukemia and AIDS-related Kaposi's sarcoma. Interferon alfa-2b, recombinant, is used to treat hairy-cell leukemia, AIDS-related Kaposi's sarcoma, chronic hepatitis B, and condylomata acuminata. Both agents may also be used to treat chronic myelocytic leukemia, renal carcinoma, superficial bladder carcinoma, non-Hodgkin's lymphomas (especially nodular, poorly differentiated types), malignant melanoma, multiple myeloma, mycosis fungoides, and papillomas. Interferon alfa-2b has also been used to treat laryngeal papillomatosis.
• Interferon alfa-n3 is used to treat condylomata acuminata.
• Sargramostim (granulocyte macrophage colony stimulating factor, or GM-CSF) is used to stimulate hematopoietic reconstitution after bone marrow transplantation.

MECHANISM OF ACTION

- A naturally occurring hormone, produced by recombinant DNA technology, epoetin alfa is one of the factors controlling the rate of erythrocyte, or RBC, production. It mimics naturally occurring erythropoietin, which is produced by the kidney, and stimulates the division and differentiation of cells within bone marrow to produce RBCs.
- Filgrastim is a glycoprotein produced by monocytes, fibroblasts, and endothelial cells and stimulates proliferation and differentiation of granulocytes, also called neutrophils.
- Sargramostim is structurally similar to filgrastim. Sargramostim promotes survival, differentiation, and production of both granulocytes and macrophages. Sargramostim induces hematopoietic cellular responses by binding to specific receptors on cell surfaces of target cells.
- The recombinant products interferon alfa-2a and interferon alfa-2b are sterile proteins produced by recombinant DNA techniques. Their mechanisms of action appear to involve direct antiproliferative action against tumor cells or viral cells to inhibit replication; they modulate host immune response by enhancing the phagocytic activity of macrophages and augmenting specific cytotoxicity of lymphocytes for target cells.
- Interferon alfa-n3 is a naturally occurring antiviral agent derived from human leukocytes. It attaches to membrane receptors and causes cellular changes, including increased protein synthesis.

ABSORPTION, DISTRIBUTION, METABOLISM, AND EXCRETION

More than 80% of a dose of recombinant interferon alfa-2a or interferon alfa-2b is absorbed after I.M. or S.C. injection. The agents appear to be metabolized in the liver and kidney, and are reabsorbed from glomerular filtrate with minor biliary elimination.

More than 80% of interferon alfa-n3 is absorbed and widely distributed. The agent is not metabolized. It is reabsorbed from glomerular filtrate with minor biliary excretion.

Distribution, metabolism, and excretion of epoetin alfa, filgrastim, and sargramostim have not been described.

ONSET AND DURATION

Epoetin alfa may be given S.C. or I.V. After S.C. administration, peak serum levels occur within 5 to 24 hours. Peak levels of interferon alfa-2a occur 3.8 hours after I.M. administration, 1 to 3 hours after S.C. injection. Peak levels of interferon alfa-2b occur 6 to 8 hours after S.C. or I.M. administration. Peak levels of sargramostim occur 2 hours after S.C. administration; the drug's half-life is about 2 hours.

ADVERSE REACTIONS

Epoetin alfa may cause iron deficiency, elevated platelet count, headache, seizure, hypertension, nausea, vomiting, diarrhea, rash, and increased clotting in arteriovenous grafts.

Filgrastim may cause thrombocytopenia, hematuria, proteinuria, alopecia, exacerbation of preexisting skin conditions (such as psoriasis), skeletal pain, fever, splenomegaly, and osteoporosis.

The recombinant interferons, interferon alfa-2a and interferon alfa-2b, may cause CNS reactions, including dizziness, confusion, paresthesia, lethargy, depression, nervousness, irritability, and fatigue. Cardiovascular reactions to these agents include hypotension or hypertension, chest pain, arrhythmias, CHF, and edema. GI reactions include anorexia, nausea, diarrhea, and vomiting. Patients may also experience rash, dry skin, pruritus, partial alopecia, or urticaria. Other reactions may include pharyngitis and flulike symptoms (fever, headache, chills, muscle aches).

Interferon alfa-n3 may cause dizziness, light-headedness, dyspepsia, heartburn, vomiting, nausea, mild to moderate flulike syndrome, arthralgia, back pain, and malaise.

Sargramostim may cause blood dyscrasias and hemorrhage, various GI reactions (nausea, vomiting, diarrhea, anorexia, hemorrhage, and stomatitis), liver damage, and urinary tract disorder and abnormal kidney function.

PROTOTYPE: BIOLOGICAL RESPONSE MODIFIERS

INTERFERON ALFA-2A, RECOMBINANT
(int er fear′ on al′ fa)
Roferon-A
Classification: biological response modifier
Pregnancy risk category C

How supplied
INJECTION: 3 million IU/vial; 18 million IU/multiple-dose vial

Indications and dosage
Treatment of hairy-cell leukemia
ADULTS: for induction, 3 million IU S.C. or I.M. daily for 16 to 24 weeks; maintenance, 3 million IU S.C. or I.M. three times a week.

Treatment of AIDS-related Kaposi's sarcoma
ADULTS: for induction, 36 million IU S.C. or I.M. daily for 10 to 12 weeks; maintenance, 36 million IU S.C. or I.M. three times a week.

Contraindications and precautions
Recombinant interferon alfa-2a is contraindicated in patients with known hypersensitivity to interferon alfa, mouse immunoglobulin, or any component of the product. It should not be used to treat visceral AIDS-related Kaposi's sarcoma associated with rapidly progressive or life-threatening disease. Use with caution in patients with severe preexisting cardiac disease, severe renal or hepatic disease, seizure disorders, or compromised CNS function. Also use caution when administering recombinant inter-

feron alfa-2a to patients with myelosuppression or when used in combination with other agents known to cause myelosuppression.

Adverse reactions

BLOOD: leukemia, mild thrombocytopenia.

CNS: dizziness, confusion, paresthesia, numbness, lethargy, depression, nervousness, difficulty in thinking or concentrating, insomnia, sedation, apathy, anxiety, irritability, fatigue, vertigo, gait disturbances, poor coordination.

CV: hypotension, chest pain, **arrhythmias,** palpitations, syncope, **CHF,** hypertension, edema.

EENT: visual disturbances, dryness or inflammation of the oropharynx, rhinorrhea, sinusitis, conjunctivitis, earache, eye irritation, rhinitis.

GI: anorexia, nausea, diarrhea, vomiting, abdominal fullness, abdominal pain, flatulence and constipation, hypermotility, gastric distress, dysgeusia.

GU: transient impotence.

HEPATIC: hepatitis.

RESPIRATORY: **bronchospasm,** coughing, dyspnea, tachypnea.

SKIN: rash, dryness, pruritus, partial alopecia, urticaria, flushing.

LOCAL: inflammation at injection site (rare).

OTHER: *flulike syndrome (fever, fatigue, myalgia, headache, chills, arthralgia),* diaphoresis, hot flashes, excessive salivation, cyanosis.

Interactions

Blood dyscrasia-causing medications, bone marrow depressants, or radiation: increased bone marrow depressant effects. Monitor for increased toxicity; dosage reduction may be required.

CNS depressants: enhanced CNS depression. Use with caution.

Live virus vaccines: may potentiate replication of vaccine virus, increase adverse effects, and decrease patient's antibody response. Postpone elective vaccinations.

Theophylline, aminophylline, and other methylxanthines: may substantially increase the half-life of these drugs, perhaps by interfering with drug-metabolizing enzymes. Monitor for toxicity. Dosage reduction may be required to offset drug accumulation.

Nursing considerations

Assessment

• Review the patient's history for a condition that contraindicates the use of recombinant interferon alfa-2a.

• Obtain a baseline assessment of the patient's disease and his immune-response status before initiating interferon alfa-2a therapy.

• Be alert for common adverse reactions.

• Evaluate the patient's and family's knowledge about interferon alfa-2a therapy.

Planning (Nursing Diagnoses)

Potential nursing diagnoses for the patient receiving recombinant interferon alfa-2a include:

• Injury related to potential adverse drug reactions.

Italicized adverse reactions are common   Boldfaced adverse reactions are life-threatening

• Altered health maintenance related to flulike syndrome caused by recombinant interferon alfa-2a.
• Knowledge deficit related to interferon alfa-2a therapy.

Implementation
Preparation and administration
— When preparing this drug for injection, take special precautions because of potential for carcinogenicity and mutagenicity. Use of a biological containment cabinet is recommended. Do not shake vials.
— Store drug in refrigerator.
— Give, and review with the patient, the manufacturer's patient information sheet before administering the first dose. Because of the possibility of severe or even fatal adverse reactions, patients should be informed not only of the benefits of therapy but also of the risks involved.
— Administer by S.C. route in patients with platelet counts below 50,000/mm^3.
— Do not switch to another brand; different brands of interferon may not be equivalent and may require different dosage.
— Administer at bedtime to minimize daytime drowsiness.

Monitoring
— Monitor the effectiveness of recombinant interferon alfa-2a therapy by regularly assessing for improvement in patient's disease status.
— Monitor the patient for adverse drug reactions.
— Monitor for flulike symptoms. Almost all patients experience these at the beginning of therapy, but they should diminish with continued therapy.
— Neurotoxicity and cardiotoxicity are more common in elderly patients, especially those with underlying CNS or cardiac impairment. Regularly monitor for adverse CNS reactions, such as decreased mental status and dizziness, and for signs of CHF.
— Also monitor blood pressure; BUN, ALT, AST, LDH, alkaline phosphatase, serum bilirubin, creatinine, and uric acid levels; WBC count and differential, hematocrit, and platelet count; and ECG. Interferon alfa-2a may decrease hemoglobin and hematocrit, as well as WBC, platelet, and neutrophil counts; increase prothrombin and partial thromboplastin time; and increase serum levels of AST, ALT, LDH, alkaline phosphatase, calcium, phosphorus, and fasting glucose. These effects are dose-related and reversible; recovery occurs within several days or weeks after withdrawal of interferon alfa-2a.
— Monitor the patient's fluid intake. Patient should be well hydrated, especially during initial stages of treatment.
— Monitor the patient for drug interactions.
— Monitor the patient's compliance with interferon alfa-2a therapy.
— Periodically reevaluate the patient's and family's knowledge about interferon alfa-2a.

Intervention

—If the patient develops a severe adverse reaction, notify the doctor. Expect that dosage may be reduced by one half or that therapy may be discontinued until reactions subside.

—Provide supportive care for flulike symptoms. Before next dose, premedicate with acetaminophen to minimize symptoms.

—If the patient develops a persistent headache, notify the doctor; dosage reduction may be needed.

—If the patient develops fluid depletion, watch for hypotension and provide supportive care, and encourage the patient to increase fluid intake.

—If the patient develops thrombocytopenia, take precautions to minimize the risk of bleeding: exercise extreme care in performing invasive procedures; inspect injection site and skin frequently for signs of bruising; limit frequency of I.M. injections; and test urine, emesis fluid, stool, and secretions for occult blood.

—Keep all members of the health care team informed of the patient's response to the drug.

Patient teaching

—Inform the patient and family about recombinant interferon alfa-2a, including the dosage, frequency, action, and adverse reactions.

—Explain the disease process and rationale for therapy.

—Stress the importance of drinking extra fluids to prevent hypotension from fluid loss.

—Instruct the patient in proper oral hygiene during treatment, because the bone marrow suppressant effects of interferon alfa-2a may lead to microbial infection, delayed healing, and gingival bleeding. The agent may also decrease salivary flow.

—Advise the patient not to take a missed dose or to double the next dose. Instead, he should check with the doctor for further instructions after missing a dose.

—Teach patients who will self-administer interferon alfa-2a how to prepare and administer the injection and how to use a disposable syringe. Give them information on drug stability.

—Emphasize the need to follow doctor's instructions about taking and recording temperature, and how and when to take acetaminophen. Tell the patient to avoid aspirin and excessive alcohol use because they may increase the risk of GI bleeding.

—Warn the patient not to have any immunization without doctor's approval and to avoid contact with persons who have taken oral poliovirus vaccine. Because interferon alfa-2a may decrease antibody response and potentiate replication of vaccine viruses, the patient is at special risk for infection during therapy.

—Tell the patient that interferon alfa-2a may cause temporary loss of some hair. Normal hair growth should return when agent is withdrawn.

—Warn the patient against driving or other hazardous tasks requiring alertness until response to medication is known.

— Advise the patient to seek medical approval before taking OTC medications for colds, coughs, allergies, and similar disorders.

— Explain that interferon alfa-2a commonly causes flulike symptoms and that patient may need to take acetaminophen before each dose.

— Tell the patient not to change brands of interferon without consulting the doctor, because a change in dosage may result.

— Advise patient that laboratory tests will be performed before and periodically during therapy. Such tests will include a CBC with differential, platelet count, blood chemistry and electrolyte studies, liver function tests, and if the patient has a preexisting cardiac disorder or advanced cancer, ECGs.

— Advise mothers of infants that drug is usually not recommended during breast-feeding because of the potential for serious adverse reactions in breast-fed infants.

— Tell the patient to notify the nurse or doctor if adverse reactions develop or questions arise about interferon alfa-2a therapy.

Evaluation

In the patient receiving recombinant interferon alfa-2a, appropriate evaluation statements include:

• Patient exhibits few or no adverse reactions.
• Patient manages flulike symptoms effectively.
• Patient and family state an understanding of interferon alfa-2a therapy.

SELECTED MAJOR DRUGS: BIOLOGICAL RESPONSE MODIFIERS

DRUG, INDICATIONS, AND DOSAGES	SPECIAL PRECAUTIONS
epoetin alfa (Epogen, Procrit) *Anemia from reduced production of endogenous erythropoietin, end-stage renal disease—* **Adults:** dosage is individualized. Starting dose is 50 to 100 units/kg I.V. three times weekly. (Nondialysis patients with chronic renal failure may receive the drug S.C. or I.V.) Reduce dosage when target hematocrit is reached or if the hematocrit rises more than 4 points in any 2-week period. Increase dosage if hematocrit does not increase by 5 to 6 points after 8 weeks of therapy. Maintenance dosage is usually 25 units/kg three times weekly. *Adjunctive treatment of HIV-infected patients with anemia secondary to zidovudine therapy—* **Adults:** 100 units/kg I.V. or S.C. three times weekly for 8 weeks or until target hematocrit is reached.	• Contraindicated in patients with uncontrolled hypertension. Reduce dosage in patients who exhibit a rapid rise in hematocrit (more than 4 points in any 2-week period) because of the risk of hypertension.
interferon alfa-2b (Intron A) *Hairy-cell leukemia—* **Adults:** 2 million units/m² I.M. or S.C. three times a week.	• Contraindicated in patients with known hypersensitivity to interferon alfa or any component of the injection.

(continued)

SELECTED MAJOR DRUGS: BIOLOGICAL RESPONSE MODIFIERS
continued

DRUG, INDICATIONS, AND DOSAGES	SPECIAL PRECAUTIONS
interferon alfa-2b *(continued)* *Condylomata acuminata (genital or venereal warts)—* **Adults:** 1 million units/lesion intralesionally three times a week for 3 weeks. *AIDS-related Kaposi's sarcoma—* **Adults:** 30 million units/m² S.C. or I.M. three times a week.	• Use cautiously in patients with debilitating medical conditions, such as cardiovascular or pulmonary disease, or diabetes mellitus with risk of ketoacidosis; in patients with coagulation disorders or severe myelosuppression; or during pregnancy or breast-feeding. • Use cautiously because of the risk of carcinogenesis, mutagenesis, or impaired fertility.
interferon alfa-n3 (Alferon-N) *Condylomata acuminata—* **Adults:** 0.05 ml/lesion intralesionally twice weekly for 8 weeks. Dosage should not exceed 0.5 ml (2.5 million units)/session.	• Contraindicated in patients with known hypersensitivity to interferon alfa and in patients with a history of anaphylactic reactions to mouse immunoglobulin, eggs, or neomycin.

SELF-TEST

1. Elmer Horn, age 24, has AIDS-related Kaposi's sarcoma, for which he receives recombinant interferon alfa-2a. Which of the following adverse reactions is most commonly associated with this therapy?
   a. Stomatitis
   b. Alopecia
   c. Flulike syndrome
   d. Photosensitivity

2. Mr. Horn asks the nurse when he should administer the drug. The nurse should reply:
   a. in the morning immediately upon rising.
   b. anytime during the day.
   c. with meals.
   d. at bedtime.

3. When teaching Mr. Horn, the nurse explains that interferon alfa-2a is:
   a. produced by recombinant DNA techniques.
   b. a naturally occurring hormone.
   c. a naturally occurring antiviral agent derived from human leukocytes.
   d. a lymphokine.

Check your answers on page 1075.

CHAPTER 77

OPHTHALMIC ANTI-INFECTIVES

bacitracin zinc ✦ boric acid ✦ chloramphenicol
chlortetracycline hydrochloride ✦ ciprofloxacin ✦ erythromycin
gentamicin sulfate ✦ idoxuridine ✦ natamycin ✦ neomycin sulfate
norfloxacin ✦ oxytetracycline ✦ polymyxin B sulfate ✦ silver nitrate 1%
sulfacetamide sodium ✦ sulfisoxazole ✦ tetracycline hydrochloride
tobramycin ✦ trifluridine ✦ vidarabine

OVERVIEW

- Ophthalmic anti-infectives are used locally in the eye to combat infection. Only drugs that are nonirritating and possess adequate lipid solubility to penetrate corneal membranes may be used in the eye.

MAJOR USES

- Ophthalmic anti-infectives are used to treat susceptible bacteria causing corneal ulcers, blepharitis, blepharoconjunctivitis, acute meibomianitis, and dacryocystitis.
- Tetracycline and erythromycin are indicated for prophylaxis of ophthalmia neonatorum due to *Neisseria gonorrhoeae* or *Chlamydia trachomatis*. Other antibiotics, including bacitracin, chloramphenicol, chlortetracycline, ciprofloxacin, gentamicin, neomycin, norfloxacin, oxytetracycline, polymyxin B sulfate, sulfacetamide, and sulfisoxazole, are indicated for conjunctivitis, corneal ulcer, and other superficial ocular infections due to susceptible microorganisms and as adjunctive treatment in systemic sulfonamide treatment of trachoma.
- Silver nitrate is used in weak solutions (1%) as a germicide and astringent for mucous membranes. The germicidal action is due to precipitation of bacterial proteins by liberated silver ions. As a 1% solution, it is used for the prevention of gonorrheal ophthalmia neonatorum. Higher concentrations (10% or more) are used as chemical cauterizing agents and should never be used in the eye. Do not administer silver nitrate with sulfonamides because these drugs are incompatible.
- Natamycin is active against various yeasts and filamentous fungi. It is indicated for fungal blepharitis, conjunctivitis, and keratitis caused by susceptible organisms.
- Idoxuridine, trifluridine, and vidarabine are topical antivirals. Idoxuridine is used for the treatment of herpes simplex keratitis. Trifluridine and vidarabine are used to treat primary keratoconjunctivitis and recurrent epithelial keratitis due to herpes simplex virus types 1 and 2. Vidarabine

GLOSSARY

Blepharitis: inflammation of the lash follicles and meibomian glands of the eyelids.
Conjunctivitis: inflammation of the conjunctiva.
Dacryocystitis: infection of the lacrimal sac.
Keratitis: inflammation of the cornea.
Meibomianitis: inflammation of the sebaceous glands located on the posterior margin of each eyelid.
Tonometry: indirect measurement of intraocular pressure by determining the resistance of the eyeball to indentation by an applied force.

is also effective for superficial keratitis caused by herpes simplex virus that has not responded to topical idoxuridine or when toxic or hypersensitivity reactions to idoxuridine have occurred. To ensure stability, idoxuridine solutions should not be mixed with other medications.

- Boric acid is used to soothe and cleanse the eye. It is applied as an irrigant after tonometry, gonioscopy, foreign body removal, or the instillation of fluorescein.

MECHANISM OF ACTION

- Bacitracin may be bactericidal or bacteriostatic, depending on the drug's concentration at the site of infection and the infecting organism's susceptibility.
- Chloramphenicol, erythromycin, and the tetracyclines are usually bacteriostatic but may be bactericidal in high concentrations or against highly susceptible organisms.
- Ciprofloxacin, gentamicin, neomycin, norfloxacin, polymyxin B sulfate, and tobramycin are usually bactericidal. These drugs appear to inhibit protein synthesis.
- Silver nitrate is bacteriostatic.
- Natamycin appears to be fungicidal.
- Idoxuridine exerts its activity through incorporation into DNA and prevention of DNA replication.
- The exact mechanisms of action of trifluridine and vidarabine are unknown but appear to involve inhibition of viral replication.
- Sulfonamides exert a bacteriostatic effect by competing with PABA to restrict the synthesis of folic acid, which bacteria require for growth.

ABSORPTION, DISTRIBUTION, METABOLISM, AND EXCRETION

Ophthalmic solutions and gels penetrate the cornea and are found in varied concentrations in the aqueous humor. Systemic absorption does not appear to occur after instillation. Idoxuridine is poorly absorbed after instillation into the eye. Absorption of gentamicin, neomycin, and tobramycin is greatest when the cornea is abraded. Chloramphenicol may be absorbed into the aqueous humor; the degree of penetration varies with the dosage form and the frequency of application. Aqueous humor concentrations are highest with frequent application of chloramphenicol ophthalmic ointment; the possibility of systemic absorption after ophthalmic application should be considered.

ONSET AND DURATION

Frequency and duration of dosage is specific for each product. General guidelines are as follows: For acute infections—1 to 2 drops (solution) every 15 to 30 minutes to start, with the frequency gradually reduced as the infection is controlled; ½" ribbon (ointment) every 3 to 4 hours until improvement, with reduced treatment before discontinuation. For moderate infections—1 to 2 drops (solution) four to six times daily or more often as needed; ½" ribbon (ointment) two to three times daily.

ADVERSE REACTIONS

These agents produce various local reactions. Sensitivity reactions include transient irritation, burning, stinging, itching, angioneurotic edema, urticaria, and vesicular and maculopapular dermatitis. Sensitization from topical use of an anti-infective may contraindicate later systemic use in serious infections.

Products containing neomycin may cause cutaneous and conjunctival sensitization.

Ciprofloxacin can precipitate in the ulcerated cornea. Onset of crystallization occurs within 1 to 7 days after start of therapy. Ciprofloxacin has also caused foreign body sensation, itching, conjuctival hyperemia, corneal staining, bad taste in the mouth, keratitis, lid edema, eyelid margin crusting, tearing, photophobia, corneal infiltrates, nausea, and decreased vision.

Norfloxacin has caused conjunctival hyperemia, photophobia, and bitter taste in the mouth.

Systemic reactions may also occur. Prolonged or frequent intermittent use of ocular chloramphenicol has produced adverse hematologic reactions, including aplastic anemia. Tetracycline has caused dermatitis and photosensitivity; tobramycin has caused localized ocular toxicity and hypersensitivity, eyelid itching, eyelid swelling, and conjunctival erythema; gentamicin has caused mydriasis and conjunctival paresthesia.

Reported systemic reactions to norfloxacin include conjunctival hyperemia, photophobia, and bitter taste in the mouth.

Sulfonamide medications have produced severe sensitivity reactions in patients with no prior history of sulfonamide hypersensitivity. These reactions include rare occurrences of Stevens-Johnson syndrome, bone marrow depression, exfoliative dermatitis, toxic epidermal necrolysis, and photosensitivity.

Use of anti-infectives, especially for prolonged or repeated therapy, may result in bacterial or fungal overgrowth of nonsusceptible organisms.

SULFACETAMIDE SODIUM 10%
(sul fa see' ta mide)
Bleph-10 Liquifilm, Cetamide, Sodium Sulamyd 10%, Sulf-10

SULFACETAMIDE SODIUM 15%
Isopto-Cetamide, Sulfacel-15

SULFACETAMIDE SODIUM 30%
Sodium Sulamyd 30%
Classification: ophthalmic anti-infective
Pregnancy risk category C

How supplied
OPHTHALMIC OINTMENT: 10%
OPHTHALMIC SOLUTION: 10%, 15%, 30%

Indications and dosage
Inclusion conjunctivitis, corneal ulcers, trachoma, chlamydial infection
ADULTS AND CHILDREN: instill 1 to 2 drops of 10% solution into lower conjunctival sac q 2 to 3 hours during day, less often at night; or instill 1 to 2 drops of 15% solution into lower conjunctival sac q 1 to 2 hours initially, increasing interval as condition responds; or instill 1 drop of 30% solution into lower conjunctival sac q 2 hours. Instill ½″ to 1″ of 10% ointment into conjunctival sac q.i.d. and h.s. May use ointment at night along with drops during the day.

Contraindications and precautions
Sulfacetamide is contraindicated in patients with known hypersensitivity to sulfonamides.

Adverse reactions
EYE: slowed corneal wound healing (ointment), pain on instillation (solution), headache or brow pain, photophobia.
OTHER: hypersensitivity (including itching or burning), overgrowth of nonsusceptible organisms, **anaphylaxis, Stevens-Johnson syndrome**.

Interactions
Local anesthetics (procaine, tetracaine), PABA derivatives: decreased sulfacetamide action. Wait 30 minutes to 1 hour after instilling anesthetic or PABA derivative before instilling sulfacetamide.
Silver preparations: precipitate formation. Avoid using together.

Nursing considerations
Assessment
• Review the patient's history for a condition that contraindicates the use of sulfacetamide.

Boldfaced adverse reactions are life-threatening

• Obtain a baseline assessment of the patient's ophthalmic infection before initiating sulfacetamide therapy.
• Be alert for common adverse reactions.
• Evaluate the patient's and family's knowledge about sulfacetamide therapy.

Planning (Nursing Diagnoses)

Potential nursing diagnoses for the patient receiving sulfacetamide include:
• Potential for infection related to ineffectiveness of sulfacetamide.
• Pain related to administration of sulfacetamide eye drops.
• Altered health maintenance related to sulfacetamide-induced adverse reactions.
• Knowledge deficit related to sulfacetamide therapy.

Implementation

Preparation and administration

—Instill 1 to 2 drops into the lower conjunctival sac.
—If using the ointment form of the drug, instill $\frac{1}{2}''$ to $1''$ of ointment into the conjunctival sac.
—A combination of drops and ointment may be prescribed for nighttime use; if so, drops must be administered before the ointment form.
—Be aware that the instillation of the drops may cause momentary pain.
—Separate by 30 minutes to 1 hour the instillation of a local anesthetic, such as procaine or tetracaine, and sulfacetamide.
—Do not touch the tip of the eyedropper to the eye or surrounding tissue.
—Keep the eyedropper clean.
—Do not allow solution to get on clothing because it may stain.
—Store the medication tightly closed and in a light-resistant container away from heat.
—Do not use any discolored (dark brown) solutions.
—Administer eye drops using the following procedure: Wash your hands; remove as much purulent exudate as possible from the lid before instilling the drug; position the patient's head back and to the side (with the unaffected eye up), with his eyes open and looking up; pull down the lower eyelid; and instill the drops in the conjunctival sac. Be careful and gentle, especially when the patient's eyes are irritated.
—If more than one kind of eye drop is prescribed, allow at least 5 minutes between each instillation.

Monitoring

—Monitor the effectiveness of therapy by regularly examining the patient's eye for signs of improvement, such as decreased redness, swelling, and discharge.
—Monitor for hypersensitivity reaction.
—Monitor for pain in the eye at time of administration and for brow pain or headache.
—Monitor the patient for adverse drug reactions.
—Monitor for photophobia and sensitivity to light.

—Monitor for Stevens-Johnson syndrome.

—Monitor the patient for drug interactions.

—Regularly reevaluate the patient's and family's knowledge about sulfacetamide therapy.

Intervention

—Hold drug and notify the doctor if itching or burning occurs.

—Do not administer with silver preparations.

—Administer a mild analgesic for headache, as prescribed and needed.

—Institute safety precautions if infection interferes with vision.

—Keep all members of the health care team informed of the patient's response to the drug.

Patient teaching

—Instruct the patient and family about sulfacetamide, including the dosage, frequency, action, and adverse reactions.

—Warn the patient that eye drops may burn slightly.

—Warn the patient to avoid sharing washcloths and towels with other family members because it can spread the infection to other persons.

—Tell the patient to watch for signs of sensitivity, such as itching lids, swelling, or constant burning.

—Tell the patient to stop the drug immediately and notify the doctor if he develops signs of sensitivity.

—Instruct the patient on the correct instillation of eye drops as follows: He should wash hands before and after administering the ointment or solution; not touch the tip of the dropper to the eye or surrounding tissues; and not lay the dropper down or touch it to any surface that might contaminate it. The patient should apply light finger-pressure on the lacrimal sac for 1 minute after instilling the drops.

—Emphasize the importance of complying with the directions on the prescription and of proper instillation.

—If more than one type of eye drop is prescribed, tell the patient to wait at least 5 minutes between each instillation.

—Warn the patient that the solution may stain clothing.

—Tell the patient to store the drug in a tightly closed, light-resistant container away from heat.

—Tell the patient not to use the solution if it is discolored (dark brown).

—Tell the patient not to share eye medication with family members or others. A family member who develops the same symptoms should contact the doctor.

—Tell the patient that he may experience some photophobia and should minimize it by wearing sunglasses and avoiding prolonged exposure to sunlight.

—Tell the patient to notify the nurse or doctor if adverse reactions develop or questions arise about sulfacetamide therapy.

Evaluation

In the patient receiving sulfacetamide, appropriate evaluation statements include:

• Patient's ophthalmic infection is resolved.
• Patient's pain is minimal upon administration of sulfacetamide.
• Patient does not experience serious adverse reactions.
• Patient and family state an understanding of sulfacetamide therapy and demonstrate correct administration technique.

SELECTED MAJOR DRUGS: OPHTHALMIC ANTI-INFECTIVES

DRUG, INDICATIONS, AND DOSAGES	SPECIAL PRECAUTIONS
bacitracin *Ocular infections—* **Adults and children:** apply small amount of ointment into conjunctival sac several times daily or p.r.n. until favorable response is observed.	• Contraindicated in patients with known hypersensitivity to any of the drug's components. • Use cautiously in patients with hereditary predisposition to antibiotic hypersensitivity.
boric acid *For irrigation after tonometry, gonioscopy, foreign body removal, or use of fluorescein; used to soothe and cleanse the eye—* **Adults:** apply 5% or 10% ointment p.r.n.	• Contraindicated in patients with eye lacerations. • Administer cautiously to patients who are sensitive to mercury. Drug should not be used with a wetting solution for contact lenses or other eye-care products containing polyvinyl alcohol.
gentamicin sulfate (Gentacidin) *External ocular infections (conjunctivitis, keratoconjunctivitis, corneal ulcers, blepharitis, blepharoconjunctivitis, meibomianitis, and dacryocystitis) caused by susceptible organisms, especially* Pseudomonas aeruginosa, Proteus, Klebsiella pneumoniae, Escherichia coli, *and other gram-negative organisms—* **Adults and children:** instill 1 to 2 drops in eye q 4 hours. In severe infections, may use up to 2 drops hourly. Or apply ointment to lower conjunctival sac b.i.d. or t.i.d.	• Contraindicated in patients with known hypersensitivity to aminoglycosides. • Use cautiously in patients with impaired renal function.
polymyxin B sulfate *Used alone or in combination with other agents for treating corneal ulcers resulting from infection caused by* Pseudomonas *or other gram-negative organisms—* **Adults and children:** instill 1 to 3 drops of 0.1% to 0.25% solution (10,000 to 25,000 units/ml) q 1 hour. Increase interval according to patient response; or up to 10,000 units subconjunctivally daily by doctor. Do not exceed 2 million units daily.	• Contraindicated in patients with epithelial herpes simplex keratitis, vaccinia, varicella, and various other viral diseases of the cornea and conjunctiva; mycobacterial infection of the eye; fungal diseases of ocular structures; or known hypersensitivity to any of the drug's components. • Administer cautiously; prolonged use may result in glaucoma or increase the risk of secondary ocular infections.

(continued)

SELECTED MAJOR DRUGS: OPHTHALMIC ANTI-INFECTIVES *continued*

DRUG, INDICATIONS, AND DOSAGES	SPECIAL PRECAUTIONS
silver nitrate 1% *Prevention of gonorrheal ophthalmia neonatorum—* **Neonates:** cleanse lids thoroughly; instill 1 drop of 1% solution into each eye.	• Contraindicated in patients with known hypersensitivity to any of the drug's components. • Use 1% solution cautiously because cauterization of the cornea and blindness may result, especially with repeated applications.
vidarabine (Vira-A Ophthalmic) *Acute keratoconjunctivitis, superficial keratitis, and recurrent epithelial keratitis resulting from herpes simplex viruses types I and II—* **Adults and children:** instill ½″ ointment into lower conjunctival sac five times daily at 3-hour intervals.	• Contraindicated in patients with known hypersensitivity to the drug. • Administer cautiously; drug may produce a temporary visual haze.

COMPARING OPHTHALMIC ANTI-INFECTIVE COMBINATIONS

TRADE NAME AND CONTENT	SPECIAL CONSIDERATIONS
Cortisporin Ophthalmic Ointment polymyxin B sulfate 10,000 units, bacitracin zinc 400 units, neomycin sulfate 0.35%, and hydrocortisone 1%	• Combines the antimicrobial actions of polymyxin B, bacitracin zinc, and neomycin with the anti-inflammatory effect of hydrocortisone. • Contraindicated in patients with epithelial herpes simplex keratitis (dendritic keratitis), vaccinia, varicella, and various other viral diseases of the cornea and conjunctiva; mycobacterial infection of the eye; fungal diseases of ocular structures; or known hypersensitivity to any of the drug's components; and after uncomplicated removal of a corneal foreign body. • Use cautiously during pregnancy or breast-feeding and with prolonged use.
Cortisporin Ophthalmic Suspension polymyxin B sulfate 10,000 units, neomycin sulfate 0.35%, and hydrocortisone 1%	• Combines the antimicrobial actions of polymyxin B and neomycin with the anti-inflammatory effect of hydrocortisone. • Contraindicated in patients with epithelial herpes simplex keratitis (dendritic keratitis), vaccinia, varicella, and various other viral diseases of the cornea and conjunctiva; mycobacterial infection of the eye; fungal diseases of ocular structures; or known hy-

COMPARING OPHTHALMIC ANTI-INFECTIVE COMBINATIONS
continued

TRADE NAME AND CONTENT	SPECIAL CONSIDERATIONS
Cortisporin Ophthalmic Suspension *(continued)*	persensitivity to any of the drug's components; and after uncomplicated removal of a corneal foreign body. • Use cautiously during pregnancy or breast-feeding and with prolonged use.
Neotal polymyxin B sulfate 5,000 units, neomycin sulfate 5 mg, and bacitracin zinc 400 units	• Combines the antimicrobial actions of polymyxin B, neomycin, and bacitracin zinc. • Contraindicated in patients with known hypersensitivity to any of the drug's components. • Use cautiously with prolonged use.
Polysporin Ophthalmic Ointment polymyxin B sulfate 10,000 units and bacitracin zinc 500 units	• Combines the antimicrobial action of polymyxin B with the antimicrobial action of bacitracin zinc. • Contraindicated in patients with known hypersensitivity to any of the drug's components. • Use cautiously during prolonged use.

SELF-TEST

1. Mark Cameron came to the ophthalmologist because of pain in his eye. His doctor diagnosed corneal ulcers and prescribed sulfacetamide, an ophthalmic anti-infective solution. The nurse should know that the patient's eye drops would be instilled:
   a. in the inner canthus of the eye.
   b. in the outer corner of the eye.
   c. in the lower conjunctival sac.
   d. in the upper corner of the eye nearest the nose.

2. If Mr. Cameron's doctor also prescribed a local anesthetic (such as procaine) for instillation into the eye, the nurse would administer these eye drops:
   a. 30 minutes to 1 hour apart.
   b. at the same time.
   c. after discontinuing the anti-infective agent.
   c. 15 minutes apart.

3. Patient teaching for Mr. Cameron should *not* include which of the following remarks?

a. Warn patient not to share washcloths or towels with family members.

b. The drug may cause itching and burning, but this is normal.

c. It is extremely important to follow the directions for this drug as prescribed.

d. If other eye drops are prescribed, wait at least 5 minutes between each instillation.

Check your answers on page 1075.

OPHTHALMIC ANTI-INFLAMMATORY AGENTS

dexamethasone ◆ dexamethasone sodium phosphate ◆ diclofenac sodium
fluorometholone ◆ flurbiprofen sodium ◆ medrysone ◆ prednisolone acetate
prednisolone sodium phosphate ◆ suprofen

OVERVIEW

- Topical corticosteroids exert an anti-inflammatory action, suppressing aspects of the inflammatory process, such as hyperemia, cellular infiltration, vascularization, and fibroblastic proliferation. These drugs inhibit the inflammatory response if the cause is mechanical, chemical, or immunologic. Anti-inflammatory agents should not be used to treat ocular tuberculosis or acute superficial herpes simplex, keratitis, fungal diseases of ocular structures, varicella, or most other viral diseases of the cornea and conjunctiva. Medrysone should not be used in iritis and uveitis.

MAJOR USES

- Topical corticosteroids are effective in acute inflammatory conditions of the conjunctiva, sclera, cornea, lids, iris, ciliary body, and anterior segment of the globe and in ocular allergic conditions.
- Specific indications include the following: allergic conjunctivitis; nonspecific superficial keratitis; superficial keratitis; herpes zoster keratitis; iritis; cyclitis; selected infective conjunctivitis; corneal injury from chemical, radiation, or thermal burns; penetration of foreign bodies; and suppression of graft rejection following keratoplasty. Difficult cases of anterior segment eye disease, especially those that involve deeper ocular structures, require systemic therapy.
- Flurbiprofen and suprofen are used for the inhibition of intraoperative miosis. Flurbiprofen has additional unlabeled uses for the topical treatment of cystoid macular edema, inflammation after cataract surgery, and uveitis syndromes.
- Diclofenac is used to treat postoperative inflammation after cataract extraction.

MECHANISM OF ACTION

- These drugs are thought to act through potentiation of epinephrine vasoconstriction, stabilization of lysosomal membranes, retardation of

GLOSSARY

Glaucoma: eye disorder characterized by increased intraocular pressure.

Hyperemia: increased blood flow to an area, causing redness and increased warmth.

Iritis: inflammation of the iris.

Keratoplasty: excision of an opaque portion of the cornea.

macrophage movement, prevention of kinin release, inhibition of lymphocyte and neutrophil function, inhibition of prostaglandin synthesis, and, in prolonged use, decreased antibody production. Decreased scarring with clearer corneas after topical corticosteroid therapy results from inhibition of fibroblastic proliferation and vascularization.

- Flurbiprofen and suprofen are thought to act through inhibition of an enzyme essential in the biosynthesis of prostaglandins, which mediate certain kinds of intraocular inflammation.

ABSORPTION, DISTRIBUTION, METABOLISM, AND EXCRETION

Although these drugs are used for their local effects, most of them will penetrate the cornea and result in significant systemic absorption. Once absorbed, they are highly protein-bound (99%). They are metabolized in the liver and excreted in the urine as inactive metabolites.

ONSET AND DURATION

Onset and duration of corticosteroid eye drops is highly variable. They may be used hourly in severe disease. In mild conditions, 1 or 2 drops or a thin application of ointment can be used every 4 to 12 hours, depending on the product and severity of the inflammation. In both severe and mild conditions, the dosage is tapered to discontinuation as the condition improves. Duration of treatment varies with the type and severity of the condition and may extend from a few days to several weeks, depending on the response. Relapse may occur if therapy is reduced rapidly.

Treatment with nonsteroidal anti-inflammatory agents usually begins 2 or 3 hours before surgery when they are used to produce intraoperative miosis. Diclofenac therapy to treat postoperative inflammation after cataract extraction usually begins 24 hours after surgery. Its anti-inflammatory effect lasts about 6 hours. Therapy is continued for 2 weeks.

ADVERSE REACTIONS

Ocular reactions to ophthalmic anti-inflammatory agents may include glaucoma with optic nerve damage; visual acuity and field defects; posterior subcapsular cataract formation; secondary ocular infection from pathogens, including herpes simplex; perforation of the globe; exacerbation of viral or fungal corneal infections; transient stinging and burning at instillation and keratitis (with diclofenac); and sensitivity to bright light (with dexamethasone and prednisone). Among these agents, fluoro-metholone and medrysone are the least likely to cause increased intraocular pressure with long-term use.

Systemic reactions are associated with extensive use. Flurbiprofen is embryocidal and may cause increased bleeding tendencies and delayed wound healing.

Note: Because oral doses of diclofenac and suprofen can cause maternal and fetal adverse reactions, monitor use of these agents in ophthalmic dosing forms.

PROTOTYPE: OPHTHALMIC ANTI-INFLAMMATORY AGENTS

DEXAMETHASONE SODIUM PHOSPHATE
(dex a meth' a sone)
Decadron Phosphate, Maxidex
Classification: ophthalmic anti-inflammatory agent
Pregnancy risk category C

How supplied
OPHTHALMIC OINTMENT: 0.05%
OPHTHALMIC SOLUTION: 0.1%

Indications and dosage
Uveitis; iridocyclitis; inflammatory conditions of eyelids, conjunctiva, cornea, and anterior segment of globe; corneal injury from chemical or thermal burns or penetration of foreign bodies; allergic conjunctivitis
ADULTS AND CHILDREN: instill 1 to 2 drops of 0.01% suspension or 0.1% solution into lower conjunctival sac. In severe disease, drops may be used hourly, tapering to discontinuation as condition improves. In mild conditions, drops may be used up to four to six times daily or ointment applied q.i.d. As condition improves, taper dosage to b.i.d., then to once daily. Treatment may extend from a few days to several weeks.

Contraindications and precautions
Dexamethasone is contraindicated in patients with acute superficial herpes simplex (dendritic keratitis); vaccinia, varicella, or other fungal or viral diseases of cornea and conjunctiva; ocular tuberculosis; or any acute, purulent, untreated infection of the eye. Use cautiously in corneal abrasions because these may be infected (especially with herpes) and in glaucoma (any form) because of possibility of increasing intraocular pressure (glaucoma medications may need to be increased to compensate).

Adverse reactions
EYE: increased intraocular pressure; thinning of cornea; interference with corneal wound healing; increased susceptibility to viral or fungal corneal infection; corneal ulceration, glaucoma exacerbations, cataracts, defects in visual acuity and visual field, optic nerve damage (with excessive or

long-term use); mild blurred vision; *burning, stinging, or redness of eyes; watery eyes.*
OTHER: systemic effects and adrenal suppression with excessive or long-term use.

Interactions
None significant.

Nursing considerations

Assessment
- Review the patient's history for a condition that contraindicates the use of dexamethasone.
- Obtain a baseline assessment of the patient's ophthalmic inflammatory condition before initiating dexamethasone therapy.
- Be alert for common or serious adverse reactions.
- Evaluate the patient's and family's knowledge about dexamethasone therapy.

Planning (Nursing Diagnoses)
Potential nursing diagnoses for the patient receiving dexamethasone include:
- Sensory/perceptual alterations (visual) related to ineffectiveness of dexamethasone dosage regimen to relieve inflammation.
- Potential for infection related to increased susceptibility to viral or fungal corneal infection caused by dexamethasone use.
- Knowledge deficit related to dexamethasone therapy.

Implementation

Preparation and administration
— Shake the suspension before using.
— If using the ointment form of the drug, instill ½″ to 1″ of ointment into lower conjunctival sac.
— An eye pad may be used with the ointment form of the drug.
— Instillation of eye drops may cause momentary discomfort.
— Do not touch tip of the eyedropper to the eye or surrounding tissue.
— Keep the eyedropper clean.
— Administer the eye drops correctly, using the following procedure: Wash your hands; remove as much purulent exudate as possible from the eyelid before instilling the medication; position the patient's head back and to the side (with the unaffected eye up), with his eyes open and looking up; pull down the lower eyelid; and instill the drops in the lower conjunctival sac. Be careful and gentle, especially when the patient's eyes are irritated.

Monitoring
— Monitor the effectiveness of therapy by regularly examining the patient's eyes for signs of improvement, for example, decreased redness and swelling.

Italicized adverse reactions are common

— Monitor the patient's reaction to dexamethasone with follow-up ophthalmic examination that includes measurement of intraocular pressure, especially with high dosage or prolonged use.

— Monitor the patient for adverse reactions to dexamethasone.

— Monitor for visual changes.

— Monitor for eye infections because of increased susceptibility to viral or fungal corneal infection with dexamethasone use.

— Monitor for localized reactions: burning, stinging, or redness of eyes.

— Monitor for adrenal suppression with excessive or long-term use.

— Regularly reevaluate the patient's and family's knowledge about dexamethasone therapy.

Intervention

— Withhold drug and notify the doctor if corneal ulceration, eye infection, or other serious adverse reactions occur.

— Be prepared to administer ophthalmic anti-infectives if a viral or fungal corneal infection occurs.

— Institute safety precautions if visual disturbances occur.

— Keep all members of the health care team informed of the patient's response to the drug.

Patient teaching

— Instruct the patient and family about dexamethasone, including the dosage, frequency, action, and adverse reactions.

— Warn the patient to call the doctor immediately and to discontinue the drug if visual acuity changes or visual field diminishes.

— Warn the patient that eye drops might cause some discomfort.

— Warn the patient to avoid sharing washcloths and towels with other family members because this can spread eye infection to others.

— Teach the patient how to instill the drug into the eye correctly: He should wash his hands before and after administering the drug, not touch the dropper tip to the eye or surrounding tissue, and should apply light finger-pressure on the lacrimal sac for 1 minute after instillation.

— Warn the patient not to use leftover medication for a new eye inflammation. This may cause serious problems.

— Tell the patient not to share his eye medications with family members. A family member who develops similar symptoms should contact the doctor.

— Tell the patient to shake the suspension before using.

— Tell the patient to notify the nurse or doctor if adverse reactions develop or questions arise about dexamethasone therapy.

Evaluation

In the patient receiving dexamethasone, appropriate evaluation statements include:

• Patient shows no signs of eye inflammation.

• Patient shows no signs of eye infection.

• Patient and family state an understanding of dexamethasone therapy and demonstrate proper administration technique.

SELECTED MAJOR DRUGS: OPHTHALMIC ANTI-INFLAMMATORY AGENTS

DRUG, INDICATIONS, AND DOSAGES	SPECIAL PRECAUTIONS
fluorometholone (FML S.O.P.) *Inflammatory and allergic conditions of cornea, conjunctiva, sclera, and anterior uvea—* **Adults and children:** instill 1 to 2 drops in conjunctival sac b.i.d. to q.i.d. May use q 1 hour during first 1 to 2 days if needed. Alternatively, apply thin strip of ointment to conjunctiva q 4 hours, decreasing to once daily to t.i.d. as inflammation subsides.	• Contraindicated in patients with vaccinia, varicella, acute superficial herpes simplex (dendritic keratitis), or other fungal or viral eye diseases; ocular tuberculosis; or any acute, purulent, untreated eye infection. • Use cautiously in corneal abrasions because they may be contaminated (especially with herpes).
flurbiprofen (Ocufen) *Inhibition of intraoperative miosis—* **Adults:** instill 1 drop approximately q 30 minutes, beginning 2 hours before surgery. Give a total of 4 drops.	• Contraindicated in patients with epithelial herpes simplex keratitis. • Because this drug is an NSAID, use cautiously in patients who may be allergic to aspirin and other NSAIDs. • Use cautiously in patients with bleeding tendencies and in those who are receiving medications that may prolong clotting times.
medrysone (HMS Liquifilm Ophthalmic) *Allergic conjunctivitis, vernal conjunctivitis, episcleritis, ophthalmic epinephrine sensitivity reaction—* **Adults and children:** instill 1 drop in conjunctival sac b.i.d. to q.i.d. May use q 1 hour during first 1 to 2 days if needed.	• Contraindicated in patients with vaccinia, varicella, acute superficial herpes simplex (dendritic keratitis), or other fungal or viral eye diseases; ocular tuberculosis; iritis; uveitis; or any acute, purulent, untreated eye infection. • Use cautiously in corneal abrasions because they may be contaminated (especially with herpes).
prednisolone (Pred-Fort) **prednisolone sodium phosphate (Inflamase Ophthalmic)** *Inflammation of palpebral and bulbar conjunctiva, cornea, and anterior segment of globe—* **Adults and children:** instill 1 to 2 drops of 0.12% to 1% suspension (acetate) or 0.125% to 1% solution (phosphate) in conjunctival sac. In severe conditions, may be used hourly, tapering to discontinuation as inflammation subsides. In mild conditions, may be used up to four to six times daily.	• Contraindicated in patients with acute, untreated, purulent ocular infections; acute superficial herpes simplex (dendritic keratitis), vaccinia, varicella, or other viral or fungal eye diseases; or ocular tuberculosis. • Use cautiously in corneal abrasions because they may be contaminated (especially with herpes).

COMPARING OPHTHALMIC ANTI-INFLAMMATORY COMBINATIONS

TRADE NAME AND CONTENT	SPECIAL CONSIDERATIONS
Maxitrol Ointment **Maxitrol Ophthalmic Suspension** dexamethasone 0.1%, neomycin sulfate 0.35%, and polymyxin B sulfate 10,000 units	• Combines the anti-inflammatory action of dexamethasone with the anti-infective actions of neomycin and polymyxin B. • Contraindicated in patients with epithelial herpes simplex keratitis (dendritic keratitis), vaccinia, varicella, and various other viral diseases of the cornea and conjunctiva; mycobacterial infection of the eye; fungal diseases of ocular structures; or known hypersensitivity to any of the drug's components; and after uncomplicated removal of a corneal foreign body. • Use cautiously during prolonged administration.
NeoDecadron Ophthalmic Ointment dexamethasone sodium phosphate 1% and neomycin sulfate 0.35%	• Combines the anti-inflammatory action of dexamethasone with the anti-infective action of neomycin. • Contraindicated in patients with epithelial herpes simplex keratitis (dendritic keratitis), vaccinia, varicella, and various other viral diseases of the cornea and conjunctiva; mycobacterial infection of the eye; fungal diseases of ocular structures; or known hypersensitivity to any of the drug's components; and after uncomplicated removal of a corneal foreign body. • Use cautiously during prolonged administration.

SELF-TEST

1. Irma Walker, age 57, developed allergic conjunctivitis after using a new eye makeup. To relieve her red, watery, itchy eyes, her doctor prescribed dexamethasone 2 drops of 0.1% solution to be instilled into each lower conjunctival sac six times daily. Before instructing Mrs. Walker about this drug, the office nurse checked her medical history for contraindications. Which of the following conditions contraindicates the use of dexamethasone?
   a. Ocular tuberculosis
   b. Refractory disturbances
   c. Glaucoma
   d. Corneal abrasions

2. The nurse instructed Mrs. Walker to avoid excessive use of the drug and to use only as directed. Which of the following adverse reactions could result from excessive use of dexamethasone?
   a. Optic nerve damage
   b. Increased intraocular pressure
   c. Corneal ulceration
   d. Miosis

3. Later in the day, Mrs. Walker called the nurse to say she is too afraid to have her husband apply the eye drops, fearing he will poke her eyes with the dropper. Her doctor changed the prescription to an ointment form with a q.i.d. dosage schedule. How much ointment should Mr. Walker apply?
   a. Scant amount of ointment in each conjunctival sac
   b. ¼″ to ½″ of ointment in each conjunctival sac
   c. ½″ to 1″ of ointment in each conjunctival sac
   d. 2″ of ointment in each conjunctival sac

Check your answers on page 1076.

CHAPTER 79

MIOTICS

acetylcholine chloride ◆ carbachol ◆ demecarium bromide
echothiophate iodide ◆ isoflurophate ◆ physostigmine salicylate
pilocarpine hydrochloride ◆ pilocarpine nitrate

OVERVIEW

- Miotics are topical drugs that cause pupillary constriction (miosis). They are used in chronic ophthalmic conditions and in surgical procedures for ocular disorders.

MAJOR USES

- Miotics are used to treat open-angle and narrow-angle glaucoma. They are also therapeutic in iridectomy, anterior segment surgery, and other ocular surgery. When used with mydriatics, they prevent adhesions after ocular surgery.

MECHANISM OF ACTION

- Acetylcholine, carbachol, and pilocarpine (cholinergics) cause contraction of the sphincter muscles of the iris, resulting in miosis. They also produce ciliary spasm, deepening of the anterior chamber, and vasodilation of conjunctival vessels of the outflow tract.
- Demecarium, echothiophate, isoflurophate, and physostigmine (cholinesterase inhibitors) inhibit the enzymatic destruction of acetylcholine by inactivating cholinesterase. This leaves acetylcholine free to act on the effector cells of the iridic sphincter and ciliary muscles, causing pupillary constriction and accommodation spasm.

ABSORPTION, DISTRIBUTION, METABOLISM, AND EXCRETION

Little is known about the pharmacokinetics of these agents. Because small amounts of the drugs are applied locally to the eye, they usually do not produce measurable blood levels. However, some systemic absorption is possible with all agents except acetylcholine. Significant systemic absorption may cause adverse reactions, including hypersalivation, nausea, vomiting, and bronchospasm. Among all the drugs, demecarium and echothiophate are most likely to produce adverse systemic reactions when used excessively.

Because acetylcholine is a naturally occurring neurotransmitter, its metabolic fate has been well studied. Acetylcholine is metabolized by acetylcholinesterase and is broken down finally into choline and acetic acid. Choline is then taken up by the presynaptic neuron and reused in the

GLOSSARY

Iridectomy: surgical incision of part of the iris.
Miosis: contraction of the pupil.
Miotic: ophthalmic agent used to cause pupil constriction.

synthesis of more acetylcholine; acetic acid dissipates in extracellular fluid.

ONSET AND DURATION

The onset of action of acetylcholine is rapid, usually within seconds of application. Its effects last 10 to 20 minutes. Carbachol and pilocarpine act within 10 to 30 minutes, peak in 2 to 4 hours, and last 4 to 8 hours. Physostigmine begins to act in 10 to 30 minutes, and its effects last 12 to 48 hours. The other cholinesterase inhibitors are long-acting agents, with effects lasting from 3 to 10 days (demecarium) to 1 to 4 weeks (echothiophate and isoflurophate).

ADVERSE REACTIONS

The topically applied miotics produce similar adverse reactions, which are usually more severe with the long-acting cholinesterase inhibitors. Pilocarpine is generally well tolerated. Adverse reactions to the other agents may be reduced by starting with the lowest concentration, gradually increasing dosage, and administering the daily dose at bedtime.

The most common reactions are painful ciliary spasm, blurred vision, and poor vision in low light. Other adverse ocular reactions may include burning, lacrimation, pain, headache, photophobia, twitching of the eyelids, conjunctival congestion, and lacrimal passage stenosis.

Miotics may cause iris cysts, anterior chamber hyperemia, and activation of iritis or uveitis, but these reactions are more common with long-acting cholinesterase inhibitors.

Hypersensitivity reactions, such as allergic conjunctivitis, dermatitis, or keratitis, occur more frequently with physostigmine.

Systemic toxicity may occur with frequent or prolonged topical use of miotics and is more frequent with long-acting miotics. These reactions result from parasympathetic stimulation and include nausea, vomiting, diarrhea, and cramps. Frequent urination, excessive salivation, sweating, pallor, cyanosis, and bronchoconstriction have also been reported. Systemically absorbed miotics have precipitated asthmatic attacks and cardiac arrest after vagal stimulation during surgery. Severe miotic toxicity may cause tremor, muscle weakness, cardiac arrhythmias, hypotension, CNS excitation and depression, confusion, ataxia, seizures, and coma.

Miotics should be discontinued, at least temporarily, if they cause systemic reactions.

PILOCARPINE HYDROCHLORIDE
(pye loe kar' peen)
*Adsorbocarpine, Isopto Carpine, Miocarpine†, Ocusert Pilo, Pilocar,
Pilocel, Pilomiotin, Pilopine HS, Pilopt‡*

PILOCARPINE NITRATE
Pilagan
Classification: miotic
Pregnancy risk category C

How supplied
hydrochloride
OPHTHALMIC SOLUTION: 0.25%, 0.5%, 1%, 2%, 3%, 4%, 5%, 6%, 8%, 10%
OPHTHALMIC GEL: 4%
RELEASING-SYSTEM INSERT: 20 mcg/hr, 40 mcg/hr
nitrate
OPHTHALMIC SOLUTION: 1%, 2%, 4%

Indications and dosage
Primary open-angle glaucoma
ADULTS: instill 1 to 2 drops daily to q.i.d. in eye, as directed by doctor. Or
may apply 4% gel (Pilopine HS) daily.
   Alternatively, apply one Ocusert Pilo system (20 or 40 mcg/hour) q 7
days.

Emergency treatment of acute narrow-angle glaucoma
ADULTS AND CHILDREN: 1 drop of 2% solution q 5 minutes for three to six
doses, followed by 1 drop q 1 to 3 hours until intraocular pressure is
controlled.

Contraindications and precautions
Pilocarpine is contraindicated in acute iritis, acute inflammatory disease
of anterior segment of eye, and secondary glaucoma. Use cautiously in
bronchial asthma and hypertension.

Adverse reactions
EYE: *suborbital headache, myopia, ciliary spasm, blurred vision, conjunctival irritation, lacrimation, changes in visual field, brow pain.*
GI: nausea, vomiting, abdominal cramps, diarrhea, salivation.
OTHER: **bronchiolar spasm, pulmonary edema,** hypersensitivity.

Interactions
Carbachol and echothiophate: additive effect. Don't use together.
*Ophthalmic belladonna alkaloids (such as atropine and scopolamine) and
cyclopentolate:* decreased antiglaucoma effects of pilocarpine; mydriatic
effects of these agents blocked by pilocarpine. Don't use together.
Phenylephrine: decreased dilation by phenylephrine. Don't use together.

---

†Available in Canada only   ‡Available in Australia only
Italicized adverse reactions are common   Boldfaced adverse reactions are life-threatening

Nursing considerations

Assessment

- Review the patient's history for a condition that contraindicates the use of pilocarpine.
- Obtain a baseline assessment of the patient's glaucoma, including type and which eye (or both) is affected, before initiating pilocarpine therapy.
- Be alert for common adverse reactions.
- Evaluate the patient's and family's knowledge about pilocarpine therapy.
- Evaluate the elderly patient's ability to self-administer eye drops.

Planning (Nursing Diagnoses)

Potential nursing diagnoses for the patient receiving pilocarpine include:
- Sensory/perceptual alterations (visual) related to ineffectiveness of pilocarpine dosage regimen to lower intraocular pressure.
- Potential for injury related to pilocarpine-induced blurred vision.
- Knowledge deficit related to pilocarpine therapy.

Implementation

Preparation and administration

—Use proper instillation technique.

—The drug may be administered with other drugs.

—The drug is available in different concentrations. Make sure the correct drug dosage has been confirmed before administration.

—Instill the gel form of the drug at bedtime because it will blur the patient's vision.

—The Ocusert Pilo system is inserted every 7 days at bedtime. It should be placed in the upper or lower conjunctival sac.

—If the Ocusert Pilo system falls out of the patient's eye during sleep, rinse the system in cool tap water and reposition it in the patient's eye.

—The Ocusert Pilo system should be stored in the refrigerator.

—Instillation of drops may cause momentary discomfort.

—Do not touch tip of the eyedropper to the eye or surrounding tissue.

—Keep the eyedropper clean.

—Administer the eye drops correctly, using the following procedure: Wash your hands; position the patient's head back and to the side (with the unaffected eye up), with his eyes open and looking up; pull down the lower eyelid; and instill the drops in the lower conjunctival sac.

Monitoring

—Monitor the effectiveness of therapy by regularly having the patient's intraocular pressure checked.

—Monitor for drug-induced visual changes, such as blurred vision or changes in visual field.

—Monitor local reactions, such as suborbital headache, myopia, ciliary spasm, conjunctival irritation, lacrimation, and brow pain.

—Monitor the patient for adverse drug reactions.

—Monitor hydration status if adverse GI reactions occur.

—Monitor pulmonary status for evidence of bronchospasm or pulmonary edema.

—Monitor the patient for hypersensitivity reactions.

—Monitor the patient for drug interactions.

—Monitor the patient's compliance with pilocarpine therapy.

—Regularly reevaluate the patient's and family's knowledge about pilocarpine therapy.

Intervention

—Withhold drug and notify the doctor if hypersensitivity develops.

—Keep an anticholinergic agent (such as atropine) readily available in case the patient has a severe systemic response to pilocarpine.

—Institute safety precautions if visual disturbances occur.

—Obtain an order for an antiemetic or antidiarrheal as needed.

—Withhold drug and notify the doctor if bronchospasm or pulmonary edema occurs. Be prepared to treat according to the doctor's instructions.

—Keep all members of the health care team informed of the patient's response to the drug.

Patient teaching

—Instruct the patient and family about pilocarpine, including the dosage, frequency, action, and adverse reactions.

—Warn the patient that vision will be temporarily blurred, that miotic pupil may make surroundings appear dim and reduce peripheral field of vision, and that transient brow ache and myopia are common at first; assure the patient that adverse reactions subside 10 to 14 days after therapy begins.

—Tell the patient that, if the Ocusert Pilo system falls out of the eye during sleep, he should wash his hands, then rinse Ocusert in cool tap water and reposition it in the eye.

—Tell the patient to use caution in night driving and other activities in poor illumination because miotic pupil diminishes side vision and illumination.

—Stress importance of complying with prescribed medical regimen.

—Reassure the patient that adverse reactions will subside.

—Teach the patient who can manage self-administration how to instill the drug into the eye correctly: He should wash his hands before and after administering the drug, should not touch the dropper tip to the eye or surrounding tissue, and should apply light finger-pressure on the lacrimal sac for 1 minute after instillation to minimize systemic absorption.

—Tell the patient to notify the nurse or doctor if adverse reactions develop or questions arise about pilocarpine therapy.

Evaluation

In the patient receiving pilocarpine, appropriate evaluation statements include:

• Patient's intraocular pressure is normal.

• Patient does not experience injury as a result of visual disturbance.

• Patient and family state an understanding of pilocarpine therapy and demonstrate proper administration technique.

SELECTED MAJOR DRUGS: MIOTICS

DRUG, INDICATIONS, AND DOSAGES	SPECIAL PRECAUTIONS
acetylcholine (Miochol) *Anterior segment surgery—* **Adults and children:** doctor gently instills 0.5 to 2 ml of 1% solution into anterior chamber of eye.	• Contraindicated in patients with known hypersensitivity to the drug and in those in whom miosis is undesirable (for example, those with acute iritis). • Administer cautiously to patients with acute cardiac failure, bronchial asthma, peptic ulcer, hyperthyroidism, GI spasm, urinary tract obstruction, or Parkinson's disease.
carbachol (Miostat, Isopto Carbachol) *Ocular surgery (to produce pupillary miosis)—* **Adults:** doctor gently instills 0.5 ml (intraocular form) into anterior chamber for production of satisfactory miosis. It may be instilled before or after securing sutures. *Open-angle glaucoma—* **Adults:** instill 1 drop (topical form) into eye daily, b.i.d., t.i.d., or q.i.d.	• Contraindicated in patients with acute iritis or corneal abrasion. • Use cautiously in patients with acute heart failure, bronchial asthma, peptic ulcer, hyperthyroidism, GI spasm, urinary tract obstruction, or Parkinson's disease.
demecarium (Humorsol) *Angle-closure glaucoma after iridectomy, primary open-angle glaucoma—* **Adults:** instill 1 drop of 0.125% or 0.25% solution daily or b.i.d. *Treatment of accommodative esotropia (uncomplicated)—* **Adults:** instill 1 drop of 0.125% or 0.25% solution daily for 2 to 3 weeks, then reduce to 1 drop q 2 days for 3 to 4 weeks. After reevaluation, 1 drop once or twice weekly to once q 2 days as determined by patient's condition. Reevaluate q 4 to 12 weeks, adjusting dose as needed. Discontinue after 4 months if dose required is 1 drop q 2 days. *Diagnostic use—* **Adults:** 1 drop daily for 2 weeks, then 1 drop q 2 days for 2 to 3 weeks.	• Contraindicated in patients with bronchial asthma, pronounced bradycardia and hypotension, Down's syndrome, seizure disorder, spastic GI disturbances, angle-closure glaucoma before iridectomy, Parkinson's disease, uveitis, marked vagotonia, MI, or a history of retinal detachment. • Administer cautiously to patients with chronic angle-closure glaucoma; repeated administration may cause reduced serum concentration of electrolytes and cholinesterase with resultant systemic effects; also use cautiously in children and in pregnant or breast-feeding women.
echothiophate (Phospholine Iodide) *Primary open-angle glaucoma, conditions obstructing aqueous outflow—* **Adults and children:** instill 1 drop of 0.03% to 0.125% solution into conjunctival sac daily. Maximum is 1 drop b.i.d. Use lowest possible dosage to continuously control intraocular pressure. *Diagnosis of accommodative esotropia—* **Adults:** instill 1 drop of 0.03% to 0.125% solution daily or every other day h.s.	• Contraindicated in patients with narrow-angle glaucoma, seizure disorder, vasomotor instability, parkinsonism, iodide hypersensitivity, active uveal inflammation, bronchial asthma, spastic GI conditions, urinary tract obstruction, peptic ulcer, severe bradycardia or hypotension, vascular hypertension, MI,

SELECTED MAJOR DRUGS: MIOTICS *continued*

DRUG, INDICATIONS, AND DOSAGES	SPECIAL PRECAUTIONS
echothiophate *(continued)*	or a history of retinal detachment. • Use cautiously in patients routinely exposed to organophosphate insecticides; may cause nausea, vomiting, and diarrhea, progressing to muscle weakness and respiratory difficulty. Use cautiously in patients with myasthenia gravis receiving anticholinesterase therapy.
isoflurophate (Floropyrl) *Antiglaucoma agent—* **Adults:** apply thin strip of ointment to conjunctiva once q 3 days to t.i.d. *Treatment of accommodative esotropia (uncomplicated); diagnostic—* **Adults:** apply thin strip of ointment to conjunctiva h.s. for 2 weeks. *Treatment of accommodative esotropia—* **Adults:** apply thin strip of ointment to conjunctiva h.s. for 2 weeks, then once weekly to once q 2 days, depending on patient's condition, for 2 months. If patient cannot be maintained on q-2-days dosage, discontinue drug.	• Contraindicated in patients with bronchial asthma, pronounced bradycardia and hypotension, Down's syndrome, seizure disorder, spastic GI disturbances, angle-closure glaucoma before iridectomy, Parkinson's disease, uveitis, marked vagotonia, MI, or a history of retinal detachment. • Use cautiously in patients with chronic angle-closure and narrow-angle cautiously because of the risk of carcinogenesis, mutagenesis, and impairment of fertility; use with caution in children and in pregnant and breast-feeding women.
physostigmine (Eserine Sulfate, Isopto-Eserine) *Open-angle glaucoma—* **Adults and children:** 1 drop of 0.25% to 0.5% solution b.i.d. to t.i.d. or thin strip of ointment daily to t.i.d.	• Contraindicated in patients with intolerance to physostigmine, active uveitis, or corneal injury. • Administer cautiously due to possibility of hypersensitivity in an occasional patient. Keep atropine injection on hand because it is an antagonist and antidote for physostigmine.

COMPARING MIOTIC COMBINATIONS

TRADE NAME AND CONTENT	SPECIAL CONSIDERATIONS
E-Pilo P_1E_1 P_2E_1 P_3E_1 P_4E_1 P_6E_1 epinephrine bitartrate 1% and pilocarpine hydrochloride 1%, 2%, 3%, 4%, or 6%	• Combine the mydriatic action of epinephrine with the miotic action of pilocarpine. • Contraindicated in patients with acute iritis, acute inflammatory disease of anterior segment of eye, secondary or narrow-angle glaucoma, or shallow anterior chamber. • Use cautiously in patients with diabetes mellitus, hypertension, Parkinson's disease, hyperthyroidism, aphakia, cardiac disease, bronchial asthma, or cerebral arteriosclerosis and in elderly or pregnant patients.
Isopto-P-ES pilocarpine hydrochloride 2% and physostigmine salicylate 0.25%	• Combines the miotic actions of pilocarpine and physostigmine. • Contraindicated in patients with acute iritis, acute inflammatory disease of anterior segment of eye, secondary glaucoma, active uveitis, corneal injury, or known intolerance to physostigmine. • Use cautiously in patients with bronchial asthma and hypertension.

SELF-TEST

1. Scott Evans, age 70, has primary open-angle glaucoma of the left eye. The nurse's major responsibility becomes patient teaching. The *most* important teaching concern is:
   a. to be sure the patient knows how to instill the drug.
   b. to assess the patient's physical ability and his present knowledge about the drug.
   c. to assess the eye.
   d. to instruct the patient about the drug's mechanism of action.

2. The doctor orders pilocarpine 0.5% 1 drop b.i.d. in the left eye. The nurse should stress to Mr. Evans the importance of:
   a. increasing the drops used if eye pain develops.
   b. instilling the drug in the outer corner of the eye.
   c. not touching the tip of the dropper to the eye or with his hands.
   d. taking the drug only when he develops visual changes.

3. Because Mr. Evans complains that it's difficult to give himself eye drops several times a day, his doctor prescribes an Ocusert Pilo system to be used every 7 days. An important thing to teach Mr. Evans about this form of the drug is:

a. what to do if the Ocusert Pilo system falls out.
b. the importance of applying the system upon arising in the morning.
c. the possibility of hypersensitivity with prolonged use.
d. the importance of sterilizing the system in hot water before each use.

Check your answers on page 1076.

CHAPTER 80

MYDRIATICS

atropine sulfate ✦ cyclopentolate hydrochloride ✦ epinephrine bitartrate
epinephrine hydrochloride ✦ epinephryl borate
homatropine hydrobromide ✦ phenylephrine hydrochloride
scopolamine ✦ tropicamide

OVERVIEW

• Both anticholinergics (atropine, cyclopentolate, homatropine, scopolamine, and tropicamide) and adrenergics (epinephrine, epinephryl, and phenylephrine) produce mydriasis (pupillary dilation) when applied topically to the eye. In addition, the anticholinergics produce cycloplegia (paralysis of accommodation).

MAJOR USES

• Atropine, homatropine, and scopolamine are used in acute inflammation of the iris (iritis) or of the iris, ciliary body, and choroid (uveitis).
• Cyclopentolate, phenylephrine, and tropicamide are used in diagnostic procedures.
• The epinephrine salts are used with or without miotics to lower intraocular pressure in open-angle glaucoma.

MECHANISM OF ACTION

• Anticholinergics block acetylcholine, leaving the pupil under the unopposed influence of its sympathetic or adrenergic nerve supply. This causes the pupil to dilate. Relaxation of the ciliary muscle allows the lens to flatten.
• Adrenergics dilate the pupil by contracting the dilator muscle of the pupil.

ABSORPTION, DISTRIBUTION, METABOLISM, AND EXCRETION

Anticholinergics can be systemically absorbed, causing adverse reactions, particularly in children and elderly patients. Adverse reactions, such as dry mouth and tachycardia, are most common after instillation of atropine, scopolamine, and cyclopentolate.

Penetration by adrenergics is heightened during surgical procedures and in the traumatized eye. Adrenergics are systemically absorbed less often than anticholinergics. Repeated instillation of phenylephrine (10% solution) may exacerbate hypertension.

GLOSSARY

Accommodation: adjustment of the eyes for vision at various distances.
Cycloplegia: ciliary muscle paralysis.
Mydriasis: extreme dilation of the pupil
Uveitis: acute inflammation of the iris, ciliary body, and choroid.

ONSET AND DURATION

Atropine produces mydriasis in 30 to 40 minutes; dilation can last 12 to 14 days before complete recovery. The drug causes cycloplegia within a few hours; this effect lasts 2 weeks or more before complete recovery.

Cyclopentolate produces mydriasis (in 15 to 30 minutes) that lasts up to 24 hours. It also produces cycloplegia (in 15 to 45 minutes) that lasts up to 24 hours. Homatropine has a shorter duration of action than atropine. Cycloplegia begins in 30 to 90 minutes, and recovery takes 10 to 48 hours. Maximal cycloplegia occurs within 1 hour; recovery is in 1 to 3 days. Tropicamide produces maximal dilation in 20 to 25 minutes after application and cycloplegia that lasts about 20 minutes. Recovery is complete in about 6 hours.

Epinephrine salts produce mydriasis within minutes after instillation; dilation lasts several hours. Epinephrine lowers intraocular pressure for variable lengths of time. The maximal interval is 4 to 8 hours; recovery occurs in 12 to 24 or more hours. About 5 minutes after administration, epinephrine also causes vasoconstriction that lasts 1 hour. Phenylephrine (2.5% solution) produces dilation within minutes after instillation. Maximal dilation occurs in 15 to 50 minutes and lasts up to 3 hours. Scopolamine produces maximal dilation within 40 minutes after instillation; recovery occurs in 3 to 7 days. Maximal cycloplegia, which begins in 10 to 30 minutes, occurs within 30 to 45 minutes. Complete recovery may take several days.

ADVERSE REACTIONS

Atropine, cyclopentolate, homatropine, scopolamine, and tropicamide may all increase intraocular pressure and are contraindicated in patients with angle-closure glaucoma. These agents may also produce blurred vision, eye dryness, photophobia, contact dermatitis, and ocular congestion. Systemic reactions may include flushing, tachycardia, fever, ataxia, irritability, confusion, somnolence, hallucinations, seizures, and behavioral changes in children.

Epinephrine preparations frequently cause local reactions: burning, stinging, lacrimation, pain, and rebound conjunctival hyperemia. Systemic reactions may include palpitations, tachycardia, cardiac arrhythmias, hypertension, headache, trembling, pallor, and faintness. Phenylephrine also causes frequent ocular reactions: burning, stinging, blurred vision, reactive hyperemia, dermatitis, brow ache, and iris floaters. Systemic reactions include tachycardia, cardiac arrhythmias, hypertension, pallor, sweating, and trembling. These effects are most common with the 10% solution and can be minimized by using the 2.5% solution.

ATROPINE SULFATE
(a′ troe peen)
Atropisol, Atropt‡, Isopto Atropine
Classification: mydriatic
Pregnancy risk category C

How supplied
OPHTHALMIC OINTMENT: 0.5%, 1%
OPHTHALMIC SOLUTION: 1%, 2%, 3%

Indications and dosage
Acute iritis; uveitis
ADULTS AND CHILDREN: instill 1 drop of 1% solution or small amount of ointment daily to b.i.d.

Cycloplegic refraction
ADULTS: instill 1 to 2 drops of 1% solution 1 hour before refracting.
CHILDREN: instill 1 to 2 drops of 0.5% to 1% solution in each eye b.i.d. for 1 to 3 days before eye examination and 1 hour before refraction, or instill small amount of ointment daily or b.i.d. for 2 to 3 days before examination.

Contraindications and precautions
Atropine is contraindicated in angle-closure glaucoma (narrow-angle). Use cautiously in infants, children, and elderly or debilitated patients. Children with blond hair and blue eyes, patients with Down's syndrome, or those with brain damage may be more susceptible to atropine or experience higher incidence of adverse reactions.

Adverse reactions
EYE: ocular congestion in long-term use, conjunctivitis, contact dermatitis, edema, *blurred vision, discomfort upon instillation,* eye dryness, photophobia.
SYSTEMIC: flushing, dry skin, dry mouth, fever, tachycardia, abdominal distention in infants, ataxia, irritability, confusion, somnolence.

Interactions
None significant.

Nursing considerations
Assessment
• Review the patient's history for a condition that contraindicates the use of atropine.
• Obtain a baseline assessment of iritis before initiating atropine therapy.
• Be alert for common adverse reactions.

‡Available in Australia only
Italicized adverse reactions are common

• Evaluate the patient's and family's knowledge about atropine therapy.

Planning (Nursing Diagnoses)

Potential nursing diagnoses for the patient receiving atropine include:

• Sensory/perceptual alterations (visual) related to atropine-induced blurred vision.
• Potential for injury related to atropine-induced ocular or adverse systemic reactions.
• Knowledge deficit related to atropine therapy.

Implementation

Preparation and administration

— If the drug is used for refraction, it should be administered 1 hour before the procedure.
— Administer form of drug correctly, *always* verifying first that the patient does not have angle-closure glaucoma; also ask the patient about signs of glaucoma (increased intraocular pressure, ocular pain, headaches, progressive blurred vision) before administration.

Monitoring

— Monitor the effectiveness of therapy by regularly examining the eye for dilation.
— Monitor the patient for adverse drug reactions.
— Monitor the patient for ocular congestion during long-term atropine use.
— Monitor vital signs for systemic reactions, such as fever or tachycardia.
— Observe skin and oral mucous membranes for dryness.
— Monitor for adverse CNS reactions, such as ataxia, irritability, confusion, or somnolence.
— Monitor infants for abdominal distention.
— Regularly reevaluate the patient's and family's knowledge about atropine therapy.

Intervention

— Withhold drug and notify the doctor if the patient experiences adverse reactions.
— Institute safety precautions because atropine will cause blurred vision and may cause CNS reactions, such as ataxia or confusion.
— Protect the patient from bright lights because of photophobia.
— Treat adverse ocular reactions as indicated.
— Encourage the patient to use lotion on dry skin and to relieve mouth dryness with ice chips or sugarless candy or chewing gum.
— Keep all members of the health care team informed of the patient's response to the drug.

Patient teaching

— Instruct the patient and family about atropine, including the dosage, frequency, action, and adverse reactions.
— Warn the patient that his vision will be temporarily blurred.

— Tell the patient that dark glasses will ease the discomfort of photophobia.

— Warn the patient that this medication is hazardous and should be stored as a poison.

— Tell the patient to call the doctor if ocular pain, headache, or progressive blurring of vision, or a combination of these reactions, develops.

— Warn the patient to avoid driving and other hazardous activities that require alertness until the temporary visual impairment caused by this drug wears off.

— Teach the patient how to instill the drug: He should wash his hands before and after administering the solution, not touch the dropper or tip of the tube to the eye or surrounding tissue, and apply light finger-pressure on the lacrimal sac for 1 minute after the instillation.

— Advise the patient to relieve dry mouth with sugarless hard candy or chewing gum or ice chips and to relieve dry skin with lotion.

— Tell the patient to notify the nurse or doctor if adverse reactions develop or questions arise about atropine therapy.

Evaluation

In the patient receiving atropine, appropriate evaluation statements include:

• Patient's pupils are dilated.

• Patient does not experience injury as a result of atropine-induced ocular or systemic reactions.

• Patient and family state an understanding of atropine therapy and demonstrate correct application technique.

SELECTED MAJOR DRUGS: MYDRIATICS

DRUG, INDICATIONS, AND DOSAGES	SPECIAL PRECAUTIONS
cyclopentolate (Cyclogyl) *Diagnostic procedures requiring mydriasis and cycloplegia—* **Adults:** instill 1 drop of 1% solution in eye, followed by 1 more drop in 5 minutes. Use 2% solution in heavily pigmented irises. **Children:** instill 1 drop of 0.5%, 1%, or 2% solution in each eye, followed in 5 minutes with 1 drop 0.5% or 1% solution, if necessary.	• Contraindicated in patients with narrow-angle glaucoma. • Use cautiously in elderly patients and in children with spastic paralysis.
epinephrine bitartrate (Epitrate) **epinephrine hydrochloride (Epifrin)** **epinephryl borate (Epinal)** *Open-angle glaucoma—* **Adults:** instill 1 to 2 drops of 1% or 2% bitartrate solution in eye with frequency determined by tonometric readings (once q 2 to 4 days up to q.i.d.), or instill 1 drop of 0.5%, 1%, or 2% hydrochloride solution (or 0.5% or 1% epinephryl borate solution) in eye b.i.d.	• Contraindicated in patients with shallow anterior chamber or narrow-angle glaucoma. • Use cautiously in patients with diabetes mellitus, hypertension, Parkinson's disease, hyperthyroidism, aphakia (eye without lens), cardiac disease, or cerebral arteriosclerosis; and

SELECTED MAJOR DRUGS: MYDRIATICS *continued*

DRUG, INDICATIONS, AND DOSAGES	SPECIAL PRECAUTIONS
epinephrine *(continued)* *During surgery—* **Adults:** instill 1 or more drops of 0.1% solution up to three times.	in elderly patients or pregnant women.
homatropine (Isopto Homatropine) *Cycloplegic refraction—* **Adults and children:** instill 1 to 2 drops of 2% or 5% solution in eye; repeat in 5 to 10 minutes, if needed, for two or three doses. *Uveitis—* **Adults and children:** instill 1 to 2 drops of 2% or 5% solution in eye up to q 3 to 4 hours.	• Contraindicated in patients with narrow-angle glaucoma. • Use cautiously in infants and elderly or debilitated patients; in children with blond hair and blue eyes; in patients with cardiac disease; or in those with increased intraocular pressure.
phenylephrine (Prefrin Liquifilm) *Mydriasis (without cycloplegia)—* **Adults and children:** instill 1 drop of 2.5% or 10% solution in eye before examination. *Mydriasis and vasoconstriction—* **Adults and adolescents:** instill 1 drop of 2.5% or 10% solution in eye; repeat in 1 hour if needed. **Children:** instill 1 drop of 2.5% solution in eye; repeat in 1 hour if needed. *To relieve eye redness—* **Adults:** instill 1 to 2 drops of 0.12% solution in eye daily up to q.i.d. *Chronic mydriasis—* **Adults and adolescents:** instill 1 drop of 2.5% or 10% solution in eye b.i.d. or t.i.d. **Children:** instill 1 drop of 2.5% solution in eye b.i.d. or t.i.d. *Posterior synechia (adhesion of iris)—* **Adults and children:** instill 1 drop of 10% solution in eye.	• Contraindicated in patients with narrow-angle glaucoma and in soft contact lens use. • Avoid 10% solution and use cautiously in patients with marked hypertension and cardiac disorders and in children with low body weight.
scopolamine (Isopto Hyoscine) *Cycloplegic refraction—* **Adults:** instill 1 to 2 drops of 0.25% solution in eye 1 hour before refraction. **Children:** instill 1 drop of 0.25% solution or ointment b.i.d. for 2 days before refraction. *Iritis, uveitis—* **Adults:** instill 1 to 2 drops of 0.25% solution daily, b.i.d., or t.i.d. **Children:** instill 1 drop daily to t.i.d.	• Contraindicated in patients with shallow anterior chamber or narrow-angle glaucoma. • Use cautiously in patients with cardiac disease and increased intraocular pressure and in elderly patients.

COMPARING MYDRIATIC COMBINATIONS

TRADE NAME AND CONTENT	SPECIAL CONSIDERATIONS
Cyclomydril Ophthalmic cyclopentolate hydrochloride 0.2% and phenylephrine hydrochloride 1%	• Combines the anticholinergic action of cyclopentolate with the adrenergic action of phenylephrine to dilate the pupil. • Contraindicated in patients with narrow-angle glaucoma or in use of soft contact lenses. • Use cautiously in patients with marked hypertension or cardiac disorders; in children with low body weight or spastic paralysis; and in elderly patients.
Murocoll-2 scopolamine hydrobromide 0.3% and phenylephrine hydrochloride 10%	• Combines the anticholinergic action of scopolamine with the adrenergic action of phenylephrine. • Contraindicated in patients with shallow anterior chamber or narrow-angle glaucoma and in use of soft contact lenses. • Use cautiously in patients with cardiac disease, increased intraocular pressure, and marked hypertension; in children with low body weight; and in elderly patients.

SELF-TEST

1. Before routine eye examination, Jeremy Martin, age 50, received 1 drop of atropine in each eye. Why was atropine used in this situation?
   a. To constrict the pupil
   b. To anesthetize the pupil
   c. To dilate the pupil
   d. To reveal irregular borders of the pupil, if present

2. How soon after atropine instillation can the examination begin?
   a. 15 minutes
   b. 30 minutes
   c. 1 hour
   d. Immediately

3. After instructing Mr. Martin about the most likely reaction to atropine, the nurse may advise him to:
   a. try to sleep at least 8 to 10 hours per night.
   b. avoid driving or other hazardous activities.
   c. monitor fluid intake.
   d. stop reading for at least 24 hours.

Check your answers on page 1076.

CHAPTER 81

MISCELLANEOUS OPHTHALMICS

betaxolol hydrochloride ◆ levobunolol hydrochloride ◆ metipranolol
timolol maleate

OVERVIEW
• Drugs used to treat primary open-angle glaucoma, the most common type
of glaucoma, include various agents with different mechanisms of action.
Beta-adrenergic blockers, for example, can be used alone or with other
agents. They offer an advantage over pilocarpine or epinephrine by not
affecting pupil size or accommodation. Beta blockers do not have
significant membrane-stabilizing (local anesthetic) actions or intrinsic
sympathomimetic activity. They reduce elevated and normal intraocular
pressure with or without glaucoma. Betaxolol is a cardioselective agent;
the others are noncardioselective.

MAJOR USES
• The miscellaneous ophthalmic agents are used in the treatment of ocular
hypertension and chronic open-angle glaucoma.

MECHANISM OF ACTION
• The exact mechanism whereby miscellaneous ophthalmics produce ocular antihypertensive action is not known, but it may involve reduction
of aqueous humor production. A slight increase in aqueous humor
outflow facility has been reported with timolol and metipranolol.

ABSORPTION, DISTRIBUTION, METABOLISM, AND EXCRETION
The extent of ocular and systemic absorption after ophthalmic application
is unclear; however, some systemic absorption can occur. Distribution into
human ocular tissues and fluids is unclear, but results of animal studies
demonstrate that the drug is distributed rapidly throughout ocular tissues
and fluids, including the cornea, iris, ciliary body, and aqueous humor.
The metabolic fate and elimination characteristics after ocular instillation
in humans are unknown.

ONSET AND DURATION
Reduction in intraocular pressure is usually evident within 1 hour, reaches
a maximum within 2 to 6 hours, and may persist for up to 24 hours after
instillation. Some reduction in intraocular pressure may persist for up to a

GLOSSARY

Cardioselective: having greater activity on heart tissue than on other tissue.

Chronic open-angle glaucoma: occurs when pupil in an eye with a narrow angle between the iris and cornea dilates gradually, causing the folded iris to block the outflow of aqueous humor from the anterior chamber.

week or longer after the drug is discontinued. In patients with open-angle glaucoma or ocular hypertension, the maximal reduction of intraocular pressure occurs after approximately 2 to 3 weeks of use.

ADVERSE REACTIONS

The most frequent reactions to ocular hypotensive agents are mild ocular stinging or burning and discomfort at instillation of the solution. Blepharoconjunctivitis, blepharitis, decreased visual acuity, conjunctivitis, iridocyclitis, band keratopathy, erythema, itching sensation, decreased corneal sensitivity, and tearing have also been reported.

As noncardioselective beta blockers, levobunolol, metipranolol, and timolol can produce systemic CV and pulmonary reactions after topical application to the eye. They can substantially affect blood pressure and heart rate in some patients and cause pulmonary effects, such as bronchoconstriction and increased airway resistance. Betaxolol has low potential for causing systemic effects. Tolerance to the intraocular hypotensive effect may develop with prolonged use of levobunolol, but reduction of intraocular pressure may remain stable for 2 to 3 years. In patients with diabetes mellitus, beta blockers may mask the signs and symptoms of hypoglycemia; in patients with thyroid dysfunction, these agents may mask clinical signs of hyperthyroidism, such as tachycardia. Headache, depression, nausea, and insomnia have also been reported. Occasionally, timolol that was instilled in one eye reduced the intraocular pressure in both eyes.

PROTOTYPE: MISCELLANEOUS OPHTHALMICS

TIMOLOL MALEATE
(tye′ moe lole)
Timoptic
Classification: miscellaneous ophthalmic
Pregnancy risk category C

How supplied
OPHTHALMIC SOLUTION: 0.25%, 0.5%

Indications and dosage

Chronic open-angle glaucoma, secondary glaucoma, aphakic glaucoma, ocular hypertension

ADULTS: initially, instill 1 drop of 0.25% solution b.i.d. in each eye; reduce to 1 drop daily for maintenance. If patient doesn't respond, instill 1 drop of 0.5% solution b.i.d. in each eye. If intraocular pressure is controlled, dosage may be reduced to 1 drop daily in each eye.

Contraindications and precautions

Timolol is contraindicated in patients with known hypersensitivity to the drug, severe bradycardia, overt cardiac failure, second- or third-degree AV block or cardiogenic shock, bronchial asthma, allergic bronchospasm, or severe COPD. Use cautiously in patients with impaired hepatic or renal function, coronary insufficiency, diabetes mellitus, and emphysema or other pulmonary disease.

Adverse reactions

CNS: headache, depression, fatigue.
CV: slight reduction in resting heart rate.
EYE: minor irritation. Long-term use may decrease corneal sensitivity.
GI: anorexia.
OTHER: apnea in infants, evidence of beta blockade and systemic absorption (hypotension, bradycardia, syncope, exacerbation of asthma, and CHF).

Interactions

General anesthetics, fentanyl: excessive hypotension. Monitor patient closely.
Propranolol, metoprolol, other oral beta-adrenergic blockers: increased ocular and systemic effect. Use together cautiously.

Nursing considerations

Assessment

- Review the patient's history for a condition that contraindicates the use of timolol.
- Obtain a baseline assessment of the patient's intraocular pressure before initiating timolol therapy.
- Be alert for serious adverse reactions resulting from systemic absorption and beta blockade.
- Evaluate the patient's and family's knowledge about timolol therapy.

Planning (Nursing Diagnoses)

Potential nursing diagnoses for the patient receiving timolol include:
- Potential for injury related to ineffectiveness of timolol.
- Altered health maintenance related to timolol-induced adverse reactions.
- Knowledge deficit related to timolol therapy.

Implementation

Preparation and administration

—Dosage adjustment may be necessary for a patient with renal or hepatic impairment.

—Patients receiving ophthalmic timolol may need to discontinue the drug 48 hours before surgery because systemic absorption of the drug does occur. However, this practice remains controversial.

Monitoring

—Monitor the effectiveness of therapy by regularly having the patient's intraocular pressure measured.

—Monitor for evidence of beta blockade and systemic absorption (hypotension, bradycardia, syncope, exacerbation of asthma, and CHF).

—Monitor the patient for adverse drug reactions.

—Examine the eyes for irritation; long-term use may decrease corneal sensitivity.

—Monitor infants for apnea.

—Monitor the patient for drug interactions.

—Regularly reevaluate the patient's and family's knowledge about timolol therapy.

Intervention

—Alert the doctor if evidence of beta blockade and systemic absorption occurs; expect to discontinue timolol and replace with a different agent. Also be prepared to treat adverse reactions, such as acute asthma or CHF, as indicated.

—Keep all members of the health care team informed of the patient's response to the drug.

Patient teaching

—Instruct the patient and family about timolol, including the dosage, frequency, action, and adverse reactions.

—Teach the patient the proper method of eye drop administration. Warn the patient to wash his hands, not to touch the dropper to the eye or surrounding tissue, and to apply light finger-pressure to the lacrimal sac after administration to decrease systemic absorption.

—Warn the patient to be careful when touching the eye. Inform the patient that long-term use may decrease corneal sensitivity.

—Teach the patient how to recognize signs of beta blockade resulting from systemic absorption and to report them to the doctor promptly.

—Tell the patient to notify the nurse or doctor if adverse reactions develop or questions arise about timolol therapy.

Evaluation

In the patient receiving timolol, appropriate evaluation statements include:
• Patient's intraocular pressure is normal.
• Patient does not exhibit adverse reactions.
• Patient and family state an understanding of timolol therapy and demonstrate correct application technique.

SELECTED MAJOR DRUGS: MISCELLANEOUS OPHTHALMICS

DRUG, INDICATIONS, AND DOSAGES	SPECIAL PRECAUTIONS
betaxolol (Betoptic) *Chronic open-angle glaucoma and ocular hypertension—* **Adults:** instill 1 drop of 0.5% solution b.i.d. in eyes.	• Contraindicated in patients with sinus bradycardia, greater than first-degree AV block, cardiogenic shock, or overt heart failure.
levobunolol (Betagan) *Chronic open-angle glaucoma and ocular hypertension—* **Adults:** instill 1 drop daily or b.i.d. in eyes.	• Contraindicated in patients with bronchial asthma, severe COPD, sinus bradycardia, second- and third-degree AV block, cardiac failure, or cardiogenic shock. • Use cautiously in patients with chronic bronchitis and emphysema, diabetes mellitus, or hyperthyroidism.

SELF-TEST

1. Rodney Jackson, age 53, has chronic open-angle glaucoma and takes timolol 1 drop daily in each eye. The nurse reminds Mr. Jackson to be alert for signs and symptoms of beta blockade. Which of the following reactions occurs with timolol-induced beta blockade?
   a. Tachycardia
   b. Bradycardia
   c. Hypertension
   d. Seizures

2. To prevent systemic absorption of timolol through the nasolacrimal duct, the nurse should instruct Mr. Jackson to:
   a. apply finger-pressure over the punctum at the internal canthus for 5 minutes.
   b. hold the head down for 2 minutes after instilling the eye drops.
   c. apply light finger-pressure over the lacrimal sac after instilling the eye drops.
   d. rub the eyes gently for about 1 minute after instilling the eye drops.

3. Which of the following drugs can cause excessive hypotension when used with timolol?
   a. Fentanyl
   b. Digoxin
   c. Chloral hydrate
   d. Ampicillin

Check your answers on page 1076.

OTICS

Anti-infectives
chloramphenicol ✦ colistin sulfate ✦ neomycin sulfate ✦ polymyxin B sulfate

Ceruminolytic
carbamide peroxide

OVERVIEW
• Otics are used for local treatment of ear problems.
• Otics are classified primarily into two groups: anti-infectives and ceruminolytics.

MAJOR USES
• Chloramphenicol, colistin, neomycin, and polymyxin B are used for their antibacterial actions.
• Carbamide peroxide is used to remove accumulated cerumen (earwax) and to treat superficial bacterial infections of the external auditory canal.
• Otic suspensions are used to treat infections associated with mastoidectomy and fenestration.

MECHANISM OF ACTION
• Antibiotics treat infections caused by susceptible microorganisms. Chloramphenicol is primarily bacteriostatic and acts by inhibition of protein synthesis. It may be bactericidal in high concentrations or against highly susceptible organisms. Colistin is bactericidal. Neomycin acts by disruption of bacterial protein synthesis.
• Carbamide peroxide is a source of hydrogen peroxide and nascent oxygen. By releasing oxygen, carbamide has a mechanical loosening effect on cerumen (earwax) that has been softened by anhydrous glycerol.

ABSORPTION, DISTRIBUTION, METABOLISM, AND EXCRETION
Topical otics are not significantly absorbed from the ear canal, and their absorption, distribution, metabolism, and excretion have not been determined. However, because adverse reactions have followed administration of some of these drugs (specifically, chloramphenicol), some systemic absorption must occur.

GLOSSARY

Cerumen: earwax.
Ceruminolytic: agent that has a mechanical loosening effect on cerumen.
Mastoidectomy: removal of mastoid bone in middle ear.
Otic: pertaining to the ear.

ONSET AND DURATION

Onset and duration of action varies. Anti-infective dosage ranges from 1 to 4 drops instilled three or four times daily.

Dosages for the ceruminolytics can be adjusted as needed. Usual dosage is 5 to 10 drops instilled into the external ear canal. The drops should remain in the ear for at least 15 minutes. Dosing can be scheduled twice daily for up to 4 days, or longer if needed.

ADVERSE REACTIONS

Signs of local irritation include itching or burning, angioneurotic edema, urticaria, and vesicular and maculopapular dermatitis. With prolonged or repeated use of anti-infectives, superinfection can occur. Chloramphenicol requires special caution because bone marrow hypoplasia (including fatal aplastic anemia) has been reported after local application of chloramphenicol.

PROTOTYPE: ANTI-INFECTIVES

CHLORAMPHENICOL
(klor am fen′ i kole)
Chloromycetin Otic, Sopamycetin
Classification: anti-infective
Pregnancy risk category C

How supplied
OTIC SOLUTION: 0.5%

Indications and dosage
External ear canal infection
ADULTS AND CHILDREN: 2 to 3 drops t.i.d. or q.i.d. into ear canal.

Contraindications and precautions
Chloramphenicol is contraindicated in patients with minor infections (such as influenza, throat infections, and colds) or as prophylaxis against infection because potential toxicity may outweigh therapeutic benefit. It is also

contraindicated in patients with known hypersensitivity or a history of toxic reaction to the drug. Administer cautiously to infants and to patients with renal or hepatic dysfunction, acute intermittent porphyria, or G6PD deficiency because of potential for adverse hematopoietic effects.

Adverse reactions
LOCAL: pruritus, burning, urticaria, vesicular or maculopapular dermatitis.
SYSTEMIC: sore throat, angioedema, **blood dyscrasia**.
OTHER: overgrowth of nonsusceptible organisms.

Interactions
None significant.

Nursing considerations
Assessment
• Review the patient's history for a condition that contraindicates the use of chloramphenicol.
• Obtain a baseline assessment of the patient's ear infection before initiating chloramphenicol therapy.
• Be alert for common or serious adverse reactions.
• Evaluate the patient's and family's knowledge about chloramphenicol therapy.

Planning (Nursing Diagnoses)
Potential nursing diagnoses for the patient receiving chloramphenicol include:
• Pain related to ineffectiveness of chloramphenicol to relieve infection.
• Potential for infection related to chloramphenicol-induced overgrowth of nonsusceptible organisms.
• Knowledge deficit related to chloramphenicol therapy.

Implementation
Preparation and administration
— Know the proper technique for administration of ear drops.
— Avoid touching the ear with the dropper.
— Avoid prolonged use.

Monitoring
— Monitor the effectiveness of therapy by regularly assessing the patient's degree of discomfort and inspecting ear canal for decreasing signs of redness, swelling, and drainage, if originally present.
— Monitor the patient's hearing.
— Monitor for superinfection, such as continued pain, inflammation, and fever.
— Monitor the patient for adverse drug reactions, especially for sore throat (an early sign of toxicity).
— Monitor culture and sensitivity results of any drainage.
— Regularly reevaluate the patient's and family's knowledge about chloramphenicol therapy.

Intervention

—Reculture persistent drainage.
—Alert doctor if sore throat occurs or superinfection is suspected.
—Keep all members of the health care team informed of the patient's response to the drug.

Patient teaching

—Instruct the patient and family about chloramphenicol, including the dosage, frequency, action, and adverse reactions.
—Instruct the patient to follow the directions for use as prescribed. The drops should be administered for 3 to 4 days to be effective.
—Tell the patient to call the doctor if redness, pain, or swelling persists or if a sore throat develops.
—Tell the patient to avoid touching the ear with the dropper.
—Instruct the patient on the proper administration of ear drops.
—Tell the patient to notify the nurse or doctor if adverse reactions develop or questions arise about chloramphenicol therapy.

Evaluation

In the patient receiving chloramphenicol, appropriate evaluation statements include:
• Patient's culture and sensitivity test is negative, and patient has no signs or symptoms of infection.
• Patient shows no signs of superinfection.
• Patient and family state an understanding of chloramphenicol therapy and demonstrate correct application technique.

PROTOTYPE: CERUMINOLYTIC

CARBAMIDE PEROXIDE
(kar′ ba mide per ox′ ide)
Debrox◊
Classification: ceruminolytic
Pregnancy risk category C

How supplied
OTIC SOLUTION: 6.5% carbamide in glycerin or glycerin and propylene glycol

Indications and dosage
Impacted cerumen
ADULTS AND CHILDREN: 5 to 10 drops b.i.d. into ear canal for 3 to 4 days.

Contraindications and precautions
Carbamide is contraindicated in perforated eardrum.

Adverse reactions

None reported.

Interactions

None significant.

Nursing considerations

Assessment

• Review the patient's history for a condition that contraindicates the use of carbamide peroxide.
• Obtain a baseline assessment of the patient's impacted cerumen before initiating carbamide peroxide therapy.
• Evaluate the patient's and family's knowledge about carbamide peroxide therapy.

Planning (Nursing Diagnoses)

Potential nursing diagnoses for the patient receiving carbamide peroxide include:
• Sensory/perceptual alterations (auditory) related to ineffectiveness of carbamide peroxide.
• Knowledge deficit related to carbamide peroxide therapy.

Implementation

Preparation and administration

— Avoid touching ear with dropper.
— Instill ear drops using proper technique.

Monitoring

— Monitor the effectiveness of therapy by inspecting ear canal to see if cerumen has been removed.
— Regularly reevaluate the patient's and family's knowledge about carbamide peroxide therapy.

Intervention

— Remove cerumen remaining after instillation by using a soft rubber-bulb otic syringe to gently irrigate the ear canal with warm water.
— Withhold drug and notify the doctor if redness, pain, or swelling occurs.
— Keep all members of the health care team informed of the patient's response to the drug.

Patient teaching

— Instruct the patient and family about carbamide peroxide, including the dosage, frequency, action, and adverse reactions.
— Teach the patient how to use product correctly.
— Tell the patient to call the doctor if inflammation or irritation persists.
— Warn the patient not to use otic preparation for more than 4 consecutive days and to avoid contact with eyes.

— Instruct the patient to keep otic solution in ear for at least 15 minutes by tilting head sideways or putting cotton in ear.
— Tell the patient to notify the nurse or doctor if adverse reactions develop or questions arise about carbamide peroxide therapy.

Evaluation

In the patient receiving carbamide peroxide, appropriate evaluation statements include:

• Patient's ear canal is clear and patient can hear at baseline level.
• Patient and family state an understanding of carbamide peroxide therapy and demonstrate proper administration technique.

SELECTED MAJOR DRUG: OTIC

DRUG, INDICATION, AND DOSAGES	SPECIAL PRECAUTIONS
polymyxin B (Aerosporin) *Superficial bacterial infections of the external auditory canal; infections following mastoidectomy or infections of fenestration cavities caused by organisms susceptible to antibiotics—* **Adults:** 4 drops t.i.d. or q.i.d. in the affected ear. **Infants and children:** 3 drops t.i.d. or q.i.d. in the affected ear.	• Contraindicated in patients with known hypersensitivity to any of the drug's components and in those with herpes simplex, vaccinia, or varicella infections. • Administer cautiously to patients with perforated eardrum and with chronic otitis media because of the risk of ototoxicity.

COMPARING OTIC COMBINATIONS

TRADE NAME AND CONTENT	SPECIAL CONSIDERATIONS
Cortisporin Otic neomycin sulfate 5 mg/ml, polymyxin B sulfate 10,000 units/ml, and hydrocortisone 1%	• Combines the antimicrobial actions of neomycin and polymyxin B with the anti-inflammatory action of hydrocortisone. • Contraindicated in patients with known hypersensitivity to any of the drug's components and in those with herpes simplex, vaccinia, or varicella infections. • Use cautiously during prolonged administration and in pregnant or breast-feeding women.

(continued)

COMPARING OTIC COMBINATIONS *continued*

TRADE NAME AND CONTENT	SPECIAL CONSIDERATIONS
Coly-Mycin S Otic neomycin sulfate 3.3 mg/ml, colistin sulfate 3 mg/ml, hydrocortisone acetate 10 mg/ml, and thonzonium bromide 0.05%	• Combines the antimicrobial actions of neomycin and colistin with the anti-inflammatory action of hydrocortisone and the surface-active action (promotes tissue contact) of thonzonium. • Contraindicated in patients with known hypersensitivity to any of the drug's components and in those with herpes simplex, vaccinia, or varicella infections. • Use cautiously in patients with perforated eardrum or chronic otitis media.

SELF-TEST

1. Vincent Anderson, age 56, sought medical attention because of ear pain. Examination revealed a severe external ear canal infection. After obtaining a culture of the drainage, his doctor prescribed otic chloramphenicol, 3 drops q.i.d. into affected ear canal. The office nurse checked Mr. Anderson's medical history before instructing him about the drug. Which of the following conditions requires cautious use of chloramphenicol?
   a. Renal dysfunction
   b. CV disease
   c. Endocrine disorders
   d. Obstructive respiratory disease

2. The nurse should tell Mr. Anderson to call his doctor if he develops:
   a. dizziness.
   b. diarrhea.
   c. sore throat.
   d. palpitations.

3. Melanie Morrison, age 39, complained of decreased hearing during a routine physical examination. The doctor observed impacted cerumen in both ear canals and therefore prescribed 5 drops of carbamide peroxide b.i.d. into each ear canal. Mrs. Morrison was scheduled for a follow-up examination in 4 days to determine effectiveness. What may be necessary if cerumen is still present at the follow-up visit?
  a. 3 more days of carbamide peroxide therapy as prescribed above
  b. Increase in dosage to 10 drops for 4 more days
  c. Irrigation of ear canals
  d. Use of different ceruminolytic

Check your answers on page 1077.

CHAPTER 83

NASAL AGENTS

Local vasoconstrictors
ephedrine sulfate ✦ epinephrine hydrochloride ✦ naphazoline hydrochloride
oxymetazoline hydrochloride ✦ phenylephrine hydrochloride
propylhexedrine ✦ tetrahydrozoline hydrochloride
xylometazoline hydrochloride

Anti-inflammatory agents
beclomethasone ✦ dexamethasone sodium phosphate ✦ flunisolide

OVERVIEW
- Nasal agents, decongestants and corticosteroids, are used to relieve acute and chronic congestion caused by bacterial and viral microorganisms and allergy-producing agents.
- Nasal agents are classified primarily into two groups: local vasoconstrictors and anti-inflammatory agents.

MAJOR USES
- Nasal decongestants, the sympathomimetic vasoconstrictors, are used to relieve membrane congestion in acute conditions, such as hay fever, allergic rhinitis, vasomotor rhinitis, acute coryza, sinusitis, and the common cold. They are also used as adjuncts in middle ear infections because they decrease congestion around the eustachian tube. Used in nasal inhalers, they may relieve ear blockage and pressure pain during air travel.
- Epinephrine is used locally to control superficial bleeding. It can also be applied topically as a nasal decongestant, but it has a short duration of action, and other long-acting sympathomimetics are more commonly used for this purpose. Phenylephrine also has a short duration of action, and rebound congestion occurs frequently with both epinephrine and phenylephrine.
- Tetrahydrozoline 0.1% is contraindicated in children under age 6; 0.05% solution, in infants under age 2. Naphazoline should be used cautiously in patients with glaucoma. Sympathomimetics should be administered cautiously to patients with hypertension, hyperthyroidism, diabetes mellitus, CV disease, increased intraocular pressure, or prostatic hyperplasia.
- The anti-inflammatory agents beclomethasone and flunisolide are used for symptomatic relief of seasonal or perennial rhinitis when treatment with antihistamines and decongestants is ineffective. Beclomethasone is also used to manage nasal polyposis, primarily to prevent recurrence of nasal polyps after surgical removal. Dexamethasone is used intranasally

to relieve inflammatory nasal conditions and nasal polyps, except those polyps originating in the sinuses.

MECHANISM OF ACTION

- Nasal decongestants are sympathomimetic amines applied directly to nasal membranes. Some stimulate alpha-adrenergic receptors of vascular smooth muscle, leading to intense vasoconstriction when applied directly to mucous membranes; others have alpha and beta activity.
- Epinephrine and phenylephrine act on the alpha-adrenergic sites to effect vasoconstriction. The exact mechanism of action of naphazoline, oxymetazoline, propylhexedrine, tetrahydrozoline, and xylometazoline has not been conclusively determined. However, they produce constriction and shrinkage of the mucous membranes, promoting drainage, improving ventilation, and relieving the stuffy feeling.
- The anti-inflammatory agents are corticosteroids. They decrease inflammation by several mechanisms: they produce a local vasoconstriction effect, prevent IgE and most cell-mediated allergic reactions, stabilize most cells, and inhibit migration of inflammatory cells into nasal tissue.

ABSORPTION, DISTRIBUTION, METABOLISM, AND EXCRETION

Epinephrine is rapidly absorbed with some systemic distribution. Duration of action is short (approximately 1 hour). After topical application of naphazoline solution to the nasal mucous membranes, local vasoconstriction usually occurs within 10 minutes and may persist for 2 to 6 hours. Information on the distribution and elimination of the drug in humans is not available.

Although the anti-inflammatory agents are intended for local use, some systemic absorption is inevitable. These drugs are metabolized in the liver; metabolites are excreted primarily in the urine.

ONSET AND DURATION

Most vasoconstrictors act within a few minutes of application and their effects last from 4 to 6 hours. The effects of oxymetazoline and xylometazoline may last for up to 12 hours. The effects of the anti-inflammatory agents become more pronounced with regular daily use.

Use topical vasoconstrictors only in acute disease and not longer than 3 to 5 days. The usual dose is 2 to 3 drops or sprays, no more than every 3 hours for the drops or 4 to 6 hours for the spray.

ADVERSE REACTIONS

Mild, transient stinging is common after topical application. Systemic effects are less likely, but may follow excessive use.

Rebound congestion may occur. Patients ages 60 and over are more likely to experience adverse reactions to sympathomimetics. Insomnia, dizziness, weakness, and tremor may occur. Epinephrine can cause nervousness and restlessness, but it produces less CNS stimulation than ephedrine.

PHENYLEPHRINE HYDROCHLORIDE
(fen ill ef' rin)
Alconefrin 12◊, Alconefrin 25◊, Alconefrin 50◊, Doktors◊, Duration◊,
Neo-Synephrine◊, Nostril◊, Rhinall◊, Rhinall-10◊, Sinex◊, St. Joseph
Measured Dose Nasal Decongestant◊

Classification: local vasoconstrictor
Pregnancy risk category C

How supplied
NASAL JELLY: 0.5%◊
NASAL SOLUTION◊: 0.125%, 0.16%, 0.2%, 0.25%, 0.5%, 1%

Indications and dosage
Nasal congestion
ADULTS: 1 to 2 drops or sprays of 0.125% to 1% solution; apply jelly or spray to nasal mucosa.
CHILDREN AGES 6 TO 12: 1 to 2 drops or sprays of 0.25% solution.
CHILDREN UNDER AGE 6: 2 to 3 drops or sprays of 0.125% solution.
Drops, spray, or jelly can be given q 4 hours p.r.n.

Contraindications and precautions
Phenylephrine is contraindicated in narrow-angle glaucoma. Use cautiously in hyperthyroidism, hypertension, diabetes mellitus, or ischemic cardiac disease because systemic absorption may occur.

Adverse reactions
CNS: headache, tremor, dizziness, nervousness.
CV: palpitations, tachycardia, **premature ventricular contractions, hypertension, pallor.**
EENT: *transient burning, stinging;* dryness of nasal mucosa; rebound nasal congestion may occur with continued use.
GI: nausea.

Interactions
None significant.

Nursing considerations
Assessment
• Review the patient's history for a condition that contraindicates the use of phenylephrine.
• Obtain a baseline assessment of the patient's nasal congestion before initiating phenylephrine therapy.
• Be alert for common adverse reactions.
• Evaluate the patient's and family's knowledge about phenylephrine therapy.

◊ Available OTC
Italicized adverse reactions are common   Boldfaced adverse reactions are life-threatening

Planning (Nursing Diagnoses)

Potential nursing diagnoses for the patient receiving phenylephrine include:

- Altered health maintenance related to ineffective phenylephrine dosage regimen.
- Decreased cardiac output related to phenylephrine-induced tachycardia.
- Knowledge deficit related to phenylephrine therapy.

Implementation

Preparation and administration

— Have the patient gently blow his nose before administration. Tilt his head back, instill the drops or spray, and have the patient maintain this position for a few minutes to ensure distribution of the drug.

Monitoring

— Monitor the effectiveness of therapy by regularly noting if nasal congestion is relieved.
— Observe for rebound nasal congestion when drug is discontinued.
— Monitor vital signs for tachycardia, irregular heartbeat, and hypertension.
— Monitor the patient for adverse drug reactions.
— Observe nasal passages for evidence of dryness.
— Monitor the patient for adverse CNS reactions, such as headache, tremor, dizziness, and nervousness.
— Monitor hydration status if nausea persists or becomes severe.
— Regularly reevaluate the patient's and family's knowledge about phenylephrine therapy.

Intervention

— Notify the doctor if nasal congestion is not relieved or serious adverse reactions, such as tachycardia, occur.
— Institute safety precautions if adverse CNS reactions occur.
— Obtain an order for an antiemetic if nausea persists or becomes severe.
— Keep all members of the health care team informed of the patient's response to the drug.

Patient teaching

— Instruct the patient and family about phenylephrine, including the dosage, frequency, action, and adverse reactions.
— Tell the patient not to exceed the recommended dose.
— Teach the patient how to administer the medication. The patient should blow his nose before instilling the medication and hold his head erect to minimize swallowing.
— Advise the patient to rinse the dropper with hot water after use and to dry with a clean towel. Emphasize that only one person should use the dropper bottle or nasal spray.
— Tell the patient to notify the nurse or doctor if adverse reactions develop or questions arise about phenylephrine therapy.

Evaluation
In the patient receiving phenylephrine, appropriate evaluation statements include:
• Patient's nasal congestion is relieved.
• Patient's heart rate remains within normal limits.
• Patient and family state an understanding of phenylephrine therapy and demonstrate correct application technique.

PROTOTYPE: ANTI-INFLAMMATORY AGENTS

BECLOMETHASONE DIPROPIONATE
(be kloe meth' a sone)
Aldecin Aqueous Nasal, Beconase AQ Nasal Spray, Beconase Nasal Inhaler, Vancenase AQ Nasal Spray, Vancenase Nasal Inhaler
Classification: anti-inflammatory agent
Pregnancy risk category C

How supplied
NASAL AEROSOL: 42 mcg/metered spray, 50 mcg/metered spray‡
NASAL SPRAY: 0.024%, 50 mcg/metered spray‡

Indications and dosage
Relief of symptoms of seasonal or perennial rhinitis; prevention of recurrence of nasal polyps after surgical removal
ADULTS AND CHILDREN OVER AGE 12: 1 spray (42 mcg) in each nostril b.i.d. to q.i.d. (total dosage is 168 to 336 mcg daily). Most patients require 1 spray in each nostril t.i.d. (252 mcg daily).
Not recommended for children under age 12.

Contraindications and precautions
Use beclomethasone cautiously, if at all, in patients with active or quiescent respiratory tract tubercular infections or those with untreated fungal, bacterial, or systemic viral infections, or ocular herpes simplex infections. Use cautiously in patients who have recently had nasal septal ulcers or nasal surgery or trauma.

Adverse reactions
CNS: headache.
EENT: *mild transient nasal burning and stinging,* nasal congestion, sneezing, epistaxis, watery eyes.
GI: nausea and vomiting.
OTHER: development of nasopharyngeal fungal infections.

Interactions
None significant.

‡Available in Australia only
Italicized adverse reactions are common

Nursing considerations

Assessment
- Obtain a baseline assessment of nasal inflammation before initiating beclomethasone therapy.
- Be alert for common adverse reactions.
- Evaluate the patient's and family's knowledge about beclomethasone therapy.

Planning (Nursing Diagnoses)
Potential nursing diagnoses for the patient receiving beclomethasone include:
- Altered health maintenance related to ineffectiveness of beclomethasone.
- Pain related to administration of beclomethasone.
- Knowledge deficit related to beclomethasone therapy.

Implementation

Preparation and administration
— Have the patient gently blow his nose before administration. Tilt his head back, instill the aerosol or spray, and have the patient maintain the position for a few minutes to ensure distribution of the drug.

Monitoring
— Monitor the effectiveness of therapy by regularly asking the patient about nasal irritation and inspecting nasal cavities for signs of inflammation.
— Monitor for mild transient nasal burning and stinging at application.
— Monitor the patient for adverse drug reactions.
— Monitor for fungal infections.
— Monitor hydration status if nausea and vomiting occur.
— Regularly reevaluate the patient's and family's knowledge about beclomethasone therapy.

Intervention
— Be aware that beclomethasone is not effective for active exacerbations. Nasal decongestants or oral antihistamines may be needed instead.
— If symptoms don't improve within 3 weeks or if nasal irritation persists, the patient should stop the drug and notify the doctor.
— Obtain an antiemetic order if nausea and vomiting occur.
— Keep all members of the health care team informed of the patient's response to the drug.

Patient teaching
— Instruct the patient and family about beclomethasone, including the dosage, frequency, action, and adverse reactions.
— Warn the patient not to exceed the prescribed dosage. The drug must be used regularly to be effective.
— Tell the patient that the therapeutic effect of this drug is not immediate. Most patients achieve benefits within a few days, but some need 2 to 3 weeks of treatment for maximum benefits.

— Instruct the patient to call the doctor if symptoms don't improve within 3 weeks or if nasal irritation persists.

— Teach the patient good nasal and oral hygiene.

— Instruct the patient how to administer the drug: Shake the container and invert; after clearing the nasal passages, tilt the head back, insert the nozzle into the nostril, pointing away from the septum; while holding the other nostril closed, inspire and spray; shake the container again and repeat in the other nostril.

— Tell the patient to notify the nurse or doctor if adverse reactions develop or questions arise about beclomethasone therapy.

Evaluation

In the patient receiving beclomethasone, appropriate evaluation statements include:

• Patient's rhinitis is relieved, and patient's nasal passages are not inflamed.

• Patient does not experience local burning and stinging when beclomethasone is applied.

• Patient and family state an understanding of beclomethasone therapy and demonstrate correct application technique.

SELECTED MAJOR DRUGS: NASAL AGENTS

DRUG, INDICATIONS, AND DOSAGES	SPECIAL PRECAUTIONS
Anti-inflammatory agents	
dexamethasone (Decadron Phosphate Turbinaire) *Allergic or inflammatory conditions, nasal polyps—* **Adults:** 2 sprays b.i.d. or t.i.d. in each nostril. Maximum is 12 sprays daily. **Children ages 6 to 12:** 1 or 2 sprays b.i.d. in each nostril. Maximum is 8 sprays daily. Each spray delivers 0.1 mg dexamethasone sodium phosphate equal to 0.084 mg dexamethasone.	• Contraindicated in patients with cutaneous tuberculosis and fungal and herpetic lesions. • Use cautiously in patients with diabetes mellitus, peptic ulcer, or tuberculosis because systemic absorption can activate disease.
flunisolide (Nasalide) *Relief of symptoms of seasonal or perennial rhinitis—* **Adults:** starting dose is 2 sprays (50 mcg) b.i.d. in each nostril. Total dosage is 200 mcg daily. If necessary, dose may be increased to 2 sprays t.i.d. in each nostril. Maximum total dosage is 8 sprays daily in each nostril (400 mcg daily). **Children ages 6 to 14:** starting dose is 1 spray (25 mcg) t.i.d. in each nostril or 2 sprays (50 mcg) b.i.d. in each nostril. Total dosage is 150 to 200 mcg daily. Maximum total dosage is 4 sprays daily in each nostril (200 mcg daily). Not recommended for children under age 6.	• Contraindicated in patients with known hypersensitivity to any of the drug's ingredients. • Use cautiously, if at all, in patients with active or quiescent respiratory tract tubercular infections or in those with untreated fungal, bacterial, or systemic viral or ocular herpes simplex infections. • Use cautiously in patients who have recently had nasal septal ulcers, nasal surgery, or trauma.

SELECTED MAJOR DRUGS: NASAL AGENTS *continued*

DRUG, INDICATIONS, AND DOSAGES	SPECIAL PRECAUTIONS

Local vasoconstrictors

ephedrine (Efedron Nasal Jelly ◇, Va-tro-nol Nose Drops ◇)
Nasal congestion —
Adults and children: 3 to 4 drops of 0.5% solution or apply a small amount of jelly to nasal mucosa. Use no more frequently than q 4 hours.

• Contraindicated in patients with CV disease, hyperthyroidism, or hypertension and in those with known hypersensitivity to the drug or its components.
• Use cautiously in patients with hyperthyroidism, coronary artery disease, hypertension, or diabetes mellitus because systemic absorption can occur.

epinephrine (Adrenalin Chloride)
Nasal congestion, local superficial bleeding —
Adults and children: 0.1% solution applied to oral or nasal mucosa.

• Contraindicated in patients with narrow-angle glaucoma, shock, or organic brain damage; in those undergoing general anesthesia or local anesthesia; and during labor.
• Use cautiously in patients with hyperthyroidism, coronary artery disease, hypertension, or diabetes mellitus because systemic absorption can occur.

naphazoline (Privine ◇)
Nasal congestion —
Adults: 2 drops or sprays of 0.05% solution q 3 to 4 hours to nasal mucosa.
Children ages 6 to 12: 1 to 2 drops or sprays of 0.05% solution to nasal mucosa. Repeat q 3 to 6 hours p.r.n. Use no longer than 3 to 5 days.

• Contraindicated in patients with narrow-angle glaucoma.
• Use cautiously in patients with hyperthyroidism, heart disease, hypertension, or diabetes mellitus because systemic absorption can occur.

oxymetazoline (Afrin ◇ , Neo-Synephrine 12 Hour ◇)
Nasal congestion —
Adults and children over age 6: 2 to 4 drops or sprays of 0.05% solution b.i.d. to nasal mucosa.
Children ages 2 to 6: apply 2 to 3 drops 0.025% solution b.i.d. to nasal mucosa. Use no longer than 3 to 5 days. Dosage for younger children has not been established.

• Contraindicated in patients with narrow-angle glaucoma or known hypersensitivity to any components of the preparation.
• Use cautiously in patients with hyperthyroidism, cardiac disease, hypertension, or diabetes mellitus because systemic absorption can occur.

tetrahydrozoline (Tyzine)
Nasal congestion —
Adults and children over age 6: 2 to 4 drops of 0.1% solution or spray q 4 to 6 hours p.r.n. to nasal mucosa.
Children ages 2 to 6: 2 to 3 drops of 0.05% solution q 4 to 6 hours p.r.n. to nasal mucosa.

• Contraindicated in patients with narrow-angle glaucoma.
• Use cautiously in patients with hyperthyroidism, hypertension, cardiac disease, or diabetes mellitus because systemic absorption can occur.

(continued)

◇ Available OTC

SELECTED MAJOR DRUGS: NASAL AGENTS *continued*

DRUG, INDICATIONS, AND DOSAGES	SPECIAL PRECAUTIONS
Local vasoconstrictors *(continued)*	
xylometazoline (Otrivin ◇ , Sine-Off Nasal Spray ◇) *Nasal congestion—* **Adults and children over age 12:** 2 to 3 drops or 1 to 2 sprays of 0.1% solution q 8 to 10 hours to nasal mucosa. **Children under age 12:** 2 to 3 drops or 1 spray of 0.05% solution q 8 to 10 hours to nasal mucosa.	• Contraindicated in patients with narrow-angle glaucoma. • Use cautiously in patients with hyperthyroidism, cardiac disease, hypertension, diabetes mellitus, and advanced arterio-sclerosis because systemic absorption can occur.

◇ Available OTC

COMPARING NASAL COMBINATIONS

TRADE NAME AND CONTENT	SPECIAL CONSIDERATIONS
Dristan Nasal ◇ phenylephrine hydrochloride 0.5% and pheniramine maleate 0.2%	• Combines the vasoconstriction action of phenylephrine with the histamine antagonistic action of pheniramine. • Contraindicated in patients with narrow-angle glaucoma. • Use cautiously in hyperthyroidism, hypertension, diabetes mellitus, and cardiac disease because systemic absorption can occur.
4-Way Fast Acting ◇ phenylephrine hydrochloride 0.5%, naphazoline hydrochloride 0.05%, and pyrilamine maleate 0.2%	• Combines the vasoconstriction actions of phenylephrine and naphazoline with the histamine antagonistic action of pyrilamine. • Contraindicated in patients with narrow-angle glaucoma. • Use cautiously in hyperthyroidism, hypertension, diabetes mellitus, and cardiac disease because systemic absorption can occur.
Myci-Spray ◇ phenylephrine hydrochloride 0.25% and pheniramine maleate 0.15%	• Combines the vasoconstriction action of phenylephrine with the histamine antagonistic action of pheniramine. • Contraindicated in patients with narrow-angle glaucoma. • Use cautiously in hyperthyroidism, hypertension, diabetes mellitus, and cardiac disease because systemic absorption can occur.

◇ Available OTC

SELF-TEST

1. Laura Jones has seasonal rhinitis for which her doctor prescribed beclomethasone (Beconase) 1 spray b.i.d. in each nostril and phenylephrine (Neo-Synephrine) 1 spray daily in each nostril. What is the rationale for treating seasonal rhinitis with beclomethasone?
   a. Beclomethasone relieves inflammation.
   b. Beclomethasone relieves congestion.
   c. Beclomethasone relieves allergic response.
   d. Beclomethasone relieves nasal pain.

2. The nurse should warn Miss Jones about which common adverse reaction to beclomethasone?
   a. Palpitations
   b. Tachycardia
   c. Nervousness
   d. Nasal burning

3. When administering phenylephrine the nurse must be aware that:
   a. this drug can be used by the patient as needed.
   b. the medication is not a prescription drug and may be shared by all infected family members.
   c. the drug is used for nasal congestion.
   d. the drug can be administered to a 10-year-old child.

Check your answers on page 1077.

CHAPTER 84

LOCAL ANTI-INFECTIVES

Bacteriostatic agents
chloramphenicol ✦ chlortetracycline hydrochloride ✦ erythromycin
mafenide acetate ✦ meclocycline sulfosalicylate ✦ nitrofurazone
tetracycline hydrochloride

Bactericidal agents
bacitracin ✦ gentamicin sulfate ✦ neomycin sulfate

Fungicidal agents
amphotericin B ✦ carbol-fuchsin solution ✦ ciclopirox olamine
clotrimazole ✦ econazole nitrate
gentian violet (methylrosaniline chloride) ✦ haloprogin
miconazole nitrate 2% ✦ silver sulfadiazine ✦ terconazole

Fungistatic agents
clioquinol ✦ nystatin ✦ tolnaftate
undecylenic acid and zinc undecylenate

Antiviral agent
acyclovir

OVERVIEW

- Local anti-infectives are widely used to treat local bacterial, fungal, and viral infections. They are classified into five categories: bacteriostatic, bactericidal, fungicidal, fungistatic, and antiviral agents. Bacteriostatic and fungistatic drugs suppress growth of microorganisms; bactericidal antibiotics and fungicidal agents destroy them.
- Bacteriostatic antibiotics include chloramphenicol, chlortetracycline, erythromycin, mafenide, meclocycline, nitrofurazone, and tetracycline. Bactericidal antibiotics include bacitracin, gentamicin, and neomycin.
- The effectiveness of antifungal agents depends on concentration: most of them are fungistatic at low concentrations or against some organisms, but fungicidal at higher concentrations or against other organisms. Fungistatic drugs include clioquinol, nystatin, tolnaftate, and undecylenic acid and zinc undecylenate. Agents generally considered fungicidal are amphotericin B, carbol-fuchsin, ciclopirox olamine, clotrimazole, econazole nitrate, gentian violet, haloprogin, miconazole, and silver sulfadiazine.
- Acyclovir is an antiviral agent.

GLOSSARY

Antiviral: capable of killing a virus.
Bactericidal: capable of killing bacteria.
Bacteriostatic: tending to restrain the development or reproduction of bacteria.
Cream: semisolid emulsion of oil in water or water in oil; usually used as a base.
Fungicidal: capable of killing fungi.
Fungistatic: tending to restrain the development or reproduction of fungi.
Lotion: suspension of powder and water that requires shaking before application; usually provides a protective, drying, or cooling effect.
Ointment: semisolid oil-based preparation for external application; usually has an occlusive effect.
Paste: semisolid preparation usually made by incorporating fine powder into an ointment; usually used as a protectant.
Powder: substance made up of an aggregation of small particles; usually produces a drying effect.

MAJOR USES

- Bactericidal and bacteriostatic agents are used to treat bacterial infections caused by susceptible organisms and responsive to local therapy.
- Fungicidal and fungistatic agents are used to treat fungal infections caused by susceptible organisms and responsive to local therapy.
- Acyclovir, a topical antiviral, is used to treat herpes simplex virus infections.

MECHANISM OF ACTION

- Bacitracin acts by inhibiting cell-wall synthesis; the other bactericidal and bacteriostatic agents act primarily by disrupting protein synthesis of bacterial ribosomes.
- Amphotericin B, econazole, miconazole, terconazole, and nystatin act mainly by altering the permeability of the cell membrane. Fungistatic agents act primarily by removing diseased tissue (softening and dissolving the horny layer of the epidermis).
- Acyclovir inhibits herpesvirus DNA synthesis by interfering with the action of viral DNA polymerase.

ABSORPTION, DISTRIBUTION, METABOLISM, AND EXCRETION

Most topical anti-infectives, in the absence of inflammation, undergo minimal systemic absorption; however, absorption increases when they're applied to large areas of denuded or inflamed skin. Applied externally, anti-infectives generally penetrate quickly and easily into the skin.

Gentamicin and neomycin are systemically absorbed to a greater extent than the other anti-infectives, and special caution is needed with their use.

Gentamicin cream may be absorbed more readily than the ointment, with up to 2% to 5% of the drug appearing in urine.

ONSET AND DURATION
The onset of action of local anti-infectives is rapid—usually within minutes. The fungistatic agents that remove diseased tissue have a more prolonged onset of action than other antifungals. Therapeutic benefit may not appear for 1 to 3 weeks. Duration of action of local anti-infectives is limited because they're often inactivated by components of blood, pus, and exudates. They should generally be applied often (three to six times a day) after the skin is cleansed of adherent crusts and debris.

ADVERSE REACTIONS
All local anti-infective agents may cause burning, local rashes, pruritus, and hypersensitivity reactions. When applied to extensive abraded areas, some local anti-infectives may cause systemic toxicity; others may do so even if applied in small areas, in certain at-risk patients. For example, bacitracin and neomycin can cause nephrotoxicity and ototoxicity. Application of large amounts of neomycin and gentamicin can cause hearing loss. Chloramphenicol may cause blood dyscrasia, and silver sulfadiazine may cause neutropenia in 3% to 5% of patients receiving extensive applications.

PROTOTYPE: BACTERIOSTATIC AGENTS

MAFENIDE ACETATE
(ma' fe nide)
Sulfamylon
Classification: local bacteriostatic agent
Pregnancy risk category C

How supplied
CREAM: 8.5%

Indications and dosage
Adjunctive treatment of second- and third-degree burns
ADULTS AND CHILDREN: apply $\frac{1}{16}''$ thickness of cream daily or b.i.d. to cleansed, debrided wounds. Reapply p.r.n. to keep burned area covered.

Contraindications and precautions
Mafenide is contraindicated in patients with known hypersensitivity to the drug and to sulfonamides. Use with caution in burn patients with acute renal failure.

Adverse reactions
BLOOD: eosinophilia; rarely, increased serum chloride level.
SKIN: pain, burning, rash, itching, swelling, hives, erythema, blisters,

facial edema.
OTHER: metabolic acidosis.

Interactions
None significant.

Nursing considerations
Assessment
• Review the patient's history for a condition that contraindicates the use of mafenide.
• Obtain a baseline assessment of the area of skin with second- or third-degree burns before therapy.
• Be alert for common adverse reactions.
• Evaluate the patient's and family's knowledge about mafenide therapy.

Planning (Nursing Diagnoses)
Potential nursing diagnoses for the patient receiving mafenide include:
• Impaired skin integrity related to potential ineffectiveness of mafenide to alleviate infection.
• Potential for infection related to improper application of mafenide.
• Knowledge deficit related to mafenide therapy.

Implementation
Preparation and administration
— If ordered, obtain culture and sensitivity report on involved area before administering initial dose.
— Read orders and drug label carefully.
— Cleanse and debride burn area before applying mafenide.
— Wear sterile gloves and use sterile technique when applying mafenide.
— Apply a thin layer of the drug over the entire surface of burn area. Keep area covered with mafenide cream at all times.
— Dressings are usually not necessary; however, if ordered, use a thin layer of dressing.
— Chart the administration of the drug and related observations.

Monitoring
— Monitor the effectiveness of mafenide therapy by regularly inspecting involved areas of skin.
— Monitor the patient for hypersensitivity reaction, which may present with severe and prolonged pain.
— Monitor the patient for adverse drug reactions.
— Monitor acid-base balance, especially in patients with pulmonary or renal dysfunction.
— Monitor vital signs and wound appearance for signs and symptoms of infection.
— Monitor CBC and differential, and platelet count; BUN, serum creatinine, and electrolyte levels; liver function tests; and urinalysis.
— Monitor serum drug levels.

—Periodically reevaluate the patient's and family's knowledge about mafenide.

Intervention

—Hold dose and notify the doctor if hypersensitivity or other adverse reactions occur.

—Bathe or shower patient daily; if possible, administer whirlpool therapy, because it aids in wound debridement.

—Use reverse isolation to prevent infection of affected area.

—Keep bed linens and patient's clothing from adhering to affected areas by using foot cradles and keeping wound exposed if possible.

—Medicate the patient for pain before dressing changes.

—Keep all members of the health care team informed of the patient's response to the drug.

Patient teaching

—Inform the patient and family about mafenide, including the dosage, frequency, action, and adverse reactions.

—Instruct the patient and family to cleanse involved area before applying a thin layer of drug over the entire surface using sterile technique.

—Teach the patient and family how to identify and report signs and symptoms of infection in the involved area.

—Tell the patient and family to use the entire prescription of mafenide, exactly as prescribed, even if wound appears to heal.

—Tell the patient to notify the nurse or doctor if adverse reactions develop or questions arise about mafenide therapy.

Evaluation

In the patient receiving mafenide, appropriate evaluation statements include:

• Patient's burns appear healed on inspection, with decreased areas of involvement.

• Patient demonstrates no signs or symptoms of infection.

• Patient and family state an understanding of mafenide therapy.

PROTOTYPE: BACTERICIDAL AGENTS

BACITRACIN
(ba' si tray sin)
Baciguent, Cacitin
Classification: local bactericidal agent
Pregnancy risk category C

How supplied

OINTMENT: 500 units/g

Indications and dosage
Topical infections, impetigo, abrasions, cuts, and minor burns or wounds
ADULTS AND CHILDREN: apply thin film b.i.d. or t.i.d., or more often, depending on severity of condition.

Bacitracin is contraindications and precautions
Bacitracin is contraindicated in patients with known hypersensitivity to the drug, and for use in the external ear canal in patients with perforated eardrum. Use with caution in patients with known hypersensitivity to neomycin (cross-sensitivity possible), renal disease (drug is nephrotoxic), or multiple sclerosis (systemically absorbed drug may prolong or increase neuromuscular blockade).

Adverse reactions
LOCAL: stinging, rashes, and other allergic reactions; itching, burning, swelling of lips or face.
SYSTEMIC: possible with extensive use for prolonged periods—nephrotoxicity, ototoxicity; **allergic reactions**; tightness in chest, hypotension.

Interactions
None significant.

Nursing considerations
Assessment
• Review the patient's history for a condition that contraindicates the use of bacitracin.
• Obtain a baseline assessment of involved areas of skin before therapy.
• Be alert for common adverse reactions.
• Evaluate the patient's and family's knowledge about bacitracin therapy.

Planning (Nursing Diagnoses)
Potential nursing diagnoses for the patient receiving bacitracin include:
• Impaired skin integrity related to ineffectiveness of bacitracin to alleviate infection.
• Potential for infection related to improper administration of bacitracin.
• Knowledge deficit related to bacitracin therapy.

Implementation
Preparation and administration
— Read orders and drug label carefully.
— Obtain a wound specimen for culture and sensitivity testing before initial application of bacitracin. First dose may be given before results are obtained.
— If applying drug to external ear canal, inspect eardrum for perforation before administration. Drug should not be used if eardrum is perforated.
— Cleanse area before each application of bacitracin, using the cleansing agent specified by the doctor. Remove all crusts and debride the wound before applying the drug.
— Wear sterile gloves and use sterile technique if skin breaks are present.

—Apply a thin layer of bacitracin over entire surface of involved area.

—Chart the administration of the drug and related observations.

Monitoring

—Monitor the effectiveness of bacitracin therapy by regularly assessing involved areas of skin.

—Monitor temperature and pulse (for infection) and BP (for hypotension).

—Monitor the patient for adverse drug reactions.

—Monitor results of culture and sensitivity tests of wound drainage for overgrowth of nonsusceptible organisms with prolonged use.

—Periodically reevaluate the patient's and family's knowledge about bacitracin.

Intervention

—Discontinue the drug and notify the doctor if severe adverse reactions or hypersensitivity develops.

—Use reverse isolation if necessary to prevent infection.

—Keep the patient's bed linens and clothing from adhering to affected area by using a foot cradle and keeping wound exposed if possible.

—If necessary, medicate patient for pain before administering the drug.

—Keep all members of the health care team informed of the patient's response to the drug.

Patient teaching

—Inform the patient and family about bacitracin, including the dosage, frequency, action, and adverse reactions.

—Tell the patient and family to cleanse affected area before each application of bacitracin and to apply the drug in a thin layer that covers the entire surface area involved; teach them sterile technique.

—Teach the patient and family how to identify and report signs of infection or hypersensitivity reactions.

—Tell the patient and family to use the entire prescription of bacitracin, even if lesions appear to have healed.

—Tell the patient and family not to share drug with others.

—Tell the patient to notify the nurse or doctor if adverse reactions develop or questions arise about bacitracin therapy.

Evaluation

In the patient receiving bacitracin, appropriate evaluation statements include:

• Patient's skin appears to be healing, with diminished areas of skin involvement.

• Patient demonstrates no signs or symptoms of infection.

• Patient and family state an understanding of bacitracin treatment.

MICONAZOLE NITRATE
(mi kon' a zole)
Micatin◊, Monistat-Derm Cream and Lotion, Monistat 7 Vaginal Cream◊, Monistat 7 Vaginal Suppository◊, Monistat 3 Vaginal Suppository
Classification: imidazole antifungal agent
Pregnancy risk category C

How supplied
CREAM: 2%◊
LOTION: 2%◊
POWDER: 2%◊
SPRAY: 2%◊
VAGINAL CREAM: 2%◊
VAGINAL SUPPOSITORIES: 100 mg◊, 200 mg

Indications and dosage
Tinea pedis, tinea cruris, tinea corporis, tinea versicolor, cutaneous candidiasis (moniliasis), infections from common dermatophytes
ADULTS AND CHILDREN: apply or spray sparingly b.i.d. for 2 to 4 weeks.
Vulvovaginal candidiasis
WOMEN: insert 1 applicatorful or suppository (Monistat 7) intravaginally h.s. for 7 days; repeat course if necessary. Alternatively, insert suppository (Monistat 3) intravaginally h.s. for 3 days.

Contraindications and precautions
Miconazole is contraindicated in patients with known hypersensitivity to the drug. Do not use vaginal suppository form with latex condoms or contraceptive diaphragms.

Adverse reactions
LOCAL: isolated reports of irritation, burning, maceration; with vaginal cream, vulvovaginal burning, itching, or irritation.

Interactions
None significant.

Nursing considerations
Assessment
- Review the patient's history for conditions that contraindicate the use of miconazole.
- Obtain a baseline assessment of involved skin or vulvovaginal areas before therapy.
- Be alert for common adverse reactions.
- Evaluate the patient's and family's knowledge about miconazole therapy.

Planning (Nursing Diagnoses)

Potential nursing diagnoses for the patient receiving miconazole include:
- Impaired skin integrity related to ineffectiveness of miconazole to treat fungal infection.
- Pain related to adverse reactions to miconazole.
- Knowledge deficit related to miconazole therapy.

Implementation

Preparation and administration

— Obtain specimen for culture and sensitivity test before first application of drug. In vulvovaginitis, potassium hydroxide smear or culture is necessary to confirm candidiasis (moniliasis) and to rule out other organisms. First dose may be given before culture and sensitivity test results are known.

— Read orders and drug label carefully.

— Cleanse affected area before each application of miconazole, using the cleansing agent specified by the doctor.

— Use wound and skin precautions when administering the drug on broken skin. Use sterile technique to prevent secondary infections.

— For skin application, apply thin layer over entire surface of affected area. Do not use occlusive dressings unless specified.

— For vaginal application, insert suppository or vaginal cream high into the vagina with the applicator provided. Have the patient remain recumbent for a few minutes to retain medication in the vagina and increase local absorption.

— Chart administration of drug and related observations.

Monitoring

— Monitor the effectiveness of miconazole therapy by regularly assessing involved areas.

— Monitor the patient for adverse drug reactions.

— Monitor the amount and characteristics of vaginal discharge.

— Monitor the patient for pain, such as burning with application.

— Periodically reevaluate the patient's and family's knowledge about miconazole.

Intervention

— Discontinue use and notify the doctor if hypersensitivity reaction occurs.

— To prevent staining of clothing, loosely cover skin areas treated with miconazole, and provide women using vaginal cream or suppositories with sanitary pads.

— Keep all members of the health care team informed of the patient's response to the drug.

Patient teaching

— Inform the patient and family about miconazole, including the dosage, frequency, action, and adverse reactions.

—Tell the patient and family to apply the entire prescription of miconazole exactly as ordered, even if skin lesions appear to have healed or vulvovaginal symptoms dissipate.

—Teach the patient and family how to identify and report signs of hypersensitivity or secondary infection.

—Instruct the patient and family to cleanse skin area before each application of drug and to apply in a thin layer over entire involved area.

—Instruct patients using the vaginal forms not to use tampons during therapy with miconazole. Suggest the use of sanitary pads to prevent staining of clothing. Tell these patients to avoid douching unless ordered by doctor.

—Instruct the patient to carefully insert vaginal suppository or cream with applicator provided high into the vagina and to remain recumbent for a few minutes to enhance absorption of medication.

—Advise patients with vulvovaginal candidiasis to avoid sexual intercourse during therapy and to advise sexual partners to seek treatment.

—Teach the patient to use good hand washing technique before and after application of miconazole.

—Tell the patient not to share the drug with others.

—Tell the patient to notify the nurse or doctor if adverse reactions develop or questions arise about miconazole therapy.

Evaluation
In the patient receiving miconazole, appropriate evaluation statements include:
• Patient's skin appears healed on inspection, with decreased area of skin involvement.
• Patient is free of pain and discomfort.
• Patient and family state an understanding of miconazole therapy.

PROTOTYPE: ANTIVIRAL AGENT

ACYCLOVIR
(ay sye′ kloe ver)
Zovirax
Classification: synthetic antiviral agent
Pregnancy risk category C

How supplied
OINTMENT: 5%

Indications and dosage
Initial herpes genitalis; limited, non-life-threatening mucocutaneous herpes simplex virus infections in immunocompromised patients
ADULTS AND CHILDREN: apply sufficient quantity to adequately cover all lesions q 3 hours six times daily for 7 days.

Contraindications and precautions

Acyclovir is contraindicated in patients with known hypersensitivity to the drug or those who develop a chemical intolerance to any component of the product.

Adverse reactions

LOCAL: transient burning and stinging, rash, pruritus.

Interactions

None reported.

Nursing considerations

Assessment

• Review the patient's history for a condition that contraindicates the use of acyclovir.
• Obtain a baseline assessment of areas of skin involvement, severity, and distribution of lesions before therapy.
• Be alert for common adverse reactions.
• Evaluate the patient's and family's knowledge about acyclovir therapy.

Planning (Nursing Diagnoses)

Potential nursing diagnoses for the patient receiving acyclovir include:
• Impaired skin integrity related to ineffectiveness of acyclovir to alleviate infection.
• Pain related to burning and stinging caused by application of acyclovir.
• Knowledge deficit related to acyclovir therapy.

Implementation

Preparation and administration

— Read orders and drug label carefully.
— If necessary, medicate patient for pain before applying drug. Herpes lesions are characteristically tender and sensitive to contact.
— Use wound and skin precautions when applying drug.
— Although dose varies with lesion size, apply approximately ½" ribbon of ointment for every 4" square of surface area. Cover all lesions thoroughly.
— Chart administration of drug and related observations.

Monitoring

— Monitor the effectiveness of acyclovir therapy by regularly inspecting involved skin areas.
— Monitor the patient for hypersensitivity reactions.
— Monitor the patient for adverse drug reactions.
— Monitor for signs of secondary infection caused by scratching.
— Periodically reevaluate the patient's and family's knowledge about acyclovir.

Intervention

— Have the patient's fingernails cut short, and discourage scratching.
— Keep all members of the health care team informed of the patient's response to the drug.

Patient teaching
—Inform the patient and family about acyclovir, including the dosage, frequency, action, and adverse reactions.
—Instruct the patient and family to seek treatment as soon as signs and symptoms of an acute herpes outbreak occur.
—Teach the patient and family to apply acyclovir ointment in sufficient quantities to all involved areas. Stress the importance of continuing the treatment for as long as the doctor specifies, even after the lesions appear to be healed.
—Teach the patient and family to prevent spread of the infection to others and to other body parts by wearing a glove or finger cot when applying ointment, using good hand washing technique, and not sharing ointment with others.
—Emphasize that acyclovir alone will not prevent the spread of herpes infection.
—Tell the patient to avoid scratching and irritation of lesions. Suggest wearing loose-fitting clothing.
—Tell the patient and family to avoid getting the drug in or around eye.
—Teach the patient and family how to identify and report signs of secondary infection or hypersensitivity reactions.
—Instruct patients with genital herpes to refrain from sexual contact as long as lesions are present, because acyclovir will not prevent the spread of herpes to others. Instruct patients to advise sexual partners to seek treatment.
—Encourage women with genital herpes to have annual Pap smears to check for cervical cancer.
—Instruct the patient to notify the doctor if no improvement is seen after 7 days.
—Tell the patient to notify the nurse or doctor if adverse reactions develop or questions arise about acyclovir therapy.

Evaluation
In the patient receiving acyclovir, appropriate evaluation statements include:
• Patient's skin shows healing on inspection, with diminished lesions.
• Patient is free of pain and discomfort.
• Patient and family state an understanding of acyclovir therapy.

SELECTED MAJOR DRUGS: LOCAL ANTI-INFECTIVES

DRUG, INDICATIONS, AND DOSAGES	SPECIAL PRECAUTIONS
Bacteriostatic agents	
chloramphenicol (Chloromycetin) *Superficial skin infections caused by susceptible bacteria—* **Adults and children:** after thorough cleansing, apply t.i.d. or q.i.d.	• Contraindicated in patients with known hypersensitivity to any component. • Administer cautiously. Prolonged use may cause overgrowth of nonsusceptible organisms, including fungi.
chlortetracycline hydrochloride (Aureomycin ◇) *Superficial infections of the skin caused by susceptible bacteria—* **Adults and children:** rub into affected area b.i.d. or t.i.d.	• Contraindicated in patients allergic to wool. • Administer cautiously. Prolonged use may cause overgrowth of nonsusceptible organisms.
erythromycin (Akne-Mycin, A/T/S, C-Solve-2 M, Erycette, Erygel) *Superficial skin infections caused by susceptible organisms; acne vulgaris—* **Adults and children:** after cleansing affected area, apply t.i.d. or q.i.d.	• Contraindicated in patients with known hypersensitivity to any component. • Use cautiously in pregnant or breast-feeding women.
meclocycline sulfosalicylate (Meclan) *Acne vulgaris—* **Adults and adolescents:** apply to affected area b.i.d.	• Contraindicated in patients with known hypersensitivity to any component or to any other tetracycline. • Use cautiously in patients sensitive to formaldehyde and in pregnant or breast-feeding women.
nitrofurazone (Furacin) *Adjunctive treatment of second- and third-degree burns (especially when resistance to other antibiotics and sulfonamides occurs); prevention of skin allograft rejection—* **Adults and children:** apply directly to lesion daily or every few days, depending on severity of burn.	• Contraindicated in patients with known hypersensitivity to any component. • Use cautiously in patients with known or suspected renal impairment.
tetracycline hydrochloride (Topicycline) *Acne vulgaris—* **Adults and children over age 12:** apply generously to affected areas b.i.d. until skin is thoroughly covered.	• Contraindicated in patients with known hypersensitivity to tetracycline. • Use cautiously in children under age 11 and in pregnant or breast-feeding women.

◇ Available OTC

SELECTED MAJOR DRUGS: LOCAL ANTI-INFECTIVES *continued*

DRUG, INDICATIONS, AND DOSAGES	SPECIAL PRECAUTIONS

Bactericidal agents

gentamicin sulfate (Garamycin, G-Myticin)
Primary and secondary bacterial infections, superficial burns, skin ulcers, infected insect bites and stings, infected lacerations and abrasions, wounds from minor surgery—
Adults and children over age 1: rub in small amount gently t.i.d. or q.i.d., with or without gauze dressing.

• Contraindicated in patients with known hypersensitivity to any component.
• Administer cautiously because excessive use may lead to resistant organisms. Avoid use on large skin lesions or over a wide area because of possible systemic toxic effects.

neomycin sulfate (Myciguent ◇)
Topical bacterial infections, minor burns, wounds, skin grafts; after surgical procedures; primary pyodermas, pruritus, trophic ulcerations, otitis externa—
Adults and children: rub in small quantity gently b.i.d., t.i.d., or as directed.

• Contraindicated in patients with impaired renal function unless risk to benefit ratio has been assessed. Do not use on more than 20% of the body surface.
• Administer cautiously. Prolonged use, especially of combinations that contain corticosteroids, may result in overgrowth of nonsusceptible organisms.

Fungicidal agents

amphotericin B (Fungizone)
Cutaneous or mucocutaneous candidal infections—
Adults and children: apply liberally b.i.d., t.i.d., or q.i.d. for 1 to 3 weeks; up to several months for interdigital lesions and paronychias.

• Contraindicated in patients with known hypersensitivity to amphotericin or any component of the formulation.

carbol-fuchsin solution
Tinea, dermatophytosis, skin infections—
Adults and children: apply liberally once daily to b.i.d.

• Contraindicated in patients with known hypersensitivity to any component.

ciclopirox olamine (Loprox)
Tinea pedis, tinea cruris, tinea corporis, and tinea versicolor; cutaneous candidiasis—
Adults and children over age 10: massage gently into the affected and surrounding areas b.i.d., in the morning and evening.

• Contraindicated in patients with known hypersensitivity to any component. Do not use with occlusive dressings.
• Use cautiously in children under age 10 and in pregnant or breast-feeding women.

clotrimazole (Gyne-Lotrimin Cream ◇, Lotrimin, Lotrimin AF ◇, Mycelex, Mycelex OTC ◇)
Superficial fungal infections (tinea pedis, tinea cruris, tinea corporis, tinea versicolor, candidiasis)—
Adults and children: apply thinly and massage into affected and surrounding area, morning and evening, for 1 to 8 weeks.

• Contraindicated in patients with known hypersensitivity to the drug.
• Use cautiously in hepatic impairment because abnormal liver function tests have been reported.

(continued)

SELECTED MAJOR DRUGS: LOCAL ANTI-INFECTIVES *continued*

DRUG, INDICATIONS, AND DOSAGES	SPECIAL PRECAUTIONS
Fungicidal agents *(continued)*	

clotrimazole *(continued)*
Candidal vulvovaginitis—
Women: insert 1 applicatorful or 1 tablet intravaginally h.s. daily for 7 to 14 days. Alternatively, insert 2 tablets (100 mg) once daily for 3 consecutive days or 1 tablet (500 mg) one time only h.s.
Oropharyngeal candidiasis—
Adults and children: dissolve lozenge in mouth five times daily for 14 consecutive days.

• Use with caution intravaginally during first trimester of pregnancy because of possible adverse effects on the fetus.

---

econazole nitrate (Spectazole)
Tinea pedis, tinea cruris, and tinea corporis; cutaneous candidiasis—
Adults and children: apply sufficient quantity to cover affected areas b.i.d., in the morning and evening.
Tinea versicolor—
Adults and children: apply once daily.

• Contraindicated in patients with known hypersensitivity to any component.
• Use with caution in pregnant or breast-feeding women.

---

gentian violet (methylrosaniline chloride) (Genapax)
Superficial infections of skin; lesions, except ulcerative lesions of face, particularly Candida albicans —
Adults and children: apply with swab b.i.d. or t.i.d. Keep affected area clean, dry, and exposed to air to prevent spread of infection.
Vaginal fungal infections—
Adults: insert 1 tampon intravaginally for 3 to 4 hours once daily to b.i.d. for 12 days. An additional tampon may be used overnight for resistant infections.

• Contraindicated in patients with ulcerative lesions of the face. Do not use with occlusive dressings.
• Administer cautiously. Tattooing of the skin may occur if applied to granulation tissue.

---

haloprogin (Halotex)
Superficial fungal infections (tinea pedia, tinea cruris, tinea corporis, tinea manuum, and tinea versicolor)—
Adults and children: apply liberally b.i.d. for 2 to 3 weeks.

• Contraindicated in patients with known hypersensitivity to any component.
• Use cautiously in children and in pregnant or breast-feeding women.

---

silver sulfadiazine (Silvadene)
Prevention and treatment of wound infection, especially for second- and third-degree burns—
Adults and children: apply 1/16″ thickness of cream to cleansed and debrided burn wound, then apply daily or b.i.d.

• Contraindicated in premature and newborn infants during first month of life. (Drug may increase possibility of kernicterus.)
• Use with caution in patients with known hypersensitivity to sulfonamides.

SELECTED MAJOR DRUGS: LOCAL ANTI-INFECTIVES *continued*

DRUG, INDICATIONS, AND DOSAGES	SPECIAL PRECAUTIONS

Fungistatic agents

clioquinol (Vioform ◇)
Inflamed skin conditions, including eczema, athlete's foot, and other fungal infections; cutaneous or mucocutaneous mycotic infections caused by Candida species (monilia) —
Adults and children over age 2: apply a thin layer b.i.d. or t.i.d., or as directed. Continue for 1 week after cessation of symptoms.

• Contraindicated in patients with known hypersensitivity to iodine or iodine-containing preparations, and in those with tuberculosis, vaccinia, and varicella.

---

nystatin (Mycostatin, Nilstat, O-V Statin)
Infant eczema, pruritus ani and vulvae, localized forms of candidiasis —
Adults and children: apply to affected area b.i.d. for 2 weeks.
Vulvovaginal candidiasis —
Adults: 1 vaginal tablet daily or b.i.d. for 14 days.

• Contraindicated in patients with known hypersensitivity to any component. Do not use with occlusive dressings.

---

tolnaftate (NP-27 ◇ , Tinactin ◇ , Ting ◇)
Superficial fungal infections of the skin caused by common pathogenic fungi, tinea pedis, tinea cruris, tinea corporis, tinea versicolor —
Adults and children: ¼" to ½" ribbon of cream or 3 drops of lotion to cover about the size of one hand; same amount of cream or 3 drops of lotion to cover the toes and interdigital webs of one foot; or a sufficient amount of gel, powder, or spray to cover affected area. Apply and massage gently into skin b.i.d. for 2 weeks, up to 6 weeks.

• There are no contraindications or precautions to this drug.

---

undecylenic acid and zinc undecylenate (Cruex ◇ , Desenex ◇)
Athlete's foot and ringworm of the body exclusive of nails and hairy areas —
Adults and children: apply b.i.d. to thoroughly cleansed area.

• Contraindicated in children under age 2 except under direct medical supervision.

◇ Available OTC

COMPARING ANTI-INFECTIVE COMBINATIONS

TRADE NAME AND CONTENT	SPECIAL CONSIDERATIONS
Myco II **Mycobiotic II** **Mycogen II** **Mycolog II** **Myco-Triacet II** **Mytrex** **NGT** **Tristatin II** nystatin 100,000 units/g and triamcinolone acetonide 0.1%	• Combines the antifungal action of nystatin with the anti-inflammatory action of the topical corticosteroid triamcinolone acetonide. • Contraindicated in patients with known hypersensitivity to any component. Many preparations contain preservatives that cause allergic contact dermatitis in some patients. • Usually well tolerated when applied locally; however, some patients have experienced an acnelike eruption after use of these drugs. Discontinue the drug if local irritation occurs.
Neomixin ◇ **Neosporin** ◇ **Triple Antibiotic** ◇ bacitracin 400 units/g, neomycin sulfate 0.5%, and polymyxin B sulfate 5,000 units/g	• Combines the antimicrobial efficacy of three antibiotics in a topical ointment. • Contraindicated in patients with known hypersensitivity to any of the components. • Usually associated with little toxicity; however, some patients have experienced anaphylactic reactions to these three drugs when administered systemically. Cross-sensitivity has occurred with neomycin and bacitracin.

◇ Available OTC

SELF-TEST

1. Jennifer Green has second-degree burns, which are being treated with mafenide (Sulfamylon) cream 8.5%. The nurse understands that this medication is a:
   a. bactericidal agent.
   b. bacteriostatic agent.
   c. fungistatic agent.
   d. fungicidal agent.

2. Virginia Bates developed vulvovaginal candidiasis, for which her doctor prescribed miconazole (Monistat 7) vaginal suppositories, to be inserted intravaginally daily at bedtime. Mrs. Bates asked how long she will need to take the medication. What should the nurse tell her?
   a. 3 days
   b. 7 days
   c. 10 days
   d. 14 days

3. Don Sutton has a superficial skin infection that followed an abrasion on his hand. His doctor ordered culture and sensitivity tests and bacitracin ointment 500 units/g t.i.d. The nurse should:
 a. start the bacitracin immediately.
 b. obtain the sample for culture and sensitivity tests before the initial application of the bacitracin.
 c. wait for the results of culture and sensitivity tests before initiating bacitracin treatment.
 d. understand that the sequence of carrying out the doctor's orders has no impact on the patient's care.

4. Amelia Zonderman's discharge orders include acyclovir ointment (Zovirax) 5% to be applied to genital herpes lesions. Which of the following should the nurse include in her discharge teaching?
 a. The patient can discontinue use of the acyclovir when the lesions decrease in number.
 b. She cannot transfer the virus while she applies the acyclovir.
 c. Acyclovir will not prevent the spread of herpes to others.
 d. Recurrence of the herpes infection cannot occur after treatment with acyclovir.

Check your answers on page 1077.

CHAPTER 85

SCABICIDES AND PEDICULICIDES

benzyl benzoate lotion ✦ crotamiton
lindane (gamma benzene hexachloride) ✦ malathion ✦ permethrin
pyrethrins

OVERVIEW

- Scabicides and pediculicides destroy the most common parasitic arthropods that infest man.
- Persistent itching after adequate therapy indicates either continued infestation, slow-resolving hypersensitivity, or irritation from the drug. Laundering or dry-cleaning all contaminated linens and clothing is essential to eradicate infestations. Commercial sprays can be used to decontaminate furniture or rugs that may harbor the parasites.

MAJOR USES

- These drugs eradicate parasitic arthropod infestations such as scabies and pediculosis. They're used against *Sarcoptes scabiei* (scabies), *Pediculus humanus* var. *capitis* (head louse), *Pediculus humanus* var. *corporis* (body louse), and *Phthirus pubis* (crab louse). One application is usually enough to kill adult forms, but repeated applications are necessary to destroy nits.

MECHANISM OF ACTION

- Lindane appears to inhibit neuronal membrane function in arthropods.
- Pyrethrins acts as a contact poison that disrupts the parasite's nervous system, resulting in the paralysis and death of the parasite. Pyrethrins is mixed with piperonyl butoxide, which inhibits the parasite's ability to detoxify pyrethrins.
- The mechanism of action of the other scabicides and pediculicides is unknown.

ABSORPTION, DISTRIBUTION, METABOLISM, AND EXCRETION

Lindane is absorbed through intact skin when applied topically. Absorption through skin is usually greatest when the drug is applied to face, scalp, neck, axillae, scrotum, or damaged skin.

No information is available on systemic absorption of the other scabicides and pediculicides. Lindane is stored in body fat, metabolized in the liver, and eliminated in urine and feces.

GLOSSARY

Pediculicide: drug that kills lice.
Pediculosis: infestation of the body or scalp by lice.
Scabicide: drug that destroys the itch mite.
Scabies: disease caused by *Sarcoptes scabiei*, the itch mite, characterized by intense itching of the skin and excoriation from scratching.

ONSET AND DURATION

Onset of action of all the scabicides and pediculicides is immediate. Duration of action is limited. The scabicide or pediculicide must be reapplied, if necessary, according to product information.

ADVERSE REACTIONS

All of these agents may cause itching, irritation, mild erythema, rash, or hypersensitivity reactions; a local burning sensation is common.

Lindane can also cause adverse CNS reactions ranging from dizziness to seizures. Lindane penetrates human skin, which accounts for its systemic reactions. These neurotoxicities are more severe in young patients and with repeated use.

PROTOTYPE: SCABICIDES AND PEDICULICIDES

LINDANE
(lin' dane)
gBh†, Kwell, Kwellada†, Scabene
Classification: scabicide and pediculicide
Pregnancy risk category C

How supplied
CREAM: 1%
LOTION: 1%
SHAMPOO: 1%

Indications and dosage
Parasitic infestation (scabies, pediculosis)
ADULTS AND CHILDREN: scrub entire body with soap and water. Then apply thin layer of cream or lotion over entire skin surface (with special attention to folds, creases, interdigital spaces, and genital area) for scabies, or to hairy areas for pediculosis. After 12 hours, wash off drug. If second application is needed, wait 1 week before repeating. Alternatively, apply shampoo undiluted to affected area and work into lather for 4 to 5 minutes. Rinse thoroughly and rub with dry towel.

Contraindications and precautions
Lindane is contraindicated for application on raw or inflamed skin.

Adverse reactions
CNS: dizziness, seizures.
SKIN: irritation with repeated use.

Interactions
None significant.

Nursing considerations

Assessment
- Review the patient's history for a condition that contraindicates the use of lindane.
- Obtain a baseline assessment of skin and hair for degree of infestation before therapy.
- Be alert for common adverse reactions.
- Evaluate the patient's and family's knowledge about lindane therapy.

Planning (Nursing Diagnoses)
Potential nursing diagnoses for the patient receiving lindane include:
- Impaired skin integrity related to ineffectiveness of lindane.
- Potential for injury related to adverse CNS reactions to lindane.
- Knowledge deficit related to lindane therapy.

Implementation

Preparation and administration
— Before treatment, wash the patient's entire body with soap and water. Pat dry and allow body to cool before application.
— Wear gloves to avoid systemic absorption and infestation when administering.
— To apply shampoo, use a sufficient amount to wet hair and scalp (30 ml for short hair; 45 ml for medium-length hair; 60 ml for long hair). Work into a lather for 4 to 5 minutes. Rinse thoroughly and rub with a dry towel. When hair is dry, use a fine-toothed comb dipped in white vinegar to remove remaining nits or nit shells. Lindane shampoo may be used to disinfect combs and brushes to prevent spread of infestation.
— Chart the administration of drug and related observations.

Monitoring
— Monitor the effectiveness of lindane therapy by regularly assessing the skin and hair for degree of infestation.
— Monitor for hypersensitivity to the drug.
— Monitor the patient for adverse drug reactions.
— Monitor the patient for seizures and dizziness.
— Monitor the patient's family and close contacts (such as sexual partners) for infestation.
— Periodically reevaluate the patient's and family's knowledge about lindane.

Intervention

—If a hypersensitivity reaction to lindane occurs, immediately wash off the drug and notify the doctor.

—Have the patient's fingernails cut short to minimize skin trauma from scratching.

—Apply cool, moist compresses to relieve itching.

—Maintain seizure and safety precautions if adverse CNS reactions occur.

—Keep all members of the health care team informed of the patient's response to the drug.

Patient teaching

—Inform the patient and family about lindane, including the dosage, frequency, action, and adverse reactions.

—Instruct the patient to avoid repeated use of lindane (more than once per week) because it may cause toxicity.

—Tell the patient that itching may persist for several weeks after treatment.

—Instruct the patient to launder all recently worn clothing, linens, and towels in very hot water to prevent reinfestation.

—Tell the patient to notify all close contacts and inspect all family members for infestation.

—Warn the patient to avoid hazardous activities that require mental alertness if dizziness occurs.

—Tell the patient to notify the nurse or doctor if adverse reactions develop or questions arise about lindane therapy.

Evaluation

In the patient receiving lindane, appropriate evaluation statements include:
• Patient's skin and hair reveal no evidence of infestation on inspection.
• Patient does not experience injury as a result of adverse CNS reactions.
• Patient and family state an understanding of lindane therapy.

SELECTED MAJOR DRUGS: SCABICIDES AND PEDICULICIDES

DRUG, INDICATIONS, AND DOSAGES	SPECIAL PRECAUTIONS
benzyl benzoate lotion *Parasitic infestation (scabies,* Phthirus pubis *)*— **Adults and children:** first, scrub entire body with soap and water. Remove scales or crusts. Then apply the lotion undiluted over entire body, except the face and scalp, while still damp. Be sure to apply around nails. Let dry. Apply second coat on the most involved areas. Bathe after 24 hours.	• Contraindicated when skin is raw or inflamed. • Use cautiously in patients in isolation and in hospitals; use linen-handling precautions until treatment is completed.

(continued)

SELECTED MAJOR DRUGS: SCABICIDES AND PEDICULICIDES
continued

DRUG, INDICATIONS, AND DOSAGES	SPECIAL PRECAUTIONS
crotamiton (Eurax) *Parasitic infestation (scabies)—* **Adults and children:** scrub entire body with soap and water. Then, apply a thin layer of cream over entire body, from chin down (with special attention to folds, creases, interdigital spaces, and genital area). Apply second coat in 24 hours. Wait additional 48 hours, then wash off. *Itching—* **Adults and children:** apply locally b.i.d. or t.i.d.	• Contraindicated when skin is raw or inflamed, in patients who develop sensitivity or are allergic to it, or in those who manifest a primary irritation response to topical medications. • Use cautiously in patients at risk for carcinogenesis, mutagenesis, or impaired fertility; in children; and in pregnant women.
permethrin (Elimite, Nix ◇) *Infestation with* Pediculus humanus capitis *(head lice) and nits—* **Adults and children:** use after hair has been washed with shampoo, rinsed with water, and towel-dried. Apply a sufficient amount (25 to 50 ml) of liquid to saturate the hair and scalp. Allow to remain on hair for 10 minutes before rinsing off with water.	• Contraindicated in patients with known hypersensitivity to pyrethrins or chrysanthemums. • Use cautiously in patients at risk for carcinogenesis, mutagenesis, or impaired fertility; in children; and in pregnant or breast-feeding women.
pyrethrins (R&C ◇ , RID ◇) *Infestations of head, body, and pubic (crab) lice and their nits—* **Adults and children:** apply to hair, scalp, or other infested area until entirely wet. Allow to remain for 10 minutes, but no longer. Wash thoroughly with warm water and soap, or shampoo. Remove dead lice and nits with fine-toothed comb. Treatment may be repeated, if necessary, but don't exceed two applications within 24 hours. May repeat in 7 to 10 days to kill newly hatched lice.	• Contraindicated when skin is raw or inflamed, or in patients allergic to ragweed. • Use cautiously in infants and small children.

◇ Available OTC

SELF-TEST

1. Karen Turner seeks medical treatment of scabies. The doctor orders application of lindane cream 1% to all skin surfaces from neck to toes. After the treatment Mrs. Turner continues to complain about itching. The nurse should:
   a. reapply the lindane cream treatment.
   b. advise the patient to apply some moisturizing lotion.
   c. explain that itching may continue for several weeks after treatment.
   d. recognize that continued itching signifies lice infestation.

2. Mrs. Turner should be informed that adverse reactions to lindane may include:
   a. seizures.
   b. hypertension.
   c. hyperglycemia.
   d. dehydration.

3. The nurse should teach Mrs. Turner to prevent reinfestation by:
   a. reapplying the lindane cream every 3 days for 2 weeks.
   b. laundering all recently worn clothes and linens in very hot water.
   c. keeping hair cut short.
   d. avoiding use of soap when bathing for 3 days after application.

Check your answers on page 1077.

CHAPTER 86

TOPICAL CORTICOSTEROIDS

amcinonide ◆ betamethasone ◆ betamethasone benzoate
betamethasone dipropionate ◆ betamethasone valerate
clobetasol proprionate ◆ clocortolone pivalate ◆ desonide
desoximetasone ◆ dexamethasone ◆ dexamethasone sodium phosphate
diflorasone diacetate ◆ flumethasone pivalate ◆ fluocinolone acetonide
fluocinonide ◆ fluorometholone ◆ flurandrenolide ◆ halcinonide
hydrocortisone ◆ hydrocortisone acetate ◆ hydrocortisone valerate
methylprednisolone acetate ◆ triamcinolone acetonide

OVERVIEW

- Topical corticosteroids reduce inflammation, constrict blood vessels, and occasionally relieve itching. Their potency depends on the drug, the method of application, and the degree of penetration. The base or vehicle of the drug may also affect its release and therefore its potency. Ointments furnish the most complete penetration of the skin by the drug; gels, creams, and lotions are less penetrating, in descending order. Topical corticosteroids reduce inflammation without curing the underlying disease; use them with caution.
- After the drug is applied to the affected site, it may be covered by an occlusive dressing held in place by tape. The dressing facilitates the drug's absorption through the skin. It protects the adjacent unaffected skin from abrasion, rubbing, discoloration, and chemical irritation. It also acts as a mechanical splint for fissured skin and prevents medication from being removed by washing or rubbing against clothing.

MAJOR USES

- Topical corticosteroids are used to treat acute and chronic inflammatory dermatoses; psoriasis; atopic and infantile eczema; pruritus ani and vulvae; neurodermatitis; and contact, seborrheic, and exfoliative dermatitis.
- Occlusive dressings are used with topical corticosteroids in the medical management of psoriasis or such resistant conditions as localized neurodermatitis or lichen planus.
- Creams are useful for wet lesions; lotions, for areas subject to chafing (axillae, feet, or groin); and ointments, for dry, scaly lesions.

MECHANISM OF ACTION

- Exactly how these drugs work is unknown. Some investigators believe that topical corticosteroids attach to tissue receptors, decreasing membrane permeability and inhibiting release of toxins. They may also control the rate of protein synthesis.
- The actions of topical corticosteroids on the inflammatory process include inhibition of edema, fibrin deposition, capillary dilation, migration of leukocytes into the inflamed area, and phagocytic activity. They may also moderate later inflammatory developments such as capillary and fibroblast proliferation and deposition of collagen.
- Corticosteroid-induced vasoconstriction decreases extravasation of blood, swelling, and itching.
- The drugs also act as antimitotics, reducing cell multiplication in psoriasis.

ABSORPTION, DISTRIBUTION, METABOLISM, AND EXCRETION

Corticosteroids are absorbed through the skin, and absorption varies markedly with the area of the body on which the drugs are applied. If the skin is well hydrated, absorption will be increased four to five times. Inflamed or damaged skin also allows increased penetration. Occlusive dressings retain perspiration, causing hydration of the stratum corneum; they increase absorption significantly (up to a hundred times) and may cause systemic adverse reactions.

These drugs enter the circulation and are metabolized primarily in the liver. The metabolites are excreted in urine.

ONSET AND DURATION

Topical corticosteroids begin to act within 30 minutes after application. Because their action lasts only 4 to 6 hours, they should be applied two to four times daily.

ADVERSE REACTIONS

Topical corticosteroids usually cause few systemic reactions. However, prolonged use or application over extensive areas, especially with use of occlusive dressings, can cause reactions related to suppression of the adrenal-pituitary axis and excessive steroid activity (Cushing's syndrome and glycosuria).

Significant adverse reactions to normal use include skin atrophy, miliaria, striae, and secondary infections. Other reactions include burning, itching, irritation, acneiform eruptions, dermatitis, hypopigmentation, and hypertrichosis.

HYDROCORTISONE
(hye droe kor′ ti sone)
*Acticort, Aeroseb-HC, Carmol HC, Cetacort, Cort-Dome, Cortef◊,
Cortinal, Cortizone 5◊, Cortril, Cremesone, Delacort, Dermi Cort◊,
Dermolate◊, Ecosone, Hi-Cor, Hycortole, Hydrocortex, Hytone,
Ivocort, Orabase-HCA, Penecort, Proctocort, Rocort, Squibb-HC‡,
Unicort*

HYDROCORTISONE ACETATE
*Cortaid◊, Cortef, Corticreme†, Cortifoam, Dermacort‡, Epifoam,
MyCort Lotion, Proctofoam-HC*

HYDROCORTISONE VALERATE
Westcort Cream

Classification: topical corticosteroid
Pregnancy risk category C

How supplied
hydrocortisone
AEROSOL: 0.5%
CREAM: 0.25%◊, 0.5%◊, 1%, 2.5%
GEL: 1%
LOTION: 0.125%, 0.25%, 0.5%◊, 1%, 2%, 2.5%
OINTMENT: 0.5%◊, 1%, 2.5%
TOPICAL SOLUTION: 1%
hydrocortisone acetate
CREAM: 0.5%◊
LOTION: 0.5%◊
OINTMENT: 0.5%◊, 1%
RECTAL FOAM: 90 mg/application
hydrocortisone valerate
CREAM: 0.2%
OINTMENT: 0.2%

Indications and dosage
*Inflammation of corticosteroid-responsive dermatoses; adjunctive
topical management of seborrheic dermatitis of scalp; may be safely
used on face, groin, armpits, and under breasts*
ADULTS AND CHILDREN: after cleansing affected area, apply cream, gel,
lotion, ointment, or topical solution sparingly daily to q.i.d. To administer
aerosol, shake can well and direct spray onto affected area from a distance
of 6″ (15 cm). Apply for only 3 seconds to avoid freezing tissues. Apply
to dry scalp after shampooing; no need to massage or rub medication into
scalp after spraying. Apply daily until acute phase is controlled, then
reduce dosage to one to three times a week as needed to maintain control.

---

†Available in Canada only   ‡Available in Australia only   ◊ Available OTC

To administer the rectal form, shake can well and give 1 applicatorful daily to b.i.d. for 2 to 3 weeks, then every other day as necessary.

Contraindications and precautions

Topical hydrocortisone is contraindicated in patients with known hypersensitivity to any component of the preparation. Use cautiously in patients with viral skin diseases, such as varicella, vaccinia, or herpes simplex; fungal infections; or bacterial skin infections.

Adverse reactions

SKIN: burning, itching, irritation, dryness, folliculitis, hypertrichosis, hypopigmentation, acneiform eruptions, allergic contact dermatitis; with occlusive dressings—maceration of skin, secondary infection, atrophy, striae, miliaria.

Interactions

None significant.

Nursing considerations

Assessment

- Review the patient's history for a condition that contraindicates the use of topical hydrocortisone.
- Obtain a baseline assessment of skin for extent and severity of inflammatory dermatoses before therapy.
- Be alert for common adverse reactions.
- Evaluate the patient's and family's knowledge about hydrocortisone therapy.

Planning (Nursing Diagnoses)

Potential nursing diagnoses for the patient receiving hydrocortisone include:
- Impaired skin integrity related to ineffectiveness of hydrocortisone to treat inflammatory dermatoses.
- Potential for infection related to hydrocortisone therapy.
- Knowledge deficit related to hydrocortisone therapy.

Implementation

Preparation and administration

— Read order and drug labels carefully.
— Wear gloves when administering drug.
— Before applying, gently wash the patient's skin. Apply a thin layer and rub in gently.
— When treating hairy sites, part hair and apply directly to lesion.
— To apply an occlusive dressing (only if ordered by doctor), apply cream heavily, then cover with a thin, pliable, nonflammable plastic film; seal to adjacent normal skin with hypoallergenic tape.
— To minimize adverse reactions, use occlusive dressing intermittently. Don't leave in place longer than 16 hours each day. Occlusive dressings should not be used in the presence of infection or on weeping or exudative lesions.

—For patients with eczematous dermatitis who may develop irritation with adhesive material, hold dressing in place with gauze, elastic bandage, or stockings.

—Notify the doctor and remove occlusive dressing if fever develops.

—Aerosol preparation contains alcohol and may produce irritation or burning in open lesions when administered. When using on the face, cover the patient's eyes and warn against inhalation of the spray. To avoid freezing tissues, do not spray longer than 3 seconds or closer than 6″ (15 cm).

—Treatment should be continued for a few days after clearing of lesions to prevent recurrence.

—Chart the administration of the drug and related observations.

Monitoring

—Monitor the effectiveness of topical hydrocortisone therapy by regularly assessing skin for extent and severity of inflammation.

—Monitor for hypersensitivity reaction to hydrocortisone.

—Monitor the patient for adverse drug reactions.

—Monitor for evidence of secondary infection.

—Periodically reevaluate the patient's and family's knowledge about hydrocortisone.

Intervention

—Withhold the drug and notify the doctor if hypersensitivity reaction or infection occurs.

—Have the patient's fingernails cut short to minimize skin trauma from scratching.

—Apply cool, moist compresses to involved areas to relieve itching and burning.

—Use hypoallergenic tape, gauze, stockings, or elastic bandage to secure occlusive dressings.

—Keep all members of the health care team informed of the patient's response to the drug.

Patient teaching

—Inform the patient and family about hydrocortisone, including the dosage, frequency, action, and adverse reactions.

—Instruct the patient to cleanse involved area before applying hydrocortisone in a thin layer to cover the entire surface.

—Teach the patient how to apply an occlusive dressing.

—Teach the patient and family how to recognize signs of a hypersensitivity reaction or infection. Advise them to discontinue the drug and notify the doctor immediately if they occur.

—Instruct the patient to complete the entire treatment regimen as prescribed, even if the lesions appear to have healed.

—Tell the patient and family not to share the hydrocortisone prescription with others and not to administer topical hydrocortisone to children under age 2 without a doctor's order.

— Tell the patient to notify the nurse or doctor if adverse reactions develop or questions arise about hydrocortisone therapy.

Evaluation

In the patient receiving hydrocortisone, appropriate evaluation statements include:
• Patient's skin reveals decreased or suppressed inflammation on inspection.
• Patient demonstrates no signs of infection.
• Patient and family state an understanding of hydrocortisone therapy.

SELECTED MAJOR DRUGS: TOPICAL CORTICOSTEROIDS

DRUG, INDICATIONS, AND DOSAGES	SPECIAL PRECAUTIONS
amcinonide (Cyclocort) *Inflammation of corticosteroid-responsive dermatoses —* **Adults and children:** apply a light film to affected areas b.i.d. or t.i.d. Cream should be rubbed in gently and thoroughly until it disappears.	• Contraindicated in patients with known hypersensitivity to any component of the preparation. • Use cautiously in patients with viral skin diseases, such as varicella, vaccinia, or herpes simplex; fungal infections; or bacterial skin infections.
betamethasone benzoate (Benisone, Uticort) **betamethasone dipropionate (augmented) (Diprolene)** **betamethasone dipropionate (Alphatrex Diprosone)** **betamethasone valerate (Betatrex, Valisone)** *Inflammation of corticosteroid-responsive dermatoses —* **Adults and children:** after cleansing affected area, apply cream, lotion, spray, or gel sparingly daily to q.i.d.	• Contraindicated in patients with known hypersensitivity to any component of the preparation. • Use cautiously in patients with viral skin diseases, such as varicella, vaccinia, or herpes simplex; fungal infections; or bacterial skin infections.
clocortolone pivalate (Cloderm) *Inflammation of corticosteroid-responsive dermatoses, such as atopic dermatitis, contact dermatitis, seborrheic dermatitis —* **Adults and children:** apply cream sparingly to affected areas once daily to q.i.d. and rub in gently.	• Do not use in children under age 12. • Use cautiously in patients with viral skin diseases, such as varicella, vaccinia, or herpes simplex; fungal infections; or bacterial skin infections.
desonide (DesOwen, Tridesilon) *Adjunctive therapy of inflammation in acute and chronic corticosteroid-responsive dermatoses —* **Adults and children:** after cleansing affected area, apply cream or lotion sparingly b.i.d. to q.i.d.	• Contraindicated for use near eyes, mucous membranes, or in the ear canal. • Use cautiously in patients with viral skin diseases, such as varicella, vaccinia, or herpes simplex; fungal infections; or bacterial skin infections.

(continued)

SELECTED MAJOR DRUGS: TOPICAL CORTICOSTEROIDS *continued*

DRUG, INDICATIONS, AND DOSAGES	SPECIAL PRECAUTIONS
desoximetasone (Topicort) *Inflammation of corticosteroid-responsive dermatoses*— **Adults and children:** after cleansing affected area, apply cream, gel, or ointment sparingly once daily to b.i.d.	• Contraindicated in patients with known hypersensitivity to any component of the preparation. • Use cautiously in patients with viral skin diseases, such as varicella, vaccinia, or herpes simplex; fungal infections; or bacterial skin infections.
dexamethasone (Aeroseb-Dex, Decaderm, Decaspray) **dexamethasone sodium phosphate (Decadron Phosphate)** *Inflammation of corticosteroid-responsive dermatoses*— **Adults and children:** after cleansing affected area, apply cream, gel, or aerosol sparingly b.i.d. To use aerosol on scalp, shake can well and apply to dry scalp after shampooing. Hold can upright. Slide applicator tube under hair so that it touches scalp. Spray while moving tube to all affected areas. Spraying should take about 2 seconds. Inadequately covered areas may be spot sprayed. Don't massage medication into scalp or spray forehead or eyes.	• Contraindicated in patients with systemic fungal infections or known hypersensitivity to any component. • Use cautiously in patients with viral skin diseases, such as varicella, vaccinia, or herpes simplex; fungal infections; or bacterial skin infections.
diflorasone diacetate (Florone, Flutone, Maxiflor, psorcon) *Inflammation of corticosteroid-responsive dermatoses*— **Adults and children:** after cleansing affected area, apply ointment daily to t.i.d., or apply cream b.i.d. to q.i.d. Apply sparingly in a thin film.	• Contraindicated in patients with known hypersensitivity to any component. • Use cautiously in patients with viral skin diseases, such as varicella, vaccinia, or herpes simplex; fungal infections; or bacterial skin infections. • Use very cautiously in young children because this is a high-potency corticosteroid.
fluocinolone acetonide (Fluocet, Fluonid, Flurosyn, Synalar, Synemol) *Inflammation of corticosteroid-responsive dermatoses*— **Adults and children over age 2:** after cleansing affected area, apply cream, ointment, or solution sparingly b.i.d. to q.i.d. Treat multiple or extensive lesions sequentially, applying to only small areas at any one time.	• Contraindicated in patients with known hypersensitivity to any component. • Use cautiously in patients with viral skin diseases, such as varicella, vaccinia, or herpes simplex; fungal infections; or bacterial skin infections.
fluocinonide (Lidemol†, Lidex, Lidex-E, Topsyn) *Inflammation of corticosteroid-responsive dermatoses*— **Adults and children:** after cleansing affected area, apply cream, ointment, solution, or gel sparingly t.i.d. or q.i.d.	• Use cautiously in patients with viral skin diseases, such as varicella, vaccinia, or herpes simplex; fungal infections; or bacterial skin infections.

†Available in Canada only

SELECTED MAJOR DRUGS: TOPICAL CORTICOSTEROIDS *continued*

DRUG, INDICATIONS, AND DOSAGES

SPECIAL PRECAUTIONS

flurandrenolide (Cordran, Cordran SP, Cordran Tape, Drenison†)
Inflammation of corticosteroid-responsive dermatoses—
Adults and children: after cleansing affected area, apply cream, lotion, or ointment sparingly b.i.d. or t.i.d. Apply tape q 12 to 24 hours. Before applying tape, cleanse skin carefully, removing scales, crust, and dried exudates. Allow skin to dry for 1 hour before applying new tape. Shave or clip hair to allow good contact with skin and comfortable removal. If tape ends loosen prematurely, trim off and replace with fresh tape. The incidence of adverse reactions is lowest if tape is replaced q 12 hours, but it may be left in place for 24 hours if well tolerated and adhering satisfactorily.

• Use cautiously in patients with viral skin diseases, such as varicella, vaccinia, or herpes simplex; fungal infections; or bacterial skin infections.

halcinonide (Halciderm, Halog)
Inflammation of acute and chronic corticosteroid-responsive dermatoses—
Adults and children: after cleansing affected area, apply cream, ointment, or solution sparingly b.i.d. or t.i.d.

• Contraindicated in patients with known hypersensitivity to any component.
• Use cautiously in patients with viral skin diseases, such as varicella, vaccinia, or herpes simplex; fungal infections; or bacterial skin infections.

methylprednisolone acetate (Medrol)
Inflammation of corticosteroid-responsive dermatoses—
Adults and children: after cleansing affected area, apply ointment daily to q.i.d.

• Contraindicated for intrathecal administration, in systemic fungal infections, and in patients with known hypersensitivity to any component.
• Use cautiously in patients with viral skin diseases, such as varicella, vaccinia, or herpes simplex; fungal infections; or bacterial skin infections.

triamcinolone acetonide (Aristocort, Kenalog, Kenalone‡)
Inflammation of corticosteroid-responsive dermatoses—
Adults and children: after cleansing affected area, apply aerosol, cream, lotion, or ointment sparingly b.i.d. to q.i.d. To administer aerosol, shake can well and direct spray onto affected area from a distance of approximately 6″ (15 cm); apply for only 3 seconds.

• Contraindicated in patients with known hypersensitivity to any component.
• Use cautiously in patients with viral skin diseases, such as varicella, vaccinia, or herpes simplex; fungal infections; or bacterial skin infections.

†Available in Canada only   ‡Available in Australia only

SELF-TEST

1. Martin Jerrold has chronic dermatoses on his leg. His doctor orders hydrocortisone cream 1%. Which of the following responses will this drug produce?
   a. Anti-inflammatory
   b. Antiviral
   c. Bactericidal
   d. Bacteriostatic

2. Before applying hydrocortisone cream, Mr. Jerrold's nurse should:
   a. shave the involved skin surface.
   b. apply peroxide.
   c. wash the involved skin surface.
   d. apply a warm soak.

3. Systemic absorption of topical hydrocortisone is more likely with:
   a. a diet high in fat.
   b. a secondary infection.
   c. limited body-surface treatment.
   d. use of occlusive dressings.

4. Mr. Jerrold's temperature is elevated. On inspection, the involved area on his leg appears red and warm and has a white, foul-smelling exudate. The nurse should:
   a. give 2 acetaminophen (Tylenol) tablets.
   b. stop the hydrocortisone therapy and notify the doctor.
   c. clean off the exudate with warm compresses.
   d. apply ice packs to the site.

Check your answers on pages 1077 and 1078.

CHAPTER 87

ANTIGOUT AGENTS

Uricosurics
probenecid ✦ sulfinpyrazone

Miscellaneous antigout agents
allopurinol ✦ colchicine

OVERVIEW
- Gout, a hereditary disease involving an error in metabolism, leads to hyperuricemia and the formation of monosodium urate crystals. Deposits of these monosodium urate crystals in and around a joint cause the inflammation and resultant pain of the disease. Gout is best treated with a uricosuric, such as probenecid and sulfinpyrazone, or other antigout agents, such as allopurinol and colchicine.
- The antigout agents are classified into two groups: uricosurics and miscellaneous antigout agents.

MAJOR USES
- The two major uricosurics, probenecid and sulfinpyrazone, are primarily used to prevent or control the frequency of gouty arthritis attacks. Probenecid has also been used to diagnose parkinsonian syndrome and mental depression.
- The other antigout agents are commonly prescribed to treat acute attacks of gout. Allopurinol is used to treat primary gout and gout associated with blood disorders, such as leukemia and polycythemia, cancer, and cancer chemotherapy. Colchicine is used to relieve acute attacks of gouty arthritis and to prevent recurrent gouty arthritis.

MECHANISM OF ACTION
- The uricosurics act to increase uric acid excretion in the urine by competitively inhibiting the active resorption of uric acid at the proximal convoluted tubules of the kidney. By promoting a decreased serum urate level, they reduce tophi formation and chronic joint destruction. The goal of uricosuric therapy is to reduce the frequency of acute episodes of gouty arthritis.
- Probenecid also blocks active secretion of penicillins into the urine. It is used to prolong high serum drug levels during antibiotic therapy.
- Allopurinol lowers serum and urine uric acid levels by inhibiting xanthine oxidase, the enzyme that catalyzes the formation of uric acid from xanthine.

GLOSSARY

Gout: condition caused by abnormal purine metabolism, characterized by an increased serum uric acid level, acute arthritic episodes, and formation of chalky urate deposits in the joints.

Hyperuricemia: excess uric acid in the blood.

Inflammation: tissue response to injury, characterized by pain, heat, redness, edema and, sometimes, loss of function.

Tophi: chalky urate deposits in the tissue around joints that typically occur in individuals with gout.

Uricosuric: agent that promotes uric acid excretion.

• Colchicine appears to reduce the inflammatory response by leukocytes to monosodium urate crystals deposited in joint tissues.

ABSORPTION, DISTRIBUTION, METABOLISM, AND EXCRETION

The uricosurics are absorbed rapidly and completely from the GI tract. Distribution is widespread throughout the body, with 75% to 95% of probenecid and 98% of sulfinpyrazone being protein-bound. The uricosurics are metabolized in the liver and primarily excreted in the urine. Only small amounts are excreted in the feces.

After oral administration, up to 90% of allopurinol is absorbed. It is metabolized in the liver. Allopurinol's inactive metabolite alloxanthine is distributed throughout tissue fluid, with the exception of the brain. Allopurinol is excreted primarily in the urine.

Colchicine, like allopurinol, is well absorbed after oral administration, and is metabolized in the liver. Colchicine is distributed to various tissues throughout the body, with the highest concentration found in leukocytes. It is excreted in the feces.

ONSET AND DURATION

Onset of action of the uricosurics is rapid—within 30 minutes after oral administration. The duration of action of the uricosurics ranges from 4 to 6 hours but may last as long as 10 hours. Allopurinol appears in the plasma 30 to 60 minutes after oral administration. It peaks in 2 to 6 hours and has a duration of 2 to 3 days. Colchicine achieves a peak plasma concentration within 30 minutes to 2 hours. The pain of an acute gout attack is relieved 12 to 48 hours after oral administration and 4 to 12 hours after I.V. administration. The duration of action varies.

ADVERSE REACTIONS

Although the uricosurics are usually well tolerated, some adverse reactions can occur. The most frequent adverse reactions to probenecid are headache and GI distress, including anorexia, nausea, and vomiting. Other adverse reactions include flushing, dizziness, urinary frequency, sore gums, and anemia. The most common adverse reactions to sulfinpyrazone include nausea, dyspepsia, GI pain, and GI blood loss.

Some patients taking uricosurics may develop uric acid calculi—usually on initiation of therapy. Acute gout attacks and hypersensitivity reactions may also occur.

The most common adverse reaction to allopurinol is a maculopapular rash. Adverse GI reactions may also occur. Less common reactions include hematopoietic changes.

The most common adverse reactions to orally administered colchicine include nausea, vomiting, abdominal discomfort, and diarrhea. These GI symptoms are an early sign of toxicity and require discontinuation of the drug until these symptoms disappear (usually for 24 to 48 hours). Other adverse reactions primarily affect the skin, cardiovascular system, and hematopoietic system.

PROTOTYPE: URICOSURICS

PROBENECID
(proe ben'e sid)
Benemid, Benn, Benuryl†, Probalan, Robenecid
Classification: uricosuric
Pregnancy risk category B

How supplied
TABLETS: 500 mg

Indications and dosage
Treatment of hyperuricemia of gout, gouty arthritis
ADULTS: 250 mg P.O. b.i.d. for first week, then 500 mg P.O. b.i.d., to maximum of 2 g daily. Maintenance dosage is 500 mg P.O. daily for 6 months.

Adjunct to penicillin or cephalosporin therapy
ADULTS AND CHILDREN OVER 50 KG: 500 mg P.O. q.i.d.
CHILDREN AGES 2 TO 14 UNDER 50 KG: initially, 25 mg/kg P.O., then 40 mg/kg in divided doses q.i.d.

Single-dose treatment of gonorrhea
ADULTS: 3.5 g ampicillin P.O. with 1 g probenecid P.O. given together; or 1 g probenecid P.O. 30 minutes before dose of 4.8 million units of aqueous penicillin G procaine I.M., injected at two different sites.

Contraindications and precautions
Probenecid is contraindicated in patients with known hypersensitivity to the drug and in children under age 2. It is not recommended in persons with known blood dyscrasia or uric acid renal calculi. Don't use with penicillin in patients with known renal impairment.

Use with caution in patients with a history of peptic ulcer.

Adverse reactions

BLOOD: hemolytic anemia.
CNS: *headache,* dizziness.
CV: hypotension.
GI: *anorexia, nausea, vomiting,* gastric distress.
GU: urinary frequency, renal colic, uric acid calculi.
SKIN: dermatitis, pruritus, alopecia.
OTHER: flushing, sore gums, fever, acute gout attacks.

Interactions

Indomethacin: decreased indomethacin excretion. Expect to administer lower indomethacin dose.
Methotrexate: decreased methotrexate excretion. Expect to administer lower methotrexate dose. Serum levels should be determined.
Oral antidiabetic agents: enhanced hypoglycemic effect. Monitor blood glucose levels closely. Dosage adjustment of antidiabetic agent may be required.
Salicylates: high doses inhibit uricosuric effect of probenecid, causing urate retention. Do not use together.

Nursing considerations

Assessment

• Review the patient's history for a condition that contraindicates the use of probenecid.
• Obtain a baseline assessment of the patient's gout attacks before therapy.
• Be alert for common adverse reactions.
• Evaluate the patient's and family's knowledge about probenecid therapy.

Planning (Nursing Diagnoses)

Potential nursing diagnoses for the patient receiving probenecid include:
• Potential for injury related to ineffectiveness of dosage regimen.
• Altered health maintenance related to adverse reactions.
• Pain (headache) related to adverse reactions to probenecid.
• Knowledge deficit related to probenecid therapy.

Implementation

Preparation and administration

— When used for hyperuricemia associated with gout, probenecid has no analgesic or anti-inflammatory actions, and no effect on acute attacks; start therapy after attack subsides. Because the drug may increase the frequency of acute attacks during the first 6 to 12 months of therapy, expect to administer concomitant prophylactic doses of colchicine or an NSAID during the first 3 to 6 months of probenecid therapy.
— Give with food, milk, or prescribed antacids to lessen GI upset.
— Remember that lower doses are indicated in elderly patients.

Monitoring

— Monitor the effectiveness of probenecid therapy by regularly assessing frequency of gouty arthritis attacks.
— Monitor the patient for adverse drug reactions.

—Monitor for headache.

—Monitor blood pressure for hypotension and temperature for fever.

—Monitor BUN and serum creatinine levels closely; drug is ineffective in patients with severe renal insufficiency.

—Monitor uric acid levels and adjust dosage to the lowest dose that maintains normal uric acid levels.

—Monitor CBC for evidence of hemolytic anemia.

—Monitor hydration status if adverse GI reactions occur.

—Monitor the patient's intake and output so that patient maintains minimum daily output of 2 to 3 liters.

—Monitor the patient for drug interactions.

—Monitor diagnostic test results. Probenecid may produce false-positive results on urine glucose tests with copper sulfate (Clinitest), but not with tests that use the glucose enzymatic method (Clinistix, Tes-Tape). It decreases urinary excretion of 17-ketosteroids, sulfobromophthalein sodium (BSP), aminohippuric acid, and iodine-related organic acids.

—Periodically reevaluate the patient's and family's knowledge about probenecid.

Intervention

—Notify the doctor if the patient's uric acid level increases. Expect to alkalinize urine with sodium bicarbonate or potassium citrate as ordered by doctor. These measures will prevent hematuria, renal colic, urate calculi development, and costovertebral pain.

—Maintain adequate hydration with high fluid intake to prevent formation of uric acid calculi.

—If the patient develops persistent GI distress, notify the doctor and expect to decrease dosage.

—If the patient develops a headache, obtain an order for a mild analgesic, such as acetaminophen. Avoid salicylate analgesics, which may prolong bleeding time.

—If the patient develops other adverse reactions, notify the doctor for appropriate therapy and provide supportive care as appropriate.

—In diabetic patients, perform urine glucose tests using glucose enzymatic reagent (Clinistix, Tes-Tape).

—Keep all members of the health care team informed of the patient's response to the drug.

Patient teaching

—Inform the patient and family about probenecid, including the dosage, frequency, action, and adverse reactions.

—Explain the disease process and rationale for therapy.

—Tell the patient and family that the drug must be taken regularly as ordered or gout attacks may result. Tell the patient not to discontinue drug without medical advice. Advise him to visit the doctor regularly so uric acid can be monitored and dosage can be adjusted if necessary. Lifelong therapy may be required in patients with hyperuricemia.

—Advise the patient to restrict foods high in purine: anchovies, liver, sardines, kidneys, sweetbreads, peas, and lentils.

—Tell the patient that probenecid may increase frequency, severity, and length of acute gout attacks during the first 6 to 12 months of therapy. Prophylactic colchicine or another anti-inflammatory agent is given during the first 3 to 6 months.

—Tell the patient with gout to avoid alcohol because it increases the urate level.

—Advise diabetic patients to perform urine glucose tests with a glucose enzymatic reagent (Clinistix, Tes-Tape).

—Warn the patient not to use drug for pain or inflammation and not to increase dose during gout attack.

—Tell the patient to drink eight to ten glasses of fluid daily and to take drug with food to minimize GI upset.

—Advise female patients considering breast-feeding that it is unknown whether probenecid is excreted in breast milk. An alternative feeding method is recommended during therapy with probenecid.

—Tell the patient to notify the nurse or doctor if adverse reactions develop or questions arise about probenecid therapy.

Evaluation

In the patient receiving probenecid, appropriate evaluation statements include:

• Patient is free of gout attacks.
• Patient experiences no adverse reactions and maintains normal health maintenance status.
• Patient is free of pain (headache).
• Patient and family state an understanding of probenecid therapy.

PROTOTYPE: MISCELLANEOUS ANTIGOUT AGENTS

COLCHICINE
(kol′chi seen)
Colchicine MR†, Colgout‡, Colsalide, Novocolchicine†
Classification: antigout agent
Pregnancy risk category C

How supplied
TABLETS: 0.5 mg (gr $\frac{1}{120}$), 0.6 mg (gr $\frac{1}{100}$) as sugar-coated granules
INJECTION: 1 mg (gr $\frac{1}{60}$)/2 ml

Indications and dosage
Prophylactic or maintenance therapy of acute attacks of gout
ADULTS: 0.5 or 0.6 mg P.O. daily; 1 to 1.8 mg P.O. daily for more severe cases.

---

†Available in Canada only   ‡Available in Australia only

To prevent attacks of gout in patients undergoing surgery
ADULTS: 0.5 to 0.6 mg P.O. t.i.d. 3 days before and 3 days after surgery.

To treat acute gout, acute gouty arthritis
ADULTS: initially, 1 to 1.2 mg P.O., then 0.5 or 0.6 mg P.O. q 1 hour, or 1 to 1.2 mg P.O. q 2 hours until pain is relieved or until nausea, vomiting, or diarrhea ensues. Alternatively, give 2 mg I.V. followed by 0.5 mg I.V. q 6 hours if necessary. Total I.V. dosage over 24 hours (one course of treatment) not to exceed 4 mg.

Note: Give I.V. by slow I.V. push over 2 to 5 minutes. Avoid extravasation. Don't dilute colchicine injection with dextrose 5% injection or any other fluid that might change pH of colchicine solution. If lower concentration of colchicine injection is needed, dilute with 0.9% sodium chloride solution or sterile water for injection and administer over 2 to 5 minutes by direct injection. Do not dilute with a solution that contains a bacteriostatic agent. Preferably, inject into the tubing of a free-flowing I.V. solution. However, if diluted solution becomes turbid, don't inject.

Familial Mediterranean fever suppression
ADULTS: for acute attack, give 0.6 mg P.O. hourly for four doses, then q 2 hours for four doses on the first day, followed by 1.2 mg P.O. q 12 hours for 2 days. Maintenance dosage is 0.5 to 0.6 mg P.O. b.i.d. to t.i.d.

Antiosteolytic treatment
ADULTS: 0.6 mg P.O. t.i.d. Instruct patient in proper oral hygiene, including the use of a toothbrush, dental floss, and toothpicks.

Contraindications and precautions
Colchicine is contraindicated in patients with serious GI, renal, or cardiac disorders; blood dyscrasia; and hypersensitivity to the agent. It should be used cautiously in patients with early signs of GI, renal, or cardiac disorders, because it may exacerbate them. Use with caution in elderly or debilitated patients.

Adverse reactions
BLOOD: **aplastic anemia and agranulocytosis** with prolonged use; nonthrombocytopenic purpura.
CNS: peripheral neuritis.
GI: *nausea, vomiting, abdominal pain, diarrhea.*
SKIN: urticaria, dermatitis.
LOCAL: severe local irritation if extravasation occurs.
OTHER: alopecia.

Interactions
Alcohol, loop diuretics: may impair efficacy of colchicine prophylaxis. Don't use together.
Phenylbutazone: may increase risk of leukopenia or thrombocytopenia. Avoid concomitant use.
Vitamin B_{12}: impaired absorption of orally administered vitamin B_{12}. Separate administration times.

Italicized adverse reactions are common   Boldfaced adverse reactions are life-threatening

Nursing considerations

Assessment
- Review the patient's history for a condition that contraindicates the use of colchicine.
- Obtain a baseline assessment of the patient's gout attacks before therapy.
- Be alert for common adverse reactions.
- Evaluate the patient's and family's knowledge about colchicine therapy.

Planning (Nursing Diagnoses)
Potential nursing diagnoses for the patient receiving colchicine include:
- Potential for injury related to inadequate colchicine dosage.
- Noncompliance (medication administration) related to adverse reactions.
- Knowledge deficit related to colchicine therapy.

Implementation

Preparation and administration

— Store the drug in a tightly closed, light-resistant container, away from moisture and high temperatures.
— Review baseline laboratory studies, including CBC, which should precede therapy and be repeated periodically.
— Do not administer I.M. or S.C.; severe local irritation occurs.
— Give direct I.V. injection by slow I.V. push over 2 to 5 minutes or inject into tubing of a free-flowing I.V. with compatible I.V. fluid. Avoid extravasation. Do not dilute colchicine injection with dextrose 5% injection or any other fluid that might change pH of colchicine solution. If lower concentration of colchicine injection is needed, dilute with sterile water for injection or 0.9% sodium chloride solution. However, if diluted solution becomes turbid, do not inject.
— Remember that to avoid cumulative toxicity, a course of oral colchicine should not be repeated for at least 3 days; a course of I.V. colchicine should not be repeated for several weeks.
— As maintenance therapy, give with meals to reduce GI reactions.

Monitoring

— Monitor the effectiveness of colchicine therapy by regularly assessing for relief of the patient's gout attacks.
— Monitor the patient for adverse drug reactions.
— Monitor hydration status if adverse GI reactions occur.
— Monitor intake and output.
— During prolonged use, monitor patient's CBC for evidence of aplastic anemia.
— If administering drug I.V., monitor I.V. injection site for signs of extravasation or phlebitis.
— Monitor the patient for drug interactions.
— Monitor diagnostic test results. Colchicine therapy may increase alkaline phosphatase, AST (SGOT), and ALT (SGPT) levels and may decrease serum carotene, cholesterol, and thrombocyte values. Colchi-

cine may cause false-positive results on urine tests for RBCs or hemoglobin.
— Periodically reevaluate the patient's and family's knowledge about colchicine.

Intervention

— Discontinue drug as soon as gout pain is relieved or at the first sign of GI symptoms (anorexia, nausea, vomiting, or diarrhea) or weakness. First sign of acute overdosage may be GI symptoms, followed by vascular damage; muscle weakness, and ascending paralysis. Delirium and seizures may occur without the patient losing consciousness.
— If extravasation or phlebitis occurs during I.V. use, notify the doctor and apply heat or cold to relieve the discomfort.
— If the patient becomes noncompliant, discuss reasons why and suggest methods patient may use to help maintain compliance.
— Keep all members of the health care team informed of the patient's response to the drug.

Patient teaching

— Inform the patient and family about colchicine, including the dosage, frequency, action, and adverse reactions.
— Explain the disease process and rationale for therapy.
— Instruct the patient to keep colchicine readily available so that it can be taken as soon as symptoms of an acute gout attack occur.
— Advise patient to report rash, sore throat, fever, unusual bleeding, bruising, fatigue, weakness, numbness, or tingling.
— Tell patient to discontinue colchicine as soon as gout pain is relieved or at the first sign of nausea, vomiting, stomach pain, or diarrhea. Advise patient to report persistent symptoms.
— Instruct the patient to avoid alcohol during colchicine therapy, because alcohol may inhibit drug action.
— Tell the patient to notify the nurse or doctor if adverse reactions develop or questions arise about colchicine therapy.

Evaluation

In the patient receiving colchicine, appropriate evaluation statements include:
• Patient has relief from gout attacks.
• Patient remains compliant with colchicine therapy.
• Patient and family state an understanding of colchicine therapy.

SELECTED MAJOR DRUGS: ANTIGOUT AGENTS

DRUG, INDICATIONS, AND DOSAGES	SPECIAL PRECAUTIONS

Uricosuric

sulfinpyrazone (Anturane)
Maintenance therapy for common gout; reduction, prevention of joint changes and tophi formation—
Adults: 100 to 200 mg P.O. b.i.d. first week, then 200 to 400 mg P.O. b.i.d. Maximum dosage is 800 mg daily.
Inhibition of platelet aggregation, increase of platelet survival time in treatment of thromboembolic disorders, angina, myocardial infarction, transient cerebral ischemic attacks, peripheral arterial atherosclerosis—
Adults: 200 mg P.O. q.i.d.

• Contraindicated in patients with known hypersensitivity to pyrazole derivatives (including oxyphenbutazone and phenylbutazone); active peptic ulcer; gouty nephropathy; urolithiasis or urinary obstruction; bone marrow suppression; azotemia or hyperuricemia secondary to cancer chemotherapy, radiation, or myeloproliferative neoplastic diseases; or blood dyscrasia and during or within 2 weeks after gout attack.
• Use cautiously in patients with diminished hepatic or renal function.

Miscellaneous antigout agent

allopurinol (Alloremed‡, Capurate†, Lopurin, Zyloprim)
Gout, primary or secondary to hyperuricemia; gout secondary to diseases such as acute or chronic leukemia, polycythemia vera, multiple myeloma, and psoriasis—
Dosage varies with severity of disease; can be given as single dose or divided, but doses larger than 300 mg should be divided.
Adults: mild gout, 200 to 300 mg P.O. daily; severe gout with large tophi, 400 to 600 mg P.O. daily. Same dosage for maintenance in secondary hyperuricemia.
Hyperuricemia secondary to malignancies—
Children ages 6 to 10: 300 mg P.O. daily or in divided doses t.i.d.
Children under age 6: 50 mg P.O. t.i.d.
Impaired renal function—
Adults: 200 mg P.O. daily if creatinine clearance is 10 to 20 ml/minute; 100 mg P.O. daily if creatinine clearance is less than 10 ml/minute; 100 mg P.O. more than 24 hours apart if creatinine clearance is less than 3 ml/minute.
To prevent acute gout attacks—
Adults: 100 mg P.O. daily; increase at weekly intervals by 100 mg without exceeding maximum dose (800 mg), until serum uric acid falls to 6 mg/100 ml or less.
To prevent uric acid nephropathy during cancer chemotherapy—
Adults: 600 to 800 mg P.O. daily for 2 to 3 days, with high fluid intake.
Recurrent calcium oxalate calculi—
Adults: 200 to 300 mg P.O. daily in single dose or divided doses.

• Contraindicated in patients with known hypersensitivity to the drug and in those with idiopathic hemochromatosis.
• Use cautiously in patients with cataracts and hepatic or renal disease.

†Available in Canada only   ‡Available in Australia only

SELF-TEST

1. William Oxmoor, age 50, is receiving probenecid (Benemid) as maintenance therapy for chronic gouty arthritis. He tells the nurse that he has had headaches since beginning the therapy. The nurse should advise him to:
   a. discontinue the medication.
   b. take aspirin to relieve the headache.
   c. take acetaminophen to relieve the headache.
   d. notify the doctor immediately.

2. The uricosurics are used to:
   a. treat acute gouty arthritis attacks.
   b. treat gout associated with blood dyscrasia.
   c. treat primary gout.
   d. control the frequency of gouty arthritis attacks.

3. Jay Greene, age 45, is receiving colchicine (Colchicine MR). He tells the nurse that he drinks beer on a daily basis. The nurse should advise him:
   a. to avoid alcohol during colchicine therapy.
   b. to drink the beer 1 hour after taking the drug.
   c. to drink the beer 1 hour before taking the drug.
   d. that there is no interaction between beer and colchicine.

Check your answers on page 1078.

CHAPTER 88

OXYTOCICS AND TOCOLYTICS

Oxytocics

carboprost tromethamine ✦ dinoprostone ✦ ergonovine maleate
methylergonovine maleate ✦ oxytocin, synthetic injection
oxytocin, synthetic nasal solution

Tocolytics

magnesium sulfate ✦ ritodrine hydrochloride ✦ terbutaline sulfate

OVERVIEW

- Oxytocics stimulate the smooth muscle of the uterus. They are especially useful in the last stage of labor (stage III), in which the placenta is sloughed and expelled. Oxytocics should usually be avoided in stages I and II because they increase the risk of uterine rupture.
- Tocolytics inhibit uterine contractions in preterm labor.

MAJOR USES

- Carboprost and dinoprostone induce therapeutic abortion in the second trimester.
- Ergonovine and methylergonovine correct postpartum uterine atony. Ergonovine, methylergonovine, and oxytocin control postpartum bleeding.
- Oxytocin induces labor or intensifies uterine contractions at term. Oxytocin, synthetic nasal preparation, stimulates contraction of the myoepithelium in the mammary glands, facilitating milk ejection in lactating females.
- Magnesium sulfate, ritodrine, and terbutaline are used to inhibit uterine contractions in preterm labor.

MECHANISM OF ACTION

- The prostaglandins carboprost and dinoprostone produce strong, prompt contractions of uterine smooth muscle, possibly mediated by calcium and cyclic 3′, 5′-adenosine monophosphate (cyclic AMP). Endocrine levels also influence contractions. These drugs promote cervical dilation and softening and exert uterine effects by direct stimulation of the myometrium.

GLOSSARY

Eclampsia: severe complication of pregnancy characterized by seizures, coma, hypertension, edema, and proteinuria.
Preeclampsia: complication of late pregnancy characterized by hypertension, proteinuria, and edema.
Tocolytic: drug that inhibits uterine contractions, labor, or childbirth.

- The ergot alkaloids ergonovine and methylergonovine increase motor activity of the uterus by direct stimulation. A gravid uterus responds markedly even to small doses.
- Oxytocin may act as a hormone in its potent and selective stimulation of uterine and mammary gland smooth muscle. It produces uterine contractions of the same intensity, duration, and frequency as those of spontaneous labor. Oxytocin may stimulate contractions of uterine smooth muscle by increasing the sodium permeability of uterine myofibrils.
- Magnesium sulfate's mechanism of tocolytic action is unknown. The current theory holds that magnesium sulfate competes with calcium in uterine smooth muscle, preventing calcium from triggering uterine contractions.
- The beta agonists ritodrine and terbutaline interact with beta receptors in the uterus. This stimulates release of adenylate cyclase, increasing the production of cyclic AMP, which causes an increased uptake and sequestration of intracellular calcium. The final result is inhibition of uterine smooth muscle contractions, with decreased intensity and frequency of contractions.

ABSORPTION, DISTRIBUTION, METABOLISM, AND EXCRETION

Carboprost and dinoprostone diffuse slowly into maternal blood after administration and are widely distributed in the maternal and fetal tissues. They concentrate in the fetal liver and are rapidly metabolized in the maternal lungs and liver. They're excreted within 24 hours, mainly in urine.

Ergonovine and methylergonovine are rapidly absorbed after oral or I.M. administration and are slowly metabolized in the liver. Metabolism in neonates may be prolonged.

Oxytocin is inactivated by trypsin in the GI tract; therefore, the drug is administered parenterally. Oxytocin is distributed to extracellular fluid, and small amounts may reach the fetal circulation. The drug has a short half-life (3 to 5 minutes), which is even shorter in late pregnancy and lactation. The liver and kidneys destroy most of the drug. Only small amounts are excreted unchanged in urine.

After oral administration, terbutaline and ritodrine are absorbed from the GI tract, with a bioavailability of 30% to 50% and 30%, respectively. Both agents cross the placenta and appear in breast milk. Ritodrine and terbutaline are metabolized in the liver.

Magnesium sulfate is administered I.V. and distributed widely. All tocolytics and their metabolites are excreted in urine; 90% to 98% of a magnesium sulfate dose is excreted in urine, the remainder in feces.

ONSET AND DURATION

Carboprost and dinoprostone begin to act promptly. Their action is dose-dependent, with sensitivity increasing at term. Contractions usually begin within 10 to 15 minutes after administration and may continue 10 to 30 minutes after the drug is stopped. In most patients, abortion occurs within 30 hours.

Ergonovine and methylergonovine produce uterine contractions immediately after I.V. administration and within 5 to 15 minutes after oral or I.M. administration. Contractions may continue for 3 or more hours after oral or I.M. administration and 45 minutes after I.V. administration. Small doses produce increased contractions followed by a normal degree of relaxation; larger doses produce more forceful contractions but increase resting tonus.

Oxytocin produces uterine contractions within several minutes; they continue 2 to 3 hours.

After I.V. administration, tocolytics have a rapid onset of action. Ritodrine reaches a peak concentration level after 50 minutes; terbutaline, in 30 to 60 minutes. Terbutaline has a duration of action of 1.5 to 4 hours; magnesium sulfate, 30 minutes. The therapeutic blood level for magnesium sulfate is 6 mEq/liter. When this level falls, uterine contractions may recur.

After oral administration, ritodrine has an onset of 30 to 60 minutes and reaches peak concentration in 30 to 60 minutes. Oral terbutaline has an onset of 30 minutes and reaches peak concentration in 2 hours. Ritodrine's half-life is 15 to 17 hours after I.V. administration and 12 to 20 hours after oral administration.

ADVERSE REACTIONS

Maternal adverse reactions to oxytocin include anaphylactic reactions, postpartum hemorrhage, cardiac arrhythmia, fatal afibrinogenemia, nausea, vomiting, premature ventricular contractions, increased blood loss, pelvic hematoma, and maternal death from oxytocin-induced water intoxication. Fetal arrhythmias, permanent CNS or brain damage, or death have resulted from uterine motility.

Ergonovine and methylergonovine may both cause nausea and vomiting, but this is not very common. They may also elevate blood pressure.

Carboprost and dinoprostone most commonly cause GI reactions, usually vomiting, and less often diarrhea and nausea. Other reactions are rare: dinoprostone causes headache, hypotension, and chills in 10% of patients.

Tocolytics cause many minor adverse reactions and several that can be severe, including cardiovascular reactions, electrolyte imbalances, and seizures.

Most adverse reactions to the beta agonists ritodrine and terbutaline are extensions of their actions. Common maternal adverse reactions to these agents include an increase in heart rate by 20 to 40 beats/minute, increased cardiac output, hypotension, hyperglycemia, increased insulin secretion, increased free fatty acid release, hypokalemia, anxiety, headache, nausea, vomiting, nervousness, and tremor. They also can cause hypersensitivity reactions, such as pulmonary edema, chest tightness or pain, arrhythmias, palpitations, acute CHF, and hypertensive crisis.

Because these agents cross the placenta, the fetus may receive pharmacologic doses of these drugs. If therapy fails to delay delivery, the neonate may experience adverse reactions, including increased heart rate, hypotension, and hypocalcemia as well as hypersensitivity reactions, including respiratory depression, paralytic ileus, and pulmonary edema (rare).

Adverse reactions to magnesium sulfate typically depend on the drug's dosage, the rapidity of administration, and the serum magnesium level. A woman who receives magnesium sulfate may give birth to a neonate with hypermagnesemia, hypotonia, or CNS or respiratory depression.

PROTOTYPE: OXYTOCICS

OXYTOCIN, SYNTHETIC INJECTION
(ox i toe' sin)
Pitocin, Syntocinon
Classification: oxytocic

How supplied
INJECTION: 5 units/0.5 ml in 0.5-ml ampules; 10 units/ml in 1-ml ampules, syringes, and multiple-dose vials

Indications and dosage
Induction or stimulation of labor
ADULTS: initially, 1 ml (10 units) in 1,000 ml of dextrose 5% injection or 0.9% sodium chloride solution I.V. infused at 1 to 2 milliunits/minute. Increase rate at 15- to 30-minute intervals until normal contraction pattern is established. Maximum dosage is 1 to 2 ml (20 milliunits)/minute. Decrease rate when labor is firmly established.

Reduction of postpartum bleeding after expulsion of placenta
ADULTS: 10 to 40 units added to 1,000 ml of dextrose 5% in water (D_5W) or 0.9% sodium chloride solution, infused at a rate necessary to control bleeding, usually 10 to 20 milliunits/minute. Also, 1 ml (10 units) I.M. can be given after delivery of the placenta.

Incomplete or inevitable abortion
ADULTS: 10 units of oxytocin in 500 ml of 0.9% sodium chloride solution or dextrose 5% in 0.9% sodium chloride solution, infused at 10 to 20 milliunits/minute.

Contraindications and precautions
Oxytocin is contraindicated in patients with known hypersensitivity to the drug and in the following conditions: cephalopelvic disproportion, unfavorable fetal positions or presentations, obstetric emergencies that may require surgical intervention, fetal distress when delivery is not imminent, or hypertonic uterine patterns. It is also contraindicated for prolonged use in uterine inertia or severe toxemia and when vaginal delivery is not indicated.

Except in unusual circumstances, oxytocin should not be administered in patients with borderline cephalopelvic disproportion, previous major surgery in the cervix or uterus, grand multiparity, or invasive cervical carcinoma. Its use should also be avoided in premature births.

Adverse reactions
Maternal—
BLOOD: **afibrinogenemia**; may be related to increased postpartum bleeding.
CNS: **subarachnoid hemorrhage** resulting from hypertension; **seizures** or **coma** resulting from water intoxication.
CV: hypotension; increased heart rate, systemic venous return, and cardiac output; **arrhythmias**.
GI: nausea, vomiting.
OTHER: hypersensitivity, tetanic contractions, abruptio placentae, impaired uterine blood flow, pelvic hematoma, increased uterine motility, **anaphylaxis**.
Fetal—
BLOOD: hyperbilirubinemia.
CV: bradycardia, tachycardia, **premature ventricular contractions**.
OTHER: **anoxia, asphyxia**.

Interactions
Cyclopropane anesthetics: less pronounced bradycardia; hypotension. Advise anesthesiologist of oxytocin therapy
Thiopental anesthetics: delayed induction reported. Advise anesthesiologist of oxytocin therapy.
Vasoconstrictors: severe hypertension if oxytocin is given to patient receiving caudal block anesthetic containing a vasoconstrictor (such as epinephrine). Separate administration times by at least 4 hours.

Nursing considerations
Assessment
• Review the patient's history for a condition that contraindicates the use of oxytocin, such as cephalopelvic disproportion or other significant obstetric abnormality.

- Obtain a baseline assessment of the patient's pregnancy and labor status or amount of postpartum bleeding before initiating oxytocin therapy.
- Be alert for serious adverse reactions.
- Evaluate the patient's and family's knowledge about oxytocin therapy.

Planning (Nursing Diagnoses)
Potential nursing diagnoses for the patient receiving oxytocin include:
- Potential for maternal injury related to adverse drug reactions.
- Potential for fetal injury related to adverse drug reactions.
- Knowledge deficit related to oxytocin therapy.

Implementation
Preparation and administration
— Prepare a solution containing 10 milliunits/ml by adding 10 units of oxytocin to 1 liter of 0.9% sodium chloride solution or D₅W. Prepare one containing 20 milliunits/ml by adding 10 units of oxytocin to 500 ml of 0.9% sodium chloride solution or D₅W.
— Use to induce or reinforce labor only when pelvis is known to be adequate, when vaginal delivery is indicated, when fetal maturity is assured, and when fetal position is favorable. Should be used only in hospital where critical care facilities and doctor are immediately available.
— Never administer oxytocin simultaneously by more than one route.
— Don't give by I.V. bolus injection. Oxytocin must be administered by infusion; give by piggyback infusion so the drug may be discontinued without interrupting the I.V. line. Use an infusion pump.
— Rotate the oxytocin solution container gently to distribute the drug throughout the solution during I.V. administration.
— Routine I.M. use is not recommended, but units may be given I.M. after delivery of placenta to control postpartum uterine bleeding.
— Have magnesium sulfate (20% solution) available for relaxation of the myometrium.

Monitoring
— Monitor the effectiveness of therapy by regularly assessing the patient's labor contractions or decrease in amount of postpartum bleeding.
— Monitor the patient for adverse drug reactions.
— Monitor and record uterine contractions, heart rate, blood pressure, intrauterine pressure, fetal heart rate, and character of blood loss every 15 minutes.
— Monitor fluid intake and output because oxytocin may produce an antidiuretic effect. During long infusions, watch for signs of water intoxication.
— Monitor the patient for drug interactions.
— When administering an oxytocin challenge test, monitor fetal heart rate and uterine contractions immediately before and during infusion. If fetal heart rate does not change during test, repeat in 1 week. If late deceleration in fetal heart rate is noted, the doctor may decide to deliver the baby.

— Periodically reevaluate the patient's and family's knowledge about oxytocin.

Intervention

— If contractions occur less than 2 minutes apart and contraction pressure is above 50 mm Hg, or if contractions last 90 seconds or longer, stop the infusion, turn the patient on her side, and notify the doctor.
— If the patient experiences any adverse reaction, stop the infusion and notify the doctor immediately for appropriate therapy. Provide supportive care as indicated.
— Keep all members of the health care team informed of the patient's response to the drug.

Patient teaching

— Inform the patient and family about oxytocin, including the dosage, frequency, action, and adverse reactions.
— Tell the patient to notify the nurse or doctor if adverse reactions develop or questions arise about oxytocin therapy.

Evaluation

In the patient receiving oxytocin, appropriate evaluation statements include:
• Patient experiences no adverse reactions.
• Fetus experiences no adverse reactions.
• Patient and family state an understanding of oxytocin therapy.

PROTOTYPE: TOCOLYTICS

RITODRINE
(ri′toe dreen)
Yutopar
Classification: tocolytic
Pregnancy risk category B

How supplied

TABLETS: 10 mg
INJECTION: 10 mg/ml in 5-ml ampules, 15 mg/ml in 10-ml vials and syringes

Indications and dosage
Management of preterm labor
WOMEN: dilute 150 mg in 500 ml of fluid, yielding a final concentration of 0.3 mg/ml. Usual initial dose is 0.1 mg/minute I.V., increased gradually according to the results by 0.05 mg/minute, until desired result is obtained. Effective dosage range is 0.15 to 0.35 mg/minute.

Note: I.V. infusion should be continued for 12 to 24 hours after contractions have stopped. Oral maintenance therapy begins with one 10-mg tablet approximately 30 minutes before termination of I.V. therapy. Usual dosage for first 24 hours of oral maintenance is 10 mg q 2 hours. Thereafter, usual dosage is 10 to 20 mg P.O. q 4 to 6 hours. Total daily dosage should not exceed 120 mg.

Contraindications and precautions

Ritodrine is contraindicated before the 25th week of pregnancy; in maternal or fetal conditions in which continuation of pregnancy is hazardous; in patients with antepartum hemorrhage that demands immediate delivery, eclampsia and severe preeclampsia, intrauterine fetal death, chorioamnionitis, maternal cardiac disease, pulmonary hypertension, maternal hyperthyroidism, uncontrolled maternal diabetes mellitus, preexisting maternal conditions that would be seriously affected by a betamimetic drug; and in patients with known hypersensitivity to any component of the product.

Adverse reactions

CNS: nervousness, anxiety, headache, tremor.
CV: *dose-related alterations in blood pressure*, palpitations, **pulmonary edema**, tachycardia, ECG changes.
GI: nausea, vomiting.
METABOLIC: hyperglycemia, hypokalemia.
SKIN: rash, erythema.

Interactions

Beta blockers: may inhibit ritodrine's action. Avoid concurrent administration.
Corticosteroids: may produce pulmonary edema in mother. When these drugs are used concomitantly, monitor patient closely.
Inhalational anesthetics: potentiate adverse cardiac effects, arrhythmias, hypotension. Monitor patient closely.
Sympathomimetics: additive effects. Use together cautiously.

Nursing considerations

Assessment

- Review the patient's history for a condition that contraindicates the use of ritodrine, such as eclampsia or antepartum hemorrhage.
- Obtain a baseline assessment of the patient's pregnancy status before initiating ritodrine therapy.
- Be alert for serious adverse reactions.
- Evaluate the patient's and family's knowledge about ritodrine therapy.

Planning (Nursing Diagnoses)

Potential nursing diagnoses for the patient receiving ritodrine include:
- Potential for injury related to dosage inadequate to manage preterm labor.
- Noncompliance (oral medication administration) related to adverse reactions.
- Knowledge deficit related to ritodrine therapy.

Implementation

Preparation and administration

— Prepare I.V. solution by diluting 150 mg ritodrine in 500 ml of dextrose 5% injection, 10% Dextran 40 in sodium chloride injection, 10% invert sugar solution, Ringer's injection, or Hartmann's solution to produce a solution containing 300 mcg (0.3 mg) of ritodrine per milliliter.

— Do not use ritodrine I.V. if solution is discolored or contains a precipitate. Do not use solution more than 48 hours after preparation.

— Control infusion rate by use of a microdrip chamber I.V. infusion set or an infusion control device.

Monitoring

— Monitor the effectiveness of ritodrine therapy by regularly assessing for suppression of preterm labor.

— Monitor the patient for adverse drug reactions.

— Because cardiovascular responses are common and more pronounced during I.V. administration, cardiovascular status—including maternal pulse rate and blood pressure, and fetal heart rate—should be closely monitored. A maternal tachycardia of over 140 beats/minute or persistent respiratory rate of over 20 breaths/minute may be a sign of impending pulmonary edema.

— Monitor blood glucose levels during ritodrine infusions, especially in diabetic patients.

— To prevent circulatory overload, monitor amount of I.V. fluids.

— Monitor the patient for drug interactions.

— Monitor the patient's uterine activity. Ritodrine decreases the intensity and frequency of uterine contractions.

— Monitor diagnostic test results because I.V. administration of ritodrine elevates plasma insulin and glucose levels and decreases plasma potassium concentrations (values usually return to normal within 24 hours after drug is stopped).

— If the patient is taking ritodrine orally, monitor her compliance with therapy.

— Monitor neonate for increased heart rate, hypotension, and hypovolemia.

— Periodically reevaluate the patient's and family's knowledge about ritodrine.

Intervention

— Discontinue the drug if pulmonary edema develops.

— Place the patient in left lateral recumbent position to reduce risk of hypotension.

— Ritodrine may uncover previously unknown cardiac pathology. Sinus bradycardia may follow drug withdrawal. If patient is symptomatic, be prepared to provide supportive care.

— Maternal tachycardia or decreased blood pressure usually reverses with a dosage reduction. But in 1% of patients, persistent reactions require discontinuation of the drug.

—If the neonate develops adverse reactions, such as increased heart rate, hypotension, and hypovolemia, notify the doctor immediately.

—Keep all members of the health care team informed of the patient's response to the drug.

Patient teaching

—Inform the patient and family about ritodrine, including the dosage, frequency, action, and adverse reactions.

—Advise the patient of need for frequent vital signs and uterine monitoring.

—Caution the patient not to stop taking the drug without medical approval.

—Advise the patient to keep scheduled follow-up appointments and to report any adverse reactions promptly.

—If the patient is discharged with oral therapy, emphasize the need for compliance with therapy and teach methods to help patient remember to take drug as prescribed.

—Tell the patient to notify the nurse or doctor if adverse reactions develop or questions arise about ritodrine therapy.

Evaluation

In the patient receiving ritodrine, appropriate evaluation statements include:

• Patient's preterm labor is managed appropriately and patient experiences no injury.

• Patient remains compliant with oral medication administration therapy.

• Patient and family state an understanding of ritodrine therapy.

SELECTED MAJOR DRUGS: OXYTOCICS AND TOCOLYTICS

DRUG, INDICATIONS, AND DOSAGES	SPECIAL PRECAUTIONS
Oxytocics	
carboprost (Hemabate, Prostin/15M) *Abort pregnancy between 13th and 20th weeks of gestation—* **Women:** initially, 250 mcg deep I.M. Subsequent doses of 250 mcg should be administered at intervals of 1½ to 3½ hours, depending on uterine response. Dose may be increased to 500 mcg if contractility is inadequate after several 250-mcg doses. Total dose should not exceed 12 mg. *Postpartum hemorrhage caused by uterine atony that has not responded to conventional management—* **Women:** 250 mcg deep I.M.	• Contraindicated in pelvic inflammatory disease or active cardiac, pulmonary, renal, or hepatic disease. • Use cautiously in patients with a history of asthma; hypertension; CV, renal, or hepatic disease; anemia; jaundice; diabetes; seizure disorders; or previous uterine surgery.

(continued)

SELECTED MAJOR DRUGS: OXYTOCICS AND TOCOLYTICS *continued*

DRUG, INDICATIONS, AND DOSAGES	SPECIAL PRECAUTIONS

Oxytocics *(continued)*

ergonovine (Ergotrate)
Prevent or treat postpartum or postabortion hemorrhage from uterine atony or subinvolution—
Women: 0.2 mg I.M. q 2 to 4 hours, for a maximum of five doses; or 0.2 mg I.V. (only for severe uterine bleeding or other life-threatening emergency) over 1 minute while blood pressure and uterine contractions are monitored. I.V. dose may be diluted to 5 ml with 0.9% sodium chloride injection. After initial I.M. or I.V. dose, may give 0.2 to 0.4 mg P.O. q 6 to 12 hours for 2 to 7 days. Decrease dosage if severe uterine cramping occurs.

• Contraindicated for induction or augmentation of labor, before delivery of placenta, in threatened spontaneous abortion, and in patients with allergy or known hypersensitivity to ergot preparations.
• Use cautiously in patients with hypertension, cardiac disease, venoatrial shunts, mitral valve stenosis, obliterative vascular disease, sepsis, and hepatic or renal impairment.

methylergonovine (Methergine)
Prevent and treat postpartum hemorrhage caused by uterine atony or subinvolution—
Women: 0.2 mg I.M. q 2 to 4 hours for maximum of five doses; or 0.2 mg I.V. (only for excessive uterine bleeding or other emergencies) over 1 minute while blood pressure and uterine contractions are monitored. I.V. dose may be diluted to 5 ml with 0.9% sodium chloride solution. After initial I.M. or I.V. dose, may give 0.2 to 0.4 mg P.O. q 6 to 12 hours for 2 to 7 days. Decrease dose if severe cramping occurs.

• Contraindicated for induction of labor; before delivery of placenta; in patients with hypertension, toxemia, or known hypersensitivity to ergot preparations; and in threatened spontaneous abortion.
• Use cautiously in patients with sepsis, obliterative vascular disease, or hepatic, renal, or cardiac disease.

Tocolytics

magnesium sulfate
Acute treatment of preeclampsia and eclampsia—
Women: 2 to 4 g (4 to 8 ml of 50% solution) loading dose given by slow I.V. bolus (over 5 minutes). Maintenance dosage is 1 to 2 g hourly as a constant infusion. Prepare by adding 8 ml of 50% solution to 250 ml dextrose 5% in water.
Hypomagnesemia—
Adults: 1 g, or 8.12 mEq, of 50% solution (2 ml) I.M. q 6 hours for four doses, depending on serum magnesium level. In severe hypomagnesemia (serum magnesium 0.8 mEq/liter or less, with symptoms), give 6 g, or 50 mEq, of 50% solution I.V. in 1 liter of solution over 4 hours. Subsequent doses depend on serum magnesium levels.
Magnesium supplementation in hyperalimentation—
Adults: 8 to 24 mEq I.V. daily added to hyperalimentation solution.
Children over age 6: 2 to 10 mEq I.V. daily added to hyperalimentation solution.
  Each 2 ml of 50% solution contains 1 g or 8.12 mEq magnesium sulfate.

• Contraindicated in impaired renal function, myocardial damage, or heart block, and in actively progressing labor.
• Use parenteral magnesium with extreme caution in patients receiving digitalis preparations. Treating magnesium toxicity with calcium in such patients could cause serious alterations in cardiac conduction; heart block may result.

SELECTED MAJOR DRUGS: OXYTOCICS AND TOCOLYTICS *continued*

DRUG, INDICATIONS, AND DOSAGES	SPECIAL PRECAUTIONS

Tocolytics *(continued)*

magnesium sulfate *(continued)*
Hypomagnesemic seizures —
Adults: 1 to 2 g (as 10% solution) I.V. over 15 minutes, then 1 g I.M. q 4 to 6 hours, based on patient response and serum magnesium level.
Seizures secondary to hypomagnesemia in acute nephritis —
Adults: 0.2 ml/kg of 50% solution I.M. q 4 to 6 hours, p.r.n., or 100 mg/kg of 10% solution I.V. very slowly. Titrate dosage according to serum magnesium level and seizure response.
Paroxysmal atrial tachycardia —
Adults: 3 to 4 g I.V. (as 10% solution) over 30 seconds with close monitoring of ECG.

terbutaline (Brethine)
Premature labor —
Adults: initially, 10 mcg/minute I.V. Titrate to a maximum dose of 80 mcg/minute. Maintain I.V. dosage at minimum effective dose for 4 hours. Maintenance therapy until term: 2.5 mg P.O. q 4 to 6 hours.
Relief of bronchospasm in patients with reversible obstructive airway disease —
Adults and children over age 12: 5 mg P.O. t.i.d. at 6-hour intervals. Maximum dosage is 15 mg daily. If adverse reactions occur or for children ages 12 to 15, dosage may be reduced to 2.5 mg P.O. t.i.d.; maximum dosage is 7.5 mg daily. Alternatively, 0.25 mg S.C. repeated in 15 to 30 minutes; maximum dosage is 0.5 mg q 4 hours. Or 2 inhalations q 4 to 6 hours with 1 minute between inhalations.

- Contraindicated in patients with known hypersensitivity to the drug or other sympathomimetics.
- Use cautiously in patients with diabetes, hypertension, hyperthyroidism, or cardiac disease (especially when associated with arrhythmias).

SELF-TEST

1. Beth Edwards has experienced preterm labor. Her doctor prescribes ritodrine. The usual initial I.V. infusion dose of ritodrine to manage preterm labor is:
  a. 0.01 mg/minute.
  b. 0.1 mg/minute.
  c. 1 mg/minute.
  d. 10 mg/minute.

2. The usual initial I.V. infusion rate of oxytocin, synthetic injection, to induce labor is:
   a. 0.01 to 0.02 milliunits/minute.
   b. 0.1 to 0.2 milliunits/minute.
   c. 1 to 2 milliunits/minute.
   d. 10 to 20 milliunits/minute.

3. Mary Johnson, age 28, has been receiving oxytocin, synthetic injection, to induce labor. Which of the following adverse reactions should the nurse monitor for, especially during long infusions?
   a. Hyperglycemia
   b. Water intoxication
   c. Pulmonary edema
   d. Atrial fibrillation

Check your answers on page 1078.

CHAPTER 89

GOLD SALTS

auranofin ✦ aurothioglucose ✦ gold sodium thiomalate

OVERVIEW

- Gold salts are administered to suppress or prevent arthritis and synovitis. Their effectiveness for such use was clearly established in 1960, 40 years after their introduction for treating rheumatoid arthritis. The most significant disadvantage of using the gold salts is the long time required—weeks to months of treatment before any therapeutic benefit is noted. For this reason, gold salts are not the mainstay of arthritis therapy.

MAJOR USES

- Gold salts are used to suppress or prevent—but not cure—arthritis or synovitis. They are usually reserved for patients with moderate to severe disease, and most clinicians will reserve their use until other anti-inflammatory agents have been tried for 3 to 4 months.

MECHANISM OF ACTION

- The exact mechanism by which these compounds work is not known. However, they may work by inhibiting lysosomal enzymes, decreasing vessel permeability, or decreasing phagocytosis.

ABSORPTION, DISTRIBUTION, METABOLISM, AND EXCRETION

The absorption of the injectable gold salts (gold sodium thiomalate and aurothioglucose) after I.M. injection is unknown. Twenty-five percent of oral gold (auranofin) is absorbed after administration.

After I.M. administration, gold salts are widely distributed throughout the body, with highest concentrations in the adrenal glands, kidneys, and synovial membranes. Auranofin is 60% bound to plasma protein; the parenteral forms are 95% bound.

The metabolism of the gold salts is not completely understood; however, their excretion is well documented. Over 10 days, 4% to 5% of an oral auranofin dose is eliminated in the urine, and 70% to 75% in the feces. This increases to 15% and 85%, respectively, in 6 months. After parenteral administration, 30% is excreted in the feces; 70% in the urine.

ONSET AND DURATION

Onset of action is 1 to 2 hours for auranofin; 2 to 6 hours for aurothioglucose and gold sodium thiomalate. The long half-life of the

GLOSSARY

Lysosome: minute cellular body containing hydrolytic enzymes that are released after injury to the cell.
Phagocytosis: engulfment of microorganisms, cells, or foreign particles by reticuloendothelial cells, polymorphonuclear leukocytes, monocytes, or macrophages.
Rheumatoid arthritis: autoimmune disease characterized by connective tissue inflammation, especially in the muscles and joints.

parenteral forms allows once-weekly injections. On the other hand, oral administration requires daily dosing.

ADVERSE REACTIONS

On an average, one-third of patients receiving gold therapy experience adverse reactions, which may occur during therapy or several months after therapy has stopped. Toxicity is a result of the cumulative body content of gold, not the plasma levels. For this reason, patients receiving gold via I.M. injection are more likely to experience adverse reactions.

The most common adverse reaction is diarrhea, which occurs in approximately 50% of patients receiving auranofin. Signs of hematologic toxicity, such as neutropenia and thrombocytopenia, may occur and require careful monitoring.

The most common reaction to injectable gold is dermatitis. Pruritus usually precedes the dermatitis and is a warning of a cutaneous reaction.

Other adverse reactions may include stomatitis (the second most common reaction to injectable gold), metallic taste, pulmonary infiltrates, renal toxicity, and anaphylactoid reactions (sweating, faintness, flushing, headaches, and dizziness).

PROTOTYPE: GOLD SALTS

AURANOFIN
(au rane′ oh fin)
Ridaura
Classification: gold salt
Pregnancy risk category C

How supplied
CAPSULES: 3 mg

Indications and dosage
Rheumatoid arthritis
ADULTS: 6 mg P.O. daily, administered either as 3 mg b.i.d. or 6 mg once daily. After 6 months, may be increased to 9 mg P.O. daily.

Contraindications and precautions

Auranofin is contraindicated in patients with a history of gold-induced disorders, including anaphylactic reactions, necrotizing enterocolitis, pulmonary fibrosis, exfoliative dermatitis, bone marrow aplasia, or other severe hematologic disorders.

Adverse reactions

BLOOD: thrombocytopenia (with or without purpura), **aplastic anemia, agranulocytosis,** leukopenia, eosinophilia.
GI: *diarrhea,* abdominal pain, *nausea, vomiting,* stomatitis, enterocolitis, anorexia, metallic taste, dyspepsia, flatulence.
GU: proteinuria, hematuria, nephrotic syndrome, glomerulonephritis.
HEPATIC: jaundice, elevated liver enzyme levels.
RESPIRATORY: interstitial pneumonitis.
SKIN: rash, pruritus, dermatitis, **exfoliative dermatitis.**

Interactions

Phenytoin: may increase phenytoin blood levels. Monitor for toxicity.

Nursing considerations

Assessment

- Review the patient's history for a condition that contraindicates the use of auranofin, such as anaphylactic reactions or any gold-induced disorder.
- Obtain a baseline assessment of the patient's rheumatoid arthritis before initiating auranofin therapy.
- Be alert for common adverse reactions.
- Evaluate the patient's and family's knowledge about auranofin therapy.

Planning (Nursing Diagnoses)

Potential nursing diagnoses for the patient receiving auranofin include:
- Altered health maintenance related to ineffectiveness of dosage regimen.
- Diarrhea related to adverse GI reactions to auranofin.
- Knowledge deficit related to auranofin therapy.

Implementation

Preparation and administration
— Store at controlled room temperature and in a light-resistant container.
— When switching from injectable gold, start auranofin at 6 mg P.O. daily.

Monitoring
— Monitor the effectiveness of auranofin therapy by regularly assessing the status of the patient's rheumatoid arthritis.
— Monitor the patient for adverse drug reactions.
— Monitor the patient's CBC and platelet count for adverse blood reactions.
— Monitor for diarrhea. Monitor hydration status if adverse GI reactions occur.
— Monitor renal and hepatic function studies for abnormalities.
— Monitor respiratory status for interstitial pneumonitis.

—Monitor the patient for drug interactions.

—Monitor diagnostic test results. Limited data suggest that auranofin may enhance the patient's reaction to tuberculin skin tests.

—Periodically reevaluate the patient's and family's knowledge about auranofin.

Intervention

—Notify the doctor and expect to discontinue the drug if the patient's platelet count falls below 100,000/mm^3; if hemoglobin drops suddenly; if granulocytes are below 1,500/mm^3, and if leukopenia (WBC count below 4,000/mm^3) or eosinophilia (eosinophils greater than 75%) occurs.

—If the patient develops diarrhea, notify the doctor and obtain an order for an antidiarrheal agent.

—If the patient becomes noncompliant with therapy, discuss reasons why and offer methods patient may use to maintain compliance, such as "cues" to remember to take medication.

—Regularly monitor results of urinalysis. If proteinuria or hematuria is detected, discontinue drug because it can produce a nephrotic syndrome or glomerulonephritis.

—If the patient develops other adverse reactions, notify the doctor and expect to provide supportive care.

—Keep all members of the health care team informed of the patient's response to the drug.

Patient teaching

—Inform the patient and family about auranofin, including the dosage, frequency, action, and adverse reactions.

—Explain the disease process and rationale for therapy.

—Emphasize the importance of monthly follow-up to monitor patient's platelet count.

—Reassure the patient that beneficial drug effect may be delayed as long as 3 months. However, if response is inadequate after 3 months and maximum dosage has been reached, the doctor will probably discontinue auranofin.

—Encourage the patient to take the drug as prescribed and not to alter the dosage schedule.

—Tell the patient to continue taking this drug if he experiences mild diarrhea, the most common adverse reaction; however, if he notes blood in his stool, he should contact the doctor immediately.

—Tell the patient to continue taking concomitant drug therapy, such as NSAIDs, if prescribed.

—Advise the patient to report any rashes or other skin problems immediately. Pruritus often precedes dermatitis and should be considered a warning of impending skin reactions. Any pruritic skin eruption while a patient is receiving auranofin should be considered a reaction to this drug until proven otherwise. Therapy is stopped until reaction subsides.

—Tell the patient that stomatitis is often preceded by a metallic taste. Advise him to report this symptom to his doctor immediately. Recommend careful oral hygiene during therapy.

—Auranofin is prescribed only for selected rheumatoid arthritis patients. Warn the patient not to give the drug to others.

—Give the patient a copy of the patient information insert supplied by the manufacturer.

—Tell the patient to notify the nurse or doctor if adverse reactions develop or questions arise about auranofin therapy.

Evaluation

In the patient receiving auranofin, appropriate evaluation statements include:

• Patient's rheumatoid arthritis signs and symptoms are relieved.

• Patient's bowel habits remain normal, and patient experiences no diarrhea.

• Patient and family state an understanding of auranofin therapy.

SELF-TEST

1. Joy Benner, age 69, is receiving auranofin for rheumatoid arthritis. For which of the following common adverse reactions should the nurse monitor?
   a. Diarrhea
   b. Cardiac arrhythmias
   c. Constipation
   d. Edema

2. By which of the following actions may a gold salt relieve rheumatoid arthritis?
   a. It acts primarily as an analgesic.
   b. It provides anti-inflammatory effects.
   c. It inhibits lysosomal enzymes.
   d. It reverses rheumatoid arthritis deformation.

3. When reviewing Mrs. Benner's blood studies, the nurse discovers that her platelet count is 175,000/mm³. The nurse should:
   a. notify the doctor immediately.
   b. discontinue the drug.
   c. double the dosage.
   d. do nothing—the platelet count is normal.

Check your answers on page 1078.

CHAPTER 90

DIAGNOSTIC SKIN TESTS

Candida and *Trichophyton* extracts ✦ coccidioidin ✦ diphtheria toxin
histoplasmin ✦ mumps skin test antigen ✦ skin test antigens, multiple
tuberculin purified protein derivative (PPD)
tuberculosis multiple-puncture tests

OVERVIEW
- Diagnostic skin tests are used to determine the presence of allergy, detect infection, and evaluate cell-mediated immunity.

MAJOR USES
- The tuberculin tests are used to aid in the diagnosis of tuberculosis.
- Diphtheria toxin is used to determine serologic immunity to diphtheria.
- Coccidioidin is used to help in diagnosing coccidioidomycosis and in differentiating this disease from other mycotic and bacterial infections, such as histoplasmosis.
- Histoplasmin is used infrequently to aid diagnosis of histoplasmosis and to differentiate it from other mycotic or bacterial infections, and to aid interpretation of radiographs that show pulmonary infiltration or calcification.
- *Candida* and *Trichophyton* extracts are used for the desensitizing treatment of mycotic skin infections.
- Mumps skin test antigen is used to assess immunocompetency; however, the FDA has required further investigation to confirm its effectiveness.
- Multiple skin test antigens consist of seven delayed hypersensitivity skin test antigens and a negative control (glycerin). The seven antigens are tetanus toxoid antigen, diphtheria toxoid antigen, *Streptococcus* antigen, old tuberculin, *Candida* antigen, *Trichophyton* antigen, and *Proteus* antigen. These multiple antigens are used to test for nonresponsiveness to antigens by means of delayed hypersensitivity.

MECHANISM OF ACTION
- All of these skin tests produce some form of induration if the reaction is positive. A positive reaction mainly indicates past infection.
- The reaction to *Candida* indicates presence of intact cellular immunity; to diphtheria toxin/Shick test, lack of circulating diphtheria antitoxin or, after full immunization, an antibody immunodeficiency; to *Trichophyton* and mumps, presence of intact cellular immunity.

GLOSSARY

Allergy: hypersensitivity reaction to intrinsically harmless antigens.
Antigen: substance, usually a protein, that causes formation of an antibody and reacts specifically with that antibody.
Cell-mediated immunity: mechanism of acquired immunity characterized by the dominant role of small T-cell lymphocytes.
Induration: hardening of tissue, particularly the skin, from edema, inflammation, or infiltration.

ABSORPTION, DISTRIBUTION, METABOLISM, AND EXCRETION

Not applicable.

ONSET AND DURATION

A positive response to diagnostic skin tests is noted within 24 to 72 hours. At this time, extent of induration determines significance of the reaction.

ADVERSE REACTIONS

For most patients receiving diagnostic skin tests, reactions are limited to erythema at the injection site. However, after the tuberculin or histoplasmin test, highly sensitive individuals may develop vesiculation, ulceration, or necrosis at the site. Patients receiving *Candida* and *Trichophyton* extracts should expect a mild burning immediately after the injection. This sensation will subside in 10 to 20 seconds.

PROTOTYPE: DIAGNOSTIC SKIN TESTS

TUBERCULIN PURIFIED PROTEIN DERIVATIVE (PPD)

(too ber′ kyoo lin)
Aplisol, PPD-stabilized Solution (Mantoux test), Tubersol
Classification: diagnostic skin test
Pregnancy risk category C

How supplied

INJECTION (INTRADERMAL): 1 tuberculin unit/0.1 ml in 1-ml vials, 5 tuberculin units/0.1 ml in 1- and 5-ml vials, 250 tuberculin units/0.1 ml in 1-ml vials

Indications and dosage
Diagnosis of tuberculosis; evaluation of immunocompetence in patients with cancer, malnutrition

ADULTS AND CHILDREN: initially, 1 tuberculin unit (0.1 ml of appropriate solution) intradermally into flexor surface of the forearm. Use tuberculin syringe with 26G or 27G ½″ needle. Retest with 5 tuberculin units and, if negative, 250 tuberculin units. If there is still no response, the individual is nonreactive.

Contraindications and precautions

Tuberculin PPD should not be administered to persons with a history of positive reaction to these agents.

Adverse reactions

LOCAL: pain, pruritus, vesiculation, ulceration, necrosis.
SYSTEMIC: **anaphylaxis**, Arthus reaction.

Interactions

None significant.

Nursing considerations

Assessment

- Review the patient's history for a condition that contraindicates the use of tuberculin PPD, such as a history of a positive reaction to this test.
- Obtain a baseline assessment of the patient's history of tuberculin skin testing before the test.
- Be alert for serious adverse reactions, especially anaphylaxis.
- Evaluate the patient's and family's knowledge about tuberculin testing.

Planning (Nursing Diagnoses)

Potential nursing diagnoses for the patient tested with tuberculin PPD include:

- Potential for injury related to improper administration.
- Noncompliance (test reading) related to length of time required before test is read.
- Knowledge deficit related to tuberculin PPD testing.

Implementation

Preparation and administration

— Obtain history of allergies and reactions to skin tests.
— Consider that reactions to the tuberculin PPD test may be depressed or suppressed for as long as 4 to 6 weeks in individuals who have received concurrent or recent immunization with certain virus vaccines (for example, measles or influenza), in those who are receiving corticosteroids or immunosuppressive agents, in malnourished patients, and in those who have had viral infections (rubeola, influenza, mumps, and probably others).
— Keep epinephrine for injection 1:1,000 available.
— If reaction is positive, further testing is needed to confirm diagnosis. Report all known cases of tuberculosis to the appropriate public health agency.
— Administer intradermally. S.C. injection invalidates test results. Bleb (6 to 10 mm in diameter) must form on skin at intradermal injection site. If bleb does not appear, retest at a site at least 5 cm from the initial site.
— Strongly positive test results can result in scarring at test site.

—Never give initial test with second test strength (250 tuberculin units). Use that strength only when a patient has a negative response to a 5-tuberculin unit test but has signs and symptoms of tuberculosis.

Monitoring

—Monitor the effectiveness of test by evaluating induration 48 to 72 hours after administering tuberculin PPD. An induration of 10 mm or greater is a significant reaction in patients who are not suspected of having tuberculosis and who have not been exposed to active tuberculosis. An induration of 5 mm or greater is significant in patients who are suspected of having tuberculosis or who have recently been exposed to active tuberculosis. A reaction of 2 mm or greater may be considered significant in infants or children. The amount of induration at the site, not the erythema, determines the significance of the reaction.

—Monitor the patient for adverse drug reactions.

—Monitor for pain or itching at the test site.

—Monitor induration at the test site.

—Periodically reevaluate the patient's and family's knowledge about tuberculin testing.

Intervention

—If the patient develops pain or itching at the test site, apply cold packs or obtain an order for a topical corticosteroid.

—If the patient develops anaphylaxis, notify the doctor immediately. Prepared to administer epinephrine. Provide supportive care, as indicated.

—Keep a record of the administration technique, manufacturer and tuberculin lot number, date and location of administration, date test is read, and the size of the induration in millimeters.

—Keep all members of the health care team informed of the patient's response to the drug.

Patient teaching

—Inform the patient and family about testing with tuberculin PPD.

—Advise the patient that the test results must be read 48 to 72 hours after test is performed. Arrange follow-up appointment.

—Explain to the patient that the induration will disappear in a few days.

—Tell the patient to notify the nurse or doctor if adverse reactions develop or questions arise about the tuberculin PPD test.

Evaluation

In the patient tested with tuberculin PPD, appropriate evaluation statements include:

• Patient experiences no injury to properly administered test.

• Patient returns to have test read 48 to 72 hours after administration.

• Patient and family state an understanding of testing with tuberculin PPD.

SELECTED MAJOR DRUGS: DIAGNOSTIC SKIN TESTS

DRUG, INDICATIONS, AND DOSAGES	SPECIAL PRECAUTIONS
coccidioidin (Spherulin) *Suspected coccidioidomycosis; to assess cell-mediated immunity—* **Adults and children:** 0.1 ml of 1:100 dilution intradermally into the flexor surface of the forearm. Use tuberculin syringe with 26G or 27G ½″ needle. In persons nonreactive to this form, repeat test using 1:10 dilution.	• Contraindicated in patients with known hypersensitivity to thimerosal or other mercuric compounds because thimerosal is a component of this preparation; also in patients with erythema nodosum because these patients have a high incidence of severe reactions.
histoplasmin (Histolyn-CYL) *Suspected histoplasmosis; to assess cell-mediated immunity—* **Adults and children:** 0.1 ml intradermally into the flexor surface of the forearm. Use tuberculin syringe with 26G or 27G ½″ needle.	• Contraindicated in patients with a history of positive reaction because of risk of severe reaction. • Administer cautiously because of risk of allergies and reactions to skin tests.
mumps skin test antigen (MSTA) *To assess cell-mediated immunity—* **Adults and children:** 0.1 ml intradermally into the flexor surface of the forearm. Use tuberculin syringe with 26G or 27G ½″ needle.	• Contraindicated in patients with known hypersensitivity to skin tests; to eggs, feathers, and chicken; and to thimerosal or other mercuric compounds because thimerosal is a component of this preparation. • Administer cautiously. Reactions to this test may be depressed or suppressed for as long as 4 to 6 weeks in individuals who have received concurrent or recent immunization with certain virus vaccines, in those who are receiving corticosteroids or immunosuppressive agents, in malnourished patients, and in those who have had viral infections.
tuberculosis multiple-puncture tests **old tuberculin (Mono-Vacc Test, Tuberculin Old Tine Test)** **purified protein derivative (Aplitest, Sclavo-Test, Tuberculosis Purified Protein Derivative Tine Test)** *Screening for tuberculosis—* **Adults and children:** after cleaning skin thoroughly with alcohol, make skin taut on flexor surface of forearm and press points firmly into selected site. Hold device at injection site for about 3 seconds. This will ensure stabilizing of the dried tuberculin B in tissue lymph.	• Contraindicated in known tuberculin-positive reactors. • Administer cautiously. Reactions to this test may be depressed or suppressed for as long as 4 to 6 weeks in individuals who have received concurrent or recent immunization with certain virus vaccines, in those who are receiving corticosteroids or immunosuppressive agents, in malnourished patients, and in those who have had viral infections or miliary tuberculosis.

SELF-TEST

1. Tim Walker, age 21, is required by his new employer to have a physical examination, including diagnostic skin testing with tuberculin PPD. Diagnostic skin tests may be administered to:
  a. treat infection.
  b. treat an allergy.
  c. determine if cell-mediated immunity is intact.
  d. determine if passive immunity is intact.

2. Mr. Walker's test with tuberculin PPD will be administered:
  a. intradermally.
  b. interdermally.
  c. subcutaneously.
  d. intramuscularly.

3. Mr. Walker developed a significant reaction to the test. A significant reaction is one in which the induration measures:
  a. 1 mm.
  b. 2 mm.
  c. 5 mm.
  d. 10 mm or greater.

Check your answers on page 1078.

ANSWERS TO SELF-TEST QUESTIONS

Chapter 1

1. (b) Rationale: Pharmacodynamics is the study of the mechanism of action of drugs.

2. (c) Rationale: Factors affecting the pharmacologic response of drug therapy include age; gender; weight; genetic, pathologic, or immunologic factors; psychological factors; environmental factors; time of administration; tolerance; cumulative drug effects; and drug interactions.

3. (c) Rationale: Half-life is the time required for the blood drug concentration to decrease by half.

Chapter 2

1. (c) Rationale: Enteric-coated tablets resist breakdown from stomach acid so they can reach the intestine before dissolving.

2. (a) Rationale: In each state, a nurse practice act defines the legal scope of nursing practice in all areas, including drug dispensation, prescription, and administration.

3. (b) Rationale: The maximum volume that should be injected subcutaneously is 2 ml.

Chapter 3

1. (a) Rationale: Patient risk factors for adverse drug reactions include multiple drug therapy, a history of reactions, pathologic factors, age, genetic predisposition, and gender.

2. (d) Rationale: The most common allergic reaction to a drug is a maculopapular rash.

3. (b) Rationale: A pharmacodynamic interaction occurs when one drug changes the activity of other drugs, producing additive or antagonistic effects. In this case, theophylline is being antagonistic toward phenytoin's therapeutic effects.

Chapter 4

1. (a) Rationale: Socioeconomic status (patient's age, educational level, occupation, and insurance coverage) helps determine appropriate teaching strategies to utilize and identify factors that could influence compliance with the prescribed drug therapy.

2. (b) Rationale: The statement "The patient states the importance of taking the antibiotic as prescribed" can be measured, making it possible for the nurse to know if the outcome criterion has been met.

3. (b) Rationale: The evaluation step of the nursing process determines if the outcome criteria have been met.

Chapter 5

1. (c) Rationale: Metronidazole is irritating to the GI tract and tends to cause anorexia and nausea. Taking it with meals reduces this adverse reaction.

2. (a) Rationale: A furry tongue is a sign of *Candida* infection. Metronidazole is associated with overgrowth of nonsusceptible organisms, particularly *Candida.*

3. (c) Rationale: Sexually transmitted diseases require that both partners be treated or they will reinfect each other. Absence of symptoms is not unusual in males, so it cannot be used as an indicator of absence of infection.

Chapter 6

1. (c) Rationale: Absorption is best on an empty stomach, but nausea and vomiting from GI irritation are also common and taking the drug with food may decrease their likelihood.

2. (a) Rationale: Common adverse reactions associated with piperazine include headache, vertigo, nausea, and vomiting.

3. (c) Rationale: The only clear confirmation of success in therapy is the absence of worms.

Chapter 7

1. (b) Rationale: I.V. amphotericin B prescribed as a 0.25 mg/kg dose requires administration by slow infusion over 6 hours.

2. (a) Rationale: Adverse reactions to amphotericin B include muscle weakness and abnormal renal function with hypokalemia.

3. (c) Rationale: The nurse should monitor the patient's vital signs every 30 minutes for at least 4 hours after the start of an I.V. infusion of amphotericin B.

Chapter 8

1. (d) Rationale: To prevent infection, a blood level of the drug should be present before exposure. Since the incubation period lasts for up to 35 days after exposure, the drug needs to be continued past that time. These dates provide protection outside those parameters.

2. (c) Rationale: Magnesium and aluminum salts and kaolin with pectin decrease GI absorption of chloroquine.

3. **(c) Rationale:** Although children should be treated prophylactically, their doses are significantly lower than those of adults. Prevention of accidental ingestion is critical. Fatalities have occurred when children have taken as few as 3 to 4 adult-dose tablets.

Chapter 9

1. **(c) Rationale:** Rifampin may produce a red-orange discoloration of urine, feces, saliva, sweat, and tears. If Mr. Johnson wears contact lenses, he may need to substitute eyeglasses during therapy to avoid permanently staining the contact lenses.

2. **(d) Rationale:** Food may delay absorption of rifampin. If GI distress occurs, drug may be taken with meals or an antacid may be taken 1 hour before administration.

3. **(d) Rationale:** In general, therapy for tuberculosis should be continued for 6 to 9 months or until at least 6 months have elapsed from conversion of sputum to culture negativity.

Chapter 10

1. **(c) Rationale:** Nephrotoxicity is a predictable adverse reaction to aminoglycoside therapy. Serum creatinine levels are the most reliable measure of renal function.

2. **(b) Rationale:** Aminoglycosides accumulate in the kidneys, which is their site for excretion. Increased fluid intake reduces the time the kidney is exposed to the drug by increasing glomerular filtration rate.

3. **(a) Rationale:** The time to draw the peak level is 30 minutes after completing the infusion. Peak concentrations are therapeutic when they are between 4 and 12 mcg/dl. Trough levels above 2 mcg/ml are associated with increased nephrotoxicity.

Chapter 11

1. **(c) Rationale:** Food may interfere with absorption. Ampicillin is stable in gastric juices and well absorbed after oral administration on an empty stomach.

2. **(b) Rationale:** Diarrhea is an adverse reaction to ampicillin. It is usually advisable to contact the health care provider before adding any new drug to a treatment regimen, including OTC drugs.

3. **(c) Rationale:** Cephalosporins and penicillins often have cross-allergenicity.

Chapter 12

1. **(b) Rationale:** I.V. ceftazidime should be infused over 30 minutes to prevent pain and irritation.

2. **(a) Rationale:** Penicillins and cephalosporins may have cross-sensitivity.

3. (d) Rationale: Cephalexin is well absorbed orally. GI distress is common and can be relieved by administration with food.

Chapter 13

1. (a) Rationale: Drug effectiveness is reduced when taken with milk or other dairy products, food, antacids, sodium bicarbonate, or iron products.

2. (c) Rationale: Permanent discoloration of the teeth of the infant as well as enamel defects and retarded growth are possible.

3. (a) Rationale: Outdated or deteriorated tetracycline has been associated with reversible nephrotoxicity (Fanconi's syndrome).

Chapter 14

1. (b) Rationale: Sulfonamides competitively inhibit dihydrofolate reductase. This mechanism blocks folic acid synthesis and therefore production.

2. (c) Rationale: The patient should increase his daily fluid intake to prevent crystalluria.

3. (d) Rationale: Co-trimoxazole P.O. is administered every 12 hours for 10 to 14 days.

Chapter 15

1. (b) Rationale: Ciprofloxacin should be used cautiously in CNS disorders and in patients who are at an increased risk for seizures.

2. (c) Rationale: Seizures are an adverse reaction seen with quinolone therapy.

3. (a) Rationale: Antacids should be taken at least 2 hours after taking ciprofloxacin.

Chapter 16

1. (c) Rationale: Zidovudine should be taken every 4 hours around the clock.

2. (a) Rationale: Zidovudine may cause severe bone marrow depression, resulting in anemia.

3. (b) Rationale: Acetaminophen and co-trimoxazole may impair hepatic metabolism of zidovudine, increasing the drug's toxicity.

Chapter 17

1. (b) Rationale: For best absorption, the drug should be taken with a full glass of water 1 hour before or 2 hours after meals.

2. (c) Rationale: Erythromycin may allow overgrowth of nonsusceptible bacteria or fungi.

3. (d) Rationale: Venous irritation and thrombophlebitis can occur after I.V. administration of erythromycin gluceptate or erythromycin lactobionate.

Chapter 18

1. (b) Rationale: Drug-induced aplastic anemia limits chloramphenicol use to treatment of serious infections only.

2. (d) Rationale: Nitrofurantoin may cause false-positive results in urine glucose tests that use the copper sulfate reduction method.

3. (c) Rationale: Diarrhea along with mucus and blood in the stools should alert the nurse to the development of pseudomembranous colitis.

Chapter 19

1. (c) Rationale: The loading dose of digoxin in adults under age 65 is 0.5 to 1 mg I.V. or P.O. in divided doses over 24 hours.

2. (b) Rationale: Digoxin does not cause hearing disturbances.

3. (b) Rationale: The patient should be taught to monitor pulse rate daily.

4. (a) Rationale: Nifedipine increases digoxin blood levels when administered concurrently.

5. (c) Rationale: I.V. digoxin should be infused slowly over at least 5 minutes to avoid adverse reactions.

Chapter 20

1. (a) Rationale: Moricizine must be used with extreme caution in patients with sick sinus syndrome because the drug may cause sinus bradycardia or sinus arrest.

2. (a) Rationale: Neutropenia is more likely to occur with the sustained-release forms of procainamide.

3. (c) Rationale: The initial dose of lidocaine is administered as an I.V. bolus at 25 to 50 mg/minute followed by a continuous infusion of 1 to 4 mg/minute.

4. (a) Rationale: Patients requiring a reduced dosage of lidocaine include the elderly, patients weighing under 50 kg, or those with CHF or renal or hepatic disease.

5. (b) Rationale: In many severely ill patients, seizures may be the first sign of lidocaine toxicity.

6. (b) Rationale: Therapeutic serum levels of flecainide range from 0.2 to 1 mcg/ml.

7. (c) Rationale: Full therapeutic effect of flecainide may take 3 to 5 days.

8. (c) Rationale: Slow I.V. push of propranolol should not exceed 1 mg/minute.

9. (c) Rationale: Amiodarone may increase serum digoxin levels, thus predisposing the patient to digitalis toxicity.

10. (d) Rationale: Verapamil may be repeated in 30 minutes if no response occurs to the initial dose.

Chapter 21

1. (d) Rationale: Nitrates such as nitroglycerin produce relief of angina by reducing the heart's oxygen demand (consumption).

2. (c) Rationale: Headache is a common adverse reaction to nitroglycerin therapy.

3. (b) Rationale: The liquid in the oral capsule can be withdrawn by puncturing the capsule with a needle; then instill the drug into the buccal pouch.

4. (d) Rationale: Beta blockers such as nadolol reduce the heart's oxygen demand by blocking catecholamine-induced increases in heart rate, blood pressure, and force of myocardial contraction.

Chapter 22

1. (a) Rationale: Antihypertensives are used to lower blood pressure in patients whose diastolic blood pressure averages 90 to 95 mm Hg or more.

2. (b) Rationale: Atenolol is classified as a beta-adrenergic blocker.

3. (a) Rationale: Atenolol blocks beta stimulation. All are mechanisms of action of antihypertensives, but atenolol works by beta blockade.

4. (d) Rationale: The initial dose of methyldopa may be increased after the first 48 hours of therapy and thereafter every 2 days as needed. Maximum recommended daily dosage is 3 g.

5. (d) Rationale: Assist with position changes especially when the patient moves from a seated or lying position to a standing position. If the patient develops orthostasis, assist him back into a more supine position.

6. (d) Rationale: The initial dose of prazosin should be given at bedtime to prevent "first-dose" syncope.

7. (b) Rationale: Prazosin is used to treat mild to moderate hypertension, whereas minoxidil is used to treat severe hypertension.

8. (a) Rationale: Phentolamine mesylate is used to treat extravasation.

9. (d) Rationale: Antacids decrease captopril's effect and should be administered at a separate time.

10. **(a) Rationale:** 500 mg trimethaphan camsylate should be diluted in 500 ml dextrose 5% in water to yield a concentration of 1 mg/ml I.V.

Chapter 23

1. **(a) Rationale:** The usual adult dosage for papaverine is 60 to 300 mg P.O. one to five times daily, so the order of 300 mg P.O. b.i.d. is within therapeutic dosage range.

2. **(b) Rationale:** Headache is a common adverse reaction associated with papaverine use.

3. **(c) Rationale:** Papaverine must be used cautiously in patients with glaucoma because it can make the condition worse.

Chapter 24

1. **(a) Rationale:** Antilipemics are indicated when total cholesterol levels are greater than 300 mg/dl.

2. **(b) Rationale:** A patient on antilipemic therapy also needs to be instructed on proper dietary management as part of the treatment regimen.

3. **(c) Rationale:** Lovastatin should be administered with the evening meal.

Chapter 25

1. **(b) Rationale:** Aspirin should be used cautiously in patients with a vitamin K deficiency because bleeding would be more difficult to control in such patients. Vitamin K is necessary for clotting.

2. **(d) Rationale:** Taking aspirin with meals or milk helps to prevent GI tract irritation or distress.

3. **(c) Rationale:** Adverse reactions associated with this drug include headache, vertigo, nausea, and skin rash.

4. **(c) Rationale:** Acetaminophen dosage must vary with the child's age, to ensure effectiveness and avoid severe liver damage that can occur with toxic doses. A child ages 4 to 5 should receive 240 mg/dose.

5. **(a) Rationale:** Diflunisal should not be used with acetaminophen because it increases acetaminophen blood levels, thereby increasing the patient's risk of liver damage.

Chapter 26

1. **(c) Rationale:** Adverse reactions to ibuprofen include CNS effects such as drowsiness and dizziness. The other diagnoses do not reflect adverse reactions commonly associated with this drug.

2. **(a) Rationale:** NSAIDs produce adverse renal effects by reducing renal prostaglandin synthesis. Decreased renal function may cause fluid retention which, in turn, may exacerbate CHF or hypertension.

3. (b) Rationale: Ibuprofen should be taken with food or milk to minimize adverse GI reactions.

Chapter 27

1. (c) Rationale: Respiratory depression is a potentially lethal reaction to morphine. These depressant effects may be more severe because of additive effects of perioperative drugs such as anesthetics and antiemetics.

2. (b) Rationale: Administering morphine to a patient with alcoholism requires extreme caution because liver damage from alcohol use may be present and alter the metabolism of morphine.

3. (a) Rationale: The patient should begin to feel pain relief at onset of action, which is within 20 minutes.

4. (d) Rationale: Urine retention, a possible reaction to morphine, predisposes the patient to a urinary tract infection.

Chapter 28

1. (c) Rationale: Medication should never be left at a patient's bedside unless ordered by the doctor.

2. (a) Rationale: Elderly patients may experience paradoxical excitement after receiving secobarbital.

3. (b) Rationale: Chloral hydrate is contraindicated in patients with known hypersensitivity to chloral hydrate or trichloroethanol and in patients with marked hepatic or renal impairment.

4. (c) Rationale: The first dose of flurazepam may not be therapeutically effective; however, active metabolites of the drug tend to accumulate with repeated doses over time, thereby increasing the probability that succeeding doses will be more effective.

5. (b) Rationale: The recommended dosage of flurazepam for adults over age 65 is 15 mg P.O. h.s.

Chapter 29

1. (b) Rationale: The minimum infusion time for an I.V. bolus of phenytoin is 1 minute for a 50-mg dose. The minimum infusion time for a 900-mg dose is 18 minutes.

2. (b) Rationale: Phenytoin will precipitate if mixed with solutions other than 0.9% sodium chloride. Flush I.V. lines with 0.9% sodium chloride solution before and after injecting I.V. phenytoin to avoid precipitation.

3. (a) Rationale: Phenytoin can cause gingival hyperplasia. Regular dental examinations and oral prophylaxis may be helpful in preventing, detecting, and treating this adverse reaction.

4. (b) Rationale: Phenobarbital is contraindicated during breast-feeding. A patient who wants to breast-feed her infant will need an alternative anticonvulsant.

5. (c) Rationale: Patient may take carbamazepine with food to minimize GI distress.

6. (d) Rationale: Valproate sodium is contraindicated in patients with hepatic dysfunction.

7. (d) Rationale: When used to treat status epilepticus, diazepam may be repeated every 5 to 10 minutes to a maximum total dose of 60 mg.

Chapter 30

1. (d) Rationale: Foods high in tryptophan or tyramine pose a risk of hypertensive crisis in a patient receiving MAO inhibitors. Cheese, especially aged cheeses, contain tyramine and, therefore, should be avoided during treatment with tranylcypromine.

2. (d) Rationale: Patient will be less troubled by the sedative and anticholinergic reactions of tranylcypromine if taken at bedtime.

3. (a) Rationale: This drug often requires 2 to 4 weeks of therapy.

4. (c) Rationale: The maximum dosage of fluoxetine hydrochloride is 80 mg daily.

5. (b) Rationale: Elderly or debilitated patients and patients with renal or hepatic dysfunction may require lower dosages or less frequent dosing.

Chapter 31

1. (b) Rationale: The order should be questioned because, as written, it exceeds the recommendations for frequency and total daily dosage for alprazolam. The usual starting dose of alprazolam in elderly patients is 0.25 mg b.i.d. or t.i.d.

2. (b) Rationale: Alcohol increases the CNS depressant effects of alprazolam and can cause excessive sedation and CV collapse.

3. (b) Rationale: The parenteral form of the drug is for I.M. use only with the Z-track technique. Injection into a large muscle is recommended to prevent accidental intravascular injection and to minimize local tissue injury.

4. (b) Rationale: Dosage should be decreased in elderly patients because aging can alter the metabolism and excretion of this drug.

5. (d) Rationale: Adverse CNS reactions associated with hydroxyzine hydrochloride use include drowsiness and involuntary motor activity.

Chapter 32

1. **(a) Rationale:** The antipsychotic effect of chlorpromazine is attributed to the drug's ability to block postsynaptic dopamine receptors in the brain.

2. **(d) Rationale:** Regular liver function tests are recommended during long-term use because the drug may cause cholestatic jaundice or liver damage.

3. **(a) Rationale:** Tardive dyskinesia, a neurologic syndrome characterized by abnormal muscle movement, has been associated with long-term use of high doses of antipsychotic agents.

4. **(d) Rationale:** Maximum daily dosage of haloperidol is 100 mg.

5. **(a) Rationale:** Neuroleptic malignant syndrome, a rare disorder resembling severe parkinsonism, carries a 10% mortaltiy rate.

Chapter 33

1. **(c) Rationale:** Lithium is almost entirely excreted through the kidneys as unchanged lithium ions.

2. **(d) Rationale:** Toxicity usually occurs when therapeutic lithium blood levels exceed 1.5 mEq/liter.

3. **(b) Rationale:** A diabetes-insipidus–like syndrome causing polyuria and polydypsia may occur in up to one-half of the patient's receiving lithium.

4. **(c) Rationale:** Common adverse CNS reactions include lethargy, fatigue, muscle weakness, headache, mental confusion, and hand tremor.

5. **(c) Rationale:** The syrup form of lithium is supplied as 300 mg/5 ml.

Chapter 34

1. **(b) Rationale:** Caffeine accentuates the stimulating effects of amphetamine sulfate and increases the hyperactivity that the medication can cause.

2. **(a) Rationale:** Antacids, sodium bicarbonate, and acetazolamide increase the renal reabsorption of amphetamine sulfate, enhancing its effect and increasing the risk of adverse reactions.

3. **(b) Rationale:** Because amphetamine sulfate therapy causes weight loss, less insulin may be required. Therefore, insulin dosage may need to be adjusted to prevent hypoglycemia.

Chapter 35

1. **(b) Rationale:** Severe CNS reactions such as hallucinations may require dosage reduction or withdrawal of the drug.

2. **(a) Rationale:** Antacids are known to increase the absorption of levodopa.

3. **(a) Rationale:** Initial dosage of benztropine mesylate for parkinsonism is 0.5 to 1 mg. Dosage is then adjusted to meet individual requirements with usual maintenance dosage at 1 to 2 mg daily.

Chapter 36

1. **(a) Rationale:** Adverse GI reactions may be reduced by taking drug with milk or food.

2. **(c) Rationale:** Test dose of I.V. edrophonium will aggravate drug-induced weakness but will temporarily relieve weakness caused by disease.

3. **(d) Rationale:** Atropine will reverse cholinergic effects on muscles. Have atropine injection readily available and be prepared to give as ordered in case of adverse reactions.

4. **(c) Rationale:** Bethanechol is used to prevent and treat postoperative urine retention and abdominal distention.

Chapter 37

1. **(c) Rationale:** Atropine is administered preoperatively to diminish secretions and block cardiac vagal reflexes.

2. **(d) Rationale:** Atropine is contraindicated in narrow-angle glaucoma, obstructive uropathy, obstructive disease of the GI tract, myasthenia gravis, paralytic ileus, intestinal atony, unstable CV status in acute hemorrhage, and toxic megacolon. Use cautiously in patients with Down's syndrome because they may be more sensitive to the drug.

3. **(a) Rationale:** Many of the adverse effects of atropine, such as dry mouth and constipation, are an extension of the drug's pharmacologic activity and may be expected.

Chapter 38

1. **(b) Rationale:** Dose of 2 to 10 mcg/kg/minute stimulate beta-adrenergic receptors. $Beta_1$ receptors when stimulated increase the rate and force of myocardial contraction.

2. **(d) Rationale:** Monitor blood pressure, cardiac output, pulse rate, urine output, and extremity color and temperature often during infusion.

3. **(b) Rationale:** If extravasation occurs, stop infusion immediately and call doctor. He may want to counteract the effect by infiltrating the area with 5 to 10 mg phentolamine and 10 to 15 ml 0.9% sodium chloride solution.

Chapter 39

1. **(a) Rationale:** Reserpine is contraindicated in patients with depression.

2. **(b) Rationale:** Reserpine should be taken with a meal to minimize adverse GI reactions.

3. **(c) Rationale:** Adverse CV reactions associated with guanethidine sulfate include orthostatic hypotension, bradycardia, CHF, and arrhythmias.

Chapter 40

1. **(d) Rationale:** Cyclobenzaprine reduces transmission of impulses from the spinal cord to the skeletal muscles and produces skeletal muscle relaxation.

2. **(b) Rationale:** Patient teaching for the patient receiving cyclobenzaprine includes warning the patient to avoid activities that require alertness until CNS effects of drug are known. Drowsiness and dizziness usually subside after 2 weeks.

3. **(a) Rationale:** Drowsiness is commonly associated with cyclobenzaprine.

Chapter 41

1. **(c) Rationale:** Pancuronium bromide is used as an adjunct to anesthesia to induce skeletal muscle relaxation.

2. **(b) Rationale:** The most serious adverse effect of pancuronium is prolonged dose-related apnea.

3. **(a) Rationale:** Plastic syringes may be used to administer pancuronium. Do not store medication in plastic syringe.

Chapter 42

1. **(b) Rationale:** Diphenhydramine is one of the most sedating antihistamines available and is frequently used as a hypnotic.

2. **(b) Rationale:** Antihistamine injections should be administered deep I.M. into a large muscle and injection sites should be rotated to prevent irritation.

3. **(c) Rationale:** Antihistamine should be discontinued four days before allergy skin testing to preserve the accuracy of the tests and prevent false-negative results.

Chapter 43

1. **(d) Rationale:** Epinephrine should be used with extreme caution in patients with long-standing bronchial asthma and emphysema who have developed degenerative heart disease.

2. **(b) Rationale:** Total inhalations of ipratropium should not exceed 12 in 24 hours.

3. **(d) Rationale:** Of the four drugs listed theophylline is the one which should provide the symptomatic relief for the patient with emphysema and chronic bronchitis.

Chapter 44

1. **(d) Rationale:** This patient has a persistent nonproductive cough of 4 weeks' duration and many other general symptoms that could result in any one of several diagnoses. The nurse should know that an order for a drug that will suppress the cough would not be appropriate when the cough may be a valuable diagnostic sign.

2. **(a) Rationale:** Antitussive drugs are prescribed for nonproductive coughs.

3. **(d) Rationale:** Expectorants are prescribed for their mechanism of action, which is to increase production of respiratory tract fluids to help liquefy and reduce the viscosity of thick, tenacious secretions.

4. **(b) Rationale:** After opening acetylcysteine (Mucomyst) the vial should be stored in the refrigerator, and the medication in the vial should be used in 96 hours.

5. **(c) Rationale:** Before administering a mucolytic, an antitussive, or an expectorant, the nurse needs to obtain a baseline assessment of the patient's respiratory system, noting the type and frequency of the cough, lung sounds, and the amount, color, and type of respiratory secretions. Without a baseline, treatment cannot be correctly evaluated.

Chapter 45

1. **(a) Rationale:** Antacids' onset of action is generally immediate.

2. **(a) Rationale:** Patients taking magnesium hydroxide as an antacid may develop diarrhea from the drug's laxative effects.

3. **(b) Rationale:** Aluminum hydroxide may cause enteric-coated drugs to be released prematurely in the stomach; therefore, separate doses by 1 hour.

Chapter 46

1. **(c) Rationale:** Digestants promote digestion in the GI tract.

2. **(a) Rationale:** For young children, mix powders with applesauce and give with meals.

3. **(c) Rationale:** Adequate replacement of the pancreatin decreases the number of bowel movements and improves the consistency of the stool.

Chapter 47

1. **(d) Rationale:** Diphenoxylate increases smooth muscle tone in the GI tract, inhibits motility and propulsion, and diminishes digestive secretions.

2. **(a) Rationale:** Antidiarrheals that contain atropine may exhibit adverse anticholinergic reactions, including urine retention.

3. **(a) Rationale:** Withhold the drug and consult the doctor if the patient with acute nonspecific diarrhea shows no improvement in 48 hours.

Chapter 48

1. **(a) Rationale:** An emollient laxative is the drug of choice for patients who should not strain during defecation.

2. **(b) Rationale:** Stimulant laxatives may increase peristalsis by direct effect on the smooth muscle of the intestine.

3. **(d) Rationale:** Taking the liquid (not the syrup) in milk, fruit juice, or infant formula will help mask its bitter taste.

Chapter 49

1. **(d) Rationale:** An antiemetic may cause drowsiness as an adverse reaction. While taking the drug, the patient should not drive or operate equipment that could prove to be hazardous and possibly result in injury.

2. **(a) Rationale:** Alcohol is contraindicated for patients receiving antiemetics. Drowsiness caused by the antiemetic, plus the CNS depressant effect from the alcohol, may cause dangerous adverse reactions for the patient.

3. **(d) Rationale:** Prochlorperazine is toxic to the skin. The nurse should be extremely careful when preparing this drug and should wash it off immediately if it contacts her skin.

Chapter 50

1. **(c) Rationale:** The three physical concerns listed are all normal after the administration of the drug and actually indicate the success of the drug therapy.

2. **(c) Rationale:** Anticholinergics inhibit GI smooth muscle contraction and delay gastric emptying, thus enhancing the action of antacids.

3. **(a) Rationale:** Drug should be given 30 minutes to 1 hour before meals and at bedtime.

Chapter 51

1. **(b) Rationale:** By forming a barrier at the ulcer site, sucralfate protects the ulcer, allowing it to heal.

2. **(d) Rationale:** The H_2-receptor antagonists block the stimulant action of histamine on the acid-secreting parietal cells of the stomach.

3. **(d) Rationale:** Antacids should not be administered within 1 hour of H_2-receptor antagonist administration because decreased absorption of the H_2-receptor antagonist may occur.

Chapter 52

1. (d) Rationale: Corticosteroids should not be discontinued abruptly. Increased dosage of a corticosteroid may be required during times of increased stress such as surgery.

2. (a) Rationale: Corticosteroids prevent a normal inflammatory response and may mask signs of infection.

3. (b) Rationale: A common adverse reaction to fludrocortisone acetate is sodium and water retention.

Chapter 53

1. (c) Rationale: Adverse androgenic reactions in females include acne, edema, oily skin, weight gain, hirsuitism, clitoral enlargement, and decreased or increased libido.

2. (c) Rationale: Adverse androgenic reactions in males include testicular atrophy, oligospermia, decreased ejaculatory volume, postpubertal impotence, gynecomastia, and epididymis.

3. (d) Rationale: Anabolic steroids are erroneously considered a low-risk way to enhance athletic ability.

Chapter 54

1. (a) Rationale: Patients should be taught breast self-examination because estrogen therapy can alter breast tissue.

2. (a) Rationale: Adverse cardiopulmonary reactions include pulmonary embolism, thrombophlebitis, thromboembolism, hypertension, edema, increased risk of stroke, and MI.

3. (a) Rationale: Potential CV reactions to progesterone include hypertension, thrombophlebitis, pulmonary embolism, and edema.

4. (b) Rationale: Correct dosage is important for effective birth control.

Chapter 55

1. (c) Rationale: Menotropins mimic follicle-stimulating hormone in inducing follicular growth and luteinizing hormone in aiding follicular maturation.

2. (b) Rationale: A serious adverse reaction associated with menotropins therapy is ovarian enlargement with pain and abdominal distention.

3. (a) Rationale: The use of menotropins in sexually active women can result in multiple births.

Chapter 56

1. (a) Rationale: Oral antidiabetic agents are added if weight maintenance, diet, and exercise fail to achieve adequate blood glucose control.

2. **(b) Rationale:** Glyburide administered once daily should be taken at breakfast to minimize GI reactions.

3. **(b) Rationale:** Signs and symptoms of hypoglycemia include a rapid onset of nervousness, shakiness, and confusion.

4. **(b) Rationale:** In patients with adequate glycogen stores, glucagon raises the blood glucose, reversing the effect of insulin.

Chapter 57

1. **(d) Rationale:** With thyroid hormone replacement therapy, hypothyroid symptoms should decrease as body metabolism returns to within normal limits.

2. **(d) Rationale:** An overdosage of levothyroxine sodium may commonly be exhibited by nervousness, insomnia, tremor, tachycardia, palpitations, arrhythmias, or angina pectoris.

3. **(a) Rationale:** I.V. phenytoin may cause free thyroid release in the presence of levothyroxine sodium.

Chapter 58

1. **(c) Rationale:** Adverse GI reactions to thyroid hormone antagonists include nausea, vomiting, and diarrhea.

2. **(d) Rationale:** Patient should be taught the symptoms of hypothyroidism that reflect drug overdosage and of hyperthyroidism that reflect ineffectiveness of current dosage regimen.

3. **(a) Rationale:** Methimazole inhibits the oxidation of iodine in the thyroid gland, blocking iodine's ability to combine with tyrosine to form levothyronine.

Chapter 59

1. **(b) Rationale:** Desmopressin acetate should be used with caution in patients with coronary artery insufficiency or hypertensive CV disease.

2. **(a) Rationale:** Adverse drug reactions associated with desmopressin acetate include headache, slight rise in blood pressure at high dosage, nasal congestion, rhinitis, nausea, vulval pain, and flushing.

3. **(a) Rationale:** Patient should clear nasal passages before administering drug to clear surface area for absorption of drug.

Chapter 60

1. **(b) Rationale:** Calcitonin is contraindicated in patients with an allergy to the gelatin diluent used to prepare the drug.

2. **(a) Rationale:** Administering calcitonin at bedtime may help to minimize adverse GI reactions.

3. (c) Rationale: Epinephrine is used to treat a systemic allergic reaction that may occur because the hormone calcitonin is a protein.

Chapter 61

1. (d) Rationale: The combination of furosemide and an aminoglycoside antibiotic increases the risk for development of ototoxicity, a potential adverse reaction of both drugs.

2. (a) Rationale: Hydrochlorothiazide may begin to work within 3 to 4 days but may take 3 to 4 weeks to become fully effective.

3. (d) Rationale: Spironolactone is often combined with other diuretic agents because of its potassium-sparing effect. With increased retention of potassium, hyperkalemia may develop if intake of potassium is high.

4. (c) Rationale: Mannitol increases the osmolality and eventually the volume of the plasma. If the patient's urine output doesn't increase, circulatory overload may occur.

Chapter 62

1. (a) Rationale: Ammonium chloride is contraindicated in severe hepatic dysfunction.

2. (b) Rationale: Sodium bicarbonate extravasation can cause tissue necrosis and sloughing. The most effective treatment is to elevate the extremity, apply heat, and, sometimes, to inject lidocaine or hyaluronidase.

3. (c) Rationale: Patients receiving sodium bicarbonate should be monitored for an overdose manifested as metabolic alkalosis.

Chapter 63

1. (b) Rationale: With therapeutic doses of iron salts, symptoms of iron deficiency usually improve within 2 to 3 days.

2. (b) Rationale: Common adverse reactions associated with ferrous sulfate use include nausea, constipation, and black stools.

3. (a) Rationale: Vitamin C, found in orange juice, may increase iron absorption; this is considered a beneficial drug interaction.

Chapter 64

1. (b) Rationale: Heparin sodium begins to act immediately, with peak effects occurring within minutes. Although heparin cannot dissolve existing clots it can prevent new ones from forming. Thrombophlebitis predisposes the patient to clot formation.

2. (c) Rationale: The partial prothrombin time is used to measure heparin's therapeutic effects.

3. (a) Rationale: Oral anticoagulants require 1 to 3 days to produce a therapeutic effect.

Chapter 65

1. **(b) Rationale:** A repeat dose of albumin 5% may be given in 30 minutes, as needed.

2. **(a) Rationale:** Vascular overload is the most common and serious adverse reaction associated with administration of albumin 5%, especially after rapid infusion.

3. **(a) Rationale:** Effectiveness of therapy will be reflected in the improvement of the patient's vital signs, intake and output, and laboratory tests such as serum protein and electrolyte levels, hemoglobin, and hematocrit.

Chapter 66

1. **(a) Rationale:** Streptokinase is used to dissolve (lyse) clots by activating plasminogen and converting it to plasmin.

2. **(b) Rationale:** Serious adverse reactions associated with streptokinase use include bleeding and hypersensitivity reactions, including anaphylaxis.

3. **(b) Rationale:** Active internal bleeding is a known contraindication to streptokinase therapy.

Chapter 67

1. **(c) Rationale:** Leukopenia is a common adverse reaction caused by cyclophosphamide therapy and requires close monitoring of the WBC count (part of the CBC).

2. **(b) Rationale:** Cyclophosphamide is contraindicated in patients with serious bacterial, viral, or fungal infections, especially varicella-zoster infections.

3. **(c) Rationale:** The patient should drink at least 3 liters/day to prevent hemorrhagic cystitis.

Chapter 68

1. **(a) Rationale:** Fluorouracil inhibits DNA synthesis.

2. **(c) Rationale:** Nausea, vomiting, and diarrhea occur in 30% to 50% of patients receiving fluorouracil.

3. **(d) Rationale:** Fluorouracil must be used cautiously in patients with impaired hepatic or renal function, a history of high dose pelvic irradiation, previous use of alkylating agents, or widespread tumor involvement of the bone marrow.

Chapter 69

1. **(d) Rationale:** Cardiac arrhythmias, decreased cardiac output, and irreversible cardiomyopathy are common complications of doxorubicin therapy.

2. (b) Rationale: Infiltration of doxorubicin may lead to local cellulitis and tissue sloughing.

3. (a) Rationale: Urine will turn an orange to red color for 1 to 2 days as a result of the presence of the drug in the urine.

Chapter 70

1. (c) Rationale: Tamoxifen may cause retinopathy, corneal changes, and changes in visual acuity.

2. (c) Rationale: Tamoxifen may compound hypercalcemia from bone metastases.

3. (b) Rationale: Tamoxifen acts as an estrogen antagonist.

Chapter 71

1. (b) Rationale: Vincristine causes neurotoxicity that affects the deep tendon reflexes.

2. (d) Rationale: Vincristine is given I.V. push or as an I.V. infusion in 50 ml of diluent over 15 minutes. Never give I.M., subcutaneously, or intrathecally.

3. (b) Rationale: Vincristine may cause acute bronchospasms.

Chapter 72

1. (b) Rationale: Common adverse reactions to cyclosporine include nephrotoxicity, tremor, gum hyperplasia, hypertension, and hirsutism.

2. (d) Rationale: Immunosuppressants are used primarily in combination with corticosteroids to prevent or treat organ transplant rejection.

3. (b) Rationale: The drug may be mixed with milk, chocolate milk, or orange juice, then administered immediately. Do not allow drug to stand before administering to patient.

Chapter 73

1. (a) Rationale: Vaccines and toxoids provide acquired immunity.

2. (a) Rationale: Poliovirus vaccine is administered orally. Under no circumstances should this vaccine be administered parenterally.

3. (c) Rationale: The preferred I.M. injection site in adults and children is the deltoid or midlateral thigh.

Chapter 74

1. (d) Rationale: Black widow spider venom is neurotoxic and may cause respiratory paralysis and seizures.

2. (b) Rationale: Use tetanus antitoxin, equine, only when tetanus immune globulin is not available.

3. (b) Rationale: Antitoxins and antivenins provide passive immunity.

Chapter 75

1. **(b) Rationale:** Immune serums provide passive immunity against various infectious diseases or suppress antibody formation.

2. **(c) Rationale:** If it occurs, serum sickness commonly develops within 6 to 12 days after receiving antirabies serum, equine.

3. **(a) Rationale:** Anaphylaxis is a life-threatening adverse reaction that may occur immediately after administration of antirabies serum because it is derived from horses.

Chapter 76

1. **(c) Rationale:** Almost all patients experience flulike symptoms at the beginning of therapy with interferons.

2. **(d) Rationale:** Administer at bedtime to minimize daytime drowsiness.

3. **(a) Rationale:** Interferon alfa-2a is a sterile protein produced by recombinant DNA techiques.

Chapter 77

1. **(c) Rationale:** The correct site of instillation of ophthalmic anti-infective eye drops is the lower conjunctival sac.

2. **(a) Rationale:** There should be 30 minutes to 1 hour between the instillation of a local anesthetic, such as procaine or tetracaine, and the anti-infective.

3. **(b) Rationale:** Itching lids, swelling, or constant burning is a sign of sensitivity and not normal. Tell the patient to stop the drug immediately and notify the doctor.

Chapter 78

1. **(a) Rationale:** Dexamethasone is contraindicated in ocular tuberculosis, as well as acute superficial herpes simplex, vaccinia, varicella, or other fungal or viral diseases of cornea and conjunctiva, or any acute purulent, untreated infection of the eye.

2. **(a) Rationale:** Optic nerve damage can occur with excessive or long-term use of dexamethasone.

3. **(c) Rationale:** When using the ointment form of dexamethasone, $1/2''$ to $1''$ of the ointment should be instilled into each inflamed conjunctival sac.

Chapter 79

1. **(b) Rationale:** For a 70-year-old patient, the nurse would first need to assess the patient's physical ability to handle the administration of the drug, then to assess the patient's current knowledge and begin to develop a teaching plan for this patient. Without this assessment, the nurse could not continue to properly educate this patient.

2. (c) Rationale: Touching the eye with the tip of the dropper can cause eye damage; touching the tip of the dropper with his hands can transmit bacteria or other organisms and result in an infection.

3. (a) Rationale: If the Ocusert Pilo system falls out of the eye during sleep, the patient should wash his hands, rinse the system in cool tap water, and reposition the system in the eye.

Chapter 80

1. (c) Rationale: Atropine is a mydriatic given to dilate the pupil so the doctor may be better able to visualize the internal eye structures.

2. (c) Rationale: A mydriatic prescribed for refraction examination is administered 1 hour before the examination.

3. (b) Rationale: Dry mouth is an expected adverse reaction to this drug; the patient should be advised to chew sugarless hard candy or gum.

Chapter 81

1. (b) Rationale: Signs and symptoms of beta blockade include bradycardia, hypotension, syncope, exacerbation of asthma, and CHF.

2. (c) Rationale: The patient should be told to apply light finger-pressure over the lacrimal sac after instillation to prevent systemic absorption.

3. (a) Rationale: Fentanyl and general anesthetics can cause excessive hypotension if used concurrently with timolol.

Chapter 82

1. (a) Rationale: Chloramphenicol should be administered cautiously to patients with renal or hepatic dysfunction, acute intermittent porphyria, or G6PD deficiency and to infants.

2. (c) Rationale: Sore throat should be reported because it may be an early sign of toxicity.

3. (c) Rationale: Irrigation of ear canals may be necessary to aid removal of cerumen following carbamide peroxide therapy.

Chapter 83

1. (a) Rationale: Beclomethasone is an anti-inflammatory agent.

2. (d) Rationale: Mild transient nasal burning and stinging is a common adverse reaction to beclomethasone.

3. (c) Rationale: Phenylephrine is a local vasoconstrictor used to treat nasal congestion that occurs in conditions such as seasonal rhinitis.

Chapter 84

1. (b) Rationale: Mafenide acetate suppresses the growth of bacterial cells and therefore is bacteriostatic.

2. (b) Rationale: Miconazole nitrate in the form of Monistat 7 vaginal suppository must be used for 7 days; a repeat course may be necessary.

3. (b) Rationale: Culture and sensitivity tests should precede start of the bacitracin because the medication could affect test results. The first dose may be given before receiving the results.

4. (c) Rationale: Acyclovir is not a cure and does not prevent the spread of herpes to others.

Chapter 85

1. (c) Rationale: Although lindane can alleviate parasitic infestation (scabies, pediculosis), itching may persist for several weeks after treatment.

2. (a) Rationale: Adverse CNS reactions associated with lindane include seizures and dizziness.

3. (b) Rationale: Reinfestation can be minimized if the patient launders all recently worn clothes in very hot water.

Chapter 86

1. (a) Rationale: Topical corticosteroids reduce inflammation.

2. (c) Rationale: Before applying hydrocortisone cream, the skin surface should be cleaned.

3. (d) Rationale: Systemic absorption is especially likely with occlusive dressings (up to a hundred times).

4. (b) Rationale: Secondary infection is a common adverse reaction to hydrocortisone therapy and requires discontinuation of therapy.

Chapter 87

1. (c) Rationale: The patient may use acetaminophen to relieve the headache, a common adverse reaction to probenecid; aspirin or any product containing salicylate should be avoided.

2. (d) Rationale: The uricosurics are used primarily to prevent or control the frequency of gouty arthritis attacks.

3. (a) Rationale: The patient should avoid alcohol during colchicine therapy because it may inhibit the drug's action.

Chapter 88

1. (b) Rationale: The usual initial dose of ritodrine is 0.1 mg/minute.

2. (c) Rationale: Initially infuse at a rate of 1 to 2 milliunits/minute.

3. (b) Rationale: During long infusions, watch for signs of water intoxication.

Chapter 89

1. (a) Rationale: Diarrhea is a common adverse reaction to gold salt therapy.

2. **(c) Rationale:** Although the exact mechanism is not known, a gold salt may inhibit lysosomal enzymes, decreasing vessel permeability or decreasing phagocytosis.

3. **(d) Rationale:** The nurse should do nothing because the platelet count is normal. If it falls below 100,000/mm³, the nurse should notify the doctor and expect to discontinue the drug.

Chapter 90

1. **(c) Rationale:** Diagnostic skin tests are used to determine the presence of allergy, to diagnose infection, or to see if cell-mediated immunity is intact.

2. **(a) Rationale:** The drug is administered intradermally into the flexor surface of the forearm.

3. **(d) Rationale:** An induration of 10 mm or greater is significant in patients who are not suspected of having tuberculosis or who have recently been exposed to active tuberculosis.

INDEX

---

t refers to a table; boldfaced page numbers refer to prototype drug entries

---

t refers to a table; boldfaced page numbers refer to prototype drug entries

---

t refers to a table; boldfaced page numbers refer to prototype drug entries

liothyronine sodium, 755t
liotrix, 750, 757t
lipid, 324t
lipoatrophy, 733t
lipodystrophy, 733t
lipohypertrophy, 733t
lipolysis, 733t
lipoprotein, 324t
Liquaemin Sodium, 818-822
Liquiprin, 341-344
lisinopril, 282, 285t, 306t
Lithane, 467-471
Lithicarb, 467-471
lithium carbonate, 466, **467-471**
lithium citrate, 466, **467-471**
Lithizine, 467-471
Lithobid, 467-471
Lithonate, 467-471
Lithotabs, 467-471
Lixolin, 571-575
local anti-infectives, 988-1004
combination, comparison of, 1004t
local vasoconstrictors (nasal), 978, 980-982, 985-986t
Lodine, 353t
Lodrane, 571-575
Loestrin 21 1/20, 723t
Loestrin 21 1.5/30, 723t
Lofene, 616-619
Logen, 616-619
Lomanate, 616-619
Lomotil, 616-619
Lomustine, 843
Lonavar, 697-699
Loniten, 311t
Lonox, 616-619
loop diuretics, 777, 787-791, 796t
Lo/Ovral, 723t
loperamide hydrochloride, 614, 620t
Lopid, 331t
Lopressor, 278t, 307t
Lopressor HCT 50/25, 312t
Lopressor HCT 100/25, 312t
Loprox, 1001t
Lopurin, 1030t
lorazepam, 441, 449t
Lorelco, 331t
lotion, 19t
Lotrimin, 1001-1002t
Lotrimin AF, 1001-1002t
Lo-Trol, 616-619
lovastatin, 317, 325t, **328-330**
Low-Quel, 616-619
Lowsium, 604t
loxapine hdyrochloride, 452, 455t
loxapine, succinate, 452, 455t
lozenges, 19t
Lozol, 794t

L-thyroxine sodium, 750, 752-755
Lucrin, 874t
Ludiomil, 438t
Lugol's Solution, 762t
Luminal, 389t, 399-402
Luminal Sodium, 399-402
Lupron, 874t
Lupron Depot, 874t
Lurselle, 331t
Lutrepulse, 730t
lymphocyte immune globulin, 883, 889t
lymphoma, 844t
lypressin, 764, 769-770t
Lysosome, 1046t
Lyspafen, 620t

M

Maalox Plus (Extra Strength), 605t
Macrodantin, 212-215
mafenide acetate, 988, **990-992**
magaldrate, 596, 604t
Magnacef, 142-144
magnesium hydroxide, 596, **600-602**
magnesium oxide, 596, 604t
magnesium salicylate, 333, 344t
magnesium salts, 622, 629t
magnesium sulfate, 1032, 1042-1043t
magnesium trisilicate, 596, 604t
malaria, 85t
malathion, 1006
Malogen, 694-697
Malotuss, 586-588
Mandol, 147t
mania, 425t
mannitol, 777, **791-793**
MAO inhibitors. See Mono-amine oxidase inhibitors.
Maox, 604t
maprotiline hydrochloride, 424, 427t, 438t
Marazide, 794t
Marezine, 647t
Marplan, 437t
Marzine, 647t
mastoidectomy, 971t
Matulane, 867t
Maxair, 577t
Maxidex, 943-945
Maxiflor, 1018t
Maxitrol Ointment, 947t
Maxitrol Ophthalmic Suspension, 947t
Maxzide, 798t
Maxzide-25, 798t
Mazanor, 477t
Mazepine, 416-419

mazindol, 472, 477t
measles, mumps, and rubella virus (MMR) vaccine, live, 891, 901t
measles (rubeola) and rubella virus vaccine, live attenuated, 891
measles (rubeola) virus vaccine, live attenuated, 891, 901-902t
Measurin, 336-339
Mebaral, 419t
mebendazole, 68, 72t
mecamylamine hydrochloride, 282, 286t, 310t
mechlorethamine hydrochloride, 843, 850t
Meclan, 1000t
meclizine hydrochloride, 632, 634t, **636-638**
meclocycline sulfosalicylate, 988, 1000t
Meclofen, 354t
meclofenamate, 348, 354t
Meclomen, 354t
meclozine hydrochloride, 636-638
Meda Cap, 341-344
Meda Tab, 341-344
medical history, 52
medication history, 52, 54
Medipren Caplets, 350-352
Medipren Tablets, 350-352
Mediquell, 588-590
Medrol, 688t, 1019t
medroxyprogesterone acetate, 703, 722t
medrysone, 941, 946t
medulloblastome, 853t
mefenamic acid, 348, 354t
mefloquine hydrochloride, 84, 90t
Mefoxin, 149-150t
Megace, 874t
Megacillin, 130t
megestrol acetate, 868, 874t
Megostat, 874t
meibomianitis, 932t
Mellaril, 463-464t
melphalan, 843
Menest, 719t
Meni-D, 636-638
meningitis, 94t
meningitis vaccine, 891, 902t
Menomune-A/C, 902t
menotropins, 726, **728-730**
mepenzolate bromicde, 649, 658t
meperidine hydrochloride, 358, 361t, 370t
mephentermine sulfate, 512, 516t
mephenytoin, 393, 395t, 420t

Serpasil-Esidrix #1, 533t
Serpazide, 314t, 533-534t
Sertan, 419t
serum sickness, 38t, 917t
sex, pharmacologic response
    and, 4
side effect, 37
Silvadene, 1002t
silver nitrate 1%, 931, 938t
silver sulfadiazine, 988, 1002t
simethicone, 604t
Sinemet, 490t
Sine-Off Nasal Spray, 986t
Sinequan, 438t
Sinex, 980-982
Skelaxin, 539-540t
skeletal muscle relaxants, 535-
    540
skin test antigens, multiple,
    1050
SleepEze 3, 552-555
Slo-bid Gyrocaps, 571-575
Slo-Phyllin, 571-575
Slow-Fe, 811-813
SMZ-TMP, 166-169
socioeconomic status, 54
Soda Mint, 604t
sodium bicarbonate, 596,
    604t, 800, **804-807**
sodium iodide, 758, 763t
sodium lactate, 800, 807t
sodium phosphates, 622, 630t
sodium salicylate, 333
Sodium Succinate, 206-209
Sodium Sulamyd 10%, 934-
    937
Sodium Sulamyd 30%, 934-
    937
sodium thiosalicylate, 333
Solfoton, 399-402
Solprin, 336-339
Solu-Cortef, 681-684
Solu-Medrol, 688t
solution, 19t
Soma, 539t
somatrem, 764
somatropin, 764
Sominex 2, 552-555
Somophyllin-CRT, 571-575
Somophyllin-T, 571-575
Som-Pam, 383-385
Sopamycetin, 971-973
Spasm, 536t
Spasmoban, 659t
Spastic, 536t
Spectazole, 1002t
spectinomycin hydrochloride,
    198
Spectrobid, 128t
spectrum, 165t
Spherulin, 1054t
spironolactone, 777, **784-787**
Spirotone, 784-787
Spirozide, 798t

spray, 19t
    translingual, 24t
S-P-T, 756t
Squibb-HC, 1014-1017
SSKI, 581, 591t
Stadol, 372t
stanozolol, 691, 701t
Staphcillin, 129t
Statex, 362-365
status epilepticus, 394t
Stelazine, 464t
Stemetil, 639-644
Sterol, 76t
Stevens-Johnson syndrome
    as adverse drug reaction, 40
Stimate, 766-769
St. Joseph for Children, 588-
    590
St. Joseph Measured Dose
    Nasal Decongestant, 980-982
stomatitis, 853t
Strema, 91t
Streptase, 837-840
streptokinase, 835, **837-840**
streptomycin sulfate, 93, 99t,
    101, 109-110t
streptozocin, 843, 850t
stroke volume, 223t
strong iodine solution, 762t
Stulex, 625-627
subcutaneous route, 26t, 29-
    30
Sublimaze, 368t
sublingual route, 24t
    absorption and, 9t
substrate, 2t
succinimide derivatives, 410-
    412
succinylcholine chloride, 542,
    547-548t
sucralfate, 662, **670-672**
Sucrets Cough Control For-
    mula, 588-590
Sudafed, 522-523t
Sudafed Plus, 558t
Sufenta, 371t
sufentanil citrate, 358, 361t,
    371t
Sulcrate, 670-672
Sulf-10, 934-937
Sulfacel-15, 934-937
sulfacetamide sodium 10%,
    931, **934-937**
sulfacetamide sodium 15%,
    931, **934-937**
sulfacetamide sodium 30%,
    931, **934-937**
sulfadiazine, 164, 173t
sulfafurazole, 169-172
sulfamethizole, 173t
Sulfamethoprim, 164, 166-
    169
Sulfamethoprim DS, 166-169
sulfamethoxazole, 164, 173t

sulfamethoxazole-
    trimethoprim, 166-169
Sulfamylon, 990-992
sulfapyridine, 164
sulfasalazine, 164, 174t
sulfinpyrazone, 1021, 1030t
sulfisoxazole, 164, **169-172**,
    931
sulfonamides, 164-174
    combination, comparison of,
    174t
sulfonylureas, 742-744, 747-
    748t
    action of, comparison of, 737t
sulindac, 348, 356t
Sulmeprim, 166-169
sulphafurazole, 169-172
summation, 7
Sumycin, 157-160
Supasa, 336-339
superinfection, 102t, 133t
Supeudol, 371t
Suppap, 341-344
suppository, 25t
Suprax, 150-151t
Supres, 302-305
suprofen, 941
Surfak, 625-627
Surmontil, 439t
suspension, 25t
Sus-Phrine, 520-521t, 564-
    568
sustained-release tablet, os-
    motic pump, 24t. See also
    extended-release.
Sustaire, 571-575
sympathetic nervous system,
    513t
sympatholytic agents, 526t.
    See also Centrally acting
    sympatholytics.
sympathomimetic agent, 513t
Synalar, 1018t
Synarel, 731t
Synemol, 1018t
synergism, 7
Synophylate, 571-575
Synthroid, 752-755
Synthrox, 752-755
Syntocinon, 1035-1039
syrup, 24t
systemic acidifier, 801t
systemic alkalinizer, 801t
systole, 223t
systolic blood pressure, 283t

T

T_3, 75o. See also liothyronine
    sodium.
T_4, 750, 752-755
tablet, 23t
    buccal, 24t
    coated, 23t
    enteric-coated, 23t

---

t refers to a table; boldfaced page numbers refer to prototype drug entries

Uritol, 787-791
Urocarb Liquid, 499-501
Urocarb Tablets, 499-501
Urodine, 339-341
Uro Gantanol, 174t
Urogesic, 339-341
urokinase, 835, 841t
Uro-Mag, 604t
Uroplus DS, 166-169
Uroplus SS, 166-169
Urozide, 781-784
urticaria, 38t, 551t
Uticort, 1017t
uveitis, 959t

V

vaccines, 891-896, 899-904t
vaginal route, 33
Valadol, 341-344
Valcote, 413-415
Valisone, 1017t
Valium, 402-405, 449t
Valorin, 341-344
Valpin 50, 656t
valproate sodium, 393, 395t, **413-415**
valproic acid, 393, 395t, **413-415**
Valrelease, 402-405
Vamate, 443-445
Vancenase AQ Nasal Spray, 982-984
Vancenase Nasal Inhaler, 982-984
Vancocin, 218-221
vancomycin hydrochloride, 198, **218-221**
Vanquish Caplets, 346t
Vansil, 72t
varicella-zoster immune globulin, 916, 922t
Vascor, 279t
vascular resistance, peripheral, 283t
Vaseretic, 312t
vasoconstrictors, 318t
   local (nasal), 978, 980-982, 985t-986t
Vasodilan, 321t
vasodilators, 282, 317-321
   in antihypertensive combinations, 533-534t
   as antihypertensives, 302-305, 311t
   actions of, 287t
Vasomotor, 318t
vasopressin, 764, 770t
Vasotec, 306t
Vasotec I.V., 306t
Va-tro-nol Nose Drops, 985t
Vazepam, 402-405
Veetids, 130t
Velban, 881t
Velbe, 881t

Velosef, 146-147t
Velosulin, 735t, 737-741
Velosulin Human, 737-741
Velosulin Insuject, 737-741
Venoglobulin-1, 920-921t
Venom, 908t
Ventolin, 520t
VePesid, 881t
Veradil, 255-258
verapamil hydrochloride, 231, 235t, **255-258**, 264, 280t, 282
Veriga, 69-72
Vermirex, 69-72
Vermizine, 69-72
Vermox, 72t
Vibramycin, 161t
Vicks Formula 44D, 594t
vidarabine, 931, 938t
vidarabine monohydrate, 182, 190t
vinblastine sulfate, 876, 881t
vinca alkaloids, 876, 877-881
Vincasar PFS, 877-881
Vincent's Powders, 336-339
vincristine sulfate, 876, **877-881**
Vioform, 1003t
Viokase, 611t
Vira-A, 190t
Vira-A Ophthalmic, 938t
Virazole, 189-190t
Viridium, 339-341
virus, 183t
Viscid, 582t
Visken, 308t
Vistacon-50, 443-445
Vistaject, 443-445
Vistaquel 50, 443-445
Vistaril, 443-445
Vistazine 50, 443-445
Vivol, 402-405
Voltaren, 352t
vomiting, 633t
VP-16, 876. *See also* etoposide.
VZIG, 916, 922t

W

warfarin sodium, 816, **823-826**
Warfilone Sodium, 823-826
wax-matrix tablet, 24t
Wehdryl-10, 552-555
Wehdryl-50, 552-555
weight
   adverse drug reaction and, 39
   pharmacologic response and, 4
Wellbutrin, 439t
Westcort Cream, 1014-1017
Win-Kinase, 841t
Winsprin Capsules, 336-339
Winstrol, 701t

withdrawal syndrome, 6
Wyamycin-E, 192-196
Wyamycin-S, 192-196
Wycillin, 130t
Wygesic, 373t
Wytensin, 310t

X

Xanax, 446-448
X-Prep Liquid, 629t
Xylocaine, 242-245
Xylocard, 242-245
xylometazoline hydrochloride, 978, 986t

Y

yellow fever vaccine, 891, 904t
YF Vax, 904t
Yodoxin, 66t
Yomesan, 72t
Yutopar, 1038-1041

Z

Zadine, 555t
Zanosar, 850t
Zantac, 675t
Zarontin, 410-412
Zaroxolyn, 795t
Zefazone, 147-148t
Zestoretic, 312t
Zestril, 306t
Zetran, 402-405
zidovudine, 182, **185-189**
Zinacef, 150t
Zofran, 645-647
Zoladex, 874t
ZORprin, 336-339
Zovirax, 189t, 997-999
Zyloprim, 1030t